AF807900

Bioethics

4TH EDITION

Bioethics

4TH EDITION

VOLUME I

A–B

Bruce Jennings
EDITOR IN CHIEF

MACMILLAN REFERENCE USA
A part of Gale, Cengage Learning

GALE
CENGAGE Learning®

Farmington Hills, Mich • San Francisco • New York • Waterville, Maine
Meriden, Conn • Mason, Ohio • Chicago

GALE
CENGAGE Learning

Bioethics, 4th Edition

Bruce Jennings, *Editor in Chief*

© 2014 Gale, Cengage Learning

WCN: 01-100-101

ALL RIGHTS RESERVED. No part of this work covered by the copyright herein may be reproduced, transmitted, stored, or used in any form or by any means graphic, electronic, or mechanical, including but not limited to photocopying, recording, scanning, digitizing, taping, Web distribution, information networks, or information storage and retrieval systems, except as permitted under Section 107 or 108 of the 1976 United States Copyright Act, without the prior written permission of the publisher.

For product information and technology assistance, contact us at
Gale Customer Support, 1-800-877-4253.
For permission to use material from this text or product,
submit all requests online at **www.cengage.com/permissions.**
Further permissions questions can be emailed to
permissionrequest@cengage.com

While every effort has been made to ensure the reliability of the information presented in this publication, Gale, a part of Cengage Learning, does not guarantee the accuracy of the data contained herein. Gale accepts no payment for listing; and inclusion in the publication of any organization, agency, institution, publication, service, or individual does not imply endorsement of the editors or publisher. Errors brought to the attention of the publisher and verified to the satisfaction of the publisher will be corrected in future editions.

LIBRARY OF CONGRESS CATALOGING-IN-PUBLICATION DATA

Bioethics / Bruce Jennings, editor in chief — 4th edition.
p. ; cm. —
Preceded by Encyclopedia of bioethics / edited by Stephen G. Post. 3rd ed. c2004.
Includes bibliographical references and index.
ISBN 978-0-02-866205-3 (set : alk. paper) — ISBN 978-0-02-866206-0 (v. 1 : alk. paper) — ISBN 978-0-02-866207-7 (v. 2 : alk. paper) — ISBN 978-0-02-866208-4 (v. 3 : alk. paper) — ISBN 978-0-02-866209-1 (v. 4 : alk. paper) — ISBN 978-0-02-866210-7 (v. 5 : alk. paper) — ISBN 978-0-02-866211-4 (v. 6 : alk. paper) — ISBN 978-0-02-866212-1 (e-book)
I. Jennings, Bruce, 1949– editor of compilation. II. Encyclopedia of bioethics. Preceded by (work): III. Title
[DNLM: 1. Bioethical Issues—Encyclopedias—English. 2. Ethics, Clinical—Encyclopedias—English. 3. Ethics, Medical—Encyclopedia—English. WB 13]

QH332
174.203—dc23 2014002548

Gale, a part of Cengage Learning
27500 Drake Rd.
Farmington Hills, MI 48331-3535

ISBN-13: 978-0-02-866205-3 (set)
ISBN-13: 978-0-02-866206-0 (vol. 1)
ISBN-13: 978-0-02-866207-7 (vol. 2)
ISBN-13: 978-0-02-866208-4 (vol. 3)
ISBN-13: 978-0-02-866209-1 (vol. 4)
ISBN-13: 978-0-02-866210-7 (vol. 5)
ISBN-13: 978-0-02-866211-4 (vol. 6)

This title is also available as an e-book.
ISBN-13: 978-0-02-866212-1
Contact your Gale, a part of Cengage Learning, sales representative for ordering information.

Printed in Mexico
1 2 3 4 5 6 7 18 17 16 15 14

Editorial Board

EDITOR IN CHIEF

Bruce Jennings

Director of Bioethics, Center for Humans and Nature

ASSOCIATE EDITORS

Lisa Eckenwiler

Associate Professor of Philosophy, Departments of Philosophy and Health Administration and Policy, George Mason University

Gregory E. Kaebnick

Research Scholar, Director of the Editorial Department, and editor of the Hastings Center Report *and* Bioethics Forum, *The Hastings Center*

Barbara Koenig

Professor, Department of Social and Behavioral Sciences, Institute for Health and Aging, University of California, San Francisco

Sheldon Krimsky

Lenore Stern Professor of Humanities and Social Sciences, School of Arts and Sciences, Tufts University

Carol Zicklin Professor of Philosophy, Brooklyn College

Adjunct Professor, Department of Family Medicine and Community Health, Tufts University School of Medicine

Stephen R. Latham

Director, Interdisciplinary Center for Bioethics,
Yale University

Mark R. Mercurio

Professor of Pediatrics (Neonatology) and Director, Program for Biomedical Ethics, Yale School of Medicine

Chair, Yale–New Haven Children's Hospital Ethics Committee

Director, Yale Pediatrics Ethics Program

CONSULTING EDITORS

Joseph J. Fins

E. William Davis, Jr. M.D. Professor of Medical Ethics, Chief of the Division of Medical Ethics, and Professor of Medicine, Public Health, and Medicine in Psychiatry, Weill Cornell Medical College

Senior Attending Physician and Director of Medical Ethics, New York–Presbyterian Weill Cornell Medical Center

Adjunct Faculty Member, Rockefeller University, and Senior Attending Physician at the Rockefeller University Hospital

Bruce D. White

Director of Alden March Bioethics Institute, Albany Medical College

Professor, Center for Biomedical Ethics Education and Research, Albany Medical College

Professor of Pediatrics, Albany Medical College

FOUNDING EDITOR

Warren T. Reich

Distinguished Professor of Religion and Ethics, Theology Department, Georgetown University

Editorial and Production Staff

PROJECT EDITORS

Alja Kooistra
Andrea Henderson

ASSISTING PROJECT EDITORS

Larry Baker
Jelena Krstović
Rebecca Parks
Carol A. Schwartz

MANUSCRIPT EDITORS

Anne Davidson
Jessica Hornik Evans
Gretchen Gordon
Teresa Jesionowski
Jean Fortune Kaplan
Uma Kukathas
Marcia Merryman-Means
Laura Patchkofsky
David E. Salamie
Maria Sheler-Edwards

PROOFREADERS

Kim Greenwell
Carol Holmes
Teresa Jesionowski
Uma Kukathas
Kathy Wilson Peacock
Amy L. Unterburger

INDEXER

Andriot Indexing, LLC

PRODUCT DESIGN

Kristine Julien

SENIOR BUYER

Evi Seoud

BUYER

Rita Wimberley

PERMISSIONS

Bill Smith Group

COMPOSITOR

PreMediaGlobal

ASSOCIATE PUBLISHER

Hélène G. Potter

Contents

Preface

At the time of the first publication of the *Encyclopedia of Bioethics* in 1978, the then fledgling field of bioethics was neither well defined nor widely recognized. Warren T. Reich, Senior Research Scholar with the Kennedy Institute of Ethics at Georgetown University, undertook to develop a major reference work that would contribute significantly to the establishment of bioethics as a field by integrating historical background, current issues, future implications, ethical theory, and comparative cultural and religious perspectives. Professor Reich became the editor in chief for the first edition, which was published in four volumes. It was immediately acknowledged as a landmark work defining the field. The essential vision of a synthetic and comprehensive reference work for this interdisciplinary field endured and guided two subsequent editions published in 1995 and 2006—and inspired the current edition as well.

The *Encyclopedia of Bioethics* received the American Library Association's 1979 Dartmouth Medal for outstanding reference work of the year and since then has garnered widespread critical acclaim. Over the years the field of bioethics has grown enormously through the establishment of educational programs in bioethics and medical humanities, from the high school to the doctoral level. The field's growth has also been fueled by widespread mass media attention and involvement with legislative, judicial, and public policy affairs. Ultimately, the growth and influence of bioethics rest on a burgeoning corpus of scholarly research and policy analysis emanating from centers and departments of major research universities and medical schools worldwide, independent research institutes, several professional journals, and the work of many professional associations such as the International Association of Bioethics and the American Society for Bioethics and the Humanities. Amid these developments over nearly forty years, the *Encyclopedia of Bioethics* has been a constant, a trustworthy point of departure for further study, an anchor for the breadth and depth of the knowledge that bioethics offers society.

The new fourth edition has followed in the footsteps of its predecessors except that it has grown to six volumes, and it has a new title, *Bioethics*. Following the examples set by Reich; Stephen G. Post, who was editor in chief of the third edition; and their editorial colleagues and contributors, this new edition maintains an interdisciplinary, historical, and multicultural perspective and reflects the changing orientations and lines of inquiry in the field. Its contributors offer a thoughtful self-awareness concerning the bioethics enterprise and provide an assessment of new trends in the field and of areas in need of further philosophical and practical refinement. *Bioethics* is a work at the interface of biology, technology, health care, and ethics. The fast pace of biotechnological development, changes in the health care delivery system, and the emergence of important new voices in a rapidly expanding field pose challenges for any comprehensive reference work. This new edition has made every effort to keep pace with such change and to reflect the global growth of bioethics.

DEVELOPMENT OF THE FOURTH EDITION

Bioethics has retained broad coverage of essential topic areas, including key concepts in the discourse of bioethics; ethical theory; religious ethics; the social sciences; the health care system; clinical practice and decision making; mental health and behavioral issues; sexuality and gender; fertility and human reproduction; genetics and biotechnology; organ and tissue transplantation and artificial organs; death and dying; population issues; public health; environmental ethics; and biomedical and behavioral research, to list just a few.

Of the 569 entries in the fourth edition, 221 are newly written and published for the first time. Just over 100 of these address topics not included in previous editions, and the rest offer new treatments of previous topics. Eighty-two of the new entries are addenda to "classic" entries that are reprinted without much change from the third edition. The balance of entries have been carefully updated and revised, often by the original authors. A handful of entries are reprinted with bibliography updates, and 14 dealing with the history and religious traditions of medicine and medical ethics appear in an appendix. For all revisions, whenever possible we went back to the articles' original authors, and many agreed to bring their earlier articles up to date. In those cases where the original authors were not available, another expert on that topic was engaged.

The Appendices, found in volume six, consist of (1) a group of articles on historical perspectives on medicine, ethics, and health care, (2) a listing of historical and contemporary codes, oaths, and directives related to bioethics, with links to the primary documents, (3) a listing of additional resources in bioethics, (4) a listing of key legal cases in bioethics, and (5) an annotated bibliography of literature and health care, including a filmography of works related to bioethics themes.

ACKNOWLEDGMENTS

Seventeen years passed between the first and second editions of the *Encyclopedia*, and nearly a decade passed between the second and third. Slightly less than a decade has elapsed between editions three and four. The fact that there is a recurring need to take a new look at the entire field once every ten years or so attests to the continuing vitality and activity within bioethics, as well as to the pace of scientific, technological, and social change surrounding issues in ethics and the life sciences.

In 2011 I was honored to assume the position of editor in chief, knowing full well that I could—and would need to—rely on the support and good counsel of Warren Reich, Stephen Post, and the wide range of scholars and colleagues with whom they had worked so successfully. This expectation has more than been fulfilled, and I want to express my gratitude to them and my admiration for what they achieved. How Professor Reich created this work from scratch I will never fully comprehend. All I can say is thank goodness I have been able to stand on foundations that others had already established. When I entered the field of bioethics in 1980, it was not common, as it is today, to take an advanced degree in "bioethics" per se. I myself learned on the job, so to speak. When I began work on *Bioethics* I certainly did not have an encyclopedic knowledge of the field; having read and edited over 500 wonderfully thoughtful and informative articles, I now feel I almost do. I will confess to Professors Reich and Post that I had never read their editions from cover to cover. If I had done so in my youth, I would have been the better for it.

One of the things that led me to undertake this assignment was the opportunity to think about the landscape of the field as a whole. I was especially intrigued by the challenge of identifying new topics that should be given more attention in bioethics, and to encourage that future work by including discussions of these topics in the standard reference work of the field. That has been a very gratifying undertaking. The other thing was the chance to assemble a team of colleagues for the editorial board. Our field is rich with talent, expertise, and personality, but I feel particularly fortunate to have secured the collaboration of the individuals who agreed to join the board of associate editors and consulting editors of the fourth edition of *Bioethics*. Working with them has been one of the high points of my career. The thousands of hours they have devoted to preparing this edition are exceeded only by the tens of thousands of hours put in by the hundreds of authors who have contributed the articles.

Editorial Board. The development of this fourth edition of *Bioethics* was facilitated by a new editorial board consisting of Lisa Eckenwiler, Gregory E. Kaebnick, Barbara Koenig, Sheldon Krimsky, Stephen R. Latham, and Mark R. Mercurio. These scholars were selected because their insight and expertise—in medicine, science, law, social science, history, philosophy, and education—were essential to achieve the goals of the new edition. I aimed and was successful at recruiting colleagues who are unusually broad in their intellectual scope and interests and who care deeply about the service that bioethics can provide to enhance human rights and justice and to alleviate suffering. The editor in chief and the editorial board were responsible for the intellectual planning of the fourth edition, including all decisions about contents and authorship, as well as for reviewing and approving all manuscripts.

Consultants. Joseph J. Fins and Bruce D. White served as editorial consultants and reviewed selected articles. Naomi Scheinerman updated article bibliographies and developed materials for various appendices. Therese Jones and Delese Wear edited and provided new material for the annotated bibliography of literature and health care.

Publishing Staff. The day-to-day work of preparing the fourth edition entailed close collaboration with the publisher's team in New York and Michigan. None of this work would have been possible without a publisher able to efficiently implement the intellectual plan. The Macmillan team commissioned all the articles, maintained contact with all authors, coordinated reviews, copyedited all manuscripts, checked revised manuscripts and bibliographies, and prepared all materials for production. In particular, Hélène G. Potter, Associate Publisher, Macmillan Reference USA, an imprint of Cengage Learning, provided vision and managerial insight for the development of the fourth edition—as well as many thoughtful perspectives. Similarly, Alja Kooistra and Andrea Henderson, Senior Content Project Editors, Macmillan Reference USA, an imprint of Cengage Learning, provided excellent leadership in implementing all the operational aspects of the project.

Bruce Jennings

Editor in Chief, Fourth Edition

January 14, 2014

Introduction

In his introduction to the first edition of the *Encyclopedia of Bioethics*, editor in chief Warren T. Reich defined bioethics as "the systematic study of human conduct in the area of the life sciences and health care, insofar as this conduct is examined in the light of moral values and principles." This definition has shaped the previous three editions of the *Encyclopedia of Bioethics* (1978, 1995, and 2004) and provides the jumping-off point for this new fourth edition, now simply called *Bioethics*. The scope of this formulation depends on what one includes in "the life sciences," the definition and the determinants of health, and the methods of ethics. The fourth edition, like its predecessors, treats these matters broadly and has a capacious conception of the scope of bioethics.

THE INVENTION OF BIOETHICS

The word *bioethics* was coined nearly half a century ago, notably by Van Rensselaer Potter in *Bioethics: Bridge to the Future* (1971). Behind the term stood the idea of encouraging public and professional reflection on two new and serious topics, which were, in the words of Stephen G. Post, editor in chief of the third edition, (1) "the responsibility to maintain the generative ecology of the planet, upon which life and human life depends," and (2) "the future implications of rapid advances in the life sciences with regard to potential modifications of a malleable human nature." In the beginning these two aspects of bioethics were intertwined; later they tended to diverge, as the field of environmental ethics worked on the first, while bioethics attended to the second, focusing on the so-called biological revolution, which involved innovations in medically assisted reproduction (test-tube babies), genetic components of disease and diagnostic genetic testing and population screening, and aspects of behavior modification and control (as popularized by the novel and film *A Clockwork Orange*).

In addition, the scope and focus of bioethics were influenced by the long-standing traditions of professional medical ethics, by advances in technology with powerful applications in clinical medicine, such as organ transplantation, and by ethical awareness of problems and abuses arising in the conduct of biomedical research using human beings as experimental subjects. New clinical capabilities created the need for explicit choice and decision, which were not resolvable on the basis of scientific or medical information alone. Such choices provoked ethical dilemmas—they involved personal and social values, religious convictions, and ethical and legal rights and obligations. It is perhaps revealing that when the Hastings Center, a pioneering bioethics research institute, began in 1969, the first research groups formed there were in the areas of death and dying, behavior control, genetic testing, and population control.

Medicine, the law, and ethics began to converge. Those who specialized in moral philosophy and political theory were ready to contribute because at precisely this same time the academic study of ethics was moving away from abstract conceptual analysis and toward public policy and practical application, as evidenced by the launching in 1972 of an influential new journal, *Philosophy and Public Affairs*.

In the mid-1970s in the United States, with cognate events occurring from time to time in other countries, research ethics broke into the headlines because of various abuses involving medical research and in response the National Commission for the Protection of Human Subjects of Biomedical and Behavioral Research was formed. Research ethics issues recalled the terrible legacy of the Nazi era and the unethical medical experiments documented during the Nuremberg Doctor Trials in the late 1940s. In 1966 an influential article in the *New England Journal of Medicine* by Henry Knowles Beecher called attention to questionable research practices that were then commonplace. (In the 1990s disturbing questions also arose in connection with research on the effects of radiation conducted in the United States after World War II.)

Clinical ethics followed suit with the controversy concerning mechanical life-sustaining technology (as in the case of Karen Ann Quinlan, whose parents wanted their permanently and irreversibly unconscious daughter to be allowed to die) and the paternalistic refusal of physicians to honor the wishes of a competent patient (as in the case of Dax Cowart, who had been severely burned and explicitly attempted to refuse continued life-sustaining, but extremely painful, treatment). In 1974 a documentary film about the Cowart case titled *Please Let Me Die* was widely shown. Quinlan's case got publicity worldwide when the New Jersey Supreme Court affirmed the right to refuse medical treatment in 1976. In addition to technological interventions involving life support, clinical ethics controversies also arose from advances in neurological testing that permitted a new whole-brain criteria for the declaration of death and in surgical and medical advances that permitted organ transplantation.

With this impetus and background, for over forty years bioethics has effectively addressed a range of issues having to do with justice, power, technology, and life. As it developed early in English-speaking countries, it has tended to reflect Anglo-American styles of philosophical and legal reasoning. And substantively, bioethics is most at home in the realm of liberal individualism. Its ethical vocabulary is made up of concepts such as self-interest, social utility, individual well-being based on health and choice, respect for the autonomy of persons, human rights, and equity or fair sharing in social benefits and burdens. The analytic style and substantive theory of the philosopher John Rawls in his major work, *A Theory of Justice* (1971), was important in setting the early tone of bioethics in this regard, as was the paradigmatic influence of *Principles of Biomedical Ethics* (1979) by Tom L. Beauchamp and James F. Childress, which developed an ethical framework initially established in the context of human subject research in the Belmont Report of the National Commission. Various ethical traditions in the medical profession and in religious traditions, especially the long history of Roman Catholic teachings on medical ethics, were also vitally important and influential in contemporary bioethics.

Bioethics engages with moral philosophy (and its cognate disciplines such as political and social philosophy, jurisprudence, and theological ethics) to provide a basic normative conceptual framework. Bioethics also engages with actually existing values, norms, and cultural belief systems. It should meet actors and institutions where they are, but it cannot just leave them there: change in assumptions, commitments, understanding, and action is the entire point of the enterprise. If it is not critical, bioethics can become apologetic and ideological.

THE DISCOURSE OF BIOETHICS

The discourse of bioethics is a sensitive indicator of the social context in which it germinates because the basic subject matter of this discourse—the human experience and meaning of health and illness—moves so fluidly from the most intimate, personal needs and experiences to the broadest social, systemic, and policy questions. Pain makes policy vivid and compelling; suffering makes systems come alive as tangible social agents rather than as intellectual constructs or abstractions. Every society needs to have a discourse with which to affirm and to contest power, equality, individual and group identity, knowledge, duty, and trust. Actually, societies need not merely one such discourse but several layered and overlapping ones. Repressive and stagnant societies tend to flatten and winnow this discursive array; more dynamic and open societies tend toward more diversity and argumentative conflict.

As mentioned above, in its early days bioethics was given impetus by a sudden burst of new possibilities in medicine and molecular biology, the biological revolution of the 1960s. A source of worry was a possible cultural lag between ethics and law, on one hand, and scientific knowledge and technology, on the other. The latter changes much more rapidly than the former. Therefore our repositories of value—ethics, cultural mores, religion, the law—were unable to guide and govern the use of science. Individuals were confronted with unprecedented choices in reproduction, in plumbing the body's genetic secrets, in postponing or avoiding death. Physicians were becoming facilitators of these new powers and ranges of choice. Investors sought to profit from them, governments sought to regulate them. But all were acting without a legal road map or an ethical compass. Bioethics was invented, so to speak, in order to respond to this lag. Those skilled in ethical discernment and calibration should anticipate scientific developments and adopt safeguards and procedures of review proactively, before problematic technologies become institutionally embedded and vested interests form to protect them. Bioethics should not merely react to a scientific *fait accompli*. And neither should it respond with knee-jerk rejection nor with thoughtless affirmation and permissiveness.

In retrospect, however, one can see that this mission of bioethics tended to overlook two things: history—the systemic interconnection of several problems with which it dealt seriatim—and the subtle cultural effects of technology. The problems raised by biomedical technology, such as, for example, the use of in vitro fertilization (IVF) to produce eugenic "designer children," were viewed as logical or moral puzzles to be solved by governance and social planning. (In the event, some countries, such as the United Kingdom, publicly regulated IVF; others, such as the United States, relegated it to the commercial marketplace.) This was a Solomonic bioethics, applying wisdom to individual disputes that came before it. Those in bioethics did not generally see this problem in any broader historical narrative of modernization and social change. Scholarship on the same issues in other fields, such as science, society, and technology studies or disability studies, did more along these lines than bioethics.

Moreover, the field of bioethics did not always recognize the conceptual baggage carried by its central motifs and problem definitions. The notion of a lag effect between two social systems flows out of a structural-functionalist orientation in sociology that has been taken to task by many social theorists for being ahistorical. From an anthropological point of view, bioethics also did not inquire with sufficient nuance into the dynamics of cultural response to behavioral innovation or comprehend the varieties of ways in which values are given cultural meaning.

However pointed such criticisms may be, bioethics persevered and often succeeded in framing issues, both in the media and in the thinking of professionals and policy makers, in certain ways. The bioethics puzzle and the lag effect were then solved using the following steps:

1. *Identifying moral principles, ideals, or standards*. Universal ethical principles make up a commonsense or "good reasons" morality. This is taken to be both rationally authoritative and widely accepted in the broader society, at least implicitly and by those most articulate and morally self-aware. Its principles are the touchstones for deducing justifiable conduct in particular situations.

2. *Assessing practice or behavior in the light of principles.* The conduct that emerges from the new biomedical knowledge and technology (such as the so-called technological imperative, the objectification of the person, and genetic engineering) is then assessed in light of the normative standards deduced from the general ethical principles.

3. *Suggesting policies or procedures to bring practice into line with principle.* Finally, regulation and governance of the new technology are proposed so that the morally beneficial conduct it induced would be promoted and the morally harmful conduct it induced would be minimized.

This pattern of discourse was widely endorsed over time by political and professional leaders and was welcomed into the precincts of law, policy, and clinical practice. For some, especially those who were unalloyed supporters of new technology and those who resented any incursion into professional self-sovereignty, the voice of bioethics was resisted or at best condescended to. But overall, bioethics gained a strong measure of legitimacy from the professional establishment, the philanthropic sector, and the media from roughly the late 1970s on.

THE REFERENCE IN THE FIELD

There is no doubt that bioethics succeeded in injecting a higher standard of ethical propriety and self-consciousness into medicine and health care, certainly into medical research with human subjects (and later into the care and use of animals in research) and important areas of health law, but also into clinical practice and public policy. Nonetheless, bioethics did not powerfully challenge or threaten the biomedical establishment with this pattern of discourse and analysis. The explanation for this, I believe, is precisely that bioethics discourse did not cut deeply into the workings of institutional, political, and economic power. It scrutinized the human and social consequences of the use of science and technology up to a point but no further. Many reasons can be adduced—the need to gain entry into certain professional, governmental, and financial citadels, the need to retain academic respectability by not becoming too activist or radical, and personal and temperamental factors of those self-selected individuals who entered the field.

I simply would add the proposition that, factors such as those aside, the character of the analysis and the remedies contained in much of bioethics discourse over the years has been shaped from within and delimited by the conceptual frameworks that bioethicists (whether they be physicians, nurses, lawyers, philosophers, or social scientists) brought to bear on the troubles they identified. To be sure, the field of bioethics today is becoming more self-reflective and critically aware of the conceptual limitations of its own discourse, but this is a relatively recent trend, prompted often by the work of feminists, philosophers working out of nonanalytic traditions, social scientists, and others who are able to adopt an external stance on mainstream bioethics. Included in the articles that are new to this edition of *Bioethics* are numerous entries focused on particular ethical and philosophical concepts. We have commissioned articles on such concepts to supplement cognate articles revised and updated from previous editions in order to broaden *Bioethics*'s engagement with the essential working vocabulary of the field. New articles along these lines include "Authenticity," "Biocentrism versus Anthropocentrism," "Biopolitics," "Epistemic Injustice," "Exploitation," "Genetic Citizenship," "Global Justice," "Liberty," "Naturalism," "Oppression," "Reductionism," "Social Constructionism," "Solidarity," and "Vulnerability."

I offer these remarks on the development and what I take to be the mainstream orientation of the field as a way of introducing what this new edition of *Bioethics* has to offer. Although not laid out as schematically as I have done here, a great many of the articles in this edition implicitly follow the working of the pattern—identify principle; assess practice; recommend process to align practice with principle—through the discussion of the topic in question. This can be seen across the entire body of articles, from access to health care and adoption through divided loyalties in mental health care and impaired professionals to privacy in health care and surrogate decision making. What is instructive about this is precisely that it is not a formulaic analysis but rather an exploration of three main realms: the logic of theoretical reasoning about universal values and norms; the nuance and complexity of making judgments and interpretations of general values in the light of specific cultural and social circumstances and situations; and the pragmatic considerations of devising measures to organize and control human behavior in accordance with considerations of efficiency, enforceability, and fairness.

If some work in bioethics is insufficiently aware historically and culturally, we have tried to craft articles that do not make that mistake. This edition, like previous ones, embraces cross-cultural approaches, the history of medicine and bioethics, comparative religious and philosophical ethics, and global perspectives. A common thread running through many, if not most, of the articles is the degree to which our contemporary theories of ethics and bioethics evolve from particular social, cultural–religious, and historical contexts. Virtually every major spiritual and faith tradition's outlook on bioethical issues is represented in this edition, as they have been in the prior ones. If some work in bioethics is overly individualistic, there is an answering voice in many articles that explore the roots of freedom and autonomy in relationship and community. Some of these articles focus on particular concepts such as care ethics, community and communitarianism, narrative, solidarity, and trust. Traditional dichotomies are often confronted and questioned. When it comes to ideas, at least, many articles here, on the basis of reason and evidence, afflict the comfortable. This edition of *Bioethics* does not overlook or play down questions of power in the realm of science, technology, and health. Ethical dilemmas are often indicative of underlying structural, institutional, and systemic inequality and injustice. Again, these themes are explored in numerous articles relating to public health, inequality and exploitation, racism, and issues having to do with child welfare, gender, and sexuality.

In 2014 the field of bioethics is one that has changed and is changing. Three major developments are particularly salient among a range of articles in this edition. These are professionalization, disciplinary rigor, and international expansion and the recognition of a global perspective.

Bioethics is becoming more "professionalized" as many now take primary degrees in bioethics, as distinct from studying some other discipline first and then coming into bioethics issues from another intellectual home. Nonetheless, I would guess that a majority of the contributing authors to the fourth edition of *Bioethics* still would not call themselves "bioethicists" as a first impulse. Many of those with the greatest knowledge and expertise on bioethics topics come to them because of those topics' intrinsic interest and importance but have other intellectual identities and label themselves in different ways. A number of articles explicitly take up themes of professionalization and governance within the field of bioethics itself, including entries on bioethics professionalism, the ethics of bioethics, the sociology, anthropology, and politics of bioethics, and developments in clinical ethics consultation.

The field is also becoming more "disciplinary" in the sense that it is more conscious of its methodological approaches and conventional requirements of scholarship, and it is more oriented than it once was toward an audience of fellow specialists and practitioners. For many in the field today, career advancement requires conformity to grant-seeking strategies and quantitative research. There are signs that the "two cultures"—as C. P. Snow called the divide between the sciences and the humanities—is becoming a factor in the culture of bioethics itself. Interdisciplinary work is always vulnerable to charges of dilettantism and a lack of rigor. On the other hand, disciplinary specialization can weaken the kind of serious, even passionate, ethical concern and social engagement that has so animated the field of bioethics over the years. Articles on bioethics methods generally and empirical methodology specifically, those that look at the field from social scientific perspectives, and those that study the patterns of discourse, ideological disagreement, and legitimation—all make note of intellectual, occupational, and economic forces affecting the field of bioethics and emerging internal divisions in it.

Finally, the field is becoming more international as nations all over the world develop their own educational and research structures devoted to bioethics and as regional and international bodies such as the Council of Europe and the World Health Organization fund and sponsor important bioethics research and policy analysis. These developments are perfectly understandable and appropriate in the wake of new developments in the biomedical sciences and economic and commercial interests surrounding biotechnology, not to mention widespread interest among the general public in many nations. Studies on the use of genetically modified food, technology transfer and patenting, and research in the area of synthetic biology are three examples of international bioethics collaboration. And one should not discuss international bioethics without mentioning what has sadly but undeniably been a major factor in the growth of international interest in bioethics, the worldwide HIV/AIDS pandemic. Many articles focus on AIDS and human rights issues. There are also country-by-country reviews of bioethics research, education, and regulation in virtually every region of the world.

Indeed, the international aspects of bioethics have increased the relatively scant attention that bioethics in the past has paid to population health and public health policy and practice. Influenza pandemics, and all-hazard types of public health emergency preparedness, have demonstrated that matters previously understood from a domestic, national perspective need to be viewed more broadly; old questions need to be asked in new ways. Articles in this edition that address this topic are more numerous than in previous editions, including entries on global justice, globalization and health, cross-border medical travel, health justice, and a variety of human rights entries, as well as those on pandemic, climate change, and multinational research.

In the years ahead international bioethics will take another step and become global bioethics. This is necessary because the questions of power, justice, science, technology, and health with which bioethics fundamentally deals today have no geographical boundaries, and the legal sovereignty of separate nation-states is more of a hindrance than a help in managing and regulating the bioeconomy of the world today. These global problems seem to be particularly challenging, and perhaps beyond the ken of existing forms of international cooperation. The record thus far in managing global climate change certainly does not make one sanguine in this regard.

NEW POINTS OF EMPHASIS

Bioethics now includes a total of 108 articles on topics new to this edition. In addition to those previously mentioned, it contains new articles on such topics as "Abortion: Hindu Perspectives," "Abuse of Health Care Workers," "Biodiversity Conservation," "Cognitive Impairment/Traumatic Brain Injury," "Hospitals, Ethical Issues in the Governance of," "Humanitarian Relief," "Nuclear Weapons," and "Pedagogy of Bioethics."

Several topics have received expanded emphasis in this edition. One is a greater focus on public health and public health ethics and on matters closely linked to public health policy and response, such as infectious disease and environmental health, and emergency preparedness. Another is health policy and policy bioethics. At a time of significant health policy innovation and reform in the United States and many European countries, numerous articles in this volume are devoted to those topics and to improvements in health care quality, comparative effectiveness research, and economic sustainability and justice, both domestic and global.

Aging, chronic illness, and long-term care also receive concerted attention. Changing attitudes and policies toward abortion internationally are surveyed. An emphasis is given to new developments in biotechnology, genetics, and reproduction, and end-of-life care is thoroughly discussed, with more expansive coverage of palliative care, again both domestic and global.

Finally, this edition of *Bioethics* envisions greater communication in the future with the field of environmental ethics in terms of its philosophies and theories (biocentrism and ecocentrism), scientific fields (ecology, conservation biology, evolutionary biology), and policy problems (climate change, biodiversity loss, environmental health hazards, freshwater, the ecological and health effects of technology, urbanization, agricultural practices, and the like). Areas like posthumanism and transhumanism, advances in neuroscience, nanotechnology, and synthetic biology are topics where a creative engagement between bioethics and environmental ethics should prove to be quite interesting. This will put the "bios" back into bioethics in a new way, and may bring us back full circle to thinkers like Van Rensselaer Potter.

ORGANIZATION OF *BIOETHICS*

Entries are arranged alphabetically. Some entries comprise several subentries. For example:

Care: I. History of the Notion of Care

Care: II. Historical Precedents for an Ethic of Care in Health Care

Care: III. Care Ethics

Care: IV. Care and Society/Public Policy

The reader wishing to study ethical aspects of care and caregiving would do well to read all four of these interlocking articles.

Cross-references are provided for each article. However, for a complete perspective on the thematic relationships between articles, please see the "Topical Outline" at the beginning of the first volume, following the list of contributors.

The bibliographies following each article are an important resource. These were prepared by the authors or otherwise updated with approval by the editor in chief. The bibliographies are necessarily selective rather than exhaustive given the volume of significant new books and articles relevant to each article.

The appendices contained in the sixth volume are of great value to students and researchers. In the past they have been reprints of primary source documents. In keeping with our digital research environment, the current edition provides electronic links to many documents rather than reprinting the documents themselves. This section of the work includes: (1) a group of articles on historical perspectives on medicine, ethics, and health care, (2) a listing of historical and contemporary codes, oaths, and directives related to bioethics, with links to the primary documents, (3) a listing of additional resources in bioethics, (4) an annotated list of key legal cases in bioethics, and (5) an annotated bibliography of literature and health care, including a filmography of works related to bioethics themes.

Bioethics has always been a distinctive reference work because it includes so many voices and theoretical and disciplinary orientations in an effort to foster dialogue, prevent the narrowing of the field, and engage a wide international readership.

A special effort has been made to keep these volumes free from technical jargon. The articles should be accessible to students at the high school, college, and graduate levels, as well as to interested lay readers. They are written in such a manner as to be authoritative for professionals wishing to gain a clear perspective on how ideas have evolved.

A special effort has also been made to ensure that this new edition of *Bioethics* lives up to the example of its predecessors in being an exemplar of civic discourse. By this I mean that within each article and for the body of articles taken as a whole, we have strived to offer discussions that are clearly reasoned, evidence-based and diligently researched, respectful and open to serious engagement with opposing views, open to difference and plurality, free from objectifying stereotype or stigma, and ardent in their vision of justice and moral possibility. Many of the finest contributors to the field of bioethics are represented in these pages. These are men and women actively engaged in the service of others through voluntary associations or professional practice. As appropriate to the assignment they have undertaken for *Bioethics*, they often move beyond the mere exposition of the essential inventory of existing thoughts on a topic to argue persuasively for a normative viewpoint. Indeed, I hope that those who read these volumes will be motivated by a sense of responsibility and service, as well as by intellectual curiosity.

THE PRESENCE OF THE FUTURE

One way to look at an academic encyclopedia in any field is to see it as a comprehensive repository of the current state of knowledge and scholarly discussion in that field or discipline. This is the idea of an encyclopedia as a mirror. A reference work of that sort is of great utility and value, to be sure. Another way to view an encyclopedia, however, is to see it not only as a repository but as a publication that expands and develops the field beyond its current position. Such an encyclopedia reflects what is behind but also illuminates what lies ahead. This is the idea of the encyclopedia as a lamp. As such, an encyclopedia can be a creative intellectual force in the dynamic of the field, inspiring new lines of research and new questions and theoretical perspectives that are currently underdeveloped in the mainstream.

The philosopher Thomas Hobbes remarked that only the present is real because the past is gone and the future does not yet exist. Closer to the truth, I believe, is the novelist Marcel Proust's idea that the past exists through memory, the future exists through imagination, and the present is largely constituted by the interplay of memory and imagination. My notion is that perhaps the main calling of bioethics now is to muster the moral imagination necessary to sense the presence of the future. If we can manage that, then we may be able to grasp the fact that we bear a moral responsibility for what we are doing toward the well-being and the life conditions of others—others living now and close to us, yes, but also those living far away and those who are not yet alive.

As editor in chief, I hope that at least in a modest way this fourth edition of *Bioethics* will serve as a lamp. I also hope that readers of these volumes become more knowledgeable about the presence of the past and more sentient about the presence of the future and its profound ethical demands on all of us.

Bruce Jennings

Editor in Chief, Fourth Edition

January 14, 2014

Articles

*An * indicates that the article appears in the appendix "Historical Perspectives on Medicine, Ethics, and Health Care."*

B

VOLUME 2

C

VOLUME 3

F

G

H

Contributors

*An * indicates that the article appears in the appendix "Historical Perspectives on Medicine, Ethics, and Health Care."*

Donald C. Ainslie

Associate Professor, Department of Philosophy, University of Toronto

PRINCIPLISM

Sandra L. Alfano

Research Scientist, General Internal Medicine, and Chair, Human Investigation Committee II and IV, Yale University School of Medicine

COMMUNITY-BASED PARTICIPATORY RESEARCH

Anita L. Allen

Henry R. Silverman Professor of Law and Professor of Philosophy, University of Pennsylvania Law School

ABORTION: III. LEGAL AND REGULATORY ISSUES

PRIVACY IN HEALTH CARE

Kirk C. Allison

Director, Program in Human Rights and Health, University of Minnesota School of Public Health

HUMAN GENOME PROJECT

Darrel W. Amundsen

Professor of Classics, Western Washington University

EUROPE: I. ANCIENT GREECE AND ROME*

EUROPE: II. EARLY CHRISTIANITY*

EUROPE: III. MEDIEVAL CHRISTIANITY*

NEAR AND MIDDLE EAST: ANCIENT NEAR EAST*

Gerard F. Anderson

Professor, Departments of Health Policy and Management and International Health, Bloomberg School of Public Health

Professor of Medicine, School of Medicine, Johns Hopkins University

HEALTH CARE SYSTEMS

Martha W. Anderson

Executive Vice President, Donor Services Division, Musculoskeletal Transplant Foundation

TISSUE BANKING AND TRANSPLANTATION, ETHICAL ISSUES IN

Matthew Anderson

Assistant Professor of Family and Social Medicine, Albert Einstein College of Medicine

SOCIAL MEDICINE

Georgia J. Anetzberger

President, National Committee for the Prevention of Elder Abuse

ABUSE, INTERPERSONAL: III. ELDER ABUSE

George J. Annas

Professor and Chair, Department of Health Law, Bioethics, and Human Rights, Boston University Schools of Public Health, Law, and Medicine

HUMAN RIGHTS

PATIENTS' RIGHTS: I. ORIGIN AND NATURE OF PATIENTS' RIGHTS

Paul S. Appelbaum

Dollard Professor of Psychiatry, Medicine & Law, Department of Psychiatry

College of Physicians & Surgeons, Columbia University

MENTAL INSTITUTIONS, COMMITMENT TO

Pat Armstrong

Professor of Sociology, York University

ABUSE, INTERPERSONAL: IV. ABUSE OF HEALTH CARE WORKERS

Peter S. Arno

Professor, Center for Long Term Care Research and Policy, New York Medical College

LONG-TERM CARE: IV. FINANCING, US AND INTERNATIONAL

Robert M. Arnold

Leo H. Creip Chair of Patient Care, Department of Medicine; Director, Palliative Care Service; Director of the Institute for Doctor-Patient Communication, University of Pittsburgh

Medical Director Palliative and Supportive Care Institute of University of Pittsburgh Medical Center

ADVANCE DIRECTIVES AND ADVANCE CARE PLANNING

BIOETHICS EDUCATION: I. MEDICINE

INFORMED CONSENT: IV. CLINICAL ASPECTS OF CONSENT IN HEALTH CARE

Mila A. Aroskar

Professor Emerita, Center for Bioethics, University of Minnesota

BIOETHICS EDUCATION: II. NURSING

Adrienne Asch

Edward and Robin Milstein Professor of Bioethics, Wurzweiler School of Social Work, Yeshiva University

Director, Center for Ethics at Yeshiva University

DISABILITY: III. MODELS OF

Richard Ashcroft

Professor of Bioethics, School of Law, Queen Mary, University of London

EUROPE, BIOETHICS IN: IV. UNITED KINGDOM

Mark P. Aulisio

Professor of Bioethics, Case Western Reserve University

Director, Center for Biomedical Ethics, MetroHealth System

CLINICAL ETHICS: I. DEVELOPMENT, ROLE, AND METHODOLOGIES

CLINICAL ETHICS: II. ETHICS COMMITTEES AND ETHICS CONSULTATION

DOUBLE EFFECT, PRINCIPLE OR DOCTRINE OF

Osman Bakar

Deputy CEO, International Institute of Advanced Islamic Studies—Malaysia

Emeritus Professor of Philosophy, University of Malaya

ABORTION: VII. ISLAMIC PERSPECTIVES

Robert Baker

William D. Williams Professor of Philosophy, Union College

Founding Director and Professor of Bioethics, Union Graduate College and Icahn Mount Sinai Bioethics Program

MEDICAL CODES AND OATHS

John D. Banja

Professor, Department of Rehabilitation Medicine, and Medical Ethicist, Center for Ethics at Emory University

Director, Ethics Section: Atlanta Clinical and Translational Science Institute

NEUROETHICS

NEUROETHICS AND FREE WILL

REHABILITATION MEDICINE

Joanne Trautmann Banks

Professor of Humanities and English, College of Medicine, Pennsylvania State University

LITERATURE AND HEALTH CARE

Michael Barber

Professor of Philosophy, Saint Louis University

PHENOMENOLOGY

David Barnard

Miles J. Edwards Chair in Professionalism and Comfort Care, Center for Ethics in Health Care, Oregon Health and Science University

END-OF-LIFE CARE

Margaret Pabst Battin

Professor, Department of Philosophy and Division of Medical Ethics and Humanities, University of Utah

POPULATION POLICIES, STRATEGIES FOR FERTILITY CONTROL IN SUICIDE

Michele Battle-Fisher

Instructor, Wright State University Boonshoft School of Medicine, Community Health

MINORITIES AS RESEARCH SUBJECTS [ADDENDUM]

Ronald Bayer

Center for the History and Ethics of Public Health, Mailman School of Public Health, Columbia University

AIDS: I. PUBLIC HEALTH ISSUES

Corrine Bayley

St. Joseph Health System, Orange, CA

HOSPITAL, CONTEMPORARY ETHICAL PROBLEMS OF THE

Françoise Baylis

Professor and Canada Research Chair in Bioethics and Philosophy, Novel Tech Ethics, Faculty of Medicine, Dalhousie University

AMERICA, BIOETHICS IN: II. CANADA

Dan E. Beauchamp

Emeritus Professor, Health Policy, Management, and Behavior, School of Public Health, University at Albany, State University of New York

PUBLIC HEALTH: III. PHILOSOPHY

PUBLIC HEALTH: IX. LIFESTYLES

Tom L. Beauchamp

Professor of Philosophy, Department of Philosophy and Kennedy Institute of Ethics, Georgetown University

INFORMED CONSENT: I. HISTORY OF INFORMED CONSENT

INFORMED CONSENT: II. MEANING AND ELEMENTS

PATERNALISM

Jonathan Beever

Doctoral Student, Department of Philosophy, Purdue University

BIOCENTRISM VERSUS ANTHROPOCENTRISM

Elizabeth A. Behnke

Creator, Study Project in Phenomenology of the Body

BODY: I. EMBODIMENT IN THE PHENOMENOLOGICAL TRADITION [ADDENDUM]

Emily Smith Beitiks

Assistant Director, Paul K. Longmore Institute on Disability, San Francisco State University

BIOPOLITICS

Catherine Belling

Associate Professor, Medical Humanities and Bioethics, Northwestern University Feinberg School of Medicine

LITERATURE AND HEALTH CARE [ADDENDUM]

Solomon R. Benatar

Emeritus Professor of Medicine, University of Cape Town, Professor, Dalla Lana School of Public Health and Joint Centre for Bioethics, University of Toronto

AFRICA, BIOETHICS IN: II. SOUTH AFRICA

Martin Benjamin

Department of Philosophy, Michigan State University

CONSCIENCE

Alina Bennett

Doctoral Candidate, Institute for the Medical Humanities, University of Texas Medical Branch at Galveston

MENTAL HEALTH SERVICES: II. ETHICAL ISSUES

Jessica Berg

Professor of Law and Bioethics, Department of Bioethics, Case Western Reserve University

INFORMED CONSENT: V. LEGAL AND ETHICAL ISSUES OF CONSENT IN HEALTH CARE [ADDENDUM]

Nancy Berlinger

Research Scholar, The Hastings Center

IMMIGRANTS, ACCESS TO HEALTH CARE

James L. Bernat

Louis and Ruth Frank Professor of Neuroscience, Professor of Neurology and Medicine, Geisel School of Medicine, Dartmouth College

MEDICAL EDUCATION [ADDENDUM]

Erin Berry-Bibee

Family Planning Fellow and Instructor, Department of Gynecology and Obstetrics, Emory University School of Medicine

ABORTION: I. MEDICAL PERSPECTIVES [ADDENDUM]

Barbara Bowles Biesecker

Associate Investigator, Social and Behavioral Branch, National Human Genome Research Institute, National Institutes of Health

GENETIC COUNSELING, PRACTICE OF

Anne-Emanuelle Birn

Professor, Dalla Lana School of Public Health and Centre for Critical Development Studies, University of Toronto

PUBLIC HEALTH: VIII. SOCIAL DETERMINANTS OF HEALTH

Anne H. Bishop

Professor of Nursing Emeritus, Lynchburg College

NURSING, PROFESSION OF

NURSING, THEORIES AND PHILOSOPHY OF

Bela Blasszauer

Scientific Adviser, Institute of Family Medicine, University of Pécs, Hungary

EUROPE, BIOETHICS IN: VIII. CENTRAL AND EASTERN EUROPE

Sidney Bloch

Emeritus Professor, Department of Psychiatry, University of Melbourne

PSYCHIATRY, ABUSES OF

Samuel W. Bloom

Professor of Sociology and Community Medicine, Mount Sinai School of Medicine

PROFESSIONAL-PATIENT RELATIONSHIP: I. SOCIOLOGICAL PERSPECTIVES

Joachim Boldt

Associate Professor, Department of Medical Ethics and the History of Medicine, University of Freiburg

SYNTHETIC BIOLOGY

John Bongaarts

Vice President and Distinguished Scholar, Population Council

POPULATION POLICIES, DEMOGRAPHIC ASPECTS OF

Kathleen M. Boozang

Associate Dean and Professor of Law, Seton Hall Law School Center for Health and Pharmaceutical Law and Policy

HOSPITALS, ETHICAL ISSUES IN THE GOVERNANCE OF

Kevin Borrup

Associate Director, Injury Prevention Center, Connecticut Children's Medical Center Assistant Professor, Department of Pediatrics, University of Connecticut School of Medicine

INJURY AND INJURY CONTROL [ADDENDUM]

Charles L. Bosk

Professor of Sociology, and Professor of Anesthesiology and Critical Care, Perelman School of Medicine, University of Pennsylvania

Senior Fellow, Leonard Davis Institute of Health Economics, University of Pennsylvania

HEALTH AND DISEASE: II. SOCIOLOGICAL PERSPECTIVES

MISTAKES, MEDICAL

Renee D. Boss

Assistant Professor, Department of Pediatrics, Division of Neonatology, Johns Hopkins School of Medicine, Johns Hopkins Berman Institute of Bioethics

INFANTS, ETHICAL ISSUES WITH [ADDENDUM]

Jeffrey R. Botkin

Chair, Division of Medical Ethics and Humanities, Department of Internal Medicine, University of Utah

CIRCUMCISION, MALE

Scott Bottenfield

Retired

TISSUE BANKING AND TRANSPLANTATION, ETHICAL ISSUES IN

Melissa M. Bottrell

Chief for Integrated Ethics, National Center for Ethics in Health Care, Department of Veterans Affairs

HEALTH CARE, QUALITY IMPROVEMENT

Ivy Bourgeault

Canadian Institutes of Health Research Chair in Health Human Resources, Institute of Population Health, University of Ottawa

HEALTH CARE, WORKER MIGRATION

Marilyn J. Boxer

Professor of History Emerita, Department of History, San Francisco State University

WOMEN, HISTORICAL AND CROSS-CULTURAL PERSPECTIVES

Gert H. Brieger

Professor Emeritus, Department of the History of Medicine, Institute of the History of Medicine, Johns Hopkins University

MEDICINE, PROFESSION OF

Dan W. Brock

Frances Glessner Lee Professor of Medical Ethics, Department of Global Health and Social Medicine, Harvard Medical School

LIFE-SUSTAINING TREATMENT AND EUTHANASIA: I. ETHICAL ASPECTS OF

PUBLIC POLICY AND BIOETHICS

SURROGATE DECISION MAKING

Howard Brody

University of Texas Medical Branch

COMMERCIALISM IN SCIENTIFIC RESEARCH

HEALTH CARE, DELIVERY OF

PATIENTS' RESPONSIBILITIES: I. DUTIES OF PATIENTS

PLACEBO

Courtenay R. Bruce

Assistant Professor of Medicine and Medical Ethics, Center for Medical Ethics and Health Policy, Baylor College of Medicine

BIOETHICS: II. KEY CASES IN

Jennifer A. Bulcock

Department of Philosophy, Rice University

HEALTH AND DISEASE: II. SOCIOLOGICAL PERSPECTIVES [ADDENDUM]

HEALTH AND DISEASE: IV. PHILOSOPHICAL PERSPECTIVES

MEDICINE, PHILOSOPHY OF

Chester R. Burns

James Wade Rockwell Professor of Medical History, Institute for the Medical Humanities, University of Texas Medical Branch

UNITED STATES: THE COLONIAL PERIOD THROUGH THE NINETEENTH CENTURY*

Jeffrey P. Burns

Chief of Critical Care Medicine and Edward and Barbara Shapiro Chair of Critical Care Medicine, Division of Critical Care Medicine, Department of Anesthesiology, Perioperative, and Pain Medicine, Boston Children's Hospital/ Harvard Medical School

DNR (DO NOT RESUSCITATE)

Lisa Sowle Cahill

J. Donald Monan Professor, Department of Theology, Boston College

ABORTION: V. ROMAN CATHOLIC PERSPECTIVES

Bethany C. Calkins

University of Rochester Medical Center, Center for Ethics, Humanities, and Palliative Care

PHYSICIAN-ASSISTED DYING/ HASTENED DEATH

J. Baird Callicott

University Distinguished Research Professor and Regents Professor of Philosophy, University of North Texas

ENVIRONMENTAL ETHICS: I. OVERVIEW

ENVIRONMENTAL ETHICS: III. LAND ETHICS

Samantha Jane Calvert

University of Birmingham

ANIMAL WELFARE AND RIGHTS: II. VEGETARIANISM [ADDENDUM]

Nigel M. de S. Cameron

Managing Director, Center for Policy on Emerging Technologies

CHRISTIANITY, BIOETHICS IN

Courtney S. Campbell

Hundere Professor in Religion and Culture, School of History, Philosophy, and Religion, Oregon State University

CLONING: III. RELIGIOUS PERSPECTIVES [ADDENDUM]

MORMONISM (CHURCH OF JESUS CHRIST OF LATTER-DAY SAINTS), BIOETHICS IN

Lisa Campo-Engelstein

Assistant Professor, Alden March Bioethics Institute & Department of OBGYN, Albany Medical College

EMBRYO AND FETUS: II. EMBRYO RESEARCH

Norman L. Cantor

Professor of Law and Justice, Nathan L. Jacobs Scholar Emeritus, Rutgers University School of Law

LIFE, QUALITY OF: III. QUALITY OF LIFE IN LEGAL PERSPECTIVE

Arthur L. Caplan

Director, Division of Medical Ethics, New York University Langone Medical Center

REPRODUCTIVE TECHNOLOGIES: IX. IN VITRO FERTILIZATION AND EMBRYO TRANSFER

Alexander Morgan Capron

University Professor and Scott H. Bice Chair in Healthcare Law, Policy and Ethics, Gould School of Law, University of Southern California

DEATH, DEFINITION AND DETERMINATION OF: II. LEGAL ISSUES IN PRONOUNCING DEATH

LAW AND BIOETHICS

Michele A. Carter

Professor, Institute for the Medical Humanities, University of Texas Medical Branch at Galveston

MENTAL HEALTH SERVICES: II. ETHICAL ISSUES

Amy Case

Palliative Medicine Fellowship Program Director and Assistant Professor of Medicine, University at Buffalo School of Medicine and Biomedical Sciences

Director of Palliative Medicine, Veterans Administration Western New York Healthcare System

HOSPICE AND PALLIATIVE CARE: PROFESSIONAL EDUCATION

Christine K. Cassel

President and Chief Executive Officer, ABIM and ABIM Foundation

HEALTH CARE INSTITUTIONS

Eric J. Cassell

Emeritus Professor of Public Health, Weill Medical College, Cornell University

Adjunct Professor of Medicine, Faculty of Medicine, McGill University

MEDICINE, ART OF

PAIN AND SUFFERING

Peter Caws

University Professor of Philosophy and Professor of Human Sciences, George Washington University

PSYCHOANALYSIS AND DYNAMIC THERAPIES

Kathy Cerminara

Professor of Law, Nova Southeastern University Shepard Broad Law Center

RIGHT TO DIE: POLICY AND LAW

Tod Chambers

Associate Professor of Medical Humanities and Bioethics and of Medicine, Medical Humanities and Bioethics Program, Northwestern University, Feinberg School of Medicine

BIOETHICS: III. DISCOURSE IN POSTMODERNISM

Louisa E. Chapman

Division of Notifiable Diseases and Healthcare Information, Public Health Surveillance and Informatics Program Office, Office of Surveillance, Epidemiology, and Laboratory Support, Centers for Disease Control and Prevention

XENOTRANSPLANTATION

Christopher Key Chapple

Doshi Professor of Indic and Comparative Theology, Loyola Marymount University

JAINISM, BIOETHICS IN

R. Alta Charo

Warren P. Knowles Professor of Law and Bioethics, University of Wisconsin Law School

REPRODUCTIVE TECHNOLOGIES: IV. LEGAL AND REGULATORY ISSUES

Frank A. Chervenak

Given Foundation Professor and Chairman, Department of Obstetrics and Gynecology, Weill Medical College of Cornell University

CHILDBIRTH, MEDICAL PROCEDURES IN

SELECTIVE TERMINATION/REDUCTION OF MULTIPLE PREGNANCY

James F. Childress

University Professor, John Allen Hollingsworth Professor of Ethics, Institute for Practical Ethics and Public Life, University of Virginia

AUTONOMY [ADDENDUM]

METAPHOR AND ANALOGY

Mildred K. Cho

Professor (Research) of Pediatrics, Stanford Center for Biomedical Ethics

RESEARCH ETHICS CONSULTATION

Larry R. Churchill

Ann Geddes Stahlman Chair of Medical Ethics, Center for Biomedical Ethics and Society, Vanderbilt University

BENEFICENCE

Ellen Wright Clayton

Professor of Pediatrics and Law, Center for Biomedical Ethics and Society, Vanderbilt University

CHILDREN: II. RIGHTS OF CHILDREN [ADDENDUM]

GENETIC TESTING AND SCREENING: II. NEWBORN GENETIC SCREENING

Cynthia B. Cohen

Faculty Affiliate, Kennedy Institute of Ethics, Georgetown University

REPRODUCTIVE TECHNOLOGIES: V. GAMETE DONATION

REPRODUCTIVE TECHNOLOGIES: VIII. ETHICAL ISSUES

David Cohen

Professor, Obstetrics and Gynecology and Chief, Section of Reproductive Endocrinology and Infertility, University of Chicago Center for Reproductive Medicine and Fertility

REPRODUCTIVE TECHNOLOGIES: I. INTRODUCTION

Robert L. Cohen

Clinical Assistant Professor, Department of Medicine, New York University School of Medicine

PRISONERS, HEALTH CARE ISSUES OF

Felicia Cohn

Bioethics Director, Kaiser Permanente Orange County, CA

ABUSE, INTERPERSONAL: II. ABUSE BETWEEN DOMESTIC PARTNERS

Rachel Cohon

Professor, Department of Philosophy, University at Albany, State University of New York

DISABILITY: I. ETHICAL AND SOCIETAL PERSPECTIVES

Ronald Cole-Turner

H. Parker Sharp Professor of Theology and Ethics, Pittsburgh Theological Seminary

EMBRYO AND FETUS: V. RELIGIOUS PERSPECTIVES

James Colgrove

Associate Professor of Sociomedical Sciences, Mailman School of Public Health, Columbia University

PUBLIC HEALTH: I. HISTORY [ADDENDUM]

Harold J. Cook

Professor of History, Brown University

EUROPE: IV. RENAISSANCE AND ENLIGHTENMENT*

Brian Cooke

Associate Professor, University of Florida Department of Psychiatry

EXPERT TESTIMONY

Steven S. Coughlin

Adjunct Professor of Epidemiology, Department of Epidemiology, Emory University

PUBLIC HEALTH: VI. RESEARCH

Jonathan K. Crane

Raymond F. Schinazi Junior Scholar in Bioethics and Jewish Thought, Center for Ethics, Emory University

JUDAISM, BIOETHICS IN [ADDENDUM]

Ronald E. Cranford

Professor of Neurology, University of Minnesota, Twin Cities

DEATH, DEFINITION AND DETERMINATION OF: I. CRITERIA FOR DEATH

Megan Crowley-Matoka

Assistant Professor, Medical Humanities and Bioethics, Feinberg School of Medicine, Northwestern University

BODY: III. COMMODIFICATION OF

Thomas J. Csordas

Professor of Anthropology, University of California, San Diego

BODY: II. CULTURAL AND RELIGIOUS PERSPECTIVES

Charles M. Culver

Professor of Medical Education, Barry University

ELECTROCONVULSIVE THERAPY

Amy T. Cunningham

Program Manager, ABIM Foundation

HEALTH CARE INSTITUTIONS

Abdallah S. Daar

Professor of Public Health Sciences and of Surgery, and Senior Scientist, Sandra Rotman Centre, University Health Network and University of Toronto Fellow, Stellenbosch Institute for Advanced Study, Wallenberg Research Centre at Stellenbosch University

XENOTRANSPLANTATION

Ariella Rabin Dagi

Lecturer, Massachusetts Institute of Technology

SELF-EXPERIMENTATION

T. Forcht Dagi

Professor, School of Medicine, Dentistry and Biomedical Sciences, Queen's University Belfast, Northern Ireland

Visiting Professor, Division of Medical Ethics, Department of Global Health and Social Medicine, Harvard Medical School

SELF-EXPERIMENTATION

Clare Dalton

Matthews Distinguished University Professor of Law, Northeastern University, Boston, MA

SEXUALITY, LEGAL APPROACHES TO

Barbara J. Daly

The Gertrude Perkins Oliva Professor in Oncology Nursing and Clinical Ethics Director, University Hospitals, Cleveland, OH

NURSING, PROFESSION OF

Marcy Darnovsky

Executive Director, Center for Genetics and Society

BIOPOLITICS

Kurt Darr

Professor of Health Services Management and Leadership, School of Public Health and Health Services, George Washington University

HEALTH SERVICES MANAGEMENT ETHICS

Rebecca Darrah

Frances Payne Bolton School of Nursing, Case Western Reserve University

GENETIC TESTING AND SCREENING: VI. PEDIATRIC GENETIC TESTING

Rahul Peter Das

Professor and Head, South Asia Department, Oriental Institute, Martin-Luther-Universität Halle-Wittenberg

HINDUISM, BIOETHICS IN

Anne J. Davis

Professor Emerita, School of Nursing, University of California, San Francisco

BIOETHICS EDUCATION: II. NURSING

Dena S. Davis

Professor, Religion Studies, Lehigh University

AUTHORITY IN RELIGIOUS TRADITIONS

Angus Dawson

Professor of Public Health and Head of Medicine, Ethics, Society and History, University of Birmingham, UK

PUBLIC HEALTH: XII. PREVENTION AND PROMOTION

VACCINATION AND IMMUNIZATION

Kenneth Allen De Ville

East Carolina University

COMMERCIALISM IN SCIENTIFIC RESEARCH

Raymond De Vries

Professor, Center for Bioethics and Social Sciences and Medicine, University of Michigan Medical School

BIOETHICS: VIII. SOCIOLOGY OF

Maurice A. M. de Wachter

Bioethics Consultant, Brussels, Belgium

EUROPE, BIOETHICS IN: III. THE BENELUX COUNTRIES

William E. Deal

Severance Professor of the History of Religion, Department of Religious Studies, Case Western Reserve University

ABORTION: VIII. BUDDHIST PERSPECTIVES

BUDDHISM, BIOETHICS IN

Matthew DeCamp

Assistant Professor, Johns Hopkins Berman Institute of Bioethics and Division of General Internal Medicine

BIOETHICS: VI. RESEARCH METHODS IN

Ralph Dell

Professor of Pediatrics, College of Physicians & Surgeons, Columbia University

Chair, Health Sciences Institutional Animal Care and Use Committee

ANIMAL RESEARCH: III. LAW AND POLICY

Ann M. Dellinger

Team Leader, Motor Vehicle Injury Prevention Team, National Center for Injury Prevention and Control, Centers for Disease Control and Prevention

INFANTS, PUBLIC POLICY AND LEGAL ISSUES

Madeline H. deLone

Exceutive Director, The Innocence Project

PRISONERS, HEALTH CARE ISSUES OF

Arthur R. Derse

Director, Center for Bioethics and Medical Humanities, Julia and David Uihlein Professor of Medical Humanities, and Professor of Bioethics and Emergency Medicine, Institute for Health and Society, Medical College of Wisconsin

PEDAGOGY OF BIOETHICS

Prakash N. Desai

Professor Emeritus of Clinical Psychiatry, Department of Psychiatry, University of Illinois at Chicago

SOUTH ASIA, BIOETHICS IN

Douglas S. Diekema

Professor, Department of Pediatrics, University of Washington School of Medicine

Director of Education, Treuman Katz Center for Pediatric Bioethics, Seattle Children's Research Institute

CIRCUMCISION, MALE [ADDENDUM]

PEDIATRICS, PUBLIC HEALTH ISSUES IN

RELIGIOUS OBJECTIONS TO MEDICAL CARE

Kris Dierickx

Professor of Medical Ethics, Centre for Biomedical Ethics and Law, Catholic University, Louvain, Belgium

EUROPE, BIOETHICS IN: III. THE BENELUX COUNTRIES [ADDENDUM]

Susan Dodds

Professor of Philosophy and Dean of Faculty of Arts, University of Tasmania

VULNERABILITY

Kenneth J. Doka

Professor of Gerontology, Graduate School, College of New Rochelle

Senior Consultant, Hospice Foundation of America

GRIEF, ETHICAL IMPLICATIONS OF

David J. Doukas

William Ray Moore Endowed Chair of Family Medicine and Medical Humanism, and Professor, Department of Family and Geriatric Medicine, University of Louisville

Director, Division of Medical Humanism and Ethics, and Codirector, Interdisciplinary Master of Arts: Bioethics and Medical Humanities, University of Louisville

BIOETHICS EDUCATION: I. MEDICINE

Derek Doyle

Founding Member and Adviser, International Association for Hospice and Palliative Care

END-OF-LIFE CARE

James F. Drane

James F. Drane Bioethics Institute, Edinboro University of Pennsylvania

ALTERNATIVE THERAPIES: II. ETHICAL AND LEGAL ISSUES

Alan Drengson

Department of Philosophy, University of Victoria

ENVIRONMENTAL ETHICS: II. DEEP ECOLOGY

Theresa Drought

Bioethics Director, Kaiser Permanente, Woodland Hills, CA

BIOETHICS EDUCATION: II. NURSING

Nancy N. Dubler

Consultant for Ethics, New York City Health and Hospitals Corporation

Professor Emerita of Bioethics, Albert Einstein College of Medicine

FERTILITY CONTROL: III. LEGAL AND REGULATORY ISSUES

PRISONERS, HEALTH CARE ISSUES OF

James M. DuBois

Professor of Medicine, Division of General Medical Sciences, and Director of the Center for
Clinical Research Ethics, Institute for Clinical and Translational Science, Washington University in St. Louis

MENTALLY DISABLED AND MENTALLY ILL PERSONS: II. RESEARCH ISSUES [ADDENDUM]

Denise M. Dudzinski

Associate Professor, Department of Bioethics and Humanities, University of Washington School of Medicine

HOSPITAL, CONTEMPORARY ETHICAL PROBLEMS OF THE [ADDENDUM]

John Duffy

Professor Emeritus, University of Maryland

PUBLIC HEALTH: I. HISTORY

Thomas Patrick Duffy

Professor of Medicine, Yale University School of Medicine

MEDICINE, PROFESSION OF [ADDENDUM]

Joseph Dumit

Professor and Director of Science and Technology Studies, University of California, Davis

COMMERCIALISM IN SCIENTIFIC RESEARCH [ADDENDUM]

Troy Duster

Chancellor's Professor and Senior Fellow, Warren Institute on Law and Social Policy, University of California, Berkeley

EUGENICS: II. ETHICAL ISSUES

Allen R. Dyer

Professor of Psychiatry and Behavioral Sciences, George Washington University

ADVERTISING AND MARKETING IN HEALTH CARE

DIVIDED LOYALTIES IN MENTAL HEALTH CARE

Thomas Eich

Professor of Islamic Studies, University of Hamburg

NEAR AND MIDDLE EAST, BIOETHICS IN: III. ARAB WORLD [ADDENDUM]

POPULATION ETHICS: IV. ISLAMIC PERSPECTIVES [ADDENDUM]

Bernice S. Elger

Professor of Ethics and Health Law, Institute for Biomedical Ethics, Faculty of Medicine and Faculty of Science, University of Basel

PRISONERS AS RESEARCH SUBJECTS

Carl Elliott

Center for Bioethics. University of Minnesota

MENTALLY DISABLED AND MENTALLY ILL PERSONS: II. RESEARCH ISSUES

Kevin C. Elliott

Lyman Briggs College and Department of Fisheries and Wildlife and Department of Philosophy, Michigan State University

ENVIRONMENTAL HEALTH ETHICS

J. Ronald Engel

Fellow, Center for Humans and Nature

SUSTAINABILITY

H. Tristram Engelhardt Jr.

Professor, Department of Philosophy, Rice University

Professor Emeritus, Department of Medicine, Baylor College of Medicine

HEALTH AND DISEASE: IV. PHILOSOPHICAL PERSPECTIVES

MEDICINE, PHILOSOPHY OF

Pedro Laín Entralgo

PROFESSIONAL-PATIENT RELATIONSHIP: HISTORICAL PERSPECTIVES*

Phyllis Griffin Epps

University of Houston

GENETIC DISCRIMINATION

Alexandre Erler

Research Associate, Oxford Uehiro Centre for Practical Ethics, University of Oxford

AUTHENTICITY

Liza Eshilian-Oates

Regional Physician Leader, Southern California Kaiser Permanente Family Violence Prevention Program

ABUSE, INTERPERSONAL: II. ABUSE BETWEEN DOMESTIC PARTNERS

John L. Esposito

Professor of Religion and International Affairs and of Islamic Studies, Georgetown University

POPULATION ETHICS: IV. ISLAMIC PERSPECTIVES

Richard J. Evans

Regius Professor of History, University of Cambridge

EPIDEMICS

Ruth R. Faden

Professor of Bioethics, Johns Hopkins Berman Institute of Bioethics, Johns Hopkins University

INFORMED CONSENT: I. HISTORY OF INFORMED CONSENT

INFORMED CONSENT: II. MEANING AND ELEMENTS

Charles J. Fahey

Program Officer, Milbank Memorial Fund Researcher, Loretto Institute for the Frail Elderly

CHRONIC ILLNESS

Jonathan M. Fanaroff

Associate Professor of Pediatrics, Case Western Reserve University School of Medicine

Director, Rainbow Center for Pediatric Ethics, Rainbow Babies and Children's Hospital, University Hospitals Case Medical Center, Cleveland, OH

MISTAKES, MEDICAL [ADDENDUM]

PEDIATRICS, OVERVIEW OF ETHICAL ISSUES IN

Margaret A. Farley

Gilbert L. Stark Professor Emerita, Yale University Divinity School

SEXUAL ETHICS

Ellyn Farrelly

Genetic Counselor, South Bay Regional Genetics Center, Santa Clara Valley Medical Center

GENETIC COUNSELING, ETHICAL ISSUES IN [ADDENDUM]

Sarah M. Fayad

Assistant Professor, Department of Psychiatry, University of Florida College of Medicine

PSYCHOSURGERY: II. MEDICAL AND HISTORICAL ASPECTS OF [ADDENDUM]

Ellen K. Feder

Associate Professor, Department of Philosophy and Religion, American University

SEXUAL IDENTITY

David M. Feldman

Rabbi Emeritus, Jewish Center of Teaneck

POPULATION ETHICS: V. JEWISH PERSPECTIVES

Gary B. Ferngren

Professor, School of History, Philosophy, and Religion, Oregon State University

NEAR AND MIDDLE EAST: ANCIENT NEAR EAST*

Joseph J. Fins

E. William Davis, Jr. M.D. Professor of Medical Ethics, Chief of the Division of Medical Ethics, and Professor of Medicine, Public Health, and Medicine in Psychiatry, Weill Cornell Medical College

Senior Attending Physician and Director of Medical Ethics, New York-Presbyterian Weill Cornell Medical Center

Adjunct Faculty Member, Rockefeller University, and Senior Attending Physician at the Rockefeller University Hospital

DEEP BRAIN STIMULATION

VEGETATIVE AND MINIMALLY CONSCIOUS STATES

Gary S. Fischer

Associate Professor of Medicine and Vice Chair for Quality Improvement and Patient Safety, Department of Medicine, University of Pittsburgh

ADVANCE DIRECTIVES AND ADVANCE CARE PLANNING

Leonard M. Fleck

Professor, Center for Ethics and Humanities in the Life Sciences, College of Human Medicine, Michigan State University

GENETIC CITIZENSHIP

GENETICS AND HUMAN BEHAVIOR: II. PHILOSOPHICAL AND ETHICAL ISSUES

MANAGED CARE [ADDENDUM]

Alan R. Fleischman

Clinical Professor of Pediatrics, Clinical Professor of Epidemiology and Population Health, Albert Einstein College of Medicine

GENETIC TESTING AND SCREENING: VI. PEDIATRIC GENETIC TESTING [ADDENDUM]

Andrew Flescher

Associate Professor of Preventive Medicine, Stony Brook University

FREEDOM AND FREE WILL

Mary Beth Foglia

National Center for Ethics in Health Care, Department of Veterans Affairs

Affiliate Faculty, Department of Bioethics and Humanities, School of Medicine, University of Washington

HEALTH CARE, QUALITY IMPROVEMENT

David P. Folsom

University of California, San Diego, Department of Psychiatry, Division of Geriatric Psychiatry

PSYCHOPHARMACOLOGY

James W. Fossett

Associate Professor, Department of Public Administration and Policy, University at Albany and Rockefeller Institute of Government

MEDICAID

Gregory L. Fowler

Affiliate Associate Professor, Department of Public Health and Preventive Medicine, Oregon Health and Science University

HUMAN GENOME PROJECT

Daniel M. Fox

President Emeritus, Milbank Memorial Fund

CHRONIC ILLNESS

Renée C. Fox

Professor Emerita, Sociology Department, Annenberg Professor Emerita of the Social Sciences, University of Pennsylvania

ORGAN TRANSPLANTS, SOCIOCULTURAL ASPECTS OF

Joel E. Frader
Professor in Pediatrics-Academic General Pediatrics and Primary Care and Medical Humanities and Bioethics, Feinberg School of Medicine, Northwestern University
MISTAKES, MEDICAL

Leslie P. Francis
Distinguished Alfred C. Emery Professor of Law and Distinguished Professor of Philosophy, University of Utah
DISABILITY: II. LEGAL ISSUES
PANDEMICS

Arthur W. Frank
Professor of Sociology, University of Calgary
HEALING

Sarah Franklin
Professor and Chair of Sociology, University of Cambridge
LIFE

Sara T. Fry
Retired Henry Luce Professor of Nursing Ethics, Boston College of Nursing
NURSING ETHICS

K.W.M. Fulford
Fellow of Saint Catherine's College and Member of the Philosophy Faculty, University of Oxford
Emeritus Professor of Philosophy and Mental Health, University of Warwick
Editor, *Philosophy, Psychiatry, and Psychology*
MENTAL ILLNESS: I. DEFINITION, USE, AND MEANING

Robert C. Fuller
Professor of Religious Studies, Bradley University
ALTERNATIVE THERAPIES: I. SOCIAL HISTORY

Atwood D. Gaines
Departments of Anthropology, Bioethics, Nursing, and Psychiatry and Schools of Nursing and Medicine, Case Western Reserve University
MENTAL ILLNESS: II. CULTURAL PERSPECTIVES
RACE AND RACISM

Michael J. Garland
Professor Emeritus, Department of Public Health and Preventive Medicine and Center for Ethics in Health Care, Oregon Health and Science University
HEALTH INSURANCE

Daniel R. George
Assistant Professor, Department of Humanities, Penn State College of Medicine
ECOLOGICAL BIOETHICS

Karen G. Gervais
Director, Minnesota Center for Health Care Ethics, St. Olaf College
Visiting Professor of Philosophy, St. Olaf College
DEATH, DEFINITION AND DETERMINATION OF: III. PHILOSOPHICAL AND THEOLOGICAL PERSPECTIVES
MANAGED CARE

Mohammed Ghaly
Professor of Islamic Law and Biomedical Ethics, Center for Islamic Legislation and Ethics (CILE), Hamad Bin Khalifa University, Qatar Foundation
ABORTION: VII. ISLAMIC PERSPECTIVES [ADDENDUM]

Raanan Gillon
Emeritus Professor of Medical Ethics, Department of Primary Care and Public Health, Imperial College London
EUROPE, BIOETHICS IN: IV. UNITED KINGDOM

Richard M. Glass
Contributing Editor, *Journal of the American Medical Association*
Clinical Professor of Psychiatry, University of Chicago
SCIENTIFIC PUBLISHING

Linda MacDonald Glenn
Assistant Professor, Alden March Bioethics Department, Albany Medical Center
EMBRYO AND FETUS: IV. FETAL RESEARCH

Shimon M. Glick
Professor Emeritus, Ben Gurion University of the Negev
NEAR AND MIDDLE EAST, BIOETHICS IN: IV. ISRAEL

Mark S. Gold
Donald Dizney Eminent Scholar, Distinguished Professor, and Chair of Psychiatry, Department of Psychiatry, College of Medicine, University of Florida
ADDICTION AND DEPENDENCE
EXPERT TESTIMONY

Aaron Goldenberg
Assistant Professor, Department of Bioethics, Case Western Reserve University
Associate Director, Center for Genetic Research, Ethics, and Law, Case Western Reserve University
GENETIC TESTING AND SCREENING: II. NEWBORN GENETIC SCREENING [ADDENDUM]

Dominic Golding
Associate Teaching Professor, Interdisciplinary and Global Studies Division, Worcester Polytechnic Institute
RISK AND RISK ASSESSMENT

Kenneth W. Goodman
Professor and Director, Bioethics Program, University of Miami
INFORMATICS, BIOMEDICAL

Jami Lynn Goodwin
Project Manager, Heart and Vascular Center, Barnes Jewish Hospital, University College, Washington University in St. Louis
BIOETHICS COMMISSIONS, HISTORY OF

Susan Dorr Goold
Professor of Internal Medicine and Health Management and Policy, Center for Bioethics and Social Sciences in Medicine, University of Michigan
TRUST [ADDENDUM]

Deborah R. Gordon
University of California, San Francisco, Department of Anthropology, History, and Social Medicine
HEALTH AND DISEASE: III. ANTHROPOLOGICAL PERSPECTIVES [ADDENDUM]

Elisa J. Gordon
Research Associate Professor, Feinberg School of Medicine, Northwestern University
HEALTH AND DISEASE: III. ANTHROPOLOGICAL PERSPECTIVES
HOSPITAL, CONTEMPORARY ETHICAL PROBLEMS OF THE

Lawrence O. Gostin
Center for Law and the Public's Health, Georgetown University
DISABILITY: II. LEGAL ISSUES

Anna Gotlib
Assistant Professor, Department of Philosophy, Brooklyn College, City University of New York
SUBJECTIVITY

Fionnuala Gough
School of Law, University of Manchester
EUROPE, BIOETHICS IN: V. REPUBLIC OF IRELAND

Diego Gracia
Emeritus Professor of History of Medicine and Bioethics, Complutense University of Madrid
EUROPE, BIOETHICS IN: II. SOUTHERN EUROPE

Teresa Gracia
MD, Master in Bioethics, Hospital Universitario 12 de Octubre
EUROPE, BIOETHICS IN: II. SOUTHERN EUROPE

Frank P. Grad
Columbia University
PUBLIC HEALTH: II. LAW

Jonathan Granoff
President, Global Security Institute
Adjunct Professor, International Law, Widener University School of Law
NUCLEAR WEAPONS

Michael J. Green
Professor, Departments of Humanities and Medicine, Penn State College of Medicine
Chair, Hospital Ethics Committee, Penn State College of Medicine
BIOETHICS EDUCATION: I. MEDICINE

Ronald M. Green
Eunice & Julian Cohen Professor for the Study of Ethics and Human Values, Department of Religion, Dartmouth College
POPULATION ETHICS: III. INTRODUCTION TO RELIGIOUS TRADITIONS

Merwyn R. Greenlick
Oregon State Representative (House District 33)
Professor Emeritus, Department of Public Health and Preventive Medicine, School of Medicine, Oregon Health and Science University
HEALTH INSURANCE

John A. Grim
Senior Lecturer and Research Scholar, Yale School of Forestry and Environmental Studies and Yale Divinity School, Yale University
NATIVE AMERICAN RELIGIONS, BIOETHICS IN

Michael A. Grodin
Department of Health Law, Bioethics, and Human Rights, Boston University School of Public Health
NAZI LEGACY AND BIOETHICS

Jeremy Gruber
President, Council for Responsible Genetics
GENETIC DISCRIMINATION [ADDENDUM]

Anita Guerrini
Horning Professor in the Humanities and Professor of History, Oregon State University
ANIMAL RESEARCH: I. HISTORICAL ASPECTS

Tee L. Guidotti
Vice-President for Health/Safety/ Environment and Sustainability, Medical Advisory Services
OCCUPATIONAL HEALTH AND SAFETY: I. ETHICAL ISSUES

Jyotsna Agnihotri Gupta
Assistant Professor, Gender and Diversity, University of Humanistic Studies, Utrecht, Netherlands
ABORTION: IX. HINDU PERSPECTIVES

Michael K. Gusmano
Research Scholar, The Hastings Center
Associate Professor of Health Policy and Management, New York Medical College
ACCESS TO HEALTH CARE
HEALTH POLICY IN THE UNITED STATES
IMMIGRANTS, ACCESS TO HEALTH CARE

Frederic W. Hafferty
Professor of Medical Education and Associate Director, Program in Professionalism and Ethics, Mayo Clinic
PROFESSIONAL-PATIENT RELATIONSHIP: I. SOCIOLOGICAL PERSPECTIVES [ADDENDUM]

Susanne B. Haga
Institute for Genome Sciences and Policy, Duke University
PHARMACOGENOMICS

Daniel E. Hall
Assistant Professor, Department of Surgery, University of Pittsburgh School of Medicine
Staff Surgeon, Veterans Administration Pittsburgh Healthcare System
INFORMED CONSENT: IV. CLINICAL ASPECTS OF CONSENT IN HEALTH CARE

Robert T. Hall
West Virginia State University
ORGANIZATIONAL ETHICS IN HEALTH CARE

Ann B. Hamric
Professor, Associate Dean of Academic Programs, School of Nursing, Virginia Commonwealth University
NURSING ETHICS [ADDENDUM]

Jaydee Hanson
Policy Director for the International Center for Technology Assessment, Washington, DC
PRECAUTIONARY PRINCIPLE

Stanley S. Harakas

Archbishop Iakovos Professor of Orthodox Theology Emeritus, Holy Cross Greek Orthodox School of Theology

EASTERN ORTHODOX CHRISTIANITY, BIOETHICS IN

POPULATION ETHICS: VII. EASTERN ORTHODOX CHRISTIAN PERSPECTIVES

Julie Harris

Staff Scientist, Division of Research, Kaiser Permanente, Oakland, CA

Assistant Adjunct Professor, Institute on Health and Aging, University of California, San Francisco

GENETIC TESTING AND SCREENING: III. POPULATION SCREENING

GENETIC TESTING AND SCREENING: IV. PUBLIC HEALTH CONTEXT

WHOLE GENOME SEQUENCING

Beverly Wildung Harrison

Caroline Williams Beaird Professor of Ethics, Union Theological Seminary in New York

ABORTION: VI. PROTESTANT PERSPECTIVES

Jacqueline Hart

Graduate Faculty at Health Advocacy Program, Sarah Lawrence College

HEALTH AND DISEASE: II. SOCIOLOGICAL PERSPECTIVES

Hassan Hathout

Director of Outreach, Islamic Center of Southern California

NEAR AND MIDDLE EAST, BIOETHICS IN: III. ARAB WORLD

Stanley M. Hauerwas

Gilbert T. Rowe Distinguished Professor Emeritus of Theology and Ethics, Duke Divinity School

VIRTUE AND CHARACTER

Joseph M. Hawes

University of Memphis

CHILDREN: I. HISTORY OF CHILDHOOD

J. Bryan Hehir

Parker Gilbert Montgomery Professor of the Practice of Religion and Public Life, John F. Kennedy School of Government, Harvard University

POPULATION ETHICS: VI. ROMAN CATHOLIC PERSPECTIVES

Michael J. Herkov

Associate Professor and Chief of Forensic and Addiction Medicine, College of Medicine, University of Florida

ADDICTION AND DEPENDENCE

D. Micah Hester

Chief, Division of Medical Humanities, University of Arkansas for Medical Sciences

PRAGMATISM

David Heyd

Department of Philosophy, Hebrew University of Jerusalem

OBLIGATION AND SUPEREROGATION

Kenneth Einar Himma

Part-Time Lecturer, University of Washington School of Law

LAW AND MORALITY

N. Ray Hiner

University of Kansas, Lawrence

CHILDREN: I. HISTORY OF CHILDHOOD

F. Russell Hittinger

William K. Warren Professor of Catholic Studies, Research Professor of Law, University of Tulsa

NATURAL LAW

Anita Ho

Associate Professor, Centre for Applied Ethics, University of British Columbia

Director, Ethics Services, Providence Health Care, Vancouver, BC

EPISTEMIC INJUSTICE

Angela Roddey Holder

Duke University Medical Center

INFORMED CONSENT: V. LEGAL AND ETHICAL ISSUES OF CONSENT IN HEALTH CARE

Stephen Holland

Departments of Philosophy and Health Sciences, University of York, UK

PUBLIC HEALTH: IV. ETHICS

Suzanne Holland

John B. Magee Professor of Science and Values, Professor of Religion, University of Puget Sound

HOMOSEXUALITY, RELIGIOUS PERSPECTIVES

Dennis Hollinger

President and Colman M. Mockler Distinguished Professor of Christian Ethics, Gordon-Conwell Theological Seminary

Distinguished Fellow, Center for Bioethics and Human Dignity

LIFE, SANCTITY OF

C. Christopher Hook

Associate Professor of Medicine, Division of Hematology and Internal Medicine, Mayo Clinic, Rochester, MN

NANOTECHNOLOGY

TRANSHUMANISM AND POSTHUMANISM

Jonathan P. Horenstein

Business Practices Officer, Oakwood Healthcare Inc.

CORPORATE COMPLIANCE

Allan V. Horwitz

Board of Governors Professor of Sociology, Department of Sociology, Rutgers University

MENTAL HEALTH SERVICES: I. SETTINGS AND PROGRAMS

Rachel L. Hulkower

Georgia State University College of Law

AIDS: II. HEALTH CARE AND RESEARCH ISSUES

Paul W. Humphreys

Professor, Corcoran Department of Philosophy, University of Virginia

SCIENCE, PHILOSOPHY OF

Matthew R. Hunt

Assistant Professor, School of Physical and Occupational Therapy, McGill University

Researcher, Centre for Interdisciplinary Research in Rehabilitation

HUMANITARIAN RELIEF

NGOS IN HEALTH CARE

Rodney J. Hunter

Professor Emeritus of Pastoral Theology, Emory University

PASTORAL AND SPIRITUAL CARE AND HEALTH CARE CHAPLAINCY

John Huss

Associate Professor, Philosophy, University of Akron

BIOLOGY, PHILOSOPHY OF [ADDENDUM]

Michael Hutchins

Executive Director/CEO, Wildlife Society

Adjunct Associate Professor, Graduate Program in Sustainable Development and Conservation Biology, University of Maryland

Affiliate Professor, Department of Environmental Science and Policy, George Mason University

ANIMAL WELFARE AND RIGHTS: V. ZOOS AND ZOOLOGICAL PARKS

Insoo Hyun

Associate Professor of Bioethics and Philosophy, Department of Bioethics, Case Western Reserve University School of Medicine

EMBRYO AND FETUS: III. EMBRYONIC STEM CELL RESEARCH

Sara Iden

Columbia University

ABORTION: I. MEDICAL PERSPECTIVES

Ana S. Iltis

Associate Professor, Department of Philosophy and Director, Center for Bioethics, Health and Society, Wake Forest University

PRIVACY AND CONFIDENTIALITY IN RESEARCH

Kirsten Jacobson

Associate Professor of Philosophy, University of Maine

HEALTH AND DISEASE: V. THE EXPERIENCE OF HEALTH AND ILLNESS

Alison M. Jaggar

Departments of Philosophy and Women and Gender Studies, University of Colorado at Boulder

HUMAN NATURE

Andrew Jameton

Professor, College of Public Health, University of Nebraska Medical Center

AMERICA, BIOETHICS IN: I. UNITED STATES

GREEN DESIGN OF HOSPITALS/IMPACT

INFORMATION DISCLOSURE, ETHICAL ISSUES OF

Dale Jamieson

Professor of Environmental Studies, New York University

Director, Center for Bioethics

CLIMATE CHANGE

Lynn A. Jansen

Oregon Health and Science University, Center for Ethics in Health Care

STEWARDSHIP

Nancy S. Jecker

Professor, Department of Bioethics and Humanities, School of Medicine, University of Washington

AGING AND THE AGED: I. SOCIETAL AGING

AGING AND THE AGED: II. HEALTH CARE FOR THE AGING

JUSTICE

Bruce Jennings

Director of Bioethics, Center for Humans and Nature

LIBERTY

PUBLIC HEALTH: X. EMERGENCY PREPAREDNESS AND RESPONSE

Dilip V. Jeste

Estelle and Edgar Levi Chair in Aging; Director, Sam and Rose Stein Institute for Research in Aging; Distinguished Professor of Psychiatry and Neurosciences; Director of Education, Clinical and Translational Research Institute; Chief, Geriatric Psychiatry Division, University of California, San Diego

PSYCHOPHARMACOLOGY

L. Syd M. Johnson

Assistant Professor of Philosophy, Department of Humanities, Michigan Technological University

ABORTION: II. ETHICAL PERSPECTIVES

Sandra H. Johnson

Professor Emerita of Law and Health Care Ethics, Center for Health Law Studies, Saint Louis University School of Law

HEALTH CARE PROFESSIONALS, LEGAL REGULATION OF

Josephine Johnston

Director of Research, Research Scholar, The Hastings Center

REPRODUCTIVE TECHNOLOGIES: VII. SPERM, OVA, AND EMBRYOS [ADDENDUM]

Albert R. Jonsen

Senior Ethics Scholar, Program in Medicine and Human Values, California Pacific Medical Center, San Francisco

AMERICA, BIOETHICS IN: I. UNITED STATES

BIOETHICS: I. HISTORY OF

CASUISTRY

Eric T. Juengst

Director, UNC Center for Bioethics, University of North Carolina at Chapel Hill

DNA IDENTIFICATION

ENHANCEMENT USES OF MEDICAL TECHNOLOGY

GENETIC TESTING AND SCREENING: III. POPULATION SCREENING

Jeffrey Kahn

Robert Henry Levi and Ryda Hecht Levi Professor of Bioethics and Public Policy, Berman Institute of Bioethics, Johns Hopkins University

Department of Philosophy, University of Minnesota

ANIMAL RESEARCH: III. LAW AND POLICY

ORGAN AND TISSUE PROCUREMENT: II. ETHICAL AND LEGAL ISSUES REGARDING LIVING DONORS

Andrea Kalfoglou

Assistant Professor, Health Administration and Policy Program, Department of Sociology and Anthropology, University of Maryland, Baltimore County

MATERNAL-FETAL RELATIONSHIP: I. MEDICAL ASPECTS [ADDENDUM]

Rosalie A. Kane

Professor, Division of Health Services Research and Policy, School of Public Health, University of Minnesota

LONG-TERM CARE: I. CONCEPTS AND POLICIES

Marshall B. Kapp

Director, Center for Innovative Collaboration in Medicine and Law, and Professor, Department of Geriatrics, Florida State University College of Medicine and College of Law

AGING AND THE AGED: III. RESEARCH ETHICS

IMPAIRED PROFESSIONALS

Katrina Karkazis

Senior Research Scholar, Center for Biomedical Ethics, Stanford University

SEX REASSIGNMENT

Jay Katz

Professor, Yale University Law School

INFORMED CONSENT: V. LEGAL AND ETHICAL ISSUES OF CONSENT IN HEALTH CARE

Maureen Kelley

University of Alabama at Birmingham

CONTRACTARIANISM AND BIOETHICS

M. Lynne Kesel

Clinical Veterinarian, Laboratory Animal Resources, Colorado State University

VETERINARY ETHICS

Daniel J. Kevles

Stanley Woodward Professor of History, Yale University

EUGENICS: I. HISTORICAL ASPECTS

John F. Kilner

Director of Bioethics Programs, Franklin and Dorothy Forman Chair of Christian Ethics and Theology, and Professor of Bioethics and Contemporary Culture, Trinity International University

HEALTH CARE RESOURCES, ALLOCATION OF: I. MACROALLOCATION

HEALTH CARE RESOURCES, ALLOCATION OF: II. MICROALLOCATION

HUMAN DIGNITY

Rihito Kimura

Professor Emeritus of Bioethics and Law, School of Human Sciences, Waseda University

JAPAN, BIOETHICS IN

Nancy M. P. King

Professor, Department of Social Sciences & Health Policy and Wake Forest Institute for Regenerative Medicine, Wake Forest School of Medicine

Co-Director, Center for Bioethics, Health, & Society and Graduate Program in Bioethics, Wake Forest University

PRIVACY AND CONFIDENTIALITY IN RESEARCH

Kenneth Kipnis

Professor, Department of Philosophy, University of Hawaii at Manoa

PUBLIC HEALTH: XI. EMERGENCY ALLOCATION OF RESOURCES AND ALTERED STANDARD OF CARE

Russell Kirkland

Professor, Department of Religion, University of Georgia

TAOISM, BIOETHICS IN

Joseph Mistuo Kitagawa

Professor Emeritus, University of Chicago

JAPAN: EARLY JAPAN THROUGH THE NINETEENTH CENTURY*

Arthur Kleinman

Esther and Sidney Rabb Professor of Medical Anthropology and Cross-Cultural Psychiatry, Harvard University

MEDICINE, ANTHROPOLOGY OF

Lonnie D. Kliever

Chair, Department of Religious Studies, Southern Methodist University

DEATH: IV. WESTERN RELIGIOUS THOUGHT

Andrew Knight

Associate Professor of Welfare and Ethics, Ross University School of Veterinary Medicine, St. Kitts, West Indies

ANIMAL WELFARE AND RIGHTS: IV. PET AND COMPANION ANIMALS [ADDENDUM]

Eric D. Kodish

Professor and Chairman, Department of Bioethics, Cleveland Clinic Foundation, Lerner College of Medicine, Case Reserve University

CANCER, ETHICAL ISSUES RELATED TO DIAGNOSIS AND TREATMENT

GENETIC TESTING AND SCREENING: VI. PEDIATRIC GENETIC TESTING

PEDIATRICS, OVERVIEW OF ETHICAL ISSUES IN

Barbara A. Koenig

Professor, Department of Social and Behavioral Sciences, Institute for Health and Aging, University of California, San Francisco

BIOETHICS: IX. ANTHROPOLOGY OF

DEATH: I. CULTURAL PERSPECTIVES

Loretta M. Kopelman

Professor Emeritus, Department of Bioethics and Interdisciplinary Studies, Brody School of Medicine, East Carolina University

Faculty Affiliate, Kennedy Institute of Ethics, Georgetown University

CHILDREN: III. HEALTH CARE AND RESEARCH ISSUES

CIRCUMCISION, FEMALE: II. CULTURAL AND ETHICAL ASPECTS

RESEARCH METHODOLOGY: II. CONTROLLED CLINICAL TRIALS

RESEARCH POLICY: II. RISK AND VULNERABLE GROUPS

Andrew M. Kopolow

Senior Project Manager, United Health Care

Adjunct Faculty, College of Health Care Sciences, University of Phoenix

Board of Directors, Arizona Association for Healthcare Quality

CORPORATE SOCIAL RESPONSIBILITY IN HEALTH

Louis E. Kopolow

Clinical Assistant Professor of Psychiatry, Department of Psychiatry and Behavioral Sciences, George Washington University School of Medicine

Director, Potomac Grove Psychiatry and Clinical Research Center, Gaithersburg, MD

Distinguished Life Fellow of American Psychiatric Association

CORPORATE SOCIAL RESPONSIBILITY IN HEALTH

PATIENTS' RIGHTS: II. MENTAL PATIENTS' RIGHTS

Greg Koski

Associate Professor, Department of Anesthesia, Critical Care, and Pain Medicine, and Senior Scientist, James Mongan Institute for Health Policy, Massachusetts General Hospital

President and Cofounder, Alliance for Clinical Research Excellence and Safety, Cambridge, MA

RESEARCH POLICY: I. GENERAL BACKGROUND

STUDENTS AS RESEARCH SUBJECTS

Olayinka A. Koso-Thomas

University of Nairobi, Kenya

CIRCUMCISION, FEMALE: I. HISTORICAL OVERVIEW

Sheldon Krimsky

Lenore Stern Professor of Humanities and Social Sciences, School of Arts and Sciences, Tufts University

Carol Zicklin Professor of Philosophy, Brooklyn College

Adjunct Professor, Department of Family Medicine and Community Health, Tufts University School of Medicine

DNA IDENTIFICATION [ADDENDUM]

Mark G. Kuczewski

Director, Health Sciences Division, Neiswanger Institute for Bioethics and Health Policy

Professor of Medical Ethics, Loyola University Chicago

COMMUNITY AND COMMUNITARIANISM

Patricia C. Kuszler

Professor of Law, School of Law, University of Washington

INFANTS, PUBLIC POLICY AND LEGAL ISSUES

Ronald Labonté

Professor, Canada Research Chair in Globalization and Health Equity, Institute of Population Health, University of Ottawa

CROSS-BORDER MEDICAL TRAVEL

H. Richard Lamb

Professor Emeritus of Psychiatry, Keck School of Medicine, University of Southern California

INSTITUTIONALIZATION AND DEINSTITUTIONALIZATION

John D. Lantos

Professor of Pediatrics, University of Missouri–Kansas City

Director, Children's Mercy Hospital Bioethics Center, Kansas City, MO

ABUSE, INTERPERSONAL: I. CHILD ABUSE

INFANTS, MEDICAL ASPECTS AND ISSUES IN THE CARE OF

PARENTAL AUTHORITY

David R. Larson

Professor of Religion, School of Religion, Loma Linda University

INFANTICIDE

Stephen R. Latham

Director, Interdisciplinary Center for Bioethics, Yale University

ANIMAL RESEARCH: III. LAW AND POLICY [ADDENDUM]

RESEARCH POLICY: I. GENERAL BACKGROUND [ADDENDUM]

Paul Lauritzen

Professor, Department of Theology and Religious Studies, John Carroll University

CLONING: III. RELIGIOUS PERSPECTIVES

Michael Lavin

Psychologist, Department of Army

SMOKING

Karen Lebacqz

Professor Emerita of Theological Ethics, Pacific School of Religion, Berkeley, CA

SEXUAL ETHICS AND PROFESSIONAL STANDARDS

Drew Leder

Professor of Philosophy, Loyola University Maryland

HEALTH AND DISEASE: V. THE EXPERIENCE OF HEALTH AND ILLNESS

Susan E. Lederer

Robert Turell Professor of the History of Medicine and Bioethics, Department of Medical History and Bioethics, University of Wisconsin School of Medicine and Public Health

MILITARY PERSONNEL AS RESEARCH SUBJECTS

Sandra Soo-Jin Lee

Senior Research Scholar, Stanford Center for Biomedical Ethics, Stanford University

GENETICS AND RACIAL MINORITIES

Kimberly Leighton

Assistant Professor, Department of Philosophy, American University

ADOPTION

Aaron D. Levine

Associate Professor, School of Public Policy, Georgia Institute of Technology

REPRODUCTIVE TECHNOLOGIES: V. GAMETE DONATION

Carol Levine

Director, Families and Health Care Project, United Hospital Fund

FAMILY CAREGIVING

RESEARCH METHODOLOGY: III. SUBJECTS

RESEARCH POLICY: III. SUBJECTS

Robert J. Levine

Professor of Medicine and Senior Fellow, Interdisciplinary Center for Bioethics, Yale University

INFORMED CONSENT: III. CONSENT ISSUES IN HUMAN RESEARCH

INSTITUTIONAL REVIEW BOARDS

Barry S. Levy
Adjunct Professor of Public Health, Tufts University School of Medicine
Past President, American Public Health Association
WARFARE: I. INTRODUCTION [ADDENDUM]
WARFARE: II. MEDICINE AND WAR
WARFARE: IV. CHEMICAL AND BIOLOGICAL WEAPONS

Joan Liaschenko
Professor, Center for Bioethics and School of Nursing, University of Minnesota
CARE: IV. CARE AND SOCIETY/ PUBLIC POLICY
NURSING, THEORIES AND PHILOSOPHY OF [ADDENDUM]

Evelyn Liberman
Department of Health Law, Bioethics, and Human Rights, Boston University School of Public Health
NAZI LEGACY AND BIOETHICS

Judith Lichtenberg
Professor of Philosophy and Adjunct Professor of Law, Georgetown University
POPULATION POLICIES, MIGRATION AND REFUGEES IN

Charles W. Lidz
Research Professor of Psychiatry, University of Massachusetts Medical School
COERCION
INFORMED CONSENT: IV. CLINICAL ASPECTS OF CONSENT IN HEALTH CARE

Victor Lidz
Professor, Department Psychiatry, Drexel University College of Medicine
DEATH: V. DEATH IN THE WESTERN WORLD [ADDENDUM]

Hilde Lindemann
Professor, Department of Philosophy, Michigan State University
FAMILY AND FAMILY MEDICINE
FEMINISM
NATURALISM
REPRODUCTIVE TECHNOLOGIES: VI. CONTRACT PREGNANCY

Andrew Linzey
Faculty of Theology and Religion, University of Oxford
ANIMAL WELFARE AND RIGHTS: II. VEGETARIANISM
ANIMAL WELFARE AND RIGHTS: IV. PET AND COMPANION ANIMALS

John D. Loike
Director for Special Programs, Center for Bioethics, Columbia University
PERSONALIZED MEDICINE

Robin W. Lovin
Director of Research, Center of Theological Inquiry
ETHICS: V. RELIGION AND MORALITY

Florencia Luna
Independent Researcher, Consejo Nacional de Investigaciones Científicas y Técnicas (CONICET)
Director of Bioethics Program, Facultad Latinoamericana de Ciencias Sociales (FLACSO)
AMERICA, BIOETHICS IN: III. LATIN AMERICA [ADDENDUM]

B. Andrew Lustig
Holmes Rolston III Professor of Religion and Science, Department of Religion, Davidson College
RELATIVISM, CULTURAL AND ETHICAL

Anne Drapkin Lyerly
Duke University Medical Center
ABORTION: I. MEDICAL PERSPECTIVES

Niels Lynöe
Professor of Medical Ethics, Karolinska Institutet, Stockholm, Sweden
EUROPE, BIOETHICS IN: VII. NORDIC COUNTRIES

Anne Lyren
Strategic Advisor, Quality Program, University Hospital Rainbow Babies and Children's Hospital, Cleveland, OH
Associate Professor, Pediatrics, Case Western Reserve University School of Medicine
PEDIATRICS, OVERVIEW OF ETHICAL ISSUES IN

M. Therese Lysaught
Professor, Institute of Pastoral Studies, Neiswanger Institute for Bioethics, Stritch School of Medicine, Loyola University Chicago
HUMAN GENE TRANSFER RESEARCH

Catriona Mackenzie
Professor of Philosophy, Department of Philosophy, Macquarie University
Director, Macquarie University Research Centre for Agency, Values and Ethics
VULNERABILITY

Barbara MacKinnon
Professor of Philosophy, University of San Francisco, Retired
CLONING: II. REPRODUCTIVE

Ruth Macklin
Professor, Department of Epidemiology and Population Health, Albert Einstein College of Medicine
RESEARCH, MULTINATIONAL

Andreas-Holger Maehle
Professor of History of Medicine and Medical Ethics, Department of Philosophy, University of Durham
EUROPE: V. NINETEENTH-CENTURY CONTINENTAL EUROPE*

David Magnus
Thomas A. Raffin Professor in Medicine and Biomedical Ethics, Stanford Center for Biomedical Ethics
BIOLOGY, PHILOSOPHY OF

José Alberto Mainetti
Instituto de Bioética y Humanidades Médicas de la Fundación Mainetti, Centro Oncologico de Excelencia
AMERICA, BIOETHICS IN: III. LATIN AMERICA

Mary A. Majumder
Assistant Professor of Medicine and Medical Ethics, Center for Medical Ethics and Health Policy, Baylor College of Medicine
Methodist Hospital System Biomedical Ethics Program, Houston, TX
BIOETHICS: II. KEY CASES IN
REPRODUCTIVE TECHNOLOGIES: VIII. ETHICAL ISSUES [ADDENDUM]

Terry L. Maple
Director, Georgia Tech Center for Conservation and Behavior
Director Emeritus, Zoo Atlanta
ANIMAL WELFARE AND RIGHTS: V. ZOOS AND ZOOLOGICAL PARKS

Jonathan Marks
Professor, Department of Anthropology, University of North Carolina at Charlotte
HUMAN GENOME DIVERSITY PROJECT

Stephen P. Marks
François-Xavier Bagnoud Professor of Health and Human Rights, Department of Global Health and Population, Harvard School of Public Health
RIGHTS

Theodore R. Marmor
Professor Emeritus of Public Policy and Management and Professor Emeritus of Political Science, School of Management, Yale University
HEALTH POLICY AND POLITICS
MEDICARE

Patricia A. Marshall
Professor of Bioethics and Anthropology, Department of Bioethics, Case Western Reserve University
BIOETHICS: IX. ANTHROPOLOGY OF
DEATH: I. CULTURAL PERSPECTIVES

Zubin Master
Assistant Professor, Alden March Bioethics Institute, Albany Medical College
Research Associate, Health Law Institute, University of Alberta
EMBRYO AND FETUS: II. EMBRYO RESEARCH

Alexandre Mauron
Professor, Institute of Biomedical Ethics, Faculty of Medicine, University of Geneva
EMBRYO AND FETUS: I. DEVELOPMENTS FROM FERTILIZATION TO BIRTH

Thomas May
Associate Professor of Bioethics and Medical Humanities, Center for Bioethics and Medical Humanities, Medical College of Wisconsin
CONSCIENCE, RIGHTS OF

William E. May
Michael J. McGivney Professor of Moral Theology, Pontifical John Paul II Institute for Marriage and the Family, Catholic University of America
DEATH: IV. WESTERN RELIGIOUS THOUGHT [ADDENDUM]
NATURAL LAW [ADDENDUM]

Jennifer B. McCormick
Assistant Professor of Biomedical Ethics, Division of General Internal Medicine and Health Care Policy Research and Biomedical Ethics Program, Mayo Clinic
TRANSLATIONAL RESEARCH, ETHICS OF

Laurence B. McCullough
Dalton Tomlin Chair in Medical Ethics and Health Policy, Center for Medical Ethics and Health Policy, Baylor College of Medicine, Houston, TX
CHILDBIRTH, MEDICAL PROCEDURES IN
LONG-TERM CARE: II. NURSING HOMES
SELECTIVE TERMINATION/ REDUCTION OF MULTIPLE PREGNANCY

Summer Johnson McGee
Associate Professor, Department of Public Management, College of Business, University of New Haven
BIOETHICS COMMISSIONS, HISTORY OF

Sheelagh McGuinness
University Fellow, School of Law, University of Birmingham
EUROPE, BIOETHICS IN: V. REPUBLIC OF IRELAND

W. H. McLeod
Professor Emeritus, University of Otago
SIKHISM, BIOETHICS IN

Dominique S. McMahon
Postdoctoral Fellow, Munk School of Global Affairs, University of Toronto
REGENERATIVE MEDICINE

John McMillan
Professor, Bioethics Centre, University of Otago
ELECTROCONVULSIVE THERAPY [ADDENDUM]
REPRODUCTIVE TECHNOLOGIES: II. SEX SELECTION

David Mechanic
René Dubos University Professor, Institute for Health, Health Care Policy and Aging Research, Rutgers University
MEDICINE, SOCIOLOGY OF

Thomas W. Meeks
Assistant Clinical Professor, Division of Geriatric Psychiatry, University of California, San Diego
Veterans Administration, San Diego Medical Center
PSYCHOPHARMACOLOGY

Maxwell J. Mehlman
Distinguished University Professor, Arthur E. Petersilge Professor of Law, and Director of the Law-Medicine Center, Case Western Reserve University School of Law
Professor of Biomedical Ethics, Case Western Reserve University School of Medicine
MALPRACTICE, MEDICAL
WARFARE: V. SOLDIER ENHANCEMENT

Curt Meine
Senior Fellow, Center for Humans and Nature
Senior Fellow, Aldo Leopold Foundation
BIODIVERSITY CONSERVATION

Alan Meisel
Professor of Law and Psychiatry and Dickie, McCamey, and Chilcote Professor of Bioethics, University of Pittsburgh School of Law
RIGHT TO DIE, POLICY AND LAW

Edgardo Menvielle
Director, Gender and Sexuality Development Program, Children's National Medical Center
Associate Professor of Psychiatry and Behavioral Sciences, George Washington University
SEXUAL IDENTITY

Paul T. Menzel
Professor of Philosophy Emeritus, Pacific Lutheran University
ECONOMIC CONCEPTS IN HEALTH CARE

Harold Merskey
Professor Emeritus of Psychiatry, University of Western Ontario
PSYCHOSURGERY: I. ETHICAL ASPECTS OF

Barret Michalec
Assistant Professor of Sociology, University of Delaware
PROFESSIONAL-PATIENT RELATIONSHIP: I. SOCIOLOGICAL PERSPECTIVES [ADDENDUM]

Steven H. Miles
Professor and Maas Family Endowed Chair in Bioethics, University of Minnesota Center for Bioethics
Professor, Department of Medicine, University of Minnesota Medical School
OPPRESSION
WARFARE: VI. TORTURE

Barbara D. Miller
Professor of Anthropology and International Affairs and Director, Institute for Global and International Studies, Elliott School of International Affairs, George Washington University
POPULATION ETHICS: IX. HINDU PERSPECTIVES

Bruce L. Miller
Professor Emeritus, Department of Philosophy, Michigan State University
AUTONOMY

Jennifer E. Miller
Residential Fellow, Edmond J. Safra Center for Ethics, Harvard University
PERSONALIZED MEDICINE

Timothy S. Miller
Professor of History, Salisbury University
HOSPITAL, MEDIEVAL AND RENAISSANCE HISTORY OF THE*

Nancy Milliken
Director, UCSF National Center of Excellence in Women's Health
Vice Dean and Professor of Clinical Obstetrics, School of Medicine, University of California, San Francisco
MATERNAL-FETAL RELATIONSHIP: I. MEDICAL ASPECTS

Carl Mitcham
Professor, Liberal Arts and International Studies, Colorado School of Mines
TECHNOLOGY: II. PHILOSOPHY OF MEDICAL TECHNOLOGY

Richard W. M. Momeyer
Department of Philosophy, Miami University
DEATH: III. WESTERN PHILOSOPHICAL THOUGHT

Kathryn Montgomery
Julia and David Uihlein Professor Emeritus of Medical Humanities and Bioethics and Professor Emeritus of Medicine, Northwestern University Feinberg School of Medicine
NARRATIVE

Jonathan D. Moreno
David and Lyn Silfen University Professor, Perelman School of Medicine, and Professor of Medical Ethics, History and Sociology of Science, and Philosophy, University of Pennsylvania
BIOETHICS: X. POLITICS OF
BIOTERRORISM
CONSENSUS, ROLE AND AUTHORITY OF

E. Haavi Morreim
College of Medicine, University of Tennessee Health Science Center
CONFLICT OF INTEREST
LIFE, QUALITY OF: II. QUALITY OF LIFE IN HEALTH CARE ALLOCATION

Daniel R. Morrison
Assistant Professor of Sociology, Seaver College, Pepperdine University
SCIENCE, TECHNOLOGY, AND SOCIETY STUDIES

Mary Beth Morrissey
Fellow and Faculty Director, Global Healthcare Innovation Management Center, Fordham University Graduate School of Business Administration
MEDICAL FUTILITY [ADDENDUM]
PHENOMENOLOGY
SOCIAL CONSTRUCTIONISM

Jacob Moses
New Media Director, The Hastings Center
BIOETHICS EDUCATION: IV. PUBLIC EDUCATION

Alvin H. Moss
Department of Medicine, Section of Nephrology, and Center for Health Ethics and Law, West Virginia University
DIALYSIS, KIDNEY

Arno G. Motulsky
Professor Emeritus of Medicine and Genome Sciences, University of Washington
GENETICS AND ENVIRONMENT IN HUMAN HEALTH

Timothy F. Murphy
Professor of Philosophy in the Biomedical Sciences, University of Illinois College of Medicine at Chicago
GENDER IDENTITY

Robert F. Murray Jr.
Professor of Pediatrics and Child Health, Howard University College of Medicine
GENETIC COUNSELING, ETHICAL ISSUES IN

David F. Musto
Professor of Child Psychiatry, Child Study Center, and Professor of the History of Medicine, Yale School of Medicine
HARMFUL SUBSTANCES, LEGAL CONTROL OF

Carol C. Nadelson
Clinical Professor, Brigham and Women's Hospital, Harvard Medical School
WOMEN AS HEALTH PROFESSIONALS, HISTORICAL ISSUES OF*

Michael Nair-Collins

Assistant Professor, Department of Medical Humanities and Social Sciences, Florida State University College of Medicine

IMPAIRED PROFESSIONALS

Jeckoniah O. Ndinya-Achola

Professor, University of Nairobi, Kenya

AFRICA, BIOETHICS IN: I. SUB-SAHARAN AFRICA

James Nelson

Professor, Department of Philosophy, Michigan State University

ETHICS: III. METAETHICS

FAMILY AND FAMILY MEDICINE

REPRODUCTIVE TECHNOLOGIES: VI. CONTRACT PREGNANCY

Nora Y. Ng

Research Assistant, Yale Schools of Medicine and Public Health, Yale University

GLOBAL JUSTICE

Michael Nias

Assistant Professor, Department of Psychiatry, University of Florida

ADDICTION AND DEPENDENCE

Nathan Nobis

Assistant Professor of Philosophy, Morehouse College

ANIMAL WELFARE AND RIGHTS: I. ETHICAL PERSPECTIVES ON THE TREATMENT AND STATUS OF ANIMALS [ADDENDUM]

Malkah T. Notman

Clinical Professor of Psychiatry, Cambridge Health Alliance, Harvard Medical School

WOMEN AS HEALTH PROFESSIONALS, HISTORICAL ISSUES OF*

David Novak

J. Richard and Dorothy Shiff Chair of Jewish Studies as Professor of the Study of Religion and Professor of Philosophy, University of Toronto

JUDAISM, BIOETHICS IN

Vivian-Lee Nyitray

Dean, Yuanjing Academy, Yitong College, Chongqing University of Posts and Telecommunication, China

CONFUCIANISM, BIOETHICS IN

John C. Oakley

Acting Assistant Professor of Neurology, University of Washington

PSYCHOSURGERY: II. MEDICAL AND HISTORICAL ASPECTS OF

Justin Oakley

Associate Professor and Deputy Director, Centre for Human Bioethics, Monash University

AUSTRALIA AND NEW ZEALAND, BIOETHICS IN

Michelle Oberman

Professor of Law, Santa Clara University School of Law

MATERNAL-FETAL RELATIONSHIP: III. LEGAL AND REGULATORY ISSUES

Thomas W. Ogletree

Frederick Marquand Professor Emeritus of Theological Ethics, Yale Divinity School

RESEARCH METHODOLOGY: III. SUBJECTS

Douglas P. Olsen

Associate Professor, College of Nursing, Michigan State University

NURSING, PROFESSION OF [ADDENDUM]

Gilbert S. Omenn

Professor of Internal Medicine, Human Genetics, and Public Health, University of Michigan

Director, University of Michigan Center for Computational Medicine and Biology

GENETICS AND ENVIRONMENT IN HUMAN HEALTH

Gerald M. Oppenheimer

Professor of Clinical Sociomedical Sciences, Mailman School of Public Health, Columbia University

PUBLIC HEALTH: I. HISTORY [ADDENDUM]

Daniel G. Orenstein

Fellow and Adjunct Professor of Law, Public Health Law and Policy Program, Sandra Day O'Connor College of Law, Arizona State University

PUBLIC HEALTH: II. LAW

Kelly Ormond

Associate Professor, Department of Genetics and Stanford Center for Biomedical Ethics, Stanford School of Medicine

GENETIC COUNSELING, ETHICAL ISSUES IN [ADDENDUM]

David T. Ozar

Professor, Department of Philosophy, Loyola University Chicago

BIOETHICS: IV. PROFESSIONALISM IN

DENTISTRY

PROFESSION AND PROFESSIONAL ETHICS

Jordan Paradise

Associate Professor of Law, Seton Hall University Law School

HUMAN GENOME ANALYSIS/RETURN OF RESULTS

Lisa S. Parker

Associate Professor, Center for Bioethics and Health Law, University of Pittsburgh

INFORMED CONSENT: VI. ISSUES OF CONSENT IN MENTAL HEALTH CARE

Susan Parry

Department of Philosophy, Hennepin Technical College

Department of Philosophy, University of Minnesota

ANIMAL RESEARCH: III. LAW AND POLICY

MENTALLY DISABLED AND MENTALLY ILL PERSONS: II. RESEARCH ISSUES

ORGAN AND TISSUE PROCUREMENT: II. ETHICAL AND LEGAL ISSUES REGARDING LIVING DONORS

Talcott Parsons

Harvard University

DEATH: V. DEATH IN THE WESTERN WORLD

Assya Pascalev

Associate Professor of Philosophy, Department of Community and Family Medicine, Howard University College of Medicine

ETHICS: II. TASK OF ETHICS

OCCUPATIONAL HEALTH AND SAFETY: II. OCCUPATIONAL HEALTH CARE PROVIDERS

Pasquale Patrizio

Professor and Director, Yale University Fertility Center, Department of Obstetrics, Gynecology and Reproductive Sciences

REPRODUCTIVE TECHNOLOGIES: IX. IN VITRO FERTILIZATION AND EMBRYO TRANSFER

Merril Pauls

Director of Ethics and the Humanities, Faculty of Medicine, Department of Emergency Medicine, University of Manitoba, Canada

ABORTION: VI. PROTESTANT PERSPECTIVES [ADDENDUM]

Edmund D. Pellegrino

Senior Research Scholar, Kennedy Institute of Ethics

Professor Emeritus of Medicine and Medical Ethics, Georgetown University

MEDICAL EDUCATION

Joy Penticuff

Retired Professor and Founding Director, Concordia Bachelor of Science in Nursing Program, Concordia University Texas

BIOETHICS EDUCATION: II. NURSING [ADDENDUM]

Brea L. Perry

Associate Professor, Department of Sociology, University of Kentucky

MENTAL HEALTH SERVICES: I. SETTINGS AND PROGRAMS

Elizabeth Peter

Associate Professor, Lawrence S. Bloomberg Faculty of Nursing and Member, Joint Centre for Bioethics, University of Toronto

CARE: IV. CARE AND SOCIETY/ PUBLIC POLICY

NURSING, THEORIES AND PHILOSOPHY OF [ADDENDUM]

Philip J. Peters Jr.

Ruth L. Hulston Professor of Law, University of Missouri School of Law

FUTURE GENERATIONS, REPRODUCTIVE TECHNOLOGIES AND OBLIGATIONS TO

William Petersen

Ohio State University

POPULATION ETHICS: I. HISTORY OF POPULATION THEORIES

Varduhi Petrosyan

Associate Professor, College of Health Sciences, American University of Armenia

HEALTH CARE SYSTEMS

Trisha Buchanan Phillips

Associate Professor, Department of Political Science, West Virginia University

EXPLOITATION

Sean Philpott

Center for Bioethics and Clinical Leadership, Union Graduate College

RESEARCH, UNETHICAL

Diane M. Plantz

Assistant Professor of Pediatrics, University of Missouri–Kansas City School of Medicine

PARENTAL AUTHORITY

Michael S. Policar

Associate Clinical Professor of Obstetrics, Gynecology, and Reproductive Sciences, University of California, San Francisco

FERTILITY CONTROL: I. MEDICAL ASPECTS

Thaddeus Mason Pope

Director, Health Law Institute, Hamline University School of Law

DEATH PENALTY [ADDENDUM]

LIFE, QUALITY OF: III. QUALITY OF LIFE IN LEGAL PERSPECTIVE [ADDENDUM]

Roy Porter

Wellcome Institute for the History of Medicine at University College, London

EUROPE: VI. NINETEENTH-CENTURY GREAT BRITAIN*

Stephen G. Post

Director, Center for Medical Humanities, Compassionate Care, and Bioethics, Stony Brook University School of Medicine

DEMENTIA

Kathleen E. Powderly

Director, John Conley Division of Humanities in Medicine, State University of New York, Downstate Medical Center, Brooklyn, NY

FERTILITY CONTROL: II. SOCIAL AND ETHICAL ISSUES

Madison Powers

Senior Research Scholar, Kennedy Institute of Ethics, and Professor of Philosophy, Georgetown University

SOCIAL JUSTICE

Nancy Press

Professor, School of Nursing, and Department of Public Health and Preventive Medicine, School of Medicine, Oregon Health and Science University

GENETIC TESTING AND SCREENING: I. REPRODUCTIVE GENETIC TESTING

Ivor Pritchard

Senior Advisor to the Director, Office for Human Research Protections, US Department of Health and Human Services

STUDENTS AS RESEARCH SUBJECTS

Jeffrey M. Prottas

Professor, Heller School for Social Policy and Management, Brandeis University

ORGAN AND TISSUE PROCUREMENT: I. MEDICAL AND ORGANIZATIONAL ASPECTS

Bernard G. Prusak

Associate Professor of Philosophy and Director of the McGowan Center for Ethics and Social Responsibility, King's College

FUTURE GENERATIONS, REPRODUCTIVE TECHNOLOGIES AND OBLIGATIONS TO [ADDENDUM]

Ruth B. Purtilo

Professor Emerita, Department of Interdisciplinary Studies, MGH Institute of Health Professions

BIOETHICS EDUCATION: III. OTHER HEALTH PROFESSIONS

PROFESSIONAL-PATIENT RELATIONSHIP: II. ETHICAL ISSUES

TEAMS, HEALTH CARE

Renzong Qiu

Professor of Philosophy, Institute of Philosophy and Center for Applied Ethics, Chinese Academy of Social Sciences

CHINA, BIOETHICS IN

Kimberly A. Quaid
Indiana University School of Medicine, Department of Medical and Molecular Genetics
GENETIC TESTING AND SCREENING: V. PREDICTIVE GENETIC TESTING

Timothy Quill
Professor of Medicine, Psychiatry, and Medical Humanities, University of Rochester School of Medicine and Dentistry
Director, Center for Ethics, Humanities, and Palliative Care
PHYSICIAN-ASSISTED DYING/ HASTENED DEATH

Raymond Raad
Chief Resident, Department of Psychiatry, Weill Cornell / New York Presbyterian Medical Center
MENTAL INSTITUTIONS, COMMITMENT TO

Arti K. Rai
Elvin R. Latty Professor of Law, Duke University
PATENTING ORGANISMS AND BASIC RESEARCH

Pinit Ratanakul
Associate Professor, College of Religious Studies, Mahidol University
POPULATION ETHICS: X. BUDDHIST PERSPECTIVES
SOUTHEAST ASIA, BIOETHICS IN

Mary C. Rawlinson
Professor, Department of Philosophy, Stony Brook University
CROSS-BORDER REPRODUCTIVE TRAVEL

Frederic G. Reamer
Professor, School of Social Work, Rhode Island College
SOCIAL WORK, PROFESSION OF

Tom Regan
Professor Emeritus of Philosophy, North Carolina State University
ANIMAL WELFARE AND RIGHTS: I. ETHICAL PERSPECTIVES ON THE TREATMENT AND STATUS OF ANIMALS

Warren Thomas Reich
Distinguished Professor of Religion and Ethics, Theology Department, Georgetown University
CARE: I. HISTORY OF THE NOTION OF CARE
CARE: II. HISTORICAL PRECEDENTS FOR AN ETHIC OF CARE IN HEALTH CARE

Stanley Joel Reiser
Adjunct Professor, University of Texas, Health Science Center of Houston, School of Public Health, Austin Regional Campus
Clinical Professor, George Washington University, School of Medicine and Health Sciences
TECHNOLOGY: I. HISTORY OF MEDICAL TECHNOLOGY

Arnold Relman
Professor Emeritus of Medicine and Social Medicine, Harvard Medical School
PROFIT AND COMMERCIALISM

David B. Resnik
Bioethicist and Chair, Institutional Review Board, National Institute of Environmental Health Sciences, National Institutes of Health
ENVIRONMENTAL HEALTH ETHICS
GENETIC ENGINEERING, HUMAN

Rosamond Rhodes
Professor of Medical Education and Director of Bioethics Education, Icahn School of Medicine at Mount Sinai, Graduate Center, City University of New York, and Union Graduate College
HUMAN MICROBIOME

Sarah S. Richardson
Assistant Professor, Department of the History of Science and Committee on Studies of Women, Gender, and Sexuality, Harvard University
REDUCTIONISM

Günter B. Risse
Professor Emeritus, Department of Anthropology, History and Social Medicine, University of California, San Francisco
HOSPITAL, MODERN HISTORY OF THE*

Laura Weiss Roberts
Katherine and Stanley McCormick Professor and Chair, Department of Psychiatry and Behavioral Sciences, Stanford University School of Medicine
DIVIDED LOYALTIES IN MENTAL HEALTH CARE

John A. Robertson
Vinson and Elkins Chair, University of Texas School of Law
REPRODUCTIVE TECHNOLOGIES: VII. SPERM, OVA, AND EMBRYOS

Wendy A. Rogers
Professor of Clinical Ethics, Department of Philosopy, Macquarie University and Australian School of Advanced Medicine
VULNERABILITY

Michael L. Roitero
University of Detroit Mercy
CORPORATE COMPLIANCE

Bernard E. Rollin
University Distinguished Professor, Colorado State University
ANIMAL WELFARE AND RIGHTS: VI. ANIMALS IN AGRICULTURE AND FACTORY FARMING

Holmes Rolston III
University Distinguished Professor, Department of Philosophy, Colorado State University
ANIMAL WELFARE AND RIGHTS: III. WILDLIFE CONSERVATION AND MANAGEMENT
ENDANGERED SPECIES AND BIODIVERSITY

Robin Room
Director, Center for Alcohol Policy Research, Turning Point Professor, Melbourne School of Population and Global Health, University of Melbourne
ALCOHOL AND OTHER DRUGS IN A PUBLIC HEALTH CONTEXT

Julie Rosenbaum
Associate Professor, Section of General Medicine, Department of Medicine, Yale University School of Medicine
PHARMACEUTICS, ISSUES IN PRESCRIBING [ADDENDUM]

Allan Rosenfield
Columbia University
ABORTION: I. MEDICAL PERSPECTIVES

Lainie Friedman Ross
Carolyn and Matthew Bucksbaum Professor of Clinical Ethics, MacLean Center for Clinical Medical Ethics, University of Chicago
INFORMATION DISCLOSURE, ETHICAL ISSUES OF [ADDENDUM]

ORGAN AND TISSUE PROCUREMENT: I. MEDICAL AND ORGANIZATIONAL ASPECTS [ADDENDUM]

ORGAN AND TISSUE PROCUREMENT: II. ETHICAL AND LEGAL ISSUES REGARDING LIVING DONORS [ADDENDUM]

Sue V. Rosser
Provost and Vice President for Academic Affairs, San Francisco State University
BIAS, RESEARCH

David J. Rothman
Bernard Schoenberg Professor of Social Medicine; Professor, History; Director, Center for the Study of Society and Medicine; Director, Center for Medicine as a Profession, Columbia University
RESEARCH, HUMAN: HISTORICAL ASPECTS

Jennifer Prah Ruger
Associate Professor, Yale Schools of Medicine and Public Health, Yale University
GLOBAL JUSTICE

Michael Ruse
Lucycle T. Werkmeister Professor, Department of Philosophy, Florida State University
HUMAN EVOLUTION

Maura A. Ryan
John Cardinal O'Hara, CSC, Associate Professor of Christian Ethics, Department of Theology, University of Notre Dame
REPRODUCTIVE TECHNOLOGIES: IV. LEGAL AND REGULATORY ISSUES [ADDENDUM]

Jeremy A. Sable
University of California, San Diego, Department of Psychiatry, Division of Geriatric Psychiatry
PSYCHOPHARMACOLOGY

Abdulaziz Sachedina
Professor and Endowed IIIT Chair in Islamic Studies, Department of Religious Studies, George Mason University
ISLAM, BIOETHICS IN

NEAR AND MIDDLE EAST, BIOETHICS IN: II. IRAN

John Z. Sadler
Professor of Psychiatry and Clinical Science, The Daniel W. Foster, M.D. Professor of Medical Ethics, University of Texas Southwestern Medical Center at Dallas
MENTAL ILLNESS: III. ISSUES IN DIAGNOSIS

Mark Sagoff
Professor, Institute for Philosophy and Public Policy, George Mason University
AGRICULTURE AND BIOTECHNOLOGY

ENVIRONMENTAL POLICY AND LAW

Nil Sari
Professor, Cerrahpasa Medical School, Istanbul University
NEAR AND MIDDLE EAST, BIOETHICS IN: I. TURKEY

Valerie B. Satkoske
Assistant Professor, Center for Bioethics and Health Law, University of Pittsburgh
INFORMED CONSENT: VI. ISSUES OF CONSENT IN MENTAL HEALTH CARE

Franziska Satzinger
PhD Candidate, Dalla Lana School of Public Health, University of Toronto
PUBLIC HEALTH: VIII. SOCIAL DETERMINANTS OF HEALTH

Todd L. Savitt
Department of Bioethics and Interdisciplinary Studies, East Carolina University
MINORITIES AS RESEARCH SUBJECTS

Kenneth F. Schaffner
University Professor of History and Philosophy of Science, University Professor of Philosophy, University Professor of Psychology, and Professor of Psychiatry, University of Pittsburgh
GENETICS AND HUMAN BEHAVIOR: I. SCIENTIFIC AND RESEARCH ISSUES

RESEARCH METHODOLOGY: I. CONCEPTUAL ISSUES

Renie Schapiro
Director of Public Health Integrative Cases, Medical Education Office, University of Wisconsin School of Medicine and Public Health
TISSUE BANKING AND TRANSPLANTATION, ETHICAL ISSUES IN

Naomi Scheinerman
Research Assistant, The Hastings Center
REPRODUCTIVE TECHNOLOGIES: VII. SPERM, OVA, AND EMBRYOS [ADDENDUM]

Ari Schick
Michigan State University
DISABILITY: III. MODELS OF

Jan Schildmann
Head of the NWR-Junior Research Group, Institute for Medical Ethics and History of Medicine, Ruhr University Bochum
EUROPE, BIOETHICS IN: VI. GERMAN-SPEAKING COUNTRIES AND SWITZERLAND [ADDENDUM]

Thomas F. Schindler
University of Detroit Mercy
LABOR UNIONS IN HEALTH CARE

Angela J. Schneider
School of Kinesiology, Faculty of Health Sciences, Western University
SPORTS, BIOETHICS OF

Bettina Schöne-Seifert
Professor and Executive Director, Institute for Ethics, History and Theory of Medicine, University of Münster
EUROPE, BIOETHICS IN: VI. GERMAN-SPEAKING COUNTRIES AND SWITZERLAND

HARM

Francis Schrag
Professor Emeritus of Educational Policy Studies, University of Wisconsin–Madison
CHILDREN: II. RIGHTS OF CHILDREN

Ted Schrecker
Professor of Global Health Policy, School of Medicine, Pharmacy, and Health, Durham University
GLOBALIZATION AND HEALTH

Udo Schüklenk
Ontario Research Chair in Bioethics and Public Policy, Department of Philosophy, Queen's University
UTILITARIANISM

Larry D. Scott
Professor, Division of Gastroenterology, Hepatology, and Nutrition, Department of Internal Medicine, University of Texas Medical School at Houston
ARTIFICIAL NUTRITION AND HYDRATION

John R. Scudder Jr.
Lynchburg College
NURSING, THEORIES AND PHILOSOPHY OF

Jackie Leach Scully
Professor of Social Ethics and Bioethics, School of Geography, Politics and Sociology, Newcastle University
DISABILITY: I. ETHICAL AND SOCIETAL PERSPECTIVES [ADDENDUM]

George E. Seidel Jr.
University Distinguished Professor, Animal Reproduction and Biotechnology Laboratory, Colorado State University
CLONING: I. SCIENTIFIC BACKGROUND

Michael J. Selgelid
Professor and Director, Centre for Human Bioethics, Monash University
PUBLIC HEALTH: VII. HEALTH SURVEILLANCE

Lesley A. Sharp
Ann Whitney Olin Professor in Anthropology, Barnard College
Senior Research Scientist in Sociomedical Sciences, Mailman School of Public Health, Columbia University
ORGAN TRANSPLANTS, SOCIOCULTURAL ASPECTS OF [ADDENDUM]

Richard R. Sharp
Director of Bioethics Research, Cleveland Clinic
GENETICS AND ENVIRONMENT IN HUMAN HEALTH

Virginia A. Sharpe
National Center for Ethics in Health Care, Veterans Health Administration
Center for Clinical Bioethics, Georgetown University Medical Center
BIOETHICS: V. ETHICS OF

Nancy Sherman
Professor, Philosophy Department, Georgetown University
EMOTIONS

Alexandra E. Shields
Harvard/MGH Center on Genomics, Vulnerable Populations, and Health Disparities, Massachusetts General Hospital and Harvard Medical School
PHARMACOGENOMICS

Margrit Shildrick
Linköping University, Tema Genus
CONTINENTAL PHILOSOPHY

Kristin Shrader-Frechette
O'Neill Family Professor of Philosophy and Concurrent Professor of Biological Sciences, University of Notre Dame
HAZARDOUS WASTES AND TOXIC SUBSTANCES

Miriam Shuchman
Chair, Research Ethics Board, Women's College Hospital, Toronto, ON
MENTALLY DISABLED AND MENTALLY ILL PERSONS: I. HEALTH CARE ISSUES

Victor W. Sidel
Distinguished University Professor of Social Medicine Emeritus, Montefiore Medical Center and Albert Einstein College of Medicine
Adjunct Professor of Public Health, Weill Cornell Medical College
SOCIAL MEDICINE
WARFARE: I. INTRODUCTION [ADDENDUM]
WARFARE: II. MEDICINE AND WAR
WARFARE: IV. CHEMICAL AND BIOLOGICAL WEAPONS

Tomas Jose Silber
Director, Pediatric Ethics Program and Adolescent Medicine Fellowship Program, Children's National Medical Center
Professor of Pediatrics, George Washington University
PEDIATRICS, ADOLESCENTS

Laura A. Siminoff
Professor and Chair, Department of Social and Behavioral Health, School of Medicine, Virginia Commonwealth University
BIOETHICS: VII. EMPIRICAL METHODS IN

Christian M. Simon
Associate Professor of Internal Medicine, University of Iowa Carver College of Medicine
CANCER, ETHICAL ISSUES RELATED TO DIAGNOSIS AND TREATMENT

Peter Singer
Ira W. Decamp Professor of Bioethics, University Center for Human Values, Princeton University
Laureate Professor, School of Historical and Philosophical Studies, University of Melbourne
ANIMAL RESEARCH: II. PHILOSOPHICAL ISSUES

I. J. Singh
Professor Emeritus, Department of Anatomical Sciences, New York University
SIKHISM, BIOETHICS IN [ADDENDUM]

Jacquelyn Slomka
Assistant Professor, Frances Payne Bolton School of Nursing, Case Western Reserve University
SMOKING

Michael A. Slote
UST Professor of Ethics, University of Miami
ETHICS: I. HISTORY OF ETHICS

Roberta M. Snow
Professor and Chair, Department of Management, West Chester University
ORGANIZATIONAL ETHICS IN HEALTH CARE [ADDENDUM]

Mildred Z. Solomon
President and CEO, The Hastings Center
Clinical Professor of Anaesthesia, Harvard Medical School
COMPARATIVE EFFECTIVENESS RESEARCH AND IMPLEMENTATION SCIENCE

W. David Solomon
Associate Professor, Department of Philosophy, University of Notre Dame
ETHICS: IV. NORMATIVE ETHICAL THEORIES

Tom Sorell
Professor of Politics and Philosophy, University of Warwick
DEATH PENALTY

Colin L. Soskolne
Professor of Epidemiology, School of Public Health, University of Alberta
Visiting Fellow, Faculty of Health, University of Canberra
PUBLIC HEALTH: V. METHODS

Michelle Spektor
Research Associate, Presidential Commission for the Study of Bioethical Issues
BIOETHICS: X. POLITICS OF

Sandro Spinsanti
Institute for the Social Study of the State, Rome
EUROPE, BIOETHICS IN: I. INTRODUCTION

Justin Stein
Doctoral Candidate, Department for the Study of Religion, University of Toronto
ALTERNATIVE THERAPIES: I. SOCIAL HISTORY

Bonnie Steinbock
Professor of Philosophy, University at Albany, State University of New York and Union Graduate College Online Bioethics Program
MATERNAL-FETAL RELATIONSHIP: II. ETHICAL ISSUES

Nathaniel Stewart
Attorney, Washington, DC
CLONING: III. RELIGIOUS PERSPECTIVES
FERTILITY CONTROL: III. LEGAL AND REGULATORY ISSUES
SEXUALITY, LEGAL APPROACHES TO

Robyn I. Stone
Executive Director, LeadingAge Center for Applied Research
LONG-TERM CARE: III. HOME CARE [ADDENDUM]

Christine Straehle
Associate Professor, Graduate School of Public and International Affairs, University of Ottawa
POPULATION POLICIES, MIGRATION AND REFUGEES IN [ADDENDUM]

Christina W. Strong
Principal, Law Office of Christina W. Strong General Counsel, New Jersey Organ and Tissue Sharing Network
TISSUE BANKING AND TRANSPLANTATION, ETHICAL ISSUES IN

Karsten J. Struhl
Department of Philosophy, John Jay College of Criminal Justice, City University of New York
HUMAN NATURE

Jeremy Sugarman
Harvey M. Meyerhoff Professor of Bioethics and Medicine, Berman Institute of Bioethics and Division of General Internal Medicine, Johns Hopkins University
BIOETHICS: VI. RESEARCH METHODS IN
RESEARCH POLICY: III. SUBJECTS

Mark D. Sullivan
Professor of Psychiatry and Behavioral Sciences, University of Washington, Seattle
MENTAL HEALTH THERAPIES

Daniel P. Sulmasy
Kilbride-Clinton Professor of Medicine and Ethics Department of Medicine and Divinity School, University of Chicago
Associate Director, MacLean Center for Clinical Medical Ethics, University of Chicago
BIOETHICS: VI. RESEARCH METHODS IN

Judith P. Swazey
President, Acadia Institute
ORGAN TRANSPLANTS, SOCIOCULTURAL ASPECTS OF

Nathanael Symeonides
Ecumenical Officer & Director of Inter-Orthodox Affairs, Greek Orthodox Archdiocese of America
Professor of Orthodox Christian Ethics, St. Vladimir's Orthodox Theological Seminary, Fordham University
EASTERN ORTHODOX CHRISTIANITY, BIOETHICS IN [ADDENDUM]

Godfrey B. Tangwa
Professor of Philosophy, University of Yaounde 1 and Cameroon Bioethics Initiative
AFRICA, BIOETHICS IN: I. SUB-SAHARAN AFRICA [ADDENDUM]

Torbjørn Tännsjö
Kristian Claëson Professor of Practical Philosophy, Stockholm University, Sweden
EUROPE, BIOETHICS IN: VII. NORDIC COUNTRIES

Carol A. Tauer
Visiting Professor, Center for Bioethics, University of Minnesota
EMBRYO AND FETUS: II. EMBRYO RESEARCH

Holly Taylor
Associate Professor, Johns Hopkins Bloomberg School of Public Health, Core Faculty, Johns Hopkins Berman Institute of Bioethics
RESEARCH METHODOLOGY: III. SUBJECTS [ADDENDUM]

Şerife Tekin

Assistant Professor, Department of Philosophy and Religious Studies, Daemen College, New York

MENTAL HEALTH, MEANING OF MENTAL HEALTH [ADDENDUM]

NEAR AND MIDDLE EAST, BIOETHICS IN: I. TURKEY [ADDENDUM]

Ruud H. J. ter Meulen

University of Bristol, School of Social and Community Medicine, Centre for Ethics in Medicine

SOLIDARITY

Michael D. Teret

Johns Hopkins University

INJURY AND INJURY CONTROL

Stephen P. Teret

Professor, Department of Health Policy and Management, Johns Hopkins University

Director, Center for Law and the Public's Health

INJURY AND INJURY CONTROL

Angela K. Thachuk

Department of Philosophy, University of Alberta

MENTAL ILLNESS: IV. BIOMEDICAL MODELS

Jon C. Tilburt

Associate Professor of Biomedical Ethics and Medicine, Mayo Clinic

SHARED DECISION MAKING

Michael J. Toole

Deputy Director, Burnet Institute

Professor, Department of Epidemiology and Preventive Medicine, Monash University, Melbourne, Australia

WARFARE: III. PUBLIC HEALTH AND WAR

Joan Tronto

Professor, Department of Political Science, University of Minnesota

CARE: III. CARE ETHICS

Robert D. Truog

Professor of Medical Ethics, Anesthesiology, and Pediatrics, Harvard Medical School

Senior Associate, Critical Care Medicine, Children's Hospital, Boston, MA

Executive Director, Institute for Professionalism and Ethical Practice

PEDIATRICS, INTENSIVE CARE IN

Seth Tuler

Associate Teaching Professor, Interdisciplinary and Global Studies Division, Worcester Polytechnic Institute

RISK AND RISK ASSESSMENT

James A. Tulsky

Professor of Medicine and Nursing and Chief, Duke Center for Palliative Care, Duke University

ADVANCE DIRECTIVES AND ADVANCE CARE PLANNING

Bryan S. Turner

Presidential Professor of Sociology, Department of Sociology, The Graduate Center, The City University of New York

BODY: II. CULTURAL AND RELIGIOUS PERSPECTIVES [ADDENDUM]

Yoram Unguru

Pediatric Hematologist/Oncologist, Berman Institute of Bioethics, Johns Hopkins University

CANCER, ETHICAL ISSUES RELATED TO DIAGNOSIS AND TREATMENT

Paul U. Unschuld

Director, Institut für Geschichte der Medizin

CHINA: PRE-REPUBLICAN CHINA*

Bernard Unti

Senior Policy Adviser, Humane Society of the United States

ANIMAL RESEARCH: II. PHILOSOPHICAL ISSUES

Gavin Van Horn

Director, Cultures of Conservation, Center for Humans and Nature

FOOD

Gerard Vanderhaar

Professor of Peace and Religious Studies, Christian Brothers University

WARFARE: I. INTRODUCTION

Harold Y. Vanderpool

Professor Emeritus, History and Philosophy of Medicine, Institute for the Medical Humanities, University of Texas Medical Branch

LIFE-SUSTAINING TREATMENT AND EUTHANASIA: II. HISTORICAL ASPECTS OF

Marian A. Verkerk

Professor, Ethics of Care, University Medical Center Groningen

NATURALISM

A. M. Viens

Lecturer, Southampton Law School, University of Southampton

Research Fellow, Institute for Medical Ethics and History of Medicine, Ruhr-University Bochum

POPULATION ETHICS: I. HISTORY OF POPULATION THEORIES

POPULATION ETHICS: II. NORMATIVE APPROACHES

Deborah Viola

Associate Professor, Center for Long Term Care Research and Policy, New York Medical College

LONG-TERM CARE: IV. FINANCING, US AND INTERNATIONAL

Benedetto Vitiello

Chief, Child and Adolescent Treatment and Preventive Intervention Research Branch, National Institute of Mental Health

Adjunct Professor, Department of Psychiatry, Johns Hopkins University

CHILDREN: IV. MENTAL HEALTH ISSUES

Jochen Vollmann

Director, Institute for Medical Ethics and History of Medicine, Ruhr University Bochum

EUROPE, BIOETHICS IN: VI. GERMAN-SPEAKING COUNTRIES AND SWITZERLAND [ADDENDUM]

Dietrich von Engelhardt
Medizinische Universität Lübeck, Lübeck, Germany
EUROPE, BIOETHICS IN: I. INTRODUCTION
HEALTH AND DISEASE: I. HISTORY OF THE CONCEPTS

Lance Wahlert
Assistant Professor, Department of Medical Ethics and Health Policy, Perelman School of Medicine, University of Pennsylvania
GENDER

Paul Waldau
Associate Professor, Anthrozoology, Canisius College
ANIMAL WELFARE AND RIGHTS: VII. POLICIES AND ORGANIZATIONS

Bailus Walker
Professor of Environmental and Occupational Medicine and Toxicology, Department of Community and Family Medicine, Howard University College of Medicine
OCCUPATIONAL HEALTH AND SAFETY: II. OCCUPATIONAL HEALTH CARE PROVIDERS

William J. Wall
Professor of Surgery, Schulich School of Medicine and Dentistry, Western University
ORGAN TRANSPLANTS, MEDICAL OVERVIEW OF

Edwin R. Wallace IV
Research Professor of Bioethics and Medical Humanities, University of South Carolina
MENTAL HEALTH, MEANING OF MENTAL HEALTH

Ernest Wallwork
Professor, Department of Religion, Syracuse University
PSYCHOANALYSIS AND DYNAMIC THERAPIES [ADDENDUM]
SEXUAL BEHAVIOR, MEDICAL CONTROL OF

James J. Walter
Austin and Ann O'Malley Chair in Bioethics, The Bioethics Institute, Loyola Marymount University
LIFE, QUALITY OF: I. QUALITY OF LIFE IN CLINICAL DECISIONS

James W. Walters
Professor of Religion, Loma Linda University
MORAL STATUS

Herbert E. Ward
Associate Professor and Vice Chair, Department of Psychiatry, University of Florida College of Medicine
PSYCHOSURGERY: II. MEDICAL AND HISTORICAL ASPECTS OF [ADDENDUM]

Karen J. Warren
Macalester College
ENVIRONMENTAL ETHICS: IV. ECOFEMINISM

Rueben Warren
Director, National Center for Bioethics in Research and Health Care, Tuskegee University
OCCUPATIONAL HEALTH AND SAFETY: II. OCCUPATIONAL HEALTH CARE PROVIDERS

Sebastian Wäscher
Researcher, Institute for Medical Ethics and History of Medicine, Ruhr University Bochum
EUROPE, BIOETHICS IN: VI. GERMAN-SPEAKING COUNTRIES AND SWITZERLAND [ADDENDUM]

David Wasserman
Director of Research, Yeshiva University
DISABILITY: III. MODELS OF

Katie Watson
Assistant Professor, Medical Humanities and Bioethics Program, Feinberg School of Medicine, Northwestern University
FERTILITY CONTROL: III. LEGAL AND REGULATORY ISSUES [ADDENDUM]

Leonard J. Weber
Professor Emeritus of Ethics, University of Detroit Mercy
LABOR UNIONS IN HEALTH CARE [ADDENDUM]
PHARMACEUTICAL INDUSTRY
PHARMACEUTICS, ISSUES IN PRESCRIBING
WHISTLEBLOWING IN HEALTH CARE

Robert F. Weir
Professor Emeritus, Departments of Pediatrics and Religious Studies, University of Iowa
INFANTS, ETHICAL ISSUES WITH

David E. Weismann
Professor Emeritus, Medical College of Wisconsin
HOSPICE AND PALLIATIVE CARE: PROFESSIONAL EDUCATION

Tonia Werner
Assistant Professor and Vice Chair, Department of Psychiatry, College of Medicine, University of Florida
Director, University of Florida Forensic Institute
EXPERT TESTIMONY

Terrie Wetle
Professor, Health Services, Policy and Practice, School of Public Health, Brown University
LONG-TERM CARE: III. HOME CARE

Robert M. Wettstein
Clinical Professor of Psychiatry, University of Pittsburgh School of Medicine
COMPETENCE
INSANITY AND THE INSANITY DEFENSE

Caroline Whitbeck
Elmer G. Beamer–Hubert H. Schneider Professor Emerita of Ethics, Case Western Reserve University
TRUST

Amanda White
Montefiore Medical Center
FERTILITY CONTROL: III. LEGAL AND REGULATORY ISSUES

Gladys B. White
Adjunct Professor, Graduate Liberal Studies, Georgetown University
REPRODUCTIVE TECHNOLOGIES: III. FERTILITY DRUGS

Peter J. Whitehouse
Professor, Department of Neurology, Case Western Reserve University
ECOLOGICAL BIOETHICS

Daniel Wikler

Mary B. Saltonstall Professor of Population Ethics and Professor of Ethics and Population Health, Department of Global Health and Population, Harvard School of Public Health

PUBLIC HEALTH: IX. LIFESTYLES

Kevin W. Wildes

President, Loyola University New Orleans

HEALTH AND DISEASE: IV. PHILOSOPHICAL PERSPECTIVES

MEDICINE, PHILOSOPHY OF

Benjamin Wilfond

Director, Treuman Katz Center for Pediatric Bioethics, Seattle Children's Research Institute

Professor, Department of Pediatrics, University of Washington

GENETIC TESTING AND SCREENING: II. NEWBORN GENETIC SCREENING [ADDENDUM]

James Wilson

Lecturer in Philosophy and Health, University College London

GLOBAL HEALTH INEQUALITIES AND INEQUITIES

RESEARCH METHODOLOGY: I. CONCEPTUAL ISSUES [ADDENDUM]

William J. Winslade

James Wade Rockwell Professor of Philosophy in Medicine, Institute for the Medical Humanities, Unviersity of Texas Medical Branch

COGNITIVE IMPAIRMENT/ TRAUMATIC BRAIN INJURY

CONFIDENTIALITY

Gerald R. Winslow

Professor of Religion, School of Religion, Loma Linda University

TRIAGE

J. Philip Wogaman

Professor Emeritus of Christian Ethics, Wesley Theological Seminary, Washington, DC

POPULATION ETHICS: VIII. PROTESTANT PERSPECTIVES

Leslie E. Wolf

Professor of Law, Georgia State University College of Law

AIDS: II. HEALTH CARE AND RESEARCH ISSUES

Paul Root Wolpe

Asa Griggs Candler Professor of Bioethics and Director, Center for Ethics, Emory University

NEUROETHICS

Roger P. Worthington

Adjunct (Assistant) Professor, General Internal Medicine, Yale University

HEALTH CARE, ETHICS AND PROFESSIONALISM IN

PATIENTS' RESPONSIBILITIES: II. CO-RELATIVE RIGHTS

Matthew Wynia

Clinical Assistant Professor of Medicine, Department of Medicine, University of Chicago

MEDICINE, ART OF [ADDENDUM]

Rebecca B. Yarrison

Assistant Professor of Medicine, Pediatrics, and Nursing, Department of Internal Medicine, University of Kentucky College of Medicine

DEATH, DEFINITION AND DETERMINATION OF: I. CRITERIA FOR DEATH [ADDENDUM]

Allan Young

Marjorie Bronfman Professor in Social Studies in Medicine, McGill University

HEALTH AND DISEASE: III. ANTHROPOLOGICAL PERSPECTIVES

Katherine K. Young

Professor Emeritus of Hinduism, Faculty of Religious Studies, McGill University

DEATH: II. EASTERN THOUGHT

Stuart J. Youngner

Susan E. Watson Professor and Chair, Department of Bioethics, School of Medicine, Case Western Reserve University

CLINICAL ETHICS: II. ETHICS COMMITTEES AND ETHICS CONSULTATION

MEDICAL FUTILITY

TISSUE BANKING AND TRANSPLANTATION, ETHICAL ISSUES IN

Boris Yudin

Professor, Corresponding Member, Russian Academy of Sciences

Head, Department of Comprehensive Problems of Human Studies, Institute of Philosophy, Russian Academy of Sciences

EUROPE, BIOETHICS IN: IX. RUSSIA

Richard M. Zaner

Professor of Medicine (Medical Ethics), Emeritus, Vanderbilt University Medical Center

BODY: I. EMBODIMENT IN THE PHENOMENOLOGICAL TRADITION

Laurie Zoloth

Professor, Department of Religious Studies, Northwestern University

ABORTION: IV. JEWISH PERSPECTIVES

GENETICS AND HUMAN SELF-UNDERSTANDING

Topical Outline

The classification of articles that follows provides a thematic view of Bioethics's *contents, depicting overall coverage in various divisions of the field of bioethics. It is also intended to assist the user, whether researcher or browser, in locating articles broadly related to a given topic. Because the topic headings are not mutually exclusive, and because many entries touch on several themes and topics, many titles are listed more than once.*

ABORTION

Abortion: I. Medical Perspectives
Abortion: II. Ethical Perspectives
Abortion: III. Legal and Regulatory Issues
Abortion: IV. Jewish Perspectives
Abortion: V. Roman Catholic Perspectives
Abortion: VI. Protestant Perspectives
Abortion: VII. Islamic Perspectives
Abortion: VIII. Buddhist Perspectives
Abortion: IX. Hindu Perspectives
Autonomy
Conscience, Rights of
Double Effect, Principle or Doctrine of
Embryo and Fetus: I. Developments from Fertilization to Birth
Embryo and Fetus: II. Embryo Research
Embryo and Fetus: III. Embryonic Stem Cell Research
Embryo and Fetus: IV. Fetal Research
Embryo and Fetus: V. Religious Perspectives
Feminism
Fertility Control
Genetic Testing and Screening: I. Reproductive Genetic Testing
Harm
Healing
Homicide
Human Dignity
Infanticide
Law and Morality
Liberty
Life
Life, Sanctity of
Maternal-Fetal Relationship: I. Medical Aspects
Maternal-Fetal Relationship: II. Ethical Issues
Maternal-Fetal Relationship: III. Legal and Regulatory Issues
Medical Codes and Oaths
Medicine, Profession of
Moral Status
Nursing, Profession of
Obligation and Supererogation
Patients' Rights: I. Origin and Nature of Patients' Rights
Patients' Rights: II. Mental Patients' Rights
Population Policies, Strategies for Fertility Control in
Professional-Patient Relationship: I. Sociological Perspectives
Professional-Patient Relationship: II. Ethical Issues
Reproductive Technologies: III. Fertility Drugs
Rights
Selective Termination/Reduction of Multiple Pregnancy
Sexual Behavior, Social Control of
Virtue and Character
Women, Historical and Cross-Cultural Perspectives

ABUSE AND HARM

Abuse, Interpersonal
Bioterrorism
Circumcision, Female: I. Historical Overview
Circumcision, Female: II. Cultural and Ethical Aspects
Circumcision, Male
Coercion
Double Effect, Principle or Doctrine of
Electroconvulsive Therapy
Embryo and Fetus: I. Developments from Fertilization to Birth
Embryo and Fetus: II. Embryo Research
Embryo and Fetus: III. Embryonic Stem Cell Research
Embryo and Fetus: IV. Fetal Research
Embryo and Fetus: V. Religious Perspectives
Eugenics: I. Historical Aspects
Genetic Discrimination
Harm
Harmful Substances, Legal Control of
Infanticide
Injury and Injury Control
Malpractice, Medical
Military Personnel as Research Subjects
Minorities as Research Subjects
Mistakes, Medical
Nazi Legacy and Bioethics
Pain and Suffering
Psychiatry, Abuses of

AGING

ANIMAL WELFARE

BIOETHICS: PROFESSION AND INFLUENCE

BIOTECHNOLOGY

CHILDREN

CHRONIC ILLNESS AND LONG-TERM CARE

CLINICAL ETHICS

Pediatrics, Intensive Care in
Pediatrics, Overview of Ethical Issues in
Physician-Assisted Dying/Hastened Death
Principlism
Privacy in Health Care
Profession and Professional Ethics
Professional-Patient Relationship: I. Sociological Perspectives
Professional-Patient Relationship: II. Ethical Issues
Race and Racism
Right to Die: Policy and Law
Rights
Risk and Risk Assessment

CONCEPTS

Authenticity
Authority in Religious Traditions
Autonomy
Beneficence
Biocentrism versus Anthropocentrism
Biopolitics
Bioterrorism
Body: I. Embodiment in the Phenomenological Tradition
Care: I. History of the Notion of Care
Casuistry
Coercion
Competence
Confidentiality
Conflict of Interest
Conscience
Consensus, Role and Authority of
Death, Definition and Determination of: III. Philosophical and Theological Perspectives
Double Effect, Principle or Doctrine of
Emotions
Epistemic Injustice
Ethics: I. History of Ethics
Ethics: II. Task of Ethics
Ethics: III. Metaethics
Ethics: IV. Normative Ethical Theories
Ethics: V. Religion and Morality
Exploitation
Feminism
Freedom and Free Will
Gender
Global Justice
Harm
Healing
Health and Disease: I. History of the Concepts
Human Dignity
Human Evolution
Human Rights
Insanity and the Insanity Defense
Justice
Liberty
Life
Medical Futility
Mental Illness: I. Definition, Use and Meaning
Moral Status
Narrative
Natural Law
Naturalism
Obligation and Supererogation
Oppression
Pain and Suffering
Paternalism
Precautionary Principle
Principlism
Privacy in Health Care
Race and Racism
Reductionism
Relativism, Cultural and Ethical
Right to Die: Policy and Law
Rights
Risk and Risk Assessment
Social Constructionism
Social Justice
Social Medicine
Solidarity
Stewardship
Subjectivity
Suicide
Sustainability
Trust
Virtue and Character
Vulnerability
Warfare: VI. Torture

DEATH AND DYING

Advance Directives and Advance Care Planning
Cancer, Ethical Issues Relating to Diagnosis and Treatment
Death: I. Cultural Perspectives
Death: II. Eastern Thought
Death: III. Western Philosophical Thought
Death: IV. Western Religious Thought
Death: V. Death in the Western World
Death, Definition and Determination of: I. Criteria for Death
Death, Definition and Determination of: II. Legal Issues in Pronouncing Death
Death, Definition and Determination of: III. Philosophical and Theological Perspectives
Death Penalty
Dementia
Endangered Species and Biodiversity
End-of-Life Care
Epidemics
Grief and Bereavement
Holocaust
Homicide
Infanticide
Life-Sustaining Treatment and Euthanasia: I. Ethical Aspects of
Life-Sustaining Treatment and Euthanasia: II. Historical Aspects of
Pastoral Care and Health Care Chaplaincy
Patients' Rights: I. Origin and Nature of Patients' Rights
Patients' Rights: II. Mental Patients' Rights
Physician-Assisted Dying/Hastened Death
Suicide
Surrogate Decision Making
Warfare: I. Introduction

DECISION MAKING AND INFORMED CONSENT

Advance Directives and Advance Care Planning
Alternative Therapies
Autonomy
Beneficence
Care
Clinical Ethics
Coercion
Compassionate Love
Competence
Confidentiality
Conscience
Conscience, Rights of
Dementia
Divided Loyalties in Mental Health Care
Emotions
Epidemics
Ethics: IV. Normative Ethical Theories
Freedom and Free Will
Genetic Testing and Screening: I. Reproductive Genetic Testing
Genetic Testing and Screening: II. Newborn Genetic Screening
Genetic Testing and Screening: III. Population Screening
Genetic Testing and Screening: IV. Public Health Context
Genetic Testing and Screening: V. Predictive Genetic Testing
Genetic Testing and Screening: VI. Pediatric Genetic Testing
Healing
Health Care Professionals, Legal Regulation of
Health Care Resources, Allocation of
Health Insurance
Human Dignity
Impaired Professionals
Information Disclosure, Ethical Aspects of
Informed Consent: I. History of Informed Consent
Informed Consent: II. Meaning and Elements
Informed Consent: III. Consent Issues in Human Research
Informed Consent: IV. Clinical Aspects of Consent in Health Care
Informed Consent: V. Legal and Ethical Issues of Consent in Health Care

Informed Consent: VI. Issues of Consent in Mental Health Care
Labor Unions in Health Care
Law and Bioethics
Life, Quality of: I. Quality of Life in Clinical Decisions
Malpractice, Medical
Managed Care
Medical Codes and Oaths
Medical Education
Medicine, Art of
Medicine, Profession of
Mental Illness: Issues in Diagnosis
Mentally Disabled and Mentally Ill Persons
Mistakes, Medical
Nursing, Profession of
Nursing, Theories and Philosophy of
Nursing Ethics
Obligation and Supererogation
Pastoral Care and Health Care Chaplaincy
Paternalism
Patients' Responsibilities: I. Duties of Patients
Patients' Responsibilities: II. Co-Relative Rights
Patients' Rights: I. Origin and Nature of Patients' Rights
Patients' Rights: II. Mental Patients' Rights
Pharmaceutical Industry
Pharmaceutics, Issues in Prescribing
Placebo
Principlism
Privacy in Health Care
Profession and Professional Ethics
Professional-Patient Relationship: I. Sociological Perspectives
Professional-Patient Relationship: II. Ethical Issues
Research, Human: Historical Aspects
Research, Unethical
Responsibility
Right to Die: Policy and Law
Rights
Shared Decision Making
Social Medicine
Surrogate Decision Making
Teams, Health Care
Trust

DISEASE AND ILLNESS

Addiction and Dependence
Advance Directives and Advance Care Planning
AIDS: I. Public Health Issues
AIDS: II. Health Care and Research Issues
Cancer, Ethical Issues Related to Diagnosis and Treatment
Chronic Illness
Cross-Border Medical Travel
Dementia
Disability: I. Ethical and Societal Perspectives
Disability: II. Legal Issues
Disability: III. Models of
Genetic Testing and Screening: I. Reproductive Genetic Testing
Genetic Testing and Screening: II. Newborn Genetic Screening
Genetic Testing and Screening: III. Population Screening
Genetic Testing and Screening: IV. Public Health Context
Genetic Testing and Screening: V. Predictive Genetic Testing
Genetic Testing and Screening: VI. Pediatric Genetic Testing
Genetics and Environment in Human Health
Global Health Inequalities and Inequities
Global Justice
Globalization and Health
Health and Disease: I. History of the Concepts
Health and Disease: II. Sociological Perspectives
Health and Disease: III. Anthropological Perspectives
Health and Disease: IV. Philosophical Perspectives
Health and Disease: V. The Experience of Health and Illness
Human Genome Analysis/Return of Results
Human Genome Diversity Project
Human Genome Project
Human Microbiome
Life, Quality of: I. Quality of Life in Clinical Decisions
Life, Quality of: II. Quality of Life in Health Care Allocation
Life, Quality of: III. Quality of Life in Legal Perspective
Medicine, Anthropology of
Medicine, Art of
Medicine, Philosophy of
Medicine, Sociology of
Mental Illness: I. Definition, Use and Meaning
Mental Illness: II. Cultural Perspectives
Mental Illness: III. Issues in Diagnosis
Mental Illness: IV. Biomedical Models
Mental Institutions, Commitment to
Mentally Disabled and Mentally Ill Persons: I. Health Care Issues
Mentally Disabled and Mentally Ill Persons: II. Research Issues
Metaphor and Analogy
Pain and Suffering
Pandemics
Paternalism
Patients' Responsibilities: I. Duties of Patients
Patients' Responsibilities: II. Co-Relative Rights
Patients' Rights: I. Origin and Nature of Patients' Rights
Patients' Rights: II. Mental Patients' Rights
Personalized Medicine
Pharmacogenomics
Profession and Professional Ethics
Professional-Patient Relationship: I. Sociological Perspectives
Professional-Patient Relationship: II. Ethical Issues
Public Health: VIII. Social Determinants of Health
Regenerative Medicine
Rehabilitation Medicine
Relativism, Cultural and Ethical
Religious Objections to Medical Care
Technology: I. History of Medical Technology
Technology: II. Philosophy of Medical Technology
Tissue Banking and Transplantation, Ethical Issues in
Transhumanism and Posthumanism
Vegetative and Minimally Conscious States
Whole Genome Sequencing

ECOLOGY AND THE ENVIRONMENT

Agriculture and Biotechnology
Animal Welfare and Rights: VI. Animals in Agriculture and Factory Farming
Biodiversity Conservation
Biopolitics
Climate Change
Ecological Bioethics
Endangered Species and Biodiversity
Environmental Ethics: I. Overview
Environmental Ethics: II. Deep Ecology
Environmental Ethics: III. Land Ethics
Environmental Ethics: IV. Ecofeminism
Environmental Health Ethics
Environmental Policy and Law
Epidemics
Food
Genetics and Environment in Human Health
Global Health Inequalities and Inequities
Global Justice
Globalization and Health
Green Design of Hospitals/Impact
Harmful Substances, Legal Control of

EMBRYO AND FETUS

END-OF-LIFE CARE

ETHNICITY AND RACE

GENETICS AND GENOMICS

Genetics and Environment in Human Health
Genetics and Human Behavior: I. Scientific and Research Issues
Genetics and Human Behavior: II. Philosophical and Ethical Issues
Genetics and Human Self-Understanding
Genetics and Racial Minorities
Harm
Human Dignity
Human Nature
Metaphor and Analogy
Natural Law
Organ and Tissue Procurement
Pharmacogenomics
Reproductive Technologies: I. Introduction
Reproductive Technologies: II. Sex Selection
Reproductive Technologies: III. Fertility Drugs
Reproductive Technologies: IV. Legal and Regulatory Issues
Reproductive Technologies: V. Gamete Donation
Reproductive Technologies: VI. Contract Pregnancy
Reproductive Technologies: VII. Sperm, Ova, and Embryos
Reproductive Technologies: VIII. Ethical Issues
Reproductive Technologies: IX. In Vitro Fertilization and Embryo Transfer
Research, Human: Historical Aspects
Research, Multinational
Research, Unethical
Research Policy: I. General Background
Research Policy: II. Risk and Vulnerable Groups
Research Policy: III. Subjects
Technology: I. History of Medical Technology
Technology: II. Philosophy of Medical Technology
Transhumanism and Posthumanism

GLOBAL PERSPECTIVES

Africa, Bioethics in: I. Sub-Saharan Africa
Africa, Bioethics in: II. South Africa
America, Bioethics in: I. United States
America, Bioethics in: II. Canada
America, Bioethics in: III. Latin America
Australia and New Zealand, Bioethics in
Biopolitics
Bioterrorism
China, Bioethics in
Climate Change
Community-Based Participatory Research
Cross-Border Medical Travel
Cross-Border Reproductive Travel
Endangered Species and Biodiversity
Europe, Bioethics in: I. Introduction
Europe, Bioethics in: II. Southern Europe
Europe, Bioethics in: III. The Benelux Countries
Europe, Bioethics in: IV. United Kingdom
Europe, Bioethics in: V. Republic of Ireland
Europe, Bioethics in: VI. German-Speaking Countries and Switzerland
Europe, Bioethics in: VII. Nordic Countries
Europe, Bioethics in: VIII. Central and Eastern Europe
Europe, Bioethics in: IX. Russia
Global Health Inequalities and Inequities
Global Justice
Globalization and Health
Health Policies in International Perspectives
Human Genome Diversity Project
Humanitarian Relief
Immigrants, Access to Health Care
International Health
Japan, Bioethics in
Justice
Near and Middle East, Bioethics in: I. Turkey
Near and Middle East, Bioethics in: II. Iran
Near and Middle East, Bioethics in: III. Arab World
Near and Middle East, Bioethics in: IV. Israel
NGOs in Health Care
Race and Racism
Research, Multinational
South Asia, Bioethics in
Southeast Asia, Bioethics in
Sustainability
Warfare: I. Introduction
Warfare: II. Medicine and War
Warfare: III. Public Health and War
Warfare: IV. Chemical and Biological Weapons
Warfare: V. Soldier Enhancement
Warfare: VI. Torture
Women, Historical and Cross-Cultural Perspectives

HEALTH CARE MANAGEMENT

Advertising and Marketing in Health Care
Commercialism in Scientific Research
Conflict of Interest
Corporate Compliance
Economic Concepts in Health Care
Green Design of Hospitals/Impact
Health Care, Delivery of
Health Care, Ethics and Professionalism in
Health Care, Quality Improvement
Health Care Institutions
Health Care Resources, Allocation of: II. Microallocation
Health Care Systems
Health Insurance
Health Policy in the United States
Health Services Management Ethics
Hospital, Contemporary Ethical Problems of the
Hospitals, Ethical Issues in the Governance of
Labor Unions in Health Care
Organizational Ethics in Health Care
Pharmaceutical Industry
Pharmaceutics, Issues in Prescribing
Pharmacogenomics
Privacy in Health Care
Profit and Commercialism
Research Policy: I. General Background
Research Policy: II. Risk and Vulnerable Groups
Whistleblowing in Health Care

HEALTH LAW

Abortion: III. Legal and Regulatory Issues
Abuse, Interpersonal: I. Child Abuse
Abuse, Interpersonal: II. Abuse between Domestic Partners
Abuse, Interpersonal: III. Elder Abuse
Abuse, Interpersonal: IV. Abuse of Health Care Workers
Access to Health Care
Advance Directives and Advance Care Planning
Alternative Therapies: II. Ethical and Legal Issues
Animal Research: III. Law and Policy
Children: II. Rights of Children
Competence
Confidentiality
Conflict of Interest
Corporate Compliance
Corporate Social Responsibility in Health
Death, Definition and Determination of: II. Legal Issues in Pronouncing Death
Death Penalty
Disability: II. Legal Issues
DNA Identification
End-of-Life Care
Environmental Policy and Law
Epidemics
Expert Testimony
Fertility Control: III. Legal and Regulatory Issues

Genetic Discrimination
Harmful Substances, Legal Control of
Health Care Professionals, Legal Regulation of
Health Insurance
Impaired Professionals
Infanticide
Infants, Public Policy and Legal Issues
Information Disclosure, Ethical Issues of
Informed Consent: V. Legal and Ethical Issues of Consent in Health Care
Insanity and Insanity Defense
Law and Bioethics
Law and Morality
Life, Quality of: III. Quality of Life in Legal Perspective
Malpractice, Medical
Maternal-Fetal Relationship: III. Legal and Regulatory Issues
Mental Institutions, Commitment to
Natural Law
Organ and Tissue Procurement: II. Ethical and Legal Issues Regarding Living Donors
Patenting Organisms and Basic Research
Patients' Rights: I. Origin and Nature of Patients' Rights
Patients' Rights: II. Mental Patients' Rights
Public Health: II. Law
Public Policy and Bioethics
Reproductive Technologies: IV. Legal and Regulatory Issues
Right to Die: Policy and Law
Rights
Sexuality, Legal Approaches to
Suicide
Surrogate Decision-Making
Whistleblowing in Health Care

HEALTH POLICY AND SYSTEMS

Access to Health Care
Advance Directives and Advance Care Planning
Advertising and Marketing in Health Care
AIDS: II. Health Care and Research Issues
Alcohol and Other Drugs in a Public Health Context
Alternative Therapies: I. Social History
Alternative Therapies: II. Ethical and Legal Issues
Animal Research: III. Law and Policy
Care: I. History of the Notion of Care
Care: II. Historical Precedents for an Ethic of Care in Health Care
Care: III. Care Ethics
Care: IV. Care and Society/Public Policy
Chronic Illness
Commercialism in Scientific Research
Community and Communitarianism
Community-Based Participatory Research
Comparative Effectiveness Research and Implementation Science
Corporate Compliance
Corporate Social Responsibility in Health
Cross-Border Medical Travel
Cross-Border Reproductive Travel
Dementia
Dentistry
Dialysis, Kidney
Disability: I. Ethical and Societal Perspectives
Disability: II. Legal Issues
Disability: III. Models of
Economic Concepts in Health Care
End-of-Life Care
Enhancement Uses of Medical Technology
Environmental Policy and Law
Genetic Citizenship
Genetic Discrimination
Global Health Inequalities and Inequities
Global Justice
Globalization and Health
Health Care, Delivery of
Health Care, Ethics and Professionalism in
Health Care, Quality Improvement
Health Care, Worker Migration
Health Care Resources, Allocation of: I. Macroallocation
Health Care Resources, Allocation of: II. Microallocation
Health Care Systems
Health Insurance
Health Policy and Politics
Health Policy in the United States
Hospice and Palliative Care: Professional Education
Hospital, Contemporary Ethical Problems of the
Hospitals, Ethical Issues in the Governance of
Immigrants, Access to Health Care
Impaired Professionals
Infants, Ethical Issues with
Infants, Public Policy and Legal Issues
Informatics, Biomedical
Information Disclosure, Ethical Issues of
Injury and Injury Control
Law and Bioethics
Law and Morality
Liberty
Long-Term Care: I. Concepts and Policies
Long-Term Care: II. Nursing Homes
Long-Term Care: III. Home Care
Long-Term Care: IV. Financing, US and International
Malpractice, Medical
Managed Care
Medical Education
Mental Health Services: I. Settings and Programs
Mental Health Services: II. Ethical Issues
Nursing, Profession of
Occupational Health and Safety: I. Ethical Issues
Occupational Health and Safety: II. Occupational Health Care Providers
Organizational Ethics in Health Care
Privacy in Health Care
Profession and Professional Ethics
Professional-Patient Relationship: I. Sociological Perspectives
Professional-Patient Relationship: II. Ethical Issues
Profit and Commercialism
Psychiatry, Abuses of
Public Health: II. Law
Public Health: VII. Health Surveillance
Public Health: X. Emergency Preparedness and Response
Public Health: XI. Emergency Allocation of Resources and Altered Standard of Care
Public Policy and Bioethics
Research, Unethical
Research Policy: I. General Background
Research Policy: II. Risk and Vulnerable Groups
Research Policy: III. Subjects
Right to Die: Policy and Law
Smoking
Social Constructionism
Social Justice
Social Medicine
Social Work, Profession of
Solidarity
Technology: I. History of Medical Technology
Technology: II. Philosophy of Medical Technology
Tissue Banking and Transplantation, Ethical Issues in
Trust
Women as Health Professionals

HUMAN ENHANCEMENT

Biopolitics
Body: I. Embodiment in the Phenomenological Tradition
Body: II. Cultural and Religious Perspectives
Body: III. Commodification

HUMAN REPRODUCTION

MEDICINE

MENTAL HEALTH

NURSING

Infants, Public Policy and Legal Issues
Informed Consent: II. Meaning and Elements
Informed Consent: IV. Clinical Aspects of Consent in Health Care
Informed Consent: V. Legal and Ethical Issues of Consent in Health Care
Informed Consent: VI. Issues of Consent in Mental Health Care
Life, Quality of: I. Quality of Life in Clinical Decisions
Life, Quality of: II. Quality of Life in Health Care Allocation
Life, Quality of: III. Quality of Life in Legal Perspective
Life, Sanctity of
Life-Sustaining Treatment and Euthanasia: I. Ethical Aspects of
Life-Sustaining Treatment and Euthanasia: II. Historical Aspects of
Medical Futility
Nursing, Profession of
Nursing, Theories and Philosophy of
Nursing Ethics
Organizational Ethics in Health Care
Pain and Suffering
Parental Authority
Paternalism
Patients' Responsibilities: I. Duties of Patients
Patients' Responsibilities: II. Co-Relative Rights
Patients' Rights: I. Origin and Nature of Patients' Rights
Principlism
Privacy in Health Care
Profession and Professional Ethics
Professional-Patient Relationship: I. Sociological Perspectives
Professional-Patient Relationship: II. Ethical Issues
Right to Die: Policy and Law
Rights
Risk and Risk Assessment

PAIN AND SUFFERING

Abuse, Interpersonal: I. Child Abuse
Abuse, Interpersonal: II. Abuse between Domestic Partners
Abuse, Interpersonal: III. Elder Abuse
Abuse, Interpersonal: IV. Abuse of Health Care Workers
Aging and the Aged: I. Societal Aging
Aging and the Aged: II. Health Care for the Aging
Aging and the Aged: III. Research Ethics
Body: I. Embodiment in the Phenomenological Tradition
Body: II. Cultural and Religious Perspectives
Body: III. Commodification
Cancer, Ethical Issues Related to Diagnosis and Treatment
Chronic Illness
Coercion
Cognitive Impairment/Traumatic Brain Injury
Dialysis, Kidney
Disability: I. Ethical and Societal Perspectives
Disability: II. Legal Issues
Disability: III. Models of
Emotions
End-of-Life Care
Epidemics
Epistemic Injustice
Exploitation
Hospice and Palliative Care: Professional Education
Injury and Injury Control
Insanity and the Insanity Defense
Life, Quality of: I. Quality of Life in Clinical Decisions
Life, Quality of: II. Quality of Life in Health Care Allocation
Life, Quality of: III. Quality of Life in Legal Perspective
Pain and Suffering
Pastoral and Spiritual Care and Health Care Chaplaincy
Physician-Assisted Dying/Hastened Death
Right to Die: Policy and Law
Vulnerability

PALLIATIVE CARE AND HOSPICE

Advance Directives and Advance Care Planning
Aging and the Aged: I. Societal Aging
Aging and the Aged: II. Health Care for the Aging
Aging and the Aged: III. Research Ethics
AIDS: II. Health Care and Research Issues
Artificial Nutrition and Hydration
Authority in Religious Traditions
Autonomy
Beneficence
Cancer, Ethical Issues Related to Diagnosis and Treatment
Care: I. History of the Notion of Care
Care: II. Historical Precedents for an Ethic of Care in Health Care
Care: III. Care Ethics
Chronic Illness
Coercion
Cognitive Impairment/Traumatic Brain Injury
Competence
Confidentiality
Conflict of Interest
Conscience, Rights of
Dementia
Dialysis, Kidney
Disability: I. Ethical and Societal Perspectives
Disability: II. Legal Issues
Disability: III. Models of
DNR (Do Not Resuscitate)
Double Effect, Principle or Doctrine of
Emotions
End-of-Life Care
Family Caregiving
Grief, Ethical Implications of
Harm
Healing
Health and Disease: II. Sociological Perspectives
Health and Disease: III. Anthropological Perspectives
Health and Disease: V. The Experience of Health and Illness
Health Care, Ethics and Professionalism in
Health Care, Quality Improvement
Health Care Professionals, Legal Regulation of
Hospice and Palliative Care: Professional Education
Human Dignity
Injury and Injury Control
Life, Quality of: I. Quality of Life in Clinical Decisions
Life, Quality of: II. Quality of Life in Health Care Allocation
Life, Quality of: III. Quality of Life in Legal Perspective
Life, Sanctity of
Medical Futility
Pain and Suffering
Parental Authority
Pastoral and Spiritual Care and Health Care Chaplaincy
Paternalism
Patients' Responsibilities: I. Duties of Patients
Patients' Responsibilities: II. Co-Relative Rights
Patients' Rights: I. Origin and Nature of Patients' Rights
Pediatrics, Adolescents
Pediatrics, Intensive Care in
Pediatrics, Overview of Ethical Issues in
Physician-Assisted Dying/Hastened Death
Principlism
Privacy in Health Care
Profession and Professional Ethics
Professional-Patient Relationship: I. Sociological Perspectives
Professional-Patient Relationship: II. Ethical Issues
Right to Die: Policy and Law
Rights
Risk and Risk Assessment
Vulnerability

PHYSICIAN AID IN DYING

Advance Directives and Advance Care Planning
AIDS: II. Health Care and Research Issues

Artificial Nutrition and Hydration
Autonomy
Cancer, Ethical Issues Related to Diagnosis and Treatment
Chronic Illness
Coercion
Double Effect, Principle or Doctrine of
Emotions
Family Caregiving
Grief, Ethical Implications of
Hospice and Palliative Care: Professional Education
Human Dignity
Life, Quality of: I. Quality of Life in Clinical Decisions
Life, Quality of: II. Quality of Life in Health Care Allocation
Life, Quality of: III. Quality of Life in Legal Perspective
Life, Sanctity of
Life-Sustaining Treatment and Euthanasia: I. Ethical Aspects of
Life-Sustaining Treatment and Euthanasia: II. Historical Aspects of
Medical Futility
Pain and Suffering
Physician-Assisted Dying/Hastened Death
Right to Die: Policy and Law
Vulnerability

POPULATION POLICY AND ETHICS

Autonomy
Coercion
Environmental Ethics: I. Overview
Fertility Control: I. Medical Aspects
Fertility Control: II. Social and Ethical Issues
Fertility Control: III. Legal and Regulatory Issues
Global Health Inequalities and Inequities
Global Justice
Globalization and Health
Human Rights
Humanitarian Relief
Immigrants, Access to Health Care
Impaired Professionals
Infanticide
Paternalism
Population Ethics: I. History of Population Theories
Population Ethics: II. Normative Approaches
Population Ethics: III. Introduction to Religious Traditions
Population Ethics: IV. Islamic Perspectives
Population Ethics: V. Jewish Perspectives
Population Ethics: VI. Roman Catholic Perspectives
Population Ethics: VII. Eastern Orthodox Christian Perspectives
Population Ethics: VIII. Protestant Perspectives
Population Ethics: IX. Hindu Perspectives
Population Ethics: X. Buddhist Perspectives
Population Policies, Demographic Aspects of
Population Policies, Migration and Refugees in
Population Policies, Strategies for Fertility Control in
Race and Racism
Rights
Sustainability

PROFESSIONAL RESPONSIBILITIES AND RELATIONSHIPS

Advance Directives and Advance Care Planning
Autonomy
Beneficence
Clinical Ethics
Coercion
Competence
Conscience
Conscience, Rights of
Dementia
Ethics: IV. Normative Ethical Theories
Freedom and Free Will
Genetic Testing and Screening: I. Reproductive Genetic Testing
Genetic Testing and Screening: II. Newborn Genetic Screening
Genetic Testing and Screening: III. Population Screening
Genetic Testing and Screening: IV. Public Health Context
Genetic Testing and Screening: V. Predictive Genetic Testing
Genetic Testing and Screening: VI. Pediatric Genetic Testing
Human Dignity
Informed Consent: I. History of Informed Consent
Informed Consent: II. Meaning and Elements
Informed Consent: III. Consent Issues in Human Research
Informed Consent: IV. Clinical Aspects of Consent in Health Care
Informed Consent: V. Legal and Ethical Issues of Consent in Health Care
Informed Consent: VI. Issues of Consent in Mental Health Care
Law and Bioethics
Malpractice, Medical
Medical Codes and Oaths
Medical Ethics, History of
Medicine, Art of
Mental Illness: III. Issues in Diagnosis
Mentally Disabled and Mentally Ill Persons: I. Health Care Issues
Mentally Disabled and Mentally Ill Persons: II. Research Issues
Nursing, Profession of
Nursing Ethics
Patients' Rights: I. Origin and Nature of Patients' Rights
Patients' Rights: II. Mental Patients' Rights
Placebo
Professional-Patient Relationship: I. Sociological Perspectives
Professional-Patient Relationship: II. Ethical Issues
Research, Human: Historical Aspects
Research, Unethical
Right to Die: Policy and Law
Rights
Surrogate Decision-Making
Teams, Health Care
Trust

PUBLIC HEALTH

Access to Health Care
Advertising and Marketing in Health Care
AIDS: II. Health Care and Research Issues
Alcohol and Other Drugs in a Public Health Context
Biopolitics
Care: IV. Care and Society/Public Policy
Chronic Illness
Commercialism in Scientific Research
Community and Communitarianism
Community-Based Participatory Research
Corporate Social Responsibility in Health
Cross-Border Medical Travel
Cross-Border Reproductive Travel
Dementia
Dentistry
Disability: I. Ethical and Societal Perspectives
Disability: II. Legal Issues
Disability: III. Models of
Economic Concepts in Health Care
End-of-Life Care
Environmental Policy and Law
Food
Gender
Genetic Citizenship
Genetic Discrimination
Global Health Inequalities and Inequities
Global Justice
Globalization and Health
Health Care, Delivery of
Health Care, Worker Migration
Health Care Resources, Allocation of: I. Macroallocation

RELIGIOUS PERSPECTIVES AND TRADITIONS

RESEARCH

SEXUALITY AND GENDER

Care: III. Care Ethics
Care: IV. Care and Society/Public Policy
Circumcision, Female: I. Historical Overview
Circumcision, Female: II. Cultural and Ethical Aspects
Circumcision, Male
Feminism
Gender
Gender Identity
Homosexuality, Religious Perspectives
Reproductive Technologies: II. Sex Selection
Sex Reassignment
Sexual Behavior, Social Control of
Sexual Ethics
Sexual Ethics and Professional Standards
Sexual Identity
Sexuality, Legal Approaches to
Women, Historical and Cross-Cultural Perspectives

SOCIAL SCIENTIFIC PERSPECTIVES

Bioethics: III. Discourse in
Bioethics: IV. Professionalism in
Bioethics: V. Ethics of
Bioethics: VI. Research Methods in
Bioethics: VII. Empirical Methods in
Bioethics: VIII. Sociology of
Bioethics: IX. Anthropology of
Bioethics: X. Politics of
Biopolitics
Bioterrorism
Body: I. Embodiment in the Phenomenological Tradition
Body: II. Cultural and Religious Perspectives
Body: III. Commodification
Circumcision, Female: I. Historical Overview
Circumcision, Female: II. Cultural and Ethical Aspects
Circumcision, Male
Commercialism in Scientific Research
Community and Communitarianism
Community-Based Participatory Research
Consensus, Role and Authority of
Death: I. Cultural Perspectives
Disability: I. Ethical and Societal Perspectives
Disability: II. Legal Issues
Disability: III. Models of
Fertility Control: II. Social and Ethical Issues
Genetics and Environment in Human Health
Genetics and Human Behavior: I. Scientific and Research Issues
Genetics and Human Behavior: II. Philosophical and Ethical Issues
Genetics and Human Self-Understanding
Genetics and Racial Minorities
Global Health Inequalities and Inequities
Globalization and Health
Health and Disease: II. Sociological Perspectives
Health and Disease: III. Anthropological Perspectives
Health and Disease: V. The Experience of Health and Illness
Health Care, Delivery of
Health Care, Ethics and Professionalism in
Health Care, Worker Migration
Health Care Systems
Health Insurance
Health Policy and Politics
Health Policy in the United States
Health Services Management Ethics
Human Genome Diversity Project
Institutionalization and Deinstitutionalization
Labor Unions in Health Care
Medicine, Profession of
Medicine, Sociology of
Mental Illness: II. Cultural Perspectives
Minorities as Research Subjects
Mistakes, Medical
Organ Transplants, Sociocultural Aspects of
Professional-Patient Relationship: I. Sociological Perspectives
Profit and Commercialism
Psychiatry, Abuses of
Public Policy and Bioethics
Race and Racism
Sexual Behavior, Medical Control of
Suicide
Trust
Women, Historical and Cross-Cultural Perspectives

THEORIES AND METHODS

Bioethics: I. History of
Bioethics: III. Discourse in
Biology, Philosophy of
Biopolitics
Body: I. Embodiment in the Phenomenological Tradition
Care: III. Care Ethics
Contractarianism and Bioethics
Disability: III. Models of
Ecological Bioethics
Economic Concepts in Health Care
Environmental Ethics: I. Overview
Environmental Ethics: II. Deep Ecology
Environmental Ethics: III. Land Ethics
Environmental Ethics: IV. Ecofeminism
Ethics: I. History of Ethics
Ethics: II. Task of Ethics
Ethics: III. Metaethics
Ethics: IV. Normative Ethical Theories
Ethics: V. Religion and Morality
Feminism
Genetic Citizenship
Global Justice
Health and Disease: I. History of the Concepts
Health and Disease: II. Sociological Perspectives
Health and Disease: III. Anthropological Perspectives
Health and Disease: IV. Philosophical Perspectives
Human Dignity
Human Evolution
Human Rights
Informed Consent: I. History of Informed Consent
Informed Consent: II. Meaning and Elements
Justice
Law and Bioethics
Law and Morality
Liberty
Life
Life, Sanctity of
Medicine, Philosophy of
Metaphor and Analogy
Moral Status
Narrative
Natural Law
Naturalism
Neuroethics
Neuroethics and Free Will
Nursing, Theories and Philosophy of
Obligation and Supererogation
Paternalism
Patients' Responsibilities: I. Duties of Patients
Patients' Responsibilities: II. Co-Relative Rights
Patients' Rights: I. Origin and Nature of Patients' Rights
Patients' Rights: II. Mental Patients' Rights
Phenomenology
Postmodernism
Pragmatism
Precautionary Principle
Principlism
Public Health: III. Philosophy
Public Health: IV. Ethics
Public Health: V. Methods
Public Health: VIII. Social Determinants of Health
Public Policy and Bioethics
Race and Racism
Reductionism
Relativism, Cultural and Ethical
Rights
Risk and Risk Assessment

TRANSPLANTATION

WARFARE

A

ABORTION

This entry consists of the following:

I. MEDICAL PERSPECTIVES

Medical information and perspectives on abortion are not just data untinged by values. Throughout history, medical facts and moral values regarding abortion have been inextricably intertwined. People interested in the ethics of abortion turn to medicine and medical practitioners for the following information and perspectives:

1. whether medical knowledge clarifies the moral status of the fetus as a human being;
2. whether medical information on abortion confirms it to be safe for the woman;
3. what the medical perspectives are on performing early versus late abortions, particularly in light of controversies regarding partial birth abortion;
4. what the public health and international perspectives are on abortion.

MEDICAL KNOWLEDGE REGARDING STATUS OF THE FETUS

However much information biomedical investigation may provide regarding pregnancy, fetal development, and abortion, it cannot provide a determination as to when human life begins. The answer to that question—which deals with the moral status of the fetus—is arrived at by a process that entwines medical facts with experiences, values, religious and philosophical beliefs and attitudes, perceptions of meaning, and moral argument. Such a process extends beyond the special competency of medicine. For example, when ensoulment—an ancient criterion involving the infusion of the soul into the body of the fetus, thus conferring moral status on the fetus—occurs, medicine has never had the ability to establish. Similarly, some physicians disagree about the moral status of the fetus and the permissibility of abortion.

There is confusion about the definition of abortion. Spontaneous abortion, or what is commonly termed a miscarriage, refers to a spontaneous loss of a pregnancy before viability (at about twenty-four weeks of gestation).

Losses after that point in a pregnancy are termed *preterm deliveries* or, in the case of the delivery of a fetus who has already died, *stillbirths.* The terminology commonly used in relation to induced abortion is different. Viability is not the key point; rather, any termination of a pregnancy by medical or surgical means is termed *abortion*, regardless of the stage of the pregnancy.

SAFETY AND HARM OF THE WOMAN

There is a close tie between medical information regarding the safety of abortion practices and ethical positions on abortion. For example, at a time when abortions were frequently harmful to women—such as when legal restrictions increased recourse to untrained practitioners—opponents of abortion appealed to information on the likelihood of medical harm to the woman and risks of future pregnancies as arguments against abortion (Kunins and Rosenfield 1991). As of 2003, induced abortions performed within the first twelve weeks of pregnancy are among the safest and simplest forms of surgery. Maternal mortality ratios (number of deaths per 100,000 live births) show that both first- and second-trimester abortions performed by properly trained personnel are safer in general than carrying a pregnancy to term (Cates and Grimes 1981). As a result, ethical arguments against abortion tend to be restricted to areas other than maternal safety. Nonetheless, some aspects of medical safety and harm—including possible complications and psychological sequelae—continue to be important for ethical discourse, especially because a basic tenet of medical ethics is to avoid harm.

Possible Physical Harm. The major immediate complications of induced abortion, in order of frequency, are infection, hemorrhage, uterine perforation, and anesthesia-related complications. Overall complication rates for legal first-trimester abortions are less than 0.5 deaths per 100,000 abortions performed (compared with more than four per 100,000 in the early 1970s, before the US Supreme Court decision *Roe v. Wade* 410 U.S. 113 [1973]) permitted medically supervised abortions. Medical complications associated with induced abortion are directly related to gestational age and the type of procedure used to terminate the pregnancy. Most abortions (over 90%) in the United States are performed within the first twelve weeks of pregnancy, when abortion is safest. More serious complications may occur in procedures performed later in pregnancy.

Abortion Procedures. Information on abortion procedures often sheds light on questions of safety and on other aspects of abortion that are relevant to ethics. The most common early-trimester abortion procedure (between seven and twelve weeks' gestation) is suction curettage, in which a thin plastic tube (cannula) is inserted through the cervix and the contents of the uterus are aspirated by negative pressure vacuum. After the aspiration procedure, curettage (performed with a sharp, spoon-shaped surgical instrument called a curette) is usually performed to ensure that all fetal tissue has been removed. Complications of suction curettage procedures are rare and even when they occur are usually not serious. Many physicians consider general anesthesia an unnecessary additional risk because injection of local anesthetic into the cervix usually is effective (Grimes et al. 1979). A short course of prophylactic antibiotics is sometimes prescribed, although postabortion infection is uncommon with suction curettage. Because of its safety, suction curettage is performed most often in freestanding clinics or outpatient centers in hospitals.

At twelve to twenty weeks' gestation, the most common method used for abortion is dilation and evacuation (D&E). In this procedure a specially designed forceps is used in conjunction with vacuum aspiration to facilitate the removal of the uterine contents. Before the procedure, the cervix is dilated gradually over a number of hours by use of sponge-like materials that expand as they absorb local cervical fluids. Though still considered a minor surgical procedure, D&E is more involved and invasive than suction curettage, and a trained and skilled clinician is essential. Although it is possible to use only local anesthesia for D&E, the procedure is considerably more uncomfortable than suction curettage, and general anesthesia is often used, increasing risk. The D&E procedure can be performed in freestanding clinics, but often ambulatory surgical services in a hospital are chosen for procedures performed later in pregnancy (after the fourteenth week) because emergency care can be quickly provided in case of a complication. Informed consent procedures require discussion of the various methods of abortion and the anesthesia alternatives.

The other abortion procedure used fairly commonly in the second trimester is instillation abortion. In this procedure, instillation of a solution into the amniotic cavity through the abdomen via amniocentesis results in the death of the fetus and termination of the pregnancy. Uterine contractions signaling labor begin twelve to twenty-four hours later and culminate with the expulsion of the fetus. Anesthesia is not commonly used for instillation procedures. Discomfort varies widely among patients, usually in relation to the length of labor and the time before complete expulsion of the fetus and placenta. Serious complications can occur during instillation procedures, including inadvertent introduction of the solution into the mother's bloodstream, excessive bleeding at the time of expulsion of the fetus, and retention of the placenta. For this reason hospital admission is usually advised. Instillation procedures are used mainly for procedures beyond the twentieth week of gestation. All late-pregnancy abortion procedures carry significant risk if performed by physicians not specially trained in the technique.

A promising alternative to surgical abortion for early first-trimester terminations of pregnancy is chemical abortion. For example, the antiprogestin drug RU-486 stops the ovaries from producing progesterone, an essential hormone in the early stages of pregnancy and in implantation of the embryo. The drug is given within the first forty-nine days of a confirmed pregnancy and is used in conjunction with a prostaglandin, which produces uterine contractions and subsequent expulsion of the uterine contents. A follow-up visit is necessary eight to twelve days later to ensure that complete termination of the pregnancy has occurred.

On September 28, 2000, the US Food and Drug Administration (FDA) approved RU-486 for use in the United States. It has been distributed since November 2000 by Danco Laboratories, LLC, under the brand name Mifeprex (generic name, mifepristone). According to the FDA guidelines, the drug has been distributed only to physicians and is not available through pharmacies. Furthermore, the FDA has approved a specific regimen for the use of RU-486. Three office visits are necessary: the first for the physician to make the diagnosis and to administer the RU-486; the second, two days later, for the prostaglandin; and the third within two weeks for the final follow-up. In France, a fourth visit is required by law because a one-week delay between the diagnosis of pregnancy and the initiation of an abortion procedure is mandated. Due to the requirement of three visits (or four in France), the fact that there may be a few days before the abortion occurs and as many as ten or more days of vaginal bleeding thereafter, and because medical abortion may be more expensive than surgical abortion, many women in France and the United States prefer suction curettage (Kolata 2002). However, there is anticipation that as awareness grows, many women will prefer a medical means of abortion, not wishing to undergo surgery (albeit a minor procedure) or to be subjected to the harassment that may occur outside some facilities.

Successful termination has been found to occur in 97 percent of patients using the RU-486 regimen. The other patients need suction curettage for complete removal of the products of conception. In comparison, for surgical procedures, less than 1 percent of patients require a second curettage, in the event that the procedure was incomplete. Most women experience strong cramping after taking the prostaglandin (because the drug induces uterine contractions) and usually expel the products of conception within a few hours after receiving the prostaglandin. In France, RU-486 is therefore provided only through clinics, and the abortion often occurs during the four hours women remain in the clinic after taking the prostaglandin. However, some French physicians believe that a clinic setting is not essential.

In the United States, specific requirements for facilities providing abortion vary from state to state. Federal guidelines, however, require only that RU-486 be prescribed by or under the supervision of a physician who can diagnose the duration of pregnancy accurately, diagnose an ectopic pregnancy, and either can provide surgical intervention in cases of incomplete abortion or make arrangements to provide such care through others.

Although studies have shown the safety and effectiveness of RU-486 as a morning-after pill for use after unexpected midcycle intercourse (Ashok, Wagaarachchi, Flett, and Templeton 2001), preparations containing the hormones found in oral contraceptive pills (estrogen and progestin or progestin alone) have been approved for this purpose. Furthermore, the copper-T intrauterine device (IUD) can be inserted up to five days after unprotected intercourse to prevent pregnancy. Both emergency contraceptive pills and the IUD are readily available and remain the standard of care for postcoital contraception in the United States (American College of Obstetricians and Gynecologists [ACOG] 2001).

Availability of Abortion Providers. Obstetrician-gynecologists perform the majority of abortion procedures in the United States. Other providers, such as family practice physicians, midwives, and nurse practitioners perform a small percentage. There are serious concerns about the provision of abortion procedures in the future for several reasons. Although most obstetrician-gynecologists believe that women should have the right to choose to terminate a pregnancy, at the same time, most do not wish to perform abortions. As a result, approximately 84 percent of counties in the United States do not have an abortion facility, and the number rises to 94 percent outside metropolitan areas.

Many obstetric-gynecologic residency training programs do not offer abortion training routinely, and as a result, many graduating residents have little or no training in this area. However, there has been an increase in the number of residency programs providing training in abortion procedures. In 1996 the Accreditation Council for Graduate Medical Education required obstetric-gynecologic residency programs to include family planning and abortion training for its students, though abortion was generally still presented as an elective rather than a routine part of training. The impact of these requirements was demonstrated in a survey conducted for the National Abortion Federation. The investigators found that from 1992 to 1998, the proportion of obstetric-gynecologic residency programs that reported providing routine training in first-trimester abortion increased from 12 percent to 46 percent and that routine training in second-trimester abortion increased from 7 percent to 44 percent (Almeling, Tews, and Dudley 2000).

Even where training has taken place, the increasing incidence of harassment and even violence (including the

1993 and 1994 murders of abortion providers in Florida) has resulted in more reluctance on the part of physicians to be involved in the provision of abortion. In response to the escalating violence, Congress in 1994 enacted the Freedom of Access to Clinic Entrances Act. This statute established federal criminal penalties and civil remedies for violent, obstructionist, or damaging conduct affecting reproductive health care providers and recipients. The statute also supplemented the penalties available under then-existing federal criminal statutes such as the Hobbs Act, the Travel Act, and federal arson and firearms statutes. Rising violence and the federal response highlight serious ethical questions as to the social responsibility of professionals in this field to make certain that this procedure is available to all patients.

Possibly Harmful Effects on Subsequent Pregnancies. Questions have been raised about possible long-term harmful effects of induced abortion, especially for women who have had multiple abortions. Much of the concern centers on subsequent pregnancies, following one or more induced abortions. Medical evidence has consistently shown that a woman who has one properly performed induced abortion in the first trimester of pregnancy has the same chance of a normal outcome of a subsequent pregnancy as a woman who has never had an abortion. The evidence is less definitive for women who have had more than one induced abortion or an abortion with complications, although there is no reason to believe that additional abortion procedures, carried out by well-trained professionals will have a long-term adverse effect. Overall, in terms of medical risk, abortion procedures, particularly those carried out in the first trimester of pregnancy, are among the safest of all surgical procedures.

Psychological Effects. A much grayer area is the psychological consequences of induced abortion. It is difficult to generalize about the emotional responses of patients to pregnancy termination, but like physical complications, psychological complications may be related to the type of procedure and the gestational age at the time of termination, with earlier suction curettage theoretically leading to fewer psychological complications than later procedures. However, most studies in this area suffer from methodological problems, including a lack of consensus about symptoms, inadequate study design, and lack of adequate follow-up. Furthermore, so-called postabortion syndrome does not meet the American Psychiatric Association definition of trauma (Gold 1990).

Despite the many problems with most investigations, "the studies are consistent in their findings of relatively rare instance of negative responses after abortion and of decreases in psychological distress after abortion compared to before abortion" (Adler et al. 1990, 42). US Surgeon General C. Everett Koop (1916–2013), at the request of the White House, undertook a major assessment of the literature on this topic and concluded in a 1989 congressional hearing that "the data were insufficient … to support the premise that abortion does or does not produce a postabortion syndrome and that emotional problems resulting from abortion are minuscule from a public health perspective" (House Human Resources and Intergovernmental Relations Subcommittee of the Committee on Governmental Operations 1989, 14). Given Koop's personal opposition to abortion, the conclusions of his assessment are of particular importance.

Approximately 10 percent of induced abortions in the United States take place between twelve and twenty weeks of gestation, and less than 1 percent take place between twenty and twenty-four weeks. This means that more than 150,000 second-trimester procedures occur each year, a much larger number than in other developed nations where abortion is legal. Most would agree that decreases in the total numbers of abortions would be highly desirable, particularly decreases in second-trimester procedures. The most common reasons for these later procedures, particularly among younger teens, are indecision about termination and the failure to recognize pregnancy (or being in denial regarding pregnancy). A smaller percentage of these later abortions occur for medical or genetic reasons, which theoretically may correlate with greater psychological distress.

Although techniques such as nuchal translucency measurement with serum screening, chorionic villus sampling, and early amniocentesis have allowed earlier diagnosis, the results of more commonly used techniques of antenatal fetal diagnosis with midtrimester amniocentesis are generally not available until well into the second trimester. Choosing to terminate a pregnancy is a serious decision that is rarely made lightly. In addition to complete information about abortion procedure options, counseling should be made available to women faced with a decision about an unplanned pregnancy.

EARLY VERSUS LATE ABORTIONS: CONTROVERSIES IN MEDICINE

Medical attitudes toward abortion have constantly been shaped by medical professionals' knowledge of and attitude toward the stage of development of the fetus and its interaction with local cultural, religious, and legal ideas and beliefs. Together these factors have had great impact on medical practice. Medical practitioners often have more difficulty with late abortions than earlier ones because late abortion procedures are more difficult to perform because of the more advanced state of fetal development and because of the political climate surrounding so-called partial-birth abortion.

Before the latter half of the nineteenth century, abortions were available in the United States under the doctrines of British common law that permitted termination of a pregnancy until the time of quickening (detection of fetal movement). However, medical knowledge available at that time made it difficult to confirm a pregnancy with certainty before quickening, for it was only this detection of fetal movement that confirmed the existence of a living human fetus. Little in the historical literature describes how physicians in that era actually felt about abortions, although on the basis of the information that follows, one can assume that there were concerns about abortion.

By the second half of the nineteenth century, as scientific knowledge grew, so did the realization that fetal development occurs on a continuum, suggesting that the fetus is a living entity before fetal movement is felt. Prompted by this new medical knowledge, physicians, particularly those who were members of the newly formed American Medical Association (AMA), began openly to oppose abortion and urged its criminalization as an immoral practice. As a basis for this change, the Hippocratic oath was used to oppose abortion at any time during pregnancy.

The concept of the fetus as a human entity separate from the mother has long been the subject of ethical concern within the medical profession. The AMA principles of medical ethics permit physicians to perform abortions, provided the procedure is done in accordance both with the law and with good medical practice (Council on Ethical and Judicial Affairs 1994). In general, since the early twentieth century, especially since the US Supreme Court decision *Roe v. Wade* greatly liberalized the legal permissibility of abortion, medical practitioners have tended to place the value of the life of the mother above that of the fetus. There also has been general agreement that late abortion is permissible in cases in which medical judgment deems that the health of the mother is seriously compromised by a pregnancy. However, just as *Roe v. Wade* allowed for some restrictions on abortions after fetal viability, the medical profession has shown a reluctance to perform abortions later in pregnancy, even early in the second trimester.

In addition to facing ethical dilemmas over fetal and maternal rights, many medical professionals remain ambivalent about the morality of abortion, a conflict that is heightened both by increased technological sophistication in the field of perinatology and genetics and the political climate. Depending on the technology available to a physician and the condition of the individual fetus (gestational age and any developmental deformity), it is often possible, depending on the availability of neonatal intensive care support, to save the lives of premature babies born at twenty-seven weeks' gestation. Babies born at twenty-four to twenty-six weeks and earlier have survived with intensive neonatal intervention and support, though often with some degree of functional impairment. With abortions occasionally performed up to twenty-four weeks' gestation, one can see the conflict within medicine: fetuses that might be aborted by one group of physicians are aggressively supported as patients by another group.

Physicians who provide abortion services prefer to perform early abortions, that is, up to twelve weeks, for several reasons. First, it is generally agreed that though a fetus may exhibit primitive reflexes before twenty weeks' gestation, there is no evidence that the brain and neurological system are developed enough even at twenty-four weeks for the fetus to experience pain. Second, second-trimester techniques that might appear to be more humane or to show more respect for the fetus generally entail more danger for the woman. Third, the physicians who are committed to offering abortion procedures are intent on offering the safest procedures for the woman and regard the benefit to the woman as superseding the goal of minimizing harm to the fetus.

The debate over partial-birth abortion has presented challenges to physicians, other providers of abortion services, and proponents of a woman's right to choose to terminate a pregnancy. Legislation to ban this procedure has been proposed and debated in the US Congress, in several state legislatures, and in the US Supreme Court. However, these bans have not been constitutionally upheld because of the vagueness of the definition of partial-birth abortion (which is not a term used by medical professionals), the failure to allow physicians to protect a woman's health after a fetus becomes viable, and the application of the ban before fetal viability (Annas 1998). In March 1995, the first Partial-Birth Abortion Ban Act (HR 1833, 112th Congress) was introduced in the US Congress to make it a federal crime to perform "an abortion in which the person performing the abortion partially vaginally delivers a living fetus before killing the fetus and completing the delivery." In April 1996 President Bill Clinton vetoed the bill because of its failure to include an exception allowing the procedure to prevent serious, adverse health consequences to the mother (Clinton 1996, 643–47). Clinton vetoed a revised bill in October 1997 for the same reason (Clinton 1997, 1545). Over the interim between the two bills, medical organizations took conflicting positions.

In contrast to the AMA, which endorsed the federal bill, the ACOG executive board urged the president to veto the bill. The executive board understood the term *partial-birth abortion* to describe a method members of the ACOG would understand as intact dilation and extraction (D&X), one method of terminating a pregnancy after sixteen weeks' gestation and specifically involving the following (ACOG 1997, 2):

1. deliberate dilation of the cervix, usually over a sequence of days;
2. instrumental conversion of the fetus to a footling breech;

3. breech extraction of the body excepting the head; and
4. partial evacuation of the intracranial contents of the living fetus to effect vaginal delivery of a dead but otherwise intact fetus.

Although the committee could identify no specific circumstance in which this method would be the only option for preserving the health of the woman, it stated that "only the doctor, in consultation with the patient, based upon the woman's particular circumstances can make this decision" (ACOG 1997, 3).

Similar laws have been passed in more than two dozen states and been found unconstitutional. The most significant decision was issued by the US Supreme Court in a challenge to Nebraska's partial-birth abortion law in the case of *Stenberg v. Carhart,* 530 U.S. 914 in 2000 (Annas 2001). The case involved Leroy Carhart, a Nebraska physician who sued in federal court to have Nebraska's law declared unconstitutional because it endangered women's lives and was void because of its vagueness in that physicians could not know exactly what procedure was proscribed. Ultimately, the Supreme Court ruled on June 28, 2000, that the Nebraska law and all other laws banning partial-birth abortion were unconstitutional. The majority opinion held that the law was unconstitutional for two reasons. First, it did not provide an exception to protect the health of the woman as required by *Roe v. Wade.* Second, the law imposed an undue burden (as proscribed in *Planned Parenthood of Southeastern Pennsylvania v. Casey* 502 U.S. 1056 [1992]) because it was written so broadly as to ban not only the rarely used D&X procedures but also the D&E so commonly used to terminate pregnancies even early in the second trimester. Ultimately, the *Stenberg v. Carhart* decision reinforced the important position that women and their physicians should make the decisions regarding how abortions can most safely and satisfactorily be performed.

PUBLIC HEALTH AND INTERNATIONAL PERSPECTIVES

Abortion is widely available with varying restrictions throughout the industrialized world. There also has been a trend toward liberalization of abortion laws in many developing countries, such as in India, where abortion has been legalized, and in Bangladesh, where an early first-trimester procedure called menstrual regulation (which is really an early suction curettage) has been officially sanctioned by the government even though abortion per se has not been legalized. Abortion laws are most restrictive in Latin America, sub-Saharan Africa, and Central Asia. Many of the countries in these regions have high rates of maternal mortality, and complications of illegal abortions are one of its leading causes. According to the World Health Organization, as many as 100,000 or more maternal deaths occur each year as a result of complications of unsafe, usually illegal, abortion. Even in the United States, some illegal abortions continue to be performed in cases in which women are without the resources to obtain a legal abortion.

Although reliable incidence data are lacking as to the number of illegal abortions performed worldwide, there clearly is a strong demand for abortion, a demand that will probably always exist. As evidenced by the estimated number of women who undergo illegal abortion, most women who are determined to terminate a pregnancy will attempt to do so either by themselves or with assistance. Consequently, the public health concerns about the complications of unsafe abortion, coupled with complex issues relating to the reproductive and autonomy rights of women versus the rights of the fetus, suggest the continuing importance that the field of bioethics must give to abortion, particularly the question whether and by what means abortion should be made available equally to all persons requesting it, regardless of national citizenship, ethnic or racial identity, or economic status.

BIBLIOGRAPHY

Adler, N. E.; H. P. David; B. N. Major; et al. 1990. "Psychological Responses after Abortion." *Science* 248 (4951): 41–44.

Almeling, Rene; Laureen Tews; and Susan Dudley. 2000. "Abortion Training in U.S. Obstetrics and Gynecology Residency Programs, 1998." *Family Planning Perspectives* 32 (6): 268–71.

American College of Obstetricians and Gynecologists. 1997. *Statement on Intact Dilatation and Extraction.* Washington, DC: Author.

American College of Obstetricians and Gynecologists. 2001. *Emergency Oral Contraception.* ACOG practice bulletin number 25. Washington, DC: Author.

Annas, George J. 1998. "Partial Birth Abortion, Congress, and the Constitution." *New England Journal of Medicine* 339 (4): 279–83.

Annas, George J. 2001. "Partial Birth Abortion and the Supreme Court." *New England Journal of Medicine* 344 (2): 152–56.

Ashok, Premila W.; Prabhath T. Wagaarachchi; Gillian M. Flett; and Allan Templeton. 2001. "Mifepristone as a Late Post-Coital Contraceptive." *Human Reproduction* 16 (1): 72–75.

Berger, Gary S.; William E. Brenner; and Louis G. Keith, eds. 1981. *Second Trimester Abortion.* Boston: PSG.

Cates, Willard, Jr., and David A. Grimes, 1981. "Morbidity and Mortality of Abortion in the United States." In *Abortion and Sterilization: Medical and Social Aspects,* edited by Jane E. Hodgson, 155–80. London: Academic Press.

Clinton, William J. 1996. "Remarks on Returning without Approval to the House of Representatives Partial Birth Abortion Legislation." *Weekly Compilation of Presidential Documents,* April 10, 643–47.

Clinton, William J. 1997. "Message to the House of Representatives Returning without Approval Partial Birth Abortion Legislation." *Weekly Compilation of Presidential Documents,* October 10, 1545.

Corson, Stephen L.; Thomas V. Sedlacek; and Jerome J. Hoffman. 1986. "Suction Dilation and Evacuation." In *Greenhill's Surgical Gynecology,* 5th ed., edited by Jacob Pearl Greenhill; Stephen L. Corson; Thomas V. Sedlacek; and Jerome J. Hoffman. Chicago: Year Book.

Council on Ethical and Judicial Affairs, American Medical Association. 1994. *Code of Medical Ethics: Current Opinions with Annotations—Including the Principles of the Medical Ethics, Fundamental Elements of the Patient-Physician Relationship, and Rules of the Council on Ethical and Judicial Affairs.* Chicago: Author.

Gold, Rachel Benson. 1990. *Abortion and Women's Health: A Turning Point for America?* New York: Alan Guttmacher Institute.

Grimes, David A. 1996. "Surgical Management of Abortion." In *Te Linde's Operative Gynecology,* 8th ed., edited by John A. Rock and John D. Thompson, 477–500. Philadelphia: Lippincott-Raven.

Grimes, David A. 1998. "The Continuing Need for Late Abortions." *Journal of the American Medical Association* 280 (8): 747–50.

Grimes, David A.; Kenneth F. Schulz; Willard Cates Jr.; and C. W. Tyler Jr. 1979. "Local versus General Anesthesia: Which Is Safer for Performing Suction Curettage Abortions?" *American Journal of Obstetrics and Gynecology* 135 (8): 1030–35.

Henshaw, Stanley K. 1990. "Induced Abortion: A World Review, 1990." *Family Planning Perspectives* 22 (2): 76–89.

House Human Resources and Intergovernmental Relations Subcommittee of the Committee on Governmental Operations. 1989. *The Federal Role in Determining the Medical and Psychological Impact of Abortions on Women.* HR 329, 101st Congress, 1st session, 14.

Kolata, Gina. 2002. "Abortion Pill Slow to Win Users among Women and Their Doctors." *New York Times,* September 25.

Koop, C. Everett. 1989. *Medical and Psychological Effects of Abortion on Women.* Washington, DC: US Department of Health and Human Services.

Kunins, Hillary, and Allan Rosenfield. 1991. "Abortion: A Legal and Public Health Perspective." *Annual Review of Public Health* 12 (1): 361–82.

US Food and Drug Administration. 2000. Approval Letter for Mifepristone. September 28. Accessed September 1, 2013. http://www.accessdata.fda.gov/drugsatfda_docs/appletter/2000/20687appltr.htm

Allan Rosenfield (1995)
Columbia University

Sara Iden (1995)
Columbia University

Anne Drapkin Lyerly (2004)
Duke University Medical Center

I. MEDICAL PERSPECTIVES [ADDENDUM]

Research findings continue to support the safety of legal abortion in the United States. In 2012 Elizabeth G. Raymond and David A. Grimes published a review on the safety of first-trimester abortion compared with childbirth in the United States from 1998 to 2005. They found that the pregnancy-associated mortality rate among women who delivered live infants was 8.8 deaths per 100,000 live births and that the mortality from first-trimester abortion was 0.6 deaths per 100,000 abortions. Thus the risk of death due to childbirth is approximately fourteen times as high as that due to first-trimester abortion. Although second-trimester abortion is riskier than first-trimester abortion, the mortality rates are less than or equal to mortality rates from live birth: at thirteen to fifteen weeks of gestation, 1.7 deaths per 100,000 abortions; sixteen to twenty weeks of gestation, 3.4 deaths per 100,000 abortions; and more than twenty-one weeks of gestation, 8.9 deaths per 100,000 abortions (Bartlett et al. 2004).

First-trimester abortion options have greatly changed since the US Food and Drug Administration approved the antiprogestin drug mifepristone in combination with misoprostol as a medication abortion regimen in 2000. Although the majority of first-trimester procedures performed in the United States are still done by dilation and curettage, the percentage of early medication abortions increases each year: 16.5 percent of first-trimester abortions performed in 2009 were early medication abortions (Pazol et al. 2012). Evidence supports the use of the mifepristone and misoprostol medication abortion regimen through sixty-three days of gestation (nine weeks or less).

It is estimated that 96 percent of second-trimester abortions in the United States are by dilation and evacuation and that only 2 percent are by labor induction abortion (Pazol et al. 2012). Labor induction abortion is a process whereby medications are administered to induce uterine contractions that lead to expulsion of the fetus and the placenta. Labor induction abortion is more commonly performed later in the second trimester or in the early third trimester, for abortions with fetal anomalies, and in areas where skilled dilation and evacuation providers are not available (Borgatta, Kapp, and Society of Family Planning 2011). The practice of intrauterine instillation and routine use of a sharp curette (after either a first- or a second-trimester procedure) has fallen out of practice because those methods have been found to increase morbidity.

After a steep decline before 2005, the number of abortion providers in the United States remained steady. However, in 2008, 87 percent of the counties in the United States did not have an abortion provider. Second-trimester abortion after thirteen weeks of gestation is offered by 64 percent of abortion providers, but only 23 percent of them provide the procedure at twenty weeks or beyond (Jones and Kooistra 2011).

In 1992 in the US Supreme Court decision in the case of *Planned Parenthood of Southeastern Pennsylvania v. Casey*, the states were granted the right to enact laws that place regulations on abortion services. These laws include regulation of abortion providers, building regulations, gestational age limits, partial-birth abortion bans, state-mandated counseling, waiting periods, parental involvement for minors, limits to both private and public insurance coverage, and more (Guttmacher Institute 2013). The hypothesis of fetal pain during an abortion is the source of multiple state regulations on the upper gestational age limit for abortions and mandating medically inaccurate counseling of patients seeking abortion services. In the early twenty-first century the medical literature supports that fetuses are unlikely to feel pain before twenty-six to thirty weeks of gestation (Lee et al. 2005). The American Congress of Obstetricians and Gynecologists stated in 2005 that it knows of "no legitimate scientific information that supports the statement that a fetus experiences pain" (2005).

Globally unsafe abortion causes 13 percent of all maternal deaths and 20 percent of the total mortality and disability due to pregnancy and childbirth (Ahman and Shah 2011; World Health Organization 2012). The safety of abortion is directly related to access, which is greatly influenced by the legal status of abortion and the availability of skilled abortion providers. There is ample documented experience that laws and regulations that restrict abortion access do not lower the number of abortions performed, nor do they increase birthrates (Levine and Staiger 2004; Sedgh et al. 2012). Steps that lead to increased access to safe abortions also do not increase abortion rates, but rather "the principal effect is to shift previously clandestine, unsafe procedures to legal and safe ones" (World Health Organization 2012, 90; see also Grimes et al. 2006).

SEE ALSO *Embryo and Fetus: I. Developments from Fertilization to Birth; Fertility Control: I. Medical Aspects; Reproductive Technologies: I. Introduction; Selective Termination/Reduction of Multiple Pregnancy*

BIBLIOGRAPHY

Ahman, Elisabeth, and Iqbal H. Shah. 2011. "New Estimates and Trends regarding Unsafe Abortion Mortality." *International Journal of Gynaecology and Obstetrics* 115 (2): 121–26.

American Congress of Obstetricians and Gynecologists. 2005. "Statement on Fetal Pain and Fetal Pain Legislation." May. Washington, DC: Author. http://www.acog.org/~/media/Departments/Members%20Only/State%20Legislative%20Activities/200505FPLegislation.pdf?dmc=1&ts=20130717T1648188782 (password protected).

Bartlett, Linda A.; Cynthia J. Berg; Holly B. Shulman; et al. 2004. "Risk Factors for Legal Induced Abortion-Related Mortality in the United States." *Obstetrics and Gynecology* 103 (4): 729–37.

Borgatta, Lynn; Nathalie Kapp; and Society of Family Planning. 2011. "Clinical Guidelines: Labor Induction Abortion in the Second Trimester." *Contraception* 84 (1): 4–18.

Grimes, David A.; Janie Benson; Susheela Singh; et al. 2006. "Unsafe Abortion: The Preventable Pandemic." *Lancet* 368 (9550): 1908–19.

Guttmacher Institute. 2013. "State Policies in Brief: An Overview of Abortion Laws." September 1. http://www.guttmacher.org/statecenter/spibs/spib_OAL.pdf

Jones, Rachel K., and Kathryn Kooistra. 2011. "Abortion Incidence and Access to Services in the United States, 2008." *Perspectives on Sexual and Reproductive Health* 43 (1): 41–50.

Lee, Susan J.; Henry J. Peter Ralston; Eleanor A. Drey; et al. 2005. "Fetal Pain: A Systematic Multidisciplinary Review of the Evidence." *Journal of the American Medical Association* 294 (8): 947–54.

Levine, Phillip B., and Douglas Staiger. 2004. "Abortion Policy and Fertility Outcomes: The Eastern European Experience." *Journal of Law and Economics* 47 (1): 223–43.

Pazol, Karen; Andreea A. Creanga; Suzanne B. Zane; et al. 2012. "Abortion Surveillance: United States, 2009." *Morbidity and Mortality Weekly Report Surveillance Summaries* 61 (8): 1–44.

Planned Parenthood of Southeastern Pennsylvania v. Casey. 1992. 502 U.S. 1056 (1992).

Raymond, Elizabeth G., and David A. Grimes. 2012. "The Comparative Safety of Legal Induced Abortion and Childbirth in the United States." *Obstetrics and Gynecology* 119 (2, pt. 1): 215–19.

Sedgh, Gilda; Susheela Singh; Iqbal H. Shah; et al. 2012. "Induced Abortion: Incidence and Trends Worldwide from 1995 to 2008." *Lancet* 379 (9816): 625–32.

World Health Organization. 2012. *Safe Abortion: Technical and Policy Guidance For Health Systems.* 2nd ed. Geneva: Author.

Erin Berry-Bibee
Family Planning Fellow and Instructor, Department of Gynecology and Obstetrics, Emory University School of Medicine

II. ETHICAL PERSPECTIVES

Abortion is widely regarded as one of the most intractable problems in bioethics. Few issues in bioethics have inspired as much discussion, debate, and open conflict as abortion, in part because the abortion controversy, unlike many others in ethics, has not been limited to scholars and practitioners, but has been engaged on numerous fronts in the United States. Churches and religious organizations, politicians, the courts, and the general public have all taken a stand on abortion. In the decades since the US Supreme Court, in its 1973 *Roe v. Wade* decision, effectively legalized abortion through the second trimester of pregnancy, the conflict has not abated.

Another reason for the intractability of the abortion issue is that the views held by critics and defenders of abortion often occupy extremes. At one extreme, abortion opponents defend an absolute prohibition on abortion, calling abortion nothing less than the murder of an innocent person. At the other extreme are those who defend a woman's absolute right to abortion on demand at any time during pregnancy. Both sides engage in rhetoric and hyperbole; abortion opponents call themselves "pro-life," implying that their opponents are antilife, while abortion rights supporters call themselves "pro-choice," suggesting that antiabortionists oppose personal freedom and choice. When the battle lines are largely ideological, there is little room for rational argument. The result is that rather than search for a middle ground, both sides of the conflict have simply dug their heels in deeper.

An additional source of difficulty in reaching agreement about abortion is that the antiabortion movement in the United States has been led primarily by the Roman Catholic Church and fundamentalist Protestants, who base their opposition to abortion on fundamental religious convictions. If it is impossible to argue rationally for or against such convictions, it is no less difficult to argue about an ethical position that is deeply rooted in them.

Finally, the abortion problem is unusually difficult because the fetus is significantly unlike other entities of moral concern, and because the relationship between a fetus and a pregnant woman is unique among human relationships. The moral status of the fetus is itself a highly contested matter, such that the general moral principles that can be appealed to in other areas of human conduct and conflict do not fit cleanly into the abortion picture. Additionally, because the status of the fetus is at issue, abortion can be as much a metaphysical problem as a moral one.

The contemporary moral controversy over abortion focuses on three central issues: the moral status of the embryo or fetus, which many ethicists contend hinges on the ontological status of embryonic and fetal life; the rights conflict between pregnant women and their fetuses; and consequentialist arguments that weigh the potential for harm to women as a result of restricting or abolishing abortion against the negative consequences of terminating fetal or embryonic life.

ONTOLOGICAL AND MORAL STATUS OF THE FETUS

The question of the ontological status of the fetus can be teased apart from the question of moral status, but in the abortion debate, fetal personhood and the possession of moral rights are often assumed to go hand in hand. The term *person,* however, is ambiguous, having a legal, a descriptive, and a normative sense. To be a legal person is simply to possess legal rights. In *Roe v. Wade* (1973), the Supreme Court held that fetuses are not persons as defined by the Fourteenth Amendment of the Constitution, but declined to offer a positive thesis on personhood, acknowledging the difficulty of doing so. "We need not resolve the difficult question of when life begins. When those trained in the respective disciplines of medicine, philosophy, and theology are unable to arrive at any consensus, the judiciary, at this point in the development of man's knowledge, is not in a position to speculate as to the answer" (*Roe v. Wade* 1973). To say that something is a descriptive person is just to say that it satisfies certain criteria of personhood, such as species membership. The claim that a fetus is a person in this sense does nothing to justify the claim that killing a fetus is morally wrong unless the fetus also qualifies as a person in the normative sense. Normatively speaking, being a person means being a bearer of moral rights, including the right to life. The crucial question of fetal or embryonic personhood, as it relates to abortion, then, is whether and when the genetically human, living entity resulting from the fertilization of an ovum by a spermatozoon is a normative person, a possessor of rights. There is, however, no more consensus on the proper criteria for personhood, and whether or not fetuses can satisfy these criteria, than there is on abortion.

At one extreme of the personhood debate is the position that personhood begins at fertilization, so even very early embryos, composed of only a few cells, are persons. At the other extreme is the view that personhood does not begin until birth or even later, and so no fetus, and perhaps no infant, qualifies as a person. Between the two extremes, there are a multitude of possibilities.

One approach to personhood is the developmental view, which denies that a bright line can be drawn at any particular point in natural development when the fetus acquires moral standing. The developmental view hinges on the continuity of fetal development and the difficulty of nonarbitrarily picking out properties that qualify some fetuses, but not others, as persons. Because infants are generally regarded as persons with a right to life, and the difference between a late-term fetus and a neonate—particularly in the case of viable premature infants—is merely a matter of location, it appears that in the continuous process of embryonic and fetal development, there is no nonarbitrary place to draw a line where personhood begins. This view is in line with the intuition, shared by many on both sides of the abortion conflict, that fetal life becomes increasingly important as gestation continues, but that it is impossible to say with certainty when, exactly, a fetus becomes a person. The inherent vagueness of the developmental view is an obstacle to translating it into practical moral guidelines or public policies.

The potentiality view advances conception or fertilization as the beginning of personhood because it is the fertilized ovum, not its constituent gametes, that is considered to have the potential to develop into a human being with full moral status. As a number of critics of the potentiality criterion have observed, having the potential to become a person is not the same as being one, and it is being a person that confers moral status and rights.

As Judith Jarvis Thomson noted, "A newly fertilized ovum, a newly implanted clump of cells, is no more a person than an acorn is an oak tree" (1971, 47). In *Roe v. Wade*, the court located fetal viability as a line of demarcation, the point after which the state may have a compelling interest in protecting fetal life. Although viability is not a specific moment in the continuum of fetal development, it occurs at approximately twenty-two to twenty-five weeks' gestation, when a number of other significant developmental markers have been achieved, and is the point at which, given proper support, a fetus can potentially survive outside the womb, independently of its mother. It has taken on significance as a convenient, relatively identifiable and verifiable turning point in fetal development, when personhood plausibly begins. Fetal viability is to some extent dependent on technology—premature neonates often need considerable medical support to survive. As technological advances in neonatal care occur, it is possible that the point at which a fetus is viable may change. Some critics of the viability standard claim that personhood ought not be contingent on external facts about the state of medical technology, and therefore cannot stand as a proper criterion for personhood.

As technology has provided a better understanding of the different stages of embryonic and fetal development, criteria such as implantation (when the conceptus becomes embedded in the uterine lining), the appearance of external human form, and the presence of detectable brain-wave activity have all been advanced as criteria for personhood and rights. Traditional criteria for fetal personhood include animation, when fetal movement first occurs, and quickening, the time at which a pregnant woman first feels fetal movement. Early Christian authors wrote of ensoulment, the time at which the embryo or fetus is imbued with a soul.

Species membership, or genetic humanity, is the most lenient criterion for personhood, and the most easily verifiable. According to this criterion, any entity conceived of human parents is a member of the human species, and is therefore a person. John T. Noonan (2003), writing from a Catholic perspective, argues that the fetus acquires personhood at the moment of conception, when it receives from its parents the human genetic code. The genetic humanity standard can be regarded as both too broad and too restrictive, however. It is too broad because it implies that any living entity with the human genetic code qualifies as a human life worthy of protection. Cancer cells, sperm, and ova all have a human genetic code, and on the least-restrictive definition of genetic humanity, such cells would have a right to life, implying that if abortion is impermissible, then so is contraception and chemotherapy. Ethicists who advance a genetic humanity view generally exclude from personhood cells that lack the potential to become human beings, combining a genetic humanity standard with a potentiality principle. The genetic humanity standard can also be regarded as too restrictive because it excludes from the possibility of personhood all nonhuman beings, including some that may warrant the moral status of rights-bearers.

Mary Anne Warren (1973) argues for a very strict psychological standard of personhood, defining a person as "a full-fledged member of the moral community." Genetic humanity alone is not sufficient for personhood, according to Warren, so not all human beings are members of the moral community. Warren proposes a set of cognitive criteria that, it is claimed, everyone can and does agree are central to the concept of personhood: consciousness, the developed capacity for reasoning and problem solving, self-motivated activity, the capacity to communicate, and self-awareness. Beings that satisfy some or all of these criteria are people with a moral claim on us, whether they are human or not, for just as some human beings are not people, "there may well be people who are not human beings" (Warren 1973). Membership in the moral community requires the capacity for moral participation, in Warren's view; it would be absurd to ascribe moral obligations and responsibilities to an entity that cannot satisfy any of the cognitive or psychological criteria for moral personhood, and it is equally absurd to ascribe full moral rights to such a being. It is obvious that no fetus can satisfy any of these criteria, and it is equally obvious, Warren argues, that anything that fails to satisfy any of these criteria cannot be a person. A fully developed fetus is no more like a person than a newborn guppy, and cannot have a right to life sufficient to override a woman's right to have an abortion at any stage of pregnancy.

Critics were quick to point out that Warren's standard of personhood could not be met by infants, nor many children and adults with serious cognitive deficits, and thus would problematically justify not only abortion, but infanticide and nonvoluntary euthanasia as well. Warren responded that although a newborn infant is not a person with a right to life, and infanticide is not murder, there are utilitarian reasons for the impermissibility of infanticide. Infanticide is wrong for the same reason it is wrong to destroy great works of art or natural resources, because destroying these things deprives people of a great deal of pleasure. Moreover, most people value infants, even if their own parents do not, and would prefer that they not be destroyed. These considerations are not sufficient to override a pregnant woman's right to an abortion at any stage of pregnancy, Warren claims, but the moment of birth marks the point at which the infant's continued life no longer violates any of its mother's rights, and is thus the point at which its mother no longer has the right to determine its fate. Birth is also morally significant "because it permits the establishment of direct social relationships between the infant and other members of society" (Warren 1985, 6). Thus, although an infant may lack the intrinsic properties that ground a right to life, "its emergence into the social world makes it appropriate to treat it as if it had such a right" (Warren 1989, 56).

While Warren has been accused of offering an ad hoc solution to the problem of infanticide, Michael Tooley argues that neither abortion nor infanticide is intrinsically wrong or undesirable, and indeed, "in the vast majority of cases in which infanticide is desirable … there is excellent reason to believe that infanticide is morally permissible" (Tooley 1985, 14). Tooley's argument is that personhood requires nothing less than self-consciousness: "An organism possesses a serious right to life only if it possesses the concept of a self as a continuing subject of experiences and other mental states, and believes that it is itself such a continuing entity" (1972, 44). Tooley and Warren both explicitly reject the view that the mere potential to become a person gives the fetus any moral standing.

Don Marquis attempts to resolve the personhood standoff by starting with an unproblematic assumption: It is seriously morally wrong to kill an adult human being. Marquis concludes that what makes killing wrong is that murder deprives its victim of a life and future that is valuable. The victim of a murder is deprived of all the experiences, activities, projects, and enjoyments that would have constituted his or her future, deprived of all that he or she values, or would have come to value, in life. The loss of that valuable future, of what Marquis calls a "future like ours," is ultimately what makes killing wrong. It is also what makes abortion morally wrong, Marquis argues, because fetuses have futures of value. "The future of a standard fetus includes a set of experiences, projects, activities, and such which are identical with the futures of adult human beings and are identical with the futures of young children" (Marquis 1989, 192).

Marquis's future-like-ours account implies that it is seriously wrong to kill any being with a future of value; it is non-speciesist in that it does not claim that only human life has value or worth. Marquis's theory leaves open the possibility that other species, if they share the property of having a valuable future, have the same right to life that a human being has, and that killing members of other species would therefore be seriously morally wrong. Marquis offers no account of what a future like ours must look like, or what shared properties of an adult human future make it valuable. This point has been a focus of attack for critics, who claim that fetuses do not, indeed cannot, have futures like ours.

Marquis's future-like-ours theory, in opposition to other pro-life accounts, is compatible with the permissibility of euthanasia because it is only the loss of a valuable future—not merely the loss of a life—that makes killing wrong. The future-like-ours theory also accounts for the basic intuition that it is seriously wrong to kill young children and infants, for it is presumed they have futures of value. Personhood theories that advance psychological criteria do not straightforwardly account for the intuition or belief that killing infants and children is morally wrong, and must make appeal to other principles, such as social utility, to account for its wrongness. Appeals to social utility, however, cannot explain the wrongness of killing those who are unwanted or unnecessary.

Marquis's critics point out that he fails to provide an argument for why a fetus that is incapable of valuing its own future should count as a being that can suffer a morally relevant loss of its future. David Boonin develops an alternative future-like-ours theory that refutes the claim that every fetus has a right to life, and that abortion is in typical cases morally impermissible, on terms that critics of abortion, like Marquis, can and do accept. Boonin argues that a fetus acquires a right to life only at the point in fetal development when organized cortical brain activity is present. The "cortical criterion" is the only morally relevant criterion for moral standing and a right to life because organized cortical activity is what makes it possible to have a future like ours. "We have a future-like-ours only because we have a brain which will enable us to enjoy, in the future, the kinds of conscious experiences that make our lives distinctively valuable to us" (Boonin 2003, 126). Boonin's theory, like Marquis's, identifies a natural property that fetuses possess that makes killing them morally wrong. However, Boonin's cortical criterion narrows the category of beings with a right to life to those with a developed capacity for conscious desires: "It is because these individuals currently have desires about their futures that our desires about how to behave are not the only ones that are morally relevant" (73). Thus, Boonin's theory does not claim that no fetus ever has a right to life, but only that this right does not exist from the moment of conception, and that if, as Marquis proposes, depriving a fetus of a future like ours is the wrong-making feature of abortion, then "abortion in typical circumstances is permissible" because the typically aborted fetus lacks a future like ours (Boonin 2003, 129). If Boonin's cortical criterion is accepted, the vast majority of abortions, which take place well before the point at which fetuses can form conscious desires, are morally permissible.

A looser cognitive criterion for personhood is advanced by Baruch Brody, who appeals to the symmetry between the development of a functioning brain as the beginning of fetal humanity and the cessation of brain function as the definition of death, or the end of humanity. That is, the property whose acquisition confers the right to life is the same property that, when permanently lost, entails the loss of a right to life: the possession of a functioning brain. If the brain death theory is correct, Brody concludes, a fetus becomes a human being about six weeks after fertilization, when it has a functioning brain. After that point, abortions, except under unusual circumstances, are morally impermissible. Brody's is a significantly looser cognitive criterion than Boonin's "organized cortical activity" criterion because it makes fetal humanity dependent on the presence of early brain function, which is not sufficiently organized to support consciousness. It is not obvious why this rudimentary level of brain development is morally significant or defining, unless it is augmented with a potentiality principle. Indeed, such a level of brain function in an infant with anencephaly or an adult with brain injury would not compel the continuation of life support.

Several states have acted to resolve the matter of fetal personhood by legislative fiat. Abortion foes have acknowledged that these so-called personhood amendments are strategically designed to provoke a constitutional challenge to *Roe v. Wade*. Oklahoma's Senate Bill 1433 defines legal personhood as beginning at fertilization: "The laws of this state shall be interpreted and construed to acknowledge on behalf of the unborn child at every stage of development all the rights, privileges, and immunities available to other persons … 'unborn child' or 'unborn children' shall include all unborn children or the offspring of human beings from the moment of conception until birth at every stage of biological development" (State of Oklahoma, SB 1433). This and other personhood amendments make no reference to exceptions for abortion in the case of rape, incest, or to protect the life or health of a pregnant woman. They have also raised concerns about the chilling effect that legal personhood for fertilized embryos could have for fertility treatment, particularly in vitro fertilization, which frequently results in a number of excess, cryopreserved, fertilized embryos, and also poses a heightened risk of miscarriage. Declaring the legal personhood of a conceptus does not resolve the controversy regarding the moral personhood or status of the embryo or fetus, but it effectively limits access to abortion, as well as some contraceptives, if abortion is legally defined as killing a person.

Both proponents and opponents of abortion believe that settling the abortion controversy requires settling the question of personhood. While there is some room for agreement at either extreme, standards of personhood like Noonan's and Warren's are incommensurable, calling into question the utility of defining personhood as a route to resolving the conflict. So long as the fetus's moral standing is believed to depend on fetal personhood, however, the question of personhood will not disappear from the abortion debate.

RIGHTS CONFLICTS AND ABORTION

Most opposition to abortion is grounded in two assumptions: the first is the moral personhood and right to life of the fetus; the second assumption is that, in a conflict of rights, the right to life must trump a woman's right to privacy, choice, and bodily autonomy. Many pro-choice arguments ignore the second assumption—perhaps because it seems intuitively implausible that any other right could outweigh a right to life—and focus solely on the first assumption, either offering support for the claim that fetal personhood occurs substantially later in fetal development than conception, or arguing that the criteria for moral personhood can never be met by a fetus. Neither proposition is acceptable or defensible to abortion opponents for whom it is an article of faith that a fetus has a right to life. Thomson (1971) puts forth an argument that grants, for the sake of argument, fetal personhood from conception, but challenges the second pro-life assumption that the right to life always overrides other rights.

Thomson's argument employs an analogy that has engendered controversy among both defenders and critics of abortion. Imagine, Thomson writes, that you awake one morning to find yourself hooked up to the body of an unconscious violinist who is suffering a fatal kidney ailment. The Society of Music Lovers has kidnapped you and plugged this famous violinist into your circulatory system, so that your kidneys can be used to filter his blood. You are told that in nine months, the famous violinist will have recovered, and can be safely detached, but in the meantime, to unhook him from your body would kill him. The violinist is a person, and so he has a right to life. Your life is not endangered, but you must remain tethered to the violinist against your will for nine months, thus greatly diminishing your freedom. If his right to life guarantees him the use of your body for life support, then it is morally incumbent on you to provide it, regardless of the cost to your personal freedom. The implications for abortion are clear: The violinist is meant to be analogous to a fetus, and you and your kidneys are analogous to a pregnant woman providing life support to a fetus. If, Thomson argues, it is implausible that you are morally obligated to sustain the violinist's life at such a cost to your personal freedom, then it ought to be equally implausible that a fetus's right to life guarantees it the right to continued use of a woman's body. Thus, the fetus's right to life does not make abortion morally impermissible, for "having a right to life does not guarantee having either a right to be given the use of or a right to be allowed continued use of another person's body—even if one needs it for life itself" (Thomson 1971, 56).

If Thomson's analogy is accepted, there are serious grounds for questioning the assumption that abortion is morally impermissible if a fetus has a right to life. However, both opponents and proponents of the right to abortion have argued against the soundness of Thomson's analogy. Abortion critics claim that there is a deep, even grotesque disanalogy between a fetus and the violinist, and that Thomson fails to attend to the moral distinction between intentionally killing and letting die. Abortion, it is argued, intentionally kills a fetus, but detaching oneself from the violinist only allows the violinist to die from his kidney ailment, an act with a very different moral status than murder. Abortion proponents and opponents alike raise a responsibility objection to Thomson's argument, claiming that her conclusion only holds in cases where pregnancy results from an involuntary act. Warren criticizes Thomson's analogy on those grounds, arguing that it is too weak to provide a thorough defense of a right to abortion, allowing it only in cases of rape (Warren 1973). Since the majority of unwanted pregnancies are not the result of rape, Thomson's argument would permit abortion in only a small fraction of unwanted pregnancies. Thomson acknowledges that her argument leaves open the possibility that there may be some cases in which the unborn person acquires, tacitly or by consent, a right to the use of the mother's body, and in which abortion would be an unjust killing. But this possibility does not force the conclusion that all abortions are unjust killings. "Except in such cases as the unborn person has a right to demand it … nobody is morally required to make large sacrifices, of health, of all other interests and concerns, of all other duties and commitments, for nine years, or even for nine months, in order to keep another person alive" (Thomson 1971, 62).

It is difficult to consistently maintain the position that a fetus's right to life trumps all other rights or considerations. In cases where the life of a pregnant woman is endangered by pregnancy, only the most extreme opponents of abortion claim that because abortion is the intentional killing of an innocent person, it is still morally wrong and the mother must be allowed to die. More moderate opposition to abortion allows exceptions for the life or health of the mother, and also for cases where pregnancy results from rape or incest. There is a clear inconsistency in the rape and incest exception, however, since it makes the unborn fetus's right to life contingent on the actions of its father. Abortion opponents who grant exceptions in cases of rape and incest must, if they are consistent, explain why those fetuses have a different moral status, or a diminished right to life, compared to other fetuses, or why the right to life loses its priority to a woman's rights in those cases.

Pro-choice feminist arguments charge that most discussions of abortion place undue emphasis on fetal rights and too little emphasis on the contexts in which decisions about abortion take place. Susan Sherwin argues that traditional, nonfeminist approaches to the abortion controversy are too simplistic, considering the permissibility of abortion in isolation from the social and sexual subordination of women, and the struggle of women for control over their bodies and reproduction. Nonfeminist arguments thus mistakenly claim that the moral status of abortion turns exclusively on the moral status of the fetus (Sherwin 1992). The central moral feature of pregnancy, Sherwin argues, is that it takes place in women's bodies and profoundly affects their lives. Because fetuses have a unique physical status of dependence on particular women, they have a unique social status as well—the value of a fetus, Sherwin claims, is determined solely by the nature of its primary relationship to the woman who carries it, and "no absolute value attaches to fetuses apart from their relational status" (111). The focus on the fetus as an independent, rights-bearing entity denies pregnant women their proper roles as independent moral agents who, alone, have "the responsibility and privilege of determining a fetus's specific social status and value" (110).

Some pro-life feminists attempt to sidestep the rights controversy and argue instead that abortion is inconsistent with the goals and ideals of feminism, such as opposition to violence, and the promulgation of an ethic of caring, nurturing, and interconnectedness. Others, like Sidney Callahan (1986), argue that feminist goals cannot be achieved in a society that permits abortion. The exclusion of the unborn from the sphere of rights and protection, Callahan argues, is analogous to the exclusion of women in unjust, patriarchal systems where "lesser orders of human life are granted rights only when wanted, chosen, or invested with value by the powerful" (368). Moreover, to grant a right to abortion in the name of women's privacy or autonomy validates the view that pregnancy and child rearing are the sole responsibility of individual women, relieving men and the community from any responsibility. Thus "women will never climb to equality and social empowerment over mounds of dead fetuses" (Callahan 1986, 371). To exercise moral autonomy, Callahan argues, requires responsiveness and responsibility not only to what is wanted or chosen, but to what is unwanted and unchosen as well. Callahan makes no exceptions for pregnancy due to rape, arguing that even the involuntarily pregnant woman has "a moral obligation to the now-existing, dependent fetus whether she explicitly consented to its existence or not" (370).

Margaret Olivia Little argues that the literature on abortion deeply undersells the moral complexity of abortion, focusing too much on a thin moral assessment of its permissibility. She proposes that what is needed in the moral discussion of abortion is an ethics of gestation that addresses questions of "what it means to play a role in creating a person, how to assess responsibilities that involve sharing, not just risking, one's body and life, what follows from the fact that the entity in question is or would be one's child" (Little 2002, 493). A more complex moral interpretation must move beyond questions of metaphysical and moral status and permissibility to consider abortion's "placement on the scales of decency, respectfulness, and responsibility" (Little 2002, 492).

If fetuses are not persons, Little argues, they are nonetheless respect-worthy because they are burgeoning human lives, and abortion remains a serious matter because it involves the loss of something significant and valuable. Even if we allow that fetuses are persons, however, the important moral question is what positive duties and responsibilities, if any, pregnant women have to continue gestational assistance. Both liberal and conservative positions on the duties of parenthood assume that it is an all-or-nothing affair, and that pregnant women either have the same obligations and responsibilities to fetuses that they do to children, or that they owe nothing beyond general beneficence. But parenthood, Little claims, is more than a social role—it is, more crucially, a relationship that develops through time, interaction, and emotional intertwinement. Regardless of the view one takes on the personhood of fetuses, gestation uniquely changes the relationship a woman has to her self, bringing with it a new identity and an impending relationship with another that is not always welcome or sustainable. Thus, "assessing the moral status of abortion … is not just about assessing the contours of generic respect owed to burgeoning human life, it's about assessing the salience of impending relationship" (Little 2002, 498).

The fetus's status becomes progressively weightier as pregnancy continues, Little suggests, but until the fetus is a person, there is a moral prerogative to decline parenthood and end pregnancy because it "so thoroughly changes what we might call one's fundamental practical identity. … As profound as the respect we should have for burgeoning human life, we should acknowledge moral prerogatives over identity-constituting commitments and enterprises as profound as motherhood" (Little 2002, 498).

THE SELECTIVE ABORTION CONTROVERSY

The development of tests to prenatally diagnose genetic diseases and disorders has greatly outpaced the development of effective treatments and therapies. Through procedures such as chorionic villus sampling, which can be performed at ten weeks' gestation, and amniocentesis, available at fourteen to sixteen weeks, numerous genetic abnormalities in the fetus can be detected in utero. The tests are routinely administered to women at risk for fetal abnormalities, such as older mothers and those with a family history of genetic disorder, but they carry the risk of miscarriage. A newer, noninvasive maternal blood test for Down syndrome (trisomy 21) and trisomies 13 and 18 is nearly 99 percent accurate at detecting these aneuploidies as early as ten weeks' gestation, with few false positives and no risk to the fetus (Palomaki et al. 2012). Ultrasound, which is routinely performed throughout most pregnancies, can detect a number of abnormalities as well, including Down syndrome, and neural tube defects that can result in severe physical and cognitive disability and death. In rare instances, fetal therapy, including surgery, can correct the problems, but the overwhelming majority of pregnant women whose fetuses are found to have abnormalities are currently faced with only two options: abort the defective fetus or risk giving birth to a child that will potentially face a lifetime of disability and hardship. An estimated 92 percent of pregnancies with a prenatal diagnosis of Down syndrome are terminated. In cases where the fetus's condition will result in severe physical or mental impairment, or where it will lead to inevitable death and a short, painful life, only the most extreme opponents of abortion maintain that it is wrong to abort. Abortion moderates and supporters see those as clear cases where abortion is not only morally permissible, but in some situations, morally required. Less agreement exists regarding the abortion of fetuses with minor abnormalities, genetic predispositions to disease, and genetic diseases that are eventually lethal, but compatible with more or less normal life for many years.

Disability rights advocates oppose the routine administration of prenatal screening and the selective abortion of fetuses found to have abnormalities. Although many disability rights scholars are pro-choice, and defend a woman's right to choose abortion, they object to the use of selective abortion for fetal indications, which they argue discriminates against existing people with disabilities and sends the message to those living with disabilities that they should never have been born. This so-called expressivist argument claims that selective abortion expresses discriminatory attitudes toward the disabled and undermines efforts to create a more just, inclusive society (Asch 2000). The disability critique of abortion is novel because it is concerned only with the abortion of otherwise wanted fetuses that possess a single undesirable trait, a disability.

Controversy exists regarding the use of fertility treatments like in vitro fertilization (IVF) and superovulatory drugs, which pose a fairly high risk of multiple gestations and births. As IVF technology has improved, multiple births involving twins and triplets have become more frequent, although higher-order births are still rare. Numerous complications affecting both the pregnant woman and her offspring are associated with multiple pregnancies. The high cost and low success rate of fertility treatments contribute to the problem—with IVF, it is typical practice to implant more than the desired number of embryos in order to increase the odds of success;

superovulatory drugs, which stimulate a woman's ovaries to produce dozens of ova, afford little control over the number that will ultimately be fertilized and implanted. It is more than a little ironic that the effort to assist couples in achieving pregnancy has led to an abortion controversy over the use of selective reduction, the practice of removing some fetuses in multiple pregnancies in order to increase the chances of a healthy pregnancy and birth for the remaining fetuses. Although the procedure is not without risks—miscarriage, fetal death, and disability are known complications of selective reduction—some commentators question whether in pregnancies with a large number of fetuses—more than two or three—there is a moral imperative to reduce in order to decrease the risks to the surviving offspring. Some ethicists question the wisdom of parents who, due to religious, moral, or personal objections to abortion, refuse the option of selective reduction, thus placing their offspring at increased risk for prematurity, low birthweight, cognitive and physical disability, and death. In addition to serious ethical concerns about the risks of fertility treatments and multiple pregnancies, there are consequentialist and social justice concerns about the multimillion-dollar cost of neonatal care associated with multiple births and, in a climate of medical cost-cutting, the responsible use of limited health care dollars.

PARTIAL BIRTH ABORTION

Partial birth abortion is a nonmedical term coined by antiabortionists to describe an abortion procedure known technically as intact dilation and extraction (D&X). D&X is used primarily in second-trimester abortions, and involves partially delivering a living fetus into the birth canal, then collapsing the skull and completing delivery of a dead but otherwise intact fetus. In an amici brief to the Supreme Court, the American College of Obstetricians and Gynecologists noted that D&X involves substantially less risk of complication than other methods of abortion used during the same gestational period (*Stenberg v. Carhart*, 2000). Fewer than 5 percent of abortions performed in the United States occur in the second trimester, with the vast majority taking place in the first trimester, but when the D&X procedure was widely publicized by abortion opponents in the mid-1990s, it created immediate controversy. President Bill Clinton twice vetoed federal bills to ban partial birth abortions, but a number of state laws were passed prohibiting the procedure. A Nebraska statute that made the performance of D&X a felony was challenged in a case brought to the Supreme Court in *Stenberg v. Carhart* (2000). The court held that the Nebraska statute violated the Constitution because it lacked any exemption for the preservation of the health of the mother, and because the law's vagueness imposed an undue burden on a woman's ability to choose the more common dilation and evacuation (D&E) abortion procedure, which sometimes involves partial delivery prior to fetal dismemberment. In striking down the Nebraska ban, the court invalidated the nearly identical laws of thirty other states.

From a consistent pro-life perspective, there can be no moral difference between partial birth abortions and abortions performed using other methods. Because a second-term fetus more closely resembles an infant than does an embryo or very early fetus, publicizing graphic and often gruesome descriptions of the D&X procedure helped the pro-life cause politically, but aside from its inflammatory aspect, it contributed little to the abortion debate. Many pro-choice ethicists, however, regard later abortions of healthy fetuses as more morally serious than early abortions. When the moral permissibility of abortion depends on the criteria used to determine fetal moral status, there is an unsettled empirical question that becomes more urgent as pregnancy continues.

FETAL PAIN

Recent antiabortion activity has focused on enacting legislation that limits access to abortion, revising restrictions based on gestational age, and mandating onerous requirements, including compulsory viewing of ultrasound images and invasive transvaginal ultrasounds for women seeking abortion. Because legislatures rarely act to mandate procedural requirements of medical providers or patients, that a specific population is targeted by abortion legislation gives rise to suspicions of gender bias and discrimination.

A number of states have enacted or proposed bans on abortion after 20 weeks on grounds of a novel theory: fetal pain. While the problem of fetal pain would be easily solved by the administration of fetal anesthesia during abortion, fetal pain bans seek to prohibit any abortion procedure on the ground of fetal pain, rather than restricting women to procedures less likely to cause pain. Nebraska's statute, for example, states that its purpose is to "assert a compelling state interest in protecting the lives of unborn children from the stage at which substantial medical evidence indicates they are capable of feeling pain" (Leg Bill 1103§1[5],5 [Neb. 2010]). The bill marks that point as twenty or more weeks' "postfertilization," thus moving the date of prohibition back considerably from the viability standard established in *Roe v. Wade*. The available medical evidence, however, does not support the statute's assertion that fetuses at twenty weeks' postfertilization are capable of feeling pain. Rather, the best available evidence suggests that fetal pain "may occur in the third trimester around 29 to 30 weeks' gestational age" (Lee et al. 2005, 952). Abortion bans based on sound scientific evidence of fetal pain, then, could move the bar several weeks past the point of viability rather than before it. Much depends, however, on how "feeling pain" is defined. The conscious experience of pain, which requires cortical processing across wide areas of the brain, does not occur before twenty-nine weeks' gestation. There is evidence that a physiological "stress response" can be provoked in fetuses much earlier, and has the potential to induce adverse long-term neural developmental changes. This "anatomical and functional perception of pain develops throughout the gestational process," but the "fetal stress response must not be used to imply that the fetus perceived pain at a conscious level" (Lowery et al. 2007, 278, 279).

The moral and legal significance of pain is far from clear. The Nebraska statute claims that the state has a compelling interest not only in preventing fetal pain, but in protecting the lives of fetuses that can experience pain. It does not follow, however, that the ability to experience pain—which all sentient creatures by definition can do—confers special moral status that prohibits either inflicting pain or killing such creatures, or that the prevention of pain "is enough to justify infringing on what is avowedly a fundamental right of women to have an abortion" (Cohen and Sayeed 2001, 238). If prevention of pain to sentient beings does justify restricting fundamental rights, it would plausibly justify infringing on other, less compelling rights as well by invoking a state interest in, for example, prohibiting hunting and animal agriculture to prevent pain to wildlife and livestock.

The language of the Nebraska statute, which refers to "unborn children," may signal an intention to use the capacity to feel pain as definitive of personhood. This would force the conclusion that all pain-capable creatures are persons. Such a definition of personhood—legal or moral—would be novel, and it is not obvious why it should stand. Additionally, while the personhood of a subject provides a moral reason not to inflict pain, neither personhood, nor the capacity to feel pain, nor both together suffice to make all inflictions of pain morally impermissible. Indeed, protecting persons from harm can provide a morally compelling reason to inflict pain on them, or on others. It is thus not obvious why fetal capacity to feel pain necessarily morally compels a prohibition on abortion. If it confers any protection at all, the fetal capacity for pain would prima facie compel no more than prevention of pain, either by the use of anesthesia, analgesia, or painless methods of abortion. A fetal person who feels pain, in that case, would be entitled to the same pain prevention measures to which any other person, including a woman undergoing abortion, is entitled.

CONSEQUENTIALISM AND ABORTION

The abortion debate in the United States has primarily focused on questions of rights, to the exclusion of all other considerations. A consequentialist approach that assesses the morality of abortion in light of its good and bad consequences has the potential to resolve the rights standoff, and a number of consequentialist considerations have bearing on the abortion debate. Abortion critics have long raised fears of a slippery slope, charging that permissiveness about abortion will inevitably lead to the devaluation of human life, and a "culture of death" in which attitudes about other forms of killing, such as infanticide and euthanasia, will become more permissive. The argument depends on the assumption that the killing of a fetus is regarded as just as serious as the killing of an infant, child, or adult, and that the permissibility of one entails the permissibility of all. The culture-of-death argument, like other slippery-slope arguments, also makes an empirical claim that the evidence to date fails to support. Since abortion was legalized in the United States in 1973, there has been no slide toward permissiveness about other forms of killing. Only three states have legalized physician-assisted suicide, under strict regulation that limits the practice to competent, terminally ill patients. In all other states that have considered physician-assisted suicide or euthanasia, voters have declined to endorse it. Neither is there evidence to suggest that the killing of newborns is more common in the United States than it was before abortion was legalized, but in parts of the world where infanticide has historically been an acceptable means of eliminating unwanted offspring, the availability of abortion has not increased the incidence of infanticide, but reduced it (Kristof 1991).

The coat hanger has been a powerful symbol of the abortion rights movement, a reminder of the dangerous, sometimes deadly abortions women endured before *Roe v. Wade*. Proponents of abortion rights have substantial evidence to support the claim that legal prohibitions on abortion lead to the deaths of women through self-induced abortions or illegal, unsafe abortions performed by untrained providers. Legal abortion performed under safe and sanitary conditions is generally safer than pregnancy, but in countries where abortion is prohibited, or access is severely limited, the negative consequences of unsafe and self-induced abortions include serious complications such as sepsis, hemorrhage, genital and abdominal trauma, perforated uterus, gangrene, secondary infertility, permanent disability, and death (World Health Organization [WHO] 2008). Treatment of complications from unsafe abortions places a serious strain on the medical infrastructure of developing countries, where a disproportionate share of scarce hospital resources are expended treating abortion complications. Unsafe abortions thus compromise other maternity and emergency health services in poor countries where health care is already inadequately resourced (WHO 2008). Statistics on abortion-related mortality are especially telling: The risk of death due to unsafe abortion is 30 per 100,000 live births globally and 40 per 100,000 for developing countries. At 80 per 100,000 live births, the risk associated with unsafe abortion for the least developed countries is twice that of developing countries. The figure for sub-Saharan Africa is even higher at 90 per 100,000, which includes eastern and middle Africa at 100 per 100,000, while in western Africa the ratio is 80 per 100,000 live births (WHO 2008). Statistics on abortion-related mortality in the United States tell a very different story about safe, legal abortion: the death rate is 0.6 per 100,000 procedures, making it as safe as a penicillin injection (WHO 2008).

INTERNATIONAL PERSPECTIVES ON ABORTION

Debates about the moral status of the fetus, and the moral distinction between therapeutic and nontherapeutic, or "social" abortion occur internationally. The influence of different religious traditions around the world frequently mirrors the influence of Catholicism and Evangelical Protestantism in the West, while colonial influences sometimes play a role in how restrictive or permissive abortion laws are in postcolonial countries (Aramesh 2009). Most Muslim countries, for example, have restrictive abortion laws that permit abortion only when the life of the mother is threatened (Hedayat, Shooshtarizadeh, and Raza 2006), although some, notably Turkey, Tunisia, and the former Soviet bloc states, permit unrestricted access to abortion. The ethical guidelines on abortion in Muslim countries generally reflect the teachings of the Koran, with its detailed discussion of embryonic development. Consistent with the belief that ensoulment occurs at four months, or 120 days' gestation, abortion is forbidden after this point, except in cases where the life of the mother is threatened (Hedayat et al. 2006). This reflects the moral status with which the fetus is imbued at ensoulment. In Iran, both therapeutic and nontherapeutic abortion are permitted during the first four months of gestation (Hedayat et al. 2006); therapeutic abortions for maternal or fetal indications conforming to a prescribed list of fifty-one eligible conditions are permitted after four months, when the fetus has moral status (Hedayat et al. 2006). Both therapeutic and nontherapeutic abortion for nonmedical or social reasons such as family hardship are subject to review and interpretation by an ayatollah, or religious leader, after four months' gestation. Although the decisions of ayatollahs can vary, they recognize the moral significance of both fetal life and of maternal burdens and suffering (Aramesh 2009).

The growing influence of technology, such as prenatal ultrasound, can be seen around the world. In Brazil, a predominantly Catholic country, abortion is a crime except in cases of pregnancy due to rape or to save a woman's life. In recent years, however, there has been a liberalization of abortion laws in Brazil to permit therapeutic abortion for fetal indications, particularly anencephaly (Diniz 2007). Diniz notes that "anencephaly became the paradigm for a wider debate about human rights and reproductive rights" (2007, 65) because "for the first time, abortion was discussed in human rights terms and not as a confrontation of religious beliefs" (67). Technology that permits prenatal diagnosis of fetal anomalies has thus sparked growing debate in Brazil about the moral status of the fetus and the right to life (Diniz 2007).

Elsewhere, particularly in Asian countries, the use of ultrasound to determine the sex of a fetus has led to growing concern about the use of abortion for sex selection. The People's Republic of China and India, two countries where there is a strong, traditional, cultural preference for male offspring, have experienced alarming growth in the incidence of sex-selective abortion following fetal ultrasound. Both countries restrict ultrasound and abortion, and criminalize their use for sex selection, as a response to a growing sex imbalance. (Nepal, South Korea, and Vietnam also have prohibitions on prenatal sex selection and abortion.) Despite the prohibitions, the practices continue to be widespread, and are growing as fetal ultrasound becomes more widely available and affordable (Ganatra 2008). Prabhat Jha et al. (2011) estimate that selective abortion of female fetuses rose from less than 2 million in the 1980s to up to 6 million in the first decade of the twenty-first century, accounting for the growing sex imbalance in India. Jha et al. (2006) show approximately 500,000 "missing" female births per year, translating to some 10 million sex-selective abortions over two decades, with the ratio of girls to boys decreasing to 92 girls per 100 boys. In China, where the one-child policy exacerbates the traditional demand for boys over girls, the ratio rose steadily from 106 boys per 100 girls in 1979 to 121:100 in 2005 (Hesketh, Lu, and Wei 2011). It is estimated that in 2005, the number of males under age twenty exceeded the number of females by around 32 million (Hesketh et al. 2011). The sex imbalance has the potential to create social instability, as large numbers of men find themselves unable to form stable relationships and marry. Prohibition has thus far not achieved the desired result of preventing female feticide or restoring the sex ratio. Indeed, the imbalance appears to be growing despite prohibitions, and has spread to more affluent and well-educated populations within both India and China, where the desire for fewer children appears to have enhanced the desire for boys (Jha et al. 2006). From a consequentialist ethical perspective, the resulting sex imbalances in countries where sex selection is commonly practiced appear to justify measures to prevent female feticide.

Restrictions and prohibitions on sex-selective abortion may have negative consequences for both women and female children, however. Sex selection is a symptom of pervasive social injustice and discrimination of women, but prohibiting sex selection may put women and girls at risk of abuse and death (Dickens, Serour, and Cook 2005).Traditional methods of eliminating unwanted female children include infanticide, abandonment, and fatal neglect, and restricting access to safe sex-selective abortion can have the unintended result of exposing female children to these dire consequences. It may also expose women to unsafe, illegal abortion and the risks of repeated pregnancy and childbirth (Dickens et al. 2005), as well as the negative familial consequences of failing to produce a male child. Viewed in that light, the consequences of restricting access to sex-selective abortion are, paradoxically perhaps, more dire for women and girls than allowing widespread female feticide, and must be weighed against the overall social harms that unfettered sex selection might produce. For consequentialist reasons, many would regard abortion as preferable in those circumstances. Little observes that in cultures that openly discriminate against women and girls, giving birth to a daughter who will face rejection and disrespect can do violence to a woman's ideals of creating and parenthood: "A woman living in a country marked by poverty and gender apartheid wants to abort because she decides it would be wrong for her to bear a daughter whose life, like hers, would be filled with hardship" (2002, 499).

While some feminists have decried sex selection against females as "femicide" or "gendercide," viewed in the context of patriarchal societies where females are systematically oppressed and devalued, Julie Zilberberg argues that a woman's choice "to have a son instead of a daughter, in order that her own child will have the best possible life, is an understandable one, particularly when viewed through the lens of relational autonomy" (2007, 518). Moreover, restricting access to sex selection has the effect of decreasing women's reproductive autonomy by limiting abortion rights, which cannot be counted as a feminist advance for women (Zilberberg 2007). To the extent that sex selection is a symptom of the more fundamental problem of oppression of women, an effective solution would seek to improve the social status of women and girls and enhance their autonomy, rather than reduce their options.

In Western countries where gender equality is avowed, there is profound disagreement about the use of prenatal screening and selective abortion to select fetuses for sex, either for purposes of family "balancing" or because of personal or cultural preferences. Sex selection leaves many abortion rights defenders uneasy with the prospect of justifying a morally serious practice done for reasons regarded as trivial or patently discriminatory.

SOCIAL JUSTICE AND ACCESS TO ABORTION

Women seeking abortions currently face difficulties that are not encountered in any other area of medical care. The consolidation of the health care industry has reduced the number of hospitals that perform abortion, and the majority of abortions today take place in freestanding clinics that are often besieged by antiabortion protesters, who block entry and harass patients. Abortion clinics have been bombed and doctors who provide abortion murdered. In 2009 Dr. George Tiller was shot to death by Scott Roeder, an antiabortion extremist, while attending a church service. Before his death, Tiller was one of only three doctors nationwide to offer late-term abortions. His clinic in Wichita, Kansas, had been bombed, and his home, office, and church had been the sites of protest for years (Stumpe and Davey 2009). The use or threat of violence by antiabortion extremists has had a profound effect on access to safe abortion by contributing to a steady decline in the number of doctors willing to perform abortion. A 2011 study shows that 87 percent of US counties have no abortion provider. The figures are even starker in rural counties, 97 percent of which lack abortion providers. Thirty-five percent of US women live in counties with no provider (Jones and Kooistra 2011).

In such an atmosphere, concerns about equality and social justice arise because limited access to abortion disproportionately affects poor women (Schulman 1998). The deeply divisive moral controversy over abortion has engendered a secondary political conflict over who should pay for abortions. Federal restrictions limit Medicaid funding for abortions to those necessary to preserve a woman's life, or for pregnancies that result from rape and incest (Guttmacher Institute 2012). At the same time, state and federal welfare reform initiatives have resulted in many women and children losing welfare benefits, putting a further strain on the ability of the poorest women to procure abortions that are available to financially better-off women, and compounding the economic injustice of a health care system already rife with inequalities. When access to safe abortion depends on the ability to pay, the right to abortion exists in principle but not practice.

Equally problematic from the standpoint of justice are government policies that deny financial assistance to family-planning clinics that provide information to clients about abortion. The global gag rule imposed on international family planning groups—which sometimes provide the only health care available to poor women and their children in developing countries—prohibits those organizations from receiving funds from the US government if they discuss abortion. The rule has become a political flashpoint in the abortion debate, with Republican administrations repeatedly adopting it, and Democratic administrations rescinding it. It is incompatible with principles of justice and equality to deny women access to information about the option and availability of abortions if it means they will be denied health care services that are available to women who are wealthier or better educated.

EARLY MEDICATION ABORTION

Early medication abortion has become an integral part of abortion care in the United States and elsewhere around the world. An estimated 30 million women worldwide have used mifepristone (RU-486), and the use of early medication abortion has resulted in a higher proportion of abortions being performed earlier in gestation (Ibis Reproductive Health n.d.). In 2008, 59 percent of abortion providers in the United States offered early medication abortions, accounting for 17 percent of all nonhospital abortions and about 25 percent of abortions before nine weeks' gestation (Guttmacher Institute 2011).

Plan B, or levonorgestrel, the so-called morning after pill, is an emergency contraceptive in the form of a single-dose pill that is effective at preventing pregnancy if taken within three days of unprotected sex. The pill was approved by the Food and Drug Administration (FDA) in 2009 for over-the-counter access without a prescription for women seventeen and older, and by prescription for women sixteen and under. The pill sparked controversy in December 2011 when an FDA advisory panel recommended approval for over-the-counter access to levonorgestrel for all females of childbearing potential, determining that the drug was safe and effective in adolescent females (FDA 2011). US Department of Health and Human Services (HHS) Secretary Kathleen Sebelius, however, rejected the recommendation, arguing that there was not "enough evidence to show that those who use this medicine can understand the label and use the product appropriately" (HHS 2011). The ruling held Plan B to a higher standard of safety than any other over-the-counter medication, creating the appearance that the political abortion controversy, rather than science, was behind the decision. In April 2013 a federal court overruled the FDA's age restriction and ordered the agency to make levonorgestrel available over-the-counter without age restriction.

Plan B has also been the focus of ethical controversy involving pharmacists who claim a conscientious objection to providing a drug they claim is a form of early abortion. In 2011 President Barack Obama revised the so-called federal conscience clause, which allows health care workers to "opt out" of performing duties they find morally objectionable, such as abortion and sterilization. Critics had argued that the conscience clause was so broad and vague that it would allow workers to opt out of providing not just abortion, but also birth control, AIDS treatment, and more. President Obama's revision, intended to revert the rules to their original intent, limit what medical personnel can refuse to perform to abortion and sterilization but not the dispensing of contraceptives (NPR 2011).

Balancing respect for individual conscience with unobstructed access to abortion and reproductive health care represents an ethical dilemma for which there is no easy resolution. Conscientious objection to providing abortion can be logically extended to allow refusal to refer or counsel women seeking abortion services. Such actions can amount to denial of care, particularly for women who live in underserved communities where access to providers is limited. The Canadian Medical Association's policy on conscientious objection to induced abortion states that a physician with moral objections to abortion should not be compelled to participate, and should "advise the patient that you do not provide abortion services ... [and] you will not initiate a referral to another physician who is willing to provide this service (unless there is an emergency)" (Blackmer 2007, 1310). Such broad protections, grounded on conscience, prevent women from accessing abortion and contraceptive services, resulting in an ethical conflict between the rights of medical personnel, who control access to medical treatment, and the rights of women to make autonomous choices about their reproductive health. While such conflicts may arise in many areas of health care provision, they are particularly common in women's reproductive health care because of the moral divisiveness of abortion. Julie Cantor argues for a moral imperative to restore "selfless professionalism" in medicine, noting that, "When broadly defined, conscience is a poor touchstone; it can result in a rule that knows no bounds," and permits "conscience creep" in which "all behavior becomes acceptable" (Cantor 2009, 1485). Conscience is a burden that belongs to the individual, Cantor argues, and patients should not have to bear it for professionals who freely choose their profession: "As the gatekeepers to medicine, physicians and other health care providers have an obligation to choose specialties that are not moral minefields for them" (2009, 1485). Rather than allowing conscience to license denial of care to patients, conscience and professionalism demand that providers put the needs of patients above their own.

CAN THE ABORTION CONFLICT BE RESOLVED?

In countries where abortion is legal, and countries where it is not, millions of women make individual moral choices to end pregnancies. Some seek abortion after contraceptive failure, others because it is the only contraceptive option available to them; some choose to end their pregnancies for financial or emotional reasons, or for the well-being of their families; still others decide to terminate a desired pregnancy because of an unwelcome prenatal diagnosis, or because their child is the wrong sex, or because their own health is in jeopardy. Regardless of what courts and politicians, ethicists and religious leaders decide about abortion, there will always be unwanted pregnancies, and there will always be women willing to risk their lives and health to have abortions. Those are the facts of the matter.

The moral picture is characterized by far less clarity. Few would argue that abortion is not a morally weighty issue, but just how serious it is remains unsettled. Abortion may be an insoluble political problem in a pluralistic society where incommensurable moral and religious convictions admit of little compromise.

Several philosophers have concluded that moral agreement about abortion is likewise unachievable. Bernard Gert (2010) makes the case that our common morality does not resolve every moral problem, and abortion is one of a small number of important moral questions that must remain controversial and unresolvable. This is because, Gert argues, all of the standard positions concerning abortion are morally acceptable, and there are neither conclusive arguments that abortion is prima facie morally wrong, nor that it is morally wrong to legally prohibit it. As with other genuinely controversial moral issues, it is futile to offer philosophical arguments, or proffer moral theories, in an attempt to resolve the abortion issue (Gert 2010). In such a moral stalemate, the solution is not to argue further, or attempt to marshal new biological facts (Gert argues there are none as concerns abortion), but to "promote moral humility or tolerance in people on both sides of the issue" (Gert 2010, 42).

David DeGrazia (2012) proposes a pluralist approach to prenatal moral status, in view of what he argues is an ethical and ontological stalemate. The discussion of abortion should thus shift to political and social policy, where the balance tips in favor of liberalism regarding abortion. While a "reasonable, well-informed person" could hold either a pro-life or pro-choice position, because the pro-life position rests on three debatable assumptions about "our essence and origins … the constancy of moral status throughout one's lifetime … and the relationship between full moral status and the ethics of killing prenatal human beings," a liberal approach to policy is called for, in view of women's interests in liberty and bodily integrity (DeGrazia 2012, 18). Such a liberal policy would be largely in accordance with the "viability" criterion for abortion, because "nearly everyone agrees that a sentient infant has moral status, and it is probably at least implicit in many people's thinking that a viable fetus could already be a newborn infant and therefore should have the same full moral status. In view of these points, and out of respect for the sensibilities of those who are pro-life … the viability criterion is optimal" (DeGrazia 2012, 50).

The prognosis for resolution of the moral controversy—or even a moral compromise—over abortion is not favorable. As Simon May notes, abortion is "a poor candidate for moral compromise because the most crucial point of contention is a discrete question: either a woman has the right to abort a pregnancy … or she does not" (2005, 347). There are compelling arguments for both sides, and no middle way for the moral discourse to follow (May 2005). What is left, then, is the possibility of a social and political compromise, about which ethics has little to say.

All sides can agree that the stakes are high in abortion, and the difficulty of resolving the moral conflict should not be understated. Equally reasonable and thoughtful moral theories about abortion have produced greatly divergent conclusions. If none of these theories has yet proved immune to counterargument and criticism, if none has yet prompted a collective sigh of relief that the debate is at last over, they have all contributed to the unavoidable conclusion that the abortion controversy defies simplification and, in its uniqueness, defies easy assimilation to familiar moral principles.

SEE ALSO *Adoption; Autonomy; Conscience; Conscience, Rights of; Double Effect, Principle or Doctrine of; Embryo and Fetus: I. Developments from Fertilization to Birth; Genetic Testing and Screening: I. Reproductive Genetic Testing; Harm; Human Dignity; Infanticide; Life; Maternal-Fetal Relationship: II. Ethical Issues; Maternal-Fetal Relationship: III. Legal and Regulatory Issues; Moral Status; Population Policies, Demographic Aspects of; Women, Historical and Cross-Cultural Perspectives*

BIBLIOGRAPHY

Aramesh, Kiarash. 2009. "A Closer Look at the Abortion Debate in Iran." *American Journal of Bioethics* 9 (8): 57–58.

Asch, Adrienne. 2000. "Why I Haven't Changed My Mind about Prenatal Diagnosis: Reflections and Refinements." In *Prenatal Testing and Disability Rights*, edited by Erik Parens and Adrienne Asch, 234–58. Washington, DC: Georgetown University Press.

Blackmer, Jeff. 2007. Clarification of the CMA's Position Concerning Induced Abortion. *Canadian Medical Association Journal* 176 (9): 1310.

Boonin, David. 2003. *A Defense of Abortion*. Cambridge, UK: Cambridge University Press.

Brody, Baruch. 1975. "The Morality of Abortion." In *Contemporary Issues in Bioethics*, 5th ed., edited by Tom L. Beauchamp and LeRoy Walters, 212–21. Belmont, CA: Wadsworth.

Callahan, Sidney. 1986. "A Case for Pro-Life Feminism." In *Ethical Issues in Modern Medicine*, 5th ed., edited by Bonnie Steinbock and John D. Arras, 366–75. Mountain View, CA: Mayfield.

Cantor, Julie. 2009. "Conscientious Objection Gone Awry—Restoring Selfless Professionalism In Medicine." *New England Journal of Medicine* 360 (15): 1484–85.

Cohen, I. Glenn, and Sadath Sayeed. 2011. "Fetal Pain, Abortion, Viability, and the Constitution." *Journal of Law, Medicine and Ethics* 39 (2): 235–42.

DeGrazia, David. 2012. *Creation Ethics: Reproduction, Genetics, and Quality of Life*. Oxford: Oxford University Press.

Dickens, B. M.; G. I. Serour; R. J. Cook; et al. 2005. "Sex Selection: Treating Different Cases Differently." *International Journal of Gynecology & Obstetrics* 90:171–77.

Diniz, Debora. 2007. "Selective Abortion in Brazil: The Anencephaly Case." *Developing World Bioethics* 7 (2): 64–67.

FDA. 2010. "Mifeprex Questions and Answers." Accessed November 2, 2012. http://www.fda.gov/Drugs/DrugSafety/PostmarketDrugSafetyInformationforPatientsandProviders/ucm111328.htm?utm_source=fdaSearch&utm_medium=website&utm_term=mifeprex&utm_content=2

Ganatra, Bela. 2008. "Maintaining Access to Safe Abortion and Reducing Sex Ratio Imbalances in Asia." *Reproductive Health Matters* 16 (31, Suppl.): 90–98.

Gert, Bernard. 2010. "Moral Disagreement concerning Abortion." *Diametros* 26:23–43.

Guttmacher Institute. 2011. "Facts on Induced Abortion in the United States." Accessed November 2, 2012. http://www.guttmacher.org/pubs/fb_induced_abortion.html

Guttmacher Institute. 2012. "State Funding of Abortion under Medicaid." Accessed November 2, 2012. http://www.guttmacher.org/statecenter/spibs/spib_SFAM.pdf

Hedayat, K. M.; P. Shooshtarizadeh; and M. Raza. 2006. "Therapeutic Abortion in Islam: Contemporary Views of Muslim Shiite Scholars and Effect of Recent Iranian Legislation." *Journal of Medical Ethics* 32:652–57.

Hesketh, Therese; Li Lu; and Zhu Wei. 2011. "The Consequences of Son Preference and Sex-Selective Abortion in China and Other Asian Countries." *Canadian Medical Association Journal* 183 (12): 1374–7.

HHS. 2011. "A Statement by U.S. Department of Health and Human Services Secretary Kathleen Sebelius." Accessed November 2, 2012. http://www.hhs.gov/news/press/2011pres/12/20111207a.html

Ibis Reproductive Health. n.d. Medication Abortion. Accessed November 2, 2012. http://www.medicationabortion.com/mifepristone/index.html

Jha, Prabhat; Maya A. Kesler; Rajesh Kumar; et al. 2011. "Trends in Selective Abortions of Girls in India: Analysis of Nationally Representative Birth Histories from 1990 to 2005 and Census Data from 1991 to 2011." *Lancet* 377:1921–8.

Jha, Prabhat; Rajesh Kumar; Priya Vasa; et al. 2006. "Low Male-to-Female Sex Ratio of Children Born in India: National Survey of 1.1 Million Households." *Lancet* 367:211–18.

Jones, Rachel K., and Kathryn Kooistra. 2011. "Abortion Incidence and Access to Services in the United States, 2008." *Perspectives on Sexual and Reproductive Health* 43 (1): 41–50.

Kristof, Nicholas D. 1991. "Stark Data on Women: 100 Million Are Missing." *New York Times*, November 5, C1.

Lee, Susan J.; Henry J. Peter Ralston; Eleanor A. Drey; et al. 2005. "Fetal Pain: A Systematic Multidisciplinary Review of the Evidence." *Journal of the American Medical Association* 294 (8): 947–54.

Leg Bill 1103§1(5),5 (Neb. 2010). Accessed March 28, 2013. http://www.legislature.ne.gov/FloorDocs/101/PDF/Slip/LB1103.pdf

Little, Margaret Olivia. 2002. "The Morality of Abortion." In *Ethical Issues in Modern Medicine*, 6th ed., edited by Bonnie Steinbock, John D. Arras, and Alex John London, 275–82. New York: McGraw-Hill.

Lowery, Curtis L.; Mary P. Hardman; Nirvana Manning; et al. 2007. "Neurodevelopmental Changes of Fetal Pain." *Seminars in Perinatology* 31:275–82.

Manninen, Bertha A. 2011. "Parental, Medical, and Sociological Responsibilities: 'Octomom' as a Case Study in the Ethics of Fertility Treatments." Special issue, *Journal of Clinical Research & Bioethics* S1:1–11.

Marquis, Don. 1989. "Why Abortion Is Immoral." *Journal of Philosophy* 86 (4): 183–202.

May, Simon C. 2005. "Principled Compromise and the Abortion Controversy." *Philosophy & Public Affairs* 33 (4): 317–48.

McInerney, Peter K. 1990. "Does a Fetus Already Have a Future Like Ours?" *Journal of Philosophy* 87 (5): 264–68.

Noonan, John T., Jr. 2003. "An Almost Absolute Value in History." In *Contemporary Moral Problems,* 7th ed., edited by James E. White, 116–21. Belmont, CA: Wadsworth.

NPR. 2011. "White House Revises Bush-Era 'Conscience Clause.'" Accessed October 5, 2012. http://www.npr.org/2011/02/18/133875483/White-House-Revises-Conscience-Clause

Palomaki, Glenn; Cosmin Deciu; Edward Kloza; et al. 2012. "DNA Sequencing of Maternal Plasma Reliably Identifies Trisomy 18 and Trisomy 13 as Well as Down Syndrome: An International Collaborative Study." *Genetics in Medicine* 14 (3): 296–305.

Reiman, Jeffrey. 1998. "Abortion, Infanticide, and the Changing Grounds of the Wrongness of Killing: Reply to Don Marquis's 'Reiman on Abortion.'" *Journal of Social Philosophy* 29 (2): 168–74.

Roe v. Wade. 1973. 410 U.S. 113; 159 (1973).

"RU-486 Report Card." 2002. *Washington Post*, May 5, B06.

Schulman, Susan. 1998. "Poorer Women Affected Most as Abortion Providers Dwindle." *Buffalo News*, November 15, 1A.

Sherwin, Susan. 1992. *Patient No More.* Philadelphia: Temple University Press.

"The Shooting of Dr. Slepian." 1998. *Washington Post*, October 27, A22.

State of Oklahoma, Senate Bill 1433 (2012).

Stenberg v. Carhart. 2000. 530 U.S. 914; 120 (2000).

Stumpe, Joe, and Monica Davey. 2009. "Abortion Doctor Shot to Death in Kansas Church." *New York Times*, May 31, A1.

Thomson, Judith Jarvis. 1971. "A Defense of Abortion." *Philosophy and Public Affairs* 1 (1): 47–66.

Tooley, Michael. 1972. *Philosophy & Public Affairs* 2 (1): 37–65.

Tooley, Michael. 1985. "Response to Mary Anne Warren." *Philosophical Books* 26 (1): 9–14.

United Nations. 1996 "Maternal Mortality Figures Substantially Underestimated, New WHO/UNICEF Study Says." Accessed October 31, 2013. http://scienceblog.com/community/older/archives/L/1996/A/un960207.html

Warren, Mary Anne. 1973. "On the Moral and Legal Status of Abortion." *Monist* 57 (1): 43–61.

Warren, Mary Anne. 1985. "Reconsidering the Ethics of Infanticide." *Philosophical Books* 26 (1): 1–9.

Warren, Mary Anne. 1989. "The Moral Significance of Birth." *Hypatia* 4 (3): 46–65.

World Health Organization. 2008. "Unsafe Abortion: Global and Regional Estimates of the Incidence of Unsafe Abortion and

Associated Mortality in 2008. Sixth ed." Accessed October 31, 2013. http://www.who.int/reproductivehealth/publications/unsafe_abortion/9789241501118/en/

Zilberberg, Julie. 2007. "Sex Selection and Restricting Abortion and Sex Determination." *Bioethics* 21 (9): 517–19.

L. Syd M. Johnson (2004, 2014)
Assistant Professor of Philosophy, Department of Humanities, Michigan Technological University

III. LEGAL AND REGULATORY ISSUES

Most contemporary legal systems regulate the practice of induced abortion. Governments around the world regulate whether, when, why, and how the estimated 43 million annual abortions occur. In some countries abortion is governed primarily by national laws; in others abortion is governed mainly by state or regional laws. Belief that abortion is unsafe, irreligious, immoral, unjust, or genocidal has tended to push regulation in the direction of laws that expressly prohibit some or all abortions. Convictions that abortion can alleviate overpopulation, avert economic hardship, protect women's health, promote sex equality, or eliminate undesirable progeny have tended to produce laws that permit, guarantee, or even compel abortion. More than 75 percent of the world's population lives in countries in which abortion is legal to protect the physical health of the pregnant woman (with many living in countries in which abortion is legal to protect the woman's mental health), even in cases in which the life of the pregnant woman is not at stake.

An international survey of existing law reveals four basic patterns or models of express abortion regulation:

1. a model of prohibition,
2. a model of permission,
3. a model of prescription,
4. a model of privacy.

Under the model of prohibition, the laws of a jurisdiction punish most or all abortions as criminal offenses, as in Ireland and Indonesia. In Ireland abortions are banned other than to save the life of the pregnant woman. In other countries with prohibitory laws, such as Indonesia, Brazil, and Mali, abortions can be permitted to save the life of the pregnant woman or in cases of rape or incest. Under the model of permission, laws permit abortions that meet criteria and conditions established by the government, as in Germany, Italy, England, India, and Zambia. In Germany women face counseling and waiting period requirements for otherwise permitted early abortions. In the United Kingdom excluding Ireland, abortion for health and disability reasons is lawful up to twenty-four weeks, but a woman must obtain the approval of two medical practitioners. Under the model of prescription, laws specifically require or encourage the termination of pregnancies falling into certain specific categories, as in the People's Republic of China. Finally, under the model of privacy, laws restrain the government from enactments that criminalize or severely restrict access to medically safe abortions, as in the United States and Canada. The model of privacy treats abortion decisions as substantially a matter of private choice rather than public law. In some countries using models of permission, prescription, and privacy, including the United States, China, France, the Russian Federation, and South Africa, women are not required by law to provide officials or physicians with a state-approved reason for routine legal abortions.

Abortion law is subject to change from one era to the next. Countries under the sway of the model of prohibition in one generation have moved toward the models of permission or privacy in subsequent generations. For example, when the US Supreme Court ruled in *Roe v. Wade* (1973) that the Constitution bars statutes categorically criminalizing all abortions, it announced a national standard for state and federal law that ushered out the model of prohibition and ushered in the model of privacy. Abortion law can also change from liberal to restrictive and back again in response to political developments and judicial interpretations of constitutional principle. Thus Poland adopted more restrictive abortion laws after democratic elections in 1989; greatly liberalized its law in 1996; and then in response to an adverse constitutional court ruling overturning the permissive 1996 law, quickly revised its law in 1997. Under a 1997 act of Parliament, Poland permits abortion to protect the pregnant woman's life or health or to terminate pregnancies resulting from criminal acts or in cases of fetal abnormality. Whether US abortion law is moving from liberal to conservative is discussed later in this entry.

THE MODEL OF PROHIBITION

The model of prohibition governs official abortion policy in many African, Latin American, South Asian, and Middle Eastern countries. Most jurisdictions in Europe and North America reject the model of prohibition, permitting abortion on request, where pregnancy results from rape or incest, or where the continuation of pregnancy threatens the physical, mental, or social well-being of the woman or her fetus. Ireland, a largely Roman Catholic nation, is one of the few European countries whose laws continued beyond the 1970s to criminalize abortions either absolutely or with strictly limited exceptions. Under a 1983 amendment to the Irish constitution, Irish law permits abortion only to save the life of the woman. Overturning a ruling that a teenage rape victim who credibly threatened suicide could not travel to England for an abortion, the Irish Supreme Court found in 1992 that abortion would be permissible "if it is established as a matter of probability that there is a real and substantial risk to the life as distinct from the health of the mother, which can only be avoided by the termination of her pregnancy." The penalty for performing an illegal abortion in Ireland is severe, up to fourteen years in prison. In 2013 the Irish president signed the Protection of Life during Pregnancy Bill 2013. The slightly less prohibitive law permits abortions to prevent the death or suicide of the pregnant woman. The 2013 statute followed an unrelated controversy concerning the 2012 death of the hospital patient Savita Halappanavar, whom physicians refused to abort even though the procedure might have averted her death due to sepsis resulting from a protracted natural miscarriage.

Jurisdictions whose laws reflect the model of prohibition often assert a strong religious or humanitarian policy interest in protecting what are thought to be the rights and interests of unborn children. However, other objectives have also prompted strict abortion prohibitions. For example, during the nineteenth and twentieth centuries abortion opponents in the United States cited the need to protect pregnant women from the medical and psychological risks of abortion. There can be no doubt that unskilled, unsanitary abortion procedures are a health risk and that some women who obtain abortion services experience medical complications and emotional anguish. However, some lawyers and judges doubt that medical abortion performed during the first three months of pregnancy is less safe than pregnancy and childbirth (Rhode 1989; Tribe 1990). They similarly doubt that elective medical abortion poses a serious risk of psychological harm. Although David C. Reardon (1987, 141), among other observers, asserts that "every woman pays a psychological price for abortion," the American Psychological Association has concluded that serious emotional problems rarely result from abortion.

Countries whose populations have been ravaged by war and genocide have sometimes proscribed abortion in an effort to increase the birthrate. Strict abortion prohibition has had the additional, if only implicit, goal of reinforcing social roles. The cultural assumption that motherhood is the appropriate social role for women buttressed Joseph Stalin's 1936 abortion prohibitions, enacted to furnish the Soviet Union with "a new group of heroes" (Tribe 1990, 56). The belief that bearing children is women's natural destiny may lead some to assume that birth control and abortion are both immoral and unhealthful. After 1933 Adolf Hitler prohibited contraception and declared abortion a capital offense on the belief that birth control was unhealthful. In contrast, abortion prohibitions adopted in Germany in 1943 aimed at the "vitality of the German people" and excluded from criminality abortions performed on "racially" undesirable women (Kraiker 1988, 189).

The reach of laws prohibiting abortion can be broad. Obtaining an abortion has been subject to criminal penalty in some instances, and so too has distributing abortion information. Provisions of the famous Comstock Law enacted by the US Congress in 1873—later rescinded—outlawed abortion-related implements and information as "obscene" and "immoral" (Rhode 1989; Garrow 1998). Offenders of the Comstock Law faced imprisonment with hard labor and monetary fines. Jurisdictions prohibiting abortion generally aim at the conduct of third-party abortion providers. However, some abortion statutes also criminalize pregnant women's own conduct, making it a punishable offense to obtain or seek abortions from third parties. Legal systems rarely punish medical abortion as the full equivalent of felonious unjustified murder.

Criminalizing nonsurgical and self-induced abortion poses special problems of detection and law enforcement. Pharmaceuticals approved for other purposes, like the cancer drug methotrexate, can be used to induce abortion. Self-induced abortion has often involved risky procedures, such as inserting knitting needles, wire coat hangers, or other foreign objects through the cervix. Many self-induced abortions are detected because they end tragically in medical and police emergencies. In 1989 a health care group in California promulgated a videotape demonstrating "menstrual extraction," a nonmedical abortion technique trainers say women can learn to perform safely at home with the help of a friend. To the extent that they are workable, abortion procedures that can be performed without professional assistance fall beyond the practical reach of law.

Prohibitive abortion law requires lawmakers to define what counts as abortion and therefore what is subject to criminal penalties. The surgical and medical procedures generally in use by physicians in licensed hospitals and clinics in Europe and the United States plainly qualify as abortion. However, certain forms of birth control not viewed as abortion could conceivably fall under the scope of strict abortion prohibitions. Popularly viewed as a form of contraception, the intrauterine device (IUD) may function as a kind of abortifacient, blocking implantation of a fertilized egg rather than preventing ovulation or fertilization. The drug RU-486 (mifepristone), developed by the French biochemist Étienne-Émile Baulieu and named for its French manufacturer, Roussel Uclaf, poses a related difficulty of definition. Described by French Minister of Health Claude Levin as "the moral property of women, not just the property of the drug company" (Greenhouse 1988), RU-486 arrived on the European scene in the 1980s and in the United States in 2000. Unlike pharmaceutical contraceptives that prevent fertilization or ovulation, RU-486 blocks the successful implantation of a fertilized egg. Rejecting the popular "abortion pill" label, Baulieu has suggested that RU-486 is neither contraception nor abortion but something new—"contragestation." Still, it seems unlikely that a jurisdiction that strictly prohibits abortion would view "contragestation" as anything other than early abortion.

Abortion flourishes under regimes of prohibitive abortion law (Sachdev 1988; Whittaker 2012). In fact about half of the abortions that take place each year are illegal in the jurisdictions in which they occur. The criminal code of Bangladesh strictly prohibits most abortions, but physicians commonly induce abortion by performing a uterine evacuation procedure known as menstrual regulation on women who are many weeks pregnant. Prohibitive abortion laws commonly fall short of their stated goals and public expectations, because governments are unwilling or unable to enforce the letter of the law. The prohibitive laws that governed abortion in the United States prior to *Roe v. Wade* were enacted to preserve unborn life and women's physical and mental health (Garrow 1998). It has been argued that the aim of fetal preservation was at least partly undermined by the large number of clandestine abortions performed, notwithstanding prohibitive laws (Tribe 1990). Although in the twentieth century most abortions were illegal in much of the United States prior to 1973, American women obtained an estimated 200,000 to 1.2 million abortions each year in the 1960s and the early 1970s (Tietze, Forrest, and Henshaw 1988), compared to about 1.5 million each year throughout the 1980s and the early 1990s and 1.3 million in 1997. Reardon (1987) puts the number of abortions pre-*Roe* at 100,000 to 200,000 per year. The aim of preserving women's health may have been frustrated under the regime of prohibition, because clandestine abortions were commonplace but were not always performed by skilled practitioners in hygienic settings. This was especially true of the illegal abortions obtained by African American women, who accounted for a disproportionate number of the victims of illegal procedures. (Twenty percent of the deaths related to pregnancy and childbirth in the United States in 1965 were attributed to illegal abortions.) Legalization of abortion probably resulted in a small to moderate increase in the number of abortions, but it appears to have greatly decreased the incidence of abortion-related infertility and death.

MODEL OF PERMISSION

The model of permission became the pervasive one around the world in the twenty-first century. Under the model of permission, abortion is legally available but only with the approval of government officials or officially designated decision makers, such as administrative boards, committees, physicians, or judges. In some permission-model jurisdictions officials grant permission pro forma in nearly every case. In Norway, prior to 1975 reforms that liberalized abortion, as many as 94 percent of the requests for abortions made to abortion boards were routinely granted (Olsnes 1993). Official decision makers in permissive jurisdictions rely on a handful of factors to determine which abortions to permit and which to prohibit (Glendon 1987; Petersen 1993).

The stage of pregnancy is very frequently a factor. Officials called on to implement legal norms or exercise discretion often permit "early" abortions and prohibit "late" ones. This no doubt helps explain the statistic that 90 percent of reported abortions take place within the first three months of pregnancy. Another factor decision makers commonly consider is the woman's medical or social status. Restrictive laws require that officials deny permission to abort for reasons other than medical hardship. Liberal laws often require that officials allow abortions because pregnancy or childbirth would involve social or economic hardship for the woman. In many jurisdictions grounds for social hardship include rape, incest, or the age and marital status of the woman. The health or condition of the fetus can be a third factor in permitting or prohibiting abortion. The law may permit access to abortion on evidence that a child would be born with serious physical or mental abnormalities.

Genetic testing for the purpose of enabling parents to abort fetuses with undesirable traits is already practiced in the United States. Health care providers in some states even face "wrongful life" and "wrongful birth" lawsuits for negligent failure to offer women information needed to prevent or abort an unwanted pregnancy. With advances in prenatal testing that enable detection of the sex of a fetus, it is possible for a pregnant woman to abort selectively unwanted male or female offspring. In some instances abortion for sex selection may be tied to a desire to avoid giving birth to a child with a gender-related genetic disease. Jurisdictions that permit abortion without regard to reason presumably permit abortion for sex selection. An outlier in this regard is Vietnam, which has liberal abortion laws but forbids abortion for the reason of sex selection (Wolf et al. 2010).

For most of the twentieth century a number of countries governed abortion under highly bureaucratic versions of the model of permission (Sachdev 1988). For a time in the Eastern European countries of Hungary, Romania, Poland, and Bulgaria, abortion was lawful only if approved by a state board or committee. These countries reportedly permitted abortion in almost every case through the fourth month of pregnancy. Romania reverted to a prohibitive policy in 1966 in response to concerns about underpopulation and the health effects of multiple abortions. It prohibited most contraception and abortions for women who did not have at least four, and eventually five, children. Abortion prohibition was accompanied by a significant incidence of mortality related to illegal abortions. In the mid-1980s 86 percent of the women in Romania who died as a consequence of pregnancy or childbirth died as a result of illegal abortions, compared with, for example, 29 percent in the Soviet Union and 13 percent in Sri Lanka.

Other historical instances of the bureaucratic model of permission are the laws and administrative regulations in force in Denmark from 1939 to 1973 and in Sweden from 1939 to 1974. In Denmark local and national committees consisting of teams of social workers, physicians, and psychiatrists evaluated the applications of women seeking legal abortions. Scandinavian officials on boards or committees charged with decision making typically assessed the impact of childbirth and child care on the mental or physical health of the woman and the woman's living conditions. The Israeli Ministry of Health regulations enacted in 1978 permitted hospitals and clinics to form committees consisting of two physicians and a social worker to decide whether to grant women's abortion requests. Although living conditions, such as other children and economic hardship, were initially an authorized basis for granting abortion requests, Israel amended the law in 1980 under pressure from religious groups and in response to concerns about a declining population rate. In the early twenty-first century in Israel the vast majority of abortion requests brought to one of about forty official committees are granted. Abortions sought on maternal health or fetal disability grounds are available at no cost.

At the beginning of the twenty-first century a number of countries in Asia, South America, Europe, and North America made a woman's obtaining an abortion dependent on the approval of one or more physicians, a judge, or one or both parents. Great Britain and countries whose abortion laws were modeled on Great Britain's—Hong Kong, Zambia, and some states in Australia—are examples of places whose laws place decision making in the hands of physicians. The law of Great Britain was transformed over a great many centuries from a model of prohibition to a model of permission and even a model of privacy. Early English common law embodied the model of prohibition, at least for abortions taking place after the first few months of pregnancy. The common law proscribed abortion after quickening, about the fourth month of pregnancy, when fetal animation or ensoulment was deemed to have taken place. In 1861 the statutory abortion law of Great Britain defined as a felony any act intended to cause abortion, whether induced by the woman herself, if she were pregnant, or by others, whether or not she was in fact pregnant. The Abortion Act of 1967 abolished the nineteenth-century felony. The act's liberal provisions permit an abortion where any two medical practitioners certify in good faith that pregnancy "would involve risk to the life of the pregnant woman, or of injury to the physical or mental health of the pregnant woman or any existing children of her family, greater than if the pregnancy were terminated." Under this rule, qualifying for abortion poses no practical difficulty for women with the money to pay private physicians. As English law illustrates, the model of permission can have the distinct effect of empowering the medical and psychiatric professions to govern reproduction in accordance with their profession's internal standards of judgment.

Abortion is common in Australia, where abortion rights vary significantly from state to state and are governed both by common law and criminal statute. A liberalizing trend has been observed since the mid-1990s, when only South Australia and the Northern Territory had statutes specifically permitting some abortions. In 1998 controversy erupted over Australian abortion law when two physicians were arrested in Western Australia for violating a moribund nineteenth-century criminal statute. The doctors had performed a consensual abortion in 1996 on a Maori woman who stored the aborted fetus in her refrigerator, planning to take it to New Zealand for burial in accordance with Maori traditions. Following reforms, early abortion is available virtually on demand in some Australian states and is subject to enforced restrictions in others.

In India the Medical Termination Pregnancy Law enacted in 1971 permitted abortions that one or, if the woman is more than twelve weeks pregnant, two physicians certify. Grounds for certification are liberal. Abortion may be obtained to preclude a risk to the pregnant woman's mental or physical health or a risk of the birth of a child with serious mental or physical abnormalities. No abortions after twenty weeks are legal under the law. A woman's mental health is considered at risk in cases of economic hardship and where pregnancy resulted from failed contraception. The 1975 Abortion and Sterilization Act made many abortions lawful in the Republic of South Africa on the certification of two physicians that statutory requirements are met. The law required that where abortion was sought on grounds of risk to mental health, one of two certifying physicians be a psychiatrist willing to attest to danger of permanent mental harm. South Africa liberalized its abortion law in 1996 and 2008, making early abortion available on demand.

French law permits women to make their own judgments (early in pregnancy) about whether they are entitled to abortion on grounds of hardship. In this respect French law resembles the federal law of the United States under *Roe v. Wade*. French regulations enacted in 1975 are representative of international responses to the judicial transformation of US law with *Roe v. Wade* in 1973. Reflecting the aspirations of both the model of permission and the model of privacy, the French enactment begins with a declaration that the law guarantees respect for every human being from the beginning of life and that this principle is to be sacrificed only in case of necessity and according to specific conditions. But the law authorizes any woman who is twelve or fewer weeks pregnant to ask a physician for an abortion if she believes pregnancy or childbirth will create hardship. Moreover at any stage of pregnancy, right up to the moment of birth, abortion is lawful if two physicians, one of them from an official list, certify that continuation of pregnancy would put the woman's health in grave peril or that there is a strong possibility that the child would suffer from an incurable condition.

The French abortion law imposes numerous conditions on all abortions. Attending physicians must inform women of the medical risks of abortion and give them an official guide to the forms of assistance available to families, mothers, and children and to relevant social service organizations. Women then must consult one of the listed social services. Women wishing to proceed with abortion must confirm their request in writing after a one-week waiting period. Abortions must be performed by physicians in a public or recognized private hospital and must be reported to the regional health authorities. Hospitals must provide women who have obtained abortions with birth control information.

The model of privacy may best describe the overall aspiration of *Roe v. Wade*. However, the model of permission is arguably more descriptive of US abortion law pertaining to unemancipated minors. The Supreme Court has taken the position that minors have a constitutional right to privacy and may terminate their pregnancies without parental consent but that minors may not object on constitutional grounds to parental notification requirements and waiting periods. Individual justices on the court have argued that requiring pregnant minors to notify family members of pregnancy and abortion in effect gives veto powers to third parties in a way that is inconsistent with the spirit of *Roe v. Wade*.

Yet a majority held in *Hodgson v. Minnesota* (1990) that states providing a "judicial by-pass procedure" may attempt to involve one or both parents in minors' abortion decision making by requiring minors or their physicians to contact parents in advance of abortion. In judicial bypass procedures minors must be permitted to ask a judge to waive parental notification requirements. The judge is expected to waive the requirement if he or she determines that the minor is mature or that notification is not in the minor's best interests. Justices in the minority have objected that bypass procedures are unwarranted, because most minors notify parents or other responsible adults of pregnancy and abortion and most minors seeking judicial waiver obtain it. In addition, the practical effect of mandatory notification is that some teens will delay abortion, increasing costs and medical risks. Some justices have argued that laws requiring parental involvement place minors with abusive parents or broken homes at a disadvantage and even at mortal risk.

MODEL OF PRESCRIPTION

Under the models of permission and privacy, a government permits some or all of the abortions women want. Under the model of prescription, a government compels or virtually compels women to obtain abortions the government wants. Far-reaching compulsory abortion laws have been rare in the modern world. In the West policy makers frown on official and unofficial policies of mandatory abortion for poor and mentally incompetent women. Although health care providers reportedly recommend abortion in some instances—for example, when a pregnant woman is addicted to cocaine or infected with HIV—the US government does not officially recommend or mandate abortion for any class of pregnancy. Under a penal code adopted in 1979, Cuban law proscribes abortion performed without the permission of the woman.

In an effort to control overpopulation and protect its economy, China began adopting "planned-birth" family-planning measures in 1953. These measures aggressively encourage abortion through a system of penalties and rewards. Under the Chinese constitution, both the government and individuals are responsible for the planned-birth policy. In 1974 couples were limited to two children. Since 1979 couples wishing to bear children have been authorized to have only one child and then only after securing a government permit. Women in certain parts of the country are allowed two children under certain conditions. To encourage compliance with the family-planning measures, abortion is offered at no cost and may entitle the woman to a two-week paid leave of absence; women who have an IUD inserted or a tubal ligation along with abortion may receive additional paid leave. The effect of the planned-birth policy on the abortion rate in China is not known in the West. Despite a law against sex identification of the fetus by technical means during pregnancy, abortion for sex selection is reported (as is female infanticide). Chinese families have reportedly resorted to infanticide and selective abortion to ensure that their one-child quota is filled by a child of the culturally preferred male sex.

MODEL OF PRIVACY

Under the model of privacy, the law rarely compels abortion and permits all or virtually all abortions as long as they are performed by medically qualified persons in clinics, hospitals, or other qualified facilities. Safety is a frequent goal of legal systems characterized by the model of privacy, although safety is not necessarily suggested by "privacy" nomenclature. The Soviet Union adopted the model of privacy on safety and privacy grounds in 1920, more than a half century before the model came to dominate understandings of US law. The goal of the Soviet decree legalizing any abortion performed by a physician in a state hospital was both to keep women safe from unskilled abortionists and to secure women's freedom and equality in work, education, and marriage. In 1936 the decree was rescinded in favor of a law prohibiting abortion other than to spare the life or health of the woman or to prevent transmission of an inheritable disease. The shift back to the models of prohibition and permission seems to have been motivated by concern about declining birthrates, health effects of medical abortions, and diminished regard for marriage and childbearing. But in 1955 the Soviet law moved back toward the model of privacy, again to protect women from unskilled abortionists and to give women themselves an opportunity to decide whether to become mothers (Sachdev 1988).

In Japan abortion has been legal since the government passed the Eugenic Protection Laws in 1948 to protect women's health and deter the birth of what were considered undesirable offspring. In practice abortion is available to women in Japan on request. The law does limit abortion, but the limitations are extremely liberal: abortion is permitted when performed by designated physicians to avert mental and physical disease or abnormalities, when pregnancy results from violence, or when the woman's health would be impaired for physical or economic reasons. Functionally one can view Japan as a model of privacy jurisdiction, yet women's autonomy and equality are not the express policy objectives of its liberal abortion law. Japan follows the model of permission insofar as laws restrict abortion and have not been designed specifically to promote autonomous, private decision making. For nearly thirty years after they had been approved for use in North America and Europe, low-dose birth control pills were banned in Japan out of concerns about safety. The end of the ban in 1999 could mean that abortion will no longer function as a major form of birth control in Japan.

In the United States abortion policy since the early 1970s has been directed to women's rights. During the early 1970s the United States and a number of other countries adopted laws approximating the model of privacy. The theory that during the first trimester abortion ought to be available without any restrictions gained popularity. In effect this approach was adopted in East Germany in 1972, Denmark in 1973, Sweden in 1974, France in 1975, and Norway in 1978 (Sachdev 1988; Olsnes 1993). "Fetal viability," the point at which, in some of these countries, the interests of the woman cease to be accorded overriding weight, is variously fixed between twenty weeks and twenty-eight weeks. In Norway, under 1978 amendments to a 1975 law, a woman "shall herself make the final decision concerning termination of pregnancy provided that it is possible to perform the operation before the twelfth week of pregnancy has elapsed." After the twelfth week abortion sought for a number of medical or social indications is available on successful application to an "abortion board" (Olsnes 1993).

In *Regina v. Morgentaler* (1988) the Supreme Court of Canada found by a margin of five to two that provisions of the criminal code infringed section 7 of the Canadian Charter of Rights and Freedoms promising "life, liberty and security of the person." The Canadian justices argued that "personal security," "bodily integrity," "human dignity," and "self-respect" were threatened by interference with reproductive choices (Morton 1993). The Canadian legislature remains free to regulate abortion consistent with the *Morgentaler* decision. However, in 1990 a bill to restrict abortion access to women whose physicians certified a health-related need for the procedure failed. The government thereafter announced that it would not seek new abortion legislation.

In Canada, the United States, and other privacy-model jurisdictions, liberal abortion laws permit autonomous choices about matters that profoundly affect women's bodies, lifestyles, and equality. However, it is generally recognized that laws that decriminalize and deregulate abortion do not guarantee that every woman who desires an abortion will get one. Abortion is costly and may or may not be covered by the health insurance of women who have insurance. The US Supreme Court has repeatedly held that state and federal governments may encourage childbirth over abortion by refusing to include abortion among Medicaid and other entitlements awarded the poor. As a consequence, public funding for abortion is not available as a matter of right, publicly funded civilian and military hospitals are not required to perform abortion services, and states may prohibit physicians employed by public hospitals from performing abortions.

FOCUS: THE UNITED STATES

The Constitution of the United States does not mention the word *abortion*. However, the Supreme Court has consistently held since *Roe v. Wade* and *Doe v. Bolton* (1973)—the simultaneously decided, lesser-known companion case—that the due process clause of the Fourteenth Amendment guarantees American women a fundamental right to obtain medically safe abortions. States may not categorically ban abortion or unduly burden women's fundamental constitutional right to terminate pregnancy.

Connecticut passed the first American legislation against abortion in 1821 (Garrow 1998). At first American law did not penalize early (pre-quickening) abortions. However, between 1827 and 1860 twenty states or territories passed statutes against abortion at all stages of pregnancy. By 1868 thirty-six states or territories had antiabortion statutes in place, enforcement of which was often lax. In 1965 all fifty states treated abortion and attempted abortion at all stages of pregnancy as felonies, subject to certain exceptions. In forty-six states and the District of Columbia the relevant statutes explicitly permitted abortion to save the pregnant woman's life, and in two of the other four states a similar exception was recognized by the courts.

Between 1967 and early 1973 a dozen jurisdictions in the United States adopted somewhat permissive abortion laws patterned on the model legislation suggested in 1962 by the influential American Law Institute. These laws permitted abortion when performed by a licensed physician who determined that there was a substantial risk that pregnancy would seriously injure the physical or mental health of the woman, that the child would be born with a grave physical or mental defect, or that the pregnancy resulted from rape or incest. Almost all of the other reforming jurisdictions nevertheless sought to strengthen the institutionalization of abortion practice by stipulating that an abortion would be lawful only if performed in an accredited hospital after approval by a committee established in the hospital for that purpose.

The decriminalization of abortion on the national level lagged behind the decriminalization of contraception. In 1965 the Supreme Court decided *Griswold v. Connecticut*, holding that states may not outlaw a married woman's use of birth control. The court based its ruling on an unenumerated constitutional "right to privacy" implicit in the Bill of Rights and the Fourteenth Amendment. This same right to privacy was invoked in 1973 in *Roe v. Wade* to limit government interference with abortion. The right to privacy was and is controversial among lawyers and judges reluctant to recognize novel unenumerated rights. However, both the American Medical Association and the American College of Obstetricians and Gynecologists favored legalization of abortion. The immediate effect of *Roe v. Wade* and *Doe v. Bolton* was to invalidate the laws prohibiting abortion in every state (except perhaps the already very permissive laws adopted in 1969 and 1970 in New York, Alaska, Hawaii, and Washington).

Roe and *Doe* established four standards:

1. No law can restrict the right of a woman to have a physician abort her pregnancy during the first three months, or first trimester, of her pregnancy.
2. During the second trimester the abortion procedure may be regulated by law only to the extent that the regulation reasonably relates to the preservation and protection of maternal health.
3. At the point at which the fetus becomes "viable," a law may prohibit abortion but only subject to an exception permitting abortion whenever necessary to protect the woman's life or health (including any aspects of her physical or mental health).
4. No law may require that all abortions be performed in a hospital, or that abortions be approved by a hospital committee or by a second medical opinion, or that abortions be performed only on women resident in the state concerned.

The court in *Roe* and *Doe* concluded that the Constitution does not accord legal personhood status to the fetus. Critics of this conclusion point out that the unborn are implicitly treated as legal persons in several other areas of the law. The unborn are taken into account in the allocation of property rights and the attribution of criminal and civil responsibility. For example, the unborn can inherit property. Negligently killing or injuring a fetus can give rise to civil liability for wrongful death, wrongful birth, battery, and other torts.

Roe made clear that women were not to be ascribed a right to exclusive control over their bodies during pregnancy. Yet the case signaled that the Constitution limits the role government may play in abortion decisions. In the first decade and a half after *Roe* the court struck down numerous state abortion restrictions. States unsuccessfully attempted to control abortion through:

- advertising restrictions;
- zoning restrictions;
- record-keeping and reporting requirements;
- elaborate "informed consent" and physician-counseling requirements;
- mandatory waiting periods;
- bans on abortions for sex selection;
- the requirement of the presence of a second physician during the abortion procedure;
- the requirement that physicians employ methods of abortion calculated to save the lives of viable fetuses;
- the oversight requirement that physicians send all tissue removed during an abortion to a laboratory for analysis by a certified pathologist;
- the requirement that insurance companies offer at a lower-cost insurance that does not cover most elective abortions;
- legislating a statewide information campaign to communicate an official state policy against abortion;
- legislating criminal sanctions for physicians who knowingly abort viable fetuses;
- requirements that some or all abortions after the first trimester be performed in a hospital.

However, the Supreme Court has repeatedly validated state and federal government policies that prefer childbirth to abortion by declining to pay for the abortions of poor women entitled to welfare benefits for prenatal care and childbirth (Solinger 1998).

A major reaffirmation of *Roe*, *Thornburgh v. American College of Obstetricians and Gynecologists* (1986), held that states were not permitted to indirectly prohibit abortion by encumbering the decision to seek abortion with unnecessary regulations. A series of highly publicized court decisions handed down since 1989 appear to permit more extensive regulation of first- and second-trimester abortions than *Roe* and *Doe* seemed to contemplate. *Webster v. Reproductive Services* (1989) permitted legislation requiring viability testing and limits on publicly funded physician care. The court declined in *Webster* to decide the constitutionality of the declaration in the preamble of a Missouri statute that the "life of each human being begins at conception" and that "unborn children have protectable interests in life, health and well being," because the state had not yet sought to limit abortion by appeal to it. Encouraged by the *Webster* decision, several states and the territory of Guam sought between 1989 and 1992 to ban or discourage abortion through aggressive new regulation and enforcement. Anticipating that the Supreme Court would welcome an opportunity to overrule *Roe* in the 1990s, Guam enacted legislation prohibiting most abortion and its advocacy. A federal judge quickly declared Guam's law unenforceable under *Roe.*

In two 1990 cases critical of *Roe*, *Hodgson v. Minnesota* and *Ohio v. Akron Center for Reproductive Health*, the court upheld parental notification requirements for minors. *Rust v. Sullivan* (1991) upheld a federal "gag rule" statute, subsequently eliminated by Congress, prohibiting abortion counseling by physicians in federally supported facilities. *Planned Parenthood of Southeastern Pennsylvania v. Casey* (1992) affirmed *Roe* as the law of the land and invalidated spousal notification. However, the case upheld a twenty-four-hour waiting period as part of a state's "informed consent" procedures. *Casey* shed the trimester framework of *Roe*, opening the door to regulation at any stage of pregnancy. *Casey* also announced a weaker standard of review in abortion cases that promised to permit more state regulation. Under *Roe* abortion statutes were to be struck down if they did not further a "compelling" state interest. Under *Casey* statutes "rationally related" to a "legitimate" state interest are to be upheld, assuming they do not "unduly burden" the abortion right. The weakening of the standard of review in abortion cases after the *Casey* decision underscores that constitutional abortion law in the United States, although grounded in the model of privacy, seems also to include elements of the model of permission. For this reason it seems likely that the Supreme Court will be asked again and again to clarify the extent to which the state and federal government may restrict abortion rights. Proposed state and federal statutes, such as the Partial-Birth Abortion Ban Act of 2000 and the Born Alive Infant Protection Act of 2002, were attempts to extend legal protections to viable fetuses and curb certain abortion practices. Yet in *Stenberg v. Carhart* (2000) the court declared unconstitutional a Nebraska statute outlawing so-called partial birth abortions. The court reasoned that the broadly drafted statute lacked a constitutionally necessary exception for abortions to save the life of the woman and could be construed to rule out the dilation and evacuation procedure and the more controversial dilation and extraction or partial birth procedures. The federal Partial-Birth Abortion Ban Act of 2003 clarified the ambiguity of proscribed abortion procedures, proscribing only dilation and extraction. The 2003 act contained an exception for the life but not for the health of the woman, with a congressional finding that dilation and extraction would never be used out of a concern for the health of the woman. The constitutionality of the 2003 act was upheld in *Gonzales v. Carhart* (2007).

The US Food and Drug Administration approved the controversial drug RU-486 in 2000. State and federal lawmakers who opposed its use acted quickly but unsuccessfully to propose legislation outlawing the drug or limiting the types of physicians authorized to prescribe it. The long awaited "abortion pill" has not become the elected method of abortion for a majority of American patients and providers, although its use is consistently increasing as a percentage of overall early abortions. Notwithstanding the limited popularity of mifepristone as an abortifacient, because of *Roe* and possible nonabortion uses of the medication, it is unlikely that a blanket legislative ban on mifepristone would be found constitutional. In 2011 seven states enacted laws that require the physician prescribing a drug for abortion to be in the same room as the patient, thereby outlawing telemedicine in this medical area.

Many Americans favor regulation of abortion, though polls consistently show that most Americans believe that abortion should be legal in any circumstance or under certain circumstances. For example, a May 2013 Gallup (2013) poll showed that more than 78 percent of Americans believed that some abortions (52%) or all abortions (26%) should be legal. The Gallup poll (2013) also found significant dissatisfaction with abortion laws—40 percent of Americans were dissatisfied with current laws on abortion, and 27 percent want stricter regulation. In the 1970s and 1980s attempts were made on both sides of the abortion debate to provide a national abortion law standard for the United States by legislation. Several attempts have been made in both houses of Congress to undercut the judicial decision through legislation. One attempt, premised on the idea of states' rights, involved legislation that if adopted would have established that no right to an abortion is secured by the Constitution and therefore that the fifty states are free to adopt restrictions on abortions. A second attempt, premised on fetal personhood, would have expanded the definition of *person* under the due process and equal protection clauses of the Fifth and Fourteenth Amendments. The fetal personhood legislation would have declared that the right to personhood attaches from the moment of conception.

Supporters of *Roe* in Congress have attempted to legislate the holding of *Roe* through a federal statute. The Freedom of Choice Act was introduced in Congress several times, beginning in November 1989. Its passage by Congress would have prohibited states from enacting restrictions on the right to abortion before fetal viability. Initiatives to amend the federal Constitution to include pro-life or pro-choice strictures have not advanced far beyond the drafting table.

Two states have, in different ways, established an abortion right independent of *Roe*. With *In re T. W.* (1989) the Florida Supreme Court invalidated that state's parental consent requirement, relying on the state constitution. As a result of this decision, Florida recognized a fundamental abortion right independent of *Roe*. A Maryland referendum endorsed by voters in 1992 similarly established state abortion rights not tied to the fate of *Roe*.

In contrast to the failed efforts at federal legislation on either side of the debate in the 1970s and 1980s and to some extent consistent with the 1998 poll that showed that Americans favored further restrictions on access to abortion, state legislation in 2011, 2012, and 2013 became an increasingly common tool for those seeking to enhance regulation of access to abortion. For example, several states in 2011 enacted one or more of the following laws:

1. placing restrictions on later abortions;
2. increasing the waiting periods after an initial consultation for an abortion;
3. mandating a pre-abortion counseling protocol;
4. requiring an ultrasound prior to any abortion;
5. restricting private insurance coverage for abortion;
6. increasing regulation of clinics that provide abortion services.

As an illustration of the second and third items, South Dakota enacted a law that would require at least a seventy-two hour waiting period for an abortion after an initial consultation with a mandated counseling session at a pregnancy crisis center during the interim. As of 2013 this law was enjoined by court order. As an illustration of the third item, Indiana and Kansas require that the woman be told that the fetus is a person. As an illustration of the fourth item, five states enacted laws mandating an ultrasound prior to abortion. Ultrasound mandates (North Carolina and Texas) requiring also that the woman be shown the ultrasound and have it explained to her have been enjoined by court orders. As an illustration of the sixth item, four states enacted laws that directed state agencies to regulate clinics that provide abortion services. The Kansas health department put in place numerous clinic requirements, such as square footage and doctor privilege requirements, with a short time span of compliance, which in 2013 were enjoined by court order. After a battle in the legislature, Texas enacted a new statute in 2013 restricting most abortions to before twenty weeks and requiring enhanced clinical facilities.

The constitutional status of many of these early twenty-first century prohibitions and regulations is unclear. As noted above, some of the laws have been enjoined, yet some have not. Some of these laws have yet to be subjected to judicial scrutiny. As long as *Roe*, *Doe*, and *Casey* stand, they will provide a national abortion law standard for the United States. The test of constitutionality is whether the 2011 state laws are rationally related to a legitimate state interest and do not unduly burden women when exercising their rights.

THE IMPLICATIONS OF ABORTION LAW

The liberalization of abortion law establishes rights for women who wish to terminate their pregnancies. Contemporary abortion rights advocates construe these rights as "human rights" in some cases and rights called for by "reproductive justice" in others. Advocates who advance access to reproductive services as human rights and as reproductive justice stress that the discourse of legal privacy obscures some of the important dignitarian, egalitarian, and welfare grounds for liberal abortion policies and the substantial economic and political barriers to the exercise of meaningful safe and independent choices by women, especially women of color and women in developing countries.

The full implications of abortion rights are unclear in matters concerning:

- the use and disposal of fertilized eggs, embryos, and fetal remains;
- the enforceability of surrogate mother and surrogate gestator contracts granting third parties a legal interest in a woman's pregnancy;
- the criminalization of pregnant women's conduct;
- the tort liability of health care providers for wrongful birth and wrongful life;
- organized protest at abortion facilities. (Purdy 1996)

One legal concern is whether women who elect to abort have a familial, proprietary, or other interest in routinely aborted embryos or fetuses. State statutes typically require that abortion providers dispose of fetal remains in the way physicians dispose of other excised tissues. Yet some effort has been made to treat abortion tissues and fetuses differently either because of their possible commercial value for research into the treatment of diabetes, leukemia, Alzheimer's disease, and Parkinson's disease or because of their possible value as deceased "children." In 1984 a federal judge in Louisiana held that a statute requiring abortion providers to present patients with the option of burial or cremation was an unconstitutional burden on freedom of choice. About 90 percent of all abortions performed in the United States and in other countries are performed during the first trimester. The court implied that women might be discouraged from first-trimester abortions on the mistaken belief that extracted tissue would resemble an infant. Another legal concern is whether aborted embryos and fetuses may be sold for research purposes. American courts and legislators are unlikely to permit outright sales of abortion tissues for research purposes. Indeed federal agency policies adopted in the 1980s declared a moratorium on the use of abortion tissues derived from elective abortions partly out of concern that women might be encouraged to abort for gain. Signaling a change in policy, in 1993 President Bill Clinton, a Democrat, issued an executive order lifting the moratorium on fetal tissue research. In 2001 President George W. Bush, a Republican, reversed this move with his announcement of new federal restrictions on moneys going to human embryo–derived stem cell research. In 2009 the Democratic president Barack Obama reversed this move yet again, restoring federal funding to embryo-derived stem cell research.

Since the 1980s men and women have been parties to commercial surrogate motherhood contracts, the terms of which may purport to limit the right to abortion. Surrogacy contracts raise questions about the commercial alienability of constitutionally protected abortion rights. Surrogates sometimes conceive a child using donated sperm but can also be impregnated with an embryo created with the gametes of others in vitro. The increasingly commonplace commercial surrogacy agreements may contain provisions in which the would-be surrogate mother or gestator undertakes that she will not obtain an abortion should she become pregnant as a result of the surrogacy transactions. The 1988 *Baby M* case, which gained national attention, arose when the surrogate mother, Mary Beth Whitehead, refused to relinquish her parental rights. Under the surrogacy contract Whitehead had agreed in writing that she would "not abort the child once conceived" unless a physician determined it necessary to protect her health or "the child has been determined … to be physiologically abnormal." The Supreme Court of New Jersey refused to enforce any part of the surrogacy contract in *Baby M.* Whereas the courts of California and other jurisdictions have enforced surrogacy contracts when disputes have arisen over parenting rights and child custody, American courts have not specifically enforced a promise not to abort.

Another set of issues relates to the extent to which abortion rights may prevent the government from intervening to enjoin or punish risky behavior by pregnant women who, for example, smoke cigarettes, consume alcohol, abuse drugs, or fail to heed medical advice. In a number of isolated cases in the United States, judges have jailed pregnant women whom they suspected would abuse or neglect their fetuses. In *Ferguson v. City of Charleston* (2001) the US Supreme Court struck down a program under which a hospital tested pregnant patients for illegal narcotics use without their informed consent and reported patients who refused prescribed rehabilitation to law enforcement authorities. A somewhat different concern is the legal implications of government intervention in the event that a pregnant woman refuses a blood transfusion needed to save her life or a cesarean delivery physicians believe to be in the best medical interest of the unborn. Some view *Roe* as holding by implication that women have a broad right to control—and even abuse—their own bodies without regard to fetal well-being. Yet a plausible counterview is that *Roe* does nothing more than immunize women from prosecution for sufficiently early abortions if they choose to have them.

Abortion is controversial in many countries. Violence aimed at abortion providers has occurred both in Canada and the United States. Abortion facilities, health care providers, and even patients have been terrorized by verbal threats, bombs, anthrax, and guns. In May 1992 a bomb blast blamed on antiabortion radicals destroyed the Morgentaler abortion clinic in Toronto. Although antiabortion violence is rare in Canada, dozens of abortion clinic bombings and fires have occurred in the United States. Antiabortion activists throughout the United States have demonstrated at abortion sites to focus attention on their concerns. Generally peaceful, these demonstrations have sometimes become blockades that interfere with the ability of patients and staff to use facilities where abortions are believed to take place. Demonstrators have sometimes resorted to harassment, noise nuisance, property damage, and murder. The shooting deaths of two Florida physicians outside abortion facilities in 1993 and 1994 dramatized the conflict between protesters and clinics. Congress passed the Freedom of Access to Clinic Entrances Act of 1994 in an effort to assure freedom of access to reproduction services. The act makes obstruction and interference at places providing reproductive services a federal offense punishable by fines and imprisonment. Yet clinic entry laws addressed only one site of violence. Barnett Slepian, a New York abortion provider, was murdered in his own home in 1998. George Tiller, a prominent abortion provider, was murdered as he attended church in 2009. Because abortions are legal in the United States, official prosecutions of abortion providers for murder are extremely rare. A Philadelphia, Pennsylvania, abortion provider, Kermit Gosnell was prosecuted for multiple counts of first-degree murder and eventually sentenced to life in prison in 2013 for the deaths of three aborted viable fetuses. In a low-income African American community, Gosnell operated what was by all accounts a substandard facility that escaped the notice of public health officials for many years.

The right to abortion has been held by some state courts to provide a rationale for permitting "wrongful birth" or "wrongful life" lawsuits. In wrongful birth actions parents sue health care providers to recover for expenses and emotional distress connected with raising children with congenital abnormalities. In wrongful life actions disabled offspring sue health care providers, alleging that professional negligence caused their births into lives of pain, suffering, and extraordinary expenses. Citing *Roe*, the New Jersey Supreme Court in *Berman v. Allan* (1979) allowed a wrongful life lawsuit for professional negligence to go forward against the obstetricians of a woman who alleged that she was not offered amniocentesis and as a consequence was denied an opportunity to exercise her legal right to abort a fetus affected by Down syndrome. Pennsylvania and several other states have refused to permit wrongful birth or wrongful life suits. Permissive jurisdictions stress the fairness of compelling negligent physicians to share the economic burdens borne by the families of the disabled. However, some policy makers believe such suits imply disrespect for human life and for the right to life of disabled persons.

Abortion rights and free-speech rights clash in the context of conflicts over abortion clinic protests. Women have a legal right to seek abortion without highly offensive intrusion, physical assault, and violence. These rights come into play where, for example, protesters block access to clinics or broadcast videos of clinic patrons over the Internet or on public access television. But antiabortion protesters have a First Amendment right to freedom of speech, expression, and assembly. Citing the First Amendment in *Schenck v. Pro-Choice Network of Western New York* (1997), the Supreme Court refused to uphold an injunction that created a "floating buffer zone" with a fifteen-foot radius around persons using abortion facilities. Seeking to balance the rights of clinic users and protestors, the court in *Hill v. Colorado* (2000) upheld a statute creating a narrow, eight-foot "bubble zone" around abortion clinics as a reasonable restriction of protestors' free speech.

Following the murders of physicians who performed abortions, a federal appeals court in *Planned Parenthood of the Columbia/Willamette, Inc., et al. v. American Coalition of Life Activists et al.* (2002) held that the federal Freedom of Access to Clinic Entrances Act's definition of a violent threat extended to the circulation by antiabortion activists of "guilty posters" targeting specific abortion providers. Some federal courts have been reluctant to enjoin abortion protestors accused of actual or threatened violence on the basis of state or federal statutes, such as the Ku Klux Klan Act, not clearly enacted for that purpose. In *National Organization for Women (NOW) v. Scheidler* (1993), however, the Supreme Court determined that the federal Racketeer Influenced and Corrupt Organizations (RICO) statute could apply to a coalition of antiabortion groups alleged to be members of a nationwide conspiracy to close abortion clinics. The alleged conspirators unsuccessfully argued that RICO applies only to conspiracies in which the alleged racketeers act for the sake of economic gain rather than out of religious, moral, or political conviction. The court found that acts that did not generate income for alleged racketeers but that adversely affected businesses, such as abortion clinics, were potentially conspiratorial under the RICO statute. The victory for groups in support of abortion rights was undercut by a later Supreme Court decision, *Scheidler v. National Organization of Women, Inc.* (2003), which held that antiabortion protesters interfering with the property right of lawful abortion did not amount to racketeering acts of extortion required by the RICO statute.

In sum, the practice of abortion raises numerous legal issues in the jurisdictions that permit it. Because many individuals oppose abortion on religious and moral grounds, abortion-related questions of legal policy will remain especially complex in the United States and other pluralistic societies. In addition, should technologies for creating, preserving, and terminating human gametes, embryos, and fetuses continue to proliferate, the number of legal concerns about reproductive rights and responsibilities is as likely to expand as to contract.

SEE ALSO *Adoption; Autonomy; Conscience; Conscience, Rights of; Double Effect, Principle or Doctrine of; Embryo and Fetus: I. Developments from Fertilization to Birth; Genetic Testing and Screening: I. Reproductive Genetic Testing; Harm; Human Dignity; Infanticide; Life; Maternal-Fetal Relationship: II. Ethical Issues; Maternal-Fetal Relationship: III. Legal and Regulatory Issues; Moral Status; Population Policies, Strategies for Fertility Control in; Selective Termination/Reduction of Multiple Pregnancy; Women, Historical and Cross-Cultural Perspectives*

BIBLIOGRAPHY

Abortion Act of 1967. Ch. 87 (Eng.).

Baby M, In re. 1988. 537 A.2d 1227, 109 N. J. 396 (1988).

Berman v. Allan. 1979. 404 A.2d 8 (N.J. 1979).

Callahan, Joan C., ed. 1995. *Reproduction, Ethics, and the Law: Feminist Perspectives*. Bloomington: Indiana University Press.

Center for Reproductive Rights. 2011. "Abortion Worldwide: Seventeen Years of Reform." http://reproductiverights.org/en/document/abortion-worldwide-seventeen-years-of-reform

Doe v. Bolton. 1973. 410 U.S. 179 (1973).

Ferguson v. City of Charleston. 2001. 532 U.S. 67, 121 S. Ct. 1281, 149 L. Ed. 2d 205 (2001).

Gallup. 2013. "Abortion." http://www.gallup.com/poll/1576/Abortion.aspx

Garfield, Jay L., and Patricia Hennessey, eds. 1984. *Abortion: Moral and Legal Perspectives*. Amherst: University of Massachusetts Press.

Garrow, David J. 1998. *Liberty and Sexuality: The Right to Privacy and the Making of* Roe v. Wade. Updated ed. Berkeley: University of California Press.

Glendon, Mary Ann. 1987. *Abortion and Divorce in Western Law*. Cambridge, MA: Harvard University Press.

Gonzales v. Carhart. 2007. 550 U.S. 124 (2007).

Greenhouse, Linda, and Reva Siegel. 2011. "Before (and After) *Roe v. Wade*: New Questions about Backlash." *Yale Law Journal* 120:2028–87.

Greenhouse, Steven. 1988. "France Ordering Company to Sell Its Abortion Drug." *New York Times*, October 29, A1.

Griswold v. Connecticut. 1965. 381 U.S. 479, 483 (1965).

Guttmacher Institute. 2012. "Laws Affecting Reproductive Health and Rights: 2011 State Policy Review." http://www.guttmacher.org/statecenter/updates/2011/statetrends42011.html

Harvard School of Public Health. 2012. "Abortion Laws of the World." http://www.hsph.harvard.edu/population/abortion/abortionlaws.htm

Hill v. Colorado. 2000. 530 U.S. 703 (2000).

Hodgson v. Minnesota. 1990. 497 U.S. 417 (1990).

Johnsen, Dawn E. 1986. "The Creation of Fetal Rights: Conflicts with Women's Constitutional Rights to Liberty, Privacy, and Equal Protection." *Yale Law Journal* 95 (3): 599–625.

Kraiker, Gerhard. 1988. "Federal Republic of Germany." In *International Handbook on Abortion,* edited by Paul Sachdev, 189–206. New York: Greenwood.

Luker, Kristin. 1984. *Abortion and the Politics of Motherhood.* Berkeley: University of California Press.

Maschke, Karen J., ed. 1997. *Reproduction, Sexuality, and the Family*. New York: Garland.

McDonagh, Eileen L. 1996. *Breaking the Abortion Deadlock: From Choice to Consent*. New York: Oxford University Press.

Michel, Aaron E. 1981–1982. "Abortion and International Law: The Status and Possible Extension of Women's Right to Privacy." *Journal of Family Law* 20 (2): 241–61.

Mohr, James C. 1979. *Abortion in America: The Origins and Evolution of National Policy, 1800–1900*. New York: Oxford University Press.

Morton, Frederick. 1993. *Pro-Choice vs. Pro-Life: Abortion and the Courts in Canada*. Norman: University of Oklahoma Press.

National Organization for Women (NOW) v. Scheidler. 1993. 510 U.S. 249 (1993).

Ohio v. Akron Center for Reproductive Health. 1990. 497 U.S. 502 (1990).

Olsnes, Ragnhild. 1993. "The Right to Self Determined Abortion." In *Birth Law*, edited by Anne Hellum, 65–91. Oslo: Scandinavian University Press.

Petchesky, Rosalind P. 1990. *Abortion and Woman's Choice: The State, Sexuality, and Reproductive Freedom*. Rev. ed. Boston: Northeastern University Press.

Petersen, Kerry Anne. 1993. *Abortion Regimes*. Brookfield, VT: Dartmouth.

Planned Parenthood of Southeastern Pennsylvania v. Casey. 1992. 505 U.S. 833 (1992).

Planned Parenthood of the Columbia/Willamette, Inc., et al. v. American Coalition of Life Activists et al. 2002. U.S. App. LEXIS 9314 (9th Cir. 2002).

Purdy, Laura. 1996. *Reproducing Persons: Issues in Feminist Bioethics*. Ithaca, NY: Cornell University Press.

Reagan, Leslie J. 1998. *When Abortion Was a Crime: Women, Medicine, and Law in the United States, 1867–1973*. Berkeley: University of California Press.

Reardon, David C. 1987. *Aborted Women: Silent No More*. Chicago: Loyola University Press.

Regina v. Morgentaler. 1988. 1 SCR 30 (1988).

Rhode, Deborah L. 1989. *Justice and Gender: Sex Discrimination and the Law*. Cambridge, MA: Harvard University Press.

Richards, David A. J. 1986. *Toleration and the Constitution*. New York: Oxford University Press.

Robertson, John A. 1983. "Procreative Liberty and the Control of Contraception, Pregnancy, and Childbirth." *Virginia Law Review* 69 (3): 405–64.

Roe v. Wade. 1973. 410 U.S. 113 (1973).

Rust v. Sullivan. 1991. 500 U.S. 173 (1991).

Sachdev, Paul, ed. 1988. *International Handbook on Abortion*. New York: Greenwood.

Scheidler v. National Organization of Women, Inc. 2003. 537 U.S. 393 (2003).

Schenck v. Pro-Choice Network of Western New York. 1997. 519 U.S. 357 (1997).

Siegel, Reva. 1992. "Reasoning from the Body: A Historical Perspective on Abortion Regulation and Questions of Equal Protection." *Stanford Law Review* 44 (2): 261–381.

Siegel, Reva. 2010. "*Roe*'s Roots: The Women's Rights Claims That Engendered *Roe*." *Boston University Law Review* 90:1875–1907.

Simon, Rita J. 1998. *Abortion: Statutes, Policies, and Public Attitudes the World Over*. Westport, CT: Praeger.

Solinger, Rickie, ed. 1998. *Abortion Wars: A Half Century of Struggle, 1950–2000*. Berkeley: University of California Press.

Solomons, Michael. 1992. *Pro Life? The Irish Question*. Dublin: Lilliput.

Stenberg v. Carhart. 2000. 530 U.S. 914 (2000).

Thornburgh v. American College of Obstetricians and Gynecologists. 1986. 476 U.S. 747 (1986).

Tietze, Christopher; Jacqueline Darroch Forrest; and Stanley K. Henshaw. 1988. "United States of America." In *International Handbook on Abortion*, edited by Paul Sachdev, 473–94. New York: Greenwood.

Tribe, Laurence H. 1990. *Abortion: The Clash of Absolutes*. New York: Norton.

T. W., In re. 1989. 551 S. 2d. 1186 (Fla. 1989).

United Nations Department of Economic and Social Affairs. 2011. "World Abortion Policies: 2011." http://www.un.org/esa/population/publications/2011abortion/2011wallchart.pdf

Webster v. Reproductive Services. 1989. 492 U.S. 490 (1989).

Weddington, Sarah R. 2013. *A Question of Choice*. 40th anniversary rev. and updated ed. New York: Feminist Press of the City University of New York.

Whittaker, Andrea. 2010. *Abortion in Asia: Local Dilemmas, Global Politics*. New York: Berghahn.

Wolf, Merrill; Phan Bich Thuy; Alyson Hyman; and Amanda Huber. 2010. "Abortion in Vietnam: History, Culture, and Politics Collide in the Era of *Doi Moi*." In *Abortion in Asia: Local Dilemmas, Global Politics*, edited by Andrea Whittaker, 149–74. New York: Berghahn.

Anita L. Allen (1995, 2004, 2014)
Henry R. Silverman Professor of Law and Professor of Philosophy, University of Pennsylvania Law School

IV. JEWISH PERSPECTIVES

The Jewish discourse of medical ethics is a multi-vocal and contentious one that crosses several centuries of text, traditions, and historical norms in global communities. However, for a tradition in which so much is in contention, and in which *maklochat* (intense debates) are the normal form of reasoning, the legal and ethical norms surrounding the issue of abortion are relatively less controversial. The Jewish tradition, in general, takes a clear middle path—allowing certain abortions, in certain circumstances, for certain, specific reasons justified by rational moral appeals. Abortion is not absolutely prohibited, as in some religious traditions, nor is it understood as the murder of a fully human person. Ending a pregnancy is understood as regrettable but permissible, or even necessary, in certain instances.

HISTORICAL BACKGROUND

The discussion about reproductive ethics is part of larger discussion about the role of women, the place of families, and the vision of the human future. Thus, it is one of the earliest debates in moral systems that attend to the questions of family life, health care, and community continuity. In antiquity, pregnancy was seen as a moment for celebration but also as a time of grave risk. All early religious responses to the issue of abortion are made in that context, in which the intention is to create and maintain families, but not at the risk of the lives of mothers. As pregnancy became safer, as childhood mortality decreased, and, finally, as the possibility of prenatal diagnosis emerged, the issue of choosing when and under what conditions to have children became a matter for religious concern. Abortion, because it addresses the fundamentally metaphysical question of when life begins, will always be a religious question. For Jews, religion is not a set of external institutional events visited on occasions of crisis or celebration; it is a binding to a commanded life, in which every single daily act of practice and attention is a part of the being of the faithful person. It is the totality of life that Jewish belief is concerned with—the inescapable call of the stranger, the constancy of the demand for justice in every interaction, and the significance of minute details of daily life. The commanded life is a matrix of competing and complementary and contentious strands. There is both a temporal aspect to the matrix, in that interpretations are the result of more than 2,000 years of discourse, and an analytic aspect, in that any act can be judged in a variety of ways. An act can be prohibited but unpunished, prohibited and punished, permitted but not sanctioned, permitted and sanctioned, obligatory but with many exceptions, or obligatory in all cases. Hence, much of our understanding about abortion comes not from these texts that describe variations and exceptions, but from the far broader range of normative texts that support a pronatalist family life.

Since the twentieth century, Judaism has had four distinct branches: Orthodox, Conservative, Reform, and Reconstructionist/New Age. For Jews who are not close followers of Talmudic law (those who belong to one of the last three branches noted), the cultural and economic realities of modernity affect religious practice, social justice decisions, and personal ethical norms that tend to raise the issue of women's authority over their embodied choices and to broadly support arguments that permit abortions. Even within Orthodox Judaism, the issue of abortion and family planning has long been shaped by both historical reality and the essentially permissive tradition that permits abortion for defensible reasons. In Jewish ethics, one considers both the whole of human activity and the whole of the community when making such decisions: Women as well as men are moral agents, with responsibilities and obligations to and within a wider community. The argument for this ethical framework is found primarily in the extensive debate and exegesis of the rabbinic literature, a contentious discourse of casuistic narrative ethics that both determines and discusses the 613 commanded acts named as the *mitzvot* by the rabbis of the Talmudic period (200 B.C.E.–500 C.E.), and which continued throughout the medieval and modern period.

In the 1,500 years since the redaction of the Talmud, Jewish law has developed by an ongoing series of *responsa* to questions about the legal code discussed in the Talmud, called halacha. Difficult cases of social crisis of all types are brought before arbiters and scholars who rule on the facts of the cases, on the methodological principles of logical argument, and on certain key principles of relationships in familial, ritual, civic, and commercial spheres. Each commentator is intellectually tied to those who came previously, and is confronted by changes in context: politics, cultural shifts, and scientific understandings that were not available to previous generations. Nowhere are these shifts more evident than in the rapidly changing field of reproductive health. Nearly all commentators would agree that the concerns of the tradition are specific, and protect four principles:

1. to ensure that women are not required to have children because childbirth was seen in the Talmudic period as potentially life-threatening;
2. to ensure that the temptation to immerse oneself in a life of study is avoided, and that every man is married and in a family with children;
3. to ensure that sexuality within marriage after producing two children—the halachically required number for men—can be enjoyed without intending pregnancy under certain conditions; and
4. to allow both women and men to pursue, within limits, options for family planning based on a complex assessment of personal needs and social context.

The discursive method of Jewish ethical reasoning follows from close analysis of key texts. The method of reasoning preserves both sides of the debates within the texts, in which there is rarely a history of unanimity; rather, it is a centuries-long, global argument, as Jewish communities in different times and places, with sharply disagreeing authorities, make definitive and, in many cases, contradictory statements. A review of the development of the internal argument of the classic texts illustrates both the mutability of the tradition and the argumentative nature of the normative debate.

BIBLICAL TEXT

Abortion as such does not appear as an option for women in the biblical text. There is only one direct reference to the interruption of a pregnancy, and it is a sort of collateral damage—when a miscarriage occurs because a pregnant woman is injured as she stands near a fight: "And if men strive, and hurt a woman with child, so that her fruit depart and yet no harm follows, he shall be surely punished, according as the woman's husband will lay upon him; and he shall pay as the judges determine. But if any harm follows, you shall give life for life." (Exodus 21:22–23). The biblical text assumes the following conditions: First, that the event described—a loss of a fetus through miscarriage—which results in the abortion of the fetus—was an accidental occurrence, but was caused by a non-natural intervention; second, that the event was not in the woman's control, and that the lost fetus has a defined value (since it is, presumably, the property of the her husband); and third, that the being that is "departed" is not a fully human life in the way that the woman is a human life, for while it is clear that a crime of some sort has been committed, it is not a capital crime. What is at stake in the text is whether the woman herself is hurt, for the end of the pregnancy, while a loss, is explicitly not the loss of a life.

The rabbinic texts that emerge far later address the question of permissibility: When can a pregnancy be ended by human action? The response is found in the earliest texts of rabbinic discourse (200 B.C.E.) in the Mishnah. Although clearly it was seen as an emergency option, abortion was nevertheless clearly available and permitted under several circumstances. These commentaries interpret the biblical text noted above, but they do so with two different types of justifying exegetical arguments, both of which allow abortion in some circumstances.

RODEF ARGUMENT

The first argument posits that the fetus is in some way a danger to the woman, and thus can be aborted because of the more general rule of self-defense. This becomes articulated as the argument called the *Rodef* (pursuer). This is evident in the following proof text: "If a woman suffer hard labor in travail, the child must be cut up in her womb and brought out piecemeal, for her life takes precedence over its life; if its greater part has [already] come forth, it must not be touched, for the [claim of one] life can not supersede [that of another] life" (Mishnah 6). Here the text assumes three things: first, that abortion is a deliberate moral act; second, that the decision to abort is a joint one, made by the woman and her birth attendant, and it is somewhat in the woman's hands because she is the "sufferer," so it is her suffering that calls the question, and it must have something to do with her limits of endurance; and third, that it is a *child* that is in her womb, but not a child who counts as a *nefesh* (fully ensouled human person) until a physical event occurs—its head, or "greater part," is born. Here, abortion is permitted because a women's life is of more value than the life of a fetus.

This first argument was further developed centuries later by the medieval commentator and physician Maimonides:

> This, too, is a mitzvah: not to take pity on the life of a pursuer (*Rodef*). Therefore the Sages have ruled that when a woman has difficulty in giving birth one may cut up the child within her womb, either by drugs or by surgery, because he is like a pursuer seeking to kill her. Once his head has emerged he may not be touched for we do not set aside one life for another; this is the natural course of the world. (Maimonides 1:9)

Maimonides assumes three things: that the fetus is in fact a *nefesh, a being and not merely a part of the woman's body*; that it is a pursuing *nefesh* (*Rodef*) in other words, that it is a being that poses fatal risk to the mother; and that since a life is at stake, it is correct to to allow the killing of the *Rodef*, in this case, allowing for the abortion that would end the deadly pursuit. The basis for Maimonides's opinion that the fetus is "like a pursuer" pursuing the mother in order to kill her is his belief that the situation falls under the general law of *pikuah nefesh* (avoiding hazard to life) in the Torah (*Hiddushei Rabbi Hayyim Soloveitchik to Mishneh Torah*, Hilkhot Rotze'ah 1:9). Ben Zion Uziel in the early modern period extended this argument to include defending not just the mother's life, but also her health:

> We learn in this matter that according to the doctors, the fetus will cause its mother deafness for the rest of her life, and there is no greater disgrace than that, for it will ruin the rest of her life, make her miserable all her [life].... Therefore, it is my humble opinion that she should be permitted to abort her fetus through highly qualified doctors who will guarantee ahead of time that her life will be preserved. (Ben Zion Uziel, *Mishpetei Uziel,* Hoshen Mishpat 3:46)

Finally, Rabbi Eliezer Waldenberg in the mid-twentieth century interpreted the text to include protection of not just the woman's physical health, but also her mental health, allowing abortion in the case of a diagnosis of Tay-Sachs disease in the child:

> One should permit ... abortion as soon as it becomes evident without doubt from the test that, indeed, such a baby [Tay-Sachs baby] shall be born, even until the seventh month of her pregnancy.... If, indeed, we may permit an abortion according to the Halacha because of *great need* and because of pain and suffering, it seems that this is the classic case for such permission. And it is irrelevant in what way the pain and suffering is expressed, whether it is physical or psychological. Indeed, psychological suffering is in many ways much greater than the suffering of the flesh. (Eliezer Waldenberg, *Responsa Tzitz Eliezer*, Part 13, no. 102)

MORAL STATUS ARGUMENT

In addition to the *Rodef* justification for the permissibility for abortion, a second line of argument can be found in the text, and it is largely based on the way that Jewish tradition understands a developmental moral status as the defining feature of pregnancy, a principle that gains ground via rabbinical medical science. This tradition emerges from the debates about menstrual blood and the blood of miscarriage. Blood, like all discharges from the human body, presents a ritual problem to be adjudicated by the rabbis, because persons (both women and men) with bodily discharges need to participate in purification rituals before they can rejoin the larger community for prayer. A woman needs to know, for example, whether her bleeding is due to her normal menstrual cycle, in which case she needs to wait two weeks, then immerse herself in a ritual bath (at the *mikvah*) before resuming sexual intercourse, or due to a miscarriage, in which case she needs to wait for a longer period before immersion in the *mikvah*. A system emerged in the early rabbinic period (and was carried forward into the present) in which every questionable discharge was collected for examination by rabbinic authorities. Because examination of the expelled contents of the womb after a miscarriage during the first forty days after conception did not reveal a fetal form, the rabbinic authorities deemed that during this period, the embryo had the status of *mere water*, and thus its existence could not be counted for ritual purposes. The rulings on the permissibility of abortion followed from this understanding of moral status: Abortions during this period could not be opposed. It is for this reason that modern Israeli scientists worked to develop blood tracer tests that could detect chromosomal abnormalities within the first forty days of pregnancy—so that abortions for trisomies such as trisomy 21 (Down syndrome) or 18 (Edwards syndrome) could be allowed.

ENSOULMENT ARGUMENT

A third line of justification develops in entirely another tractate of the Mishnah (Arakin): that abortion is permitted as a health procedure, because a fetus is not an ensouled person. Not only is an embryo in the first forty days after conception considered *like water*, but even in the last trimester, the fetus has a lesser moral status—it is more akin to a part of a woman's body than a separate being: "Gemora: But that is self-evident, for it is her body! It is necessary to teach it, for one might have assumed since Scripture says 'according as the woman's husband shall lay upon him' that it [the woman's child] is the husband's property, of which he should not be deprived. Therefore, we are informed [that it is not so]" (Exodus, cited above)

This proof text introduces an argument that the fetus is simply "not a *nefesh*," and therefore is seen as a part of a woman's body. A later authority, the medieval French scholar Rashi, assumes this is valid because the fetus is not a separate being until the head is born; his argument is based on the Talmudic permission to kill a pregnant woman, even one in the late stages of pregnancy. This argument continues in later *response*. Indeed, for some commentators, it is unclear whether the child even after birth is fully independent of its mother, with it own separate being and body. For some authorities, the status of the infant remains uncertain for thirty days after birth. Mourning practices for infants reflect this lesser moral status: "Because when a child dies within thirty days (being then considered a stillborn and not mourned like a person who had died) it becomes evident only in retrospect that it was a stillborn (*nefel*) and that the period of its life was only a continuation of the vitality of its mother that remained in him" (Ben Zion Uziel 3:46).

RECENT CONCERNS

In the post-Holocaust period, a new and contradictory tradition began to develop as some commentators voiced concerns that an overly liberal abortion practice is inappropriate in the face of declining numbers of Jews, and they urged a more strongly pronatalist stand. Although this position does not emerge from classic *halachic* sources, it has nevertheless gained some ground in the contemporary period. The argument emerges from all sectors of Jewish thought. Moshe Tendler and David Bleich in the Orthodox world, and Conservative authority Elliot Dorff both advocate for a pronatalist stand, even while clearly supporting the textual realities that permit abortion under many circumstances. Dorff argues that Jews are "a people … in deep demographic trouble. We lost one-third of our numbers during the Holocaust. … The current Jewish reproductive rate among American Jews is between 1.6 and 1.7. … This social imperative has made propagation arguably the most important mitzvah of our time" (Dorff 1998).

Abortion policies also are linked to other historical and medical changes. Since 2002 extensive genetic testing has been promoted within the Jewish community, allowing for genetic screening for disease carrier status to be standard in arranged marriages for many in the Orthodox community, and to be widely used by Jewish couples of all denominations. Family planning methods have further reduced the need for abortions, which remain legal and defensible within Jewish tradition as a matter of Jewish law and practice. In Israel, abortions are legally defended as a matter of health, and the statutes protect abortion as a personal health care decision.

SEE ALSO *Authority in Religious Traditions; Ethics: V. Religion and Morality; Judaism, Bioethics in; Population Ethics: V. Jewish Perspectives*

BIBLIOGRAPHY

Abraham, Abraham. 1984. *Medical Halachah for Everyone.* New York: Feldheim Publishers.

Abrams, Daniel, and Avraham Elqayam, eds. 2000. *Kabbalah: Journal for the Study of Jewish Mystical Texts.* Los Angeles: Cherub Press.

Abrams, Judith. 1998. *Judaism and Disability.* Washington, DC: Gallaudet University Press.

Adler, Rachel. 1998. *Engendering Judaism: An Inclusive Theology and Ethics.* Philadelphia: Jewish Publications Society.

Bleich, David. 1983. *Contemporary Halakhic Problems.* Vol. 2. New York: KTAV Publishing House, Yeshiva University Press.

Brody, Baruch. 1988. *Life and Death Decision Making.* New York: Oxford University Press.

Cohen, Arthur, and Paul Mendes-Flohr, eds. 1988. *Contemporary Jewish Religious Thought: Original Essays on Critical Concepts, Movements, and Beliefs.* New York: Free Press.

Dorff, Elliot. 1998. *Matters of Life and Death: A Jewish Approach to Modern Medical Ethics.* Philadelphia: Jewish Publications Society.

Frank, Daniel, ed. 1992. *Autonomy and Judaism.* Albany: State University of New York Press.

Freedman, Benjamin. 1999. *Duty and Healing: Foundations of a Jewish Bioethic.* New York: Routledge.

Gibbs, Robert. 2000. *Why Ethics? Signs of Responsibilities.* Princeton, NJ: Princeton University Press.

Hand, Sean, ed. 1989. *The Levinas Reader.* Oxford: Basil Blackwell.

Herring, Basil. 1984. *Jewish and Halakhah for Our Time: Sources and Commentary.* New York: KTAV Publishing House, Yeshiva University Press.

Jakobovits, Immanuel. 1962. *Jewish Medical Ethics: A Comparative and Historical Study of the Jewish Religious Attitude and Its Practice.* New York: Bloch.

Levinas, Emmanuel. 1987. *Outside the Subject.* Stanford, CA: Stanford University Press.

Mackler, Aaron, ed. 2000. *Life and Death Responsibilities in Jewish Biomedical Ethics.* Elmwood Park, NJ: G & H Soho.

Meier, Levi, ed. 1986. *Jewish Values in Bioethics.* New York: Human Sciences Press.

Pence, Gregory, ed. 1998. *Classic Works in Medical Ethics: Core Philosophical Reading.* New York: McGraw-Hill.

Preuss, Julius. 1978. *Biblical and Talmudic Medicine.* New York: Sanhedrin Press.

Rosner, Fred, ed. 1990. *Medicine and Jewish Law.* Northvale, NJ: Jason Aronson.

Rosner, Fred. 1997. *Medicine in the Bible and the Talmud.* New York: KTAV Publishing House, Yeshiva University Press.

Shatz, David, and Joel Wolowelsky, eds. 2001. *The Torah U-Madda Journal.* New York: Yeshiva University Press.

Spero, Moshe Halevi. 1986. *Handbook of Psychotherapy and Jewish Ethics.* Jerusalem: Feldeim.

Zohar, Noam. 1997. *Alterations with Jewish Bioethics.* Albany: State University of New York Press.

Laurie Zoloth (2004, 2014)
Professor, Department of Religious Studies, Northwestern University

V. ROMAN CATHOLIC PERSPECTIVES

The Roman Catholic tradition has always treated abortion as a serious sin. Yet Catholic teaching on abortion has not always centered on the "right to life" of the individual fetus, nor has it always viewed all abortion as homicide. For several centuries, early abortion in particular was characterized more as a sexual sin than as killing and was condemned as an interference in the natural outcome of the reproductive process, often assuming as its context an illicit sexual liaison.

The fact that Catholic views of the precise status of the fetus as human life have changed over time and that the church's position has a philosophical rather than a religious basis are key to late-twentieth-century church teaching on abortion. That teaching is that the fetus must be treated as a person from conception onward. This teaching is not stated as a sectarian religious proposition but as a humanistic and philosophical truth to be recognized in civil laws guaranteeing appropriate protection to fetal life. Although exhortations to protect life in the womb have often been supported with religious allusions (for instance, to the will of the Creator or to the image of God in humanity), the duties to continue pregnancy and to sustain infants have been grounded primarily in the "natural law," understood as a shared human morality innate to all persons and knowable by reason.

In examining the foundations and development of the Catholic position, it is important to place modern teaching in the context of changing views of women's roles in family and society. Other factors influencing debates about Roman Catholicism and abortion are the relation of scientific knowledge about the beginnings of human life to the moral status of life; and the relation among civil law, morality, and the church as an institutional actor.

HISTORICAL DEVELOPMENT

Although Catholic claims about abortion are not narrowly religious, certain biblical and early Christian characterizations of life in the womb no doubt have contributed to an ethos in which abortion is viewed negatively. The Hebrew Scriptures (Old Testament) did not treat the killing of a fetus as the killing of an infant (Exod. 21:22), although the Greek Septuagint translation of the Hebrew (early third century B.C.E.) adds a distinction between the formed and the unformed fetus and presents abortion of the former as homicide. This distinction reflects the ancient Greek view (Aristotle) that the matter and form of any being must be mutually appropriate (the *hylomorphic theory*) and that the embryo or fetus could not have a human soul (*form*) until the body (*matter*) was sufficiently developed. Often quoting the Septuagint, patristic and medieval theologians maintained this distinction, which remained a key component of Roman Catholic discussion of abortion until at least the eighteenth century.

The Gospels do not address abortion explicitly, though the infancy narratives manifest interest in the importance of the individual before birth, at least in respect of God's will for him or her in the future (Matt. 1:18–25; Luke 1:5–45). In Paul's Letter to the Galatians (5:20) and in Revelation (9:21), condemnations of magical drugs (*pharmakeia*) associated with various forms of immorality, including promiscuity and lechery, may very likely extend to abortifacients. The connection is made clear in two early Christian texts, the Didache and the Epistle to Barnabas. "You shall not kill. You shall not commit adultery. You shall not corrupt boys. You shall not fornicate. You shall not steal. You shall not make magic. You shall not practice medicine (*pharmakeia*). You shall not slay the child by abortions (*phthora*). You shall not kill what is generated. You shall not desire your neighbor's wife" (Didache 2.2, quoted in Noonan 1970, 9).

Contraceptive and abortifacient drugs, as well as infanticide, were certainly used widely in the ancient world, not only to conceal sexual crimes, but also to limit family size and conserve property. Early Christian authors such as Tertullian, Jerome, and Augustine in the Western church, and Clement of Alexandria, John Chrysostom, and Basil in the Eastern church, repudiated these practices. They did not, however, challenge their patriarchal social context, with its requirement that female sexuality serve the good of the family and its assumption that women seeking to avoid pregnancy were usually guilty of sexual infidelity. Local councils tended to support this stand. In 303 C.E., on the Iberian Peninsula, the Council of Elvira excluded from the church for the rest of her life any woman who had obtained an abortion after adultery. In 314 the Eastern church, at the Council of Ancyra (Ankara), reduced the period of penance to ten years, although it retained the lifetime ban for voluntary homicide. Such church laws made no distinction between the formed and the unformed fetus, but Tertullian, Jerome, and Augustine considered that the sin of abortion might not be homicide until after ensoulment. (The fetus was considered by many ancient writers to receive a soul only after the body had "formed," or reached an appropriate level of development, at about three months.)

Formation of the fetus became a consideration in assigning penance in private confession during the seventh century, but it was not universally recognized in church law until the decree *Sicut ex* of Innocent III in 1211. The decree dealt with irregularity, which could be incurred for homicide. An irregularity is a canonical impediment that bars a man from receiving or exercising holy orders. Irregularities are based on defects (such as mental or physical illness) or crimes (including attempted suicide, murder, and abortion). According to the decree, irregularity would not be incurred for abortion unless the fetus was animated. Since the time of animation was identified with formation, the decree implied that only abortion of the formed fetus was considered homicide. Following Aristotle, forty and ninety days were accepted as the time of animation for the male and the female fetus, respectively. Confusion arose, however, from a parallel tradition that extended the notion of homicide not only to the abortion of the unformed fetus but also to sterilization. Both traditions claimed a factual base, the one in the premise that the "man" is contained in miniature in the male seed, and the other in Aristotle's reported observation of aborted fetuses. During the Middle Ages, the distinction between formed and unformed was generally accepted, notably by Thomas Aquinas, and only the abortion of the formed fetus was classified as homicide, even in reference to sacramental penances. Earlier abortions were not murder, but they were still forbidden as serious sins because they interfered with the procreative outcome of sexual acts.

In the early fourteenth century, the Dominican John of Naples introduced an exception, subsequently accepted by several others: it would be permissible to abort the unformed fetus in order to save the life of the mother. Later theologians, particularly Thomas Sánchez (sixteenth century), used the argument of self-defense against an unjust aggressor (so characterizing the fetus) or the principle of totality (looking on the fetus as part of the mother). In 1588 Sixtus V reaffirmed a more rigid position, classifying even sterilization as homicide, and (in the decree *Effraenatam*) making excommunication a penalty of the universal church for the sin of abortion. A modification in 1591 again limited the provision to the case of the animated fetus, at either forty or ninety days. This legislation remained in effect until 1869, when Pius IX extended it to all direct abortion. Twenty years later, the Holy Office of the Vatican declared that neither craniotomy nor any other action to destroy the fetus directly would be permitted, even if without it both mother and child would die. Until that point, the exception to save maternal life had been debated by the theologians without receiving official condemnation. While theologians sought a balance of the value of the fetus with other values, especially the life of the mother, papal legislation moved toward a reinforcement of the abortion prohibition.

A moderating influence that continues today was exerted via the *principle of double effect*. This principle, pertaining to acts that have both good and evil effects, permits a moral distinction between direct and indirect abortion. Only direct abortions are absolutely prohibited in official Roman Catholic teaching. Indirect (permitted) abortions are those operations that have as their primary effect the saving of the mother's life, with the death of the fetus a foreseen but not directly intended secondary effect. The classic example is the removal of the cancerous uterus of a woman who is pregnant. In this case, the death of the fetus is neither in itself the desired outcome of the intervention, nor even willed and caused as the means by which the woman's life is saved. The removal of the cancer, not the fetus, heals. Double effect may also be applied to the removal of a fallopian tube in the case of an ectopic pregnancy. The premise behind the justification of indirect abortion is that while the direct killing of an innocent human being is immoral, the woman's life is at least equal in value to that of her unborn offspring, so that she has no duty to assume serious risk to her own life in order to sustain the child.

CONTEMPORARY TEACHING

In his 1930 encyclical on marriage, *Casti connubii*, Pius XI affirmed the equal sacredness of mother and fetus but condemned the destruction of the "innocent child" in the womb, who can in no way be considered an "unjust assailant." (The sticking point here, of continuing interest to moralists, is whether it is necessary to have an unjust intention to qualify as an unjust aggressor, or whether unintentionally posing an unjust danger to another is sufficient. Soldiers in war, for instance, may have noble personal intentions yet validly be viewed by their opponents as unjust attackers.) The Second Vatican Council (*Gaudium et spes*, no. 51) referred to abortion and infanticide as "unspeakable crimes." The complex agenda of and challenges to current church teaching are well focused by the 1974 Vatican *Declaration on Procured Abortion*.

This document is a response to changed Western abortion laws, as well as to population measures in developing nations. Even as it resists these pressures, it adapts its message on abortion to cultural and legal contexts characterized by the emancipation of women and the need to control births. The document responds to the Western political value of free choice by asserting that "freedom of opinion" does not extend further than the rights of others, especially the right to life. It observes that while ensoulment has been debated historically, abortion has always been condemned. Most important, the document insists that human reason can and should recognize respect for human life as the most fundamental of all goods and the condition of their realization. It sees modern science as confirming that human life begins with fertilization, though allowing that science can never definitively settle what is properly a philosophical question. Still, "it is objectively a grave sin to dare to risk murder" (20) if there is doubt as to whether the fetus is fully a human person.

In its 1987 instruction, *Donum vitae* (On respect for human life), the Congregation for the Doctrine of the Faith granted that there is no scientific "proof" of when the fetus becomes a person, but the fetus must be given the benefit of the doubt (no. 69). In its 2008 document, *Dignitatis personae* (On certain bioethical questions), the status of the fetus was stated more strongly (nos. 4–5), and the use of abortifacient methods of birth control, even for rape victims, was ruled out (no. 23).

The *Declaration on Procured Abortion*, like later teaching statements, recognizes that pregnancy can pose serious burdens for the health and welfare of women, families, and children themselves. It advocates that individuals and nations exercise "responsible parenthood" by natural means of avoiding conception. It also exhorts "all those who are able to do so to lighten the burdens still crushing so many men and women, families and children, who are placed in situations to which in human terms there is no solution" (no. 23). It excludes abortion as an answer but also concludes that what is necessary "above all" is to "combat its causes" through "political action" (no. 26). In his 1995 encyclical, *Evangelium vitae* (The Gospel of life), John Paul II sees abortion as a betrayal of women's inherent nurturing role. "A mother welcomes and carries in herself another human being, enabling it to grow inside her, giving it room, respecting it in its otherness" (no. 99). Yet he recognizes that abortion can be "a painful and even shattering decision" (99). He calls on women who have had abortions to promote respect for human life by serving others in need.

The *Declaration* anticipates later efforts, notably by the US cardinal Joseph Bernardin, to advocate moral consistency on killing, in that it contrasts growing protests against war and the death penalty with the social vindication of abortion. The unborn should be included within a greater respect for life in general and be protected by more stringent social limits on killing of all kinds.

Since the causes and rates of abortion vary globally, the local Catholic Church responds differently. For instance, in India, where sex-selective abortion is illegal but practiced, the rate of female to male infants born dropped in 2011 to 914 girls per 1,000 boys. The Indian Catholic Church has established an annual day of celebration of girls; the church also campaigns against sex selection and in favor of legal prosecution of doctors who perform sex-selective abortions and promotes adoption as an alternative.

CRITICAL DEBATES

Among the debated questions regarding the Roman Catholic tradition on abortion are certainly the following. First, is it reasonable and scientifically sound to urge that the fetus be treated as a "person" from conception onward, especially if to do so will have dire consequences for the woman who bears it? While most Roman Catholic theologians assume a conservative attitude toward the value of prenatal life, not all accept that full value is present at the outset; rather, it increases in some developmental fashion, at least through the earlier stages. Several authors (McCormick 1984; Tauer 1984; Shannon and Wolter 1990) have pointed to the time of implantation, at about fourteen days, as a "line" after which individuality appears more settled (the possibility of "twinning" being past) and the chance of survival greatly magnified.

Second, is the equality of women, and the substantive legal, social, and material support for women and families enjoined by the *Declaration*, really as high on the practical pro-life agenda of Roman Catholicism as is the enactment of punitive sanctions for abortion? A deep skepticism about whether this is so gives the "abortion rights" cry of many feminists its immense symbolic value in the struggle for gender and sexual equality. While some Catholic feminists believe that sexual self-determination and effective birth control is a better way to ensure women's liberation than recourse to a form of killing, other Catholic feminists insist that the choice to terminate pregnancy must be available to women as long as a patriarchal church and society identify women's roles as reproductive and domestic in order to constrain women's moral agency and to exclude women from the range of social participation available to men.

Third, even granted that the fetus has significant value, can and should restrictive abortion laws be kept in place—or reenacted in nations that have moved toward liberalization? John Courtney Murray (1960, ch. 7) distinguishes between law and morality. Morality in principle governs all human conduct, while law pertains to the "public order," the minimum moral requirements of healthy social functioning. Modern nations vary in the degree of restraint on abortion choice they see public order as requiring (see Glendon 1987). Abortion policy debates, especially in more lenient systems like that of the United States, challenge Roman Catholicism to reshape the social consensus about the value of the unborn. Any legislation not backed by a consensus favoring enforcement will lead both to disrespect for the law and to the proliferation of unregulated extralegal alternatives. A precondition for a less permissive abortion consensus is the creation both of avenues other than "abortion rights" for the exercise of women's social and personal freedoms, and of social supports encouraging women and families to raise children. International data show that illegality of abortion does not necessarily correlate with frequency of abortion. For example, abortion rates are lower in Sweden and Germany, where abortion laws are permissive but social welfare systems are strong, than in Chile and Peru, where abortion is illegal but poverty rates are high. A 2007 study in the United States showed that abortion rates were lower in states with more generous social welfare programs for pregnant women and families (Wright and Bailey 2007).

A major point of debate within Roman Catholicism is the level of legal compromise acceptable to those who would accord the fetus more value than it is granted in law and policy. Following the principle that law and morality are not coterminous, some argue that a policy that encourages early abortion and restricts it to "hard cases" (e.g., threat to life or health, rape, incest, serious birth defects) could command enough broad support to justify it as a practical advance in the limitation of abortion. Advocates of a more stringent position insist that the full weight of the church's moral authority be marshaled behind a policy that would outlaw abortion altogether. Still others maintain that in a country with established permissive abortion laws, the most prudent course to reduce abortion is to provide better alternatives for pregnant women and families.

Finally, can the church credibly defend its antiabortion position while disallowing the most effective forms of birth control? It is relevant to this question that many nations' aspirations to economic and cultural prosperity are plagued by limited freedom for women in marriage and family and by increasing overpopulation. In the industrialized countries, the abortion controversy tends to focus on individual rights, either of the fetus or of the mother, with Roman Catholic proponents framing the issue in terms of a legally protectable right to life. In such nations, the church tends to address itself to the absolutization of private choice over what it sees as human life, and the trivialization of the abortion decision as it becomes a substitute for sexual responsibility and contraception.

However, the Roman Catholic Church is an international organization, with a substantial or growing membership in, for example, Latin America, the Philippines, and Africa. In many nations, the question of women's freedom to combine family with public vocation as the context for the abortion debate is overshadowed by dire poverty; the inaccessibility of education, adequate employment, and health care; the ambiguous economic implications of a large family in rural, agricultural settings; and the radically disadvantaged position of girls and women within the family in some traditional cultures. Especially in the absence of ready access to contraception, abortion may appear to such women, to families, and even to government agencies to be a desperate but necessary means of controlling fertility. As the 1974 *Declaration on Abortion* indicates, the global Roman Catholic position on abortion must go beyond the condemnation of abortion as murder to address personal and social situations in which abortion appears as the only viable answer to deprivation or oppression.

This is a revision and update of the entry first written by John R. Connery in 1995.

SEE ALSO *Christianity, Bioethics in; Conscience, Rights of; Embryo and Fetus: V. Religious Perspectives; Feminism; Genetic Testing and Screening: I. Reproductive Genetic Testing; Human Dignity; Moral Status; Natural Law; Population Ethics: VI. Roman Catholic Perspectives*

BIBLIOGRAPHY

Abbott, Walter M., ed. 1966. *The Documents of Vatican II: All Sixteen Texts Promulgated by the Ecumenical Council, 1962–1965.* New York: America Press.

Ashley, Benedict; Jean DeBlois; and Kevin D. O'Rourke. 2006. *Health Care Ethics: A Catholic Theological Analysis.* 5th ed. Washington, DC: Georgetown University Press.

Bernardin, Joseph. 1988. *Consistent Ethic of Life.* Lanham, MD: Sheed and Ward.

Connery, John R. 1977. *Abortion: The Development of the Roman Catholic Perspective.* Chicago: Loyola University Press.

Glendon, Mary Ann. 1987. *Abortion and Divorce in Western Law: American Failures, European Challenges.* Cambridge, MA: Harvard University Press.

Grisez, Germain G. 1970. *Abortion: The Myths, the Realities, and the Arguments.* New York: Corpus.

John Paul II. 1995. *Evangelium vitae* [The Gospel of life]. Rome: Libreria Editrice Vaticana.

Jung, Patricia Beattie, and Thomas A. Shannon, eds. 1988. *Abortion and Catholicism: The American Debate.* New York: Crossroad.

McCormick, Richard A. 1984. *Health and Medicine in the Catholic Tradition: Tradition in Transition.* New York: Crossroad.

Murray, John Courtney. 1960. *We Hold These Truths: Catholic Reflections on the American Proposition.* New York: Sheed and Ward.

Noonan, John T., Jr., ed. 1970. *The Morality of Abortion: Legal and Historical Perspectives.* Cambridge, MA: Harvard University Press.

Pius XI. 1963 [1930]. *Casti connubii.* In *Matrimony,* 219–91, translated by Michael J. Byrnes. Papal Teachings Series. Selected and arranged by the Benedictine monks of Abbaye Saint-Pierre de Solesmes. Boston: St. Paul Editions.

Shannon, Thomas A., and Allan B. Wolter. 1990. "Reflections on the Moral Status of the Pre-embryo." *Theological Studies* 51 (4): 603–26.

Tauer, Carol A. 1984. "The Tradition of Probabilism and the Moral Status of the Early Embryo." *Theological Studies* 45 (1): 3–33.

Vatican Congregation for the Doctrine of the Faith. 1974. *Declaration on Procured Abortion.* Rome: Libreria Editrice Vaticana.

Vatican Congregation for the Doctrine of the Faith. 1987. *Donum vitae* [On respect for human life]. Rome: Libreria Editrice Vaticana.

Vatican Congregation for the Doctrine of the Faith. 2009. *Dignitatis personae* [On certain bioethical questions]. Rome: Libreria Editrice Vaticana.

Wright, Joseph, and Michael Bailey. 2007. *Reducing Abortion in America: The Effect of Social and Economic Supports.* Washington, DC: Catholics in Alliance for the Common Good.

Lisa Sowle Cahill (1995, 2014)

J. Donald Monan Professor, Department of Theology, Boston College

VI. PROTESTANT PERSPECTIVES

Reviews of the history of Protestant teaching on abortion focus most often on specific comments regarding abortion in the writings of leaders of the various church reform movements in European Christianity beginning in the sixteenth century. Several of the most effectual Reformation leaders, including Martin Luther (1483–1546) and John Calvin (1509–1564), were powerful both in reconceiving church practice and in articulating reformulations of Christian theological and ethical teaching. Consequently, for many of their followers and spiritual heirs, their teaching has remained uniquely authoritative in discerning Protestant truth claims. The formal criteria for discerning Christian truth proposed by these reformers, however, are best characterized as privileging the role of Christian scripture (usually referred to by Protestants as the Old and New Testaments) in adjudicating doctrinal and moral disputes. This primacy of scripture as theological and moral norm also characterized the teaching of most other sixteenth-century reformers, including the theological leaders of the many Anabaptist movements.

Since the sixteenth century, all dissent from authoritative Roman Catholic teaching and practice, including newly emergent Christian movements, receives the label "Protestant." The rapidly growing Pentecostal movements in Latin America, indigenous Christian movements in Asia, and the African indigenous churches that have become numerically preponderant among Christians on that continent all fall under this rubric. As a result, extreme caution needs to be exercised in characterizing "Protestant" moral teaching in any contemporary moral dilemma. Even when interpreters are familiar with very diverse Protestant cultural traditions, those who identify themselves as Protestants interpret the meaning of conformity to scriptural norms in a wide variety of ways, and reveal wide differences in biblical "hermeneutics," or principles of interpretation, of sacred texts. The diversity of hermeneutical options available accounts in part for the complexity of Protestant voices on abortion today.

Before identifying contemporary Protestant hermeneutical diversity and therefore the range of existing contemporary Protestant viewpoints on abortion, it is important to clarify the cultural roots of Protestantism that shape them.

EARLY PROTESTANT VIEWS OF ABORTION

Luther's and Calvin's theological and moral reforms were shaped by their reconceptions of both the meaning of Christian life and Christian ritual practice. Neither could be said to have proposed shifts in the foundational notions of human nature embedded in late medieval Christianity. Traditional notions of human nature, including gender and human species reproduction, were not in dispute and did not shift at the time of the Reformation. What is notable among Protestant reformers is the paucity of comment on any questions about human sexuality and reproduction, including abortion. Luther, a prolific preacher and writer, did not mention abortion at all. Had he done so, he likely would have presumed its moral wrongness because he was educated as an Augustinian monk and was learned in the available theological texts of the period, including especially *Sentences* by the twelfth-century theologian Peter Lombard, which contained collations of opinions on abortion by earlier theologians. The lists included the judgments of many who associated abortion with sexual immorality, especially with adultery, and condemned the practice.

Calvin also knew this authoritative tradition that explicitly condemned abortion, as his commentaries on Genesis 38:10 make clear. His remarks on Exodus 21:22 further attest that he believed abortion to be wrong morally. Modern critical biblical exegetes agree that Exodus 21:22 is the only text in Christian scripture that explicitly refers to abortion, albeit to abortion that occurs because of injury to a pregnant woman. The issue in this passage was not elective abortion. Even so, Calvin used the occasion of comment on this text to make known his view that the fetus is already a person, a matter the text does not address.

On gender, sexuality, and reproduction, these reformers maintained continuity with earlier traditions. Both Luther and Calvin also followed what they took to be early Christian theological consensus, that divine ensoulment (i.e., the point of spiritual animation of human beings by God) of human life occurs at conception, though not all the Protestant theologians who followed them agreed. Modern conservative historical interpreters construe Calvin and Luther's views on this point as confirming their own current belief that Protestant teaching agrees with modern papal teaching, namely, that full human life occurs at conception. Caution needs to be exercised here, however. Although the majority of Protestant theologians followed the view that ensoulment occurred when the "seed" was planted in utero, their perspectives were not developed in relation to questions about human gestation. To argue that these views speak to the value of fetal life is misleading, since their opinions were developed as aspects of the theological debate about sin and salvation, and not in relation to modern embryological understanding. In any case, Protestant ritual practice suggests that commonsense norms were in fact applied to actual fetuses. Protestants, like Roman Catholics, did not practice baptism in relation to miscarriages or aborted fetuses.

MODERN PROTESTANT VIEWS ON ABORTION

Specific comment on abortion is rare in most Reformation traditions until the twentieth century. Perhaps in deference to the lack of biblical discussion, most reformers considered matters regarding the morality of abortion, like matters governing all sexual and reproductive behavior, to be ordered by human rational discernment. They were issues of "natural morality" rather than of revealed truth. Despite emphasis on recovering the meaning of Christian biblical tradition, Lutherans, Calvinists, and Anglicans (post-Roman Church of England adherents) maintained the view, long-standing in western Christianity, that much moral knowledge, including the order of human sexuality and reproduction, falls within the purview of "natural" human knowledge, that is, they are matters for rational deliberation and discernment. Contrary to the trend of modern Protestant fundamentalist biblicism in discussions of abortion, most Protestant traditions tended to embrace a type of reasoning that accepted human rational (and therefore "scientific") data as relevant to these moral judgments on these issues. The Anabaptists were often exceptions methodologically, however. They sought guidance on moral issues exclusively from scripture without reference to other sources. However, Anabaptists also stressed freedom of conscience in deliberating moral dilemmas, and often resisted fixed ecclesiastical standards on questions such as abortion. Not surprisingly, contemporary Anabaptist heirs often oppose with great adamance state-prescribed policies making abortion illegal.

It is not too much to say that Protestantism possessed neither an explicitly developed tradition of moral reasoning about abortion nor any elaborated body of teaching on the ethics of so-called medical practice until well into the nineteenth century. Reproduction in Protestant communities, as in all premodern communities, was shaped by female cultural practice and midwifery until at least the very late nineteenth century. Contemporary cultural historians agree that nearly all female subcultures encouraged some means of fertility control, and that most took recourse to abortifacients (substances that induce abortions) in extreme cases. Such methods were primitive and dangerous, however, and documentation regarding the range and scope of their use is all but nonexistent. The fact that women, and not men, both made up and knew the culture of reproduction probably limited public awareness in prevailing practices. Knowledge about available interventions in pregnancies may not have been widely shared, and such knowledge may have been quite rare among male theologians until the "medicalizing" of pregnancy and reproduction in the twentieth century. In the nineteenth century, male medical practitioners increasingly attempted to discredit midwifery, frequently on the grounds that midwives practiced abortion, but Protestant clergy in the United States showed great reluctance to support such efforts.

The major impact of the Reformation in shaping Protestant attitudes on abortion is rarely mentioned in traditional historiography. The most important influence of Protestantism in the abortion debate arose from the changes in spiritual practice initiated by Reformation Christianity; these changes in turn led to a powerful shift in how socialization into Christian faith took place. Initiation into Christianity moved from a locus in the church-based penitential system to the Christian family, which gradually became the basic social unit of Christian piety. Protestant spirituality was pervasively formed by this embrace of the family as the proper site for transmission of both faith and morals. The change engendered by the Reformation overturned celibacy not only as the proper norm for clerical life but also as the norm of optimal Christian piety. The Reformation movements made the sexually monogamous, procreation-centered family both the center of their basic community and their strongest metaphor for divine blessing. For Calvinists, explicitly from the outset, and for Lutherans, Anglicans, and Anabaptists more slowly, adherence to this form of social practice came to be taught as a Christian duty. Parents were to oversee their children's successful entrance into procreation-centered marriage literally as a mandate of faith.

This shift in the structure of Christian sociology, more than any change in explicit moral teaching, shaped subsequent moral sensibilities toward abortion among Protestants. This new emphasis on the sacerdotal character of the family reinforced the appeal of Protestant Christianity in traditionalist non-European cultures as well. Both ancient Hebraic and Jewish and pre-Protestant Christian sources had at times equated procreation and biological fertility or fruitfulness as signs of divine blessing, and such pronatalist sentiments had had some influence in earlier Christian attitudes toward abortion. However, the rise of Protestantism made such sensibilities powerful in European cultures and central to modern Christian moral sensibility about reproduction. This portended a deep suspicion regarding elective abortion when the practice became widespread and safe.

Many modern Protestants arrive at their judgments about the morality of abortion from a deep-seated sense that any pregnancy is intrinsically a sign of divine blessing and that to deny this is impious. So deep does the equation of fertility and divine blessing run in Protestant cultures that western Christianity itself has strongly reinforced traditional patriarchal norms that female "nature" is centered in and fulfilled only through maternity. Traditional Protestant cultures (those untouched by religious pluralism) tend to experience any weighing of questions about the status of fetal life as expressing a "secular" or "antireligious" mindset.

Despite the strong pronatalist disposition of traditional Protestant spirituality, however, critical historians have also noted a certain tension between Protestant teaching on abortion and Protestant pastoral practice. Even in traditionalist Protestant cultures, where moral and theological discourse is unequivocal in condemning abortion, pastoral practice is frequently far less censorious. Scattered evidence exists that Protestant priests, pastors, and elders often treated those who had abortions or administered them with a surprising degree of compassion or even leniency. There is no evidence that the practice of abortion was deemed "an unforgivable sin," as some ancient church canons insisted, or that abortion was equated with "murder" or "unjustified killing." Even among contemporary Protestant fundamentalists, historians have observed this tension between formal moral condemnation and more permissive ecclesiastical practice. Theological and moral condemnation notwithstanding, noncelibate clergy may be in touch with many of the concrete conditions and dilemmas of pregnancy and reproduction that shape women's lives. In any case, the general stance of Protestant traditionalism and of the newer, postmodernist biblical hermeneutics is toward a degree of pastoral compassion, even if abortion is starkly condemned at the formal level. All current available data suggest that the rate of recourse to abortion among women who are part of Christian communities that formally condemn abortion—Protestant traditionalist, Protestant fundamentalist, or Roman Catholic—is at least as great as it is among women who come from liberal Protestant and Jewish communities or who are nonpracticing with regard to religion.

The most typical contemporary Protestant attitude toward abortion remains a traditionalist, pronatalist negativity toward the practice, with a reluctant recognition that abortions do occur frequently, even within the Protestant communities of faith. Such cautious negativity is maintained without strong, elaborated moral justification, chiefly because the strong cultural ethos of the existing family-centered sociology of the Protestant churches gives this view such plausibility. Traditionalist consensus tends to break down, however, whenever Protestant communities are confronted with debates shaped by conflicts within the wider culture or from newly articulate dissent within these Protestant communities themselves. Such debate is now ongoing in all churches rooted in the continental Reformation. For the most part the debate reflects the divisions in biblical hermeneutics already mentioned.

Three newer hermeneutical positions appear in the abortion debate. First, there is a quite unprecedented biblical fundamentalist hermeneutic asserting itself in many Protestant cultural contexts. This new fundamentalism is developed particularly to resist change in issues involving gender, sexuality, family, and reproduction. On all of these issues, restoration of a premodern interpretation of sex/gender and the reproductive system is the primary goal. Human gender and sexual identity, this approach insists, are rooted in "nature" and in "divine decree" central to the presumed "biblical" message. Using both the language of natural law and tradition of the mandate of divine revelation as synonymous and as equally legitimated by scripture, the new fundamentalists contend that the essence of the biblical witness is the biological-religious "givenness" of male/female nature and the revealing of the proper "telos," or end, of human sexuality. Abortion is unthinkable, a violation of all of the norms of faith and morals. This hermeneutic aims to make even the discussion of abortion taboo in Protestant theological and moral discourses, to make it literally unthinkable. This approach tends to drive from the field several generations of historical-critical study by Protestant theological liberals. Previously, liberal biblical scholarship had successfully persuaded interpreters of the Bible within mainline Protestantism that interpretation of scriptural texts had to be guided by awareness of different historical times and variations among cultures. Liberals recognized that biblical worldviews do not presuppose modern ideas about the origin and nature of the universe and its inhabitants. Such considerations undergirding previous Protestant biblical interpretation, once widely accepted, are often forgotten in the wake of the force of the new fundamentalist hermeneutic.

Second, although the new fundamentalism gains force in Protestant communities, most "old-line" Protestant denominations (rooted in Europe) remain informed by historical-critical methods of scriptural interpretation and continue to speak in a voice consistent with conclusions of the earlier liberal biblical hermeneutic. Broadly speaking, these churches acknowledge that biogenetic and other scientific knowledge must be given its due in deliberating the morality of abortion. Most concede that decisions to have abortions are justified in some cases and can be consistent with biblical faithfulness. This casts several major Protestant denominations on the side of the public policy debate that supports limited legality of abortions. Although several of the old-line denominations have been strongly pressed by fundamentalists and traditionalists in their ranks to shift to antiabortion positions on public policy, Lutherans, Anglicans, Methodists, Presbyterians, and United Church of Christ denominations, among others, have maintained their public positions. Discussion of what may constitute "justifiable reasons" for choosing abortion is decidedly underdeveloped in such Protestant communions. A strong consensus prevails that supports abortions in cases of pregnancies due to sexual violence (rape and incest); in cases where the life or physical health of the mother is at stake; and, perhaps, in cases where prospective parents lack the spiritual and physical resources to rear an additional child. There are also important historical reasons why old-line liberal Protestant communities place a strong emphasis on "responsible parenthood," but that story is outside the scope of this entry. This too is an important and largely unexamined chapter in understanding Protestant views on both family planning and abortion.

Finally, in nearly all contemporary Protestant communities/cultures, another hermeneutic for interpreting the Christian abortion tradition is emerging. It may be called a *liberationist* or even a *profeminist liberationist* principle of interpretation. Although it is still a decided minority position within formalized Protestant theological-moral discourse, this hermeneutic is influencing many, especially women. It calls on Protestant theology and ethics to reformulate moral and religious judgments with special attention to concerns for women's well-being and in recognition that Christian teaching on gender, sexuality, and reproduction is embedded in a wider system of social control of women's lives. Acknowledging internal contradictions within scripture, a liberation hermeneutic refuses authority to culturally repressive male-supremacist readings of biblical texts and postscriptural theological interpretations. Like liberals, proponents of the emerging liberation hermeneutic represent a spectrum of convictions about what reasons might justify specific acts of abortion, but strongly concur that the Protestant Christian moral voice must actively advocate broad-based social change to enable women to shape their reproductive capacity. They contend that the moral evaluation of abortion must not be predicated on discourse that obscures women's full standing as moral agents or that fails to include realism about the historical pressures surrounding biological reproduction in women's lives. Among Protestants, only Unitarian/Universalists have adopted such a hermeneutic officially.

The contesting voices characterized here are most visible and most intense within Protestant Christian communities in the United States. However, analogous dynamics are at work in Protestant communities in other areas of the globe, as they are within Roman Catholic, Orthodox, and other religious communities. The struggle over which hermeneutical voice shall prevail in Protestant teaching on abortion remains unresolved.

BIBLIOGRAPHY

Brown, Peter R. L. 1988. *The Body and Society: Men, Women, and Sexual Renunciation in Early Christianity.* New York: Columbia University Press.

Cohen, Sherrill, and Nadine Taub, eds. 1989. *Reproductive Laws for the 1990s.* Clifton, NJ: Humana.

Connery, John R. 1977. *Abortion: The Development of the Roman Catholic Perspective.* Chicago: Loyola University Press.

Gordon, Linda. 1976. *Woman's Body, Woman's Right: A Social History of Birth Control in America.* New York: Grossman.

Grobstein, Clifford. 1988. *Science and the Unborn: Choosing Human Futures.* New York: Basic Books.

Harrison, Beverly Wildung. 1983. *Our Right to Choose: Toward a New Ethic of Abortion.* Boston: Beacon Press.

Jones, Jacqueline. 1986. *Labor of Love, Labor of Sorrow: Black Women, Work, and the Family from Slavery to the Present.* New York: Vintage.

Kennedy, David M. 1970. *Birth Control in America: The Career of Margaret Sanger.* New Haven, CT: Yale University Press.

McLaren, Angus. 1990. *A History of Contraception from Antiquity to the Present Day.* Oxford: Basil Blackwell.

Mohr, James. 1978. *Abortion in America: The Origins and Evolution of Public Policy: 1800–1900.* New York: Oxford University Press.

Noonan, John T., Jr., ed. 1970. *The Morality of Abortion: Legal and Historical Perspectives.* Cambridge, MA: Harvard University Press.

Olasky, Marvin. 1992. *Abortion Rites: A Social History of Abortion in America.* Wheaton, IL: Crossways.

Rich, Adrienne C. 1976. *Of Woman Born: Motherhood as Experience and Institution.* New York: Norton.

Rousselle, Aline. 1988. *Porneia: On Desire and the Body in Antiquity.* New York: Basil Blackwell.

Schneider, Jane, and Rayna Rapp, eds. 1995. *Articulating Hidden Histories: Exploring the Influence of Eric R. Wolf.* Berkeley: University of California Press.

Beverly Wildung Harrison (1995)
Caroline Williams Beaird Professor of Ethics, Union Theological Seminary in New York

VI. PROTESTANT PERSPECTIVES [ADDENDUM]

In her original entry on this topic for this publication, Beverly Wildung Harrison describes three prominent hermeneutics that emerged as Protestant denominations developed and revised their positions on abortion. These approaches continue to shape denominational debate, ecumenical discourse, and political activism.

A small number of denominations espouse a liberation hermeneutic, which calls on the church to address inequality and reject gender-biased interpretations of scripture. They view abortion as a woman's personal choice. This approach has academic credibility but little support from most Protestant denominations.

The debate between a traditional liberal biblical hermeneutic and an increasingly vocal biblical fundamentalism dominates early twenty-first-century denominational discussions and has given rise to new political activism. This is evident in North America and in Protestant churches around the world.

The traditional liberal biblical hermeneutic is embraced by mainline European denominations and is the starting point for most American denominational positions, which consider abortion a sin and reject it as a means of birth control. However, in circumstances such as rape, incest, severe fetal disabilities, or where the mother's life is at risk, virtually all accept that abortion may be a lesser evil than allowing the pregnancy to continue. Some denominations are even more permissive, allowing those most directly involved to determine whether abortion represents the lesser evil in a given situation. Given this emphasis on compassion and context, most denominations argue for reconciliation rather than condemnation. Ecclesiastical practices focus on forgiveness, and abortion is rarely addressed from the pulpit. Most Protestant denominations are not campaigning against abortion, and few oppose the funding of abortion services.

Protestant fundamentalists are challenging these views both in the denominational discourse and in the public sphere. While the number of Protestant fundamentalists is not increasing, those who hold this view are expressing themselves with greater clarity and purpose. They are also building alliances with Catholics and others who share their views.

The fundamentalist position asserts that abortion is morally "unthinkable." It represents the destruction of a human life and is sinful under all circumstances. Many Protestants who hold this view are calling on their denominations to revise their positions. They have bolstered lobby groups, such as the National Pro-Life Religious Council, and generally support legal and political efforts to limit the availability of abortion. Some examples include the passage of the federal Partial-Birth Abortion Ban Act of 2003 and various state laws imposing restrictive conditions on women who request abortions.

From a global perspective, growth in Latin American, African, and Asian churches is greatest among Protestant denominations with fundamentalist views, such as the Pentecostals. The denominational positions of these churches will likely be less tolerant of abortion than European and North American denominations, and they will be more politically active.

Protestant believers are becoming less "religious" over time, and their beliefs and practices increasingly resemble those of the general population. While it is important to understand Protestant tradition and history, it will likely play a diminishing role in the decisions and actions of Protestant patients in the future.

SEE ALSO *Christianity, Bioethics in; Embryo and Fetus: V. Religious Perspectives; Feminism; Genetic Testing and Screening: I. Reproductive Genetic Testing; Human Dignity; Moral Status; Population Ethics: VIII. Protestant Perspectives*

BIBLIOGRAPHY

Albrecht, Gloria H. 2003. "Contraception and Abortion within Protestant Christianity." In *Sacred Rights: The Case for Contraception and Abortion in World Religions*, edited by Daniel C. Maguire, 79–103. New York: Oxford University Press.

Johnston, George F. 2003. *Abortion from the Religious and Moral Perspective: An Annotated Bibliography*. Westport, CT: Praeger.

Nelson, J. Robert. 1981. "The Divided Mind of Protestant Christians." In *New Perspectives on Human Abortion*, edited by Thomas W. Hilgers, Dennis J. Horan, and David Mall, 387–404. Frederick, MD: University Publications of America.

Pew Research Center. 2011. "Global Survey of Evangelical Protestant Leaders." Pew Forum on Religion and Public Life. Accessed August 22, 2013. http://www.pewforum.org/2011/06/22/global-survey-of-evangelical-protestant-leaders/

Pew Research Center. 2013. "Religious Groups' Official Positions on Abortion." Pew Forum on Religion and Public Life. Accessed August 22, 2013. http://www.pewforum.org/2013/01/16/religious-groups-official-positions-on-abortion/

Wald, Kenneth D., and Allison Calhoun-Brown. 2011. *Religion and Politics in the United States*. 6th ed. Lanham, MD: Rowman and Littlefield.

Wilcox, Clyde. 2003. "Evangelicals and Abortion." In *A Public Faith: Evangelicals and Civic Engagement*, edited by Michael Cromartie, 101–15. Lanham, MD: Rowman and Littlefield.

Merril Pauls

Director of Ethics and the Humanities, Faculty of Medicine, Department of Emergency Medicine, University of Manitoba, Canada

VII. ISLAMIC PERSPECTIVES

Since ancient times every human society has dealt with the issue of abortion. The way each treats the issue has depended on the way each views fundamental questions of individual and societal life, such as the meaning and sanctity of human life, sexuality and gender relations, the role of marriage and family, the meaning of human freedom, and the related issues of rights and responsibilities of the individual.

THE ROLES OF MEDICINE AND LAW IN THE ISLAMIC DEBATE ON ABORTION

Islam's response to abortion during the fourteen centuries of its existence has been documented mostly in the jurisprudential works of its doctors of law and the medical writings of its physicians. Islamic perspectives on abortion have been shaped directly by both its theology and its revealed law (sharia). Because of the centrality of the latter as a practical guide in the religious and spiritual life of Muslims, however, they depend heavily on the deliberations and ethico-legal decrees (fatwas) of experts whenever practical problems arise in society. The main practical role of theology is to provide the necessary spiritual and intellectual framework within which ethico-legal debates are pursued.

Since the Divine Law of Islam refuses to make a separation between law and ethics, the traditional Muslim jurist (*faqih*) is at once an ethicist and a legal expert. The physician's duty in matters concerning abortion is to provide medical advice and recommendations befitting each individual case, as Islamic law generally permits abortion on medical and health grounds up to a certain stage of pregnancy. Close collaboration between medicine and law in Islam has generated a well-developed branch of Islamic jurisprudence that deals with many biomedical issues, including contraception and abortion.

In all cases of abortion, the physician is an important witness. The idea of the testimony of a trustworthy physician is well known in Islam, since Islamic law puts great emphasis on the idea of a trustworthy witness, whom it always defines in terms of believing in God and having a good moral character. The close rapport between medicine and law in Islam is further strengthened by the fact that this religion has produced a sizable number of jurists who either practiced medicine or at least possessed a sound general knowledge of the subject. Ibn Rushd (known by the Latin name Averröes, d. 1198), Ibn al-Nafis (d. 1288), the discoverer of the minor circulation of the blood, Ibn Ḥazm (d. 1064), Fakhr al-Dīn Rāzī (d. 1209), and in more recent times, Ḥasan al-Aṭṭar al-Khalwatī (d. 1835), a rector of the prestigious al-Azhar University in Cairo, were some of the most famous jurists–medical practitioners. Al-Shāfiī (d. 820), the founder of one of the four Sunni schools of law, is credited in traditional sources with knowledge of medicine.

Conversely, there have been many Muslim physicians who were well versed with the philosophy of the sharia and the ethical teachings of the Koran and hadiths (i.e., recorded sayings, behavior, and actions attributed to the Prophet, and in the case of the Shi'ite branch of Islam, also to the imams, their foremost spiritual leaders), but who were never recognized as jurists in the technical sense of the term. The most famous of these was Ibn Sīnā (d. 1037). These physicians were generally knowledgeable in embryology. As scholars of natural philosophy, of which psychology is a part, many of these physicians also developed a comprehensive theory of the soul that includes a treatment of the problem of identifying the stage of pregnancy when the ensoulment of the body takes place in the womb. The connection between embryology and psychology is therefore of great practical interest to Islamic law.

At ensoulment a fetus attains the legal status of a human being, with all the rights accorded by the sharia. Although Muslim jurists rely substantially on the Koran and prophetic medicine for their knowledge of embryology, they also demonstrate a positive attitude toward the scientific embryology of the philosopher–physicians, since they do not see any basic contradiction between the two sources.

THE THEOLOGICAL CONTEXT

The abortion debate in Islam takes place in a particular religious environment created by the divinely revealed teachings of the religion. These teachings are accepted by Muslims as sacred and immutable and have remained unquestioned in the debate over the centuries. The most important of these teachings concerns the meaning and purpose of human life.

Islam teaches that human life is sacred because its origin is none other than God, who is the Sacred and the ultimate source of all that is sacred. Human beings are God's noblest creatures by virtue of the fact that he has breathed his spirit into every human body, male and female, at a certain stage of its embryological development. This breathing of the divine spirit into the human fetus is called its ensoulment; it confers on the human species the status of theomorphic beings. Islam shares with Judaism and Christianity the teaching that God has created humans in his own image.

Islam teaches that a human is not just a mind–body or soul–body entity that has come into existence through an entirely physical, historical, or evolutionary process. He or she is also a spirit whose reality transcends the physical space–time complex and even the realm of the mind. This spiritual substance present in each human individual, to which Muslim philosophers and scientists refer as the most excellent part of the rational soul and which has cognitive powers to the extent of being able to know itself, God, and the spiritual realm in general, is what distinguishes humans from the rest of earthly creatures.

The Koran refers more than once to the ensoulment of the human body, almost always in the context both of describing God's creation of Adam, the first ancestor of the human race, and of affirming the superiority of humans over the rest of creation, including the angels (for example, at 15:28–30). There is also a more specific reference to the ensoulment of the human fetus that is made as part of its description of the process of pregnancy and birth. The Koranic passage quoted perhaps most often in the abortion debate is, "We [i.e., God and his cosmic agents] have created man out of an extraction of clay [the origin of semen]; then we turn it into semen and settle it in a firm receptacle. We then turn semen into a clot [literally, something that clings] which we then fashion into a lump of chewed flesh. Then we fashion the chewed flesh into bones and we clothe the bones with intact flesh. Then we develop out of it another creature. So blessed be God, the best of creators" (23:12–14).

Both ancient and modern commentators on the Koran generally agree that the last stage in the formation of the human fetus as indicated by the phrase "develop out of it another creature" mentioned in this Koranic passage refers to the ensoulment of the fetus, resulting in its transformation from animal into human life. As to exactly when the ensoulment of the fetus takes place, the Koran does not provide any information. The prophetic hadiths contain a detailed periodization of each of the different stages of fetal growth mentioned in the Koran. In theology as in law, matters on which the Koran is either silent or held to be less explicit than the hadith, the latter takes a decisive role. Thus it is the testimony of the hadith concerning the ensoulment of the fetus that has proved decisive in the formulation of Islamic theological doctrine concerning abortion.

According to one hadith, organ differentiation in the fetus does not begin to take place until six weeks after the time of fertilization. According to another, an angel who is a divine agent of ensoulment of the fetus is sent to breathe a distinctively human soul into it after 120 days of conception have passed. In his commentary on the Koranic verse on human reproduction cited above, basing his views on hadiths as well as on the findings of physicians, Jalāl al-Dīn al-Suyutī (d. 1505), an encyclopedist and author of a popular work on prophetic medicine, declared, "All wise men are agreed that no soul is breathed in until after the fourth month" (Elgood 1962, 240).

If God has given a theomorphic nature to human persons and has created them in the best of molds (Koran, 95:4), having unique faculties not enjoyed by creatures of other species, it is not without a noble purpose. According to the Koran, human beings have been created to know God and to be God's servants and representatives on Earth in accordance with his own wishes as revealed to all branches of the human family through his prophets and messengers. One of the six fundamental articles of the Islamic creed is belief in a future life—not in this world of sensual experience and mental images, but in another world whose space–time complex is entirely different from the one we currently experience.

In the Koranic view, human life does not end with death. In reality, death is only a passage between two parts of a continuous life, namely the present and the posthumous. How we fare in that future life depends on how we conduct ourselves in this present life. By leading a spiritually, ethically, and morally healthy life in this world, we will attain salvation and prosperity in the after-death life. The previously cited verse on human conception and birth is immediately preceded by a reference to life in paradise and immediately followed by a statement on the certainty of death and resurrection. Muslims understand from this and other verses that there is a grand divine scheme for humans that they have no right to disturb. On the contrary, they are to participate fully in this cosmic scheme as helpers of God in both their capacities as his servants and representatives.

Human reproduction, birth, and death are part of this grand divine scheme. Indeed, the Koranic view is that there is even a preconception phase of human existence. The Koran refers to a covenant between God and all the human souls in the spiritual world before the creation of this world. God addressed the souls collectively, asking them "Am I not your Lord?" Without hesitation they all bore witness to his Lordship, thus implying that God-consciousness is in the very nature of the human soul.

The general implication of the Islamic teachings on the meaning and purpose of life for reproduction and abortion is clear. Although reproduction is not explicitly commanded in the Koran, it does appear to be encouraged. A few hadiths are explicit in their encouragement of procreation. The most popular is the hadith that says that, on the Day of Resurrection, the Prophet would be proud of the numbers of his community compared with other communities and that he admonishes his followers to reproduce and increase in number.

One can say with certainty that the general religious climate that prevailed in Muslim societies throughout the ages even until modern times is one in which procreation is encouraged and abortion very much discouraged. Cyril Elgood (1970) observes that "in Islamic countries moral approval of the practice of abortion was not readily given," although procurement of abortion, of which there were many cases, was not necessarily considered a criminal act. When he further says that "it is almost universally recognized by civilized nations that abortion is to be practiced only on the rarest of occasions" (240), the majority of Muslims would make the spontaneous response that this is precisely the Islamic view of abortion.

If Islam encourages the propagation of the human species, then it also insists that every human life be given due protection. (Abortion, however, is not considered the ending of a human life unless ensoulment of the fetus has occurred.) One of the fundamental goals of Islamic law is the protection of human life. Islam takes a serious view of the taking of human lives (except in cases that have been legitimized by the Divine Law itself) and of all acts injurious to life. One of the five basic human rights enshrined in the sharia is the protection by the state of every human life. The Koran asserts that "whosoever kills a [single] human for other than murder or other than the corruption of the earth [i.e., war], it is as though he has killed all humankind and whosoever has saved one human, it is as though he has saved all humankind" (5:35). The phrase "other than murder" in this verse refers to justifiable homicide, like self-defense and capital punishment as prescribed under the Islamic law of equality (*qisas*).

The Islamic view of marriage and sexuality also casts a long shadow on the abortion debate. Human reproduction should take place within the framework of the sacred institution of marriage. Islam describes marriage as "half of religion" and strongly condemns sexual relations outside of marriage. The main purpose of the institution of marriage is the preservation of the human species, although Islam also recognizes the spiritual, psychological, and socioeconomic functions of marriage. That there is indeed much more to marriage than just procreation or sexual fulfillment has been amply clarified by many classical Muslim thinkers.

One of the best treatises on the wisdom of marriage in all its dimensions was composed by the prominent jurist, theologian, and Sufi, al-Ghazālī (d. 1111). This highly influential religious scholar and critic of Aristotelian philosophy defends the permissibility of married couples' practicing contraception on the ground of their need to secure a happy marriage. He goes so far as to hold that a man who fears that his wife's bearing children might affect her health or good looks, and that he might therefore begin to dislike her, should refrain from having children (Rahman 1987). Al-Ghazālī's view clearly suggests that procreation is not the sole purpose of marriage.

Islamic discussion of abortion is always related to the question of the rights and responsibilities of both the husband and the wife. One of the major issues in contemporary debate on abortion in the West concerns the rights of women to procure abortion. Islam answers the question not only by appealing to its theological doctrines on the meaning and scope of human rights and responsibilities, but also to its religious theory of conception based on revealed data and hadith teachings. The Koran stresses the idea that everything in the heavens and on earth belongs to God. Metaphysically speaking, humans do not own anything, not even their own bodies. It is God who has apportioned rights and responsibilities to males and females, husbands and wives, fathers and mothers. Men and women in Islam obtain their mutual rights through the arbitration of the Divine Law.

In general, Muslim jurists pay great attention to women's rights in the practice of contraception and the procurement of abortion. In the words of Basim F. Musallam, "One can speak of a classical Islamic opinion on contraception generally and consistently adopted in Islamic jurisprudence, regardless of school. This classical opinion was the sanction of *coitus interruptus* with a free woman provided she gave her permission" (1983, 28). A "free woman" is a nonslave and married. Islamic jurisprudence treats *coitus interruptus* under three categories, namely (1) with a wife who is a free woman; (2) with a wife who is a slave of another party; and (3) with a man's own slave or concubine. All schools of Islamic law consider *coitus interruptus* permissible. The majority of them insist on the woman's consent only if she belongs to the first category, since Islamic law recognizes her basic rights to children and sexual fulfillment. No permission is needed from a slave woman. In the case of abortion, the Hanafis granted the pregnant woman the right to abort even without her husband's permission provided she has a valid reason in the eyes of the sharia. (The Hanafis are followers of the Islamic school of law founded by the prominent jurist Abu Hanifah and are mainly found in Turkey and the Indian subcontinent.) The Koranic teaching that children are not created of the man's semen alone but of both parents together has a bearing also on Muslim discussion of the mutual rights of husband and wife in the permissibility of abortion.

ISLAMIC LAW AND ABORTION

The Islamic view of fetal development based on the Koran and hadith is central to the Muslim arguments on abortion. All Muslim jurists believe that the fetus becomes a human being after the fourth month of pregnancy. Consequently, abortion is prohibited after that stage (Musallam 1983). However, the jurists differ in their views concerning the permissibility of abortion during the first four months of pregnancy, that is, the period prior to the ensoulment of the fetus.

Jurists of the Hanafi school of law allowed abortion to be performed at any time during the four-month period. A special document compiled by five hundred Hanafi *ulamā* (religious scholars) decrees that "the woman has the right to adopt some method of obtaining abortion if quickening of the fetus has not occurred, which happens after 120 days of conception" (Abedin 1977, 121).

Most Maliki jurists, by contrast, prohibit abortion absolutely. Their main argument is that although the fetus does not become a human until after its ensoulment, one should not tamper with the natural process of conception once the semen has settled in the womb, since the semen is destined for ensoulment. A minority of Maliki jurists, however, allow abortion of a fetus up to forty days old. Other schools of Islamic jurisprudence, among both Sunnis and Shi'ites, agree with the Hanafis in their tolerance of abortion, although again they differ on the specifics.

It is important to emphasize the fact that there is a specific theological and ethico-legal context in which abortion has been permitted in Islam. Muslim jurists classify all human acts into five categories, namely (1) the obligatory (*wājib*), (2) the recommended (*mandūb*), (3) the allowable or the indifferent (*mubāh*), (4) the blameworthy or the discouraged (*makrūh*), and (5) the forbidden (*harām*). Abortion, at the most liberal level, has been placed by jurists in the third category, that of the allowable. Jurists have deliberated on the special conditions under which abortion is permitted, apart from the biological factor of ensoulment. They have also discussed cases of criminal abortion and types of penalties to be imposed on convicted wrongdoers.

Muslim jurists permit abortion mostly on medical and health grounds. One of the valid reasons often mentioned is the presence of a nursing infant. It is feared that a new pregnancy would put an upper limit on lactation. The jurists believe that if the mother could not be replaced by a wet nurse, the infant would suffer, if not die.

Contemporary Muslim society is faced with the reality that the practice of abortion is on the rise. In a number of Muslim countries, many unwanted pregnancies result from illicit sexual relations as well as from rapes. There are also related issues of birth control or family planning as a national policy, easy access to modern contraceptives, and the challenge to traditional Islamic doctrines on abortion and contraception arising from advances in genetics and biomedical technology. A well-defined Islamic response to these contemporary challenges has not yet emerged, but interest in these subjects is gaining momentum. As contemporary Muslim intellectuals and religious scholars debate these problems, traditional sources on contraception and abortion will be of immense value.

BIBLIOGRAPHY

Abedin, Saleha Mahmood. 1977. "Islam and Muslim Fertility: Sociological Dimensions of a Demographic Dilemma." Ph.D. thesis, University of Pennsylvania.

Anees, Munawar Ahmad. 1989. *Islam and Biological Futures: Ethics, Gender and Technology.* London: Mansell.

Bakar, Osman. 1991. *Tawhid and Science: Essays on the History and Philosophy of Islamic Science.* Kuala Lumpur, Malaysia: Secretariat for Islamic Philosophy and Science.

Bouhdiba, Abdelwahab. 1985. *Sexuality in Islam,* translated by Alan Sheridan. London: Routledge and Kegan Paul.

Ebrahim, Abul Fadl Mohsin. 1988. *Biomedical Issues: Islamic Perspective.* Mobeni: Islamic Medical Association of South Africa.

Elgood, Cyril. 1962. "Tibb-ul-Nabbi or Medicine of the Prophet: Being a Translation of Two Works of the Same Name." *Osiris* 14:33–192.

Elgood, Cyril. 1970. *Safavid Medical Practice; or, The Practice of Medicine, Surgery and Gynaecology in Persia between 1500* CE *and 1750* CE. London: Luzac.

Maudoodi, Abul A'la. 1968. *Birth Control: Its Social, Political, Economic, Moral, and Religious Aspects.* 3rd ed. Lahore, Pakistan: Islamic.

Musallam, Basim. 1983. *Sex and Society in Islam: Birth Control before the Nineteenth Century.* Cambridge, UK: Cambridge University Press.

Rahman, Fazlur. 1987. *Health and Medicine in the Islamic Tradition: Change and Identity.* New York: Crossroad.

Sayyid-Marsot, Afaf Lutfi, ed. 1979. *Society and the Sexes in Medieval Islam.* Malibu, CA: Undena.

Osman Bakar (1995)
Deputy CEO, International Institute of Advanced Islamic Studies–Malaysia
Emeritus Professor of Philosophy, University of Malaya

VII. ISLAMIC PERSPECTIVES [ADDENDUM]

THE CONTEMPORARY PHENOMENON OF COLLECTIVE *IJTIHĀD* (INDEPENDENT LEGAL REASONING)

Lacking direct references in the primary sources of Islam, especially the Koran and the hadith, contemporary Muslim jurists had to give an "independent legal reasoning or interpretation, known in the Islamic tradition as *ijtihād*," of what these sources would imply about emerging bioethical issues. Recognizing the complex nature of bioethics and the specialized knowledge of modern sciences required for this purpose, cotemporary jurists have been studying bioethics in cooperation with biomedical scientists. This phenomenon, known as the collective *ijtihād* (*al-ijtihād al-jamāʿī*), assumed an institutional form in the 1980s through three main organizations. The Islamic Organization for Medical Sciences (IOMS), based in Kuwait and established officially in 1984, made the most intriguing contribution. IOMS coordinates with two other authoritative organizations that pay occasional but not exclusive attention to bioethics. One is the Islamic Fiqh Academy (IFA), established in 1977, which is affiliated with the Muslim World League and based in Mecca, Saudi Arabia. The other is the International Islamic Fiqh Academy, established in 1981, based in Jeddah, Saudi Arabia, and affiliated with the Organization of Islamic Cooperation (Ghaly 2010).

By studying the collective discussions run by these organizations on abortion, one can identify the issues that contemporary Muslim jurists took over from classical Islamic law, without considerable changes, and the issues that have undergone specific changes and the role of biomedical knowledge in this respect. The main issue relevant to abortion that remained unchanged is the aforementioned understanding of ensoulment. A number of Muslim biomedical scientists argued that the beginning of human life should not be linked to ensoulment because it is a metaphysical concept that cannot be measured by physicians. They proposed measurable biological criteria, which demonstrate that life starts from the very moment of fertilization. However, this opinion was opposed by other biomedical scientists and also by the majority of Muslim jurists, who argued that clear references in the Koran and hadith to ensoulment should not be disregarded because of controversial biomedical postulations. Thus, abortion after ensoulment cannot be tolerated on any ground except when it is firmly established that pregnancy endangers the mother's life (Awadhi and Gindi 1989; Ghaly 2012).

On the other hand, information provided by biomedical scientists proved to be influential in the discussions on the possibility of inducing abortion before ensoulment. Some of the classical opinions were rejected because of their nonconformity with recent biomedical information. This holds true, for instance, to the opinion that holds that the unborn can be aborted before ensoulment, even in the absence of any compelling need, because at this stage it is nothing more than a thickened blood (*dam mun'aqid*). Biomedical scientists demonstrated that the embryo is a living being that grows and develops from the very beginning of pregnancy. Thus, both biomedical scientists and jurists agreed that abortion should always be seen as aggression against life even if it is not yet a human life and this aggression can be tolerated only if there is a valid reason in the eyes of sharia (Ghaly 2012).

Biomedical knowledge also played a decisive role in investigating specific cases to see if they can be classified as "valid reasons" to induce abortion before ensoulment. The cases of deformed fetuses, discussed by the IFA in 1990, and pregnant women infected with AIDS, discussed by the IOMS in 1993, serve as illustrative examples in this regard. Concerning the deformed fetuses, the IFA held that aborting a deformed fetus before ensoulment, at the request of the parents, is permissible on the condition that a medical report, based on clinical and laboratory investigation and drafted by a committee of specialist and trustworthy physicians, confirm that the fetus suffers serious and incurable deformations and that even if pregnancy continues and a full-term neonate is born, the newborn will undergo a miserable life full of pains for him- or herself and for the family as well (Majma' 2005) Concerning the possibility of terminating the pregnancy of women infected with AIDS, the IOMS adopted the following standpoint: "Had science been able to diagnose the disease in a fetus at an early stage [i.e., before ensoulment], that would probably be a justification of aborting that fetus in accordance with relevant rulings of Islamic Law, particularly since no remedy for this disease has been discovered yet. A physician may recommend abortion as being in the mother's interest, because pregnancy reduces the latency period of the disease and hastens its maturity" (Awadi and Jundi 2005).

We conclude this item by quoting article 63 of *The International Islamic Code for Medical and Health Ethics* issued by the IOMS in 2004, which can be seen as a standard contemporary Islamic position on abortion:

> A physician should not cause a pregnant woman to abort, unless when medical considerations call for it, the mother's health and life are being threatened. Abortion, however, is permissible before the end of the fourth month of pregnancy when it is definitely established that continued pregnancy involves a risk of a serious injury to the mother. This, however, should be confirmed by a medical committee of specialists of no less than three members, one of whom is familiar with the disease for which the termination of pregnancy is recommended. The committee members should prepare a report in which they specify the definite risk that threatens the mother's health if the pregnancy continues. When abortion is recommended, the mother and her husband or guardian should be advised of the fact and their written consent obtained. All other exceptional cases, including pregnancy resulting from rape, should be referred to the authorities of Islamic *fatwa* and legislation, and to the laws and regulations in force. (Awadi and Jundi 2005)

SEE ALSO *Embryo and Fetus: V. Religious Perspectives; Islam, Bioethics in; Near and Middle East, Bioethics in: III. Arab World; Population Ethics: IV. Islamic Perspectives*

BIBLIOGRAPHY

Awadhi, Abd El-Rahman al-, and Ahmad Raga'i al-Gindi. 1989. *Human Reproduction in Islam.* Kuwait: Islamic Organization for Medical Sciences.

Awadhi, Abd El-Rahman al-, and Ahmad Raga'i al-Gindi. 2005. *The International Islamic Code for Medical and Health Ethics.* Kuwait: Islamic Organization for Medical Sciences.

Ghaly, Mohammed. 2010. "Human Cloning through the Eyes of Muslim Scholars: The New Phenomenon of the Islamic International Religioscientific Institutions." *Zygon* 45 (1): 7–35.

Ghaly, Mohammed. 2012. "The Beginning of Human Life: Islamic Bioethical Perspectives." *Zygon* 47 (1): 175–213.

Majma' al-Fiqh al-Islāmī. 2005. *Majallat Majma' al-fiqh al-Islāmī* 5 (7). Mecca: Islamic Fiqh Academy.

Mohammed Ghaly
Professor of Islamic Law and Biomedical Ethics, Center for Islamic Legislation and Ethics (CILE), Hamad Bin Khalifa University, Qatar Foundation

VIII. BUDDHIST PERSPECTIVES

An adequate understanding of how Buddhist traditions address the practice of abortion requires two perspectives. First, what have traditional Buddhist texts said about such issues as the morality of abortion, any instances in which it might be morally acceptable, the moral status of the fetus, and the relationship between a pregnant woman and her fetus? Second, we need to account for the fact that the term *Buddhism* is a misnomer if we assume that it refers to a singular, unified set of ideas and practices. While it might be argued that there is at least a common core of ideas, specific Buddhist cultures have instantiated Buddhist thought and practice in a variety of ways. Thus, we explore how different Buddhist cultures interpret Buddhist teachings in dealing with the morality of abortion.

HISTORICAL BUDDHIST PERSPECTIVES

The Buddhist textual record clearly indicates that abortion is considered murder and thus morally problematic because of the negative karmic consequence that such an act produces. Abortion violates the first of the five precepts that both the monastic community and the laity are expected to follow and uphold: abstention from causing injury to all living beings. Early Buddhist texts made this point with regard to the behavior of monks, as evidenced from this passage from the Vinaya section of the Pali canon:

> An ordained monk should not intentionally deprive a living thing of life even if it is only an ant. A monk who deliberately deprives a human being of life, even to the extent of causing an abortion, is no longer a follower of the Buddha. As a flat stone broken asunder cannot be put back together again, a monk who deliberately deprives a human being of life is no longer a follower of the Buddha. This is something not to be done by you as long as life lasts. (Quoted in Keown 1995, 93)

Here, the fetus is understood as holding the same moral status as an adult human being.

The same text reveals a Buddhist understanding of the temporal parameters of a human life: "A human being [exists] in the interval between the first moment when mind arises in the mother's womb [that is to say] the first manifestation of consciousness (*vijñāna*), and death" (quoted in Keown 1995, 93). The term for consciousness, *vijñāna*, is central to how Buddhists traditionally understood that the embryo was a human being at conception.

The manifestation of consciousness in the embryo is part of the ongoing process known as *saṃsāra*, the Buddhist notion that sentient *beings cycle through multiple births, deaths, and rebirths until enlightenment is* attained. In order for conception to occur, what one text describes as an "intermediate being" must be present; that is, the consciousness—or mental continuum—of an individual who exists only in an interim state between death and rebirth (Keown 1995, 93). Thus, at conception, the consciousness takes physical form as a reborn sentient being.

This way of understanding conception and the embryo has two moral implications. First, it is possible to think of the embodiment of consciousness in the embryo as constituting a Buddhist equivalent of the Christian notion of ensoulment. However, equating Buddhist consciousness and Christian ensoulment is problematic because, for Buddhists, the multiple lives, deaths, and rebirths that are experienced prior to release from the samsaric cycle are a continuous whole. From an unenlightened perspective, it appears that lives are discontinuous, but this is not the case according to Buddhist teachings. Only once enlightenment, or nirvana (nirvāna), is attained can one clearly perceive the flow of constituent elements (dharmas) that appear and disappear as sentient beings move through the samsaric cycle. This continuity also contributes to the notion that an embryo or fetus is no different than a human being who is already born.

The second moral implication involves the Buddhist understanding of existence as interdependent. The concept of dependent arising (*pratītya-samutpāda*) underscores that being is a result of cause and effect, and this has implications for how we understand the nature of a fetus. From the standpoint of interdependence, a sentient being is reborn because of deleterious actions in past lives, the result of ignorance (*avidyā*) about the true nature of the universe. Until one is enlightened, desires and selfish action will keep one enmeshed in the samsaric cycle, with the attendant mental and physical suffering, or *duhkha* (*duḥkha*), that arises when one fails to grasp that existence is transitory and impermanent. Hence, the Buddhist characterization of the fetus is not wholly innocent, at least not in the way usually assumed in American culture.

The central Buddhist notion that all life is suffering—the first of the Four Noble Truths—also applies to the fetus. A mother's womb is described as something less than the idyllic environment that nurtures the fetus until its rude awakening into the world. A fourteenth-century Thai text explains the unpleasantries of fetal life:

> The baby has great trouble while it is in the mother's abdomen: the place is extremely revolting and disgusting; it is damp and full of bad smells caused by the eighty broods of worms and parasites that live there.... These worms and parasites are all mixed up in the mother's abdomen and cover the body of the fetus like a skin disease. ... Blood and lymph run down all over its body, dripping at all times; the baby is like a monkey who, when it rains, sits in the hollow of a tree clutching its fists in a sluggish and dejected way. (Quoted in Florida 2000, 140)

Such a view underscores the conflicting sense that traditional Buddhist texts have of human existence. Life is inherently unsatisfactory, suffused with the suffering that accompanies existence. To be born as a human being—or as any kind of sentient being—is by definition to have engaged in negative actions in previous lives. So, if the fetus suffers in the womb, it is not surprising. By the same token, Buddhism posits that only human beings can gain enlightenment—thereby passing out of the samsaric cycle. Thus, only human existence offers the possibility of moving beyond a world of suffering.

Despite traditional Buddhist views that abortion is murder and a violation of the first precept, there has historically been little attempt by the Buddhist monastic community to try to persuade or otherwise coerce pregnant women into rejecting abortion as a real choice in the case of an unwanted pregnancy. Implicit in this lack of intimidation is the belief that a woman's karmic consequence is her own to shape.

CONTEMPORARY BUDDHIST PRACTICES

Traditional Buddhist attitudes toward abortion and the moral status of the fetus suggest that abortion would be equally condemned in contemporary Buddhist cultures. While formally this is true, actual practices reflect significant divergences from this expectation. Perhaps surprisingly, abortions are common in countries strongly influenced by Buddhism, such as Thailand, South Korea, and Japan. Although the Buddhist establishment in these countries officially opposes abortion, Buddhist institutions have participated little in public discourse about the morality of abortion. Instead, such conversations have mostly involved medical professionals and politicians. Furthermore, new medical technologies and recent scientific discoveries about fetal development have complicated the issue. We must also take into account that the ideals of a religious tradition often take a back seat to the realities of life. Thailand and Japan provide examples of variations in how abortion is addressed in contemporary cultures influenced by Buddhism.

Abortion in Thailand. In Thailand, Buddhism permeates all aspects of life. Abortion in Thailand is prohibited by legislation, with exceptions only in circumstances such as danger to the mother's life and in instances of rape or incest. Buddhist precepts against killing and doing harm to others are used to justify this legislation. Thai Buddhists apply the first precept to the unborn because a fetus is considered a human being from conception, and often cite traditional Buddhist texts that oppose abortion.

However, orthodox Buddhist views sometimes clash with the realities of contemporary life in Thailand. In fact, abortions are performed in Thailand (although illegally), and Thais advocate different interpretations of Buddhist ethical principles to justify or deny the morality of abortion. While some Buddhists invoke the nonharm precept, others maintain that abortion—in cases such as pregnancy due to rape or incest—can contribute to positive karmic consequence if performed with selfless intention.

On the other hand, in situations where abortions might be morally justified (at least in the United States) this is not necessarily the case in Thailand. Malee Lerdmaleewong and Caroline Francis (1998) list reasons that Thais cite for seeking illegal abortions, including economic difficulties and the lack of adequate or effective contraception. Yet when a Thai woman learns her fetus is developing abnormally due to Down syndrome or some other serious disease, abortions are rarely sought (Ratanakul 1998). In such cases, women are reluctant to seek an abortion because they believe that the fetus's disease is the result of negative karmic consequence produced by both the mother and the fetus in a prior existence. To abort the fetus would only increase the negative effect (Ratanakul 1998). Fear of detrimental karmic consequence, then, is a deterrent to having an abortion.

Abortion in Japan. Japanese Buddhists do not condone abortion. Nevertheless, in Japan, Buddhism generally tolerates abortion and does not enter into public debate over its morality. However, Japanese Buddhist institutions sometimes play a significant role in assuaging the negative karmic consequence that accrues from abortion. Rather than criticizing women for choosing abortion, rituals are enacted that are aimed at easing the pain of women and their families over the karmically problematic act of aborting a fetus.

In Japan, abortion is considered a "necessary sorrow" (LaFleur 1990). That is, while never a moral good, sometimes abortion can be justified over carrying a child to term. From a Japanese perspective, it is morally problematic and socially irresponsible to bring more children into the world than a family can support and nurture. In addition, Buddhist beliefs about rebirth characterize abortion as postponing the fetus's entry into the samsaric world. Nevertheless, there are moral consequences to aborting the fetus. In order to try to rectify the negative karmic consequence that accrues from an abortion, Japanese Buddhist rituals, known as *mizuko kuyō*, are performed in order to speed the soul of the aborted fetus (*mizuko*) to a more positive rebirth. Furthermore, *mizuko kuyō* rituals are intended to comfort aborted fetuses. Such rites also serve as a way for parents to repent sexual misconduct that results in unwanted pregnancy. Repentance helps alleviate the effects of immoral behavior, especially when admitted to a Buddha or bodhisattva (enlightenment being).

Abortions are a common form of birth control in Japan. Temples devoted to *mizuko kuyō* flourish, serving the spiritual needs of both mother and aborted fetus. The bodhisattva Jizō (in Sanskrit, Ksitigarbha*;* literally "Earth Womb") is usually a focus of worship at such temples. Jizō is believed to aid sentient beings in their movement through the samsaric cycle and is especially credited with protecting deceased children as well as miscarried and aborted fetuses. At many temples throughout Japan, small statues of Jizō, representing the fetus, are dressed in children's clothing and presented with offerings of toys. Through such offerings, the negative karmic consequence of killing the fetus can be rectified.

BUDDHIST PERSPECTIVES ON ABORTION: PROSPECTS

As with many religious traditions, Buddhism has been altered by new scientific and other kinds of knowledge and by the cultural contexts in which it is embraced. These changes are particularly evident in Buddhist perspectives on abortion that have emerged in an American context. The American Zen master Robert Aitken views a woman's decision to have an abortion in this way:

> I get the impression that when a woman is sensitive to her feelings, she is conscious that abortion is killing a part of herself and terminating the ancient process, begun anew within herself, of bringing life into being. Thus she is likely to feel acutely miserable after making a decision to have an abortion. This is a time for compassion for the woman, and for her to be compassionate with herself and for her unborn child. If I am consulted, and we explore the options carefully and I learn that the decision is definite, I encourage her to go through the act with the consciousness of a mother who holds her dying child in her arms, lovingly nurturing it as it passes from life. Sorrow and suffering from the nature of samsara, the flow of life and death, and the decision to prevent birth is made on balance with other elements of suffering. Once the decision is made, there is no blame, but rather acknowledgment that sadness pervades the whole universe, and this bit of life goes with our deepest love. (1984, 21–22)

Given the Buddhist emphasis on nonharm and compassion, it is perhaps surprising that the concern here is expressed entirely from the mother's perspective. This may reflect a Buddhist interpretation filtered through an American sensibility that centers on a woman's rights. In any event, the moral and karmic consequences of an abortion are less clear than in contexts explored previously in this article.

If Aitken's (1984) view represents an attempt to make Buddhism more palatable to an American congregation, other ideas might also influence the way that at least some contemporary Buddhists—whether in the United States or in Southeast and East Asia—view bioethical issues like abortion, especially given the globalization of scientific ideas. Thus, for instance, Buddhists may have to confront a neuroscientific view that consciousness is impossible without a central nervous system, which would seem to conflict with the traditional Buddhist notion of consciousness (*vijñāna*) and its appearance in the embryo at conception.

SEE ALSO *Buddhism, Bioethics in; Embryo and Fetus: V. Religious Perspectives; Ethics: V. Religion and Morality; Future Generations, Reproductive Technologies and Obligations to; Population Ethics: X. Buddhist Perspectives*

BIBLIOGRAPHY

Aitken, Robert. 1984. *The Mind of Clover: Essays in Zen Buddhist Ethics*. San Francisco: North Point.

Barnhart, Michael G. 1998. "Buddhism and the Morality of Abortion." *Journal of Buddhist Ethics* 5: 276–97. http://blogs.dickinson.edu/buddhistethics/files/2010/04/barnh981.pdf

Florida, Robert E. 2000. "Buddhism and Abortion." In *Contemporary Buddhist Ethics*, edited by Damien Keown, 137–68. Richmond, UK: Curzon Press.

Hardacre, Helen. 1997. *Marketing the Menacing Fetus in Japan*. Berkeley: University of California Press.

Harvey, Peter. 2000. *An Introduction to Buddhist Ethics: Foundations, Values, and Issues*. Cambridge, UK: Cambridge University Press.

Hughes, James J., and Damien Keown. 1995. "Buddhism and Medical Ethics: A Bibliographic Introduction." *Journal of Buddhist Ethics* 2:105–24. http://blogs.dickinson.edu/buddhistethics/files/2010/04/Buddhism-and-Medical-Ethics.pdf

Keown, Damien. 1995. *Buddhism and Bioethics*. Basingstoke, UK: Palgrave. Reprinted in 2001.

Keown, Damien, ed. 1998. *Buddhism and Abortion*. London: Macmillan.

Keown, Damien. 2005. *Buddhist Ethics: A Very Short Introduction*. Oxford: Oxford University Press.

LaFleur, William R. 1990. "Contestation and Confrontation: The Morality of Abortion in Japan." *Philosophy East and West* 40 (4): 529–42.

LaFleur, William R. 1992. *Liquid Life: Abortion and Buddhism in Japan*. Princeton, NJ: Princeton University Press.

Lerdmaleewong, Malee, and Caroline Francis. 1998. "Abortion in Thailand: A Feminist Perspective." *Journal of Buddhist Ethics* 5:22–48. http://blogs.dickinson.edu/buddhistethics/files/2010/04/aborti1.pdf

Ratanakul, Pinit. 1986. *Bioethics: An Introduction to the Ethics of Medicine and Life Sciences*. Bangkok: Mahidol University.

Ratanakul, Pinit. 1998. "Socio-Medical Aspects of Abortion in Thailand." In *Buddhism and Abortion*, edited by Damien Keown, 53–66. London: Macmillan.

Tsomo, Karma Lekshe. 1998. "Prolife, Prochoice: Buddhism and Reproductive Ethics." Feminism and Nonviolence Studies Association. Accessed May 18, 2013. http://www.fnsa.org/fall98/tsomo.html

Tsomo, Karma Lekshe. 2006. *Into the Jaws of Yama, Lord of Death: Buddhism, Bioethics, and Death*. Albany: State University of New York Press.

William E. Deal
Severance Professor of the History of Religion, Department of Religious Studies, Case Western Reserve University

IX. HINDU PERSPECTIVES

Hinduism is a complex belief system. It is more than a religion; rather, it is a way of life. There is no single authoritative text with regard to Hinduism and its beliefs and practices, since it did not emerge as a religion at a specific point in time. The Vedas are largely a compilation of hymns composed over a vast span of time, and within the compositions in the different Vedic texts, a changing material and social order is reflected. Similarly social commentaries, which are used as authoritative classical texts for framing laws even in contemporary India, for Hindus represent a multiplicity of views and practices, given the different locations in space and time and the social backdrop in which they were written. Diversity of practice in both custom and belief is a central feature of the vastly different ways people see themselves as Hindus in contemporary India. This arises from the historical process of the origin of the Hindus who in the first place represented the people living east of the river Indus and who broadly associated with Brahmanical practices that evolved over centuries, as they came to be extended to a range of social-material formations in which people were located in vastly different forms of socioeconomic organization that itself was continuously changing. As the peasant society and culture spread to new areas, it absorbed, assimilated, subordinated, or suppressed alternate modes of belief and practice. This process was marked by both dialogue and confrontation within what was seen to be Hinduism and between Hindus and others.

The concept of Hindu dharma, the basis of ethics in Hindu society, as enshrined in classical texts makes no distinction between social and moral motivations for one's actions. In fact the two are inextricably enmeshed with each other. Hindu perspectives on the (medical) practice of abortion, including beliefs concerning the human and moral status of the fetus and the obligations of pregnant women, other family members, and society, are derived primarily from Sanskrit texts (the canonical scriptures of the Hindus) ranging from 600 B.C.E. to 600 C.E. It was in this period that the Hindu view on the moral status of the unborn in relation to abortion was developed and established (Lipner 1989), which exerts a powerful influence on the Hindu mind even in the early twenty-first century. The classical texts, tradition, and doctrine are very clear in condemning abortion. It is not only a sin but also a serious social misdeed that imperils the stability and preservation of the social order and structure, with important social and religious consequences. Although the core beliefs remain the same, Hinduism is pragmatic and flexible, adapting to changes in different eras; it does not have a singular, static, dogmatic, and perennial view on abortion and other issues concerning bioethics (Chandrasekhar 1994).

As India is a secular state, the separation of religion and state allows for secular laws on all matters governing life. Abortion has been legal in India since 1971 and is widely practiced. Hindus in general tend to support abortion in cases where the pregnant woman's life is at risk or when the fetus has a severe congenital abnormality. However, since the 1980s the liberal abortion laws have been misused to prevent unwanted females from being born. There is little public debate on abortion in general; discussion has centered mainly on sex-selective abortion and the proliferation of abortion clinics in urban areas (Visaria et al. 2007).

HINDU BELIEF SYSTEM

Hindus believe that all life is sacred; it is a spark of the divine. All creatures have a soul (*ātman*) and are manifestations of the Supreme Being (*Paramātman*), and therefore nonviolence (ahimsa) must be practiced. The doctrine of reincarnation, which sees life as a repeating cycle of birth, death, and rebirth, is basic to Hindu thinking. Belief in the eternal law of karma informs the theory of reincarnation. The individual soul reincarnates in new bodies—evolving through many births and deaths until all the karmic results, good and bad, are resolved—and progresses toward the goal of union with the Supreme Being.

The doctrine of reincarnation is used to make a strong case against abortion. If a fetus is aborted, the soul within it suffers a major karmic setback. It is deprived of the opportunities its potential human existence would have given it to earn good karma and be liberated from the cycle of birth, death, and rebirth (*moksha*). Instead it is returned immediately to the cycle. Thus abortion hinders a soul's spiritual progress, thwarting the unfolding of the karma of both the unborn and the perpetrator of the act.

THE HUMAN AND MORAL STATUS OF THE FETUS IN HINDU SCRIPTURES

According to the doctrine of reincarnation, a fetus is not developing into a person but is a person from the moment of conception. The classical texts that are relevant in this context comprise both *śruti* (the four Vedas, the Brahmanas, the Aranyakas, and the Upanishads) and *smṛti* (the Dharmasūtras; the Puranas; the Dharmaśāstras, including the works of Manu, Yājnavalkya, and Narada; and the Mahabharata) and the evolving compendiums of medical information in Ayurvedic texts, such as the Caraka Saṃhitā and Suśruta Saṃhitā. The soul and the matter that form the fetus are joined together from conception. The soul enters the womb (*garbha*) with the union of semen and (menstrual) blood at the time of conception, making the fetus a living, individual person (*jiva*). It has both a subtle body and a reborn soul, including the karmic inheritance that defines individuality and therefore personhood. "The only dramatically different approach is found in the *Garbha Upaniśad*, a minor text belonging to the second or third century C.E., which claims that the soul's descent into matter occurs only after the seventh month" (Young 2004, 54).

The growing embryo (fetus), because of its moral inviolability and physical vulnerability, deserves special protection and respect. An indication of the special status of the unborn is the multitude of rites (prescribed especially in the Ṛgveda) to be performed at different stages of pregnancy, starting with conception—*garbhādhāna* and *garbhalambhana* rites to ensure the blessing and the tutelage of the gods—and continuing with *puṃsavana* at the end of the first trimester, *garbharakṣana* in the fourth month, and *jātakarma* at the time of delivery (Laale 1996). All these rites prove not only the special status but also the special care that the embryo/fetus requires. It was commonly believed that in a relatively advanced stage of pregnancy there is conscious experience in the womb. By the ninth month the fetus was believed to have achieved very substantial awareness. According to the Garbha Upanishad, the soul remembers its past lives during the last month the fetus spends in the womb (these memories are destroyed during the trauma of birth).

The Dharmaśāstras describe rituals called *samskāras* that mark the various stages in the Hindu life cycle. Several of them protect the fetus at key stages in fetal development. The corollary of protecting the fetus is prohibiting abortion (Young 2004).

HINDUISM AND ABORTION

In Hindu dharma the social and moral principles are inextricably intertwined. From the Hindu point of view, abortion is both a social and a moral transgression. Many Hindus regard the production of offspring as a "public duty," not simply an "individual expression of personal choice" (Lipner 1989). The social imperative lies in the need to continue one's line through male heirs and the obtaining of security for ancestral rites to be performed after death (*śrāddha*).

Hindu scriptures and tradition have from the earliest times condemned the practice of abortion except when the life of the mother-to-be is in danger. Hinduism teaches that the fetus is a living, conscious person needing and deserving protection. The Sanskrit terminology regarding abortion is illustrative for the classical Hindu view on this matter. Hindu scriptures (Ṛgveda) refer to abortion as *garbha-hatya* (womb killing), *bhrūṇahan* (the killing of an embryo), and *bhrūṇahatya* (fetus murder). A distinction is made between abortion and miscarriage; the latter is called *sraṃsana* and *garbhasrāva*, referring to the falling or emission of the embryo (Lipner 1989; Chandrasekhar 1994). This differentiated terminology suggests the moral distinction between abortion and miscarriage. Whereas the former implies intention and consequently responsibility for killing an embryo or fetus, the latter is unintended and morally neutral.

The Upanishads also condemn abortion. The Kaushitaki Upanishad draws a parallel between abortion and the killing of one's parents. The Atharva Veda mentions that the fetus slayer, or *brunaghni*, is among the greatest of sinners. The Gautama Dharma Shastra considers such perpetrators to have lost caste. Losing caste was no small matter; it affected one's social viability and had serious consequences for the socioreligious standing of the family and even prospects of salvation. Another text compares abortion to the killing of a learned Brahman. The analogy implies that the embryo was a potential male who could grow up to learn the Vedas and perform sacrifices and bring great benefits to both humans and gods. Abortion is ranked alongside particularly grievous acts (the five *mahāpātakas*), such as thieving, violating one's guru's (teacher's) bed, consuming intoxicants, and matricide/patricide.

Abortion interferes with nature's arrangement to provide a soul with a new body and is therefore bound to result in unfavorable karma. It is considered a serious violation of the socioreligious order and is proscribed in Hindu tradition and philosophy. Hindu medical ethics stem from the principle of nonviolence (ahimsa). When considering abortion, a Hindu must choose the action that will do the least harm to all involved: the mother and father, the fetus and society. Abortion is a violent act toward a human being (though yet unborn), thus an infringement of the principle of nonviolence. The only situation in which abortion is morally acceptable is when the life of the pregnant woman is threatened.

Classical Hindu medical texts emphasize that the *jiva*, the individual abode of consciousness, is present from the moment of consciousness onward through the process of fetal growth. Even though all Hindu scriptures argue about protecting the embryo by all means, the Suśruta Saṃhitā (Ayurveda), a medical treatise (c. 100), stipulates what is to be done in case of serious problems during delivery (Chikitsita-sthana chapter 15, Mudhagarbha, dealing with the difficult and malpresentation of the fetus and difficult labor), describing first the various steps to be taken to attempt to save both mother and child. "If the fetus is alive, one should attempt to remove it from the womb of the mother alive" (sutra 5). If it is dead, it may be removed. In case the fetus is alive but cannot be safely delivered, surgical removal is forbidden, for "one would harm both mother and offspring. In an irredeemable situation, it is best to cause the miscarriage of the fetus, for no means must be neglected which can prevent the loss of the mother" (sutras 10–11).

However, as Hinduism is not a textual religion, unlike other major world religions, no practicing Hindu reads the classical texts to derive prescripts for individual behavior in everyday life. Nor do Hindus have a single religious leader whose injunctions must be followed. This makes the practice of religion a largely private and individual affair for one's own spiritual development and duty to one's ancestors. It may also explain the noninterference of the religious community in secular politics regarding abortion.

THE MEDICAL PRACTICE OF ABORTION

In modern-day India abortion is widely practiced by Hindus. Abortion has been legal on broad social and medical grounds since the passing of the Medical Termination of Pregnancy Act in 1971. Women have a choice between medical and surgical abortion up to twenty weeks. Unlike the struggle for legal abortion in many countries, abortion has never been a subject of public debate in India. Indian women got the right to abortion without demanding it. Abortion is allowed in the following circumstances: if the continuance of the pregnancy involves a risk to the life of the pregnant woman or injury to her physical or mental health, if the child is likely to suffer from physical or mental abnormalities, or if the pregnancy is caused by rape or the failure of a birth control device. Abortion is not part of the government's family planning program and is ostensibly only a health measure. However, in practice it is used primarily as a family planning method to terminate unwanted pregnancies.

Despite abortion being legal, the incidence of illegal abortions is alarmingly high. According to the Consortium on National Consensus for Medical Abortion in India, every year 7 million induced abortions are reported (Mittal 2012). Other sources mention that about 11 million abortions take place annually and around 20,000 women die every year due to abortion-related complications. Most abortion-related deaths are attributable to illegal abortions. At least ten times as many illegal abortions are carried out as legal ones, and at least 80 percent of women admitted to hospitals with complications have had abortions performed by unqualified practitioners. A high percentage of women seek help for abortion at a late stage of pregnancy for reasons such as internalized abortion shame, lack of confidentiality, ignorance of their legal rights to abortion and the availability of legal abortion facilities, and above all inadequate health care services.

SEX-SELECTIVE ABORTION

Modern reproductive technologies, such as preconceptional testing (through sperm sorting or sex selecting the embryo in favor of males), or prenatal sex detection of the fetus through ultrasound scanning, chorionic villus sampling (screening of placental tissue), and amniocentesis (screening of amniotic fluid) followed by abortion of female fetuses (called female feticide) are misused to prevent unwanted females from being born. These technologies provide the scientific tools to perpetuate the embedded gender bias in society (Gupta 2011).

According to the 2011 Indian decadal census figures, there are 940 females for every 1,000 males (Office of the Registrar General and Census Commissioner, India 2011). The number of girls per 1,000 boys in the under-six age group dropped significantly to 914 from 927 in 2001 (the previous census) (Office of the Registrar General and Census Commissioner, India 2001, 2011). Indiscriminate abortion of female fetuses is the reason for this skewed sex ratio. Different reasons have been cited for the widespread abortion of female fetuses, the foremost being the twofold strong familial and societal pressures on women to bear male children, given the patriarchal system of society that places a higher value on sons, and the Indian government's population policy, which puts pressure on couples to have only one or two children. The illegal promotion of ultrasound machines by business giants and the unethical money-minded radiologists and gynecologists who comply with the demand for abortions also contribute. Strong demands from women's advocacy groups led to legislation banning sex selection in Maharashtra State in May 1988. This was broadened to the Pre-natal Diagnostic Techniques Regulation and Prevention of Misuse Act of 1996 and the amended Pre-conception and Pre-natal Diagnostic Techniques (Prohibition of Sex Selection) Act of 2003, which seek to regulate the use of prenatal diagnosis for medical purposes and to prevent its misuse in India.

However, due to the lack of an effective enforcement and vigilance agency, sex selection followed by abortion has become a clandestine practice offered at exorbitant rates at clinics where quality of care cannot be guaranteed, posing an additional risk to women's health. Although sex selection has been banned since 1994, more than 10 million female fetuses have been aborted in India (Agnihotri 2000, 2003; Patel 2007). The extremely skewed under-six sex ratio in several Indian states proves that legislation does not act as a deterrent.

CONCLUSION

Hindu scriptures specifically condemn abortion. Abortion is unacceptable in the Hindu perspective, as it is seen to interfere with the natural and necessary cycle of karma and rebirth. It is thus a grave infringement on an individual's destiny toward the goal of liberation (*moksha*) and the principle of nonviolence (ahimsa). Traditional Hinduism and many modern Hindus also see abortion as a breach of the duty to secure children for genealogical continuity and to produce new members of society. Nevertheless, the secular Indian laws make abortion a legal practice, although it is often misused to eliminate the births of unwanted females.

SEE ALSO *Embryo and Fetus: V. Religious Perspectives; Ethics: V. Religion and Morality; Hinduism, Bioethics in; Population Ethics: IX. Hindu Perspectives*

BIBLIOGRAPHY

Agnihotri, Satish B. 2000. *Sex Ratio Patterns in the Indian Population: A Fresh Exploration.* New Delhi: Sage.

Agnihotri, Satish B. 2003. "Survival of the Girl Child: Tunnelling Out of the Chakravyuha." *Economic and Political Weekly* 33 (41): 4351–60.

BBC. 2009. "Hinduism and Abortion." http://www.bbc.co.uk/religion/religions/hinduism/hinduethics/abortion_1.shtml

Bloomfield, Maurice, trans. 1897. "Hymns of the Atharva-Veda." In *Sacred Books of the East*, vol. 42, translated by Maurice Bloomfield. http://www.sacred-texts.com/hin/sbe42/index.htm

Bühler, Georg, trans. 1886. "The Laws of Manu." In *Sacred Books of the East*, vol. 25, translated by Georg Bühler. http://www.sacred-texts.com/hin/manu.htm

Chandrasekhar, S. 1994. *India's Abortion Experience.* Denton: University of North Texas Press.

Coward, Harold, and Tejinder Sidhu. 2008. "Hindu and Sikh Bioethics." In *The Cambridge Textbook of Bioethics*, edited by Peter A. Singer and A. M. Viens, 403–7. Cambridge, UK: Cambridge University Press.

Crawford, S. Cromwell. 1995. *Dilemmas of Life and Death: Hindu Ethics in a North American Context.* Albany: State University of New York Press.

Grimes, John; Sushil Mittal; and Gene Thursby. 2006. "Hindu Dharma." In *Religions of South Asia: An Introduction*, edited by Sushil Mittal and Gene Thursby, 15–86. London: Routledge.

Gupta, Jyotsna Agnihotri. 2011. "Unwanted Daughters: Discrimination and Elimination of the Girl Child in India." *Tijdschrift voor Genderstudies* 14 (3): 42–57.

Jain, Sandhya. 2003. "The Right to Family Planning, Contraception, and Abortion: The Hindu View." In *Sacred Rights: The Case for Contraception and Abortion in World Religions*, edited by Daniel C. Maguire, 129–44. Oxford: Oxford University Press.

Johnston, William Robert, comp. 2013. "Historical Abortion Statistics, India." http://www.johnstonsarchive.net/policy/abortion/ab-india.html

Laale, H. Willer. 1996. "Embryology and Abortion in Indian Antiquity: A Brief Survey." *Indian Journal of History of Science* 31 (3): 233–58.

Lipner, Julius J. 1989. "The Classical Hindu View on Abortion and the Moral Status of the Unborn." In *Hindu Ethics: Purity, Abortion, and Euthanasia*, edited by Harold G. Coward, Julius Lipner, and Katherine K. Young, 41–70. Albany: State University of New York Press.

Mittal, Suneeta. 2012. "Introduction." Consortium on National Consensus for Medical Abortion in India. Accessed September 10, 2012. http://web.archive.org/web/20081120105036/http://www.aiims.edu//aiims/events/Gynaewebsite/ma_finalsite/introduction.html

Müller, Max, trans. 1879. "The Upanishads, Part I." In *Sacred Books of the East*, vol. 1, translated by Max Müller. http://www.sacred-texts.com/hin/sbe01/index.htm

Müller, Max, trans. 1884. "The Upanishads, Part II." In *Sacred Books of the East*, vol. 15, translated by Max Müller. http://www.sacred-texts.com/hin/sbe15/index.htm

Office of the Registrar General and Census Commissioner, India. 2001. "Census Data 2001." http://www.censusindia.gov.in/2011-common/census_data_2001.html

Office of the Registrar General and Census Commissioner, India. 2011. CensusInfo India 2011. http://www.devinfolive.info/censusinfodashboard/

Patel, Tulsi, ed. 2007. *Sex-Selective Abortion in India: Gender, Society, and New Reproductive Technologies.* New Delhi: Sage.

Patel, Vibhuti. 1984. "Amniocentesis and Female Foeticide: Misuse of Medical Technology." *Socialist Health Review* 1 (2): 69–71.

Visaria, Leela; Vimala Ramachandran; Bela Ganatra; et al. 2007. "Abortion Use and Practice: Evidence, Challenges, and Emerging Issues." In *Abortion in India: Ground Realities in Use and Practice*, edited by Leela Visaria and Vimala Ramachandran, 14–16. New Delhi: Routledge.

Young, Katherine K. 2004. "The Status of the Fetus in Scriptural Hinduism." In *Der Umgang mit vorgeburtlichem Leben in anderen Kulturen: Tagungsdokumentation der Jahrestagung des Nationalen Ethikrates 2003*, edited by Nationaler Ethikrat, 51–61. Berlin: Nationaler Ethikrat.

Jyotsna Agnihotri Gupta
Assistant Professor, Gender and Diversity, University of Humanistic Studies, Utrecht, Netherlands

ABUSE, INTERPERSONAL

This entry consists of the following:

I. CHILD ABUSE

Current pediatrics and social-work textbooks generally include chapters on child abuse that describe the epidemiology, clinical manifestations, differential diagnosis, and treatment of abused children. They usually discuss the legal requirement to notify state child-protection agencies of suspected abuse and may describe the investigations such reports trigger. It is accepted by most pediatricians, social workers, and laymen that investigations may result in legal actions against parents and other responsible adults. Children may be removed from their homes. Parents may have their custodial rights terminated and may face criminal charges. The entire process of diagnosis and intervention for child abuse is presented as both necessary and morally compelling.

ATTITUDES ON CHILD ABUSE

However, within this seeming consensus of moral sentiment lies a mystery. Until the twentieth century, much of what we now consider to be child abuse was regarded as morally acceptable and legally permissible. In fact, people generally argued not only that it was permissible to oppress and punish children to the point of physical abuse, but also that such abuse was necessary for the children's moral edification (Radbill 1974); thus, "Spare the rod and spoil the child." Parents and teachers had absolute authority over children's lives. They could, and did, physically and sexually abuse children with an impunity so complete that such acts were seldom recognized or acknowledged.

Twenty-first-century approaches to child abuse in the United States and many other countries reflect a radical change in our moral view of the family. Until the twentieth century, families were usually seen as small, autocratic moral universes. Parents (in most cases, fathers) could use children (and wives) as they saw fit. Children had no independent moral rights. The movement to give children rights, including the right not to be abused, required a sea change in moral sentiment. Such moral sea changes occur only rarely in human history. For example, a culture moves from a belief in monarchy to a belief in democracy. Or slavery, once seen as legal and appropriate, is made illegal and is widely viewed as immoral. These watershed events in the history of morality raise important questions about the timelessness of moral principles. In the case of child abuse, they raise questions about our view of the moral status of children. Was child abuse always wrong? If so, why was it not recognized as such until recently? Are our moral sensitivities improving over time? Or did child abuse only recently become wrong? And more generally, are our moral values timeless and immutable or are they transient, conditional, and constantly evolving?

Attitudes about parental rights and responsibilities and about the corresponding rights and duties of children have aimed to teach children to become responsible citizens of the societies in which they live. Different societies have different moral standards with regard to many aspects of life. Our society has come to restrict child abuse. At the same time, we have come to allow children to experience things that are forbidden in many other cultures. We allow schools, rather than parents, to teach children about sexual activity. We facilitate access to contraception and do not condemn early sexual activity during the teenage years. We allow teens access to the Internet, to television, and to films that show morally problematic behaviors. Many of these activities would once have been regarded as ethically dubious. In many societies, they still are. These evolving moral standards in different domains of a child's life can be seen as experiments in social policy; we are trying out different approaches to helping children become the kind of citizens we want in our society. This entry will examine our evolving societal understanding of child abuse within this framework. By doing so, the entry will highlight the evolving ethics that undergird our view of society's role in overseeing the family and protecting children from abuse.

DEFINING CHILD ABUSE

Definitions of abuse are notoriously variable, circular, or designed to leave room for interpretation on a case-by-case basis. In the United States, the Child Abuse Prevention and Treatment Act of 1974 (PL93–247) defines abuse and neglect as "the physical and mental injury, sexual abuse, negligent treatment or maltreatment of a child under the age of 18 by a person who is responsible for the child's welfare under circumstances which indicate that the child's health and welfare is harmed or threatened thereby." This federal definition may be modified by state child-protection agencies.

State definitions of child abuse vary. A particular act may or may not be considered child abuse, depending on the nature of the act itself, whether the act caused harm, whether there was or should have been prior recognition that the act would cause harm, and whether the caretaker might have prevented the harm.

In both physical and sexual abuse, different individuals or communities distinguish acceptable from unacceptable behaviors using different criteria. In physical abuse, a distinction must be made between acceptable forms of discipline or punishment and abuse. As Kim Oates (1982) points out, definitions must specify whether abuse should be defined in terms of particular actions or particular effects. He describes two children who are pushed roughly to the ground by their fathers. One falls against a carpeted floor, the other hits a protruding cupboard door. The second sustains a skull fracture, the first is uninjured. If an act must cause harm to be abuse, then the second child was clearly abused, while the first may not have been. Acts that cause no physical harm are often not classified as abuse. This is, in part, because it is generally harder to sustain criminal convictions or obtain civil sanctions when there is no evidence of physical harm. Sadly, a child who has not been physically harmed may sustain as much or more psychological harm as from actions that cause physical signs of abuse.

In sexual abuse, definitional problems also arise. Child sexual abuse is generally intrafamilial. Thus, it falls under the rubric of incest. Prohibitions against incest are universal in human societies. However, different societies and cultures define incest differently. As Goodwin noted "Parent–child nudity, communal sleeping arrangements, and tolerance for masturbation and peer sex play in children coexist with stringent incest taboos. … Mothers in many cultures use genital manipulation to soothe and pleasure infants. Some cultures prescribe the deflowering of pubertal girls by an adult male or by the father" (Goodwin 1988, 33). Such seemingly exotic cultural differences are mirrored by widely varying beliefs about appropriate and inappropriate activities within our own culture. Some parents may sleep with their children, bathe with them, or take pictures of the children naked on the beach. These activities may be seen as legal, moral, emotionally nurturing, and entirely appropriate. They may also be seen as illegal, immoral, emotionally abusive, or entirely inappropriate.

In addition to physical and sexual abuse, parents can be found culpable of child abuse based on neglect of their child. Neglect includes psychosocial neglect as well as medical neglect. Neglect is defined as failure to provide necessary care to a child. Here, too, cultural or religious differences may lead to different views of parental obligations. Christian Scientists, for example, may claim that it is appropriate not to take their sick children to a doctor, while courts may determine that such behavior constitutes neglect. Some Native Americans believe that organ transplantation is prohibited and so may refuse life-sustaining treatment for their children in liver failure. Similarly, Jehovah's Witnesses may, on the basis of their belief, seek to refuse consent for blood transfusions for their children, even if transfusions would preserve life. In situations like these, judgments must be made about the relative importance of respecting religious and cultural diversity, on the one hand, and protecting the interests of vulnerable children, on the other.

In addition to cultural differences in defining what behaviors are or are not permissible, serious moral problems arise when we attempt to determine whether, in any particular case, a behavior that is clearly not permissible has, in fact, occurred. Court cases may turn on the rules governing the collecting and presentation of evidence. Even in adult rape cases, victims have difficulty convincing juries that they have been raped. Such difficulties are compounded in child-abuse cases, where young children often cannot testify convincingly on their own behalf.

In summary, physical abuse, sexual abuse, and medical neglect of children exist along a spectrum, from obvious cruelty, exploitation, or failure to meet the child's basic needs to grayer areas of corporal punishment, sexual game playing, or differing religious views about the desirability of medical treatment. The strong moral arguments against egregious abuse of children often lose strength as the definition of abuse expands along a spectrum that includes activities that may be considered morally praiseworthy, morally acceptable, morally forgivable, or immoral but noncriminal.

REPORTING CHILD ABUSE

Most laws are vague in defining the reporting requirements for child abuse. Generally, they require reporting if someone "has reasons to believe that a child has been subjected to abuse." Such laws do not attempt to quantify the degree of suspicion, the quality of the evidence, or the likelihood of abuse that must be present to compel a report. In the crafting of such laws, the goal was to protect the people who report abuse by allowing broad latitude to individuals in defining what they mean by a "suspicion" of abuse. This approach reflects a utilitarian calculus by which it is judged better to have reports made that prove to be groundless than to allow subtle cases of abuse to go unreported. Even with such vague and permissive requirements, evidence suggests that abuse is underreported rather than overreported.

There are a number of reasons why people might not report child abuse even though they believe it to be wrong. Child abuse may be ignored because people have difficulty defining and recognizing it (Besharov 1981; Zellman 1992). It may go undiscovered because adults who are aware that a child is being abused are reticent to get involved (Dhooper, Royse, and Wolfe 1991). Or professionals may feel reticent to threaten what they perceive as a therapeutic relationship with the adult or adults involved. Reticence to report suspected child abuse may be based on the sociology of health care delivery, on respect for confidentiality in the doctor-parent relationship, on unwillingness to stigmatize parents when there is doubt about the actual occurrence of abuse, or on a desire to preserve a therapeutic relationship or avoid the perception that professionals are enemies.

Fewer reports are made by pediatricians in private practice than by pediatricians who are salaried employees of public hospitals and clinics. This likely reflects the economics of professional practice, rather than the prevalence of abusive behavior in different populations. Pediatricians in private practice are paid by the parents. They often develop long-term relationships with these adults and the children. In such situations, relationships must be based on mutual trust. Pediatricians may give adults the benefit of the doubt regarding injuries that may be associated with abuse (McCarthy 2008). They may also be fearful that child-abuse reports will be bad for business. These factors may partially explain why reports of abuse are more likely to come from hospital emergency rooms than from private doctors' offices (Badger 1989).

In addition to economic considerations, moral aspects of the doctor-parent (or other adult) relationship may impede reporting. Generally, doctors promise confidentiality. Confidentiality is important because it allows patients to confide in their doctors, which in turn allows doctors to be more accurate in their diagnoses. This promise of confidentiality may conflict, however, with a pediatrician's concern about the child's best interest. Although the law requires doctors to report suspected child abuse, reporting is quite sporadic and inconsistent (Oates 1982; Zellman 1990; Dhooper et al. 1991). Studies of pediatricians reveal that older doctors are less likely to report child abuse than are younger doctors, and males are less likely to report it than females (Kean and Dukes 1991). None of the studies that documents inconsistent reporting disentangles the economic, moral, and legal considerations that lead doctors and other child-welfare professionals to report or not to report abuse.

Reticence to report may also result from a lack of faith in the efficacy of interventions. When abuse is reported, health professionals and legal agencies need to investigate the case, evaluate the evidence, make a judgment about whether abuse occurred, and then weigh the relative risks and benefits of preserving the family against those of removing the child from it (Zellman 1990). Child-protection agencies in the United States are generally underfunded and understaffed. In times of tight budgets, they may not receive the highest legislative priority. As a result, they may be unable to carefully investigate each case, to provide counseling and supervision services to every child or family reported to them, or to ensure that children who are removed from their homes are placed in safe living situations. In some states, child-protection agencies have themselves been so unprepared to care for the children in their custody that they themselves have been found guilty of neglect. Ironically, some child-protection agencies operate under court supervision in order to protect the children in their custody. While such agencies clearly provide excellent services to most children, highly publicized cases in which they have failed to provide adequate protection may lead people to be skeptical about the efficacy of reporting.

EVALUATING THE RISKS AND BENEFITS OF INTERVENTIONS TO PREVENT CHILD ABUSE

Broadly speaking, there have been three types of interventions designed to prevent child abuse and its consequences: (1) interventions designed to prevent abuse; (2) interventions designed to deal with the psychological consequences of abuse; and (3) interventions designed to punish offenders. Methodological challenges make it difficult to evaluate how well these approaches are working.

Preventive programs are difficult to evaluate because the ethical challenges of doing research are almost insurmountable (Conte 1987). Abuse is a hidden problem. Assessing whether heightened awareness of the problem leads to increased reporting or decreased occurrence would require intrusive evaluation and follow-up for enormous numbers of people (Reppucci and Haugaard 1989; Fink and McCloskey 1990). Generally, studies focus on surrogate outcome measures, such as doctors' or children's "ability to discriminate safe from unsafe situations," rather than on actual decreases in the incidence of sexual abuse (Hazzard et al. 1991, 134).

Intervention for children who have suffered abuse requires a delicate balance between trying to protect the child, trying to help the parents, and trying to preserve the family. Parents who abuse children often have been abused themselves, and may have a higher incidence of psychiatric problems (Steele and Pollock 1974). Many parents regret their actions, desire psychiatric help, and comply with treatment programs. However, 5 to 30 percent of abused children who stay in their family are subject to further episodes of abuse (Jellinek 1992). At present, there are no reliable indicators of which parents will continue to abuse their children and which are likely to respond to therapy. Furthermore, any data that might address this issue will necessarily be probabilistic. Thus, decisions about the value of such data in an individual case will inevitably incorporate normative values about the degree of risk appropriate for a particular child facing a particular custody decision.

Programs designed to punish child abusers are driven less by considerations of the risks and benefits of interventions and more by the dictates of the legal system. Evidence against alleged abusers seldom establishes guilt beyond a reasonable doubt. As a result, criminal prosecution is rare, and conviction even rarer (Peters 1989). Furthermore, it is unclear whether stricter laws or harsher punishments decrease the incidence of child abuse. As in other areas of criminal law, the justification for criminal prosecution seems to derive more from a notion of punitive justice than from a calculation of the degree to which punishment of offenders deters potential future offenders. Debate about this issue must take place in the context of more general debates about the morality of incarceration or the potential for rehabilitation in any criminal situation.

CONCLUSION

An apparent consensus about child abuse masks profound disagreements about the proper boundaries of family privacy, the obligations of parents and health professionals, and governmental responsibility to oversee the care and nurturing of children. These disagreements are reflected in difficulties in defining child abuse, difficulties in enforcing compliance with mandatory reporting requirements, and difficulties in evaluating the effects of interventions. Thus, while the law requires that child abuse be reported if it is suspected, health professionals can create their own index of suspicion. Some providers may report ambiguous cases, while others rarely report suspected abuse at all.

Individuals who work with children must balance their legal and ethical obligations to children, to their parents or caretakers, and to society. Professionals who have a higher regard for familial privacy and parental authority may develop a stricter standard or a higher threshold for suspecting abuse, and thus may be less likely to report it. Professionals who believe more strongly in the independent rights of children may develop a lower threshold for suspecting abuse, and may thus be more likely to report it. Current legal and moral approaches, while theoretically compelling, are quite recent, and have not been thoroughly evaluated. The principle that children deserve protection and nurturance is generally accepted, but the means by which the principle is to be brought to fruition remain uncertain.

SEE ALSO *Children: I. History of Childhood; Circumcision, Female: II. Cultural and Ethical Aspects; Harm; Parental Authority; Religious Objections to Medical Care; Social Work, Profession of*

BIBLIOGRAPHY

American Academy of Pediatrics, Committee on Bioethics. 1997. "Religious Objections to Medical Care." *Pediatrics* 99 (2): 279–81.

Badger, Lee W. 1989. "Reporting of Child Abuse: Influence of Characteristics of Physician, Practice, and Community." *Southern Medical Journal* 82 (3): 281–86.

Besharov, Douglas J. 1981. "Toward Better Research on Child Abuse and Neglect: Making Definitional Issues an Explicit Methodological Concern." *Child Abuse and Neglect* 5 (4): 383–90.

Conte, Jon R. 1987. "Ethical Issues in Evaluation of Prevention Programs." *Child Abuse and Neglect* 11 (2): 171–72.

Dhooper, Surjit S.; David D. Royse; and L. C. Wolfe. 1991. "A Statewide Study of the Public Attitudes toward Child Abuse." *Child Abuse and Neglect* 15 (1–2): 37–44.

Fink, Arlene, and Lois McCloskey. 1990. "Moving Child Abuse and Neglect Prevention Programs Forward: Improving Program Evaluations." *Child Abuse and Neglect* 14 (2): 187–206.

Gilbert, Neil, ed. 1997. *Combating Child Abuse: International Perspectives and Trends (Child Welfare).* New York: Oxford University Press.

Goodwin, Jean M. 1988. "Obstacles to Policymaking about Incest: Some Cautionary Folktales." In *Lasting Effects of Child Sexual Abuse*, edited by Gail Elizabeth Wyatt and Gloria Johnson Powell, 21–37. Newbury Park, CA: Sage.

Greipp, Mary Elizabeth. 1997. "Ethical Decision Making and Mandatory Reporting in Cases of Suspected Child Abuse." *Journal of Pediatric Health Care* 11 (6): 258–65.

Hazzard, Ann; Carol Webb; Carol Kleemeier; et al. 1991. "Child Sexual Abuse Prevention: Evaluation and One-Year Follow-Up." *Child Abuse and Neglect* 15 (1–2): 123–38.

Jellinek, Michael S.; J. Michael Murphy; Francis Poitrast; et al. 1992. "Serious Child Mistreatment in Massachusetts: The Course of 206 Children through the Courts." *Child Abuse and Neglect* 16 (2): 179–85.

Kalichman, Seth C. 1999. *Mandated Reporting of Suspected Child Abuse: Ethics, Law, and Policy.* 2nd ed. Washington, DC: American Psychological Association.

Kean, Robert B., and Richard L. Dukes. 1991. "Effects of Witness Characteristics on the Perception and Reportage of Child Abuse." *Child Abuse and Neglect* 15 (4): 423–35.

Lutzker, John R., ed. 1998. *Handbook of Child Abuse Research and Treatment.* New York: Plenum Press.

McCarthy, Claire. 2008. "Doing the Right Thing: A Primary Care Pediatrician's Perspective on Child Abuse Reporting." *Pediatrics* 122 (Suppl. 1): S21–S24.

Oates, Kim. 1982. "Child Abuse: A Community Concern." In *Child Abuse—A Community Concern*, edited by Kim Oates, 1–12. London: Butterworths.

Peters, James M. 1989. "Criminal Prosecution of Child Abuse: Recent Trends." *Pediatric Annals* 18 (8): 505–6, 508–9.

Radbill, Samuel X. 1974. "A History of Child Abuse and Infanticide." In *The Battered Child*, 2nd ed., edited by Ray E. Helfer and C. Henry Kempe, 3–21. Chicago: University of Chicago Press.

Reppucci, N. Dickon, and Jeffrey J. Haugaard. 1989. "Prevention of Child Sexual Abuse: Myth or Reality." *American Psychologist* 44 (10): 1266–75.

Steele, Brandt F., and Carl Pollock. 1974. "A Psychiatric Study of Parents Who Abuse Infants and Small Children." In *The Battered Child*, 2nd ed., edited by Ray E. Helfer and C. Henry Kempe, 89–133. Chicago: University of Chicago Press.

Steinberg, Alan M.; Robert S. Pynoos; Armen K. Goenjian; et al. 1999. "Are Researchers Bound by Child Abuse Reporting Laws?" *Child Abuse and Neglect* 23 (8): 771–77.

Zellman, Gail L. 1990. "Report on Decision-Making Patterns among Mandated Child Abuse Reporters." *Child Abuse and Neglect* 14 (3): 325–36.

Zellman, Gail L. 1992. "The Impact of Case Characteristics on Child Abuse Reporting Decisions." *Child Abuse and Neglect* 16 (1): 57–74.

John D. Lantos (1995, 2014)
Professor of Pediatrics, University of Missouri–Kansas City
Director, Children's Mercy Hospital Bioethics Center, Kansas City, Missouri

II. ABUSE BETWEEN DOMESTIC PARTNERS

Interpersonal abuse between domestic partners includes a range of abusive and neglectful behaviors perpetrated by someone who is or was involved in an intimate relationship with the victim. As an ethical issue, such abuse may fundamentally be construed as the use of one person as a means to another's end of anger release contrary to commonly accepted ethical principles and societal norms related to violence, interpersonal relationships, and familial roles. There is no intrinsic or utilitarian value for such behaviors; no ethical theory supports or excuses them. As no ethical justification exists for interpersonal violence, ethical attention moves to societal response. This entry will address early twenty-first-century descriptions of interpersonal abuse between domestic partners and the prevalence of the problem as background to informed ethical, societal, and health care response.

DESCRIPTION, INCIDENCE, AND EFFECTS

Interpersonal abuse is a social, public health, and medical issue. It may be described to emphasize patterns involving power, control, conscious manipulation, or coercion by a person who is or was involved in an intimate relationship with the victim. The perpetrator uses threats, coercion, humiliation, and/or force to effect progressive social isolation, deprivation, intimidation, psychological abuse, physical abuse, and/or sexual abuse (Ristock and Timbang 2005; Institute of Medicine 2011).

Many explanatory frameworks or theories have been developed to understand and explain interpersonal abuse. They come from the fields of psychology, biology, feminism, and sociology. These theories are hampered by their focus on a single factor rather than a description that reflects the full complexity and messiness of life. A multidimensional model that includes factors that operate on multiple levels and emphasizes the interaction and dynamic interplay between the factors offers the best framework on which to begin to understand these behaviors (Mitchell and Anglin 2009). This multidimensional approach was first introduced by Jay Belsky in 1980 to describe child maltreatment and then was later applied to intimate partner violence (IPV) (Heise 1998). The social ecology model for interpersonal violence includes four nested layers with the personal or individual factors in the center, then moving out through the family, community, and society. "Individual" factors include the biological or experiential profile that the person brings to the relationship. "Family" refers to the microsystem of communication and interaction within the family unit. "Community" is the ecosystem within which the family functions; it encompasses schools, work places, the neighborhood, and peer groups. "Society" is the greater macrosystem that determines cultural norms, policies, laws, attitudes, and biases (Heise 1998; Mitchell and Anglin 2009).

Over time the terminology used to describe interpersonal violence has evolved from *domestic violence* (DV) to *intimate partner violence* in an effort to encompass more diverse relationships and gender roles, including homosexual, cohabititation, and dating relationships. The term *domestic* connotes heterosexual relationships and certain gendered roles, whereas IPV encompasses the broader context reflected in incidence studies. Patriarchal assumptions and limitations associated with the use of the term *domestic* do not address the fact that prevalence is similar in homosexual relationships. In the late 1990s nearly 40 percent of men in same-sex relationships reported experiencing at least one type of abuse (psychological, physical, or sexual), and 18 percent of men reported experiencing more than one type in the last five years (Greenwood et al. 2002). Men living with male intimate partners experience more IPV than do men who live with female intimate partners. Approximately 15 percent of the men who had lived with a man as a couple reported being raped, physically assaulted, and/or stalked by a male cohabitant, while 7.7 percent of the men who had married or lived with a woman as a couple reported such violence by a wife or female cohabitant (Tjaden and Thoennes 2000). The research regarding lesbian IPV shows prevalence estimates from 17 to 52 percent, similar to IPV experienced by women in heterosexual relationships (Ristock and Timbang 2005).

While IPV affects men and women as victims and perpetrators (Black et al. 2011), studies indicate that more women experience IPV: 24 percent of women and 12 percent of men over their lifetimes (Breiding, Black, and Ryan 2008). Research usually focuses on women's experience (Black et al. 2011). Violence against women generally has been recognized internationally as a serious human rights abuse and public health issue. Studies suggest that 1.3 million to 5.3 million women in the United States experience IPV annually (Tjaden and Thoennes 2000; National Center for Injury Prevention and Control 2003), with estimates over the life span ranging from 22 to 39 percent (Collins et al. 1999; Centers for Disease Control and Prevention 2008).

US studies in other countries also suggest high rates of IPV (Hindin, Kishor, and Ansara 2008). In one study by the World Health Organization, lifetime prevalence of physical or sexual partner violence or both varied from 15 percent to 71 percent among the ten countries studied (Garcia-Moreno et al. 2006). *The National Intimate Partner and Sexual Violence Survey: 2010 Summary Report* reports abuse by category and suggests that psychological aggression is most prevalent (experienced by 48% of women), followed by physical violence (30%), sexual violence (17%), and rape (9%) (Black et al. 2011). Victims experience a variety of health effects, including death (Brock 2002) and injuries from physical and sexual assault; sexually transmitted infections, including HIV (Wingood et al. 2001); pelvic inflammatory disease (Letourneau, Holmes, and Chasedunn-Roark 1999); unintended pregnancy (Hathaway et al. 2000); adverse effects for pregnant women and their infants (Huth-Bocks, Levendosky, and Bogat 2002; El Kady, Gilbert, Xing, and Smith 2005; Shah, Shah, and Knowledge

Synthesis Group on Determinants of Preterm/LBW Births 2010); chronic pain, neurologic disorders, gastrointestinal disorders, migraine headaches, and other physical disabilities (Campbell and Lewandowski 1997; Coker et al. 2002); post-traumatic stress disorder (Lehmann 2000); depression (Silverman and Loudon 2010); and anxiety disorders, substance abuse, and suicide (Golding 1999; Campbell 2002). Most victims, female and male, of rape, physical violence, and/or stalking by an intimate partner (69% of female victims, 53% of male victims) experienced some form of IPV for the first time before twenty-five years of age (Black et al. 2011).

Estimates suggest that IPV results in about 2 million injuries annually, with over 550,000 requiring medical attention. Annually IPV results in the loss of almost 8 million paid work days and 5.6 million days of household productivity (Tjaden and Thoennes 2000; National Center for Injury Prevention and Control 2003). Associated costs of IPV, due largely to medical services, mental health services, and lost productivity, are estimated to be between $2 billion and $7 billion during the first year after victimization (Brown, Finkelstein, and Mercy 2008). Health care costs for women experiencing persistent abuse are reported to be as much as 42 percent higher than for women who are not abused (Bonomi, Anderson, Rivara, and Thompson 2009).

Several factors put a person at increased risk for IPV. For example, experiencing violence in the family of origin, such as witnessing parental violence or being a victim of childhood physical or sexual abuse, is a well-known risk. The Adverse Childhood Experiences Study shows that among persons who had all three forms of violent childhood experiences, the risk of victimization and perpetration increased 3.5-fold for women and 3.8-fold for men (Whitfield, Anda, Dube, and Felitti 2003). Alcohol abuse is a well-documented risk factor for abuse by men against women and by women against men. Research suggests that up to 40 percent of men and 34 percent of women who were physically abusive to their partners were drinking alcohol at the time (Caetano, Schafer, and Cunradi 2001). Specific features of the relationship can increase the risk of violence. Stress between the partners, communication style, and the level of emotional attachment on the woman's part all play a role in the initiation and continuation of the abuse (Woods 1999). Anecdotal evidence suggests that a man often refrains from physical violence until a woman has made an emotional commitment to him, such as moving in together, getting engaged or married, or becoming pregnant (Crowell and Burgess 1996). School or community environments that reinforce socialization supporting sex-role stereotypes and attitudes that condone violent behaviors have higher rates of teen dating and family violence. Other institutions that have been implicated in contributing to socialization that supports violence against women are organized religion, the workplace, the US military, and the media (Crowell and Burgess 1996). Certain societal factors increase risk for victimization. Low socioeconomic status, low or no insurance coverage, partner unemployment, and low levels of partner education are among them (Kyriacou et al. 1999). It has been noted that sheltered homeless mothers have higher cumulative rates of violent abuse over their life spans than their housed counterparts (Bassuk et al. 1996; Bassuk, Melnick, and Browne 1998). The reality is that inadequate income, lack of affordable housing, and fleeing domestic violence are key factors in making women homeless.

Most victims leave the abusive relationship after some time, with an average abusive relationship lasting five years (Tjaden and Thoennes 2000). Most, about 80 percent, do not have another abusive partner (Black et al. 2011). However, there are many barriers to leaving, and leaving is a process. Safety concerns are a critical barrier. The greatest risk of being killed is at the point when the victim decides to or attempts to leave the relationship. The abuser may have threatened to kill the victim, children, pets, or others if the victim leaves. Further, there are practical considerations of general welfare, including concerns about housing, food, clothing, and medical care. Legal concerns include fear of the loss of custody of children and threats of deportation. Poor health or substance abuse may also create barriers. Religious or cultural issues, such as beliefs that a family must stay together, that divorce is not acceptable, or that the man is supposed to be in charge, may also inhibit leaving the relationship. Personal feelings, including hope that things will get better, love for a partner, fear of being alone, not believing in divorce, and belief that the abuse is deserved, are also common barriers. Emotional abuse can be particularly damaging and is often overlooked by the victim, so it is often not an impetus to leave the relationship. Though there are no physical wounds, the day-to-day abuse caused by threats, humiliation, demeaning comments, and intimidation is often more debilitating than physical injuries. Leaving a relationship may not only further jeopardize a victim's safety but also may mean leaving behind everything a person knows.

Preliminary research shows that there are a few common factors or situations that lead to a "turning point" for a woman and increase her motivation to change her situation. The need to protect others from the abuse or the abuser is a significant catalyst. Women often report the desire to protect their children as the primary motivator for leaving the relationship, but the same holds for elderly family members and even pets. An increase in severity or an escalation of the degradation and humiliation of the abuse may also lead to departure from the relationship. When a female victim realizes that the abuser can actually end her life, she is forced to reevaluate the relationship and often seeks help. Increased awareness of options, the realization that she is not alone, and access to support and resources also drive the willingness to seek change. Women report that a kind word from their doctors, meeting an IPV advocate through the criminal justice system, or simply having strangers intervene during an abuse incident is enough to help them recognize possible avenues of support. Repeated attempts to change the abuser's behavior and the subsequent disappointment may result in fatigue or burnout. Recognition that the abuser is not going to change and that the cost of the relationship is too high to bear any longer may finally motivate action. Finally, partner betrayal or infidelity often causes the female victim to question whether her commitment to the relationship is worth suffering through the abuse (Chang et al. 2010).

SOCIETAL RESPONSE

Societal response has varied by state and locality. IPV programs continue to develop across the United States and increasingly provide services to victims, professionals, and community members, including assistance services, hotlines, and education (Greenwood et al. 2002). While state laws may not explicitly address IPV, all states have passed laws making stalking a crime and have strengthened rape laws. Many states have enacted mandatory IPV reporting laws that require the reporting of specific injuries and suspected abuse or IPV for individuals being treated by a health care professional. Specific requirements vary from state to state (Durborow, Lizdas, O'Flaherty, and Marjavi 2010). The reporting requirements remain controversial and raise ethical issues with regard to the autonomy and safety of the victim. Reporting may increase danger to the victim by provoking retribution from the abuser. Consequently, victims may choose to withhold information from health care providers regarding injuries caused by IPV. Mandated reporting also limits the victim's autonomy, which may further victimize him or her and interfere with the confidential nature of provider-patient relationship. Further, law enforcement response to reporting may be variable and inconsistent, further jeopardizing the victim's trust and safety and raising questions about the value of mandatory reporting (Rodríguez, Bauer, McLoughlin, and Grumbach 1999; Rodríguez, McLoughlin, Nah, and Campbell 2001; Mitchell and Anglin 2009). While reporting requirements are well intentioned, further examination of their effect is needed.

Other laws enacted in forty-three states since 1994 prohibit insurance discrimination on the basis of IPV. These laws vary widely in scope of coverage, including types of insurance to which they apply, types of practices prohibited, protections afforded, and remedies provided. Protecting victims' confidentiality is addressed in less than half of the state laws. The US Congress addressed this issue with regard to health insurance with the passage of the Health Insurance Portability and Accountability Act HIPAA in 1996, and many states have adopted legislation to implement these federal requirements. In 2010 Congress adopted the Patient Protection and Affordable Care Act to be implemented in 2014, which would potentially give IPV victims the most protection thus far against health insurance discrimination. A federal law is important not only for comprehensive coverage for all lines of insurance but also for uniformity of protection. When victims of abuse flee to escape IPV, they may travel across state lines. The ability to maintain insurance coverage for themselves and their children is often critical to the determination as to whether one has the financial resources to leave an abusive relationship (Durborow, Lizdas, O'Flaherty, and Marjavi 2010).

In 1994 the US Congress approved the Violence against Women Act (VAWA), the first legislation to address the health care or public health approach to IPV at the federal level. VAWA was reauthorized in 2005 and again in 2012. Since VAWA was first enacted, reporting for IPV has increased as much as 51 percent (National Task Force to End Sexual and Domestic Violence against Women 2012), the number of individuals killed by an intimate partner has decreased by 34 percent for women and 57 percent for men (Tjaden and Thoennes 2000), and the rate of nonfatal IPV against women has decreased by 53 percent (Mitchell and Anglin 2009). VAWA 2005 included funding for health-related projects. VAWA Health and VAWA Prevent, authorized but not funded in 2012, capitalize on a public health approach designed both to address the needs of IPV victims and to break the cycle of intergenerational violence by focusing on effective prevention programs targeting children who have been exposed to violence and young families at risk for violence. Initiatives address health professional training to identify and respond to domestic and sexual violence, grant making to foster collaborative public health responses, research to identify effective interventions in health care settings, best practices for reducing and preventing violence, and public education and awareness campaigns. Until funding for such programs matches the magnitude of the problem, which has been described as a pandemic, progress in addressing family violence as a health issue will be limited (Cohn, Salmon, and Stobo 2002; Mitchell and Anglin 2009). Such a national public health approach to IPV is likely to better address the multifactorial nature of violence and provide a multidisciplinary approach to intervention beyond the limits of a criminal justice approach alone.

HEALTH CARE PROFESSIONAL RESPONSE

Most major health care organizations recognize violence and abuse as a health issue and have issued policy statements on the topic. The American Medical Association, the American Academy of Family Physicians, the American College of Obstetrics and Gynecology, the American Academy of Pediatrics, the American College of Emergency Physicians, the American Nurses Association, and the National Association of Social Workers, among many others, have developed detailed policies and educational materials that address IPV in terms of health care professional training and practice (Cohn, Salmon, and Stobo 2002).

Health professionals provide care for the physical and psychological problems associated with abuse and neglect, ranging from acute injuries and chronic medical conditions to psychiatric and psychological disorders. Because of their contact and relationships with actual and potential victims, health care professionals have a unique opportunity to screen for, diagnose, treat, and even prevent abuse and neglect. For some victims, health professionals may be the only individuals that a victim has contact with outside of an abusive relationship. Despite this distinct role, health professionals are often inadequately prepared to intervene effectively. Health professionals commonly report feeling insufficiently supported, ill equipped, and generally frustrated in their attempts to deal with family violence victims (Cohn, Salmon, and Stobo 2002).

Privacy, a value fundamental to medical practice, may complicate the health professional response to IPV. It is valued as both an intrinsic and an instrumental good, helpful in promoting trusting patient-clinician relationships and maximizing individual health. Yet privacy can also be harmful, functioning as an impediment to necessary care. In situations of family violence, the value on privacy may reinforce a nonintervention norm among health care professionals, perpetuating a detrimental reticence to report what might otherwise be a well-recognized public health threat (Cohn 2008). Though ample research demonstrates the extent and severity of the family violence pandemic, the issue receives insufficient practical attention in the health care setting. The ethical and practical dilemma over the proper role of privacy in situations of family violence will persist at least until the importance of health professional intervention is regularly recognized and evidence-based treatment and intervention protocols are developed and routinely implemented. This presupposes that family violence is a medical as well as a social ill that requires health care response, among other societal interventions. As health care professionals are often best situated to identify the existence of family violence, medical protocols are needed that will account for the trade-off between individual privacy protections and health benefits, directly addressing the nonintervention norm.

In addition to the privacy question, a health care professional who recognizes IPV faces several ethical decisions related to the patient's identity, safety and security, resource utilization, and economic constraints, each of which creates potential barriers to appropriate patient care that become more challenging over time. Without definitive intervention, the patient is likely to progress along a continuum of violence that increases the likelihood of additional encounters with the health care system. A progressive escalation of violence may result in increased patient visits to the emergency room or primary care clinic, with more significant consequences of abuse to the point at which the health care provider must address the patient's complex medical, social, and ethical situation (Cohn and Rudman 2004).

Though inadequate, the existing research demonstrates that health professional intervention does improve health behaviors and outcomes. For example, victims who discussed their abuse with their health care provider were more likely to use an intervention (McCloskey et al. 2006), those who were screened for abuse and referred for services reported fewer threats of violence and assaults (Tiwari et al. 2005; McFarlane, Groff, O'Brien, and Watson 2006), and brief interventions decreased poor pregnancy outcomes and encouraged victims to leave unhealthy and unsafe relationships (Miller et al. 2011).

The appropriate diagnostic coding of domestic violence is another ethical challenge to health care systems. IPV diagnosis codes are often underused or displaced by higher-paying codes (such as injury codes) that reflect the patient's symptoms rather than the cause of injury or illness (Rudman et al. 2008). This may result in underrecognition of IPV, inadequate response and follow-up, increased health care use for repeated or escalated violence, and inaccurate surveillance of the scope of the problem. As coding systems evolve with the adoption of the new *International Statistical Classification of Diseases and Related Health Problems*, additional codes will be available to better specify the problem or suspicions of IPV, which may enhance both patient care and public health reporting. This in turn may improve the recognition of IPV and response to victims' needs.

Research suggests that routine screening for IPV, documentation, and appropriate coding by health care professionals may improve identification and response to people at risk, which may result in reduced violence and improved health outcomes. Research findings and health professional organization recommendations informed the Institute of Medicine (IOM) 2011 recommendation for IPV screening and counseling as a preventive service for women. Based on the IOM report, US Department of Health and Human Services Secretary Kathleen Sebelius issued new guidelines on August 1, 2011, under the authority of the Patient Protection and Affordable Care Act to ensure that women and adolescents receive preventive health services at no additional cost to the patient. IPV screening and counseling services were among the eight new preventive health services covered by this guidance. In

August 2012 these guidelines went into effect for new health plans and those not grandfathered, with other plans to comply over time. Questions remain about optimal settings and methods for screening, but recognition of the need for confidential, safe, and supportive discussions in the health care setting explicitly underlies these guidelines. Research will continue to evaluate screening approaches, rates, and standardization and efforts to minimize adverse effects (Nelson, Bougatsos, and Blazina 2012).

CONCLUSION

Despite increasing research and interventions, IPV remains a complex social, medical, and ethical problem. With research reflecting a pandemic with myriad health effects and societal costs, greater emphasis is ethically imperative. As a multifactorial problem, no single intervention or prevention tactic is likely to be successful. Risk factors can be sorted into major categories, and interventions or prevention strategies can be applied to each. For example, witnessing marital violence as a child is an individual risk factor for future perpetration or victimization of violence. Prevention strategies for this risk factor may include the promotion of healthy stress and coping strategies by health care providers and the educational system, routine assessment for exposure to violence in health care, and the availability of shelters for victims (Mitchell and Anglin 2009). A risk factor from one's community for perpetrating partner violence is associating with peer groups that encourage violence. Public education campaigns to "denormalize" violence and model healthy relationships can work to neutralize this important risk factor (Mitchell and Anglin 2009). Further attention needs to be focused on the assessment of the victim, the perpetrator, and family dynamics to determine how best to proceed. The priority should always be on the immediate health and safety of the family and the societal impact. A partnership among health care providers, the judicial system, and community agencies is necessary to adequately assess and manage the needs of the IPV victim and to effectively address the problem more broadly.

The views expressed in this entry are those of the authors and not of Kaiser Permanente.

SEE ALSO *Family and Family Medicine; Feminism; Harm; Rights; Sexual Ethics; Women, Historical and Cross-Cultural Perspectives*

BIBLIOGRAPHY

Bassuk, Ellen L.; Sharon Melnick; and Angela Browne. 1998. "Responding to the Needs of Low-Income and Homeless Women Who Are Survivors of Family Violence." *Journal of the American Medical Women's Association* 53 (2): 57–64.

Bassuk, Ellen L.; Linda F. Weinreb; John C. Buckner; et al. 1996. "The Characteristics and Needs of Sheltered Homeless Women." *Journal of the American Medical Association* 276 (8): 640–46.

Belsky, Jay. 1980. "Child Maltreatment: An Ecological Integration." *American Psychologist* 35 (4): 320–35.

Black, Michele C.; Kathleen C. Basile; Matthew J. Breiding; et al. 2011. *The National Intimate Partner and Sexual Violence Survey: 2010 Summary Report.* Atlanta: National Center for Injury Prevention and Control, Centers for Disease Control and Prevention. Accessed August 1, 2012. http://www.cdc.gov/Violence Prevention/pdf/NISVS_Report2010-a.pdf

Bonomi, Amy E.; Melissa L. Anderson; Frederick P. Rivara; and Robert S. Thompson. 2009. "Health Care Utilization and Costs Associated with Physical and Nonphysical-Only Intimate Partner Violence." *Health Services Research* 44 (3): 1052–67.

Breiding, Matthew J.; Michele C. Black; and George W. Ryan. 2008. "Chronic Disease and Health Risk Behaviors Associated with Intimate Partner Violence: 18 U.S. States/Territories, 2005." *Annals of Epidemiology* 18 (7): 538–44.

Brock, Karen. 2002. *When Men Murder Women: An Analysis of 2000 Homicide Data.* Washington, DC: Violence Policy Center. Accessed August 1, 2012. http://www.vpc.org/studies/dv5cont.htm

Brown, Derek S.; Eric A. Finkelstein; and James A. Mercy. 2008. "Methods for Estimating Medical Expenditures Attributable to Intimate Partner Violence." *Journal of Interpersonal Violence* 23 (12): 1747–66.

Caetano, Raul; John Schafer; and Carol B. Cunradi. 2001. "Alcohol-Related Intimate Partner Violence among White, Black, and Hispanic Couples in the US." *Alcohol Research and Health* 25 (1): 58–65.

Campbell, Jacqueline C. 2002. "Health Consequences of Intimate Partner Violence." *Lancet* 359 (9314): 1331–36.

Campbell, Jacqueline C., and Linda A. Lewandowski. 1997. "Mental and Physical Health Effects of Intimate Partner Violence on Women and Children." *Psychiatric Clinics of North America* 20 (20): 353–74.

Centers for Disease Control and Prevention. 2008. "Adverse Health Conditions and Health Risk Behaviors Associated with Intimate Partner Violence: United States, 2005." *Morbidity and Mortality Weekly Report* 57 (5): 113–17.

Chang, Judy C.; Diane Dado; Lynn Hawker; et al. 2010. "Understanding Turning Points in Intimate Partner Violence: Factors and Circumstances Leading Women Victims toward Change." *Journal of Women's Health* 19 (2): 251–59.

Cohn, Felicia. 2008. "The Veil of Silence around Family Violence: Is Protecting Patient Privacy Bad for Health?" *Journal of Clinical Ethics* 19 (4): 321–29.

Cohn, Felicia, and William Rudman. 2004. "Fixing Broken Bones and Broken Homes: Domestic Violence as a Patient Safety Issue." *Joint Commission Journal on Quality and Safety* 30 (11): 636–46.

Cohn, Felicia; Mark Salmon; and John Stobo, eds. 2002. *Confronting Chronic Neglect: The Education and Training of Health Professionals on Family Violence.* Institute of Medicine and National Research Council. Washington DC: National Academies Press.

Coker, Ann L.; Keith E. Davis; Ileana Arias; et al. 2002. "Physical and Mental Health Effects of Intimate Partner Violence for Men and Women." *American Journal of Preventive Medicine* 23 (4): 260–68.

Collins, Karen S.; Cathy Schoen; Susan Joseph; et al. 1999. *Health Concerns across a Woman's Lifespan: The Commonwealth Fund 1998 Survey of Women's Health.* New York: Commonwealth Fund. Accessed August 1, 2012. http://www.commonwealthfund.org/~/media/Files/Publications/Fund%20Report/1999/May/Health%20Concerns%20Across%20a%20Womans%20Lifespan%20%20The%20Commonwealth%20Fun%201998%20Survey%20of%20Womens%20Health/Health concerns_surveyreport%20pdf

Crowell, Nancy A., and Ann W. Burgess, eds. 1996. *Understanding Violence against Women.* National Research Council. Washington, DC: National Academies Press.

Durborow, Nancy; Kristine Lizdas; Abigail O'Flaherty; and Anna Marjavi. 2010. "Compendium of State Statutes and Policies on Domestic Violence and Health Care." Family Violence Prevention Fund. Accessed August 1, 2012. http://www.futureswithoutviolence.org/userfiles/file/HealthCare/Compendium%20Final.pdf

El Kady, Dina; William M. Gilbert; Guibo Xing; and Lloyd H. Smith. 2005. "Maternal and Neonatal Outcomes of Assaults during Pregnancy." *Obstetrics and Gynecology* 105 (2): 357–63.

Garcia-Moreno, Claudia; Henrica A. F. M. Jansen; Mary Ellsberg; et al. 2006. "Prevalence of Intimate Partner Violence: Findings from the WHO Multi-Country Study on Women's Health and Domestic Violence." *Lancet* 368 (9543): 1260–69. Accessed August 1, 2012. http://www.who.int/gender/violence/who_multicountry_study/media_corner/Prevalence_intimatepartner_WHOStudy.pdf

Golding, Jacqueline M. 1999. "Intimate Partner Violence as a Risk Factor for Mental Disorders: A Meta-analysis." *Journal of Family Violence* 14 (2): 99–132.

Greenwood, Gregory L.; Michael V. Relf; Bu Huang; et al. 2002. "Battering Victimization among a Probability-Based Sample of Men Who Have Sex with Men." *American Journal of Public Health* 92 (12): 1964–69.

Hathaway, Jeanne E.; Lorelei A. Mucci; Jay G. Silverman; et al. 2000. "Health Status and Health Care Use of Massachusetts Women Reporting Partner Abuse." *American Journal of Preventive Medicine* 19 (4): 302–7.

Heise, Lori L. 1998. "Violence against Women: An Integrated, Ecological Framework." *Violence against Women* 4 (3): 262–90.

Hindin, Michelle J.; Sunita Kishor; and Donna L. Ansara. 2008. *Intimate Partner Violence among Couples in 10 DHS Countries: Predictors and Health Outcomes.* DHS Analytical Studies 18. Calverton, MD: Macro International. Accessed August 13, 2012. http://www.measuredhs.com/pubs/pdf/AS18/AS18.pdf

Huth-Bocks, Alissa C.; Alytia A. Levendosky; and G. Anne Bogat. 2002. "The Effects of Domestic Violence during Pregnancy on Maternal and Infant Health." *Violence and Victims* 17 (2): 169–85.

Institute of Medicine. 2011. "Clinical Preventive Services for Women: Closing the Gaps Consensus Report." Accessed August 10, 2012. http://www.iom.edu/Reports/2011/Clinical-Preventive-Services-for-Women-Closing-the-Gaps.aspx

Kyriacou, Demetrios N.; Deirdre Anglin; Ellen Taliaferro; et al. 1999. "Risk Factors for Injury to Women from Domestic Violence against Women." *New England Journal of Medicine* 341 (25): 1892–98.

Lehmann, Peter. 2000. "Posttraumatic Stress Disorder (PTSD) and Child Witnesses to Mother-Assault: A Summary and Review." *Children and Youth Services Review* 22 (3–4): 275–306.

Letourneau, Elizabeth J.; Melisa Holmes; and Jennifer Chase-dunn-Roark. 1999. "Gynecologic Health Consequences to Victims of Interpersonal Violence." *Women's Health Issues* 9 (2): 115–20.

McCloskey, Laura A.; Erika Lichter; Corrine Williams; et al. 2006. "Assessing Intimate Partner Violence in Health Care Settings Leads to Women's Receipt of Interventions and Improved Health." *Public Health Report* 121 (4): 435–44.

McFarlane, Judith M.; Janet Y. Groff; Jennifer A. O'Brien; and Kathy Watson. 2006. "Secondary Prevention of Intimate Partner Violence: A Randomized Controlled Trial." *Nursing Research* 55 (1): 52–61.

Miller, Elizabeth; Michele Decker; Heather McCauley; et al. 2011. "A Family Planning Clinic Partner Violence Intervention to Reduce Risk Associated with Reproductive Coercion." *Contraception* 83 (3): 274–80.

Mitchell, Connie, and Deirdre Anglin. 2009. *Intimate Partner Violence: A Health-Based Perspective.* New York: Oxford University Press.

National Center for Injury Prevention and Control. 2003. *Costs of Intimate Partner Violence against Women in the United States.* Atlanta: Centers for Disease Control and Prevention. Accessed August 1, 2012. http://www.cdc.gov/violenceprevention/pdf/IPVBook-a.pdf

National Task Force to End Sexual and Domestic Violence against Women. 2012. "VAWA Fact Sheets: Reauthorization of the Violence against Women Act; Building on Our Successes." Accessed August 14, 2012. http://4vawa.org/pages/vawa-fact-sheets

Nelson, Heidi D.; Christina Bougatsos; and Ian Blazina. 2012. "Screening Women for Intimate Partner Violence: A Systematic Review to Update the 2004 US Preventive Services Task Force Recommendation." *Annals of Internal Medicine* 156 (11): 796–808, W-279, W-280, W-281, W-282.

Ristock, Janice, and Norma Timbang. 2005. "Relationship Violence in Lesbian/Gay/Bisexual/Transgender/Queer (LGBTQ) Communities: Moving beyond a Gender-Based Framework." Violence against Women Online Resources. Accessed August 1, 2012. http://www.mincava.umn.edu/documents/lgbtqviolence/lgbtqviolence.html

Rodríguez, Michael A.; Heidi M. Bauer; Elizabeth McLoughlin; and Kevin Grumbach. 1999. "Screening and Intervention for Intimate Partner Abuse: Practices and Attitudes of Primary Care Physicians." *Journal of the American Medical Association* 282 (5): 468–74.

Rodríguez, Michael A.; Elizabeth McLoughlin; Gregory Nah; and Jacqueline C. Campbell. 2001. "Mandatory Reporting of Domestic Violence Injuries to the Police: What Do Emergency

Department Patients Think?" *Journal of the American Medical Association* 286 (5): 580–83.

Rudman, William; Susan Hart-Hester; C. Andrew Brown; et al. 2008. "Ethical Dilemmas in Coding Domestic Violence." *Journal of Clinical Ethics* 19 (4): 353–59.

Shah, Prakesh S.; Jyotsna Shah; Knowledge Synthesis Group on Determinants of Preterm/LBW Births. 2010. "Maternal Exposure to Domestic Violence and Pregnancy and Birth Outcomes: A Systematic Review and Meta-analyses." *Journal of Women's Health* 19 (11): 2017–31.

Silverman, Michael, and Holly Loudon. 2010. "Antenatal Reports of Pre-Pregnancy Abuse Is Associated with Symptoms of Depression in the Postpartum Period." *Archives of Women's Mental Health* 13 (5): 411–15.

Tiwari, A.; W. Leung; T. Leung; et al. 2005. "A Randomized Controlled Trial of Empowerment Training for Chinese Abused Pregnant Women in Hong Kong." *BJOG: An International Journal of Obstetrics and Gynaecology* 112 (9): 1249–56.

Tjaden, Patricia, and Nancy Thoennes. 2000. *Extent, Nature, and Consequences of Intimate Partner Violence: Findings from the National Violence against Women Survey.* Rockville, MD: National Institute of Justice and Centers for Disease Control and Prevention. Accessed August 1, 2012. http://www.nij.gov/pubs-sum/181867.htm

Wenzel, Suzanne L.; Joan S. Tucker; Marc N. Elliott; et al. 2004. "Physical Violence against Impoverished Women: A Longitudinal Analysis of Risk and Protective Factors." *Women's Health Issues* 14 (5): 144–54.

Whitfield, Charles L.; Robert F. Anda; Shante R. Dube; and Vincent J. Felitti. 2003. "Violent Childhood Experiences and the Risk of Intimate Partner Violence in Adults." *Journal of Interpersonal Violence* 18 (2): 166–85.

Wingood, Gina M.; Ralph J. DiClemente; Donna Hubbard McCree; et al. 2001. "Dating Violence and the Sexual Health of Black Adolescent Females." *Pediatrics* 107 (5): E72.

Woods, Stephanie J. 1999. "Normative Beliefs regarding the Maintenance of Intimate Relationships among Abused and Nonabused Women." *Journal of Interpersonal Violence* 14 (5): 479–91.

Felicia Cohn
Bioethics Director, Kaiser Permanente Orange County, California

Liza Eshilian-Oates
Regional Physician Leader, Southern California Kaiser Permanente Family Violence Prevention Program

III. ELDER ABUSE

The phenomenon known as elder abuse first appeared in the British scientific literature in 1975 (Burston 1975) to describe the physical abuse of an elderly dependent person by a caregiving family member. In the years that followed the definition expanded to include acts of commission (physical, psychological, and financial abuse) and omission (neglect) that result in harm to a person sixty-five years (in some states sixty or fifty-five years) or older by a relative or a person with whom the elder has a trusting relationship. Self-neglect and self-abuse typically are included under broad conceptualizations of elder abuse. They refer to neglectful or abusive behaviors of older persons directed at themselves that threaten their own health or safety.

Beginning in the mid-1980s the meaning attached to elder abuse expanded further to reflect a criminalization of the phenomenon. Accordingly, interest evolved in such areas as sexual assault in later life, battered older women, and fraud and scams (e.g., Ramsey-Klawsnik 1991; Harris 1996; Tueth 2000). Likewise, since the 1990s a resurgence of attention has been given to elder abuse in institutions, particularly nursing facilities. Exposure of fires and inadequate care in these settings during the 1970s fueled the enactment of federal legislation to protect residents. Investigations of resident conditions led to the identification of additional institutional elder abuse forms, like violation of rights, theft, and examples of covert or ritual abuse (e.g., Meddaugh 1993; Payne and Kovic 1995; Harris and Benson 1998; Ulsperger and Knottnerus 2011). Finally, international perspectives on elder abuse resulted in the United Nations World Assembly on Aging's delineation of still more abuse forms in 2002. Included among them are variations emanating out of social conditions in individual countries, such as political violence and armed conflict.

Throughout this period of problem recognition and definition expansion, there has been concern about the lack of universally accepted definitions and forms of elder abuse evident in either research or state laws. This deficiency results from the failure of the federal government to direct states or researchers to use standard definitions through either mandate or funding incentive and the inability to resolve various controversies surrounding elder abuse definitions. The most notable early attempts to produce common definitions are found in research led by Margaret F. Hudson (Hudson 1991; Hudson and Carlson 1999; Hudson et al. 2000). Using a national panel of elder abuse experts, Hudson developed a five-level elder abuse taxonomy with eleven related definitions. Georgia J. Anetzberger in 2012 updated the taxonomy to reflect current understanding about elder abuse. In addition, Kendon J. Conrad and his associates (2008) have used concept mapping as a technique to better characterize financial abuse and psychological abuse.

Still, there remains much diversity in how elder abuse is defined. For example, after reviewing state laws, Jeanette M. Daly and Gerald J. Jogerst (2001, 2006) concluded that no single term describes elder abuse. However, there is more similarity among definitions of elder abuse in domestic settings in adult protective services laws than for the problem in residential care settings in nursing home laws. In addition, numerous studies suggest that differences exist in defining elder abuse among cultural groups within a country as well as across countries (e.g., Anetzberger, Korbin, and Tomita 1996; Tatara 1997, 1999; Malley-Morrison 2006).

This entry focuses on elder abuse in the United States. However, where appropriate it also discusses the problem in other countries, particularly Canada and western Europe, where most of the research outside the United States has occurred.

POLICY DEVELOPMENT

In the United States interest in elder abuse was sparked by testimony on the battering of parents before a US House of Representatives subcommittee investigating family violence in 1978. The growing numbers of elderly persons in society, the rising political power of the older population, and the existing state bureaucracies for delivering protective services lent legitimacy to making elder abuse a public issue. Despite the efforts of a few representatives to pass comprehensive national legislation throughout the 1980s, Congress took no action. Nevertheless, federal agencies did incorporate elder abuse into their agendas, albeit through legislation enacted with other intents. For example, amendments to the Older Americans Act gave area agencies on aging roles in elder abuse prevention and created the National Center on Elder Abuse, enactment of the Family Violence Prevention and Services Act enabled funding for select elder abuse–related projects, and passage of the 1987 Omnibus Budget Reconciliation Act severely limited the use of physical and chemical restraints for residents of long-term care facilities because they were seen to violate human rights and potentially cause harm.

Without a national focus, knowledge base, or model statutes, the states developed their own laws, elder abuse definitions, and reporting procedures. Some used existing adult protective legislation, others domestic violence acts. Still others passed specific elder abuse laws. By the late 1980s each of the fifty states had a system in place for receiving reports and investigating, assessing, and monitoring cases. Nearly all states adopted the child abuse approach, making it mandatory for health and social service professionals and others who work with older persons to report suspected cases of abuse and neglect, subject to a fine or imprisonment or both. In the remaining states reporting is voluntary. Since the 1980s all states have revised their protective or elder abuse laws, often to clarify definitions, increase penalties for perpetrators, or criminalize certain abuse types.

Despite the widespread enactment of mandatory reporting laws, most elder abuse is not reported to authorities charged with investigating the problem. Early studies suggested that no more than one in fourteen elder abuse situations was reported to authorities (Pillemer and Finkelhor 1988; US House Select Committee on Aging 1990; National Center on Elder Abuse 1998). However, early twenty-first-century research found that underreporting may be much higher. Mark Lachs and Jacquelin Berman (2011) investigated self-reports of abuse from community-dwelling elderly residents of New York State and compared these to documented case data from such agencies as adult protective services and law enforcement. The findings indicated that only one in twenty-four instance of past year elder abuse was reported to agencies that could provide assistance, with the rate declining to one in forty-four for financial abuse.

Other policy activity has centered at the federal level. This includes convening the first National Policy Summit on Elder Abuse in 2001. More than eighty individuals and agencies from across the country identified priority recommendations to address elder abuse at multiple levels of responsibility. Some of these recommendations are evident in the first enacted comprehensive legislation to address elder abuse—the Elder Justice Act, introduced in the US Senate in 2002 and passed into law in 2010 as an amendment to the Patient Protection and Affordable Care Act. Among its many provisions, the act created the Elder Justice Coordinating Council in the US Department of Health and Human Services, established a new formula grant program for adult protective services, developed forensic capacity in abuse detection, and increased efforts to address abuse in long-term care. By 2013 funds to implement the act had not yet been appropriated.

Four agencies in the US Department of Health and Human Services and four in the US Department of Justice fund elder abuse initiatives nationwide. Together they spent $11.9 million to address the problem in fiscal year 2009 (Government Accountability Office 2011). They support activities aimed at practitioner training and public awareness (Administration on Aging, Offices of Violence against Women and for Victims of Crime), multidisciplinary coordination (Administration on Aging, Office for Victims of Crime), a uniform adult protective services administrative data system (Centers for Disease Control and Prevention), and research (National Institutes of Aging and Justice).

THEORETICAL CONSIDERATIONS

Early attempts to understand the nature of elder abuse were influenced by the child abuse model. Victims were viewed as very dependent older women mistreated by well-meaning but overburdened adult daughters. Later findings suggested that spouse abuse might be a more useful framework for study, since the individuals involved were legally independent adults. To some health researchers, however, using the family violence paradigm with its emphasis on harm, intentionality, and responsibility was counterproductive, particularly in cases that involved elders with unmet needs (Phillips 1986; Fulmer and O'Malley 1987). They recommended that elder abuse be considered from the perspective of family caregiving. None of these interpretations is sufficient in and of itself. Neither the child abuse nor the spouse abuse model considers the impact of the aging process, and the family caregiving theory cannot explain abusive situations in which the victim has no unmet physical needs. To capture the broad array of situations labeled elder abuse, attention has focused on ecology theory or on integrating multiple theories (e.g., National Research Council 2003; Biggs and Goergen 2010).

Sheena R. Horsford and her associates (2011) use ecology theory to understand elder abuse in the African American community, breaking the theory down into macro-, exo-, and microsystems and addressing elder abuse issues at each level. At the macro- and exosystem levels, risk factors like poverty and health disparities are considered along with such culturally protective factors as a strong sense of spirituality and value of the elderly. At the microsystem level, identified risk factors include caregiver/perpetrator burden, mental health problems, dependency on elders, and limited caregiving skills. Thomas Goergen and Marie Beaulieu (2010) integrate various criminology theories to explain elder abuse in its various forms and dynamics. In particular, they demonstrate the usefulness of strain and control theories when perpetrators experience life stress and are opportunistic. They also suggest that routine activity and situational action theories have application in situations of elder financial abuse or abuse and neglect by family caregivers.

RISK FACTORS AND CHARACTERISTICS

Although early studies usefully documented the existence of the problem and promoted state elder abuse policies, they were generally based on data collected from agency files; used small, unrepresentative samples; and lumped together the various forms of abuse. Therefore they provided little information on the nature and scope of elder abuse, including risk factors, victim and perpetrator characteristics, consequences, prevalence, and incidence. Because most subsequent studies have better scientific rigor, they are beginning to offer greater understanding about the problem.

Several salient risk factors emerge from the collective research on elder abuse. Those risk factors found to characterize the perpetrator include mental or emotional problems, substance abuse, hostility, and dependence on the victim. Risk factors associated with the victim include dementia, declining or poor health or functional capacity, lack of social supports, and such troublesome behavior as aggressiveness or socially inappropriate actions. Finally, situational risk factors include social isolation and shared living arrangements between the perpetrator and the victim.

Various studies distinguish risk factors by abuse form. An early illustration comes from a case comparison by Rosalie S. Wolf and her associates (1986). Perpetrators of physical/psychological abuse were more likely than perpetrators of neglect to have a history of mental illness and alcohol abuse and to be dependent on the victim for financial resources. The victims were apt to be in poor emotional health but relatively independent in the activities of daily living. In contrast, those cases involving neglect appeared to be related to the dependency needs of the victim, with the victims a source of stress for the perpetrators. Financial abuse victims typically were widowed and had few social supports. Their perpetrators had financial problems and histories of substance abuse along with desire for money. Ron Acierno and his associates (2009) conducted a nationally representative study of elder abuse in the United States and found that victim physical disability was a risk factor for financial exploitation; victim poor health, low income, and little social support were risk factors for neglect; and perpetrator mental health problems, substance abuse, and unemployment were risk factors for other abuse forms.

Few studies have examined the consequences of elder abuse. Those that have suggest that the effects of abuse infliction may have physical, behavioral, psychological, or social dimensions. In particular, victims of elder abuse seem to experience higher levels of depression than nonvictims (Pillemer and Prescott 1989; Harris 1996; Comijs et al. 1999). Furthermore, elder abuse victims are likely to die sooner (Lachs et al. 1997; Dong et al. 2009). Finally, the economic consequences of elder abuse can be significant in terms of both victim losses and intervention costs. Using a mixed-methods approach, MetLife Mature Market Institute (2011) found that financial abuse resulted in $2.6 billion in victim losses nationwide for 2008, increasing 12 percent to $2.9 billion three years later. The National Committee for the Prevention of Elder Abuse (2011) examined intervention expenses associated with three types of elder abuse cases. The costs ranged from $1,485 for social services to address a situation of self-neglect to $120,213 for medical services needed in a situation of physical abuse and neglect.

PREVALENCE AND INCIDENCE

In 1998 the National Center on Elder Abuse completed the first national incidence study on elder abuse in the United States. Using a representative sample of twenty counties in fifteen states, the study examined two data sources to identify the number of unduplicated new cases of elder abuse in a single year. The data sources were reports to adult protective services and reports from sentinels, that is, specially trained community agency personnel having frequent contact with older people. The results for 1996 suggest a national incidence rate of

551,011, with self-neglect and neglect constituting over two-thirds of all elder abuse reported.

Another decade passed before nationally representative prevalence studies were conducted in the United States. In the first study Edward Laumann and his associates (2008) surveyed community-dwelling adults ages fifty-seven to eighty-five about past year elder abuse and discovered that 9 percent reported verbal, 3.5 percent financial, and 0.2 percent physical mistreatment. In the second study Acierno and his associates (2009) interviewed 5,777 community-dwelling persons age sixty and older and 813 proxies about their past year experiences with elder abuse. Eleven percent reported at least one form, and 1.2 percent reported two or more forms of past year mistreatment.

A few national elder abuse incidence and prevalence investigations have been conducted outside the United States as well. Studies vary in operational definitions, sampling techniques, response rates, and other research factors, thereby limiting their comparability and generalizability. However, collectively they demonstrate that elder abuse is a global problem, acknowledged in every region recognized by the World Health Organization (Podnieks et al. 2010).

The following studies illustrate national prevalence research outside the United States. Simon Biggs and his associates (2009) interviewed 2,111 persons age sixty-six and older living in private households in the four countries of the United Kingdom. Among the respondents, 2.6 percent reported mistreatment by family members, close friends, or care workers, with neglect the most common form (1.1%) and sexual abuse the least common form (0.2%). Ariela Lowenstein and her associates (2009) surveyed 1,045 community-dwelling adults age sixty-five and older in Israel on past year abuse, with 18.4 percent exposed to at least one form, usually either verbal abuse or financial exploitation. Rates were similar for Jews and Arabs. Finally, Isabel I. Marmolejo (2008) interviewed 2,401 persons age sixty-four or older and 788 caregivers of dependent older people in Spain. Caregiver respondents reported past year elder abuse at a rate twice as high as that of older adult respondents (1.5% vs. 0.8%).

TREATMENT AND ETHICAL ISSUES

A number of potential conflicts face practitioners who are handling elder abuse cases. While tangible proof may be obtainable in situations involving physical and financial abuse, psychological abuse and neglect are far more difficult to verify. Because psychological abuse leaves no visible marks, it can be difficult to detect. Moreover, the effects of neglect can mirror other health problems or sometimes even the aging process itself. Symptoms of sexual abuse may elude the investigator who is not aware that old people can be so victimized. Cultural biases and lack of full knowledge about the circumstances involved in a case may lead a worker to conclude falsely that abuse has occurred. For example, belief that African American, Latino, or select other families "take care of their own" can lead a worker to conclude that informal care is preferred, when actually it may represent financial abuse, as the family attempts to keep the older person's assets intact rather than deplete them through purchase of nursing facility or home health care. The instability of the mental and physical status of the victim and/or the perpetrator and the dynamics of their relationship may add to case uncertainty. The issue of competency can be particularly troublesome. For instance, an older person with dementia may still possess social skills and appear mentally capable, when in fact impaired executive function inhibits carrying out decisions made in any effective manner. There may be resistance on the part of the victim to undergo medical assessment, or of the perpetrator to allow it, or even of the medical profession to make a decision.

An individual who under the law is mandated to report a case of suspected abuse may hesitate because the details of the situation have not been fully documented. Reporting may be seen as unnecessarily intrusive in such situations or even jeopardizing hard-won rapport established between the worker and older person. Whether the problem is civil or criminal may be unclear. Certainly, the unwillingness of the victim to press charges has been a major hindrance to intervention efforts. Even though the law may require an investigation, the older person may not wish to cooperate or to accept the services that are offered. This negative response brings the worker face-to-face with a dilemma—the interest of the state, professionals, and society in protecting vulnerable persons versus the individual's right to self-determination—in terms of ethical principles and the tension between justice, beneficence, and autonomy.

Advances in understanding the nature of elder abuse require examining the problem from many perspectives. Not only must distinctions be made among the various forms of elder abuse, but more attention must be paid to differences based on gender, race, culture, relationships, and circumstances. The growing interest in the problem among social scientists and medical personnel all over the world is important. The results of their efforts will be constructive in further building the theoretical and empirical base for successful treatment and prevention programs.

This is a revised version of the entry first written by Rosalie S. Wolf in 1995.

SEE ALSO *Dementia; Harm; Long-Term Care: I. Concepts and Policies; Long-Term Care: II. Nursing Homes; Long-Term Care: III. Home Care*

BIBLIOGRAPHY

Acierno, Ron; Melba Hernandez-Tejada; Wendy Muzzy; et al. 2009. *National Elder Mistreatment Study*. Report to the National Institute of Justice, Project #2007-WG-BX-0009. Rockville, MD: National Institute of Justice.

Anetzberger, Georgia J. 2012. "An Update on the Nature and Scope of Elder Abuse." *Generations* 36 (3): 12–20.

Anetzberger, Georgia J.; Jill E. Korbin; and Susan K. Tomita. 1996. "Defining Elder Mistreatment in Four Ethnic Groups across Two Generations." *Journal of Cross-Cultural Gerontology* 11:187–212.

Biggs, Simon, and Thomas Goergen. 2010. "Theoretical Development in Elder Abuse and Neglect." *Ageing International* 35:167–70.

Biggs, Simon; Jill Manthorpe; Anthea Tinker; et al. 2009. "Mistreatment of Older People in the United Kingdom: Findings from the First National Prevalence Study." *Journal of Elder Abuse and Neglect* 21:1–14.

Burston, Geoffrey R. 1975. "Granny-Battering." *British Medical Journal* 3 (5983): 592.

Comijs, Hannie C.; Brenda W. J. H. Penninx; Kees P. M. Knipscheer; et al. 1999. "Psychological Distress in Victims of Elder Mistreatment: The Effects of Social Support and Coping." *Journal of Gerontology: Psychological Sciences* 54B (4): P240–P245.

Conrad, Kendon J.; Madelyn Iris; John W. Ridings; et al. 2008. *Conceptualization and Measuring Financial Exploitation and Psychological Abuse of Elderly Individuals*. Report to the National Institute of Justice, Project #2006-MU-MU-0004. Rockville, MD: National Institute of Justice.

Daly, Jeanette M., and Gerald J. Jogerst. 2001. "Statute Definitions of Elder Abuse." *Journal of Elder Abuse and Neglect* 13 (4): 39–57.

Daly, Jeanette M., and Gerald J. Jogerst. 2006. "Nursing Home Statutes: Mistreatment Definitions." *Journal of Elder Abuse and Neglect* 18 (1): 19–39.

Dong, XinQi; Carlos Mendes de Leon; and Melissa Simon. 2009. "Elder Self-Neglect and Abuse and Mortality Risk in a Community-Dwelling Population." *Journal of the American Medical Association* 302 (5): 517–26.

Fulmer, Terry, and Terrence O'Malley. 1987. *Inadequate Care of the Elderly: A Health Care Perspective on Abuse and Neglect*. New York: Springer.

Goergen, Thomas, and Marie Beaulieu. 2010. "Criminological Theory and Elder Abuse Research: Fruitful Relationships or Worlds Apart?" *Ageing International* 35:185–201.

Government Accountability Office. 2011. *Elder Justice: Stronger Federal Leadership Could Enhance National Response to Elder Abuse*. Report to the Chairman, Special Committee on Aging, US Senate, GAO-11-208. Washington, DC: US Government Printing Office.

Harris, Diana K., and Michael L. Benson. 1998. "Nursing Home Theft: The Hidden Problem." *Journal of Aging Studies* 12 (1): 57–67.

Harris, Sarah B. 1996. "For Better or for Worse: Spouse Abuse Grown Old." *Journal of Elder Abuse and Neglect* 8 (1): 1–33.

Horsford, Sheena R.; José Rubén Parra-Cardona; Lori A. Post; and Larry Schiamberg. 2011. "Elder Abuse and Neglect in African American Families: Informing Practice Based on Ecological and Cultural Frameworks." *Journal of Elder Abuse and Neglect* 23 (1): 75–88.

Hudson, Margaret F. 1991. "Elder Mistreatment: A Taxonomy with Definitions by Delphi." *Journal of Elder Abuse and Neglect* 3 (2): 1–20.

Hudson, Margaret F.; Cherry Beasley; Ruth H. Benedict; et al. 2000. "Elderly Abuse: Some Caucasian-American Views." *Journal of Elder Abuse and Neglect* 12 (1): 89–114.

Hudson, Margaret F., and John R. Carlson. 1999. "Elder Abuse: Its Meaning to Caucasians, African Americans, and Native Americans." In *Understanding Elder Abuse in Minority Populations*, edited by Toshio Tatara, 187–204. Philadelphia: Brunner/ Mazel.

Lachs, Mark, and Jacquelin Berman. 2011. *Under the Radar: New York State Elder Abuse Prevalence Study; Self-Reported Prevalence and Documented Case Surveys, Final Report*. Rochester, NY: Lifespan of Greater Rochester, Weill Cornell Medical Center of Cornell University, and New York City Department for the Aging.

Lachs, Mark S.; Christianna Williams; Shelley O'Brien; et al. 1997. "Risk Factors for Reported Elder Abuse and Neglect: A Nine-Year Observational Cohort Study." *Gerontologist* 37 (4): 469–74.

Laumann, Edward O.; Sara A. Leitsch; and Linda J. Waite. 2008. "Elder Mistreatment in the United States: Prevalence Estimates from a Nationally Representative Study." *Journal of Gerontology: Social Sciences* 63B (4): S248–S254.

Lowenstein, Ariela; Zvi Eisikovits; Tava Band-Winterstein; et al. 2009. "Is Elder Abuse and Neglect a Social Phenomenon? Data from the First National Prevalence Survey in Israel." *Journal of Elder Abuse and Neglect* 21 (3): 253–77.

Malley-Morrison, Kathleen, ed. 2006. "Perspectives on Elder Abuse: Europeans and European Americans." Special issue, *Journal of Elder Abuse and Neglect* 18 (2–3).

Marmolejo, Isabel I. 2008. *Elder Abuse in the Family in Spain*. Valencia, Spain: Centro Reina Sophia para el Estudio de la Violencia.

Meddaugh, Dorothy I. 1993. "Covert Elder Abuse in the Nursing Home." *Journal of Elder Abuse and Neglect* 5 (3): 21–38.

MetLife Mature Market Institute. 2009. *Broken Trust: Elders, Family, and Finances*. New York: Metropolitan Life Insurance.

MetLife Mature Market Institute. 2011. *The MetLife Study of Elder Financial Abuse: Crimes of Occasion, Desperation, and Predation against America's Elders*. New York: Metropolitan Life Insurance.

National Center on Elder Abuse. 1998. *The National Elder Abuse Incidence Study*. Washington, DC: Author.

National Committee for the Prevention of Elder Abuse. 2011. *Examining the Costs of Elder Abuse: Three Case Studies*. Washington, DC: National Center on Elder Abuse.

National Research Council. 2003. *Elder Mistreatment: Abuse, Neglect, and Exploitation in an Aging America*. Panel to Review Risk and Prevalence of Elder Abuse and Neglect. Washington, DC: National Academies Press.

Payne, Brian K., and Richard Kovic. 1995. "An Empirical Examination of the Characteristics, Consequences, and Causes of Elder Abuse in Nursing Homes." *Journal of Elder Abuse and Neglect* 7 (4): 61–74.

Phillips, Linda R. 1986. "Theoretical Explanations of Elder Abuse: Competing Hypotheses and Unresolved Issues." In *Elder Abuse: Conflict in the Family*, edited by Karl A. Pillemer and Rosalie S. Wolf, 197–217. Dover, MA: Auburn House.

Pillemer, Karl A., and David Finkelhor. 1988. "The Prevalence of Elder Abuse: A Random Sample Survey." *Gerontologist* 28:51–57.

Pillemer, Karl A., and Denise Prescott. 1989. "Psychological Effects of Elder Abuse: A Research Note." *Journal of Elder Abuse and Neglect* 1 (1): 65–74.

Podnieks, Elizabeth; Georgia J. Anetzberger; Susannah J. Wilson; et al. 2010. "WorldView Environmental Scan on Elder Abuse." *Journal of Elder Abuse and Neglect* 22:164–79.

Ramsey-Klawsnik, Holly. 1991. "Elder Sexual Abuse: Preliminary Findings." *Journal of Elder Abuse and Neglect* 3 (3): 73–90.

Tatara, Toshio, ed. 1997. "Elder Abuse in Minority Populations." Special issue, *Journal of Elder Abuse and Neglect* 9 (2).

Tatara, Toshio, ed. 1999. *Understanding Elder Abuse in Minority Populations*. Philadelphia: Brunner/Mazel.

Tueth, Michael J. 2000. "Exposing Financial Exploitation of Impaired Elderly Persons." *American Journal of Geriatric Psychiatry* 8 (2): 104–11.

Ulsperger, Jason S., and J. David Knottnerus. 2011. *Elder Care Catastrophe: Rituals of Abuse in Nursing Homes and What You Can Do about It*. Boulder, CO: Paradigm.

US House Select Committee on Aging. 1990. *Elder Abuse: A Decade of Shame and Inaction*. Washington, DC: US Government Printing Office.

Wolf, Rosalie S.; Michael A. Godkin; and Karl A. Pillemer. 1986. "Maltreatment of the Elderly: A Comparative Analysis." *Journal of Long Term Home Health Care* 5 (4): 10–17.

Georgia J. Anetzberger (2004, 2014)
President, National Committee for the Prevention of Elder Abuse

IV. ABUSE OF HEALTH CARE WORKERS

Health care work is dangerous. Rates of absence due to illness and injury are among the highest in all industrial sectors. It is difficult to know to what extent these rates reflect the abuse experienced by the health care labor force, in part because much of the abuse is suffered in silence and is not defined as a justifiable basis for work absences. But those who work in health care are known to face physical, sexual, mental, racial, verbal, and emotional abuse.

Although discussions of abuse frequently focus on professionals, as the World Health Organization (2006) makes clear the term *health worker* includes all those employed in health services delivery. That is the definition used here. Accordingly it is important to note that a significant proportion of care work is provided by those unpaid and untrained for the task. These people too suffer from abuse, and the abuse may be even less visible and less likely to be reported than among paid workers. It is also important to note that health care work is done primarily by women and often by those from racialized groups. This distribution may well contribute to both the prevalence of abuse and the relative silence about abuse in care work. Research from Statistics Canada (2007), for example, indicates that a third of violent workplace incidents occur in health and social services, and whereas nearly 60 percent of workplace violence experienced by men was reported to the police, this was the case for only 20 percent of the violent incidents involving women.

PHYSICAL ABUSE

Physical abuse is common and visible although it is not necessarily reported, nor does it usually lead to work absences. It is most common in emergency rooms, in psychiatric wards, and in care for the elderly, although it can happen anywhere. Working alone, especially in a private home, increases the opportunities for physical assault. Residents and patients—and especially men—are the ones who most frequently physically attack, although friends and relatives can also become violent. Violence from coworkers is not unknown either. Intimate care, such as changing a diaper or bathing, offers frequent opportunities for physical assault. It is also the time when patients and residents feel the most vulnerable.

The recipients of physical violence are most often those termed either health care aides or personal support workers, but doctors, nurses, and therapists all experience violent attacks. According to the Joint Commission (2010), a US nonprofit that accredits health care organizations, incidences of physical violence against all health care employees have been increasing since the late twentieth century. As Pat Armstrong et al. (2009, 127) found in their international study of long-term residential care, physical violence against personal support workers "includes being slapped or hit with an object. It frequently involves being pinched, bitten, having one's hair pulled, being poked or spit on. Having one's wrists twisted is also common." Whereas these are the primary means residents use in nursing homes and hospital rooms, those employed in emergency services too often face assault with a range of weapons. This can also happen in nursing homes and hospital rooms when relatives or other visitors bring knives, guns, or other objects with them. The result could be death but is most often bruising, scratches, broken bones, and broken skin accompanied by fear of future assaults. In an environment where infection is common, these can have serious physical consequences.

SEXUAL ABUSE

Although the media most frequently highlight sexual abuse of patients and residents, sexual abuse of health care workers is not uncommon. Touching inappropriately is the most frequent and mildest form of sexual abuse. Workers have their breasts, buttocks, and genitals grabbed on a regular basis. Sexual comments are frequent, as are suggestive comments, jokes, and gestures. Health care workers may also experience rape, threats of rape, and sexual coercion.

Those who provide direct care are most likely to face the touching, grabbing, and comments, especially if they work in nursing homes. Women provide the bulk of such care and face the overwhelming majority of sexual abuse. But no one working in health care is immune. There is, however, a difference in physical assault in terms of who perpetuates the assault. In their survey of the literature on the sexual harassment of nurses, Sharon M. Valente and Vern Bullough (2004) report that a majority experienced sexual harassment and that most of this harassment came from doctors, followed by supervisors and coworkers. Patients, families, and visitors played smaller roles.

The consequences of sexual abuse are less visible than physical abuse but nonetheless real. Such abuse disrupts concentration on providing care and often leads to mental health problems. Some workers leave their jobs, whereas others may develop depression, resort to drugs, or stay home on sick leave.

RACISM

Like sexual abuse, racist abuse is often invisible and usually unreported in official documents. Although much of the literature exposing racism focuses on nurses, no health care worker from a racialized group is immune. Martin Stevens, Shereen Hussein, and Jill Manthorpe (2012) document the racism experienced by migrant workers in the United Kingdom. But racism is not only experienced by those at the bottom of the health care hierarchy. The King's Fund (Coker 2001) has detailed the racism against doctors in the United Kingdom, and the American Medical Association has acknowledged racial discrimination in its ranks. Patients, residents, and their families too often refuse services from doctors, therapists, and the entire range of direct care workers who are from racialized groups. Those who do accept such care may make racist comments and jokes. Colleagues and supervisors can also be sources of racism that ranges from subtle comments to obvious exclusion or physical assault. As with sexual abuse, the consequences of racism are often invisible and frequently lead to withdrawal from the job, work absences, or mental health problems.

VERBAL, MENTAL, AND EMOTIONAL ABUSE

Health care workers are yelled at and harangued. They are blamed, accused, and called names. Such verbal abuse can come from patients, residents and their families, colleagues, and supervisors. It can come from either women or men and be directed toward any provider, regardless of professional status. It is not the only cause of mental or emotional anguish but is one of them. In a Statistics Canada survey of nurses (Shields and Wilkins 2006, 135), nearly half of the respondents reported that they were emotionally abused by a patient, with more men than women saying this was the case. Visitors were the next most frequent source of such abuse, but some also came from physicians and coworkers. Mental and emotional abuse may take the form of anything from body language to shunning and bullying. The sources of these forms of abuse need not be individuals. Workers may also feel emotional abuse when conditions do not allow them to do the job they think should be done, such as changing diapers when they are wet or having the time to sit with a crying resident.

Such abuse may well help explain the higher-than-average use of medications, such as antidepressants, among both male and female providers. It does make their workloads more difficult to handle and disrupts their relationships at home. Mental and emotional abuse are the least obvious and the most difficult to document but can be nonetheless harmful to physical health. Indeed the difficulty of documenting the abuse can contribute to stress-related health consequences.

COMBATING VIOLENCE

While surveys and interviews with individual health care workers provide the evidence of widespread abuse, they also indicate that a great deal of this abuse goes unreported to officials. As Rebecca Hagey et al. (2001), for example, have documented, one reason is that the workers experience reprisals if they complain and often face unfairness in the complaint process. In an editorial on the "epidemic of violence," D. M. Gates (2004, 649) summarizes the most common reasons as "reporting is too time consuming, reporting lacks supervisory support, and reporting won't make a difference." Perhaps most significantly, health care workers and their managers too often see abuse, at least from patients and residents, as an inevitable part of health care work. However, Armstrong et al. (2009, figures 29, 30) found in their survey of nursing home workers that Canadians were over six times more likely than their Scandinavian counterparts to report that they experienced physical abuse on a daily basis, whereas half as many Canadians compared to Scandinavians said they never experienced sexual abuse. Yet the resident populations in these countries are quite similar. This study, along with others documenting considerable variation in abuse, indicates that the problem cannot be primarily attributed to the uncontrollable and inevitable actions of those who need care.

The abuse of health care workers results in physical and mental health problems for workers as well as high turnover and work absences that incur costs to employers. The abuse can undermine the capacity to provide good care and can spill over into households as workers take their abuse home. Not surprisingly, multiple strategies have been developed to address the growing problem of abuse faced by health care workers. Organizations such as the International Labour Organization (2005) and the US Occupational Safety and Health Administration (2004) have developed training manuals and prevention strategies.

These strategies depend to a large extent on how abuse is understood and where the abuse comes from. When abuse is understood as the result of the individual inadequacies of managers, supervisors, and colleagues, the focus is on training, monitoring, and reporting. It can also include new approaches to how complaints and grievances are handled. When visitors and families are seen as the problem, higher security and screening are encouraged. In the case of those who provide care in individual households, the use of electronic communications systems and regular call-ins are encouraged. When patients and residents are seen as the problem, training is often offered as the main strategy. Working in teams can also reduce violence, as a team can provide support not only for the workers but also for the patient or resident. Meaningful consultation with and among workers about both work organization and disruptive individuals can help create a more supportive environment, which in turn can help reduce the incidence of abuse.

These strategies emphasize changing individual behavior and some collective behavior. However, the comparative research by Armstrong et al. (2009) suggests that workload and worker autonomy are critical not only to understanding but also to changing the growing incidence of abuse. Patients and visitors are much more likely to get physically and verbally abusive when their needs are not being met. Employees too are more likely to abuse others when they are overworked and stressed. Moreover health care workers are more likely to feel mental and emotional abuse when they cannot do the work in the way they have been taught and in the way their experience teaches them it should be provided.

Paul Farmer (2003) and Johan Galtung (1969) use the term *structural violence* to denote the larger organization and policy factors that prevent people from reaching their potential or using their capacities. As health care organizations throughout the Western world move toward lean production and standardized care plans that mean more work and less autonomy for health care workers, incidences of abuse are increasing, and so are turnover rates and work absences. Equally important, when cost control and cost cutting are the focus, it is difficult to provide the training, the education, the support, or even the surveillance that is the basis of many prevention strategies.

CONCLUSION

Abuse of health care workers is common and increasing. It is a problem not only for workers and their employers but also for those who need and those who fund health care. Residents, patients, and visitors account for the majority of abuse. Those working in nursing homes and those providing direct care anywhere are the most likely to be abused. However, most workers experience some form of abuse, especially when they are younger and from racialized groups, and the abuse can also come from colleagues or supervisors. Prevention strategies primarily focus on changing individuals, although there is growing interest in altering managerial, organizational, and policy approaches.

SEE ALSO *Care: IV. Care and Society/Public Policy; Health Care, Worker Migration; Medicine, Profession of; Nursing, Profession of*

BIBLIOGRAPHY

Armstrong, Pat; Albert Banerjee; Marta Szebehely; et al. 2009. *They Deserve Better: The Long-Term Care Experience in Canada and Scandinavia.* Ottawa: Canadian Centre for Policy Alternatives.

Coker, Naaz, ed. 2001. *Racism in Medicine: An Agenda for Change.* London: King's Fund.

Farmer, Paul. 2003. *Pathologies of Power: Health, Human Rights, and the New War on the Poor.* Berkeley: University of California Press.

Galtung, Johan. 1969. "Violence, Peace, and Peace Research." *Journal of Peace Research* 6 (3): 167–91.

Gates, D. M. 2004. "The Epidemic of Violence against Healthcare Workers." *Occupational and Environmental Medicine* 61 (8): 649–50.

Hagey, Rebecca; Ushi Choudhry; Sepali Guruge; et al. 2001. "Immigrant Nurses' Experience of Racism." *Journal of Nursing Scholarship* 33 (4): 389–94.

Hegney, Desley; Anthony Tuckett; Deborah Parker; and Robert M. Eley. 2010. "Workplace Violence: Differences in Perceptions of Nursing Work between Those Exposed and Those Not Exposed; A Cross-Sector Analysis." *International Journal of Nursing Practice* 16 (2): 188–202.

International Labour Organization. 2005. *Framework Guidelines for Addressing Workplace Violence in the Health Sector: The Training Manual.* January 1. http://www.ilo.org/safework/info/instr/WCMS_108542/lang—en/index.htm

Joint Commission. 2010. *Preventing Violence in the Health Care Setting.* Sentinel Event Alert, issue 45. June 3. http://www.jointcommission.org/assets/1/18/SEA_45.PDF

Occupational Safety and Health Administration. 2004. *Guidelines for Preventing Workplace Violence for Health Care and Social Service Workers.* Washington, DC: Author. http://www.osha.gov/Publications/OSHA3148/osha3148.html

Rippon, Thomas J. 2000. "Aggression and Violence in Health Care Professions." *Journal of Advanced Nursing* 31 (2): 452–60.

Shields, Margot, and Kathryn Wilkins. 2006. *Findings from the 2005 National Survey of the Work and Health of Nurses.* Statistics Canada, Health Canada, and Canadian Institute for Health Information. Ottawa: Minister of Industry.

Statistics Canada. 2007. "Study: Criminal Victimization in the Workplace." *Daily*, February 16.

Stevens, Martin; Shereen Hussein; and Jill Manthorpe. 2012. "Experiences of Racism and Discrimination among Migrant Care Workers in England: Findings from a Mixed-Methods Research Project." *Ethnic and Racial Studies* 35 (2): 259–80.

Valente, Sharon M., and Vern Bullough. 2004. "Sexual Harassment of Nurses in the Workplace." *Journal of Nursing Care Quality* 19 (3): 234–41.

World Health Organization. 2006. *Health Workers*. Geneva: Author.

Pat Armstrong
Professor of Sociology, York University

ACCESS TO HEALTH CARE

The United States is the only country among the wealthy nations of the Organisation for Economic Co-operation and Development (OECD) that does not provide universal access to health care for its residents. Despite the patchwork quilt of public and subsidized private insurance, more than 47 million people living in the United States do not have health insurance. Even if the Patient Protection and Affordable Care Act (ACA) of 2010 is fully implemented, more than 20 million Americans will remain uninsured. Under the ACA, undocumented immigrants will remain ineligible for public insurance programs. There are federal, state, and local laws that recognize a public obligation to provide at least some health care to all members of society. Under the Emergency Medical Treatment and Active Labor Act of 2011, hospitals that operate emergency departments are obligated to assess the needs of patients to determine whether they need emergency care or are in active labor. If they require care, these hospitals are obligated to treat them until stable. Similarly, patients who are otherwise ineligible for public insurance may receive "emergency" Medicaid coverage to pay for health care services that address immediately life-threatening conditions. In addition, the United States has an extensive, but chronically underfunded, network of health care safety-net institutions that are designed to provide health care to those who are unable to afford it (Hall and Rosenbaum 2012).

The existence of these policies does not prevent large inequalities in access to care. People without health insurance are less likely than people with insurance to have a regular source of care (such as a primary care doctor), more likely to go without needed care, and more likely to die prematurely from conditions for which there are effective medical treatments. Beyond the financial barriers associated with a lack of insurance, there may be a variety of nonfinancial barriers to access. The supply of health care providers and other resources, the accessibility of those health care resources, and the attitudes of people working in the system to the personal characteristics of patients may all serve as barriers to access (Kullgren, McLaughlin, Mitra, and Armstrong 2011). Even among people with some form of public or private health insurance, Americans who live in low-income neighborhoods and people who do not speak English well are less likely to receive timely and appropriate care, as are racial and ethnic minorities as compared to whites. Several studies find significant black-white differences in access to the treatment of cancer and heart disease (Gusmano, Rodwin, and Weisz 2010; Hao et al. 2011; Jha et al. 2005).

In countries with universal or near universal coverage, primary care visits are relatively equitably distributed across income groups (Van Doorslaer, Masseria, and OECD Health Equity Research Group Members 2004). This is seen in countries with national health services and those with some form of national health insurance. In a national health service, which is financed primarily by general revenue taxes, most care is delivered by the government. Most primary care is provided by general practitioners with whom the government contracts, and specialty care is provided by consultants who are government employees in public hospitals. In contrast, a national health insurance system offers publicly financed social insurance to cover health care expenses. These systems are usually financed through a combination of payroll taxes and general revenue. Although some countries with a national health insurance system have a large public health care delivery system, care is often delivered by private-sector physicians and hospitals (White 1995; Gusmano et al. 2010). Lower-income residents of Australia, Canada, and New Zealand, which have national health insurance systems, and the United Kingdom, which has a national health service, are less likely to report barriers to health care than people with below-median incomes in the United States (Blendon et al. 2002).

But even among countries that provide universal coverage there are differences in access to specialty services by socioeconomic status (Roos and Mustard 1997). In Canada, a country that strives to eliminate financial barriers to care, residents of higher-income Winnipeg neighborhoods receive "substantially more" specialty and surgical care than lower-income residents (Roos and Mustard 1997, 102). In France, Germany, and England, access to some specialty health care services is significantly worse among residents of lower-income neighborhoods

(Gusmano, Weisz, and Rodwin 2009; Degos and Rodwin 2011). Inequalities in access to health care are even greater within countries outside the OECD. For example, despite remarkable economic growth since the late twentieth century, there are enormous disparities in access to health care within the People's Republic of China and India (Balarajan, Selvaraj, and Subramanian 2011; Hung, Rane, Tsai, and Shi 2012).

Are the health care inequalities described above unjust? All countries limit access to publicly funded health care services. Some ration care on the basis of ability to pay, but most countries adopt a budget mechanism to set a cap on total spending. Are such limits ever acceptable? What normative standards should be used to evaluate the performance of health care systems with regard to access? Should health care be distributed equally or according to need or should those who are worst off be given priority? Should other forms of disadvantage (e.g., poverty, or being a target of discrimination) influence the distribution of health care resources? Does the magnitude of inequalities in access matter? If we conclude that inequalities in access to health care are unjust, should we give this problem a higher priority than other social problems? Are there circumstances under which the costs of reducing or eliminating inequities in access to health care may outweigh the benefits?

RIGHTS, EQUALITY OF OPPORTUNITY, AND HUMAN FLOURISHING

Advocates for universal health care coverage often assert that health care is a human right. International law recognizes a right to health care, but the United States has not signed the United Nations (UN) conventions that explicitly recognize a right to health. According to the Universal Declaration of Human Rights, adopted in 1948 by the UN General Assembly, "Everyone has the right to a standard of living adequate for health and well-being of himself and of his family, including food, clothing, housing and medical care." In 2000 the UN Committee on Economic, Social, and Cultural Rights issued "General Comment No. 14" that asserts a "right to the highest attainable standard of health," which can be interpreted as a right to health care and other social and economic conditions that are needed for good health (Gostin 2001; Arras and Fenton 2009). Calls for treating access to health care as a human right are often based on assertions rather than arguments; one justification is that health care, in that it contributes to health, is a human right because it is one of the basic human interests "whose fulfillment is a necessary condition for living a decent or dignified human life" (Arras and Fenton 2009, 30).

Liberal arguments for providing equal access to health care focus on the relationship between health care and equality of opportunity. Norman Daniels argues that, although "equality of opportunity does not imply leveling individual differences," it is unfair if "disease and disability restricts an individual's opportunity relative to that portion of the normal opportunity range his skills and talents would have made available to him were he healthy" (1985, 33–34). To the extent that health care is able to address the conditions that limit a person's fair share of the normal opportunity range, society is obligated to provide it.

The capability approach argues that we should evaluate social arrangements, including access to health care, in terms of their impact on "functionings" or states of "being and doing," not just on the fair allocation of resources (Sen 1999; Nussbaum 2001; Powers and Faden 2008). People should be free to choose the kind of life they value. Without good health, this freedom does not exist. Health care is not intrinsically valuable, but it should be socially guaranteed because it contributes to good health, without which "no other human functionings are possible, including agency" (Ruger 2004, 1075). Human flourishing is only possible if people are in good health, so to the degree that access to health care is necessary to achieve this goal, a just society must make it available (Powers and Faden 2008).

The "instrumental" value of health care raises important questions about the relationship between health and health care. The role of health care in improving life expectancy and its impact on the social health gradient is small in comparison to actions aimed at social and environmental determinants, such as income, education, neighborhood, and occupational status (Wright and Weinstein 1998; Marmot 1999). Some scholars argue that, if we care about ensuring that people enjoy sufficient health to live a decent life, enjoy the normal opportunity range or flourish, society should focus its limited resources on addressing the social and economic determinants of health rather than worrying about access to a service that does relatively little to affect inequalities in health status (Sreenivasan 2007).

Despite this skepticism about the influence of health care on health, there is evidence that health care matters. Studies have found that, although health care expenditure has little impact on life expectancy at birth, it is associated with large reductions in infant mortality (Rodwin and Neuberg 2005; Nixon and Ulmann 2006). Other studies conclude that access to primary care leads to "better health status, lower overall mortality, lower death rates due to diseases of the heart and cancer, longer life expectancy, lower neonatal death rate, and lower low birth weight" (Shi 1994, 431). Studies that focus on specific diseases reach similar conclusions. Health care has contributed substantially, for example, to the reduction in mortality from heart disease. In England and Wales, 42 percent of the decrease in coronary heart disease (CHD) mortality between 1981 and 2000 can be attributed to medical and surgical treatments (Unal, Critchley, and Capewell 2005).

Studies from Scotland and the Netherlands reach similar conclusions about the contributions of medical and surgical interventions to the reduction of CHD mortality (Capewell, Morrison, and McMurray 1999). More broadly, health care has contributed to overall declines in avoidable mortality, defined as premature death due to conditions for which there are effective medical treatments (Weisz et al. 2007; Nolte and McKee 2008; Chau et al. 2011). Medical care has been found to improve the health of people with breast cancer, heart attacks, depression, and cataracts and of low-birth weight infants; moreover, the economic value of health gains associated with medical treatments has been found to be equal to or greater than the cost (Cutler and McClellan 2001).

COMMUNITARIAN AND POLITICAL ARGUMENTS FOR ACCESS

Communitarian arguments for providing universal access to health care focus less on the relationship between health and health care and more on the extent to which universal access contributes to mutual respect among members of a community. Along with making it possible for individuals to flourish, the universal provision of health care may enhance the capacity of a community to flourish.

In a society that aspires to be democratic, decisions should be made on the basis of deliberation. Without a minimum level of mutual respect for other human beings and other ways of life, genuine deliberation about the public good may be impossible even if the formal institutions of government attempt to facilitate it (Elkin 1987). The communal provision of social goods, such as health care and education, helps to lessen the impact of the inequality and "atomization" stemming from market interaction (Taylor 1992). Vast material inequality can, and often has, led to the moral condemnation of the poor (Katz 1990). At a minimum, social welfare policy should avoid exacerbating these material inequalities. Communal provision fosters deliberation and public-spirited thinking by reminding us that we are more than strangers bargaining with each other over the distribution of goods. An extensive welfare state involving the communal provision of some public goods is the institutional structure needed to provide balance in a society with a large market-based economy. Markets help to limit government and provide some level of freedom, but they also tend to atomize and fracture society. The communal provision of public goods works to counter this effect by creating a sense of solidarity. Communal provision of security and welfare is important because, as Michael Walzer (1983) observes, "it teaches us the value of membership" (64); as Charles Taylor (1992) argues, it fosters republican solidarity, which underpins freedom.

This argument raises important questions about membership. In countries with either a national health service or national health insurance, legal immigrants have access to publicly funded health care. In the United States, legal immigrants must wait five years before they are eligible for public health insurance programs. In most countries, undocumented immigrants are not eligible for public health insurance, even if they have lived in the country for many years.

Is it fair to exclude undocumented immigrants from publicly funded health care programs? One justification for doing so is that citizens and legal immigrants have a more legitimate claim on limited health care resources because they contribute to the society through the tax code. This argument fails to recognize that undocumented immigrants often constitute a vital, if primarily low-wage, part of the workforce. In the United States, the food production and construction industries rely heavily on this workforce. These workers pay a variety of state and local taxes, such as sales taxes. Some have payroll taxes withheld, although they are not entitled to claim Social Security or Medicare benefits. Another argument that is often used to exclude undocumented immigrants from publicly funded health care programs is that they are less deserving of health care because they have broken the law. Yet prison inmates in the United States receive publicly funded health care. It may be reasonable for countries to limit access by noncitizens to publicly funded health care services; but if a country depends on the labor of undocumented immigrants without offering them a reliable way to gain legal resident status, denying them health care and health insurance on the basis of their current status is exploitative (Carens 2008).

WHAT DOES JUSTICE REQUIRE?

If we need health care to flourish as individuals and to foster mutual respect among members of a community, how much health care do we need? The general claim that health care enjoys special moral status does not provide specific guidance on these questions.

How do we define need? Each of the normative standards articulated above seem to call, at a minimum, for providing health care that would help to avoid premature mortality. But is this sufficient to provide people with an opportunity to pursue life's goals or to flourish? How can we distinguish between needs and preferences? Few would argue that health care for a patient experiencing a heart attack is unnecessary, but does justice require public funding for a heart transplant? Most people would agree that patients diagnosed with cancer should have access to chemotherapy if oncologists believe it is medically appropriate, but should the public fund the cost of prescription medications and supplemental therapies to counteract side effects of this treatment?

In his book *Just Health Care*, Daniels argues that a "basic tier" of health care services "would include *health-care services that meet health-care needs, or at least important health-care needs—as judged by their impact on the normal opportunity range*" (emphasis in the original; 1985, 79). Although he recognizes that there may be a social obligation to provide access to additional health care services, depending on social resources available, his account of justice requires that "there should be no obstacles—financial, racial, geographical, and so on—to access to the basic tier" (1985, 79–80).

The concept of a normal opportunity range is similar to the argument presented by Daniel Callahan in *Setting Limits: Medical Goals in an Aging Society* as to why it is appropriate to limit public funding for curative medical care for older people. Callahan argues that, by the time people have reached their late seventies or eighties, "most of those opportunities which life affords people will have been achieved" (1987, 66). Both authors' arguments raise the question of how to define a normal life span or the normal opportunity range. As Robert N. Butler (2008) notes, the matter is further complicated by the possibility that new health care technologies will continue to change expectations about what is normal.

FAIR PROCESS AND ACCESS TO HEALTH CARE

Even if there is universal agreement that people are entitled to enough health care so as to enjoy the normal opportunity range, accomplish most of life's major possibilities, and flourish, universal agreement as to the precise requirements of these standards is unlikely. Jennifer Prau Ruger argues that the capability approach does not call for a particular set of health care services or a specific level of availability of care. Like the liberal justifications for access to care, the capability approach does suggest that society is obligated to help individuals achieve a level of health consistent with "minimal normal functioning"; but rather than attempting to distinguish between essential health care benefits and those that justice might not require, the capability approach emphasizes the need for a fair process to make decisions about these details (2004, 1077).

John Arras and Elizabeth Fenton designate the "attempt to spell out the demands of a universal conception of morality in particular social contexts" *institutional* human rights: "different people deliberating under different conditions will come to different conclusions as to how best to realize these demands, but they should all be working toward the same ultimate goal of providing for basic human interests" (2009, 33). Although it may be possible to reach consensus about the need to provide some access to health care, it is not clear that it is desirable or possible to impose universal criteria about how much health care ought to be financed publicly and across all societies.

Every society faces fundamental questions as to the extent to which it is appropriate to pool risks associated with poor health over the course of a lifetime. What choices should be left to the individual and what choices should be made collectively? How should we decide what constitutes a "normal opportunity range" available to members of the society? At what point would limiting public funding for health care impair functioning and constitute an unacceptable impediment to human flourishing? Answers to these questions require a legitimate political process, based on Aristotelian ideas, in which those who are affected by these decisions have the opportunity to shape them (Gutmann and Thompson 1996). Drawing on the experiences and perspectives of a greater number of people and groups not only helps policy makers learn from past mistakes and identify new solutions, it leads to decisions that are more legitimate (Lindblom 1965; Grogan and Gusmano 2007).

SEE ALSO *Aging and the Aged: II. Health Care for the Aging; AIDS: II. Health Care and Research Issues; Children: III. Health Care and Research Issues; Economic Concepts in Health Care; Family Caregiving; Global Health Inequalities and Inequities; Health Care Institutions; Health Care Systems; Health Insurance; Health Policy in the United States; Immigrants, Access to Health Care; Justice; Medicaid; Medicare; Mentally Disabled and Mentally Ill Persons: I. Health Care Issues; NGOs in Health Care; Rights; Whistleblowing in Health Care*

BIBLIOGRAPHY

Aristotle. 1912. *Politics: A Treatise on Government.* Book 3, chapter 9. Translated by William Ellis. London: J. M. Dent and Sons.

Arras, John D., and Elizabeth M. Fenton. 2009. "Bioethics and Human Rights: Access to Health-Related Services." *Hastings Center Report* 39 (50): 27–38.

Balarajan, Yarlini; S. Selvaraj; and S. V. Subramanian. 2011. "Health Care and Equity in India." *Lancet* 377 (3764): 505–15.

Blendon, Robert; Cathy Schoen; Catherine M. DesRoches; et al. 2002. "Inequities in Health Care: A Five-Country Survey." *Health Affairs* 21 (3): 182–91.

Butler, Robert N. 2008. *The Longevity Revolution: The Benefits and Challenges of Living a Long Life.* New York: PublicAffairs.

Callahan, Daniel. 1987. *Setting Limits: Medical Goals in an Aging Society.* New York: Simon and Schuster.

Capewell, Simon; C. Morrison; and John McMurray. 1999. "Contribution of Modern Cardiovascular Treatment and Risk Factor Changes to the Decline in Coronary Heart Disease Mortality in Scotland between 1975 and 1994." *Heart* 81 (4): 380–86.

Carens, Joseph H. 2008. "The Rights of Irregular Migrants." *Ethics and International Affairs* 22 (2): 163–86.

Chau, Pui Hing; Jean Woo; Kam Che Chan; et al. 2011. "Avoidable Mortality Pattern in a Chinese Population—Hong Kong, China." *European Journal of Public Health* 21 (2): 215–20.

Cutler, David M., and Mark McClellan. 2001. "Is Technological Change in Medicine Worth It?" *Health Affairs* 20 (5): 11–29.

Daniels, Norman. 1985. *Just Health Care*. Cambridge, UK: Cambridge University Press.

Degos, Laurent, and Victor G. Rodwin. 2011. "Two Faces of Patient Quality and Safety: A Franco-American Comparison." *Health Economics, Policy, Law*. May/June.

Elkin, Stephen L. 1987. *City and Regime in the American Republic*. Chicago: University of Chicago Press.

Emergency Medical Treatment and Active Labor Act. 2011. 42 U.S.C. § 1395dd (2011).

Gostin, Lawrence. 2001. "The Human Right to Health: A Right to the 'Highest Attainable Standard of Health.'" *Hastings Center Report* 31 (2): 29–30.

Grogan, Colleen M., and Michael K. Gusmano. 2007. *Healthy Voices, Unhealthy Silence: Advocacy and Health Policy for the Poor*. Washington, DC: Georgetown University Press.

Gusmano, Michael K.; Victor G. Rodwin; and Daniel Weisz. 2010. *Health Care in World Cities: New York, Paris, and London*. Baltimore, MD: Johns Hopkins University Press.

Gusmano, Michael K.; Daniel Weisz; and Victor G. Rodwin. 2009. "Achieving Horizontal Equity: Must We Have a Single Payer Health Care System?" *Journal of Health Politics, Policy and Law* 34 (4): 617–33.

Gutmann, Amy, and Dennis Thompson. 1996. *Democracy and Disagreement: Why Moral Conflict Cannot Be Avoided in Politics, and What Should Be Done about It*. Cambridge, MA: Harvard University Press.

Hall, Mark A., and Sara Rosenbaum, eds. 2012. *The Health Care "Safety Net" in a Post-Reform World*. New Brunswick, NJ: Rutgers University Press.

Hao, Yongping; Hope Landrine; Ahmedin Jemal; et al. 2011. "Race, Neighbourhood Characteristics and Disparities in Chemotherapy for Colorectal Cancer." *Journal of Epidemiology and Community Health* 65 (3): 211–17.

Hung, Li-Mei; Sarika Rane; Jenna Tsai; and Leiyu Shi. 2012. "Advancing Primary Care to Promote Equitable Health: Implications for China." *International Journal for Equity in Health* 11 (2): 2–5.

Jha, Ashish K.; Elliott S. Fisher; Zhonghe Li; et al. 2005. "Racial Trends in the Use of Major Procedures among the Elderly." *New England Journal of Medicine* 353 (7): 683–91.

Katz, Michael B. 1990. *The Undeserving Poor: From the War on Poverty to the War on Welfare*. New York: Pantheon.

Kullgren, Jeffrey T.; Catherine G. McLaughlin; Nandita Mitra; and Katrina Armstrong. 2011. "Nonfinancial Barriers and Access to Care for U.S. Adults." *Health Services Research* 47 (1, pt. 2): 462–85.

Lindblom, Charles E. 1965. *The Intelligence of Democracy: Decision Making through Mutual Adjustment*. New York: Free Press.

Marmot, Michael. 1999. "Acting on Evidence to Reduce Inequalities in Health." *Health Affairs* 18 (3): 45–46.

Nixon, John, and Philippe Ulmann. 2006. "The Relationship between Health Care Expenditure and Health Outcomes. Evidence and Caveats for a Causal Link." *European Journal of Public Health* 7 (1): 7–18.

Nolte, Ellen, and Martin McKee. 2008. "Measuring the Health of Nations: Updating an Earlier Analysis." *Health Affairs* 27 (1): 58–71.

Nussbaum, Martha C. 2001. *Women and Human Development: The Capabilities Approach*. Cambridge, UK: Cambridge University Press.

Powers, Madison, and Ruth Faden. 2008. *Social Justice: The Moral Foundations of Public Health and Health Policy*. Oxford: Oxford University Press.

Rodwin, Victor G., and Leland G. Neuberg. 2005. "Infant Mortality and Income in 4 World Cities: New York, London, Paris, and Tokyo." *American Journal of Public Health* 95 (1): 86–90.

Roos, Noralou P., and Cameron Mustard. 1997. "Variation in Health and Health Care Use by Socioeconomic Status in Winnipeg, Canada: Does the System Work Well? Yes and No." *Milbank Quartely* 75 (1): 89–111.

Ruger, Jennifer Prau. 2004. "Health and Social Justice." *Lancet* 364 (9439): 1075–80.

Sen, Amartya. 1999. *Development as Freedom*. New York: Knopf.

Shi, Leiyu. 1994. "Primary Care, Specialty Care, and Life Chances." *International Journal of Health Services* 24 (3): 431–58.

Sreenivasan, Gopal. 2007. "Health Care and Equality of Opportunity." *Hastings Center Report* 37 (2): 21–48.

Taylor, Charles. 1992. *The Ethics of Authenticity*. Cambridge, MA: Harvard University Press.

Unal, Belgin; Julia Alison Critchley; and Simon Capewell. 2005. "Modeling the Decline in Coronary Heart Disease Deaths in England and Wales, 1981–2000: Comparing Contributions from Primary Prevention and Secondary Prevention." *British Medical Journal* 331:614.

Van Doorslaer, Eddy; Cristina Masseria; and the OECD Health Equity Research Group Members. 2004. "Income-Related Inequality in the Use of Medical Care in 21 OECD Countries." OECD Working Paper. Paris: OECD. http://www.oecd.org/health/health-systems/31743034.pdf

Walzer, Michael. 1983. *Spheres of Justice: A Defense of Pluralism and Equality*. New York: Basic Books.

White, Joseph. 1995. *Competing Solutions: American Health Care Proposals and International Experience*. Washington, DC: Brookings Institution.

Wright, Janice C., and Milton C. Weinstein. 1998. "Gains in Life Expectancy from Medical Interventions: Standardizing Data on Outcomes." *New England Journal of Medicine* 339:380–86.

Michael K. Gusmano
Research Scholar, The Hastings Center

ADDICTION AND DEPENDENCE

People have been using substances since the beginning of recorded time. Ancient cultures even had gods associated with particular drugs (Dionysius, for example, was the Greek god of wine and drunkenness). However, closer reading of early manuscripts also documents the societal dark side of addiction. For example, the Bible documents how Noah, the first recorded winemaker, suffered shame and embarrassment after becoming drunk (Genesis 9:20–24). Addiction is perhaps the least discriminating of all the disease processes, with hardly a race, ethnicity, nation, or family spared its ravaging effects. This entry discusses what constitutes addiction (and dependence and tolerance), who becomes addicted and how, the epidemiology of substance abuse in society, the personal and societal consequences of addiction, the treatment of addiction, and the measures that can be taken to curb this pernicious epidemic.

WHAT IS ADDICTION?

The concept of addiction—whether to alcohol, cigarettes, drugs, or sex—is widely misunderstood. In fact the term *addiction* does not appear in the diagnostic criteria of the American Psychiatric Association's *Diagnostic and Statistical Manual of Mental Disorders* (DSM-IV-TR) (2000). The DSM-IV-TR uses such terms as *substance abuse* and *substance dependence*, but these classifications, along with addiction, are used to describe problematic substance use.

Some argue that use of alcohol or drugs is a choice and perhaps a right. A 2011 Gallup poll showed that 50 percent of Americans supported the legalization of marijuana, the highest percentage ever recorded by the poll and more than four times the percentage of those who had favored legalization (12%) when the group first began asking the question in 1969 (Gallup Politics 2011). The simple use of a substance does not constitute addiction. Statistics dating to 2010, supplied by the Substance Abuse and Mental Health Services Administration (SAMHSA) (2011), show that 70 percent of those twenty-one to twenty-five year old reported current alcohol use, but only 15 percent reported heavy use. Similarly not everyone who uses tobacco, marijuana, cocaine, or opiates becomes "addicted." What, then constitutes, addiction?

The National Institute on Drug Abuse (2010) reports that "addiction is a disease, just as diabetes and cancer are diseases." The American Society of Addiction Medicine (2013) defines addiction as being characterized by the inability to consistently abstain from a substance, impairment in behavioral control associated with substance use, craving of the substance, diminished recognition of significant problems with one's behaviors and interpersonal relationships associated with using the substance, and a dysfunctional emotional response. Addictive disease is further defined by compulsion, loss of control, and continued and repeated use despite adverse consequences. Even though a person knows the ill effects, he or she will use the addictive substance again. Thus the addict engages in repetitive and destructive use of one or more substances stemming from a biological vulnerability exposed or induced by environmental factors, such as drug taking. Addiction includes a preoccupation with the acquisition of a drug. In general when obtaining a drug plays a central role in a person's life, addiction is a concern. Many studies have shown that addicts rank finding and using their chosen drugs above work, family, religion, hunger, sex, and survival. Even when the "high" is no longer achieved, the drug and its use are paramount. Drug taking fools the brain, giving the user a false sense of accomplishment that is at odds with reality to the point that denial is common.

Because drugs cause a chronic disease in an otherwise healthy person, staying clean, or straight, becomes a daily challenge. Relapse therefore is another significant and expected part of addictive disease. It is common for addicts to have relatively long periods of abstinence intermingled with drug-use binges. Chemical addiction does not happen overnight. Addicts are not moral failures but victims of a disease.

We have a reasonably good understanding of the neurobiology of drug addiction, but there is still much debate on whether drug addicts are properly regarded as sufficiently autonomous and thus in control of their addiction such that they can be held accountable for their continued addiction or whether they have lost a degree of autonomy, such that they are unable to voluntarily refrain from further drug taking (Tieu 2010). The target for drugs of abuse is the brain, and changes in the neuroanatomy of the brain occur in all addicts and underlie the disease of addiction. Research in neuroscience has identified a specific area of the brain described as the reward center. The prefrontal cortex is used for carrying out executive functions, such as working memory, reinforcement learning, planning, adapting, inhibitory control, and integration of information for goal-directed guidance of behavior. This area of the brain is integrated with the reward system and is involved in the encoding of reward-based goals (Tieu 2010). It makes certain essential survival behaviors (such as eating, drinking, and having sex) pleasurable and reinforcing (Merlo et al. 2011) and therefore likely to be repeated. It has become evident that virtually all drugs of abuse target this area of the brain and result in neurotransmitter brain reward.

At its most basic level, then, addiction is a brain disease. All drugs of abuse achieve their pleasurable effects through their impact on neurotransmitter systems in the brain. Neurotransmitters are chemical messengers between nerve cells that are intricately involved in regulating moods. It is these transmitters (e.g., dopamine and serotonin) that are responsible for activation of the brain's innate reward system in response to such behaviors as eating and having sex. Abusive use of drugs generates increases of these neurotransmitters that dwarf those caused by natural rewards. Thus the use of the drug results in a hijacking of the reward system so that drug use becomes paramount, with the person forgoing basic human functions, such as eating and having sex, in favor of the use of the drug. Alteration of transmitters, such as dopamine and serotonin, in different parts of the brain account for not only the reward sensations associated with substance use but also the negative physical, psychological, and behavioral consequences of drug use. Research has shown that drugs of abuse can alter these neurotransmitter systems long after the person stops using the drug, changing the way neurons in the brain function and affecting mood and cognitive function. For example, marijuana use among adolescents has been shown to result in persisting cognitive deficits in verbal learning, working memory, and attention likely related to the drug's impact on hippocampal, subcortical, and prefrontal function (Hanson et al. 2010).

The problem is that the neurotransmitter changes caused by drugs far exceed those produced by natural reinforcers. Animals will press a lever for a drug injection or a puff of cocaine. Once they learn that pressing the lever gives them cocaine, they press again and again, frequently at the expense of eating and drinking, ultimately leading to death. The same is true for humans. It is not uncommon for addicts to lose family, careers, and even their lives because of their addiction. Alcoholics lose control over drinking and cannot stop. Eventually they hit a low point that requires them to make an enormous effort to regain their senses and achieve total abstinence. Thus one drink leads to more and more drinks, beyond one's ability to control (Tieu 2010).

This same part of the brain has connections to the area of the brain that controls the emotions—the limbic system. Thus drug use and addiction can be seen as a disease of brain reward with significant physical and psychological consequences. To truly understand the concept of addiction, one must look at issues of both positive and negative reinforcement. The pleasure effects of the drugs obviously result in positive reinforcement. However, continued drug use ultimately produces changes in neurotransmitter levels and a host of negative states and emotions (e.g., depression, anxiety, and fatigue). In these cases continued use of the drug leads to a decrease in these unpleasant effects and results in what is called negative reinforcement (e.g., removal of unpleasant feelings) and the subsequent return to a normal (in this case, drugged brain) state. Research has led to a new understanding of addiction that is not based solely on withdrawal effects. If addiction is understood as defined here, it is easy to see why it can be called a process: drug use produces brain changes that invite tolerance, which sets the stage for abuse, which then leads to loss of control, chemical dependence, and addiction.

The drug cocaine elucidates the addiction process (Paczynski and Gold 2011). Such drugs as cocaine trick the limbic system by triggering the reward response through the release of neurotransmitters. Cocaine use, for example, leads to the increased availability of the neurotransmitter dopamine. Dopamine causes specific nerve cells to fire, and the result is endogenous brain reward, or euphoria. Because cocaine employs brain systems normally reserved for species survival reward, users feel as if they have just accomplished something important. The euphoria and brain reward produced by cocaine make the brain view the drug as a substance critical for survival. Hence the brain asks for more cocaine, and excessive amounts of dopamine are released. Normally any surplus dopamine released by the nerve cells is reabsorbed by them; however, cocaine interferes with this reabsorption. Finally the brain's store of dopamine is depleted. With their supply of neurotransmitters depleted, cocaine users experience intense depression and cravings for more cocaine. In addition, the limbic system remembers cocaine's pleasurable response, a memory that can be triggered by talking about the drug, or by smelling it, or even through a visual stimulus, such as talcum powder. Positive rewards for negative behaviors aided or caused by environmental stimuli often have unintended social implications for the drug addict.

Given enough repetitions, drug and alcohol use become as entrenched as eating, drinking, or having sex. Furthermore the dopamine pathways have many other influences—on the hypothalamus and hormones and on the frontal lobe of the brain, the area responsible for judgment and insight. Drugs cause the addict's brain to demand more drugs, and the addict's ability to handle this demand rationally in the context of other everyday demands (such as work, family responsibilities, and concerns for their health and safety) becomes distorted. Tormented by the acquired drive for the drug, the memory of euphoria, and the denial of obvious ill consequences, the addict spirals out of control. No matter the drug of choice, the brain of an addict supports his or her becoming more irresponsible. Many times this has led to loss of control, and the addict responds with continuing or increased drug use and drug-seeking behavior.

Drug use provides a quick and powerful means of changing one's moods and sensations. In a cost-benefit analysis the user seeks the immediately gratifying effects as a benefit that outweighs the long-term cost of drug use. Other users may be influenced by physical or psychological states, such as depression, pain, or stress, which may be temporarily relieved by drug consumption. Drug use is such a powerful shaper of behavior that drug paraphernalia and virtually all of the events associated with finding and using drugs become reinforcers. A variety of nondrug factors, including psychological states, such as depression, anxiety, or environmental factors, can become so associated with drug taking that merely being depressed or seeing drug paraphernalia may trigger the urge to use drugs. Other factors may lead to positive reinforcement. For example, drug use may enhance a person's social standing, encourage approval by drug-using friends, and convey a special status to the user. Research has shown that among teens environmental factors can account for a considerable amount of the variance attributed to the decision to use or abstain from alcohol (Rose et al. 2001a).

The complexity of the body and the brain means that no simple answer for the cause of addiction will be found. However, researchers are using sophisticated diagnostic examinations to uncover more information in an attempt to better understand the effects of drugs on the brain (Gold et al. 2009). It is doubtful that these procedures will provide a definitive, simple answer to the cause of addiction, but the information gleaned from them may result in more effective treatment and prevention strategies.

What Is Dependence? What is meant by *dependence*? Is there a real distinction between dependence and addiction, or is the difference only semantic? Examination of the DSM-IV-TR criteria for substance dependence shows that the criteria for addiction cited herein (e.g., compulsive use, loss of control, and continued use despite adverse consequences) are included in the dependence criteria. However, the substance dependence criteria incorporate the additional factors of tolerance and withdrawal. Thus traditional distinctions that viewed dependence as a stage below addiction, where the choice to continue taking drugs or drinking alcohol can be stopped if the person really wants to stop, may be of limited utility (Kleiman 1992).

In any event once a person's drug use progresses from abuse to dependence, the capacity for voluntary control is significantly limited. The addicted brain becomes an impaired brain because the original drug-free condition has been replaced by a drug-present new normality. As the drug policy expert Mark A. R. Kleiman (1992) explains, people act and make decisions differently when they are intoxicated than when they are sober. Making such decisions as having another round of drinks, Kleiman points out, may lead to more bad choices. The nature of the drug—to reduce inhibition when intoxicated—brings about drugged choices.

What Is Tolerance? Tolerance may occur when the brain redefines normal and resets that level of feeling as the result of continued drug use. When a person takes drugs in the pursuit of pleasurable feelings, the brain resets to require larger quantities of the drug to obtain the same desired pleasurable effect that previously required smaller drug amounts. In other words, it takes more and more just to feel normal.

The emphasis on drug reward in the addiction process paves the way for other conditions, such as eating disorders and even sexual or gambling disorders, to be considered addictions. Eating disorders in particular share common behavioral symptoms, biological reward pathways, high relapse rates, and treatment strategies with other forms of substance abuse. Motivation is best understood in terms of affinitive versus aversive motivation, where the former involves behavior directed toward achieving pleasure and the latter involves behavior directed away from unpleasantness (Tieu 2010). More research is necessary to establish the legitimate inclusion of sexual and gambling behaviors with other expressions of addiction.

Withdrawal. Significant evidence supports the role of dopamine in the reward process, but the neuroanatomy of withdrawal is not as clearly defined. However, a wide variety of abused drugs, with apparently little in common pharmacologically, have similar withdrawal effects in certain areas of the brain. Patients addicted to opiates, benzodiazepines, nicotine, and alcohol have all had their withdrawal symptoms treated effectively with clonidine, a medication that works in an area of the brain called the locus coeruleus.

Unlike opiate and alcohol withdrawal, symptoms of cocaine withdrawal are relatively mild and disappear quickly. This dearth of withdrawal symptoms helps explain the episodic pattern of use reported by many cocaine addicts: periods of intense bingeing alternate with intervals of abstinence. The intense craving and high relapse rate associated with cocaine use appear to derive more from a desire to repeat a pleasurable experience than to avoid the discomfort of withdrawal. In fact for all drugs reward may be more important than withdrawal in the persistence of addiction and relapse in that successful treatment of withdrawal has not generally improved recovery.

WHO BECOMES ADDICTED?

Drug and alcohol abuse and dependence cut across all geographic, ethnic, and social boundaries (Graham et al. 2011; Degenhardt and Hall 2012). Data show differential rates of abuse and dependence among various ethnic groups. For example, SAMHSA 2010 data indicate lower rates of abuse among some ethnic groups (e.g., Asians at 4.1%), but there was little difference among whites (8.9%), Hispanics (9.7%), or blacks (8.2%) (SAMHSA 2011). As noted, not everyone who uses drugs or alcohol becomes addicted to the substance. What, then, leads some people to use a substance occasionally and others to spiral into addiction? The process is complicated and not yet completely understood, but data are emerging to help us further understand this addiction process.

Clearly there are individual differences, mostly involving brain chemistry, that place certain individuals at increased risk for addiction. No "addiction gene" has been found, and it seems unlikely that such a gene will ever be found (Buckland 2008). Nonetheless, genetic factors do seem to play a role in a person's risk of addiction in general and addiction to only a specific substance. For example, some individuals who take an opiate will experience the analgesic effects of the drug and even negative side effects, such as somnolence and nausea. Other people, however, experience energy and a sense of well-being from opiate medications, thus increasing their risk for misuse and addiction. Genetic factors account for approximately 50 percent of the risk associated with drug addiction (Buckland 2008; Urbanoski and Kelly 2011). However, that means that half of the risk of addiction is associated with other factors.

Research has shown that a number of environmental factors either are protective against abuse or increase the likelihood of addiction. For example, rates of use of illicit drugs and alcohol in the past month were lower for adolescents who agreed or strongly agreed with the statement that religious beliefs are important in their lives (7.9%) than for those adolescents who disagreed with the statement (16.6%). Similarly only 4.4 percent of adolescents who perceived strong parental disapproval for trying marijuana once or twice used the drug in the past month compared with a rate of 32.8 percent among those who did not perceive such parental disapproval. Environmental events can also lead to an increase in substance use. There is evidence in the research literature strongly linking childhood neglect, physical abuse, and sexual abuse with increased substance use and abuse among adults (Swogger et al. 2011).

Who becomes addicted is a complex disease process that is best understood as a biopsychosocial model where biological, environmental, and social influences create brain disease (Tsuang et al. 2001). Research in this area is ongoing, but several findings are clear. First, genetics plays a powerful role in who becomes addicted and to what substance. For example, approximately 10 percent of the population has a preexisting biological or genetic predisposition to drug and alcohol dependency. This genetic relationship is supported by the higher likelihood that a person will have the same substance dependence as his or her identical twin (a sibling who shares the same genetic material) compared with a fraternal twin (a sibling with nonidentical genetic material). Genetic factors underlie neurotransmitter receptor patterns in the brain that predispose a person to addiction (Rose et al. 2001b). Genetic factors are important in explaining why one person can have a drink and walk away and another person cannot stop drinking until he or she passes out.

Second, there is clearly a drug effect. That is, all drugs affect reward properties of the brain, but the pharmacological properties of some drugs are more addictive than others. Almost anyone can become addicted to some substances, such as cocaine or narcotics, regardless of genetic predisposition, if he or she uses the substance frequently for a long time.

Third, environmental factors and drug-use expectancies (i.e., motivation and intent) also play a role in the addiction process (Jang et al. 2001). For example, rarely do cancer patients become addicts despite taking powerful doses of narcotic pain medication. Similarly, an estimated 20 percent of American soldiers in Vietnam became addicted to heroin, but 90 percent were able to give up heroin once they returned from Vietnam, an outcome rate much higher than typically seen among heroin users (Robins 1993). Drugs are powerful conditioners shaping behavior and responses.

EPIDEMIOLOGY OF SUBSTANCE USE

Substance use does not discriminate; it is prevalent throughout American society and affects all demographic groups. National Survey on Drug Use and Health 2010 data indicate that 22.6 million Americans (8.9% of the population aged twelve and older) used an illicit drug in the month prior to the survey (SAMHSA 2011). Marijuana was the most commonly used drug (6.9%, or 17.4 million people). National rates for use of other drugs were lower: cocaine (0.6%), hallucinogens (0.5%), and inhalants (0.7%). Approximately 140,000 Americans (0.2%) are heroin users. MDMA, commonly known as Ecstasy, use between 1999 and 2000 increased by almost 25 percent to 6.4 million persons. This figure declined over time, and in 2010 there were 695,000 Ecstasy users (0.3%).

Total sales of illicit drugs in the United States reached $100 billion in 2006. This makes the sale of illicit drugs as large a business as a top ten company on the Fortune 500 list.

There is a relationship between a number of demographic factors (such as age, gender, and ethnicity) and particular substance use patterns. For example, 2010 SAMHSA data indicated that the highest rate of illicit drug use occurs among eighteen- to twenty-year-olds (23.1%) (SAMHSA 2011). Certainly youth is associated with drug use, with 16.6 percent of sixteen- to seventeen-year-olds, 9.3 percent of fourteen- to fifteen-year-olds, and 4 percent of twelve- to thirteen-year-olds reporting illicit drug use within the past month. However, illicit drug use is seen among all age groups, with 7.2 percent of fifty- to fifty-four-year-olds, 4.1 percent of fifty-five- to fifty-nine-year-olds, and 2.7 percent of sixty- to sixty-four-year-olds admitting to illicit drug use within the previous month (the thirty days prior to taking the survey).

Drug use does not show any racial or ethnic discrimination. SAMHSA data on persons aged twelve and older indicate similar rates of past-month use of illicit

Table 1. Total Expenditures on Cocaine, Heroin, Methamphetamines, and Marijuana (US billion dollars)

	2000	2001	2002	2003	2004	2005	2006
Cocaine	$34.6	$35.0	$35.9	$40.1	$37.2	$37.9	$37.8
Heroin	$11.9	$12.3	$12.7	$12.1	$11.5	$10.8	$11.0
Methamphetamines	$11.7	$11.6	$12.5	$13.4	$15.7	$17.4	$17.9
Marijuana	$25.2	$25.2	$35.7	$36.9	$30.3	$33.5	$33.7
Total	**$83.4**	**$84.1**	**$96.8**	**$102.5**	**$94.7**	**$99.6**	**$100.4**

SOURCE: Office of National Drug Control Policy, "Table ES. 3: Total Expenditures on Cocaine, Heroin, Metamphetamine, and Marijuana ($ Billions)," *What America's Users Spend on Illegal Drugs, 2000–2006* (Washington, DC: Executive Office of the President, 2012), 13.

drugs among African Americans (10.7%), whites (9.1%), and Hispanics (8.1%), with only Asians (3.5%) using at a lower rate (SAMHSA 2011). Rates of illicit drug use indicate generally higher rates of use by males (11.2%) than females (6.8%), but this difference evaporates among younger users: 10.4 percent of twelve- to seventeen-year-old males and 9.8 percent of twelve- to seventeen-year-old females report past-month illicit drug use, perhaps serving as a harbinger for less differentiation between genders in future generations.

Alcohol, however, is the most popular overused substance. The 2010 SAMHSA data indicate that over half (51.8%) of Americans aged twelve and older reported using alcohol (SAMHSA 2011). Use patterns among various age groups are similar to those seen with illicit drugs, with those twenty-one to twenty-five years old reporting the highest rate of use (70%). The rates of alcohol use in older groups are higher than those for illicit drugs. For example, 51.6 percent of sixty- to sixty-four-year-olds reported current alcohol use. Racial data indicate a higher rate of current use among whites (56.7%) compared with blacks (42.8%), Hispanics (41.8%), and Asians (38.4%). Gender patterns mimic those for illicit drugs, with men in general using at higher rates than women (57.4% vs. 46.5%, respectively); that difference disappears in the subset of twelve- to seventeen-year-olds (13.7% vs. 13.5%, respectively).

Even though studies have confirmed an encouraging decline in the number of illicit drug users, substance abuse continues to be a national problem. The 2010 National Survey on Drug Use and Health states that over 22.6 million Americans are users of illicit drugs. One of the major problems with combating this national problem according to the annual survey conducted by the University of Michigan Monitoring the Future study (Johnston et al. 2012), speaks to the early age many youths start using licit and illicit prescription and psychotherapeutic drugs. We have raised a nation of young drug users and abusers.

PERSONAL AND SOCIETAL CONSEQUENCES OF SUBSTANCE USE

Since 1990 trauma victims (such as those in automobile accidents) seen in emergency rooms have tested positive for the presence of drugs (such as cocaine and opiates) in increasing numbers. This increase approaches several hundredfold.

Ecstasy use among adolescents jumped almost 25 percent between 1999 and 2000. In 2010, 1.7 percent of eighth graders, 3 percent of tenth graders, and 5.3 percent of high school seniors had used Ecstasy in their lifetimes (Johnston et al. 2012). Increased use has resulted in a dramatic increase in emergency room visits (Center for Behavioral Health Statistics and Quality, SAMHSA 2010).

It is obvious that pharmaceuticals have overtaken illicit drugs as the largest cause of emergency room visits. Most of these are cases where the prescription medication is taken by someone other than the intended receiver of the drug. Diversion of prescription medication is a growing problem. The third-largest cause is alcohol in combination with other drugs.

Despite concerted efforts at education and interdiction, drug use is still commonplace in the United States. The business community is so concerned about substance abuse and dependence that drug screening of prospective employees has become commonplace. The majority of Fortune 500 companies have a drug-testing program. Drug testing is the norm in the US armed forces, and many court cases in the early twenty-first century are examining whether and when the government has the right to test its employees. In 2002 in *Board of Education of Independent School District No. 92 of Pottawatomie*

Table 2. Misused or Abused Drugs Most Commonly Involved in Emergency Department (ED) Visits, 2009

Drugs	Number of ED Visits	Number of ED Visits per 100,000 Population
Illicit drugs	973,591	317.1
Cocaine	422,896	137.7
Marijuana	376,467	122.6
Heroin	213,118	69.4
Pharmaceuticals	1,244,679	405.4
Narcotic pain relievers	397,160	129.4
Oxycodone products	175,949	57.3
Hydrocodone products	104,490	34.0
Antianxiety/insomnia drugs	433,600	141.2
Benzodiazepines	373,328	121.6
Antidepressants	104,940	34.2
Alcohol in combination with other drugs	519,650	169.3
Underage drinking	199,429	227.2

SOURCE: Adapted from Center for Behavioral Health Statistics and Quality, Substance Abuse and Mental Health Services Administration 2010.

County v. Earls the US Supreme Court held that drug testing of students is a reasonable means of preventing and deterring drug use among schoolchildren and is not a violation of Fourth Amendment rights.

The death toll from health problems caused by smoking is staggering. A study published in the *Journal of the American Medical Association* in 2000 estimated that almost 400,000 Americans die each year from smoking-related illnesses (Thun, Apicella, and Henley 2000). Beyond the health consequences for adults, smoking is a serious threat to young people on several levels. Despite widespread antismoking programs, 10.7 percent of teenagers smoke on a regular basis. Unfortunately many youth perceive a low risk of dangers from smoking, and others start smoking tobacco cigarettes after smoking "safe" marijuana.

Smoking is not the only potential threat from addictive substances to young people. The National Survey on Drug Use and Health 2010 estimates that 26.3 percent of twelve- to twenty-year-olds have used alcohol in the past month (SAMHSA 2011). The same survey found that 7.4 percent of the population aged twelve to seventeen had used marijuana in the preceding month, whereas 10.1 percent reported using some illicit drug during the same period.

Addiction has been called a victimless crime, but nothing could be further from the truth. Research consistently demonstrates that acts of violence against self and others, accidents, decreased productivity, health problems, and a number of other social ills have links to alcohol and drug abuse and addiction. Few people disagree that substance abuse and dependence are destructive behaviors, yet there seems to be a vast sea of confusion surrounding them. The facts are clear: addiction to and dependence on tobacco, alcohol, illicit drugs, and diverted prescription drugs are widespread and destructive. Certain behaviors, such as pathological gambling, compulsive eating, and problem patterns of sexual behavior, are also considered addictions. These findings are supported by research.

In a study of drinking consequences across eighteen colleges, Toben F. Nelson et al. (2009) found a host of negative consequences associated with heavy alcohol use. Of those students who reported "heavy drinking" (32%), 24.5 percent fell behind in schoolwork, 38.2 percent reported a blackout, 26.1 percent engaged in unplanned sexual activity, 14.1 percent damaged property, 36.8 percent drove after drinking, 7.5 percent got into trouble with police, and 39.8 percent admitted to doing something regrettable. Many students experienced more than one problem, with 25.5 percent reporting five or more different problems. Apart from the personal negative consequences associated with their alcohol use, the students' intoxication led to negative consequences for others. For example, in the same study 27.4 percent of students reported being insulted or humiliated by a drunken peer, 9.6 percent reported having been physically assaulted, 16.3 percent experienced unwanted sexual advances, and 1.3 percent were the victims of rape. Again these consequences did not occur in isolation: 56.4 percent of students endured two or more of these secondary effects. Drug use continues to be associated with criminal behavior, with as many as 33 percent of arrestees testing positive for cocaine (Hunt et al. 2012). In a study of twenty-six countries, Kathryn Graham et al. (2011) found similar negative consequences associated with substance use.

Addiction also has wide-ranging health consequences through four primary mechanisms: acute toxic effects (e.g., overdose), acute effects of intoxication (e.g., accidental injury), dependence, and chronic disease associated with use (e.g., cirrhosis). Louisa Degenhardt and Wayne Hall (2012) examined the global burden of disease associated with substance abuse. Their data indicate that drug abuse is a substantial global cause of premature mortality and morbidity. Andrew C. Darke (2006) found that cocaine users had higher rates of ventricular hypertrophy and ischemic heart disease than opioid users or non-drug-using populations. As is evident from these data, drug and alcohol abuse have serious negative health and behavioral consequences for both users and society at large.

POLYDRUG ADDICTION HAS BECOME THE NORM

The disease model of addiction is supported by the high degree of addiction produced by various drugs and the likelihood that someone addicted to one drug often will be using more than one drug. This picture of multiple-drug use plays a significant role in the treatment of addiction. Treatment strategies aimed at eliminating one specific form of addiction, such as cocaine abuse, without addressing the concurrent use of other mood-altering substances, have usually failed. The addict who abuses only one drug is rare. The Epidemiologic Catchment Area study (Regier et al. 1990) of over 20,000 respondents found that 16 percent of the general population experienced alcoholism at some point during its lifetime—with 30 percent of these alcoholics also abusing drugs. Alcoholics were indeed 3.9 times more likely than nonalcoholics to be abusing drugs. Similarly, the rates of alcohol abuse among other drug addicts were high: 36 percent of cannabis addicts, 62 percent of amphetamine addicts, 67 percent of opiate addicts, and 84 percent of cocaine addicts were also alcoholics. These studies, combined with clinical observations regarding the concurrent use of multiple substances, suggest common biological determinants for all addiction (Miller and Gold 1991).

TREATMENTS AND MEASURES TO CURB THE EPIDEMIC

Addiction is a chronic disease with a relapsing/remitting pattern. There is no "cure" for addiction, but there is the hope of "recovery." Recovery lasts for a lifetime.

The earliest (1930s) successful treatment for addiction was the twelve-steps program of Alcoholics Anonymous (AA). The success of AA, with its broad ban on all mood-altering substances, lends further support to the unified disease concept of addiction. The AA program has spawned parallel organizations, such as Narcotics Anonymous (NA) and Overeaters Anonymous (OA). These recovery programs use AA's twelve steps and twelve traditions either in their original form or by changing only the alcohol-specific references. All twelve-steps programs include admission of one's own powerlessness to control the addiction, belief in a higher power, making an inventory of one's hurtful/harmful actions, making restitution, and doing service work. By "working the program" the addict is led to the hope and freedom of recovery. The fellowship aspect of AA is a big part of its success; every member has a sponsor, someone to call in moments of weakness, "a buddy," so to speak. The meetings encourage sharing of the good and the difficulties and provide enormous support for its members.

PHARMACEUTICAL AIDS TO RECOVERY

In any discussion of pharmaceutical treatments, a few facts need to be understood. Addiction is a brain disease, and use of drugs of abuse causes neurobiological changes in the opiate and dopaminergic systems of the brain similar to that of traumatic brain injury (Gold et al. 2009). Naltrexone, a medication known previously for its efficacy in helping opiate addicts recover, has been used successfully to treat alcoholism, cocaine addiction, and eating disorders. Although naltrexone can block the effects only of opiates, it appears to be effective against other drugs of abuse primarily because of the involvement of the opiate system in reward (Gold and Merlo 2009). According to this theory, naltrexone's opiate inhibition makes other drug use less reinforcing and ultimately prevents full-blown relapse to drug use as the addict's body learns not to associate drug use with reward.

Methadone and buprenorphine are also effective medications for the treatment of opiate addiction. They suppress withdrawal symptoms and relieve cravings. In alcoholism three medications are US Food and Drug Administration approved: naltrexone, acamprosate, and disulfiram. All medications help patients disengage from drug seeking and related criminal behavior and become more receptive to behavioral treatments.

BEHAVIORAL TREATMENTS

The goal of behavioral treatments is to help patients modify their attitudes and behaviors related to drug abuse and to increase their life and coping skills. There are a wide variety of options, such as cognitive-behavioral therapy, multidimensional family therapy, motivational interviewing, and motivational incentives. These therapies can be done on an outpatient basis or can be included in residential treatment programs. However, even with involvement in a twelve-steps program and adoption of viable pharmacological therapies, such as naltrexone, addiction remains difficult to treat primarily because of poor adherence.

For an addict, drug use becomes an acquired drive state that permeates all aspects of life. Withdrawal from drug use activates separate neural pathways that cause withdrawal to be perceived as life threatening, and the subsequent physiological and psychological reactions often lead to renewed drug consumption. Drug reinforcement is so powerful that even when it is eliminated by pharmacological blockade, humans quickly identify themselves as opiate available or unavailable and change their behavior without changing their attachment to the drug and its effects. Once pharmacological intervention is discontinued, the addict will often resume self-administration.

The treatment research consensus is that time in treatment, or abstinence, or both is the greatest predictor of treatment success and may reflect the time required to reinstate pre-drug neural homeostasis, fading of the memory of euphoria and conditioned cues, and the reemergence of normal endogenous reinforcement for work, friends, shelter, food, water, and sex.

Clearly, relapse prevention (Blum and Gold 2011) and successful treatment of addiction require much more than the alleviation of withdrawal symptoms. It is well-known that patients with higher pretreatment levels of social support, employment, and productivity have a better prognosis for successful response to initial treatment and long-term abstinence. Treatment outcomes for these patients may improve because they perceive the long-term cost of drug use (loss of family or job) as outweighing the short-term benefit of drug use. Educational efforts that stress the risks associated with drug abuse help individuals avoid drug use. No pharmacological or nonpharmacological treatment strategy can match the success of prevention. Research has shown that treatment efforts and relapse prevention are especially effective among impaired professionals (i.e., health care and other professionals whose licenses are controlled by state agencies). It appears as though these individuals have access to necessary inpatient and residential care to reverse the patterns of this devastating disease. These programs use a carrot-and-stick approach and rely on abstinence verification through objective random urinalysis testing. Lessons from treatment of these patients can be used to improve the treatment of all patients with addiction.

The disease model of addiction should not be used to excuse the addict's responsibility; abuse has to begin somewhere. The addict remains culpable for the initial decision to use the drug and for continuing to use it despite adverse consequences. Nevertheless, an understanding of addiction and the addiction process allows us to comprehend the existence of addiction and why abstinence in treatment is difficult to achieve.

SEE ALSO *Alcohol and Other Drugs in a Public Health Context; Harmful Substances, Legal Control of; Health and Disease: I. History of the Concepts; Impaired Professionals; Maternal-Fetal Relationship: I. Medical Aspects; Organ Transplants, Medical Overview of; Smoking*

BIBLIOGRAPHY

American Psychiatric Association. 2000. *Diagnostic and Statistical Manual of Mental Disorders*. 4th ed. Washington, DC: Author.

American Society of Addiction Medicine. 2013. "Definition of Addiction." http://www.asam.org/for-the-public/definition-of-addiction

Blum, Kenneth, and Mark S. Gold. 2011. "Neuro-Chemical Activation of Brain Reward Meso-Limbic Circuitry Is Associated with Relapse Prevention and Drug Hunger: A Hypothesis." *Medical Hypotheses* 76 (4): 576–84.

Board of Education of Independent School District No. 92 of Pottawatomie County v. Earls. 2002. 536 U.S. 822 (2002). http://www.law.cornell.edu/supct/html/01-332.ZS.html

Buckland, Paul R. 2008. "Will We Ever Find the Genes for Addiction?" *Addiction* 103 (11): 1768–76.

Center for Behavioral Health Statistics and Quality, Substance Abuse and Mental Health Services Administration. 2010. *The DAWN Report: Highlights of the 2009 Drug Abuse Warning Network (DAWN) Findings on Drug-Related Emergency Department Visits*. Rockville, MD: Author. http://www.oas.samhsa.gov/2k10/DAWN034/EDHighlights.htm

Dackis, Charles A., and Mark S. Gold. 1990. "Biological Aspects of Cocaine Addiction." In *Cocaine in the Brain*, edited by Nora D. Volkow and Alan C. Swann, 135–54. New Brunswick, NJ: Rutgers University Press.

Darke, Andrew C. 2006. "Controlled-Release Opioids and Alcohol." *Canadian Medical Association Journal* 174 (3): 352.

Degenhardt, Louisa, and Wayne Hall. 2012. "Extent of Illicit Drug Use and Dependence, and Their Contribution to the Global Burden of Disease." *Lancet* 379 (9810): 55–70.

DuPont, Robert L.; A. Thomas McLellan; William L. White; et al. 2009. "Setting the Standard for Recovery: Physicians' Health Programs." *Journal of Substance Abuse Treatment* 36 (2): 159–71.

Gallup Politics. 2011. "Record-High 50% of Americans Favor Legalizing Marijuana Use." http://www.gallup.com/poll/150149/record-high-americans-favor-legalizing-marijuana.aspx

Gold, Mark S.; Firas H. Kobeissy; Kevin K. W. Wang; et al. 2009. "Methamphetamine- and Trauma-Induced Brain Injuries: Comparative Cellular and Molecular Neurobiological Substrates." *Biological Psychiatry* 66 (2): 118–27.

Gold, Mark S., and Lisa J. Merlo. 2009. "Addiction Research Update." *Chinese Journal of Drug Dependence* 18 (4): 249–58.

Graham, Kathryn; Sharon Bernards; Sharon C. Wilsnack; and Gerhard Gmel. 2011. "Alcohol May Not Cause Partner Violence but It Seems to Make It Worse: A Cross National Comparison of the Relationship between Alcohol and Severity of Partner Violence." *Journal of Interpersonal Violence* 26 (8): 1503–23.

Hanson, Karen L.; Jennifer L. Winward; Alecia D. Schweinsburg; et al. 2010. "Longitudinal Study of Cognition among Adolescent Marijuana Users over Three Weeks of Abstinence." *Addictive Behaviors* 35 (11): 970–76.

Hunt, Dana; Sarah Kuck Jalbert; Ryan Kling; et al. 2012. *Arrestee Drug Abuse Monitoring Program II: 2011 Annual Report*. Washington, DC: Office of National Drug Control Policy, Executive Office of the President.

Jang, Kerry L.; Philip A. Vernon; W. John Livesley; et al. 2001. "Intra- and Extra-Familial Influences on Alcohol and Drug Misuse: A Twin Study of Gene-Environment Correlation." *Addiction* 96 (9): 1307–18.

Johnston, Lloyd D.; Patrick M. O'Malley; Jerald G. Bachman; and John E. Schulenberg. 2012. *Monitoring the Future: National Results on Adolescent Drug Use; Overview of Key Findings, 2011*. Ann Arbor: Institute for Social Research, University of Michigan.

Kleiman, Mark A. R. 1992. *Against Excess: Drug Policy for Results*. New York: Basic Books.

Merlo, Lisa J.; Brian K. Ahmedani; David A. Barondess; et al. 2011. "Alcohol Consumption Associated with Collegiate American Football Pre-game Festivities." *Drug and Alcohol Dependence* 116 (1–3): 242–45.

Miller, Norman S., and Mark S. Gold. 1991. "Dependence Syndrome: A Critical Analysis of Essential Features." *Psychiatric Annals* 21 (5): 282–90.

National Institute on Drug Abuse. 2010. "What Is Drug Addiction?" In *Drugs, Brains, and Behavior: The Science of Addiction*. http://www.drugabuse.gov/publications/science-addiction/drug-abuse-addiction

Nelson, Toben F.; Ziming Xuan; Hang Lee; et al. 2009. "Persistence of Heavy Drinking and Ensuing Consequences at Heavy Drinking Colleges." *Journal of Studies on Alcohol and Drugs* 70 (5): 726–34.

Office of National Drug Control Policy. 2012. "What America's Users Spend on Illegal Drugs." http://www.whitehouse.gov/sites/default/files/page/files/wausid_report_final_1.pdf

Paczynski, Richard P., and Mark S. Gold. 2011. "Cocaine and Crack." In *Lowinson and Ruiz's Substance Abuse: A Comprehensive Textbook*, 5th ed., edited by Pedro Ruiz; Eric C. Strain; and Joyce H. Lowinson, 191–213. Philadelphia: Lippincott Williams Wilkins.

Regier, Darrel A.; Mary E. Farmer; Donald S. Rae; et al. 1990. "Comorbidity of Mental Disorders with Alcohol and Other Drug Abuse: Results from the Epidemiologic Catchment Area (ECA) Study." *Journal of the American Medical Association* 264 (19): 2511–18.

Robins, Lee N. 1993. "The Sixth Thomas James Okey Memorial Lecture: Vietnam Veterans' Rapid Recovery from Heroin Addiction; A Fluke or Normal Expectation?" *Addiction* 88 (8): 1041–54.

Rose, Richard J.; Danielle M. Dick; Richard J. Viken; et al. 2001a. "Drinking or Abstaining at Age 14? A Genetic Epidemiological Study." *Alcoholism: Clinical and Experimental Research* 25 (11): 1594–1604.

Rose, Richard J.; Danielle M. Dick; Richard J. Viken; et al. 2001b. "Gene-Environment Interaction in Patterns of Adolescent Drinking: Regional Residency Moderates Longitudinal Influences on Alcohol Use." *Alcoholism: Clinical and Experimental Research* 25 (5): 637–43.

Substance Abuse and Mental Health Services Administration. 2011. *Results from the 2010 National Survey on Drug Use and Health (NSDUH): Summary of National Findings*. Rockville, MD: Author. http://store.samhsa.gov/product/Results-from-the-2010-National-Survey-on-Drug-Use-and-Health-NSDUH-/SMA11-4658

Swogger, Marc T.; Kenneth R. Conner; Zach Walsh; and Stephen A. Maisto. 2011. "Childhood Abuse and Harmful Substance Use among Criminal Offenders." *Addictive Behaviors* 36 (12): 1205–12.

Thun, Michael J.; Louis F. Apicella; and S. Jane Henley. 2000. "Smoking vs. Other Risk Factors as the Cause of Smoking-Attributable Deaths." *Journal of the American Medical Association* 284 (6): 706–12.

Tieu, Matthew. 2010. "Understanding the Nature of Drug Addiction." *Bioethics Research Notes* 22 (1): 7–11.

Tsuang, Ming T.; Jessica L. Bar; Rebecca M. Harley; and Michael J. Lyons. 2001. "The Harvard Twin Study of Substance Abuse: What We Have Learned." *Harvard Review of Psychiatry* 9 (6): 267–79.

Urbanoski, Karen A., and John F. Kelly. 2012. "Understanding Genetic Risk for Substance Use and Addiction: A Guide for Non-geneticists." *Clinical Psychology Review* 32 (1): 60–70.

Mark S. Gold (1995, 2004, 2014)
Donald Dizney Eminent Scholar, Distinguished Professor, and Chair of Psychiatry, Department of Psychiatry, College of Medicine, University of Florida

Michael J. Herkov (2004, 2014)
Associate Professor and Chief of Forensic and Addiction Medicine, College of Medicine, University of Florida

Michael Nias (2014)
Assistant Professor, Department of Psychiatry, University of Florida

ADOLESCENT HEALTH AND MEDICINE

SEE *Pediatrics, Adolescents*

ADOPTION

Adoption as a practice of family making prompts a consideration of assumptions about what is normal and good, what it means to be related, and how we should create—and not create—children. Ethical inquiry into whether and to what extent adoption is morally permissible must take into account the interests and needs of children; the social and material conditions under which adoption becomes a possible, or even necessary, practice in domestic and international contexts; and societal attitudes, both negative and positive, toward adoption. Although it is a commonly held view that adoption is an option of last resort when sexual reproduction—or for those who can afford it, assisted reproductive technology—has failed to deliver a biological child "of one's own," a consideration of the ethical questions related to adoption leads to a more complicated picture.

ADOPTION AND WOMEN'S REPRODUCTIVE AUTONOMY

In US history, two culturally accepted narratives have long informed how people imagine a woman's decision to give up her child for adoption: (1) adoption is the consequence of a woman's free choice based on the best interests of her child, and (2) adoption is the ethical means of saving a child from a desperate situation. Many women do, in fact, make well-informed and uncoerced decisions about placing a child for adoption, and many children prior to their adoptions are in situations of desperate need. In an ethical consideration of adoption, however, it is essential to highlight the conditions that lead many women to have to surrender their children (or that lead to the removal of their children). The contexts in which children are in need of being adopted include poverty, illness, violence, and war, as well as the legacy of racism. Historically, women who experienced so-called out-of-wedlock pregnancies were regarded as "fallen," depraved, or even mentally deficient, and therefore unfit to be mothers. Being unmarried and pregnant in the first quarter of the twentieth century could qualify a woman for commitment to a mental institution with a diagnosis of sexual deviancy. Although such women were more often poor and black than wealthy and white, sex—and therefore pregnancy—outside of marriage for women was seen as evidence of mental illness across race and class differences (McWhorter 2009).

The ethics of adoption has a long-standing association with the ethics of abortion. The central themes in discussions of the ethics of abortion in the United States are the moral status of the fetus and the right of women to make reproductive health decisions. Prior to the landmark US Supreme Court decision in *Roe v. Wade* in 1973, giving up a child for adoption in the United States was the central legal option for women who did not want or were unable to enter into an ongoing parental relationship with a child. Adoption scholars have tied *Roe v. Wade* to the dramatic decrease in the number of infants surrendered for adoption, as well as increasing social acceptance of households headed by unmarried women and single mothers by choice.

The issue underlying adoption and abortion is birth control. The history of adoption as a mechanism for managing human sexual and reproductive behavior—most directly that of women—echoes many of the moral and political issues that arise in discussions of abortion (Solinger 1992, 2001). Discussions of abortion and adoption reflect the many ways in which women have or have not been autonomous in their sexual and reproductive lives. When lacking safe and reliable methods of contraception, women are exposed both to the risk of unplanned pregnancy and to judgments of sexual activity evidenced by pregnancy. Until very recently in the history of the United States and the West in general, to be pregnant and unmarried was sufficient to subject women to the societal judgment that they are morally bad and thus unfit to be mothers. The decision to have an abortion, like the decision to surrender a child for adoption, is not necessarily a matter of free choice, and historically women have undergone various degrees of coercion (Solinger 1992). Lack of support for single parenting, shame about evidence of sexual activity, sexual abuse and lack of safety, and religious and cultural double standards about sex have contributed to the conditions under which women have undergone the experience of pregnancy.

Prior to *Roe v. Wade*, terminating a pregnancy by abortion was an option most women had access to only at the hands of nonmedical practitioners. Even women who could afford physician fees, and the cost of travel to see those physicians, were often left damaged by illegal abortions. Women weighing the decision to have an abortion thus often had to consider not only religious or moral apprehensions but also the high risk of permanent physical harm from unregulated abortifacient treatments. The lack of access to safe and legal abortion was—and for many women continues to be—one of the key conditions for the development and institutionalization of adoption as a means of resolving a pregnancy where raising the child is an unwanted or unmanageable outcome. Where women have safe, legal, and morally non-punitive access to abortion and birth control, the number of children surrendered for adoption is substantively lower than where such access is impossible.

For those defending what they consider to be the right to life of the fetus, the shift away from adoption as a resolution to pregnancy represents a moral crisis. Pro-life literature commonly invokes the slogan "adoption not abortion," reflecting a stance that has influenced what information health care providers are required by law to offer to women seeking an abortion. Since Congress enacted the Adolescent Family Life Act (AFLA) in 1981, a law that tied federal funding to the promotion of adoption for pregnant teens, adoption has become a component of discussions of the politics and public policy of abortion. Moreover, the Infant Adoption Awareness Act (IAAA) of 2000 specifically designated funding for the development of curricula and other tools that would train counselors and health care providers in how to offer pregnant women information on options other than abortion. Previous federal guidelines for family planning funding under Title X already required "adoption information and referrals [be given] to pregnant women on an equal basis with other courses of action included in nondirective counseling." Critics of the adoption not abortion position contend that the view misleads women into thinking the two actions are morally comparable. A significant difference for some is that, as progenitors, birth parents are causally responsible for a child's coming into existence, a fact that holds them in a relation of moral obligation to a child, even after adoption (Porter 2012).

INTERCOUNTRY ADOPTION

Intercountry adoption (ICA), the adoption of a child by adults outside that child's nation of origin, is a practice regulated primarily by the laws and policies of the home or "providing" countries, with some regulation of immigration by the "receiving" countries. Ethical concerns regarding ICA have focused on two issues: whether and to what extent ICA can be accomplished without encouraging corruption or exploitation of providing countries by receiving countries, and whether and to what extent ICA is in children's best interests. Some argue for the abolition of ICA, contending that removing a child from her home nation violates the child's fundamental interests as it denies her access to what is referred to as heritage rights—a fundamental need to be raised by one's group or community of origin (Bainham 2003). Opponents of ICA make a human rights–based argument, relying on documents such as the United Nation's (UN) Convention on the Rights of the Child (CRC). Others maintain, also referencing the UN CRC, that ICA is ethical on the grounds that it gives some children a chance to escape from adverse conditions, such as war, poverty, and lack of available education, in their home country—or, in the case of orphans, of having no parents at all. Advocates of ICA argue that heritage rights amount to an essentialist, and thus excessively limiting, understanding of origins. Critics of ICA who are heavily invested in notions of blood or genetic kinship as the only form of "real" family face the charge that they are merely echoing the dominant view in many countries in which adopting children, in its presumed announcement of infertility, is culturally frowned upon. Expecting in-country adoption to satisfy the needs of parentless children in orphanages is thus unrealistic in countries where adoption itself is considered shameful or stigmatizing. Rather than adopting, the infertile who can afford to, in countries such as India, often opt for donor-assisted conception as donor "matching" and pregnancy can hide the fact of infertility in a way adoption cannot (Bharadwaj 2003).

Those who argue for reforming ICA point to the risk that extreme global inequities might subject impoverished families and pregnant women to exploitation by corrupt lawyers and agencies. Such agencies may contribute to the commodification of children on what is feared to be an international "baby market." Some critics argue that ICA is inherently unethical as it represents a form of child trafficking (Smolin 2004). In response to such concerns, many nations in Central and South America, for example, have outlawed adoption intermediaries, allowing only an overarching state authority to carry out adoptions. Critics of this move have countered that outlawing intermediaries in ICA in effect abolishes ICA, as most countries with large populations of children in need of parental care lack the infrastructure needed to secure a child's status as adoptable or to determine prospective adoptive parents' eligibility. India has sought to mitigate the alleged harms of ICA to children who are, in fact, in need of parents by instituting policies requiring that at least 50 percent of all children eligible for adoption be adopted by Indian citizens. Such policies seem in concert with the international regulatory document on ICA known as the Hague Intercountry Adoption Convention (1993), which, though not prohibiting international adoption, clearly supports provisions that prioritize in-country adoption over ICA, even if this results in children spending more time in facilities such as orphanages.

Other grounds for objections to ICA are the effects it might have on providing countries' broader institutions, policies, and social norms. ICA could be seen, for example, as relieving nations from developing critically needed social services for unmarried mothers or from providing benefits to extended kin willing to adopt related children. If a major ethical concern is the noncoercion of birth parents, it must also be recognized that some state policies, such as the People's Republic of China's one-child rule, encourage relinquishment or abandonment of children. Another ethical issue arises from situations in which the receiving country could seem to be endorsing the providing nation's assumptions about who is an appropriate adoptive parent. The regulations of providing nations commonly exclude some groups—for example, gay and lesbian people, unmarried women, and people with disabilities—from eligibility as adoptive parents.

TRANSRACIAL ADOPTION

As with intercountry adoptions, transracial adoption (TRA) has raised two main ethical issues: To what extent are adoptions morally permissible when the adoptive parents are recognized as being members of a "race" different from that of their adopted child? And, even if such adoption is regarded as morally permissible, to what extent might TRA be a part of unjust institutional practices? With TRA, the ethics of adoption come in contact with historic practices of racism, classism, and gender oppression. TRA compels us to ask under what systemic conditions children might become available for adoption, and how adoption might function as a means of regulating the population in terms of racist norms. In the United States, the public debate about TRA can be traced, to some extent, to concerns raised first in the 1970s and then again in the 1990s over foster care, a system in which children are placed in temporary homes until they either are returned to their birth families, are adopted, or reach the age of eighteen and exit the system. Unlike infants placed for adoption, very few children in foster care were surrendered at the will of a birth parent; commonly, they have been removed from their families by the state based on apparent evidence of neglect or abandonment and sometimes of abuse.

The majority of children in foster care in the United States, and the majority who remain in foster care because they are never adopted, are African American (Roberts 2005). Many regard this situation as a crisis, but there is strong disagreement as to the nature of the crisis and ways to resolve it. "Too little attention has been paid to why so many Black children are available for adoption in the first place" (Roberts 2005, 234).

In the 1970s those working in the area of child and family services regarded adoption as the solution to the rising number of children in foster care. For many holding this view, a key impediment to moving children into adoptive families was the policy of "matching." A persistent practice in the history of adoption, matching placed children with adoptive parents on the basis of how much the child and parents together would resemble a "normal" family (i.e., one in which the children were biologically related to their parents) (Carp 1998). Advocates of matching have historically defended it as being in the best interest of adopted children because it allowed adoption to be less obvious, and consequently would make children feel less different and promote greater family unity. As the number of African American children in foster care grew exponentially in the 1970s, the efficacy of maintaining matching in adoption was challenged.

At the time, those in favor of racial matching in adoption argued, in keeping with a 1972 statement by the National Association of Black Social Workers (NABSW), that ending it would have a deleterious effect on adopted black children. Proponents of matching pointed to two important considerations: First, although white families may be able to love and parent a black child, they cannot effectively give black children the skills they need to challenge the racism they are likely to face throughout their lives. Second, white parents may not be able to engender in black children a strong and positive identity as a black person—a quality essential for life in a socially segregated society that privileges whiteness in nearly every regard.

Sandra Patton (2000) argues that the NABSW's 1972 position on matching was misunderstood and misrepresented as equating TRA with racial genocide, a view associated with black nationalist politics. In 1994 the NABSW issued another statement emphasizing the importance of preserving African American families through better social and economic support of families in need. State-authorized removal of African American children from their families should be a last resort after at-home provision of care—which is more often made available to white families—has been exhausted.

The debate over TRA was in some sense resolved by the Multiethnic Placement Act, passed in 1994 and amended 1996, which prohibited any consideration of race in the context of adoption. But it was the passing of the Adoption and Safe Families Act in 1997 that, in response to what many saw as earlier policies' risky emphasis on reunifying families, prioritized as "paramount" the health and safety of children over any consideration of maintaining biological family ties (Patton 2000). Since the 1990s discussions of the ethics of TRA have shifted away from an either-or identity politics to recognize the needs of minority children to dwell in communities where they not marked as different, but are, at least part of the norm in terms of race or ethnicity. Concerns about the inherent harm of TRA have been replaced by an increasing focus on the need of parents in TRA families to live racially integrated lives.

The question of how to practice TRA in an ethical way remains unsettled. Critics of color-blind approaches to adoption contend that, far from being postracial, such policies inadvertently invest in whiteness as the universal. On the other hand, inadvertently positioning children of color—US- or foreign-born—to represent their race or ethnic heritage is equally problematic. As Hawley Fogg-Davis notes, "a fine line divides racial awareness and racial discrimination" (2005, 248). The philosopher Sally Haslanger, a white mother of two adopted black children, writes, "I have, in an important sense, been resocialized by my kids, and although I do not share their 'blood,' I have 'inherited' some aspects of their race" (2005, 285).

GAY AND LESBIAN ADOPTION

The norms most often guiding adoption policy replicate dominant views about what is in children's best interests, specifically in terms of what family structure can best protect and promote those interests. Views critical of permitting gay and lesbian couples to adopt children allege that the families such couples can offer, even when the couples are married, cannot meet children's essential needs. Although ongoing debates about gay and lesbian adoption seem to hinge on concerns about the sexuality of potential adoptive parents, these worries suggest broader investments in gender norms and the importance of the family in upholding them.

The question of whether gay and lesbian people should be parents at all is, in some important ways, moot. According to a 2007 study, more than one in three lesbians has given birth, and one in six gay men has fathered or adopted a child (Gates et al. 2007). The 2000 US Census indicated that 65,000 children lived with same-sex parents; by 2012 the number had risen to 110,000 (Alper 2012). In terms of adoption, an estimated 65,500 adopted children are living with a lesbian or gay parent. Gay and lesbian parents are raising 4 percent of all adopted children in the United States, and as of 2007, 14,100 foster children, or 3 percent, are living with lesbian or gay parents (Gates et al. 2007).

Opposition to gay adoption in the United States is found largely among organizations such as Focus on the Family, the Center for American Values, and Concerned Women for America. Such groups view states' legalization of gay marriage as a profound threat to the health and safety of marriage and the family, and thus of children. Using a loosely Christian-based argument connecting marriage with reproductive sex and the family with heterosexual marriage, these groups argue that when the government permits gays to adopt, it violates children's rights in two ways: first, it denies children the right to be raised with the kind of love that only a married mother and father can provide, and second, by providing children with state-sanctioned less-than-optimal families, it abandons children's best interests in the name of asserting gay rights. According to the Thomas More Law Center in Ann Arbor, Michigan, there is an "inherent distinction" at stake in the debate about gay marriage: "there are those pairs capable of engaging in the act which can produce human offspring, and those pairs which cannot" (Thomas More Law Center 2013). Such a distinction makes allies of gay and straight families formed through adoption, as both can be thought to belong to the "cannot" category.

Gay adoption advocates draw on the abundance of research that provides data contradicting fears perpetuated about gay and lesbian people as potential parents. Studies of children raised in lesbian and gay families, for example, show that such children in no statistically significant way suffer harms different from other children. National professional organizations such as the American Psychological Association (APA) echo this view: "Overall, results of research suggest that the development, adjustment, and well-being of children with lesbian and gay parents do not differ markedly from that of children with heterosexual parents" (APA 2004). In fact, a twenty-five year study of children born to lesbian parents affirmed that if there were any marked differences, these children "were rated significantly lower in social problems, rule breaking, and aggressive problems" (APA 2004). In 2011 the American Academy of Pediatrics released a statement announcing that, consistent with its mission of promoting children's health and well-being, it supports adoption by people who are willing and able to provide a home, regardless of sexual orientation; it reaffirmed this support in a 2013 statement on gay marriage.

The ultimate threat posed by gay adoption, for bioethicists like Margaret Somerville, is that it permanently "unlinks" the social and biological elements of the family. A gay family, state-sanctioned through marriage, "radically changes the primary basis of parenthood from natural or biological parenthood to legal (and social) parenthood" (2007). For Somerville, this cleavage of the natural and the social is itself a source of harm to children, a view that supports arguments not only against gay adoption, but against all modes of family making outside of the marriage of a woman and a man who have children created through unassisted heterosexual coitus. The permitting of gay marriage and adoption, she contends, will have a ripple effect as it spreads the purportedly harmful view that families need not be biologically related to be real and good for children.

ADOPTION VS. ASSISTED REPRODUCTIVE TECHNOLOGY

Couples facing difficulties conceiving sometimes turn to assisted reproductive technology (ART). Given what many deem the success of ART despite its costliness, the idea has been proposed that government should require insurance companies to cover infertility treatment for all who need it. This suggestion has been met with concern, however, that greater use of ART could have harmful consequences for children in need of adoption. Critics of expanded access to ART through government-mandated insurance view it as a biased and even harmful form of incentivization (Bartholet 1999). To the extent that such mandates lend greater support to genetic family making, they pose the risk of discouraging infertile people from adopting children awaiting the opportunity (Freund-lich 1998). Thus, because indirect government support for ART may have harmful effects on children waiting to be adopted, such mandates are not ethically permissible according to critics (De Wispelaere and Weinstock 2014).

The various objections to indirect government support of ART raise ethical questions not only about the regulation of ART but also about the ethics of policies on adoption (Hollinger 1985). Should mechanisms such as tax breaks or mandated insurance coverage be put in place that effectively subsidize one method of family making but not another? Does this represent an endorsement by the state of a preferred mode of family making? Would such mechanisms put infertile couples who would rather adopt at a disadvantage? One might also ask whether indirect financial incentives have the effect of coercing the infertile into seeking medical treatment. Individuals' infertility might be a medical condition, but it poses a relevant harm to their lives only if they want to have genetically related children. As Elizabeth Bartholet contends, "society drives the infertile away from adoption and toward efforts to reproduce with a wide array of conditioning mechanisms and regulatory structures" (Bartholet 1993, 30). Another, possibly more contestable view is that a government's duty to promote the health of all its citizens requires promoting their interests, if not equally, then at least in a way that benefits the most vulnerable. A policy that promotes in vitro fertilization (IVF) over adoption, then, if it leads to more uses of IVF and less adoption, would unethically discount the interests of children waiting to be adopted.

Some scholars question the assumptions underlying objections to government support of ART. These objections seem to give more weight to the needs and interests of adoptees than those of infertile adults who want children. Glenn Cohen and Daniel Chen (2010), criticizing what they call the "substitution theory," argue that there is no direct evidence that encouraging IVF will in fact lead to fewer adoptions. The core of the objection to mandating coverage for ART is that such a turn fails to prioritize the needs of the most vulnerable—children without parental caretakers. Cohen and Chen note that, though surely laudable, the prioritizing of children's interests requires additional justification, specifically for the premise that the burden of adopting should fall on the infertile. If there is a duty to put the interests of children without parents above the interests of adults who want to have genetically related children, then should it not be the case that no one may reproduce until all of the parentless children find homes?

Ultimately, ethical considerations underscore the importance of addressing the needs of children without parents. Joan Heifetz Hollinger cites the potential "risk of indifference" to children "who are already born but in desperate need of parents to raise them" (1985). To commit to addressing those children's needs touches on society's understanding of the family in terms of genetic relatedness. The core of the moral problem is that the infertile are not alone in their preference for children who would be genetically related to them; yet it is they who are positioned as needing to resist this generally accepted preference. To put the burden on the infertile raises the question of why the fertile, just because they are capable of reproducing, are not expected to adopt.

EMBRYO ADOPTION

Another area where government support of ARTs has raised ethical questions, especially in terms of possible effects on adoption, concerns so-called frozen "spare" embryos. There are an estimated 600,000 embryos that are being cryopreserved, a result mostly of in vitro fertilization, a fertility treatment that commonly involves producing a larger number of embryos than will be utilized to create children (Nightlight 2013). Close to 90 percent of these "supernumerary" embryos that remain in cryopreservation do so at the request of parents who wish to maintain the option of future reproductive use (Hoffman et al. 2003). Despite this fact, many worry that parents will either allow the embryos to die or opt to donate them for research. Beginning in 2002 the US Congress approved a program that would provide education to the public about the importance of what has come to be called embryo adoption. Run by the Office of Population Affairs (OPA), under the guidance of the Department of Health and Human Services (HHS), the Public Awareness Campaign on Embryo Adoption has provided nearly $24 million to organizations (as of fiscal year 2013), many of which have a religious mission aimed at encouraging parents to give up for adoption those embryos they will not be using in conceptions. According to the OPA website, the purpose of the campaign is "to educate Americans about the existence of frozen embryos (resulting from in-vitro fertilization), which may be available for donation/adoption for family building" (HHS 2013).

The ethics of the federal government subsidizing organizations promoting embryo adoption is uncertain. In addition to possibly encouraging the use of ARTs over adoption of already existing children, the campaign indirectly contributes to ongoing debates over the moral status of embryos. As noted by many who see frozen embryos as presenting a moral crisis, "adoption of this sort implicitly recognizes embryos as human beings" (Iozzio 2002). Thus, the government's promotion of embryo adoption could make morally problematic policies that permit, for example, abortion or the use of embryos in research.

The campaign actually developed out of Senate hearings on stem cell science where the issue of the number of frozen embryos in existence raised concern. Senators worried that these "spare" embryos would be donated by parents to research, thus being destroyed in the process, and advocated for the government taking an active role in encouraging adoption as the solution. Some critics of the campaign have noted how the language of embryo adoption lends support to arguments against abortion based on the purported "personhood" of embryos and fetuses, a view the campaign directly preceded (Sweet 2012).

Organizations that have received a bulk of the funding include the National Embryo Donation Center and Nightlight Christian Services. While the former defines its mission as "protecting the lives and dignity of human embryos," the latter is known for creating "Snowflakes" in 1997, the first embryo adoption program. The Snowflakes program has two aims: to assist couples in donating embryos and to help those facing infertility "give birth to their adopted child" (Nightlight 2013). In such a view, embryos not only have the dignity of being human but also should be considered as children waiting for adoption. According to the Evangelical Christian Gabriel Fluhrer, being against abortion requires, in addition to picketing, "doing the hard work of adopting the orphans around the world, whether embryos or orphans living in China" (Kapralos 2012). Bioethicists such as Sarah-Vaughan Brakman, who are in support of what they call heterologous human embryo transfer (HET), make the connection between embryo adoption and adoption clear: "the adoption paradigm provides the proper lens through which to analyze the moral issues raised by HET" (2007, 192). This view can be defended in part because like adoptees, children born through HET will not be genetically related to their parents (Widdows and MacCallum 2002). Whether this similarity is sufficient to require, for example, those seeking to "adopt" embryos be rigorously vetted in the way prospective adoptive parents are remains an issue of debate.

"GENEALOGICAL BEWILDERMENT" AND THE RIGHT TO KNOW

Adoption, as a topic for ethics, can contribute to current discussions of the management of genetic information, especially—though not only—in relation to ARTs. In particular, adoption can reveal connections between how personal identity and the family are understood as grounded in "genetics" and how genetic information is believed to be important to know. The position that adoptees have a right to know who their biological parents were has played a central role in both the history of adoption and the history of adoptees. The adoption rights movement is largely based on the belief that adoptees' right to know counters the legacy of secrecy and shame commonly associated with so-called illegitimacy. An ongoing and active project in the adoption rights movement is fighting to open sealed adoption files for adoptees who seek information on their birth parents. The goal of this project is broader than allowing adoptees to read documents or discover birth parents' names, though to be sure these are important goals for many adoptees. The open records movement represents a challenge to much of the history of adoption, in which attitudes toward women's sexuality and identity in relationship to pregnancy contributed to stigmatization, secrecy, and deception (Fessler 2007).

During the early years of formal adoption in the United States, information was shared with adoptive parents as a means of "preparing" and reassuring them. The move away from relative full disclosure toward restricting the exchange of information in adoption was coincident with a shift in the overall understanding of adoption as a mode of family making. Originally, the aim of adoption in many countries where it was formally regulated was the finding of homes for parentless children; in the pre– and post–World War II (1939–1945) era, when the rate of infertility and the desire for adopted children rose dramatically, the aim was expanded to bring parentless children and childless adults together as a "normal" family. Adoption as a mechanism for making unrelated people intelligible as a normal family—that is, as if they were related by blood—thus required not merely the creation of legal structures, but a view of children as capable of being, in a sense, reborn in and through their new families (Modell and Dambacher 1997).

During periods when this theme of rebirth was less central to the justification of adoption, more information about children was released to would-be adoptive parents. As adoption became identified with the state's ability to make adoptive families as "good" as blood-related families, adoptees became reborn in the sense of being issued new birth certificates with the adoptive parents' names listed as mother and father and the sealing of original birth certificates. This public procedure through law thus finalized the shift in the metaphysics of adoption: a child's body could become unmarked by the stigma of illegitimacy, and thus could be released from the future his biological parents as his parents would have determined for him. It was not that nurture won out over nature, but that nature could be remade through the right match.

Ethical issues surrounding adoption and the disclosure of information have resurfaced in debates over donor-assisted conception. In this form of conception, couples make use of donated sperm, ova, or embryos to conceive a child. The child so conceived typically has no access to identifying information about the donor where policies permit anonymous gamete donation. Specifically appropriating the language of rights used in the context of adoption and sealed records, some ethicists argue that people who were "donor-conceived" have a right to know the identity of the donor or donors involved, just as adoptees have a right to know who their biological parents were, because they too suffer from their ignorance about their own identity (Velleman 2005). The ethics literature on the topic of donor-assisted conception consistently refers to the debate about open records in adoption and, more specifically, the harm adoptees have suffered in their lack of knowledge about themselves, or "genealogical bewilderment."

In a 1952 article, the psychiatrist Eric Wellisch used the term *genealogical bewilderment* to describe what he saw as a disorder suffered by children, particularly children who were adopted, when they were "without genealogy." According to Wellisch, "lack of knowledge of their real parents and ancestors can be a cause of maladjustment in [adopted] children" (1952, 41). The symptoms of such maladjustment were thought to include feelings of alienation from "foster parents," tendencies to running away, and suicidal ideation. According to Wellisch, adoptees have a weakened ability to develop a coherent body image, a requirement for a complete sense of self-identity.

The justification for sealing adoption records and maintaining the confidentiality of birth mothers was the worry that, if children discovered that they were adopted, they would suffer from a kind of psychological uncertainty. Significantly, however, the purported diagnosis of genealogical bewilderment as understood by its originators applied equally to adoptees who knew and who did not know they were adopted. From Wellisch's point of view, the cause of the harm was not knowing one's genealogy rather than knowing one was adopted. H. J. Sants (1964) developed more fully the concept of genealogical bewilderment, contending that adoptees could never achieve a sense of true belonging with parents not of their own kind.

Both Wellisch and Sants considered the desire to know—or even curiosity about—birth parents a symptom of the bewilderment itself. Thus, according to the "logic" of genealogical bewilderment, adoptees who do not know they are adopted are like ticking time bombs, able to experience the effects of their bewilderment at any time. Should they show a desire to know, this interest in their genealogy could turn into a social problem, even "delinquency." According to Sants, adoptees' "concern over their lack" of knowledge will likely "at some time" become a "searching for clues. Once they have begun, their preoccupation with the task can reach disturbing proportions" (1964, 133).

The term *genealogical bewilderment* was reclaimed by several early critics of the historic secrecy of adoption who wished to bring attention to the experience of adoptees and to the need for policy change that would allow for opening adoption records so that adoptees could have access to their original birth certificates. The term has also been used by adoptees themselves in court cases involving a fight either for access to their individual adoption records or original birth certificates or for the overturning of policy preventing such access. In their attempts to gain access to information that many adoptees feel they have a right to know, adoptees have had to prove to courts that their suffering was deeply damaging.

Jean Paton, founder of Orphan Voyage, the first adoptee organization in the United States in 1953, was among the early activists speaking out on behalf of adoptees. These activists incorporated the concept of bewilderment into their understandings of what the adoptee's search for information involved. According to the adoption scholar Ellen Herman, Paton conceptualized the adoptee as in some sense defined by her desire to search. Paton believed "that the desire to know the natural parents can be the deepest and most compelling factor in an adopted child's life" (quoted in "Search and Reunion," Adoption History Project).

The work of Betty Jean Lifton, a psychologist and adoptee, drew heavily on the meaning and value of the search for adoptees. For Lifton the search represented an act of defiance and self-assertion, a claiming of one's true self: "the very idea of search and reunion is empowering.... Empowerment and reconnection are the core experiences of recovery. Healing begins when adoptees take control of their lives by making the decision to search ... as one sets out on this forbidden journey toward self" (1994, 128). The scope and value of the search for Lifton thus has a doubleness to it: at once, the desire to know reflects a deep, perhaps unhealable wound, and—yet—the search itself is a mode of claiming one's identity.

Perhaps this tension at the heart of the adoptee's desire to know is what appeals to activists in what some have referred to as the donor-conception movement (Cahn and Kramer 2011). Many arguments against anonymous gamete donation turn on the claim that knowing the identity of the donor is paramount to the well-being of someone who was donor-conceived; such criticisms of anonymous gamete donation (AGD) specifically align the experiences of the donor-conceived with those of adoptees including their right to know, their suffering from genealogical bewilderment, their history of secrecy and shame. These arguments have coincided with changes in policy on AGD. Where once anonymity was required, it is now in some places prohibited in the context of donor-assisted conception: Sweden first instituted this policy in 1984, with the United Kingdom, most of Australia, and many countries in the European Union following.

Some critics have questioned the aptness of the analogy between the harm of secrecy suffered by people who were donor-conceived and people who were adopted. Kimberly Leighton has argued that the analogy itself could be harmful to adoptees as it "geneticizes" their identities, removing the specificity that comes with being adopted (2011). The literature on the ethics of AGD, however, seems increasingly weighted toward defending the analogy, and using it to support claims for the right to know of the donor-conceived. In some contexts, people who were donor-conceived have been presented as "genetic orphans" or "gamete adoptees." A much-publicized Canadian legal case on AGD, *Pratten v. British Columbia*, rested on the very question of whether or not the harm of not knowing one's donor for a donor-conceived person was sufficiently analogous to the harm of not knowing one's birth parents for an adoptee. Writing for the Supreme Court of British Columbia, Justice Elaine Adair found that denying a donor-conceived person's right to information about her origins, in that such a right is recognized for adoptees, is a form of discrimination (2011). Adoption, as the justice noted, provides an example of the suffering that results from "alienation by whatever means of a child from a biological parent." The decision was overturned on appeal, but the widespread coverage of the case brought much attention to ethical issues surrounding donor-assisted conception and adoption, and encouraged the overall acceptance of the analogy.

CONCLUSION: PRE-ADOPTION GENETIC TESTING

Adoption continues to raise questions about what constitutes family and what is the value of genetic relatedness. If adoption is in the best interest of children who need parents, issues remain undecided regarding which adults should adopt which children and how information about adoptees should be circulated. Advances in and increased reliance on genetic medicine only complicate issues about the ethics of adoption and disclosure. Pre-adoption genetic testing (PAGT), for example, is a practice growing in acceptance where prospective adoptive parents test children for genetic disorders prior to the child's actual adoption. Whether children available for adoption should be able to be tested beyond the ethical limits observed for children with parents continues to be debated. Advocates of increased PAGT argue that, to the extent that it will help "match" the right parents to the right children, genetic testing should be permitted, if not encouraged (Jansen and Ross 2001). Critics of this view counter that such arguments risk investing in kind of genetic determinism that, as this history of adoption illustrates, is not necessarily in the best interests of children available for adoption, for adoptees, or for adoptive families. Concerns over the implications of PAGT will likely continue as explanations of psychological, intellectual, and emotional characteristics—in addition to health concerns—are increasingly framed as genetic in nature. Prospective adoptive parents may find themselves in a serious ethical dilemma when considering adoption, especially if adoption is a "second-best" option to having children to whom they are genetically related. They will need to decide to what extent testing the genetics of a child prior to adoption is in the best interests of that child and to what extent it serves the self-interests of the prospective parents. The promotion of such testing may even contribute to regulatory norms about identity, reproduction, and the family.

SEE ALSO *Abortion; Children: I. History of Childhood; Embryo and Fetus: V. Religious Perspectives; Genetic Testing and Screening: I. Reproductive Genetic Testing; Infanticide; Moral Status; Natural Law; Reproductive Technologies*

BIBLIOGRAPHY

Adoption History Project. N.d. "Search and Reunion." University of Oregon, Department of History. http://pages.uoregon.edu/adoption/topics/search&reunion.htm

Alper, Gideon. 2013. "Gay Adoption Statistics." In *The Gay Law Report*. Accessed October 2, 2013. http://www.galperlaw.com/gay-law-report/gay-adoption-statistics/

American Academy of Pediatrics. 2013a. "American Academy of Pediatrics Supports Same Gender Civil Marriage." March 21. http://www.aap.org/en-us/about-the-aap/aap-press-room/pages/American-Academy-of-Pediatrics-Supports-Same-Gender-Civil-Marriage.aspx

American Academy of Pediatrics, Committee on Psychosocial Aspects of Child and Family Health. 2013b. "Policy Statement: Promoting the Well-Being of Children Whose Parents Are Gay or Lesbian." *Pediatrics* 131 (4): 827–30.

American Psychological Association. 2004. "Sexual Orientation, Parents, and Children." http://www.apa.org/about/policy/parenting.aspx

Bartholet, Elizabeth. 1993. *Family Bonds: Adoption, Infertility, and the New World of Child Production*. Boston: Beacon Press.

Bartholet, Elizabeth. 1999. *Nobody's Children: Abuse and Neglect, Foster Drift, and the Adoption Alternative*. Boston: Beacon Press.

Bharadwaj, Aditya. 2003. "Why Adoption Is Not an Option in India: The Visibility of Infertility, the Secrecy of Donor Insemination, and Other Cultural Complexities." *Social Science and Medicine* 56:1867–80.

Brakman, Sarah-Vaughan. 2007. "Paradigms, Practices, and Politics: Ethics and the Language of Human Embryo Transfer/Donation/Rescue/Adoption." In *Pluralistic Casuistry: Balancing Moral Arguments, Economic Realities, and Political Theory*, edited by Mark Cherry and Anna Smith Iltis, 191–210. Dordrecht, Netherlands: Springer.

Cahn, Naomi R., and Wendy Kramer. 2011. "End the Anonymity." *New York Times*, September 13. http://www.nytimes.com/roomfordebate/2011/09/13/making-laws-about-making-babies/sperm-donors-should-not-be-anonymous

Cohen, I. Glenn, and Daniel L. Chen. 2010. "Trading-Off Reproductive Technology and Adoption: Does Subsidizing IVF Decrease Adoption Rates and Should It Matter?" *Minnesota Law Review* 95:485–575.

De Wispelaere, Jurgen, and Daniel Weinstock. Forthcoming. "State Regulation and Assisted Reproduction: Balancing the Interests of Parents and Children." In *Family-Making: Contemporary Ethical Challenges*, edited by Françoise Baylis and Carolyn McLeod. New York: Oxford University Press.

Fessler, Ann. 2007. *The Girls Who Went Away: The Hidden History of Women Who Surrendered Children for Adoption in the Decades before* Roe v. Wade. New York: Penguin.

Fogg-Davis, Hawley. 2005. "Racial Randomization: Imagining Nondiscrimination in Adoption." In *Adoption Matters: Philosophical and Feminist Essays*, edited by Sally Haslanger and Charlotte Witt, 247–64. Ithaca, NY: Cornell University Press.

Freundlich, Madelyn. 1998. "Supply and Demand: The Forces Shaping the Future of Infant Adoption." *Adoption Quarterly* 13:14–20.

Gates, Gary; Lee M. V. Badgett; Jennifer Ehrle Macomber; and Kate Chambers. 2007. "Adoption and Foster Care by Lesbian and Gay Parents in the United States." Publication of the Williams Institute, UCLA School of Law and the Urban Institute, Washington, DC. Accessed August 4, 2013. http://www.urban.org/UploadedPDF/411437_Adoption_Foster_Care.pdf

Haslanger, Sally. 2005. "You Mixed? Racial Identity without Racial Biology." In *Adoption Matters: Philosophical and Feminist Essays*, edited by Sally Haslanger and Charlotte Witt, 265–90. Ithaca, NY: Cornell University Press.

Haslanger, Sally, and Charlotte Witt, eds. 2005. *Adoption Matters: Philosophical and Feminist Essays*. Ithaca, NY: Cornell University Press.

Hoffman, David; Gail L. Zellman; Christine Fair; et al. 2003. "Cryopreserved Embryos in the United States and Their Availability for Research." *Fertility and Sterility* 79 (5): 1063–69.

Hollinger, Joan Heifetz. 1985. "From Coitus to Commerce: Legal and Social Consequences of Noncoital Reproduction." *University of Michigan Journal of Law Reform* 18 (4): 865–932. http://scholarship.law.berkeley.edu/facpubs/307

Iozzio, Mary Jo. 2002. "It Is Time to Support Embryo Adoption." *National Catholic Bioethics Quarterly* 2 (4): 585–93.

Jansen, Lynn, and Lainie Friedman Ross. 2001. "The Ethics of Preadoption Genetic Testing." *American Journal of Medical Genetics* 104 (3): 214–20.

Kapralos, Krista. 2012. "Evangelicals Embryo Adoption: Devout Christians Seek a Future for Thousands of Frozen Embryos." *Huffington Post*, September 9. Accessed October 2, 2013. http://www.huffingtonpost.com/2012/09/10/evangelicals-embryo-adopt_n_1871832.html?utm_hp_ref=religion

Leighton, Kimberly. 2005. "Being Adopted and Being a Philosopher: An Exploration of the 'Desire to Know' Differently." In *Adoption Matters: Philosophical and Feminist*

Essays, edited by Sally Haslanger and Charlotte Witt. Ithaca, NY: Cornell University Press.

Leighton, Kimberly. 2012. "Addressing the Harms of Not Knowing One's Heredity: Lessons from Genealogical Bewilderment." *Adoption and Culture: The Interdisciplinary Journal of the Alliance for the Study of Adoption and Culture* 3:63–107.

Lifton, Betty Jean. 1994. *Journey of the Adopted Self: A Quest for Wholeness*. New York: Basic Books.

Lifton, Betty Jean. 2008. *Lost and Found: The Adopted Experience*. Ann Arbor: University of Michigan Press.

McWhorter, Ladelle. 2009. *Racism and Sexual Oppression in Anglo-America: A Genealogy*. Indianapolis: Indiana University Press.

Modell, J., and N. Dambacher. 1997. "Making a 'Real' Family: Matching and Cultural Biologism in American Adoption." *Adoption Quarterly* 1 (2): 3–33.

National Association of Black Social Workers. 1972. "Position Statement on Trans-Racial Adoptions." Unpublished position paper, September.

National Association of Black Social Workers. 1994. "Preserving Families of African Ancestry." http://www.nabsw.org/mserver/PreservingFamilies.aspx

Nightlight Christian Adoptions. 2013. "Snowflakes Embryo Adoption and Donation." Accessed October 2, 2013. http://www.nightlight.org/snowflakes-embryo-donation-adoption/

Patton, Sandra. 2000. *BirthMarks: Transracial Adoption in Contemporary America*. New York: New York University Press.

Pratten v. British Columbia (Attorney General). 2011. BCSC 656 (CanLII). http://www.canlii.org/en/bc/bcsc/doc/2011/2011bcsc656/2011bcsc656.html

Roberts, Dorothy. 2005. "Feminism, Race, and Adoption Policy." In *Adoption Matters: Philosophical and Feminist Essays*, edited by Sally Haslanger and Charlotte Witt, 234–45. Ithaca, NY: Cornell University Press.

Sants, H. J. 1964. "Genealogical Bewilderment in Children with Substitute Parents." *British Journal of Medical Psychology* 37 (2): 133–42.

Smolin, David M. 2005. "Intercountry Adoption as Child Trafficking." *Valparaiso Law Review* 39 (2): 281–325. http://works.bepress.com/david_smolin/3

Solinger, Rickie. 1992. *Wake Up Little Susie: Single Pregnancy and Race before* Roe v. Wade. New York: Routledge.

Solinger, Rickie. 2001. *Beggars and Choosers: How the Politics of Choice Shapes Adoption, Abortion, and Welfare in the United States*. New York: Hill and Wang.

Somerville, Margaret. 2007. "Children's Human Rights and Unlinking Child-Parent Biological Bonds with Adoption, Same-Sex Marriage and New Reproductive Technologies." *Journal of Family Studies* 13 (2): 179–201.

Sweet, Craig. 2012. "Federal Funding of Embryo Donation and 'Embryo Adoption': Is It Time for the Federal Government to Reconsider Its Goals?" March 20. http://www.embryodonationblog.com/640/federal-funding-of-embryo-donation-and-embryo-adoption-is-it-time-for-the-federal-government-to-reconsider-its-goals/

Thomas More Law Center, Amicus Brief. *Hollingsworth et al. v. Perry*. 2013. US Court of Appeals for the Ninth Circuit. January 28. http://www.americanbar.org/content/dam/aba/publications/supreme_court_preview/briefs-v2/12-144_pet_amcu_tmlc-cs.authcheckdam.pdf

US Department of Health and Human Services, Office of Population Affairs (HHS). 2013. "Embryo Adoption." Accessed October 7, 2013. http://www.hhs.gov/opa/about-opa-and-initiatives/embryo-adoption/

Velleman, David J. 2005. "Family History." *Philosophical Papers* 34 (3): 357–78.

Wellisch, Eric. 1952. "Children without Genealogy: A Problem of Adoption." *Mental Health* 13:41–42.

Widdows, Heather, and Fiona MacCallum. 2002. "Disparities in Parenting Criteria: An Exploration of the Issues, Focusing on Adoption and Embryo Donation." *Journal of Medical Ethics* 28:139–42.

Kimberly Leighton
Assistant Professor, Department of Philosophy, American University

ADVANCE DIRECTIVES AND ADVANCE CARE PLANNING

Advance directives are oral or written statements in which people declare their treatment preferences in the event that they lose decision-making capacity. Advance directives may allow patients to prevent unwanted and burdensome treatments when struck by terminal illness, permanent unconsciousness, or profound mental disability. Advance directives are only one part of a process known as advance care planning, in which patients, ideally in consultation with physicians and loved ones, plan in a thoughtful and reflective manner for medical care in the event of future incapacity.

This entry discusses the various types of advance directives along with the goals of and the ethical basis for advance care planning. It explores practical problems associated with advance care planning and concludes with discussions of how advance directives are used in clinical practice and how decision makers ought to proceed in the absence of a clear advance directive.

GOALS OF ADVANCE CARE PLANNING

Advance care planning refers to any planning by patients for decision making in the event of future decisional incapacity. Although it could refer simply to signing a form in a lawyer's or a doctor's office, ideally it creates an opportunity for patients to explore their own values, beliefs, and attitudes regarding quality of life and medical interventions, particularly as they think about the end of their lives. Patients may speak with loved ones, physicians, spiritual advisers, and others during the process. This reflective work can help patients make important decisions about issues that may come up even when they still have the capacity to make decisions. When a patient loses decision-making capacity, physicians and loved ones who have been involved in the advance care planning process may feel that they know the patient's goals and values better. This allows them to make medical decisions that are likely to be consistent with the patient's values and preferences.

Advance care planning accomplishes a variety of goals for patients and families. First, patients may use the process to clarify their own values and to consider how these affect their feelings about care at the end of life. Second, patients can learn more about what they can expect as they face the end of life and about various options for life-sustaining treatment and palliative care. Third, they can gain a sense of control over their medical care and their future, obtaining reassurance that they will die in a manner that is consistent with their preferences. Finally, patients may increase the probability that loved ones and health care providers will make decisions in accordance with their values and goals.

Advance care planning may serve other goals not directly related to medical treatments. Patients may wish to relieve loved ones of the burden of decision making and to protect loved ones from having to watch a drawn-out dying process. Patients also may use the process to prepare themselves for death. Advance care planning may help one reflect more deeply about one's life—its meaning and its goals. Patients may reflect on relationships with loved ones, "unfinished business," and fears about future disability and loss of independence. In this way advance care planning may improve patients' feelings of life completion and satisfaction with their treatment in their final days.

Many people engage in advance care planning through conversations with their lawyers or loved ones and may not see any reason to involve their doctors. Nevertheless, physicians, physician extenders, nurses, chaplains, and medical social workers can play an important role in assisting patients in advance care planning.

Health care providers have their own reasons for wanting to engage their patients in advance care planning. First, providers may use these discussions to reassure patients that their wishes will be respected. This can enhance a sense of trust. Second, providers may hope that advance directives will help decrease conflict among family members and between family members and the health care team when the patient is seriously ill. Finally, they may hope that advance directives will assist them in making difficult decisions when the patient has lost decision-making capacity.

Advance care planning discussions vary depending on a patient's state of health. Patients who are in good health may benefit from selecting a health care proxy and thinking about whether there are any situations so intolerable that they would not want their lives prolonged. When patients are older or have more serious chronic illnesses, physicians may wish to begin a discussion that is broader in scope. Although many view advance care planning as an opportunity for patients to make known their "preferences" for treatment, many patients do not have firm treatment preferences. By careful exploration of patients' values, health care providers can help patients develop these preferences. Patients can be asked to talk about their goals for life, their fears about disability, their hopes for what the ends of their lives will look like, and their ideas about states worse than death. This expanded view of advance care planning allows people to think about their mortality and legacy. From such discussions, health care providers can help patients consider more specifically whether there are certain treatments that they might wish to forgo and to think about the circumstances under which they might forgo them.

When the patient's illness has progressed to its final stages, health care providers can use the groundwork from these earlier discussions to make specific plans about what is to be done when the inevitable worsening occurs. Among other things, the patient and the health care providers can decide the following: Should an ambulance be called? Should the patient come to the hospital? Which life-prolonging treatments should be employed and which should be forgone? Are there particular treatments aimed at symptomatic relief that should be employed?

TYPES OF ADVANCE DIRECTIVES

Advance care planning may lead to written documentation of the patient's wishes. Although this documentation can take the form of a physician's note documenting a discussion, patients often complete written advance directives. These are particularly important in jurisdictions with formal legal requirements about the level of evidence surrogates need to forgo treatments or in situations in which conflicts are likely.

There are two types of advance directives: proxy directives and instructional directives. Both proxy and instructional directives are invoked only if the patient has lost decision-making capacity. Proxy directives, often referred to as durable powers of attorney for health care, allow patients to specify a person or persons to make decisions. They are relatively easy for physicians and other health care providers to discuss with patients and are straightforward for patients to understand. Proxy directives, however, do not indicate the patient's wishes, preferences, or values, and used alone they do not provide any information to the decision makers about what treatments the patient might have wanted under the circumstances at hand.

Instructional directives attempt to fill this gap. These directives, often referred to as living wills, identify situations in which the patient would or would not want specified treatments. For example, a patient's directive might state that "if I am permanently unconscious or terminally ill, I would not want to undergo cardiopulmonary resuscitation." Documents vary in terms of the scenarios described and the specificity of the different treatments. Some documents use general terms such as "aggressive care," whereas others list the specific interventions in detail.

Instructional directives apply only under the circumstances specified in the document. If, for example, a patient has a directive relating to treatment in the event of permanent unconsciousness, the directive will not help in decision making if that patient has suffered a devastating stroke. Although advance directives often focus on situations in which the patient would want to forgo treatment, they sometimes state circumstances under which a patient would want aggressive treatment. Forms often include both proxy directives and instructional directives. Finally, on some forms in addition to instructions about medical interventions, people have the opportunity to provide more comprehensive information about their values and goals and more general wishes about how they should be treated as they are dying.

Instructional directives provide evidence of a patient's prior wishes, yet they require a health care provider to interpret them, make medical decisions, and write orders to implement them. Unfortunately providers frequently do not have enough time or information to decide whether a patient's directive applies to a given emergency situation, and patients receive treatments that they would not have wanted. In the United States this has led to the development of a third type of form, physician orders for life sustaining treatment (POLST), also known as medical orders for life sustaining treatment (MOLST). This document is signed by a physician and contains explicit orders regarding cardiopulmonary resuscitation (CPR) in the event of cardiopulmonary arrest and the level of care to be provided (aggressive, limited, or comfort only) under other circumstances. These forms are meant to be universally honored as physician orders in all institutional and community settings. The use of these forms is supported by law in a growing number of states.

PHILOSOPHICAL ISSUES

The ethical argument that advance directives should be honored is based on the principle of patient autonomy and is a logical extension of the doctrine of informed consent. Patients with decision-making capacity have the right to refuse treatment, even if the treatment would extend their lives. Advance directives are a means for patients to continue to exercise this right even if they lose decision-making capacity by making thoughtful and informed decisions in advance. This approach allows patients to direct that medical care be given in a way that they feel best reflects their values and goals. Because physicians generally feel that they have an ethical obligation to work to preserve life, advance directives most commonly give patients a way to tell physicians caring for them the circumstances under which they would not want to be kept alive. Alternatively some patients might use advance directives to indicate that they would want life-sustaining treatment even under conditions in which most patients would choose to decline these measures.

Advance directives also serve ethical principles other than autonomy, such as beneficence. Physicians often feel duty-bound to preserve life under almost all circumstances, regardless of quality, even if they are uncertain that this serves the patient's best interests. Encouraging a patient to engage in advance care planning is a means for a physician to safeguard the patient's best interests.

A number of objections to the use of advance directives have been noted in the literature. Some have argued that an advance directive form cannot possibly direct the care that is to be given in a real clinical situation. If a patient writes a very general form, stating, for example, that "if I have no reasonable chance of recovery, I direct that no life-sustaining treatment be used," decision makers will have to determine how much of a chance of recovery is "reasonable," how much of a recovery would be worth trying for, and what precisely are "life-sustaining" interventions. Even if one specifies a list of treatments to be forgone in a number of detailed scenarios, this too can pose problems. First of all, no matter how specific the document, it is unlikely to capture the circumstances of a real clinical situation exactly. Also patients might not truly understand the specific treatments they are listing in the document and thus run the risk of erroneously requesting or forgoing a treatment.

This objection is sound as far as it applies to advance directive documents, and it illustrates the need for a rich advance care planning process. Documents are inherently limited for the reasons suggested above. While they provide some insight into the patient's wishes, they nearly always require interpretation. If, however, the patient had engaged in discussions with doctors and proxies about his or her values, beliefs, and wishes, then decision makers will be in a better position to interpret a document and to make medical decisions with the patient's values in mind.

A related objection is the concern that patients can never know what they would want under conditions they have not experienced or that they may change their minds. There is certainly reason to be cautious in this matter. Nevertheless, advance directives apply when patients have lost decision-making capacity, often for what is anticipated to be an indefinite time. Because these patients can no longer express their preferences, the choice is either to comply with their previous wishes about treatment in a given situation or to apply some standard external to the patient (the provider's opinion or some societal consensus). Given these alternatives, it would seem most respectful to patients to rely on their previously stated wishes when making treatment decisions unless there is good reason to believe that the patient did not understand what was written in the directive. Patients also should be told that they may change their advance directives at any time.

In a 1989 article Rebecca Dresser and John A. Robertson raised another objection regarding whether advance directives should determine the medical care of a patient who has become demented. They believe that when an individual becomes severely demented, he or she may in a sense become a new person who no longer has the same thoughts, memories, attitudes, values, and beliefs of her or his "former self" who wrote the advance directive.

Now, imagine a moderately demented woman who has pneumonia. Before she developed pneumonia, she had appeared content and comfortable, chatting socially with the staff even though she is unable to recognize anyone, has severe memory loss, and needs assistance with daily activities. This woman has an advance directive stating that if she ever became moderately demented, she would not want life-saving antibiotics for pneumonia; when she wrote the directive, she said that she would find such a life intolerable. Dresser and Robertson contend that the advance directive would not apply to the "new person" who now has pneumonia. Instead of relying on the values and beliefs of a person who no longer exists, a decision should be made based on what is in the best interests of the demented person in her current state. If she appears content and able to enjoy life, Dresser and Robertson argue, she ought to be treated with antibiotics.

There is significant controversy over what to do in such a situation. Accepting Dresser and Robertson's argument would mean frustrating the desires of many people who would not want the final chapter of their lives to involve being kept alive in a demented state. And after all, the demented individual is not treated as a new person in any other way: she continues to have ownership of the property that she acquired when she was healthier; she continues to be responsible for any debts that she incurred previously; and when she dies the will that she wrote when she was of sound mind will be operative.

PRACTICAL PROBLEMS WITH ADVANCE DIRECTIVES

There are practical barriers to the use of advance directives. Although this entry describes an ideal of advance care planning in which patients first consult with loved ones and physicians and then document their wishes, most advance directives are not products of this sort of process. Patients often write advance directives when they create an estate will. They may leave the documents in safe-deposit boxes or with their lawyers. Occasionally, they will give them to family members. All too often they will not take them to their doctors or they will not have discussed its contents with people who may be in a position someday to make decisions on their behalf. Advance directives created in this manner might not be available when needed for decision making. Because there has been no discussion with physicians about life goals and values and how medicine fits into these, the physicians are deprived of critical information that is needed in interpreting the advance directives. Patients, meanwhile, might have signed documents that they do not completely understand and that are not truly in keeping with their values. The same is true for documents created in a hospital in the midst of a medical crisis. To overcome this problem, physicians need to routinely ask their patients if they have advance directives.

Furthermore, advance directives may not be available when needed. They often do not accompany patients transferred to the hospital from a nursing home. Patients may not be under the care of their regular doctors when they are hospitalized, and the hospital staff may not know about the existence of an advance directive. In addition to the federal regulations requiring hospitals to ask about advance directives, electronic medical records and registries of advance directives may also help with this problem.

Another problem is that physicians are often reluctant to raise the subject with their patients. They may be under overwhelming time constraints. They may have never been trained to discuss this issue and are not sure how to introduce the topic. They may be worried that they will give patients the impression that they are "giving up" on them or that they think they will die soon. If they have focused in past discussions on interventions rather than patient values and goals, they may have found these discussions frustrating and unhelpful.

Time constraints are difficult to overcome. Physicians could dedicate visits to discussing advance directives, but insurance companies may not pay for such a visit, and many patients may not wish to make a separate trip to the doctor for this purpose. The use of booklets and other tools to introduce the concepts involved in advance care planning may help physicians efficiently use their time to answer patients' specific questions and to guide patients through the process. Enlisting nurses and social workers to help patients with the advance care planning process may also help.

Although physicians are often worried that patients will be put off by a discussion about advance care plans, surveys in the United States show that most patients want to discuss these issues early in the course of their disease and that they think that the doctor should bring up the topic

(Johnston, Pfeifer, and McNutt 1995). Nevertheless, there will be some patients who are not ready to discuss advance directives, and health care providers must be sensitive to these patients. Advance care planning is a process that should be offered to patients, not forced upon them.

The root cause of much of physicians' reluctance stems from lack of training in how to have these discussions. With training, physicians can feel more comfortable having these discussions, can learn how to deal with patients' emotional responses, and can have effective discussions that the physician will find truly helpful in caring for patients.

CLINICAL USE OF ADVANCE DIRECTIVES

Rarely do advance directives clearly dictate the care that should be given to a patient who lacks decision-making capacity. Generally some interpretation of the document is required, a responsibility left to the named surrogate decision maker, other family members, and the health care team.

When a patient who has an advance directive lacks decision-making capacity and is seriously ill, the health care providers should discuss the situation with the named surrogate and loved ones as appropriate. Reviewing the advance directive, those involved should decide what they think the patient would have wanted under the current circumstances. People who are not used to working with advance directives often misunderstand them. For example, an advance directive may state that life-sustaining treatment should be forgone but mention only the scenario of permanent unconsciousness. If the patient under discussion has had a devastating stroke but is not permanently unconscious, the document itself may not provide much evidence of the patient's wishes. In this case it will be necessary to proceed almost as if there were no advance directive. In such situations prior discussions involving the patient, his or her loved ones, and physicians about the patient's values regarding prolongation of life would be extremely useful. For example, when the patient under discussion expressed the preference to forgo treatment in the case of permanent unconsciousness, he or she might have given reasons for this that can shed light on his or her likely preferences in the circumstances of the stroke.

Even when there seems to be an applicable advance directive, there may be disagreement among family members or between family members and the health care team regarding the patient's care. These disagreements can occur even when everyone agrees that the advance directive applies to the current circumstances. Loved ones may disagree with the content of the advance directive, believe that the patient changed her or his mind, or believe that the patient made an error. In these situations it helps to focus the decision makers on what the patient would have wanted and why the advance directive was written in the first place. Health care providers should, however, listen carefully to evidence that the patient changed her or his mind. This is a realistic possibility, and patients do not always remember to destroy the advance directive or issue a written revocation.

Other times disagreements may occur because of differing interpretations of the document. Loved ones or health care providers may disagree on the meaning of a "reasonable chance of recovery," for example. In this case as well it is helpful to try to focus decision makers on what they think the patient would have wanted.

When health care proxies make decisions that seem to clearly be at odds with a written advance directive, health care providers face a dilemma. On the one hand, the principle of autonomy would dictate that the patient's previously expressed wishes should take priority. On the other hand, it is not clear that all patients would want their proxy's or loved one's wishes overruled. Because people often write advance directives to relieve family members of the burden of decision making, the patient may not have wanted the directive followed if doing so would cause tremendous anguish. Many advance directive documents explicitly ask the patient what should be done in the event of conflict between instructions in the directive and the proxy's decisions.

When no advance directive is present, decision making often proceeds in a similar fashion. Generally the physician will initiate a discussion with those who seem closest to the patient to discuss the patient's medical situation. Physicians should then focus the family on discussing whether the patient had ever discussed similar situations and what he or she would want under the current situation. Some states have laws regarding who is the surrogate decision maker in the absence of a written durable power of attorney. In other cases the health care providers should try to determine who was closest to the patient, or it may be best to try to reach a consensus decision. Advance directives do not change this process much, but they are a mechanism for the patient to provide evidence about his or her own wishes.

GLOBAL PERSPECTIVES ON ADVANCE CARE PLANNING

The advance directive movement began in the United States. Yet even in the United States most patients do not have advance directives, and for the most part they are seldom used in other countries. The European Convention on Human Rights and Biomedicine, drafted in Oviedo, Spain, in 1997, states in article 9 that "The previously expressed wishes relating to a medical intervention by a patient who is not, at the time of the intervention, in a state to express his or her wishes shall be taken into account" (Council of Europe 1999). Nevertheless, there is wide variation in the laws regarding advance directives in Europe, with some countries making them legally binding under some circumstances and allowing people to name surrogate decision makers, other countries recognizing them but not making them binding, and still other countries having no explicit law regarding previously expressed wishes while recognizing that close family members should be involved in the medical decision making for patients who have lost decision-making capacity. There is even more variability in such laws in the non-Western world.

How advance directives are used in a country depends on cultural norms and values surrounding the importance of authority, individual autonomy, and the role of the family in determining an individual's choices. So, for example, in countries that recognize advance directives yet have a strong cultural preference for medical paternalism, the directives may have little impact on decision making. Similarly health care providers may give much more credence to family members' instructions than a patient's previously expressed wishes in countries where there is more cultural emphasis on the connectedness of families. In addition, nations' cultural, moral, and religious norms determine the range of permissible actions that may be stipulated in an advance directive. For example, in the Netherlands one can include a directive for active euthanasia, whereas in Israel the law limits patients' rights to request the withdrawal of certain life-sustaining treatments.

CONCLUSION

Advance directives provide documentation of patients' wishes for medical care in the event of future incompetence. Health care providers can assist patients in developing useful advance directives through the process of advance care planning. The goals of advance care planning will be different for patients at different stages of life and health, but the aim in all cases is to help patients articulate health-related values in a manner that can assist decision makers when the patients can no longer speak for themselves. In this manner patients' autonomy and uniqueness as individuals can be respected.

SEE ALSO *Autonomy; Beneficence; Cancer, Ethical Issues Related to Diagnosis and Treatment; Competence; Conscience, Rights of; Dementia; DNR (Do Not Resuscitate); Hospice and Palliative Care: Professional Education; Informed Consent: I. History of Informed Consent; Life-Sustaining Treatment and Euthanasia: I. Ethical Aspects of; Medical Futility; Nursing Ethics; Pain and Suffering; Right to Die: Policy and Law; Surrogate Decision Making*

BIBLIOGRAPHY

Brett, Alan S. 1991. "Limitations of Listing Specific Medical Interventions in Advance Directives." *Journal of the American Medical Association* 266 (6): 825–28.

Buchanan, Alan E., and Dan W Brock. 1990. *Deciding for Others: The Ethics of Surrogate Decision-Making.* New York: Cambridge University Press.

Council of Europe. 1999. "Convention for the Protection of Human Rights and Dignity of the Human Being with Regard to the Application of Biology and Medicine: European Convention on Human Rights and Biomedicine." http://conventions.coe.int/Treaty/Commun/QueVoulezVous.asp?NT=164&CL=ENG

Doukas, David J., and Larry B. McCullough. 1991. "The Values History: The Evaluation of the Patient's Values and Advance Directives." *Journal of Family Practice* 32 (2): 145–53.

Dresser, Rebecca, and John A. Robertson. 1989. "Quality of Life and Non-Treatment Decisions for Incompetent Patients: A Critique of the Orthodox Approach." *Law, Medicine, and Health Care* 17 (3): 234–44.

Emanuel, Linda L.; Michael J. Barry; John D. Stoeckle; et al. 1991. "Advance Directives: A Case for Greater Use." *New England Journal of Medicine* 324 (13): 889–95.

Fischer, Gary S.; James A. Tulsky; Mary R. Rose; et al. 1998. "Patient Knowledge and Physician Prediction of Treatment Preferences after Discussion of Advance Directives." *Journal of General Internal Medicine* 13 (7): 447–54.

Hickman, Susan E.; Susan W. Tolle; Kenneth Brummel-Smith; et al. 2004. "Use of the Physician Orders for Life-Sustaining Treatment Program in Oregon Nursing Facilities: Beyond Resuscitation Status." *Journal of the American Geriatrics Society* 52 (9): 1424–29.

Hofmann, Jan C.; Neil S. Wenger; Roger B. Davis; et al. 1997. "Patient Preferences for Communication with Physicians about End-of-Life Decisions." *Annals of Internal Medicine* 127 (1): 1–12.

Johnston, Sarah Coate; Mark P. Pfeifer; and Robert McNutt. 1995. "The Discussion about Advance Directives: Patient and Physician Opinions regarding When and How It Should Be Conducted." *Archives of Internal Medicine* 155 (10): 1025–30.

Kim, Soyoon; Ki-Hyun Hahm; Hyoung Wook Park; et al. 2010. "A Korean Perspective on Developing a Global Policy for Advance Directives." *Bioethics* 24 (3): 113–17.

Kolarik, Russ C.; Robert M. Arnold; Gary S. Fischer; et al. 2002. "Objectives for Advance Care Planning." *Journal of Palliative Medicine* 5 (5): 697–704.

Pascalev, Assya, and Takis Vidalis. 2010. "'Vague Oviedo': Autonomy, Culture, and the Case of Previously Competent Patients." *Bioethics* 24 (3): 145–52.

Pearlman, Robert A.; Kevin C. Cain; Donald L. Patrick; et al. 1993. "Insights Pertaining to Patient Assessments of States Worse than Death." *Journal of Clinical Ethics* 4 (1): 33–41.

Sehgal, Ashwini; Anne Galbraith; Margaret Chesney; et al. 1992. "How Strictly Do Dialysis Patients Want Their Advance Directives Followed?" *Journal of the American Medical Association* 267 (1): 59–63.

Shalev, Carmel. 2010. "Reclaiming the Patient's Voice and Spirit in Dying: An Insight from Israel." *Bioethics* 24 (3): 134–44.

Singer, Peter A.; Douglas K. Martin; James V. Lavery; et al. 1998. "Reconceptionalizing Advance Care Planning from the Patient's Perspective." *Archives of Internal Medicine* 158 (8): 879–84.

SUPPORT Principle Investigators. 1995. "A Controlled Trial to Improve Care for Seriously Ill Hospitalized Patients: The Study to Understand Prognoses and Preferences for Outcomes and Risks of Treatments (SUPPORT)." *Journal of the American Medical Association* 274 (20): 1591–98.

Tulsky, James A. 2005. "Beyond Advance Directives: Importance of Communication Skills at the End of Life." *Journal of the American Medical Association* 294 (3): 359–65.

Tulsky, James A.; Gary S. Fischer; Mary R. Rose; et al. 1998. "Opening the Black Box: How Do Physicians Communicate about Advance Directives?" *Annals of Internal Medicine* 129 (6): 441–49.

University of Zurich, European Science Foundation. 2008. *County Reports on Advance Directives.* Zurich: Institute of Biomedical Ethics, University of Zurich.

Gary S. Fischer (2004, 2014)
Associate Professor of Medicine and Vice Chair for Quality Improvement and Patient Safety, Department of Medicine, University of Pittsburgh

James A. Tulsky (2004, 2014)
Professor of Medicine and Nursing and Chief, Duke Center for Palliative Care, Duke University

Robert M. Arnold (2004, 2014)
Leo H. Criep Professor of Patient Care and Chief, Section of Palliative Care and Medical Ethics, University of Pittsburgh
Chief Medical Officer, Palliative and Supportive Institute, University of Pittsburgh Medical Center

ADVERTISING AND MARKETING IN HEALTH CARE

As the cost of health care becomes an increasing focus of attention, advertising becomes an increasing object of concern. Ideally, advertising can provide information to help consumers make informed choices. In practice it can also inflate expectations, create demand, manipulate desire, transform wants into supposed needs, and increase the use and cost of health care services. In the not too distant past, health care was understood as medical care. The activities of physicians were regulated by standards of ethics that eschewed commercialism. Although there has always been an economic aspect (usually a fee) associated with the physician-patient encounter, the revolution in the financing of health care delivery is transforming the personal doctor-patient relationship into a socially complex interaction in which physicians are cast among a multitude of providers and patients are transformed into consumers. The focus on the economics of health care underscores the commercial aspects of health care delivery both by physicians and by other providers. Though physicians and nonprofit institutions should be responsive to a service ethic, they compete in the same economic arena as for-profit organizations and often behave similarly. Furthermore, in some cases the patients are not the direct consumers; services may be purchased by employers, alliances, the state, or other contracting entities whose interests may not entirely coincide with those of patients or even necessarily the public interest.

Advertising may be judged by the standards of business ethics: truthfulness, non-deceitfulness, nonexploitativeness, and profitability. But health care is not strictly a commodity to be sold effectively with profit to the public. The care of health is also a fundamental human endeavor binding the caregiver and the care seeker in mutually reciprocal ways. Otto E. Guttentag, noting the essential human quality of health care, defined medicine as "the care of health of human beings by human beings." Lawrence J. Nelson and colleagues argued in a 1989 article that several key features distinguish caring for the sick from other commercial products: (1) patients are in a distinctive position of vulnerability and dependency on those providing the services, (2) their own self and destiny—even life—are at stake in the encounter with the provider, and (3) the relationship with the provider may become an important aspect of the healing encounter. All of these elements suggest that there are special obligations incumbent on health care providers that go beyond the usual obligations of the seller to the buyer of most commodities (de Arruda and de Arruda 1999).

Traditional prohibitions against advertising attempted to orient professionals to their service obligations by minimizing the commercialization of the encounter (Relman 1978, 2007). According to the traditional view, physicians and other professionals should obtain business by developing a reputation for quality service and getting referrals from satisfied patients and clients or others who know their work, not through any kind of self-promotion.

The major ethical issue in advertising in a market economy is truthfulness. If given adequate information, the consumer should make appropriate choices: what kind of health care, where, when, provided by whom, at what cost. A larger question concerns the justice of a market system of choice based on individual self-interest. Proponents view advertising in health care as a way to promote competition and thus reduce cost in a highly regulated industry. Opponents criticize advertising for inflating expectations and thus increasing cost. Others suggest that the quality of care has been lowered by making cost rather than quality the focus of allocation decisions (Rodning and Dacso 1987).

The high cost of health care in the United States has prompted a search for ways to reduce both the cost of medical services and the percentage of gross national product devoted to health care without appreciably lowering quality of care. Advertising is located at the crossroads between cost and quality, between regulated markets with an emphasis on quality and free markets with an emphasis on cost and choice. Regulations that provide standards for training, licensure, specialty certification, and hospital accreditation have resulted in high-quality but expensive health care. Market solutions, such as encouraging advertising to promote competition, have been seen as a way of reducing cost.

HISTORICAL BACKGROUND

Physicians participate in markets but traditionally orient themselves by ethical standards that go beyond economic behavior.

The Origins of Professionalism. Modern professional organizations, defined by their codes of ethics and regulating themselves by ethical principles, take their origin from the Aesculapian societies of the fourth century B.C.E. and in particular from the oath associated with the Greek physician Hippocrates (c. 460–c. 377 B.C.E.), which bound its members to ethical standards that did not apply to society as a whole. The Hippocratic oath emphasizes the principle of patient benefit, placing the patient at the center of the physician's attention.

By the nineteenth century, when the British Medical Association (BMA) and the American Medical Association (AMA) were founded, the concept of a profession organized around explicit standards of ethics was well established. Prohibitions against advertising were among the first professional standards, because treatments based on scientific knowledge distinguished physicians from their main competitors, itinerant nostrum salespeople promoting often dubious products with even more dubious promotional claims. Advertising was expressly prohibited as unprofessional and undignified in virtually all countries in which physicians had established their professional identities through professional associations such as the BMA and the AMA, which were organized around a code of ethics (Havighurst 1978; Dyer 1985). Although the actual license to practice is granted and regulated by the state, the task of enforcing the ethics codes falls to the professional associations or the specialty societies.

The Antitrust Challenge to the Professions. The professions have always maintained a delicate balance between altruism and economic self-interest (Jonsen 1990). As the medical profession became more scientifically effective and better organized, it enjoyed regulations (licensure, specialty certification, and accreditation) that guaranteed a virtual monopoly on health care delivery. Health care became synonymous with medical care. Although the Sherman Antitrust Act of 1890 banned monopolies, the learned professions were considered exempt from the act, which applied only to businesses. Late in the twentieth century, however, the business aspects of medicine began receiving increased attention, and the learned professions exemption ended in 1975 with the US Supreme Court's *Goldfarb v. Virginia State Bar* (1975) decision, in which Virginia lawyers were found liable to charges of price-fixing the fees charged for title searches.

The *Goldfarb* decision heralded a flurry of antitrust activity in the professional arena, most notably the 1975 suit by the Federal Trade Commission (FTC) against the AMA holding that the AMA was in restraint of trade because its code of ethics prohibited advertising. The AMA Principles of Medical Ethics then in effect (1957 version) said simply, "[A physician] shall not solicit patients," meaning that a physician should not attempt to obtain patients by deception. The 1980 revision eliminated all reference to advertising. Nonetheless, in the 1982 case *Federal Trade Commission v. American Medical Association*, the Supreme Court decided in favor of the FTC, barring the AMA from making any reference to advertising and the solicitation of patients and further prohibiting the AMA from "formulating, adopting and disseminating" any ethical guidelines without first obtaining "permission from and approval of the guidelines by the Federal Trade Commission." In essence, medicine had been redefined as a trade for the purposes of commercial regulation.

The FTC suit hinged on the questions of cost, advertising, and the mercantile aspects of medical practice. The position of the FTC was that costs were high because doctors had a monopoly on health care delivery and could thus maintain artificially high costs for their own profits. If doctors were not prohibited from advertising, it was argued, prices would come down because patients could shop for the best prices. As the FTC chairman Michael Pertschuk stated at a 1977 conference, medicine could better be controlled if it were regulated as a business rather than as a profession (cited in Rosoff 1979).

It might be argued that in the twenty-first century the traditional idea of a profession, defined by its ethics and self-regulating, no longer exists. Nonetheless, the behavior of professionals, dedicated to their work and those they serve, may well be inspired by ethical norms and may be understood by responsible practitioners as part of a social covenant with society (May 1975). Of course "health care" encompasses broadly the activities of physicians and the scores of health care professions ("providers," however understood), patients ("clients" or "consumers," however understood), technology or technological "devices," pharmaceuticals and other products, hospitals and health care institutions, and the taxes, fees, or insurances exchanged to make it all happen. Although all this is "commerce" in a very real sense, it may ultimately be misleading to think of health care as a commodity in which cost is but one of the surrogates for value. The unscrupulous will always seek their own advantage in unrestrained markets. The public "community" must be ever vigilant to define and defend the right and the good.

THE ETHICS AND GOALS OF ADVERTISING

Advertising serves two distinct and divergent objectives: on the one hand, the dissemination of information and, on the other, product differentiation, which economists define as public perception of differences between two products, even though such differences may not in fact exist.

Dissemination of information provides the facts on which rational consumers can make informed choices. In health care, information about the services provided, location, hours of service, fees charged, and languages spoken are examples of services that might be advertised. Arguments in favor of advertising in health care are based on an understanding of advertising as the dissemination of information.

Advertising also differentiates products, and the methods for doing so are more ethically problematic. How can the claim be made and justified that one product is better than another? The FTC requires that any claims of product differentiation be empirically measurable. For example, to claim that a particular mouthwash "kills germs on contact by the millions," it is necessary to be able to count killed germs. Usually advertisers attempt to differentiate products not on the basis of objective criteria about the product but by manipulating unconscious wishes and fantasies (pertaining to youth, power, beauty, sex, and affluence), associating the product with images of attractive people in beautiful surroundings. The consumer may be induced to feel anxiety about the possible consequences of making the wrong choice of detergent, antiperspirant, or health plan.

Although many physicians have shown reluctance (or an aversion) to advertising their services, health care institutions have readily accepted the imperative to advertise in an attempt to create markets, capture market share, and find niches in the marketplace. Notable in this regard is advertising directed at target populations, for example, women, cancer patients, and those needing psychiatric and substance abuse services. Truth in advertising was the concern in the early twentieth century, when the field of advertising itself attempted to follow the course of professionalism. At issue were the values that distinguished professional advertisers from retail-space merchants. The American Marketing Association established university training programs and codes of ethics that promoted the scientific ideal of detachment and statistical analysis. The scientific vision of community and definition of people as consumers replaced the older, empathic, and value-laden world in which a merchant understood what customers (not consumers) wanted and needed based on living in the same community (Christians, Schultze, and Simms 1978; Schultze 1981).

Professional advertising is illustrative because medicine's traditions of professionalism are derived from an era in which physicians participated in the life of the community in which they practiced. Knowledge of the patient as a person and the patient's life history and social situation has traditionally been deemed essential to quality care. At issue for twenty-first-century health care is whether it will be possible to preserve the values of personal care that characterized the ideals of an earlier era.

COMMODIFICATION AND COMMERCIALIZATION

Some aspects of health care are unquestionably commercial. A price must be attached to the acquisition of pills that only a doctor can prescribe. Hospital overhead (the costs of running it) becomes part of the chain of health care costs. Physicians' services (either for procedures or for time spent with a patient), though not solely commercial, entail compensation. The locus of ethical decision making shifts as the mechanism for financing shifts. Whereas physicians once made decisions on behalf of patients or with patients (according to principles of beneficence or autonomy), decisions are being made by corporations on behalf of populations or in the interest of reducing costs to populations or maximizing gain for the organizations. As this happens, marketing of goods and services becomes an investment opportunity not necessarily in the interest of conserving resources but rather in the interest of creating capital for investors.

Medicine and medical technologies are increasingly considered in economic terms as commodities. It is fashionable to think of health care as an "industry," and as such the activities of the players—doctors and patients, providers and consumers, hospitals and health care organizations, equipment manufacturers and pharmaceutical suppliers—are seen in terms of market value rather than values deriving from a personal healing encounter. Value becomes a matter of money rather than a matter of conscience. It is the job of a market economy to distribute goods and services, bringing together consumers and products. Markets may be trusted to be free (laissez-faire) to the extent that they do not violate their own frame of reference. Markets must be valued and controlled on their own terms, such as in the admonition caveat emptor (let the buyer beware). But when vast public resources are involved, public oversight is also required. Deceptive or coercive marketing practices cannot be tolerated and require regulatory restraints on market freedoms.

Direct-to-Consumer Marketing. The growing trend of direct-to-consumer marketing needs to be evaluated in terms of the integrity of the information provided and the nature of the appeals made. Informed consumers make good partners in the healing relationship. Advertisements that contain messages such as "Ask your doctor if this medication is right for you" provide little or no information about the product being promoted. Hair loss, impotence (erectile dysfunction), unhappiness, and sleeplessness are among many subjects to be discussed with physicians and for which pharmacological remedies might be expected. Once the expectation of a prescription is created, it may be harder for the physician to assess risks (such as addiction liability) or side effects versus benefits, especially if a drug company has already courted the physician with gifts ranging from pens and notepads (bearing the name of a drug) to dinners (where "information" about products is offered) to vacations in expensive resorts.

Such practices by the pharmaceuticals industry, often called Big Pharma, are rightly receiving increased scrutiny. And because of real or supposed conflicts of interests and the difficulties of maintaining appropriate "boundaries," medical schools, hospitals, and many physicians' practices are no longer allowing pharmaceutical company representatives to market (detail) physicians and students in their halls. This trend only increases the pressure to market directly to consumers, who may be even less prepared to assess the merits of the claims being made, a situation not unlike the nostrum salespeople of old (Katz, Caplan, and Merz 2003). The staggering costs of pharmaceutical research and development, passed on to people who are ill and often cannot afford their medications, raise an even more fundamental question: should there be a free market in information? As Andreas Hasman and Søren Holm wonder in a 2006 article, would the public interest be better served if development costs were "pre-competitive," with the cost information made available to all and subject to peer review and public scrutiny and accountability?

The traditional way to mediate claims made by product developers and manufacturers is through scientific research published in peer-reviewed journals. Consumers have access via the Internet to all sorts of information that does not receive such academic scrutiny (Chandra, Sikula, and Paul 2004). In the United States federal regulatory agencies, such as the Food and Drug Administration (FDA) and the FTC, are charged with evaluating the research on which such claims are made. Yet much of the research is performed or funded by the product manufacturers themselves; results that are unfavorable to the product may be suppressed, resulting in a publication bias in which only positive results are published and leading to a false (unscientific but commercially advantageous) impression of the efficacy of a particular product, as a 2001 article by Michael Otto and colleagues shows in relation to one particular disorder and class of drugs. Expensive high-technology screening tests are similarly promoted as educational information directly to consumers even though some of these tests' lack of specificity (resulting in false positives and negatives) prompts physicians to question their value, as with computed tomography scans for heart disease and cancer (Lee and Brennan 2002). The ethical standard for judging such advertisements would be the truthfulness of the claims made. But presenting such appeals as informational when they are in fact promotional is a manipulation of demand, especially when the research on which such claims are made is not presented or, even worse, when it is skewed (Wolfe 2002).

Several dramatic examples illustrate the ethical constraints that might be necessary on advertising designed to create markets. Cosmetic surgery to improve a person's subjective sense of his or her own attractiveness, for example, is medical in a way that is different from reconstructive surgery to repair a face damaged by an accident, although both involve similar skills and may be performed by the same plastic surgeon. Similarly (in an economic sense), assisted reproductive technologies, such as in vitro fertilization, may like other medical treatments relieve the distress of a childless couple, although the availability of such services may be based more on the ability to pay than on need. The assisted reproduction industry commodifies the product, a human pregnancy, in ways that are more ambiguous ethically than they are commercially (Macklin and White 1997). Technologies, such as assisted reproduction, along with the emerging genetic technologies and more established technologies, such as safe abortion, intensive care, and organ transplantation, prompt a consideration of the limits on commercialization, advertising, and marketing (Dyer 1997). As Allen Verhey (1997, 135) noted: "There are some boundaries and limits to the sphere of the marketplace. We do not want a market in which body parts are profitable; we prohibit the sale of organs, even those of the dead. We do not want babies sold at auction. Some things are not to be commodified and commercialized."

THE ONGOING ETHICAL DEBATE

It could be debated whether advertising that goes beyond dissemination of information is ever ethical, though such advertising is an accepted feature of market economies. The ethical issue for advertising is whether it is truthful and whether there can be objectively measurable standards for judging the truthfulness of its claims. A more complex problem is the way advertising plays on people's unconscious wishes and fantasies concerning sex, wealth, power, status, and perfection. The scientific basis for advertising rests on the ability to identify and manipulate such longings and fears. When one speaks of "the market" or "market forces" or "demand," one is generally talking about human wants and wishes.

Key questions facing the ethics of advertising in health care include:

What standards or regulations should be in place concerning the placement of advertisements?

Is any appeal legitimate so long as it does not mislead, make false claims, or actually harm?

Is the effectiveness of the psychology of persuasion sufficient to justify advertisements, or can some higher principle be brought to bear?

Perhaps advertising itself should be subjected to the first principle of Hippocratic ethics, *primum non nocere* (first do no harm). Or to echo the caveat of President Dwight D. Eisenhower about the "military-industrial complex," beware the medical-industrial complex. Advertising that promotes consumer choice by providing information is consistent with the ethical ideal to promote patient autonomy. Advertising that deceptively promotes the interest of the provider at the expense of the consumer cannot be ethically condoned, especially when the consumer is a patient.

SEE ALSO *Harmful Substances, Legal Control of; Medicine, Profession of; Pharmaceutical Industry; Profit and Commercialism; Public Health: IX. Lifestyles*

BIBLIOGRAPHY

Chandra, Ashish; Andrew Sikula Sr.; and David P. Paul III. 2004. "Ethical Considerations in the Marketing of E-Health Products." *Journal of Medical Marketing: Device, Diagnostic, and Pharmaceutical Marketing* 4 (2): 110–18.

Christians, Clifford G.; Quentin J. Schultze; and Norman H. Simms. 1978. "Community, Epistemology, and Mass Media Ethics." *Journalism History* 5 (2): 38–41, 65–67.

Colman, Richard D. 1989. "The Ethics of General Practice and Advertising." *Journal of Medical Ethics* 15 (2): 86–89, 93.

De Arruda, Maria Cecilia Coutinho, and Marcelo Leme de Arruda. 1999. "Ethical Standards in Advertising: A Worldwide Perspective." *Journal of Business Ethics* 19 (2): 159–69.

Dyer, Allen R. 1985. "Ethics, Advertising, and the Definition of a Profession." *Journal of Medical Ethics* 11 (2): 72–78.

Dyer, Allen R. 1988. *Ethics and Psychiatry: Toward Professional Definition*. Washington, DC: American Psychiatric Press.

Dyer, Allen R. 1997. "Ethics, Advertising, and Assisted Reproduction: The Goals and Methods of Advertising." *Women's Health Issues* 7 (3): 143–48.

Federal Trade Commission v. American Medical Association. 1982. 638 F.2d 443 (1982).

Gillon, Raanan. 1989. "Advertising and Medical Ethics." *Journal of Medical Ethics* 15 (2): 59–60, 85.

Goldfarb v. Virginia State Bar. 1975. 421 U.S. 773; 44 L.Ed.2d 572; 92 Sup. Ct. 2004 (1975).

Guttentag, Otto E. 1963. "On Defining Medicine." *Christian Scholar* 46:200–211.

Guttentag, Otto E. 1963. Personal communication.

Hasman, Andreas, and Søren Holm. 2006. "Direct-to-Consumer Advertising: Should There Be a Free Market in Healthcare Information?" *Cambridge Quarterly of Healthcare Ethics* 15 (1): 42–49.

Havighurst, Clark. 1978. "Advertising and Medical Ethics." In *Encyclopedia of Bioethics*, edited by Warren T. Reich. New York: Macmillan.

Jonsen, Albert R. 1990. *The New Medicine and the Old Ethics*. Cambridge, MA: Harvard University Press.

Katz, Dana; Arthur L. Caplan; and Jon F. Merz. 2003. "All Gifts Large and Small: Toward an Understanding of the Ethics of Pharmaceutical Industry Gift-Giving." *American Journal of Bioethics* 3 (3): 39–46.

Lee, Thomas H., and Troyen A. Brennan. 2002. "Direct-to-Consumer Marketing of High-Technology Screening Tests." *New England Journal of Medicine* 346 (7): 529–31.

Macklin, Ruth, and Gladys B. White. 1997. "Assisted Reproductive Technologies, Ads, and Ethics: Philosophical, Ethical, and Clinical Perspectives on the Use of Advertising in Reproductive Medicine." *Women's Health Issues* 7 (3): 127–31.

May, William F. "Code, Covenant, Contract, or Philanthropy." 1975. *Hastings Center Report* 5 (6): 29–38.

Morreim, E. Haavi. 1988. "A Moral Examination of Medical Advertising." *Business and Society Review* 64 (1): 4–6.

Nelson, Lawrence J.; H. Westley Clark; Robert L. Goldman; et al. 1989. "Taking the Train to a World of Strangers: Health Care Marketing and Ethics." *Hastings Center Report* 19 (5): 36–43.

Otto, Michael W.; Kimberly S. Tuby; Robert A. Gould; et al. 2001. "An Effect-Size Analysis of the Relative Efficacy and Tolerability of Serotonin Selective Reuptake Inhibitors for Panic Disorder." *American Journal of Psychiatry* 158 (12): 1989–92.

Relman, Arnold S. 1978. "Professional Directories—but Not Commercial Advertising—as a Public Service." *New England Journal of Medicine* 299 (9): 476–78.

Relman, Arnold S. 2007. "The Problem of Commercialism in Medicine." *Cambridge Quarterly of Healthcare Ethics* 16 (4): 375–76.

Rodning, Charles B., and Clifford C. Dacso. 1987. "A Physician/Advertiser Ethos." *American Journal of Medicine* 82 (6): 1209–12.

Rosoff, Arnold J. 1979. "Antitrust Laws and the Health Care Industry: New Warriors into an Old Battle." *Saint Louis University Law Journal* 23:446–490.

Schultze, Quentin J. 1981. "Professionalism in Advertising: The Origin of Ethical Codes." *Journal of Communication* 31 (2): 64–71.

Verhey, Allen. 1997. "Commodification, Commercialization, and Embodiment." *Women's Health Issues* 7 (3): 132–42.

Wolfe, Sidney M. 2002. "Direct-to-Consumer Advertising: Education or Emotion Promotion?" *New England Journal of Medicine* 346 (7): 524–26.

Allen R. Dyer (1995, 2004, 2014)

Professor, Department of Psychiatry and Behavioral Sciences, George Washington University

AFRICA, BIOETHICS IN

This entry consists of the following:

I. SUB-SAHARAN AFRICA

The geographic region of sub-Saharan Africa includes all the African countries immediately below the Sahara Desert, together with all the associated island states but excluding the Republic of South Africa. Although the latter is within the region, it is excluded from this text in view of the heavy influence that apartheid exerted on indigenous African cultures. All the countries considered are bound by the Tropic of Cancer on the north and the Tropic of Capricorn on the south. In addition to a multitude of indigenous languages, the majority of the countries are either Anglophone or Francophone; five are Lusophone (Portuguese-speaking).

Medical ethics in sub-Saharan Africa is extremely complicated and cannot be considered homogeneous in any sense. This is because the vast geographic area (almost 23 million square kilometers, or about 9 million square miles) contains forty-three independent countries with innumerable sociocultural groupings. Many of the countries are nation-states only superficially, since their borders enclose ethnic groups that have little in common with their fellow citizens, being more closely affiliated with groups in other countries. Quite apart from the matter of indigenous cultures, these countries were under the domination of European colonial powers that sought to impose their cultures upon local cultures. Some countries gained political independence only in the 1980s, and in some supposedly independent countries (Angola, Mozambique, Sudan) civil strife based on ethnic differences has raged throughout most of their independent period. The interaction between an externally introduced culture and a local one is more complicated in the field of medicine than in any other. The differences in urban-center development in East Africa and West Africa demonstrate the role that colonial power had in influencing cultural and ethical values (Larson 1989).

TRADITIONAL AND SCIENTIFIC METHODS

Some of the countries have had contact with scientifically based European medicine for fewer than fifty years and others for little more than one hundred years. The development of medical ethics in all the African countries has therefore tended to follow the existing European ethical values, principally those of France and Great Britain, the two dominant colonial powers. European medical professionals, faced with traditional African medical practice, took the position that all such medical practices and values, as well as their practitioners, were bad. Traditional African healers were considered no more than quacks and deceivers and therefore were either ignored or actively persecuted. Even the traditional midwives or "birth attendants," as they are now known, who from time immemorial have provided help to women at a most difficult time, were looked upon with disfavor. To a certain extent such attitudes were underwritten by the beliefs and practices of the colonizers' religion, Christianity. Since much of traditional healing relied on the intervention of gods and spirits, which Christians found abhorrent, the practice of traditional healing was strongly discouraged. Furthermore, European medical ethics required that European doctors not associate with practitioners whose training and beliefs differed from their own.

With the rise of black consciousness and the acceptance of the notion that blackness is not a sign of inferiority, African peoples have begun to reappropriate the medical knowledge gained over centuries by traditional medicine and medical practice. In some countries laws have been passed recognizing traditional medical practice as legal and effective. This process has been very slow. Many African medical schools still do not offer any instruction in traditional medicine, and where interest exists, it is only at a research level. Financial grants have been made for research into the methods and preparations of traditional medicine. In a few instances medical scientists are actively involved with traditional practitioners.

This new collaboration between traditional and imported medical practice is likely to be furthered by the indigenization of African churches and the improvement of the quality of their leadership. Previously, priests and ministers in the majority of churches had been inadequately trained, and they tended to assume a patronizing approach to their congregants. Now, a growing number can be considered well educated; some can even be viewed as theologians who are able to help formulate the churches' views on subjects of such crucial importance as the conflict between traditional and modern medical practice. Medical professionals in the majority of countries now feel relatively free to develop new ways of practice and to work with traditional birth attendants, herbalists, and other healers without fear of losing either the respect or the comradeship of colleagues in Europe.

Traditional and Western practices are seeing crossover training in the areas of psychiatry, childbirth, and grassroots education. Much of traditional medicine touches on the realm of psychiatry. Involvement of traditional practitioners in psychiatric treatment makes for a more humane treatment and much better integration of patients into society (Lambo 1971). Among other efforts that may be cited is the involvement of the University of Ghana Medical School in training programs for traditional birth attendants. In many countries the medical schools (Makerere University in Uganda, University of Nairobi in Kenya, and University of Yaounde in Cameroon, for example) are striving to identify relevant practices within their own societies, such as use of peer groups to educate members of their societies on health-related issues. These medical schools are, therefore, embarking on programs that identify and preserve traditional practices considered valuable (Jelliffe and Bennett 1960). In these programs, traditional practices considered harmless or beneficial are to be permitted, and those practices considered truly harmful are to be eliminated.

STANDARDS FOR MEDICAL PRACTICE

Most English-speaking countries have general medical councils or boards responsible for registration, accreditation, and supervision of medical practice. In most of these countries the boards of control are generally quite distinct from the ministries of health (Kenya Government 1977). Many of these medical councils or boards, however, have fashioned policies more responsive to western European norms and needs than to African ones. These boards have had little time to devote to the development of ethical guidelines relevant to social and cultural conditions peculiar to life within African countries. Some principles remain fundamental, however: privacy of the patient is respected, and so is confidentiality, although here and there disclosure is required by the government for various reasons, including payment for medical service, granting of sick leave by employers, and mandatory registration of births and deaths.

HEALTH CARE SERVICE

There are very few scientifically trained medical personnel in Africa. The ratio of scientifically trained doctors to population ranges from 1:3,000 in such better-off cities as Dakar (Senegal), Accra (Ghana), and Nairobi (Kenya) to 1:200,000 in some poorer rural areas, such as most of the northern region of Nigeria and all of the immediate sub-Saharan countries, including Mauritania, Mali, Burkina Faso, Niger, and Chad, which are sometimes referred to as the Sahel. There are countries within which there may not be a single specialist in any recognized field of medicine. This immediately raises the issue of what kind of medicine is most suitable in such conditions.

European medicine has developed and gained the reputation of being "one-on-one" medicine, and it also has concentrated more on curative than on preventive medicine. In Africa, on the other hand, the practice of one-on-one medicine, if it is accepted as the ideal, means excluding 80 to 90 percent or more of the population, who have no access to Western-oriented medical facilities. Such medical practice also places an inhuman load on the few medical practitioners and quickly reduces them to no more than purveyors of drugs and injections. N. R. E. Fendall (1972) sees this as the "quantity versus quality" dilemma, although not all agree with his view.

Doctors in Africa are now being asked to view their role in light of certain priorities—the first being promotive and preventive health services and the second being curative—in terms of individual patient treatment in offices or hospitals. In attempting to respond to the first priority, many have pointed out that not much can be done until medical practice is so arranged that the community is both the consumer and the provider of its own health care. This can be done only if delegation of health care to nonphysician personnel, such as traditional birth attendants and community leaders, is done on a basis of genuine need. The debate will continue, but almost all the new medical schools have agreed that doctors' training should be responsive to the needs of the community and to the organization and priorities set by ministries of health.

Many African countries depend on the use of paramedical personnel in the running of health services at the level of primary health care. Paramedics are often the only health care personnel available at this level. They include clinical officers, laboratory technologists, public-health technicians, environmental health officers, and various kinds of nurses. They are usually trained at medical training colleges, which are nonuniversity, diploma-awarding institutions established in countries including Zambia, Kenya, and Tanzania. Apart from the nurses, who take an oath at graduation, paramedical personnel are not subject to any ethically binding oath. This cadre of personnel has on occasion been the source of breaches of confidentiality.

Pharmacies and pharmacists, too, have presented new dilemmas to medical practice in Africa. The regulation of the drug supply has been the prerogative of the ministries of health and their relevant licensing bodies. In keeping with the increased number of university-trained pharmacists, there is increased licensing of private pharmacies, especially in Zaire (now the Democratic Republic of the Congo), Kenya, Cameroon, and Nigeria. Pharmacists regard themselves as trained "doctors" and dispense drugs without prescription, including drugs that have previously required doctors' prescriptions. Pharmacies also may dispense inactive drugs or drugs that have no relevance to the patient's illness (World Health Organization 1992).

THE ETHICS OF EDUCATING AND REMUNERATING DOCTORS

Medical education has had to contend with the issue of "excellence versus quantity" in the training of doctors.

Most African medical schools have felt it necessary to enroll students of the highest possible scientific caliber and to train them to internationally accepted standards. (These students are chosen based on their national high school final examination results.) The result has been that very few doctors can be graduated in any given year; but much more important, in many countries the best and sometimes the only available scientific skills are channeled into medicine, depriving other socially important areas of potential contributors. This is an ethical issue of considerable importance. In the end, many of the doctors produced choose to become specialists who can practice medicine only where they find quite sophisticated support facilities and services. Frequently they serve existing hospital needs rather than those of preventive medicine. The frustration and wastefulness of this situation underscore one of the major ethical issues on the African medical scene.

Doctors' fees have been the subject of debate in many African countries. Poverty is a major socioeconomic problem in all the countries of sub-Saharan Africa. Civil wars, political instability, ethnic violence, drought, and famine have transformed millions of already poor individuals into refugees who have fled across borders. In the midst of extensive poverty, charging fees for care raises serious ethical questions. In most of these countries, physicians are employed by the government and are not supposed to charge fees for their services. However, government pay schedules have not kept up with the cost of living, and many government doctors engage in private practice to supplement their salaries. In the late 1980s, the Kenya Medical Association considered fee schedules that would charge standard amounts for various services, without waivers or reductions for the poor. Objections were raised, and the schedule was not adopted. In Ghana, attempts have been made to adjust doctors' salaries to costs of living. In general, the costs of physicians' services, drugs, and hospitalization amid such serious deprivation deserve serious ethical scrutiny.

POPULATION, FAMILY PLANNING, AND ABORTION

Population control as advocated in the Western world unfortunately has blurred the issues of family planning and led to a debate that should have been completely unnecessary. There are two basic concepts in family planning. The first is to regulate total family size to a level that can be comfortably maintained using the available resources. The second is to space the intervals between pregnancies in order to promote the health of both mothers and children (King 1966). Many African countries rightly consider themselves underpopulated. Some, such as Gabon, Cameroon, and the Central African Republic, want much larger populations. All feel that they need development for the benefit of their people; but with very few exceptions, they refuse to admit that curbing population growth is relevant to the need for increased development.

Unfortunately, some doctors have failed to recognize the doctor's role in articulating relevant issues in family planning. Many doctors seem not to understand the medical importance of postponing pregnancies until a woman is biologically most prepared and of helping to stop reproduction when biological factors are no longer in a woman's favor. They also fail to recognize that spacing of births—which used to be practiced in Africa based either on sexual abstinence or on a geographic separation of husband and wife—is necessary to ensure the health of both mother and child. The excessive mortality in childbirth for women fourteen to forty-five years of age has not been fully appreciated by most of the medical profession in Africa (World Health Organization 1975). Even where this situation is recognized, continued adherence to inappropriate laws and practices imposed from Europe often means that family-planning services are withheld from the majority of the population in need. The Catholic Church, through its influence in the French-speaking countries, did much to prevent medical leadership in family planning. French laws passed in 1920 prohibiting contraception are still on the statute books of many French-speaking African countries, despite their repeal by France and Mali in 1972 (Wolf 1973).

In the field of contraception, the major ethical question the doctor faces is, therefore, whether he or she should encourage free provision of contraceptives by nonmedical personnel, knowing that Europe and the United States, which are the sources of these supplies, require that they be dispensed almost exclusively by doctors. The doctor must weigh the possibility of breaking outdated laws against the results of withholding such supplies from populations that have no other source.

Other serious ethical questions are raised in providing contraception to women who are not married, according to the traditional norms prevailing in their locality, or who want to practice contraception without the knowledge of their regular partner. Yet so tenuous are some of the marital relationships, so difficult is it to get some husbands into a hospital or family-planning clinic, that insistence on consent by both parties might, in the end, do an injustice to the woman. Physicians must resolve this ethical dilemma within their own national frontiers.

African societies generally do not accept abortion because they value highly the continuity of lineage; the unborn child, for example, may be a reincarnation of an ancestor. However, it would be untrue to say that abortions were not known in Africa before the arrival of white colonizers. In many African cultures, pregnancies resulting from taboo relationships or from adultery are terminated generally by women and the men are kept in the dark.

The question of abortion is now debated seriously. Many of the abortion laws in Africa are based on those of England and France, which repealed them in 1967 and 1974, respectively. However, in the majority of former British and French possessions the old laws are still on the statute books. The increasing number of illegal abortions, with their consequent mortality, morbidity, and sterility, have still not prompted the collective conscience of medical practitioners to have the laws reviewed. Zambia did review its laws and amend them in 1973, but stipulations within the new law, particularly one that the approval of two medical practitioners is required, make it unlikely to serve the majority of those in need. The Africa Regional Conference on Abortion held in Accra, Ghana, in 1973 agreed to call for a review of the laws, but little has been done.

The doctors' dilemma regarding abortion is twofold. Despite the law, increasing numbers of women risk their lives by recourse to backstreet abortionists. At the same time there are so few doctors to respond to such a wide range of needs that to make abortion laws more liberal may mean increasing the load on doctors still further. Given these problems, it is difficult to understand the view of some doctors in African countries that education, information, and services for fertility regulation should be limited.

HEALTH CARE AND RESEARCH IN THE ERA OF AIDS

The acquired immunodeficiency syndrome (AIDS), first recognized in 1981, has had the most profound impact on health care in Africa. Major concerns in health care provision are related to confidentiality, informed consent, counseling, research, drug therapy, serotesting, and care of the sick.

When AIDS was first identified as a major public-health problem and a rapidly spreading epidemic in Africa, many African governments reacted with violent denials. This behavior, which was attributed in part to the claim that AIDS originated in Africa, received support from some physicians and ministries of health. The early rapid spread of AIDS in Africa was partly a result of the fact that it was not acknowledged as a major public health problem and thus received only slow governmental response (Ndinya-Achola 1991).

Confidentiality and counseling are two components in AIDS-control programs that have received, at best, lip service in Africa. Counseling is an extension of preventive educational campaigns. At population levels these campaigns use information, education, and communication as their basic tools and public health officials as their main promoters. Counseling deals directly with the individual. The personal interaction between counselor and patient enables individuals to better understand their personal risks, to make informed decisions, and to take appropriate action.

Under ideal conditions, counseling is provided on a one-to-one basis and each case is dealt with on its own merit. Counseling also involves providing facilities that respond to the physical and emotional needs of the affected individuals and their loved ones. In Africa, AIDS counselors began to be trained in 1988; the needs of the society far exceed the number of counselors available. Much of the counseling that is provided is done by individuals who have no training. In many instances it amounts to informing an individual that he or she is infected with the AIDS virus; the health care provider is faced with the ethical question of whether to withhold information about the illness because there are no facilities to cater to individual needs.

Even where conditions are adequate and counseling facilities are available, confidentiality is a major issue because some of the trained counselors are not ethically bound to keep confidentiality. In particular, confidentiality is lacking in Africa for individuals diagnosed with AIDS. Counselors, however, are not the only health care providers ignoring confidentiality. Information regarding AIDS diagnosis often is leaked by hospital laboratory and other care staff.

BIOMEDICAL RESEARCH

Care for those with AIDS and drug therapy are two additional areas of major ethical concern. In many African settings the diagnosis of AIDS results in patient neglect because of the stigma attached to the disease. AIDS is a stigmatized disease in Africa mainly because the earliest information linked it to homosexuality, which is regarded as antisocial behavior in many parts of Africa. After it was ascertained that AIDS was being transmitted primarily by heterosexual contact, the homosexual stigma of AIDS lessened; but then AIDS became further stigmatized because of the rapid spread among heterosexuals by means of multiple sex partners and increased promiscuity. AIDS educational programs also had the inappropriate but true message that death is the final outcome. For these reasons, AIDS has had a negative impact on social interactions. Many people fear to be associated with a person with AIDS. This fear is evident even among professionals. Nurses have been a little more ethical in their approach to care of AIDS patients than physicians, perhaps because the nurses' increased contact with the patients makes them more sympathetic to the patients' plight.

During the early years of the AIDS epidemic, researchers from all over the world quickly identified populations in Africa for epidemiological studies (Van de

Perre et al. 1985; Kreiss et al. 1986; Piot et al. 1987). Clinical studies on drugs and vaccines are also being done. This research brings to the fore ethical questions about biomedical research in African countries that predated the AIDS epidemic: Should Western scientists do studies on populations that may never benefit from the results? Can appropriate informed consent be obtained in cultures that have different values? These questions are much debated within Africa and abroad (IJsselmuiden and Faden 1992). Standards of research have been improved: some medical journals, such as *East African Medical Journal,* insist that proof of informed consent be provided before articles are accepted; granting agencies in Europe and the United States require local ethical review before funding is provided; and local review boards are becoming quite strict.

One of the important contributions of biomedical research in AIDS is the development of antiretroviral drugs for treating infection caused by human immunodeficiency virus (HIV), the causative agent of AIDS. Although the available drugs do not currently offer a cure, some of them have been shown to prolong life significantly. These drugs are far too expensive for African populations. The same research groups that solicited funds for epidemiologic studies should be persuaded to do the same in order to make anti-AIDS drugs affordable for African populations. The first ten years of the AIDS epidemic had profound social, cultural, economic, and health impacts in sub-Saharan Africa. These effects included loss of social structure, orphaned children, reduced productivity, and severe depletion of health care budgets. Even if medical care or a vaccine had been made available immediately, the already large number of infected individuals would have continued to burden the society. Health care standards will be influenced by the AIDS epidemic for a long time. The decade of the 1990s was the right time for African health care services to review their programs and put in place relevant practices and resources without compromising their ethics in caring for people with AIDS.

CONCLUSION

Significant improvements are continually being made in medical training and standards of health care throughout sub-Saharan Africa. These improvements, however, are still not matched by proportionate improvement in medical ethics. Many African medical schools' curricula do not include ethics. Where it is included, the subject is still accorded very little time (usually a one-hour lecture). In order to sensitize doctors and other health care personnel on issues related to medical ethics, African medical schools and medical training colleges should be encouraged to develop curricula on ethics. It may also be necessary to sensitize populations on the subject along the same lines that disease prevention has been brought to the community level through health education.

BIBLIOGRAPHY

Aja, Egbeke. 1997. "Changing Moral Values in Africa: An Essay in Ethical Relativism." *Journal of Value Inquiry* 31 (4): 531–43.

Bryant, John H. 1969. *Health and the Developing World.* Ithaca, NY: Cornell University Press.

Feachem, Richard G., and Dean T. Jamison, eds. 1995. *Disease and Mortality in Sub-Saharan Africa.* New York: Oxford University Press.

Fendall, N. R. E. 1972. *Auxiliaries in Health Care: Programs in Developing Countries.* Baltimore: Johns Hopkins University Press.

Grant, James P. 1989. "The Bamako Initiative." In *The State of the World's Children,* by UNICEF. Oxford: Oxford University Press.

IJsselmuiden, Carel B., and Ruth R. Faden. 1992. "Research and Informed Consent in Africa: Another Look." *New England Journal of Medicine* 326 (12): 830–34.

Institute of Medical Ethics Working Party on the Ethical Implications of AIDS. 1992. "AIDS, Ethics, and Clinical Trials." *British Medical Journal* 305 (6855): 699–701.

Jelliffe, Derrick B., and F. John Bennett. 1960. "Indigenous Medical Systems and Child Health." *Journal of Paediatrics* 57 (2): 248–61.

Kasenene, Peter. 1998. *Religious Ethics in Africa.* Kampala, Uganda: Fountain.

Kenya Government. 1977. The Medical Practitioners and Dentists Act (Cap 253). *Kenya Gazette.* Nairobi: Government Printer.

King, Maurice H. 1966. "Family Planning." In *Medical Care in Developing Countries,* edited by Maurice H. King. Nairobi: Oxford University Press.

Kopelman, Loretta M. 2002. "If HIV/AIDS Is Punishment, Who Is Bad?" *Journal of Medicine and Philosophy* 27 (2): 231–43.

Kopelman, Loretta M., and Anton A. van Niekerk. 2002. "AIDS and Africa: Introduction." *Journal of Medicine and Philosophy* 27 (2): 139–42.

Kreiss, Joan K.; Davy Koech; Francis A. Plummer; et al. 1986. "AIDS Virus Infection in Nairobi Prostitutes: Spread of the Epidemic to East Africa." *New England Journal of Medicine* 314 (7): 414–18.

Lambo, T. Adeoye. 1971. "The African Mind in Contemporary Conflict." Jacques Parisot Foundation Lecture. *WHO Chronicle* 25 (8): 343–53.

Larson, A. 1989. "Social Context of Human Immunodeficiency Virus Transmission in Africa." *Reviews of Infectious Diseases* 11 (5): 716–31.

Magesa, Laurenti. 1997. *African Religion: The Moral Traditions of Abundant Life.* Maryknoll, NY: Orbis Books.

Ndinya-Achola, Jeckoniah O. 1991. "A Review of Ethical Issues in AIDS Research." *East African Medical Journal* 68 (9): 735–40.

Paris, Peter J. 1994. *The Spirituality of African Peoples: The Search for a Common Moral Discourse.* Minneapolis, MN: Fortress Press.

Piot, Peter; Joan K. Kreiss; Jeckoniah O. Ndinya-Achola; et al. 1987. "Heterosexual Transmission of HIV." *AIDS* 1 (4): 199–206.

Seidel, Gill. 1993. "The Competing Discourses of HIV/AIDS in Sub-Saharan Africa: Discourses of Rights and Empowerment vs. Discourses of Control and Exclusion." *Social Science and Medicine* 36 (3): 175–94.

Snyder, Francis G. 1974. "Health Policy and the Law in Senegal." *Social Science and Medicine* 8 (1): 11–28.

Van de Perre, Philippe; Nathan Clumeck; Michel Carael; et al. 1985. "Female Prostitutes: A Risk Group for Infection with Human T-cell Lymphotropic Virus Type III." *Lancet* 2 (8454): 524–27.

Wolf, Bernard. 1973. *Anti-contraception Laws in Sub-Saharan Francophone Africa: Sources and Ramifications.* Laws and Population Monograph Series 15. Medford, MA: Tufts University, Fletcher School of Law and Diplomacy, Law and Publication Programme.

World Health Organization. 1975. *World Health Statistics Annual, 1972,* vol. 1, *Vital Statistics and Causes of Death.* Geneva: World Health Organization.

World Health Organization. 1992. "Safe Drugs for Everyone." *World Health,* March–April, 4–6.

Jeckoniah O. Ndinya-Achola (1995)
Professor, University of Nairobi

I. SUB-SAHARAN AFRICA [ADDENDUM]

The three most significant terms marking the beginning of the twenty-first century are, arguably, biotechnology, bioethics, and globalization. Globalization has resulted in an unprecedented flow and mixing of not only people, goods, and services but also of ideas, values and, above all, information, epitomized in the incomparable informative and communicative content of the Internet. The technological revolution, which is coextensive with the Western industrial revolutions of the eighteenth and nineteenth centuries (Tangwa 1999) has clearly peaked in biotechnology in the twenty-first century. Globalization is propelled by technology and in turn drives technology, clearly indicating the technological imperatives of the present and the future. One consequence of this state of affairs is the enormous increase in the human capacity to do good or evil; hence, the rise and importance of bioethics and other moral concerns in the contemporary world. So rapid have been developments in the field of bioethics that to compare the main focal concerns, idioms, and metaphors of today with those of only two decades ago is like comparing two different languages and situations.

The HIV/AIDS pandemic that emerged in the mid-1980s and that has been described as "the world's deadliest epidemic since the Black Plague of the 14th century" (Niekerk and Kopelman 2005, 53) has revolutionized bioethics, including medical ethics, in the world at large but particularly in Africa. Since the emergence of HIV/AIDS, the epicenter of the epidemic has been in sub-Saharan Africa, an unenviable descriptive qualification that is generally combined with abject poverty, ignorance, and a plethora of other deadly epidemics or diseases. The obvious need for health research that this situation requires has led to something of a scramble for Africa on the part of industrialized Western world researchers, research organizations, and pharmaceutical companies, for a multiplicity and mixture of motives and reasons: rational self-interest, philanthropic altruism, mutually beneficial cooperation, and undisguised exploitative self-interest.

As the most powerful and dominant culture of the modern world, Western industrialized culture sets the pace and tempo of developments in nearly all domains of human activity. Western culture has overrun the globe, and its merging of medicine and the open liberal market is having important repercussions in all parts of the world today (Benatar 1998; Benatar, Gill, and Bakker 2011).

The enormous increase in health research studies on the African continent has led directly to the concern and need for health research ethics because biomedical research, apart from its positive prospects, also comes with the danger of exploiting, let alone harming, the weak, poor, and ignorant. Attempts to address this need are seen both in international regulatory guidelines—the Declaration of Helsinki (2008), the Council for International Organizations of Medical Sciences (CIOMS) International Ethical Guidelines for Biomedical Research Involving Human Beings (2002), the UNESCO Declaration on Bioethics and Human Rights (2005)—and in capacity-building initiatives on the continent (Kilama and Nyika 2009; Tangwa and Munung 2011; Chilengi et al. 2013; IJsselmuiden et al. 2012).

With funding from various sources in Europe and the United States, notably the National Institutes of Health (NIH), the Bill and Melinda Gates Foundation, the European and Developing Countries Clinical Trials Partnership (EDCTP), the World Health Organization (WHO), the Wellcome Trust, the Netherlands Ministry of Foreign Affairs, and Danish International Development Agency (DANIDA), and so on, capacity building in bioethics and especially in biomedical research ethics is being carried out across the continent of Africa by various stakeholders. These stakeholders include but are not limited to the following: the African Malaria Network Trust (AMANET), the International Research Ethics Network for Southern Africa (IRENSA), the South African Research Ethics Training Initiative (SARETI), the Pan-African Bioethics Initiative (PABIN), the Training and Resources in Research Ethics Evaluation (TRREE), the Networking for Ethics in Biomedical Research in Africa (NEBRA), the Mapping African Research Ethics Review Capacity (MARC), the Central African Network on Tuberculosis, HIV/AIDS and Malaria (CANTAM), and the Cameroon Bioethics Initiative (CAMBIN).

Bioethics is increasingly faced with the problems and issues posed by globalization. Bioethics concerns are necessarily global in nature: no single nation or group of countries can combat an epidemic like HIV/AIDS or other infectious diseases, cleanse the environment, conduct pharmacological research, prevent bioterrorism, and the like alone, without the involvement and cooperation of others. Bioethics has become necessarily a global interdisciplinary domain of concern and Africa is deeply implicated in the field's current status and future prospects. African voices and perspectives, so far inaudible, if not nonexistent, need to be heard clearly in global bioethics discourse. This discourse is currently dominated by North American, European, and Australian voices, which backed by the strategic advantages of economic, military, and technological powers, inevitably leaves little room and gives little consideration to weak voices, let alone dissenting ones, from the largely marginalized rest of the world.

BIBLIOGRAPHY

Benatar, Solomon R. 1998. "Global Disparities in Health and Human Rights." *American Journal of Public Health* 88 (2): 295–300.

Benatar, Solomon R.; Stephen Gill; and Isabella Bakker. 2011. "Global Health and the Global Economic Crisis." *American Journal of Public Health* 101 (4): 646–53. Accessed July 21, 2012. http://ajph.aphapublications.org/doi/full/10.2105/AJPH.2009.188458

Chilengi, Roma; Aceme Nyika; Godfrey B. Tangwa; et al. 2013. "Role of E-Learning in Teaching Health Research Ethics and Good Clinical Practice in Africa and Beyond." *Cambridge Quarterly of Healthcare Ethics,* 22, 110–19.

IJsselmuiden, Carel; Debbie Marais; Douglas Wassenaar; and Boitumelo Mokgatla-Moipolai. 2012. "Mapping African Ethical Review Committee Activity onto Capacity Needs: The MARC Initiative and HRWEB'S Interactive Data-Base of RECs in Africa." *Developing World Bioethics* 12 (2): 74–86.

Kilama, Wen, and Aceme Nyika, eds. 2009. "Health Research in Africa: Ethical and Practical Challenges." Special issue, *Acta Tropica* 112, Supp. 1.

Niekerk, Anton A. van, and Loretta M. Kopelman. 2005. *Ethics and AIDS in Africa: The Challenge to Our Thinking.* Walnut Creek, CA: Left Coast Press.

Tangwa, Godfrey B. 1999. "Globalisation or Westernisation? Ethical Concerns in the Whole Bio-business." *Bioethics* 13 (3–4): 218–26.

Tangwa, Godfrey B., and Nchangwi Syntia Munung. 2011. "Sprinting Research and Spot Jogging Regulation: The State of Bioethics in Cameroon." *Cambridge Quarterly of Healthcare Ethics* 20 (3): 356–66.

Godfrey B. Tangwa

Professor of Philosophy, University of Yaounde 1 and Cameroon Bioethics Initiative

II. SOUTH AFRICA

The histories of medicine and of medical ethics in South Africa are intimately linked to political, social, and economic aspects of that country's development, dominant components of which included institutionalized racial discrimination and social segregation prior to transition to a much-admired constitutional democracy in 1994. Almost two decades after a political transition that offered the potential to narrow disparities in health and achieve peace between diverse peoples, a brief review of some key political events is offered as a backdrop to the evolution of medical services and bioethics in this country, which manifests in microcosm many of the world's diverse human and health problems in the early twenty-first century.

POLITICAL BACKGROUND

During the period of the Dutch settlers (1652–1820) the indigenous Khoi-Khoi (pastoral people) and the San (hunter-gatherers) were treated with the arrogance and paternalism that for subsequent centuries epitomized European domination over blacks and exploitation through enslavement and colonial and cultural imperialism. Such attitudes, together with warfare and the introduction of new diseases (e.g., smallpox in 1713), facilitated the breakdown of the organized cultures of these indigenous peoples (Burrows 1958; Laidler and Gelfand 1971).

British annexation of the Cape (1795) and the arrival of British immigrants in Algoa Bay were followed by ninety years of conflict that included devastating wars between rival black tribes, the freeing of slaves (1833), the "importation" of Indians to work in the sugarcane fields of Natal (1860), the first Anglo-Boer War (1880), several wars against the Zulus, and the bitter second Anglo-Boer War (1899–1902), during which 26,000 Afrikaner women and children died in British concentration camps.

The British Parliamentary Act of Union (1910), which gave whites the right to self-determination, and the subsequent failure of the British to exercise their veto powers to restrain the union parliament from enacting oppressive racial laws (the Native Land Act of 1913, depriving blacks of their land, and the Native Administration Act of 1927, eliminating blacks' right to self-determination) set the scene for the growth of Afrikaner political and economic dominance. The rise to power of the Nationalist Party in 1948 was followed by the proliferation of apartheid policies, relentlessly entrenched through legislation that oppressed and dehumanized the black people of South Africa.

Black opposition evolved from powerless peaceful protest into a politically powerful process with the potential for peaceful progress. However, such progress was hampered by a growing culture of individual and group violence fueled by brutal elements within the state security forces and by internal hostilities that horrified the world (Schlemmer 1992). Intensification of black resistance, more clearly articulated demands for human rights globally, and changing foreign policy agendas progressively isolated South Africa from its previous friends and from international markets. By the 1980s economic decline, rapid population growth, urbanization, destabilization in neighboring states, the collapse of communism in Eastern Europe, and the Soviet retreat from regional disputes constituted the matrix from which arose the Nationalist Party's acceptance of the need to seek a negotiated settlement as a step toward developing a democracy (Sparks 1995).

Legislative changes since the "unbanning" of the black opposition movements in February 1990 include the repeal of the 1913 Native Land Act, the 1927 Native Administration Act, the 1950 Population Registration Act, and the 1950 Group Areas Act, which together formed a powerful core of statutory discriminatory policies. A transition period in the late 1980s and early 1990s abounded with ironies and ambiguities but ultimately led to a peacefully established constitutional democracy with a bill of rights and attempts to pursue truth and reconciliation rather than revenge (Truth and Reconciliation Commission 2003). In 2012 the African National Congress celebrated its centenary.

Early achievements in the new South Africa included stabilization of the inherited fragile economy, significant economic growth, reversal of all discriminatory legislation, rationalization of the complex bureaucracy associated with apartheid and homeland policies, and extensive new health legislation (Benatar 2004a). Against this background, the history of medicine and medical ethics in South Africa is briefly reviewed.

HISTORY OF MEDICINE

Early development of medical practice has both continued and intensified along two divergent paths, a private commercial venture predominantly for those who could afford to pay for health care and a public service for the poor, and remains a critical concern in the early twenty-first century.

The impact of apartheid and economic disparities on health care became increasingly apparent in the 1980s to many who viewed the medical care delivered by physicians with dedication and integrity (but with lack of social vision) to a limited segment of South African society (Benatar 1986; Savage and Benatar 1990; Van Rensburg and Benatar 1993). Despite the fact that in both the private and the public sectors undisputedly high standards of Western medicine were practiced by many generations of practitioners dedicated to exemplary patient care, this model of care was highly criticized by social scientists because of its specialized focus, uneven distribution, inaccessibility, and racially discriminatory characteristics.

However, it should be noted that in South Africa, as elsewhere in the world, widely applicable advances made in the treatment of individuals enthuse practitioners and the public more than medicine's ability to impact public health. For example, heart transplantation excited more interest in laboratory research, operating techniques, preventing rejection of transplants, and intensive care than did the potential to eliminate tuberculosis globally. Money is more easily raised for high-profile "rescue" medicine than for everyday medical needs and for preventive and public health medicine. Unsurprisingly, modern medical progress in South Africa has thus disproportionately advanced the health of individuals over the health of whole populations, the latter being influenced more by social, cultural, and economic conditions of life than by medical practice. The extent to which modern treatment of HIV infection and associated opportunistic infections was implemented for the benefit of tens of thousands of people is a striking exception (Fleischer, Kevaney, and Benatar 2010). The narrow focus that has long characterized modern biomedicine remains a problem for medical practice worldwide.

Deficiencies in the health care system were clearly articulated in the 1940s. The comprehensive Gluckman Commission Report on a national health service was an impressive attempt to rectify these, but its proposals were rejected, and the report lay dormant. The case for reform toward a unitary health service again became the subject of intense debate in the 1980s when health care in apartheid South Africa came under increasing criticism from the international community and the debate on universal access was resuscitated as part of the transition thrust toward a new democratic South Africa (Benatar 1986, 1988, 1990b, 1991, 1997, 2004a; "Health in South Africa" 2009).

The problems of escalating privatization and commercialization of health care were foreseen, and concern was expressed that unless the issue of universal access to health care was addressed in an economic transition, racial apartheid in health care would be replaced with economic apartheid (Benatar 1991). South Africa continues to be confronted with widening disparities in health and access to health care that are considerably aggravated by the HIV/AIDS pandemic and the spread of multi- and extra-drug-resistant tuberculosis. For example, in 2005 infant mortality rates ranged from 18 per 1,000 live births in white people to 74 per 1,000 in black people. Overall maternal mortality increased from 150 per 100,000 pregnancies in 1998 to 650 per 100,000 in 2007. These mortality statistics highlight the imperative to work toward narrowing disparities. Also there is a tenfold difference in annual per capita expenditure on the 16 percent of people covered by private medical insurance and the over 80 percent who are dependent on the public health service. Having lost the opportunity to move toward some form of universal access to health care or a national health insurance scheme in the 1980s, the renewed high aspirations for national health insurance will be difficult to implement (Benatar 2013).

As elsewhere in Africa, traditional African medicine continues to be practiced, particularly in rural areas. While black Africans have increasingly accepted Western medicine, they eclectically choose varying combinations of modern and traditional medical advice, the implications of which remain uncertain (Van Rensburg and Benatar 2001; Van Niekerk 2012).

MEDICAL ETHICS

Since the early twentieth century bioethics in South Africa has moved through several stages, as it has in other countries. Theologians played a pioneering role in reawakening an interest in bioethics, and several conferences were held in South Africa in the 1960s and the 1970s under church or theological auspices. The first, stimulated by the historic heart transplant in Cape Town in December 1967, was on the ethics of tissue transplantation (Oosthuizen 1972). Others followed on abortion, euthanasia, professional secrecy, and clinical experimentation.

An event that gave bioethics in South Africa a specific dimension was the inadequate response by medical professional bodies to the unethical manner in which state-employed medical practitioners provided professional attention to the prominent black activist Steve Biko prior to his death during detention in 1977 (Jenkins 1988; Baldwin-Ragavan 1999). Subsequent attention to ethical responsibilities toward prisoners, detainees, and hunger strikers was a gratifying response to the Biko case (Benatar 1990a; Kalk and Veriava 1991).

Other milestones that place bioethics at the intersection of the concerns of both the developed and the developing worlds include the peaceful transition to democracy with increased focus on human rights, the challenge of reducing inequity in access to health care, the complexity of resource allocation, the HIV/AIDS pandemic (initially denied by the Thabo Mbeki government but well supported in the early twenty-first century), and the ethics of medical research in a country with particular historical, geographic, and social conditions (Van Niekerk and Benatar 2011).

Bioethics Education at Medical Schools. In the late 1970s medical schools began developing modern bioethics education programs. The University of Cape Town (UCT) medical faculty initiated a course in bioethics for undergraduates in the early 1980s. The importance of transdisciplinary cooperation was recognized, and scholars from philosophy, law, sociology, and anthropology were actively included. Regular postgraduate educational activities followed, and the undergraduate program continues to be modified and developed. Several faculty symposia have been held and the proceedings published. These symposia have included theological, philosophical, and sociological debates on death and dying; resource allocation; the doctor-patient relationship; abortion and in vitro fertilization; research on humans; principles of biomedical ethics; moral reasoning; withholding and withdrawing treatment; health care of detainees; hospital ethics; the right to health care and the structure of health services; ethical considerations in relation to AIDS; teaching medical ethics; and human rights, human needs, gender, and medical ethics. Clinical consultations, research projects and many educational activities are well embedded in the everyday clinical practice of the UCT faculty of health sciences' teaching hospitals but regrettably without any full-time positions in bioethics (Benatar and Benatar 2012).

In 2007 the University of the Witwatersrand's faculty of health sciences, which was the first to begin teaching medical ethics to undergraduates in the late 1970s, created the first full-time post for a bioethicist in the country in its Division of Bioethics. The idea of an international journal focusing on bioethics issues from a developing world perspective, *Developing World Bioethics*, originated in this division (Landman and Schuklenk 2001–).

Other universities have also been active. The University of Stellenbosch has a long-standing postgraduate program in applied ethics (including medical ethics), based in the Department of Philosophy. An undergraduate educational program in bioethics has also been established by its faculty of health sciences. The law faculty at the University of Kwa-Zulu Natal has a long-standing program in medical law, ethics, and human rights. The Centre for the AIDS Program of Research in South Africa (CAPRISA) established an ethics program to provide ethical and legal advice for all of CAPRISA's projects and for organizing community outreach programs. The Nelson R. Mandela Faculty of Medicine in Kwa-Zulu Natal has appointed a full-time bioethicist. The dean of the faculty of health sciences at the University of Transkei has had a long commitment to bioethics and actively participates in national bioethics activities. Several books and many articles on bioethical topics in peer-reviewed journals have resulted from the work of local bioethics scholars (see Benatar 2012).

Ethics Institute of South Africa. The Ethics Institute of South Africa, an institution independent of all universities, and other public organizations and the private sector promotes applied ethics in South Africa. It has achieved a high profile through several empirical research projects on the ethics of doctors' business practices and ethics audits of major public hospitals.

Research Ethics. All medical schools have had research ethics committees (RECs) or institutional review boards (IRBs) for many years. Originally staffed predominantly by senior faculty who lacked formal training in ethics or research ethics, in the early twenty-first century these have widespread membership, many of whom have participated in programs aimed at building the capacity required to work effectively in RECs and in particular to review international collaborative research with a view to avoiding exploitation and enhancing benefits for research subjects and their communities.

The South African Medical Research Council first formulated guidelines on the ethics of medical research in 1979. These were subsequently updated in 1987, 1993, and 2002 (South Africa HealthInfo 2013).

In the early 2000s the minister of health appointed the Interim National Health Research Ethics Committee (INHREC) to initiate the work of the National Health Research Ethics Council. The INHREC produced a set of national guidelines for medical research and developed plans for the registration and ultimately the accreditation of all RECs in the country. The Health Act in 2004 formed the National Research Ethics Council. This council could play an important role in setting standards for research ethics committees and for ethics review and in creating a database of all clinical trials in the country (Department of Health 2004).

Generous grants to the UCT and the University of Pretoria (Southern Africa Research Ethics Initiative [SARETI]) from the National Institutes of Health in the United States through its Fogarty International Center have made highly valued contributions to capacity building in research ethics in southern Africa (Benatar and Landman 2006). For example, the UCT-funded program IRENSA trained ninety-seven midcareer health care professionals from South Africa and eight other African countries in a part-time one-year postgraduate diploma program (annually from 2003 to 2010). RECs in South Africa and other African countries have benefited from their members' participation. Additional annual two-day courses attracted almost 1,000 participants. The achievements of the IRENSA and the SARETI are of great importance in an era of rapidly expanding international collaborative research (Benatar 2004b).

CONCLUSION

There has been significant progress in bioethics in South Africa, but much remains to be done (Van Niekerk and Benatar 2011; Benatar 2012). In addition to fostering more and improved bioethics education for professionals, there is a need to ensure that ethical discourse takes cross-cultural issues into consideration and significantly contributes to both health policy making and health care practices. Resource allocation decisions are gradually being formulated with transparency and accountability and with the support of local health authorities. Given the gap in health care between what can be achieved in wealthy countries and what can actually be delivered in resource-constrained settings, open dialogue and participation in policy development could contribute to promoting more realistic professional and public expectations of what is achievable in South Africa. Formal employment positions for bioethicists will need to be created in faculties of health science in the country to sustain education, provide clinical ethics consultations, and undertake research. Increasingly, such positions will also be required in the private sector.

The greatest ethical challenges for medicine in South Africa and elsewhere arise through the erosion of professionalism by powerful market forces, the widening disparities between care available to those with resources and those without, the challenges of preventing and treating new and recrudescent infectious diseases, and the tension between the ethics of individual patient care and the ethics of public health, with its focus on whole populations and the common good. The newly developing fields of public health and global health ethics offers opportunities to augment the discourse on bioethics and to address from new perspectives the many global and local challenges facing health care in the twenty-first century (Benatar 2003; Benatar and Brock 2011).

BIBLIOGRAPHY

Baldwin-Ragaven, Laurel. 1999. *Ambulances of the Wrong Colour: Health Professionals, Human Rights, and Ethics in South Africa.* Cape Town: University of Cape Town Press.

Benatar, Solomon R. 1986. "Medicine and Health Care in South Africa." *New England Journal of Medicine* 315 (8): 527–32.

Benatar, Solomon R. 1988. "Ethics, Medicine, and Health Care in South Africa." *Hastings Center Report* 18 (4): S3–8.

Benatar, Solomon R. 1990a. "Detention without Trial, Hunger Strikes, and Medical Ethics." *Law, Medicine, and Health Care* 18 (1–2): 140–45.

Benatar, Solomon R. 1990b. "A Unitary Health Service for South Africa." *South African Medical Journal* 77 (9): 441–47.

Benatar, Solomon R. 1991. "Medicine and Health Care in South Africa: 5 Years Later." *New England Journal of Medicine* 325 (1): 30–36.

Benatar, Solomon R. 1992. "Transition towards a New South Africa." *South African Medical Journal* 81 (6): 295–98.

Benatar, Solomon R. 1997. "Health Care Reform in the New South Africa." *New England Journal of Medicine* 336:891–95.

Benatar, Solomon R. 2003. "Public Health and Public Health Ethics." *Acta Bioethica* 9 (2): 195–207.

Benatar, Solomon R. 2004a. "Health Care Reform and the Crisis of HIV and AIDS in South Africa." *New England Journal of Medicine* 351:81–92.

Benatar, Solomon R. 2004b. "Towards Progress in Resolving Dilemmas in International Research Ethics." *Journal of Law, Medicine and Ethics* 32 (4): 574–82.

Benatar, Solomon R. 2012. "Ethical Challenges for Health Care in South Africa." In *Health Care in South Africa*, 2nd ed., edited by Hendrick C. J. Van Rensburg, 653–700. Pretoria, South Africa: Van Schaik.

Benatar, Solomon R. 2013. "The Challenge of Health Disparities in South Africa." *South African Medical Journal* 103 (3) 154–55.

Benatar, Solomon R., and David Benatar. 2012. "From Medical Manners to Moral Reasoning." *South African Medical Journal* 102 (6): 406–8.

Benatar Solomon R., and Gillian Brock. 2011. *Global Health and Global Health Ethics*. Cambridge, UK: Cambridge University Press.

Benatar, Solomon R., and Willem Landman. 2006. "Bioethics in South Africa." *Cambridge Quarterly of Healthcare Ethics* 15:239–47.

Benatar, Solomon R., and Hendrick C. J. Van Rensburg. 1995. "Health Care Services in a New South Africa." *Hastings Center Report* 25 (4): 16–26.

Benatar, Solomon R., and Hendrick C. J. Van Rensburg. 2001. "Medicine in Africa: Present and Future." In *The Oxford Illustrated Companion to Medicine*, edited by Stephen Lock and John M. Last, 18–23. Oxford: Oxford University Press.

Burrows, Edmund H. 1958. *A History of Medicine in South Africa*. Cape Town: Balkema.

Department of Health. 2004. "Ethics in Health Research: Principles, Structures, and Processes." Accessed November 1, 2013. http://www.nhrec.org.za/wp-content/uploads/2008/09/ethics.pdf

Ethics Institute of South Africa. 2013. Accessed April 22, 2013. http://www.ethicsa.org

Fleischer, Theodore; Sebastian Kevaney; and Solomon R. Benatar. 2010. "Will Escalating Spending on HIV Treatment Displace Funding for Treatment of Other Diseases?" *South African Medical Journal* 100 (1): 32–34.

"Health in South Africa." 2009. *Lancet* 374. http://www.thelancet.com/series/health-in-south-africa

Jenkins, Trefor. 1988. "The Health Care of Detainees." *South African Medical Journal* 74 (9): 436–38.

Kalk, W. John, and Yusuf Veriava. 1991. "Hospital Management of Voluntary Total Fasting among Political Prisoners." *Lancet* 337 (8742): 660–62.

Laidler, Percy W., and Michael Gelfand. 1971. *South Africa: Its Medical History 1652–1898; A Medical and Social Study*. Cape Town: Struik.

Landman, Willem A., and Udo Schuklenk, eds. 2001–. *Developing World Bioethics*. Oxford: Blackwell.

Oosthuizen, Gerhardus C. 1972. *The Ethics of Tissue Transplantation*. Cape Town: Howard Timmins.

Savage, Michael, and Solomon R. Benatar. 1990. "An Analysis of Health and Health Services in South Africa." In *Critical Choices for South Africa*, edited by Robert A. Schire, 147–67. Oxford: Oxford University Press.

Schlemmer, Lawrence. 1992. "Violence: What Is to Be Done?" *South Africa International* 23:60–64.

South Africa HealthInfo. 2013. "MRC Ethics Guidelines." Accessed March 29, 2013. http://www.sahealthinfo.org/ethics/index.htm

Sparks, Alistair. 1995. *Tomorrow Is Another Country: The Inside Story of South Africa's Road to Change*. New York: Hill and Wang.

Truth and Reconciliation Commission. 2003. *Truth and Reconciliation Commission of South Africa Report*. Cape Town: Juta. Accessed February 7, 2013. http://www.info.gov.za/otherdocs/2003/trc/rep.pdf

Van Niekerk, Anton A., and Solomon R. Benatar. 2011. "The Social Functions of Bioethics in South Africa." In *Bioethics around the Globe*, edited by Catherine Myser, 134–51. Oxford: Oxford University Press.

Van Niekerk, Johannes P. 2012. "Traditional Healers Formalized?" *South African Medical Journal* 102 (3): 105–6.

Van Rensburg, Hendrick C. J., and Solomon R. Benatar. 1993. "The Legacy of Apartheid in Health and Health Care." *South African Journal of Sociology* 24 (4): 99–111.

Van Rensburg, Hendrick C. J., and Solomon R. Benatar. 2001. "The History of Medicine in Africa." In *The Oxford Illustrated Companion to Medicine*, edited by Stephen Lock and John M. Last, 14–18. Oxford: Oxford University Press.

Solomon R. Benatar (1995, 2014)
Emeritus Professor of Medicine, University of Cape Town
Professor, Dalla Lana School of Public Health and Joint Centre for Bioethics, University of Toronto

AGING AND THE AGED

This entry consists of the following:

I. SOCIETAL AGING

A society is said to age when its number of older members increases relative to its number of younger members. The societies in most of the world's industrialized nations have been aging since at least 1800. In 1800 the demographic makeup of developed countries was similar to that of many third world countries in the early 1990s, with roughly half the population under the age of sixteen and very few people living beyond age sixty. Since 1800 increases in life expectancy combined with declines in fertility rates have dramatically increased the proportion of older persons in developed nations. By contrast, the age profile in many third world countries is still heavily weighted toward younger age groups, even though the increase in the actual numbers of old people is even greater in many developing countries than it is in the developed world. What future societies will regard as distinct about population aging in the twentieth and twenty-first centuries is the rapid pace at which it has occurred. For example, the proportion of Americans aged sixty-five and over increased from 4 percent in 1900 to 12 percent in 2000 and is projected to be 20 percent in 2050 (Administration on Aging 2010). The fastest growth has occurred among the oldest old. In 1900 the proportion of the population aged eighty-five and over was just 0.2 percent, but by 2000 it was 1.5 percent, and it is projected to be 2.3 percent in 2030 and 4.3 percent in 2050 (Administration on Aging 2010). Although this entry focuses primarily on the United States, it carries important implications for global aging, especially in industrial nations experiencing similar rates of societal aging. There are distinct challenges facing elderly individuals in developing nations (Engelman and Johnson 2007).

During the time that population records have been kept, women's life expectancy has always exceeded men's. Although at younger ages there are more men than women, by old age women far outnumber men (Cassel and Neugarten 1988). In 2010 there were 132 women for every 100 men aged sixty-five and over. As sex-based disparities increase with age, in the eighty-five and over age group the ratio of women to men was 203 to 100 in 2010 (Administration on Aging 2010). Demographers predict that in the early twenty-first century this sex differential is narrowing and has begun to level off. Thus by 2050 there will be just 122 women per 100 men aged sixty-five and over and 156 women per 100 men aged eighty-five and over. However, other sex-based differences among the elderly are increasing. Thus elderly women's health is generally worse than elderly men's health, and more older women than older men are poor. Women constitute 58 percent of the population aged sixty-five and over but 75 percent of the impoverished elderly, and this percentage is rising (Tong 2002).

ETHICAL IMPLICATIONS

The rapid increase in the number of older persons relative to younger ones carries important societal implications. In the domain of health care, societal aging will increase costs and exert greater pressure to ration services. It will thus bring to the fore questions regarding a just distribution of health care between young and old. The population's aging will also alter the nature of health services by increasing the number of patients who have chronic and disabling conditions that are not life threatening. This in turn will change the nature of bioethical debates from a focus on acute life-and-death medical decisions made at a particular instant to an emphasis on ongoing and often relatively mundane problems spanning many years. Finally, societal aging portends changes for family life. Already the imbalance between young and old is placing strains on offspring who undertake caregiving responsibilities and is prompting questions about the scope and limits of filial duties. To the extent that family members play a prominent role in elder care, their role in health care decision making is a significant and vigorously debated issue.

HEALTH CARE RATIONING

Most developed nations seek to guarantee a minimum level of health care to all citizens. In the United States the Patient Protection and Affordable Care Act of 2010 expands access to care for millions of US citizens by means of an individual mandate requiring all US citizens to have health insurance or face a penalty consisting of 1 percent of income or $285 per family, whichever is greater. Other nations use a variety of means to provide citizens with health care coverage, such as direct taxation, mandatory employer and employee contributions, and affordable private insurance.

The aging of society that is occurring in most developed nations will increase health care expenditures simply because persons over the age of sixty-five consume far more health care than other age groups do. For example, in the United States persons aged sixty-five and over account for roughly 13 percent of the population but use 36 percent of the country's total personal health care expenditures exclusive of research costs. To put this in perspective, the average health care expense for elderly people is $11,089 per year, whereas it is only $3,352 per year for those between the ages of nineteen and sixty-four (Stanton 2006).

The disproportionate cost of caring for a nation's elderly makes the elderly an obvious target for health care rationing. Yet overt efforts to limit health care to the elderly have generally been met with resistance. Major international organizations, such as the European Union (2007, Article 21), the World Health Organization (2002), and the United Nations General Assembly (1948, preamble), have rejected any form of age-based discrimination and stress the equal rights of elderly people to access health care. In the United States the Patient Protection and Affordable Care Act restricts any reduction in services or increase in fees to beneficiaries of Medicare, the federal program serving the nation's elderly and disabled. Despite such resistance, public moneys to pay for health care are limited. As the Medicare trustees report of 2012 made clear, Medicare expenditures exceeded income annually between 2008 and 2012, and they were projected to continue doing so until the fund becomes exhausted in 2024 (Boards of Trustees, Federal Hospital

Insurance and Federal Supplementary Medical Insurance Trust Funds 2012). It also remains to be seen whether certain provisions of the Affordable Care Act will limit access for seniors. For example, some express concern that efforts to reduce the growth in Medicare spending by means of care coordination and disease-management programs designed to reduce avoidable hospitalizations will limit access to care for the frail elderly with multiple chronic conditions who require hospitalization (Konetzka, Karon, and Potter 2012). Implicit rationing of care to the elderly may occur even if it is not part of an explicit policy or plan to implement age-based rationing.

It is important to underscore that even if nations successfully implement efforts to contain health care costs, the elderly will nonetheless continue to claim a rising share of national economies. To address the high cost of caring for the elderly, some bioethicists propose age-based rationing. Arguments supporting age-based rationing are advanced, for example, by Norman Daniels, who in his 1988 book *Am I My Parents' Keeper? An Essay on Justice between the Young and the Old* contended that justice between the young and the old should be considered from a prudential, first-person perspective. According to this approach, when people view their lives as a whole rather than from a particular moment in time, it will sometimes be prudent to prefer a health care plan that distributes fewer services in old age in exchange for more services earlier in life. From this perspective, age-based rationing can be compatible with a principle of equality, as all are treated equally over time, reaping the benefits of access to more resources in earlier years and fewer in later life.

A somewhat different way of arguing for age-based rationing draws on the idea of "fair innings" and the related claim that no one is entitled to "extra" innings, especially when some have not yet had their fair share. For example, other things being equal, the elderly ought not receive publicly funded, life-extending medical treatment if this results in the denial of such treatments to younger individuals (Harris 1985, 1999).

Debates about the merits of age-based rationing are difficult to settle in part because of the very general and abstract nature of the concept of "equality." Different reasonable accounts can be given of how equality should be specified and whether age-based discrimination is compatible with it. Thus opponents of age-based rationing insist that equality requires that the needs and preferences of the elderly and the young alike merit equal consideration (Giordano 2005). One alternative to age-based rationing is the kind of approach to budgeting used in the United Kingdom, whose National Institute for Health and Clinical Excellence uses a complex quality-adjusted life year system to put an explicit value on a treatment's ability to extend life.

LONG-TERM CARE

Societal aging will increase the number of disabled persons and the need for long-term care, including adult day care; in-home services; and care in resident facilities, convalescent homes, and intermediate and skilled nursing facilities. Several factors will contribute to a greater need for long-term care. First, women, more than men, fill the ranks of older Americans, and older women experience a greater incidence of morbidity and disability than older men. Second, the population over the age of eighty-five constitutes the fastest-growing age group in the population, and those in this group are also the heaviest users of long-term care. More than 70 percent of those aged eighty-five and over require some kind of assistance with one or more activities of daily living. Finally, fewer offspring will be available to serve as informal caregivers for future generations of elderly persons. This is because individuals are having fewer children than those of previous generations did and greater numbers of women are joining the paid labor force.

The growing need for long-term care raises social and policy questions concerning how long-term care ought to be organized, structured, and financed. In a 2008 report the Institute of Medicine's Committee on the Future Health Care Workforce for Older Americans noted that direct-care workers, who include nurse aides, home health aides, and personal and home care aides, are very poorly paid, garner fewer benefits, work under high levels of physical and emotional stress, receive little or no training for their duties, and have high turnover rates with difficulty recruiting and retaining workers. The number of direct-care workers is insufficient to meet demand, and the gap between demand and supply is projected to increase.

By far the majority of caregiving for the elderly is done by informal caregivers. In contrast to paid, direct-care workers, informal caregivers may be family members, friends, or neighbors who render assistance based on an emotional bond or a personal relationship with an individual needing care. The most common family caregiver is a spouse or an adult daughter.

Because the work of caring for dependent people falls disproportionately on women, caregiving raises ethical questions related to justice and gender. Whether it is the care of children, disabled children and adults, or the elderly, caregiving is done predominantly by women (Kittay 1999). In the United States 89 percent of direct-care workers for the elderly are females typically between the ages of twenty-five and fifty-five, unmarried, and without college degrees, with roughly 30 percent African American and 15 percent Hispanic or Latino (Institute of Medicine, Committee on the Future Health Care Workforce for Older Americans 2008). In a 2002 article Martha Nussbaum argued that paid caregiving in particular raises justice questions regarding the exploitation of one class of women by another. Within the family, questions concerning what constitutes a fair sharing of caregiving between the sexes raises justice concerns (Jecker 2002).

From a health systems perspective, delivering high-quality care to elderly patients with multiple chronic health conditions and complex health care needs requires that health care professionals provide comprehensive assessment and evidence-based care planning and monitoring and to promote the active engagement of patients and caregivers (Boult and Wieland 2010).

FAMILY RELATIONSHIPS

The rapid aging of society will reshape relationships in the family as parent-child relationships extend over many more years and pose new challenges in later life. Although most agree that parents undertake special duties toward offspring, there are different views about whether or not grown children have corresponding duties toward aging parents. If one conceives of intergenerational relationships in terms of a social contract delineating rights and obligations, it might be thought incumbent upon older generations to avoid becoming a burden on younger generations, because the young did not agree to and may not accept such burdens. By contrast, older generations presumably consented to bear children and thus agreed to undertake the corresponding obligation to care for them.

An alternative conception of intergenerational relationships emphasizes community and solidarity rather than generational equity, leading to a very different set of conclusions. For example, if the emphasis is placed on maintaining relationships or strengthening communal bonds, a principle of reciprocity may be invoked, suggesting that adult offspring are obligated to care for their parents in light of the benefits they received from them in the past (Engelman and Johnson 2007). Alternatively a principle of gratitude might be invoked to support filial duties (Jecker 1989). A somewhat different analysis conceives of moral obligations to care for aging parents as based on the specific content of family narratives that shape people's moral identities (Nelson 2001) or on the broader idea that the web of human connection both in families and in the broader society is sustained by caregivers, including those, such as doulas, who care for caregivers (Kittay 1999). By contrast, some deny that adult offspring owe their parents anything by virtue of being their offspring, with Jane English (1991, 147), for example, defending the idea that "the duties of grown children are those of friends, and result from love between them and their parent, rather than being things owed in repayment for the parents' earlier sacrifices."

HISTORICAL AND CULTURAL PERSPECTIVES

An aging society, defined as a society in which the population of older individuals is increasing relative to the population of younger individuals, presupposes that individuals can be separated into meaningful categories of old and young. Although contemporary Western society tends to conceive of youth, adolescence, middle age, and old age as unique life stages with distinct sets of problems, this perspective is hardly universal. Indeed, early twenty-first-century conceptions of the life course are a relatively recent phenomenon. In his 1992 book *The Journey of Life: A Cultural History of Aging in America,* Thomas R. Cole traced the metaphor of life's stages to the cities of northern Europe in the sixteenth and seventeenth centuries, where the current life-stage metaphor first emerged. Picturing life as a series of ordered stages represents the life course as in conformity with the order of the universe and makes it possible for every individual to "step outside of his own life experiences and view it as a whole" (Cole 1992, 25).

Just as a society's recognition of aging reflects its historical and cultural traditions, so a society's beliefs about the meaning and value of old age bespeak its historical and cultural heritage. The social rank of elderly persons varies during different historical and culture periods depending on the perceived cost of supporting older age groups and the contributions they are thought to make (Amoss and Harrell 1981). For example, the Akamba people of Africa believe that "the older a person becomes, the more intricately interwoven that person becomes in the lives of others, and the greater the damage done if that person is removed. At the same time, the older person has wisdom—a perspective on life that comes only with age—which is considered to be a particularly important social resource" (Kilner 1984, 19). By contrast, US society has traditionally valued "pragmatism, action, power, and the vigor of youth over contemplation, reflection, experience and the wisdom of age" (Butler 1969, 243). Hence ageism (age discrimination) is especially evident in US society.

Despite different cultural conceptions of aged persons and their roles in society, anthropologists identify common biological and cultural features of aging. Thus every known society has "a named category of people who are old—chronologically, physiologically, or generationally. In every case these people have different rights, duties, privileges, and burdens from those enjoyed or suffered by their juniors" (Amoss and Harrell 1981, 3). This suggests that people in culturally distinct societies may face ethical questions unique to aging and to relationships among people of different ages.

SEE ALSO *Chronic Illness; Future Generations, Reproductive Technologies and Obligations to; Health Care Resources, Allocation of; Human Dignity; Life, Quality of: I. Quality of Life in Clinical Decisions; Long-Term Care: I. Concepts and Policies; Long-Term Care: II. Nursing Homes; Long-Term Care: III. Home Care; Natural Law; Right to Die: Policy and Law; Women, Historical and Cross-Cultural Perspectives*

BIBLIOGRAPHY

Administration on Aging. 2010. "Aging Statistics: Projected Future Growth of the Older Population." Last modified June 23, 2010. http://www.aoa.gov/aoaroot/aging_statistics/future_growth/future_growth.aspx

Amoss, Pamela T., and Stevan Harrell, eds. 1981. *Other Ways of Growing Old: Anthropological Perspectives*. Stanford, CA: Stanford University Press.

Boards of Trustees, Federal Hospital Insurance and Federal Supplementary Medical Insurance Trust Funds. 2012. "2012 Annual Report of the Boards of Trustees of the Federal Hospital Insurance and Federal Supplementary Medical Insurance Trust Funds." Accessed September 25, 2012. http://www.cms.gov/Research-Statistics-Data-and-Systems/Statistics-Trends-and-Reports/ReportsTrustFunds/Downloads/TR2012.pdf

Boult, Chad, and G. Darryl Wieland. 2010. "Comprehensive Primary Care for Older Patients with Multiple Chronic Conditions." *Journal of the American Medical Association* 304 (17): 1936–43.

Butler, Robert N. 1969. "Age-ism: Another Form of Bigotry." *Gerontologist* 9 (4, pt. 1): 243–46.

Cassel, Christine K., and Bernice L. Neugarten. 1988. "A Forecast of Women's Health and Longevity: Implications for an Aging America." *Western Journal of Medicine* 149 (6): 712–17.

Cole, Thomas R. 1992. *The Journey of Life: A Cultural History of Aging in America*. Cambridge, UK: Cambridge University Press.

Daniels, Norman. 1988. *Am I My Parents' Keeper? An Essay on Justice between the Young and the Old*. New York: Oxford University Press.

Engelman, Michal, and Summer Johnson. 2007. "Population Aging and International Development: Addressing Competing Claims of Distributive Justice." *Developing World Bioethics* 7 (1): 8–18.

English, Jane. 1991. "What Do Grown Children Owe Their Parents?" In *Aging and Ethics: Philosophical Problems in Gerontology*, edited by Nancy S. Jecker, 147–54. Clifton, NJ: Humana Press.

European Union. 2007. "Charter of Fundamental Rights of the European Union." Accessed September 27, 2012. http://eur-lex.europa.eu/LexUriServ/LexUriServ.do?uri=OJ:C:2007:303:0001:0016:EN:PDF

Giordano, Simona. 2005. "Respect for Equality and the Treatment of the Elderly: Declarations of Human Rights and Age-Based Rationing." *Cambridge Quarterly of Healthcare Ethics* 14 (1): 83–92.

Harris, John. 1985. *The Value of Life*. London: Routledge and Kegan Paul.

Harris, John. 1999. "Cardiac Surgery in the Elderly." *Heart* 82 (2): 119–20.

Institute of Medicine, Committee on the Future Health Care Workforce for Older Americans. 2008. *Retooling for an Aging America: Building the Health Care Workforce*. Washington, DC: National Academies Press.

Jecker, Nancy S. 1989. "Are Filial Duties Unfounded?" *American Philosophical Quarterly* 26 (1): 73–80.

Jecker, Nancy S. 2002. "Taking Care of One's Own: Justice and Family Caregiving." *Theoretical Medicine and Bioethics* 23 (2): 117–33.

Kilner, John F. 1984. "Who Shall Be Saved? An African Answer." *Hastings Center Report* 14 (3): 18–22.

Kittay, Eva Feder. 1999. *Love's Labor: Essays on Women, Equality, and Dependency*. New York: Routledge.

Konetzka, R. Tamara; Sarita L. Karon; and D. E. B. Potter. 2012. "Users of Medicaid Home and Community-Based Services Are Especially Vulnerable to Costly Avoidable Hospital Admissions." *Health Affairs* 31 (6): 1167–75.

Nelson, Hilde Lindemann. 2001. *Damaged Identities, Narrative Repair*. Ithaca, NY: Cornell University Press.

Nussbaum, Martha. 2002. "Introduction to the Symposium on Eva Kittay's *Love's Labor: Essays on Women, Equality, and Dependency*." *Hypatia* 17 (3): 194–99.

Stanton, Mark W. 2006. "The High Concentration of U.S. Health Care Expenditures." Research in Action 19, Agency for Healthcare Research and Quality. Accessed February 16, 2012. http://www.ahrq.gov/research/findings/factsheets/costs/expriach/index.html

Tong, Rosemarie. 2002. "*Love's Labor* in the Health Care System: Working toward Gender Equity." *Hypatia* 17 (3): 200–213.

United Nations General Assembly. 1948. "The Universal Declaration of Human Rights." Accessed September 27, 2012. http://www.un.org/en/documents/udhr/index.shtml

World Health Organization. 2002. "Active Ageing: A Policy Framework." Accessed September 27, 2012. http://whqlibdoc.who.int/hq/2002/who_nmh_nph_02.8.pdf

Nancy S. Jecker (1995, 2004, 2014)

Professor, Department of Bioethics and Humanities, School of Medicine, University of Washington

II. HEALTH CARE FOR THE AGING

How will the aging of individuals and societies affect health care and health-related goods? What challenges will societies face as individuals live longer and as the number of young people relative to older people declines? This entry addresses health care for the aging and discusses the implications of aging for individuals, families, and societies.

AGING

Individuals are living longer today than ever before. Whereas babies born in 1900 did not usually live past age fifty, life expectancy at birth now exceeds eighty-three years in Japan—the current leader—and is at least eighty-one years in several other countries (NIA/WHO 2011). Increased longevity is the result of a variety of trends, including improvements in public health, reductions in infant mortality, and the waning of infectious diseases.

Families are also aging in the sense that they are now comprised of more members in middle and older age groups and fewer infants and children. This is the result not only of increasing longevity but also of declining fertility rates. Worldwide, the number of children born per woman of childbearing years is estimated to be 2.55, which is about half the level of 5 children per woman for the period from 1950 to 1955 (UN 2007). The so-called beanpole family describes a family whose living members are from multiple generations but within each generation there are fewer members. Such a structure places more pressure on "productive" members, usually defined as those between the ages of fifteen and sixty-four, to care for "dependent" members, defined as those under age fifteen and over age sixty-four. Within families and societies the "dependency ratio," defined as the number of dependent members relative to productive members, is rising. Moreover, making sacrifices or using resources to benefit older family members may be considered problematic in a way that sacrifices for children are not (Minkler and Estes 1998).

Societies around the globe are also aging. A society is said to "age" when its number of older people increases relative to its number of younger people. While societies have been aging for as long as records have been kept, the pace of population aging has accelerated rapidly during the twentieth and twenty-first centuries. This is the result of both increasing longevity and declining fertility rates. The most rapidly aging societies are in less developed nations. Between 2010 and 2050, for example, the number of older people in less developed countries is projected to increase more than 250 percent, compared with an increase of 71 percent in developed nations during the same period (NIA/WHO 2011). Although the age profile of developing nations is currently younger than the age profile of developed nations, by mid-century the developing world is likely to reach the same stage in the process of population aging as that of the developed world today (UN 2009).

In addition to the aging of individuals, families, and societies, the population of persons sixty-five and over is itself aging. Among the elderly, the fastest-growing group is the eighty-five and over age group, which is forecast to increase 351 percent globally between 2000 and 2050 (UN 2010). As the population of older persons ages, its ranks will increasingly be filled with women, who tend to live longer than men do. Worldwide, women outnumber men by an estimated 66 million among those aged sixty years and over. Among those aged eighty years and over, women are nearly twice as numerous as men, and among centenarians women are between four and five times as numerous as men (UN 2010).

AGING AND HEALTH CARE

Aging will have a significantly impact on health care systems, social services, and economies worldwide. As people live longer, benefits, such as health care, old-age support, and pensions, will need to be paid over a longer time. Societal aging will increase the demand and cost for health care because the elderly on average consume a much greater share of health care resources in comparison with younger age groups. For example, in the United States persons aged sixty-five and over account for roughly 13 percent of the population but use 36 percent of the country's total personal health care expenditures exclusive of research costs. To put this in perspective, consider that while the average health care expense for elderly people is $11,089 per year, it is only $3,352 per year for those aged nineteen to sixty-four (HHS 2006).

Accompanying the rapid aging of societies has been what epidemiologists call an "epidemiologic transition," or a waning of infectious and acute disease and the emerging importance of chronic and degenerative diseases, such as heart disease, cancer, diabetes, and dementia. This shift in disease patterns, first identified by Abdel R. Omran (1971), is thought to occur as nations modernize and improve their social, economic, and health conditions. As more sanitary living conditions, improved medical technology, and better lifestyles reduce the spread of infectious and parasitic diseases, those saved from dying from such diseases survive into middle and older ages, where they face the elevated risk of dying from degenerative disease. While some have challenged the theory of epidemiologic transition as a universal or unidirectional theory, emphasizing instead the heterogeneity in the rate and type of transition in different times and places (Murray and Chen 1992; Fetter et al. 1997), analyses based on World Health Organization data tend to confirm the general principles of this approach (Salomon and Murray 2002).

As chronic degenerative conditions become more prevalent, health care systems will need to shift from focusing on short-term, acute interventions to managing chronic progressive conditions for people who neither get well nor improve function. This will require providing and paying for long-term-care services, such as home health care, community-based assisted-living facilities, and skilled nursing homes. In many parts of the world, public funding at present provides only minimal support for such services. In the United States, for example, unpaid caregivers, such as family members and neighbors, provide an estimated 90 percent of long-term care for the disabled (Institute of Medicine 2008). Medicare, the federal health insurance program for the elderly and the disabled, covers only short-term assisted-living stays. Long-term-care coverage under Medicaid, the federal-state program that provides means-tested health insurance for the poorest Americans, requires people to exhaust their assets to qualify. The Patient Protection and Affordable Care Act, signed into law in the United States in 2010, was originally designed to include a program of national, voluntary long-term-care insurance, known as Community Living Assistance Services and Supports (CLASS).

Although designed to be self-supporting, with monthly deductions from workers' paychecks, critics of CLASS charged that it would add to federal budget deficits. In 2011 the US Department of Health and Human Services under President Barack Obama announced that the federal government would not be implementing this program.

Structural as well as financial barriers impede the provision of high-quality care for elderly patients with chronic conditions. In the United States, the fragmentation of health care occurs when multiple decision makers are each responsible for only a fragment of a relevant set of health care decisions. Where there is no single health care professional aware of the patient's full range of health care needs and responsible for making sure that necessary and appropriate actions are taken, the quality of care a patient receives is reduced (Elhauge 2010). This problem is exacerbated by the underuse of electronic medical records and the absence of systems that interconnect electronic medical records from different providers (Hall and Schulman 2009, 2010). Fragmentation is associated with adverse outcomes, such as medical errors, as a result of a lack of effective data sharing and teamwork among health care professionals (Institute of Medicine 2000, 2007). Fragmentation is of particular concern for elderly patients, who are more likely than other age groups to suffer from multiple medical conditions. The average Medicare beneficiary, for example, sees two physicians and five specialists a year, whereas Medicare beneficiaries with chronic illnesses see an average of thirteen physicians a year (Hyman 2010). When there is a lack of direct coordination among providers treating a patient for different conditions, patients or family members often find themselves trying to coordinate care. The problem with this approach is that patients and family do not coordinate effectively; not only do they lack medical expertise, but they also lack authority over physicians and control of decision making (Elhauge 2010).

In contrast to the United States, many European countries demonstrate a more robust conception of social welfare and obligation (Moody 2007). In many European countries, norms of solidarity provide an ethical and social basis for systems of social welfare protection. By contrast, in the United States the emphasis is often placed on individual autonomy and self-sufficiency. As a result, the safety net in the United States tends to be relatively weaker. The challenge of caring for dependent elderly may be perceived in countries such as the United States not as a moral and political mandate but as a matter of individual and family responsibility. European countries are also more likely to better integrate health care, such as through national health care systems with centralized ownership and through care coordination by primary care providers.

FUTURE CHALLENGES

The demographic changes described above will raise ethical challenges for individuals, families, and societies. These include challenges related to caregiving for growing numbers of dependent elderly, conceptualizing human disability and dependency, allocating health care among age groups, and addressing clinical and policy questions related to the care of the elderly.

Caregiving for the Dependent Elderly. While many nations rely on unpaid caregivers to support the chronically ill, the sustainability of such an approach is uncertain. It assumes the availability of family members, friends, or volunteers able and willing to house, feed, and meet the medical and psychosocial needs of the chronically ill (Buhler-Wilkerson 2007). Part of the appeal of such an approach is that it represents a less costly alternative for society. Yet as a model for providing social services to the elderly it has been criticized as unrealistic. According to one analysis, the "continuing belief that women will always be available to provide such care contributes to the lack of public will necessary to address these questions thoroughly, honestly, and realistically" (Buhler-Wilkerson 2007, 613). Family caregivers often experience negative psychological, behavioral, and physiological effects on their daily lives and health. Public policies to alleviate caregiver burden, such as by providing respite care, paid family leave, or other support services for caregivers, would improve the quality of life for both caregivers and care recipients.

The sustainability of informal, unpaid caregiving in the future is rendered more difficult not only in light of changing roles for women around the globe but also in light of global trends toward having fewer children, which entails that there will be less potential care and support for older people from their families in the future. Added to this is the global change toward different generations within a family living separately, rather than together, thereby reducing the availability of in-home family caregiving. Even in societies such as Japan that have strong traditions of older parents living with their children, cohabitation of parents and children is becoming less common. Worldwide, the number and often the percentage of older people living alone are rising in most countries (NIA/WHO 2011).

Whereas caregiving in the past was associated primarily with the care of infants and small children, in the future many more recipients of caregiving will be elderly. This change in caregiving will be unprecedented. Since the beginning of recorded history, young children have always outnumbered their elders. But soon the number of people aged sixty-five and over will outnumber children under age five (NIA/WHO 2011). This change is occurring in tandem with the epidemiologic shift to chronic and degenerative diseases noted already. As a result, many people in older age groups will suffer from such conditions as stroke, diabetes, cancer, dementia, and heart disease. As these conditions progress, individuals will grow more dependent over time as their health and function deteriorate.

Understanding Disability and Dependency. These changes are likely to alter the way people think about disability and dependency. Rather than being considered a condition affecting only a minority of the population, disability may eventually come to be regarded as a condition that all humans will potentially face as they age. As the World Health Organization urges, "every human being can experience a decrement in health and thereby experience some disability. This is not something that happens to only a minority of humanity.... It [is] a universal human experience" (2002, 3). Limited mobility, frailty, and other declines in physical and cognitive functioning are becoming more pervasive at the end of life as people live to older ages. For example, the prevalence of Alzheimer's disease and other dementias is very low at younger ages, then nearly doubles with every five years of age after age sixty-five (NIA/WHO 2011).

Like the experience of disability, the experience of dependency may be construed in a new light as a result of increased longevity and societal aging. Rather than thinking of dependency as a condition affecting only a minority of the population, it can instead be seen as condition affecting all humans. Dependency at both ends of the life span, in early childhood and in old age, will become the new norm as people live to increasingly older ages. Feminists have contributed considerably to scholarship in this area by challenging the myth of individual self-reliance and by emphasizing the shared vulnerability and dependency of human beings (Kittay 1999).

Allocating Health Care Fairly among Age Groups. Another area in which demographic changes will raise new questions and ethical challenges is the allocation of health care and health-related services. Because the dollars to pay for health care are limited, it is always necessary to ask what is a just and fair allocation of finite resources. In the context of an aging society, this question becomes more urgent and gives rise to another. What would be a fair allocation of health care among age groups? This question need not imply generational opposition or competition but instead speaks to the fact that when more resources are devoted to older age groups, this places pressure on other age groups, both middle-aged wage earners and dependent youth. In this context, some policy makers and scholars have asked whether it is ever ethically justifiable to impose age-based limits on health care. Different answers to this question are possible, depending on the underlying conception of justice one holds. Many modern conceptions of justice emphasize the equal worth and dignity of all persons, irrespective of age (Fleischacker 2004). Equality, however, is a general and abstract idea that is open to different reasonable specifications. Thus, some argue that equality requires equal access to health care: if a health care resource is available to anyone, it must be equally available to anyone with similar health care needs (Gutmann 1983). An alternative interpretation of equality emphasizes equal functioning and capability, rather than equal access to resources (Nussbaum 2006). According to this interpretation, giving more resources to the old than to the young can be justified provided doing so is necessary in order to bring the elderly closer to a level of equal functioning and capability. Alternatively, the emphasis might be placed on equality in human well-being, and well-being, in turn, might be understood as encompassing health, personal security, reasoning, respect, attachment, and self-determination (Powers and Faden 2006). Finally, it could be argued that age-based limits on health care are consistent with equal respect because as people age, each person will experience both the benefits and burdens of age-based restrictions (Daniels 1988). According to this analysis, age-based discrimination is not necessarily invidious or a reflection of "ageism"—that is, negative stereotypes about elderly individuals (Butler 1969).

From a practical standpoint, scholarly debates about justice and equality do not preclude the need to make practical decisions about exactly who gets exactly what (Arrras and Fenton 2009). Moreover, despite different conceptual approaches to justice, people might agree about the practical methods for achieving a fair distribution of health care resources. For example, accountability for reasonableness is a strategy that aims to hold decision makers accountable for the reasonableness of their decisions by requiring (1) a process that is public about the grounds for a decision, (2) decisions that rest on reasons that stakeholders can agree are relevant, and (3) decisions that are open to revision in light of new evidence and arguments (Daniels and Sabin 2008a, 2008b).

Clinical and Policy Challenges of Caring for the Elderly. Finally, changes in health care will raise new clinical and policy challenges. In clinical settings, more ethical concerns will need to be faced that relate to the care of elderly people with chronic, disabling conditions. For example, how should life-extending care be used for frail, elderly persons at the end of life? What are the ethical and social implications of discharging impaired elderly patients to the home? What should be the role of family members in health care decisions for cognitively impaired elders?

At the level of public policy, there will be societal choices to be made concerning health system reforms to meet the needs of aging populations. It is estimated that the United States will need an additional 3.5 million health care workers by 2030 just to maintain the current ratio of health care workers to the population (Stone and Barbarotta 2010–2011). As the 2008 Institute of Medicine report titled *Retooling for an Aging America* makes evident, workforce shortages in health care for the elderly present a formidable challenge. Health professionals generally receive little training in the common problems of older adults, and there is a dearth of specialists, such as geriatricians, geriatric psychiatrists, geriatric nurses, geriatric social workers, and physician assistants, specializing in meeting the needs of older people. Retention rates for direct-care workers for the elderly are poor, partly because these workers earn relatively low wages and often lack benefits, such as health insurance. For example, the average home care aide in the United States earns $8.54 per hour, compared to the $7.76 paid to food counter attendants.

CONCLUSION

The future will bring unprecedented demographic change for individuals, families, and societies around the globe. Aging is nothing new for individuals, but living to older and older ages is unprecedented. Societal aging is also a long-standing condition, but it is occurring around the globe at a much quicker pace than ever before. In developing nations, where aging is occurring more rapidly, there will be less time to adjust to such changes and implement structural reforms to meet social and health care needs for elderly people. Demographers predict that there will soon be more elderly people than young people worldwide. The ethical and social implications of these changes require careful scrutiny and bold action. Bioethics can contribute to this process by articulating ethical concerns and by contributing to ethical analyses of health care decisions and policies affecting the elderly.

SEE ALSO *Access to Health Care; Artificial Nutrition and Hydration; Care; Dementia; End-of-Life Care; Family Caregiving; Health and Disease: V. The Experience of Health and Illness; Hospice and Palliative Care: Professional Education; Life-Sustaining Treatment and Euthanasia; Long-Term Care; Medicare*

BIBLIOGRAPHY

Arras, John D., and Elizabeth M. Fenton. 2009. "Bioethics and Human Rights: Access to Health-Related Goods." *Hastings Center Report* 39 (5): 27–38.

Buhler-Wilkerson, Karen. 2001. *No Place Like Home: A History of Nursing and Home Care in the United States*. Baltimore: Johns Hopkins University Press.

Buhler-Wilkerson, Karen. 2007. "Care of the Chronically Ill at Home: An Unresolved Dilemma in Health Policy for the United States." *Milbank Quarterly* 85 (4): 611–39.

Butler, Robert N. 1969. "Age-ism: Another Form of Bigotry." *Gerontologist* 9 (4, pt. 1): 243–46.

Daniels, Norman. 1988. *Am I My Parents' Keeper? An Essay on Justice between the Young and the Old*. New York: Oxford University Press.

Daniels, Norman. 2006. "Toward Ethical Review of Health System Transformations." *American Journal of Public Health* 96 (3): 447–51.

Daniels, Norman, and James E. Sabin. 2008a. "Accountability for Reasonableness: An Update." *British Medical Journal* 337:a1850.

Daniels, Norman, and James E. Sabin. 2008b. *Setting Limits Fairly: Learning to Share Resources for Health*. 2nd ed. Oxford: Oxford University Press.

Elhauge, Einer. 2010. "Why We Should Care about Health Care Fragmentation and How to Fix It." In *The Fragmentation of U.S. Health Care: Causes and Solutions*, edited by Einer Elhauge, 1–20. New York: Oxford University Press.

Fetter, Bruce; Philip R. P. Coelho; John Rogers; and Marie C. Nelson. 1997. "Forum: The Epidemiologic Transition." *Health Transition Review* 7 (2): 235–55.

Fleischacker, Samuel. 2004. *A Short History of Distributive Justice*. Cambridge, MA: Harvard University Press.

Gutmann, Amy. 1983. "A Principle of Equal Access." In *Securing Access to Health Care: A Report on the Ethical Implications of Differences in the Availability of Health Services*, by President's Commission for the Study of Ethical Problems in Medicine and Biomedical and Behavioral Research, vol. 2, 51–66. Washington, DC: US Government Printing Office.

Hall, Mark A., and Kevin A. Schulman. 2009. "Ownership of Medical Information." *Journal of the American Medical Association* 301 (12): 1282–84.

Hall, Mark A., and Kevin A. Schulman. 2010. "Property, Privacy, and the Pursuit of Integrated Electronic Medical Records." In *The Fragmentation of U.S. Health Care: Causes and Solutions*, edited by Einer Elhauge, 165–99. New York: Oxford University Press.

HHS (US Department of Health and Human Services). Agency for Healthcare Research and Quality. 2006. "The High Concentration of U.S. Health Care Expenditures." Research in Action, issue 19. Accessed March 24, 2013. http://www.ahrq.gov/research/findings/factsheets/costs/expriach/index.html

Hyman, David A. 2010. "Health Care Fragmentation: We Get What We Pay For." In *The Fragmentation of U.S. Health Care: Causes and Solutions*, edited by Einer Elhauge, 21–36. New York: Oxford University Press.

Institute of Medicine. 2000. *To Err Is Human: Building a Safer Health System*. Washington, DC: National Academy Press. Accessed March 18, 2013. http://www.nap.edu/catalog.php?record_id=9728#toc

Institute of Medicine. 2007. *Preventing Medication Errors*. Washington, DC: National Academies Press. Accessed March 18, 2013. http://www.nap.edu/catalog.php?record_id=11623#toc

Institute of Medicine, Committee on the Future Health Care Workforce for Older Americans. 2008. *Retooling for an Aging America: Building the Health Care Workforce*. Washington, DC: National Academies Press.

Kittay, Eva Feder. 1999. *Love's Labor: Essays on Women, Equality, and Dependency*. New York: Routledge.

Minkler, Meredith, and Carroll L. Estes, eds. 1998. *Critical Gerontology: Perspectives from Political and Moral Economy*. Amityville, NY: Baywood.

Moody, H. Rick. 2007. "Aging, Generational Opposition, and the Future of the Family." In *Challenges of an Aging Society: Ethical Dilemmas, Political Issues*, edited by Rachel A. Pruchno and Michael A. Smyer, 175–89. Baltimore: Johns Hopkins University Press.

Murray, Christopher J. L., and Lincoln C. Chen. 1992. "Understanding Morbidity Change." *Population and Development Review* 18 (3): 481–503.

NIA/WHO (National Institute on Aging and World Health Organization). 2011. "Global Health and Aging." Accessed April 5, 2013. http://www.who.int/ageing/publications/global_health.pdf

Nussbaum, Martha C. 2006. *Frontiers of Justice: Disability, Nationality, Species Membership*. Cambridge, MA: Belknap Press of Harvard University Press.

Olshansky, S. Jay, and A. Brian Ault. 1986. "The Fourth Stage of the Epidemiologic Transition: The Age of Delayed Degenerative Diseases." *Milbank Quarterly* 64 (3): 355–91.

Omran, Abdel R. 1971. "The Epidemiologic Transition: A Theory of the Epidemiology of Population Change." *Milbank Memorial Fund Quarterly* 49 (4): 509–38.

Powers, Madison, and Ruth Faden. 2006. *Social Justice: The Moral Foundations of Public Health and Health Policy*. Oxford: Oxford University Press.

Salomon, Joshua A., and Christopher J. L. Murray. 2002. "The Epidemiologic Transition Revisited: Compositional Models for Causes of Death by Age and Sex." *Population and Development Review* 28 (2): 205–28.

Stone, Robyn I., and Linda Barbarotta. 2010–2011. "Caring for an Aging America in the Twenty-First Century." *Generations: Journal of the American Society on Aging* 34 (4): 5–10.

UN (United Nations). 2007. "World Population Prospects: The 2006 Revision; Highlights." Accessed November 20, 2012. http://www.un.org/esa/population/publications/wpp2006/WPP2006_Highlights_rev.pdf

UN (United Nations). 2009. "World Population Ageing: 2009." Accessed April 5, 2013. http://www.un.org/esa/population/publications/WPA2009/WPA2009_WorkingPaper.pdf

UN (United Nations). 2010. "World Population Prospects: The 2010 Revision." Accessed April 5, 2013. http://esa.un.org/wpp/

World Health Organization. 2002. "Towards a Common Language for Functioning, Disability, and Health: ICF." Accessed November 19, 2012. http://www.who.int/classifications/icf/training/icfbeginnersguide.pdf

Nancy S. Jecker
Professor, Department of Bioethics and Humanities, School of Medicine, University of Washington

III. RESEARCH ETHICS

The conduct of biomedical and behavioral research involving human beings as research subjects entails a variety of ethical considerations. These considerations may become particularly complex when the research protocol potentially includes the enrollment of older individuals and even more so when the possible human subjects have some significant degree of cognitive and/or emotional impairment. This selection outlines the most salient ethical and legal issues raised by the conduct of research on older persons.

THE NEED FOR RESEARCH ON AGING POPULATIONS

Although some commentators have described biomedical and behavioral research as an ethically optional activity, only a tiny minority of citizens in the early twenty-first century would favor freezing the state of medical knowledge and practice forever in its present incarnation by forgoing further research endeavors. Continuously generating new knowledge that can be translated directly into better clinical care for patients is a core ethical objective (Naylor et al. 2012). The National Institute on Aging (2011) notes, for example, that "clinical trials are the only way to test whether a potential intervention for Alzheimer's disease is safe and effective in humans."

Moreover, progress in developing new diagnostic and therapeutic interventions that can eventually become part of standard clinical practice for preventing, curing, or ameliorating medical and psychological problems prevalent in older individuals, especially those with dementia or other sources of impairment, requires that research projects be done in which individuals suffering from the precise problems under investigation are the basic sources of data. This is explained by a leading national advocacy organization:

> Without clinical trials, there can be no better treatments, no prevention and no cure for Alzheimer's disease. Scientists work constantly to find better ways to treat diseases, but improved treatments can never become a reality without testing in clinical trials with human volunteers. Today, at least 50,000 volunteers, both with and without Alzheimer's disease, are urgently needed to participate in more than 100 actively enrolling clinical trials with human volunteers. Recruiting and retaining trial participants is now the greatest obstacle, other than funding, to developing the next generation of Alzheimer's treatments. (Alzheimer's Association 2013)

In addition to the ethical and practical imperatives to conduct research aimed at developing diagnostic and therapeutic improvements in the care of older persons, it is also essential to continuously accumulate and analyze data pertaining directly to the protection and promotion of older persons' ethical interests. Thus substantial research in the geriatrics sphere focuses on issues such as patient autonomy, self-determination, and informed consent (Suhonen et al. 2010).

RECRUITMENT ISSUES

Some have lamented the often insufficient enrollment of older people in research protocols, especially clinical trials relevant to geriatrics (Watts 2012). There are a number of possible impediments to enrolling older persons as volunteers in research projects. Among these challenges are low education backgrounds, cultural and linguistic differences between researchers and putative subjects, and rural location, although properly conducted recruitment efforts have generally successfully overcome these barriers (Wu et al. 2010; Chao et al. 2011). In addition, the primary ethical and legal catch-22 is that the very conditions that may qualify a person for eligibility as a participant in a research project (particularly one studying dementia or other aging-associated mental impairments) frequently make it impossible for that person to take part in a rational, autonomous decision-making process about his or her own participation as a research subject. This paradox notwithstanding, the hope for creating any medical advances that would benefit older persons in the future depends on successfully navigating the boundary between needed scientific discovery to improve the status quo, on the one hand, and the imperative of beneficence and nonmaleficence to protect vulnerable people against serious, avoidable harm, on the other.

RESEARCH REGULATIONS AND ETHICAL STANDARDS

Among other things, federal regulations covering biomedical and behavioral research in the United States—45 Code of Federal Regulations §46.116 (US Department of Health and Human Services 2013) and 21 Code of Federal Regulations §15.20—mandate that the institutional review board (IRB) reviewing a proposed research protocol involving the enrollment of human subjects (of any age) ensure that informed consent for participation is obtained from either the "subject or the subject's legally authorized representative" (US Department of Health and Human Services 2013). A subject's legally authorized representative is defined in the federal regulations as an "individual or judicial or other body authorized under applicable law to consent on behalf of a prospective subject." Consequently individual state statutes, regulations, and judicial decisions (which often are ambiguous or silent on this point) are the controlling legal authority.

Because the older individuals whom the researcher approaches about participation in a protocol studying some facet of dementia or another mental impairment often will themselves have significant cognitive and/or emotional deficits, we must engage in more clinical investigation and policy discussion to improve the process of assessing the mental capacity of older individuals to make their own autonomous decisions about participating in research projects (Kim 2011). Because decisional capacity frequently is situation dependent, the design of a research protocol itself may be a highly relevant consideration in evaluating whether potential human subjects are adequately able to consent to or refuse participation (Krestar et al. 2012). When the individual is reliably determined not to possess sufficient present capacity to make an autonomous choice regarding enrollment in a specific protocol, mechanisms for accomplishing acceptable surrogate decision making become very important. There is evidence that the idea of surrogate consent-based dementia research (particularly when the surrogate decision makers are family members) is broadly supported by older Americans (Kim, Kim, et al. 2011), although more as a matter of "cautious pragmatism" than of enthusiastic embrace for most people (DeVries et al. 2012). This support may be increased by involving older persons in in-depth democratic deliberation about the pertinent scientific and ethical issues (Kim, Kim, et al. 2011).

Some alternatives for effectuating surrogate consent for research participation include a proxy advance directive for research participation executed while the potential research subject still retains sufficient capacity to decide to appoint a surrogate (Kim, Karlawish, et al. 2011); research living wills or mental health advance directives with particular sections anticipating the individual's participation in future research (Brodoff 2009); reliance on family default statutes, just as they are relied on in the case of diagnostic and therapeutic interventions; informal or extralegal dependence on available family members; guardianship/conservatorship court orders that explicitly empower the guardian/conservator to make decisions about research; particular prior court orders authorizing the decisionally incapacitated person's enrollment in research projects on a case-by-case basis; and designation of a surrogate by the IRB or a long-term care facility's resident council.

In choosing whether to enroll a decisionally incapacitated older person in a research protocol, the surrogate should be guided by the substituted judgment standard, which entails knowing or being able to reasonably infer the wishes that would be expressed by the incapacitated person if that individual were able currently to formulate and communicate an autonomous choice. When it is not realistically feasible to know or infer what the incapacitated individual would wish regarding research participation, rather than engaging in unsupported speculation the surrogate should operate on the basis of the traditional best interests standard. A fallback best-interests analysis concerning the incapacitated person's possible research participation should compare the probable burdens or risks for the research subject to the possible benefits to that person and others over time coming out of the research findings.

There have been suggestions in the recent past that special, additional regulatory protections should be put into place to protect vulnerable older human volunteers from the risks of participating in research. Such safeguards might consist of greater IRB scrutiny of protocols submitted for approval when the inclusion of older human subjects is proposed, deeper IRB activity in monitoring and supervising research protocols after their initial approval, and allowing individual older participants (regardless of their present mental status) a veto power—the right to give or withhold their assent (Black et al. 2010)—even if informed surrogate consent had already been obtained. Specifically targeted regulations of this nature have not been promulgated at the federal level or enacted in most states, although there is a provision in the federal Elder Justice Act, 42 United States Code §1397k-2 (part of the 2010 Affordable Care Act), ordering that "the Secretary [of the Department of Health and Human Services] promulgate guidelines to assist researchers working in the area of elder abuse, neglect, and exploitation with issues relating to human subject protections." Due to the absence so far of specifically targeted regulations focused on age, older potential research subjects—including those who are severely decisionally compromised—continue to depend on the legal protections found in generic federal and state laws impacting human subjects research. This situation, which effectively leaves the job of imposing any appropriate special protections for older human subjects to the ethical sensitivities of the IRB that is reviewing a particular protocol submission, applies also to other countries besides the United States (Bellemare et al. 2010).

SEE ALSO *Alternative Therapies: II. Ethical and Legal Issues; Dementia; Informed Consent: III. Consent Issues in Human Research; Institutional Review Boards; Research, Unethical; Research Methodology; Research Policy: II. Risk and Vulnerable Groups*

BIBLIOGRAPHY

Alzheimer's Association Research Center. 2013. "Why Participate." Accessed April 30, 2013. http://www.alz.org/research/clinical_trials/why_participate_in_clinical_trials.asp

Bellemare, Suzanne; Gina Bravo; Carole A. Cohen; et al. 2010. "Research with Decisionally Incapacitated Older Adults: Practices of Canadian Research Ethics Boards." *IRB: Ethics and Human Research* 32 (6): 1–8.

Black, Betty S.; Peter V. Rabins; Jeremy Sugarman; and Jason H. Karlawish. 2010. "Seeking Assent and Respecting Dissent in Dementia Research." *American Journal of Geriatric Psychiatry* 18 (1): 77–85.

Brodoff, Lisa. 2009. "Planning for Alzheimer's Disease with Mental Health Advance Directives." *Elder Law Journal* 17 (2): 239–308.

Chao, Steven Z.; Ngan B. Lai; Marian M. Tse; et al. 2011. "Recruitment of Chinese American Elders into Dementia Research." *Gerontologist* 51 (supp. 1): S125–33.

DeVries, Raymond; Kerry A. Ryan; Aimee Stanczyk; et al. 2012. "Public's Approach to Surrogate Consent for Dementia Research: Cautious Pragmatism." *American Journal of Geriatric Psychiatry*. doi: 10.1016/j.jagp.2012.11.010.

Kim, Scott Y. 2011. "The Ethics of Informed Consent in Alzheimer Disease Research." *Nature Reviews: Neurology* 7 (7): 410–14.

Kim, Scott Y.; Jason H. Karlawish; Hyungjin M. Kim; et al. 2011. "Preservation of the Capacity to Appoint a Proxy Decision Maker: Implications for Dementia Research." *Archives of General Psychiatry* 68 (2): 214–20.

Kim, Scott Y.; Hyungjin M. Kim; David S. Knopman; et al. 2011. "Effect of Public Deliberation on Attitudes toward Surrogate Consent for Dementia Research." *Neurology* 77 (24): 2097–104.

Kim, Scott Y.; Hyungjin M. Kim; Kenneth M. Langa; et al. 2009. "Surrogate Consent for Dementia Research: A National Survey of Older Americans." *Neurology* 72 (2): 149–55.

Krestar, Maura L.; Wendy Looman; Sara Powers; et al. 2012. "Including Individuals with Memory Impairment in the Research Process: The Importance of Scales and Response Categories Used in Surveys." *Journal of Empirical Research on Human Research Ethics* 7 (2): 70–79.

National Institute on Aging. 2011. *2010 Alzheimer's Disease Progress Report*. Bethesda, MD: Author.

Naylor, Mary D., Jason H. Karlawish; Steven E. Arnold; et al. 2012. "Advancing Alzheimer's Disease Diagnosis, Treatment, and Care: Recommendations from the Ware Invitational Summit." *Alzheimer's and Dementia* 8 (5): 445–52.

Suhonen, Riitta; Minna Stolt; Veikko Launis; and Helena Leino-Kilpi. 2010. "Research on Ethics in Nursing Care for Older People: A Literature Review." *Nursing Ethics* 17 (3): 337–52.

US Department of Health and Human Services. 2013. "Code of Federal Regulations, Title 45, Public Welfare." Accessed April 30, 2013. http://www.hhs.gov/ohrp/humansubjects/guidance/45cfr46.html

Watts, Geoff. 2012. "Why the Exclusion of Older People from Clinical Research Must Stop." *British Medical Journal* (Overseas and Retired Doctors Edition) 344:e3445.

Wu, Bei; Eric A. Goedereis; Richard J. Crout; and Brenda Plassman. 2010. "Recruitment of Rural and Cognitively Impaired Older Adults for Dental Research." *Special Care in Dentistry* 30 (5): 193–99.

Marshall B. Kapp

Director, Center for Innovative Collaboration in Medicine and Law, Florida State University College of Medicine and College of Law

AGRICULTURE AND BIOTECHNOLOGY

Among approximately 80,000 types of plants that are known to be edible, only about 100 are cultivated intensively worldwide, and of that number fewer than 20, such as rice, maize, wheat, and rapeseed (canola), constitute 90 percent of food crops. This handful of species has been subjected to genetic manipulation for millennia, so that even before the advent of gene splicing they diverged dramatically in genotype and phenotype from their wild ancestors.

THE DISTINCTION BETWEEN CONVENTIONAL BREEDING AND GENETIC ENGINEERING

For thousands of years human beings have altered the genomes of all major crops radically and constantly to change growth and ripening characteristics, speed maturity, eliminate grain shattering, improve taste and reduce toxins, increase size, and even get rid of seeds, as in grapes and bananas. Pictures comparing the wild and cultivated types of any crop invite incredulity, because the differences are so sweeping.

Crops that are very different from each other, such as brussels sprouts, cabbage, cauliflower, and broccoli, derive from the same ancestral stock, whereas other crops, such as bread wheat and canola, are artifacts. Wheat used for bread was created when technologists about 4,000 years ago hybridized tetraploid durum wheat with an inedible goat grass. Canola (Canada oil low acid) was fabricated in the twentieth century by Canadian biologists who assaulted and pummeled by heat, radiation, and other means the genome of an inedible rape (mustard) plant. They selected mutations that eliminated toxic acids and smelly glucosinolates that had made the plentiful rapeseed oil unpalatable. Every cultivar has a story of its own about genetic manipulation and hybridization that explains its stark differences from its wild ancestors. Some of those stories, such as those of the kiwi fruit, strawberry, and tomato, suggest that one can make the agronomic equivalent of a silk purse out of a sow's ear.

To assess ethical objections to agricultural biotechnology one must distinguish concerns that apply to forced mutation, hybridization, and artificial selection generally from those that apply only to the changes—often small by comparison—associated with genetic manipulation. Because conventional breeding techniques have become more sophisticated and in principle may be able to achieve (although through a more arduous process) the same mutations that genetic manipulation accomplishes easily, the boundary between old and new biotechnologies may be hard to draw. The principal difference may be that genetic manipulation performs "outcrosses" that take advantage of the apparent fact that all life has the same origin, whereas conventional techniques cross species that are more closely related or apply pressure to a genome to induce hoped-for changes.

HEALTH RISKS AND BENEFITS OF GENETICALLY MODIFIED FOOD

Critics of genetically modified (GM) food present three kinds of arguments to suggest that it may not be good to eat (Thompson 1997). First, GM foods may produce allergic reactions because known or unknown allergens could be introduced into products people believe are safe. The food industry should and does take this problem seriously; the liability issues alone are sobering. For example, because many people are allergic to peanuts, it would be risky to introduce into other crops genes that code for a protein unique to the peanut. The argument that GM foods should be tested or screened for allergens—and this may be true of all foods—seems incontrovertible.

Second, critics contend that GM foods are not more nutritious or tasty or otherwise better for the consumer than the foods that traditionally have been available (Kneen 1999). This is largely correct. Although all kinds of crops that promise benefits to the consumer are said to be on the horizon, few have materialized. Even the highly touted vitamin A–rich "golden" rice may not be better—or cheaper or more acceptable to target consumers—than simple vitamin pills. As things stand, the benefits of GM crops go principally to farmers. Those benefits are discussed below. Time will tell whether GM foods will offer significant benefits to consumers.

Third, critics invoke the precautionary principle to argue that genetic manipulation is novel and untested: how can one be sure it is safe? (Pence 2002). Defenders of the technology answer that GM crops are hardly new; hybridization, including distant outcrossing, has been the basis of agriculture for millennia (Prakash 2001). The alterations that genetic manipulation achieves are typically more precise and therefore less extensive than those associated with conventional breeding. There is no evidence suggesting that genetic material introduced into a plant from more distant relatives is more dangerous than that introduced from closer cousins. The food product, moreover, will not be any less safe because of the placement of a few nucleotides in its DNA. The oil from GM soy or canola, indeed, will not contain in principle any DNA or protein (there could be traces) and thus will be chemically identical to that from the non-GM plant, which is itself an artifact of conventional breeding. Those who study the extent to which genomes of plant crops have been manipulated over the millennia see no reason to think that twenty-first-century techniques produce food that is inherently more dangerous (Institute of Food Technologists [IFT] 2000).

Those who make this reply do not contend that forced mutation and artificial selection—whether by conventional methods of breeding, more advanced techniques of hybridization, or genetic recombination—are always or necessarily safe. Instead, they contend that the risks are the same across all these ways of re-creating plant genomes. Techniques of embryo rescue, mutation-forcing irradiation, and the type of wide crosses that transformed varieties of nightshade into the tomato, for example, dwarf the twenty-first century's molecular methods in scope and effect.

In a conclusion typical of those of expert panels in this area, the IFT (2000, 23) stated that "crops modified by modern molecular and cellular methods pose risks no different from those modified by earlier genetic methods." Similarly, a report by the Food and Agriculture Organization of the United Nations and the World Health Organization (FAO/WHO) (1991) states:

> Biotechnology has a long history of use in food production and processing. It represents a continuum embracing both traditional breeding techniques and the latest techniques based on molecular biology. The newer biotechnological techniques, in particular, open up very great possibilities of rapidly improving the quantity and quality of food available. The use of these techniques does not result in food that is inherently less safe than that produced by conventional method.

Whether genetically manipulated crops pose significant risks to human safety or health or to the environment remains uncertain. It could be that they pose fewer risks than more traditional methods of crop production. The risks could be different. There is no clear way to test the relative riskiness of genetically manipulated crops other than to note that so far they have not differed from conventionally bred varieties enough to pay for the time of the plaintiff's bar to go after producers in tort. That does say something. As to risks to nature, it is not clear what that means. There is no way to test whether biotechnology is good or bad from an ecological point of view because science has no easy time determining what is valuable in nature from what is not.

GM AND THE FARMER

Farmers eagerly adopt GM varieties, especially herbicide-resistant soybean and insect-resistant cotton and corn, for several economic reasons. Farmers like to rotate soy with corn, for example, because soy, a legume, nourishes the soil that corn depletes. Soy is sensitive, however, to the residues of the glyphosphate herbicide that control weeds in corn. A glyphosphate-tolerant soy (Roundup Ready is the trademark under which Monsanto markets seeds resistant to that company's brand of herbicide) allows rotation, whereas an insect-resistant corn goes far toward eliminating the risk from insects. As farmers produce a more predictable crop and are able to plant more closely because they do not have to cultivate it, their harvests increase. This is a mixed blessing, however, if the resulting surpluses drive down prices. As the risks decrease, moreover, farms become a target for vertical integration by agribusiness.

In the developed world GM crops represent the latest turn in the technological treadmill with the usual consequence: glut. According to the pure theory of the treadmill, as overproduction causes crop prices to fall, farmers adopt new technology to increase yields and lower cost. The early adopters of the new technology eke out a profit by underpricing the competition, thus driving farm prices down further. Those who are late to adopt the technology go broke and sell their land to those who still operate, leading to ever-greater concentration in the industry. The survivors must adopt increasingly more efficient technology, and so the cycle continues (Cochrane 1993). A year of drought in the United States may allow producers in countries such as Brazil to take market share; the treadmill will continue toward drought-resistant crops.

In the twenty-first century, although about 593,000 Americans identify farming as their principal occupation, most of those farmers produce less than $100,000 in annual sales; only about 172,000 farmers produce the bulk of American crops. Demographers expect these numbers to continue to fall. For every full-time farmer under age thirty-five there are three over sixty-five years old. There is a lot of speculation about what agriculture will look like in the mid-twenty-first century, as science and technology continues to displace labor in the production of basic foodstuffs (Berardi and Geisler 1984). The services that are not automated may be provided by contract labor, as is the case with hogs and chickens. As technology reduces risk, there is less reason for agribusinesses, such as Monsanto, to refrain from buying up farmland and contracting its use. The "vertical integration" of agriculture, however, has yet to take place in spite of the economic forces that tend in that direction.

As biotechnology takes the risk out of agriculture, making production more predictable, farming in the traditional sense may become a "cottage" industry like glassblowing, or there may be two different kinds of agriculture: one method utterly industrialized and efficient and the other a "craft" system responsive to aesthetic, cultural, landscape, and noneconomic concerns. Large corporations may integrate food production vertically by absorbing farms. Those companies also may make and market craft food products, just as General Mills manufactures organic foods under the Cascadian Farms and Muir

Glen brands through its Small Planet Foods subsidiary. The regulations that govern the "organic" label may impose costs on production such that only the biggest corporations can muster the legal and technological resources needed to meet "sustainability" labeling requirements.

Critics protest with good reason that industrial farming by megacorporations (with genetic manipulation of seeds being only one aspect of the industrialization of agriculture) undermines the cultural, aesthetic, ethical, ecological, and landscape values and commitments that are associated with pastoralism or with the traditional farming of the agrarian past (Comstock 1987). These critics contend that the products of industrial agriculture, even if they are technically safe, are so manipulated, artificial, and unnatural that they are inherently disgusting, distasteful, demoralizing, and repellent. Even if food safety is not the issue, one can argue that food is more than nourishment; it is part of a way of life and has symbolic and aesthetic value. Genetic manipulation undermines nature and with it the value of food.

These are credible criticisms, but there is a rub. The people who make these charges generally are unwilling to grow their own food. They expect other people, such as farmers, to do it for them. Farmers do the best they can against nearly impossible economic odds. They find that they cannot provide the variety, quality, and abundance of food people demand at anything close to the prices people pay unless they take advantage of the efficiencies offered by technology. Farmers will, however, absorb the relatively higher costs of raising crops free of genetic manipulation if people are willing to pay a large enough premium for them. Just as members of religious communities—Jews who keep kosher, for example—pay a little more for food that meets their requirements, so too may people who prefer non-GM foods. ·Consumers should have an exit option with respect to GM foods; presumably, the market for organic food provides that option. The organic label, however, by no means guarantees that the ingredients were produced in pastoral or nature-friendly ways. It means only that the product meets various requirements set by the US Department of Agriculture that are subject to wrangling by many interest groups.

BOOTLEGGERS AND BAPTISTS

Environmental groups may inadvertently have served the interests of the large industrial corporations, such as Monsanto, that have come to dominate the GM seed market. Local companies, including college or university agricultural "extension" services, are quite capable of the now-routine procedures needed to develop GM seeds suited to the needs of their local farmers. Many commentators suggest, however, that by leveraging the concerns of environmentalists regarding ecological risks, corporations such as Monsanto encouraged the imposition of regulations that require extensive and expensive field testing of GM crops to ensure that they are ecologically safe, whatever that may mean. Only major corporations can afford to pay the millions of dollars these tests often require. Thus ecological safety testing of GM crops is often construed to function primarily as a bar to market entry for firms seeking to compete in their development. This kind of political alliance is often analogized to that between the Baptists and the bootleggers, both of whom supported Prohibition but for opposing reasons (Miller and Conko 2004).

In addition, environmental groups at least initially supported the further industrialization of agriculture—though they may be backing away from this in the early twenty-first century—by calling for the use of ethanol in automobile fuel as a way to cut down on carbon emissions and thus slow climate change. Regulations requiring the use of ethanol in fuel and, even more important, a subsidy of fifty-one cents per gallon paid by the federal government to producers, have turned vast landscapes into monocultures of maize, the principal feedstock for ethanol production. Many analysts have argued that producing ethanol and shipping it to market uses as much fossil fuel as it displaces—in other words, that there is little or no advantage on balance for the climate. Good environmental intentions are often easily bent by economic interests to other ends.

LABELING

Critics of GM foods may agree that they have to send a message not only through political advocacy but also through the consumer choices they make. For consumers to send a message through their choices, they must know which foods contain GM ingredients. No one questions the right of the consumer to make informed choices. Why not require that GM food be labeled to guide consumer choice?

Industry representatives offer three responses to this question. First, they observe that any manufacturer can state on a label or in advertising that its product is free of genetically modified organisms (GMOs) as long as this is true; indeed, the organic label implies as much. If the label does not say that a product is "GMO free" or "organic," the consumer can assume that it is not. The label "may contain GM ingredients," if stamped on food products, would add no information. In international forums, US representatives have appeared to be ready to accept this type of universal label or symbol. The label would underscore the fact that a product not labeled as being GMO free may contain at least some amount of an ingredient from a GM plant.

Second, to segregate commodity flows would be enormously costly. If a drop of soy oil from an engineered plant is mixed into a tank of oil from conventional soy, chemically identical to it, would that taint the whole lot? How well would the tanker have to be cleaned to remove the taint? Those who observe religious restrictions have over the centuries worked out rules to determine, for example, how milk and meat are to be separated and how plates are to be washed. Are the resources available to segregate and trace through the entire food industry flows of commodities, such as canola oil, to segregate by source substances that are nearly indistinguishable chemically? No one objects if those who wish to observe aesthetic, ceremonial, or religious distinctions do so, but this must be done at their own expense. At present purveyors of organic food pay to ensure its identity and history. Those who produce, sell, and buy ordinary products do not want the burden of that expense (IFT 2000).

Third, so many methods of genetic manipulation enter into the production of food at so many levels—bacteria that produce enzymes that catalyze fermentation are genetically engineered but are not found in the cheese, for example—that it would be a nightmare to write regulations that determine what is or is not manipulated. By comparison, to set up rules to define organic food was an exercise as difficult as squaring the circle; in a literal, biological sense all food is organic. Virtually all foods are genetically manipulated as the products of artificial selection; to say which ones are not manipulated in a relevant sense is not easy. Worse, megacorporations design for the label; lawyers and engineers find ways to make the products of industrial processes comply with any set of regulations. This is the way the food industry works. This situation frustrates those who want to get food from Mother Nature rather than from "consolidated agribusiness" (Pollan 2001).

BIOTECHNOLOGY AND THE DEVELOPING WORLD

From a global perspective, increased production of food, however efficient, will not relieve the principal causes of famine and hunger, for these forces involve powerlessness, destitution, civil war, and oppression. The road to food security lies in making governments less corrupt, reducing ethnic and racial rivalries and hatreds, ending civil wars, improving education, providing employment, and halting gender discrimination. Food security is a function of social justice. With or without the latest advances in genetic engineering, a peaceful and just world could feed its people easily.

Farmers can and will plant and harvest as much as they can sell. As the economist Amartya Sen (2000, 67) has written, "Thus food output was held back by a lack of effective demand in the market" rather than by ecological constraints on production. In other words, food is not scarce, but demand is suppressed, because many people are too poor or powerless to purchase food even at the twenty-first century's historically low prices. As Gordon Conway (2000, under "Food Security in a Globalized World") of the Rockefeller Foundation points out, however, even if global production is ample, "there could still be nearly a billion people who lie outside the market and are chronically undernourished." Conway believes that agricultural biotechnology can benefit peasants who depend on local subsistence farming. In Kenya, for example, scientists funded by Monsanto have developed a recombinant sweet potato that resists a devastating virus. Edible vaccines may be engineered into crops such as bananas. A rust-resistant cassava could make a huge difference in Africa. There is no general economic theory that shows why or how biotechnology can benefit people in developing countries. A long list of examples can be supplied, however, of the nearly miraculous potential of genetic engineering to relieve malnutrition and hunger on a crop-by-crop, problem-by-problem basis.

As the developmental economists Robin Broad and John Cavanaugh (1995–1996, 28) wrote, however, biotechnological innovations that create "substitutes for everything from vanilla to cocoa and coffee threaten to eliminate the livelihood of millions of Third World agricultural workers." Vanilla cultured in laboratories costs a fifth as much as vanilla extracted from beans and thus jeopardizes the livelihoods of tens of thousands of vanilla farmers in Madagascar. A rapeseed engineered to express high levels of laurate, an ingredient in soaps and shampoos, allows growers in Canada to take markets away from producers of palm oil in developing countries. Asian and African farmers have planted wormwood, an herb that contains artemisinic used to treat malaria. Michael Specter (2009) reported that synthetic biology, which produces DNA molecules artificially, can produce this substance at a fraction of the cost.

In general, the genetic engineering of crops leads to biosubstitution, biorelocation, and bioreplication, enabling industrialized countries to produce the equivalent of traditionally tropical products and thus cease importing those commodities from developing countries. Developing nations by virtue of the same technology may flood world markets. The technological treadmill is poised to increase commodity surpluses, especially of commodities such as cocoa and coffee that sustain the developing world, and therefore, ironically, to result in further impoverishment and further declines in demand. Rather than tending by its logic to make everyone better off, biotechnology may make wealthy countries more wealthy while taking from poor countries their monopolies of the few export commodities that once were exclusively theirs. It could also work the other way. Brazil, once regarded as a third world country, has industrialized its production so well that it challenges US supremacy in soybean production. According to the *AGProfessional* (2012) newswire, "There is a good chance that Brazil will be the world's largest soybean producer during the 2012/13 season." No one really knows which nations will surpass others in bioproduction based on biotechnology.

THE ECOLOGICAL IMPLICATIONS OF BIOTECHNOLOGY

Critics contend that GM crops are likely to have deleterious environmental effects. They argue, for example, that GM crops will lead to greater pesticide resistance among weeds and insects because genetic material from GM organisms will drift into wild varieties; plant leaves and pollen that contain Bt or other insecticides will kill nontarget species; drought tolerance, salt tolerance, cold hardiness, and other feats of genetic engineering will permit farms to expand into wild areas that formerly were not arable; and animals, particularly fish such as salmon, will hybridize with wild stocks, domesticating all of nature (Graziano 1996). Nothing will evolve free of human influence.

Although all these concerns are credible, defenders of biotechnology respond that these objections are not specific to genetic engineering but apply to agriculture and aquaculture generally. Indeed, genetic manipulation technologies may increase only slightly—or indeed decrease slightly—the relentless, total, and overwhelming impact of agriculture on the natural world. Even before the discovery of the structure of DNA, the entire midsection of the United States was turned from prairie or savanna ecosystems into amber waves of grain. To restore the prairie, ecologists have searched for native species in abandoned cemeteries and railroad rights-of-way. Modern agriculture roots out nature literally and figuratively and replaces it with monocultures that cover millions of acres. Nature is equally devastated whether those monocultures consist of conventional hybrids or GM plants.

Insecticides promote resistance whether they are sprayed on or bred into a plant. When they are sprayed from airplanes over large areas, these chemicals may kill nontarget species more extensively than they would if they were engineered into the leaves of crops. Weeds subjected to dousings of glyphosphate eventually must evolve to withstand the herbicide; the addition of herbicide resistance in crops may hasten this inevitable process somewhat. Crops that are the products of conventional breeding are no more "natural" than GM crops are. Indeed, human-caused mutation and selection have just taken longer to achieve the desired properties. These conventional hybrids—both crops and animals, including fish—can intermingle their genes with wild types if and when wild types are found.

The effect of farming on nature can be seen best in Europe, where agriculture counts as "nature," with the alternative being urban or suburban development. Americans think of nature as wilderness, although the wilderness that remains is managed, designated wilderness—a kind of botanical garden maintained in national parks. To estimate the extent to which GM plants threaten nature, one must ask what "nature" is—whether it is more than the smile of the Cheshire cat. Environmental historians, such as William Cronon (1983), state that agriculture and industry have transformed the landscape so thoroughly so many times over that it is hard to say what people are trying to protect. In addition, the pressure of *Homo sapiens* on other organisms has directed their evolution for millennia; humans are the "keystone" species that structures the natural environment that people consider wild (McKibben 1989).

HUMAN BIOTECHNOLOGY

Many of the most controversial technologies bioethicists study in medicine—artificial fertilization and cloning are obvious examples—originated in the barnyard. The genetic manipulation of animals will be the proving ground for the genetic manipulation and enhancement of human beings. What may be most interesting in the ethical study of agricultural biotechnology therefore may lie in its effort to identify something "natural"—some essence, condition, history, or pedigree—that makes an animal characteristically itself and that can be lost as a result of genetic engineering. If this essence proves elusive in the agricultural context or if it turns out that everything physically possible is equally natural, then by analogy it may not be possible to identify any limits in the nature of humans (e.g., mortality) that people may not try to transcend. Human beings may be tempted, then, to improve human qualities through germ cell engineering just as they have improved the qualities of plants and animals.

The distinction between the "natural" and the "artificial" may not survive the advance of biotechnology because everything, including the human genome, may become both. This makes the human species responsible for everything, or it greatly diminishes the "given" or contingent in nature. The ability to manipulate the human genome—as people have manipulated the genomes, say, of salmon and chickens—for many technical reasons is a long way off. Indeed, it still may be considered science fiction. Someday human beings may cultivate themselves as they do other organisms. The idea that people eventually may apply to the human genome the same techniques by which they have changed crops and livestock—now only a speculation of science fiction—could be the ultimate irony of agricultural biotechnology.

SEE ALSO *Animal Welfare and Rights: I. Ethical Perspectives on the Treatment and Status of Animals; Animal Welfare and Rights: VI. Animals in Agriculture and Factory Farming; Cloning: I. Scientific Background;*

Environmental Ethics: I. Overview; Environmental Policy and Law; Food; Technology: I. History of Medical Technology

BIBLIOGRAPHY

AG Professional. 2012. "Brazil's Soybean Production May Exceed U.S. Production." November 6. Accessed November 27, 2012. http://www.agprofessional.com/resource-centers/soybean/news/Brazils-soybean-production-may-exceed-US-production-177308741.html

Bailey, Britt, and Marc Lappe, eds. 2002. *Engineering the Farm: The Social and Ethical Aspects of Agricultural Biotechnology.* Washington, DC: Island Press.

Berardi, Gigi M., and Charles C. Geisler, eds. 1984. *The Social Consequences and Challenges of New Agricultural Technologies.* Boulder, CO: Westview Press.

Broad, Robin, and John Cavanaugh. 1995–1996. "Don't Neglect the Impoverished South." *Foreign Policy,* no. 101 (Winter): 18–35.

Cochrane, Willard W. 1993. *The Development of American Agriculture: A Historical Analysis.* 2nd ed. Minneapolis: University of Minnesota Press.

Comstock, Gary, ed. 1987. *Is There a Moral Obligation to Save the Family Farm?* Ames: Iowa State University Press.

Conway, Gordon. 2000. "Genetically Modified Crops: Risks and Promise." *Conservation Ecology* 4 (1): 2. Accessed October 15, 2012. http://www.ecologyandsociety.org/vol4/iss1/art2/

Cornell University, College of Agriculture and Life Sciences. 2012. "National Agricultural Biotechnology Council." Accessed October 15, 2012. http://nabc.cals.cornell.edu/

Cronon, William. 1983. *Changes in the Land: Indians, Colonists, and the Ecology of New England.* New York: Hill and Wang.

Food and Agriculture Organization of the United Nations and World Health Organization (FAO/WHO). 1991. "Strategies for Assessing the Safety of Foods Produced by Biotechnology: Report of a Joint FAO/WHO Consultation." Geneva: World Health Organization.

Graziano, Karen M. 1996. "Biosafety Protocol: Recommendations to Ensure the Safety of the Environment." *Colorado Journal of International Environmental Law and Policy* 7:179–96.

Institute of Food Technologists (IFT). 2000. "IFT Expert Report on Biotechnology and Foods." *Food Technology* 54 (8): 124–36.

Kneen, Brewster. 1999. *Farmageddon: Food and the Culture of Biotechnology.* Gabriola Island, BC: New Society Publishers.

McKibben, Bill. 1989. *The End of Nature.* New York: Random House.

Miller, Henry I., and Gregory Conko. 2004. *The Frankenfood Myth: How Protest and Politics Threaten the Biotech Revolution.* Westport, CT: Praeger.

National Research Council, Committee on Genetically Modified Pest-Protected Plants. 2000. *Genetically Modified Pest-Protected Plants: Science and Regulation.* Washington, DC: National Academies Press.

Paarlberg, Robert. 2000. "The Global Food Fight." *Foreign Affairs* 79 (3): 24–38.

Pence, Gregory E. 2002. *Designer Food: Mutant Harvest or Breadbasket of the World?* Lanham, MD: Rowman and Littlefield.

Pew Charitable Trusts. 2012. Pew Initiative on Food and Biotechnology. Accessed October 15, 2012. http://www.pewhealth.org/projects/pew-initiative-on-food-and-biotechnology-85899367237

Pollan, Michael. 2001. "Behind the Organic-Industrial Complex." *New York Times Magazine,* May 13.

Prakash, Channapatna S. 2001. "The Genetically Modified Crop Debate in the Context of Agricultural Evolution." *Plant Physiology* 126 (1): 8–15.

Sen, Amartya. 1994. "Population: Delusion and Reality." *New York Review of Books,* September 22: 41.

Smale, Melinda, and José Falck-Zepeda, eds. 2012. "Farmers and Researchers Discovering Biotech Crops: Experiences Measuring Economic Impacts among New Adopters." Special issue, *AgBioForum* 15 (2). Accessed October 15, 2012. http://www.agbioforum.org/

Specter, Michael. 2009. "A Life of Its Own: Where Will Synthetic Biology Lead Us?" *New Yorker,* September 28. Accessed November 26, 2012. http://www.newyorker.com/reporting/2009/09/28/090928fa_fact_specter#ixzz2DUCOS1Sr

Thompson, Paul B. 1997. *Food Biotechnology in Ethical Perspective.* London: Blackie Academic.

Union of Concerned Scientists. 2012. "Food and Agriculture." Accessed October 15, 2012. http://www.ucsusa.org/food_and_agriculture/

Mark Sagoff (2004, 2014)
Professor, Institute for Philosophy and Public Policy, George Mason University

AIDS

This entry consists of the following:

I. PUBLIC HEALTH ISSUES

At the conclusion of *Plagues and People,* a magisterial account of epidemics and their impact on history, William McNeill asserts, "Infectious disease, which antedates the emergence of humankind, will last as long as humanity itself and will surely remain, as it has been hitherto, one of the fundamental parameters and determinants of human history" (1976, 291). In the mid-1970s this observation seemed overdrawn, especially in relation to economically advanced societies, where chronic diseases had displaced infectious threats to communal well-being. Yet just five years later, McNeill's comment seemed prescient.

In June 1981, the first cases of what would ultimately be called acquired immunodeficiency syndrome (AIDS) were reported by the Centers for Disease Control (CDC). Within three years of the first CDC report, human immunodeficiency virus (HIV), the viral agent responsible for AIDS, was identified. Although those who were infected could experience a long disease-free state—50 percent remained symptom-free for up to ten years—in the end the virus attacked the immune system, resulting in a series of ultimately fatal opportunistic disorders. By the beginning of the twenty-first century, it was estimated that approximately 900,000 Americans and more than 42 million people worldwide were infected. Although found on every continent, AIDS had made its most stunning impact on Africa. Projections by the World Health Organization (WHO) forecast a grim picture, with catastrophic spread of HIV in Asia and the former Soviet Union.

EXCEPTIONALISM AND THE ETHICS OF TESTING, REPORTING, AND PARTNER NOTIFICATION

In the early and mid-1980s, at the outset of the American encounter with AIDS, it was necessary to face a set of fundamental questions: Did the history of responses to lethal infectious diseases provide lessons about how best to contain the spread of HIV? Should the policies developed to control sexually transmitted diseases or other communicable conditions be applied to AIDS? If AIDS were not to be so treated, what would justify such differential policies?

To understand the importance of these questions, it is necessary to recall that conventional approaches to public health threats typically provided a warrant, when deemed appropriate, for mandating compulsory examination and screening, breaching the confidentiality of the clinical relationship by reporting to public health registries the names of those diagnosed with "dangerous diseases," imposing treatment, and, in the most extreme cases, confining persons through the power of quarantine. To be sure, many aspects of this public health tradition, forged at the outset of the twentieth century, had been modulated over the decades, in part because of changes in the patterns of morbidity and mortality.

Nevertheless, it was the specter of the historically coercive aspects of the public health tradition that most concerned proponents of civil liberties and advocates of gay rights and bioethics as they considered the potential direction of public health policy in the presence of AIDS, a disease that so disproportionately affected disfavored groups—gay men, drug users, the poor in minority communities. In place of the conventional approach to public health threats, there emerged an alternative view—broadly defined as exceptionalism (Bayer 1991)—that took as its starting point the need to craft policies that were persuasive rather than coercive, which viewed the protection of the rights of those who were infected as integral rather than as antagonistic to the goals of disease prevention. For those who advanced this new perspective, privacy and confidentiality were to be accorded great importance. In all, the goal was to avoid measures and practices that might be counterproductive, which might "drive the epidemic underground" by inspiring fear and distrust rather than fostering engagement between public health officials and those most at risk. How the exceptionalist perspective with its commitment to noncoercive approaches to HIV affected policy is most clearly illustrated in the debates over HIV testing, reporting of HIV, and partner notification efforts.

At a global level the exceptionalist perspective was framed in the diction of human rights. It is one of the remarkable and significant consequences of the AIDS epidemic that out of the context of enormous suffering and death there emerged a forceful set of ideas linking the domains of health and human rights. At first, the effort centered on the observation that protecting individuals from discrimination and unwarranted intrusions on liberty were, contrary to previous epidemics, crucial to protecting public health and interrupting the spread of HIV. But in fairly short order, the scope of the health and human rights perspective expanded dramatically to focus on the ways in which the most fundamental social arrangements rendered individuals and communities vulnerable to HIV. Racial and ethnic minorities, those who were marginalized, and women were at risk because of their subordinate status. In the face of such an understanding, nothing short of social change could be adequate to the challenge posed by the AIDS epidemic (Oppenheimer, Bayer, and Colgrove 2002). Jonathan Mann, who led the WHO's first efforts on AIDS, played a central and defining role in the elaboration of these ideas.

HIV TESTING

From the moment of its introduction in 1985, the HIV test became the subject of intense debate. Fear that those identified as having HIV might be subject to discrimination and stigma; concern about how the diagnosis of HIV infection, in the absence of effective therapy, could produce unbearable psychological burdens; and a belief that testing had little to do with behavioral change led AIDS activists generally, and gay leaders specifically, to adopt a posture of hostility and/or skepticism regarding the test. On the other hand, many public health officials believed that the identification of infected persons could play a crucial role in fostering behavioral change. Out of their confrontations emerged a broad consensus that, except in a very few well-defined circumstances, people should be tested only with their informed, voluntary, and specific consent (Bayer 1989).

Much of the early discussion of HIV testing occurred in the context of extreme therapeutic limits. And indeed in the epidemic's early years the primary function of testing was as an adjunct to prevention efforts. By 1990, as a result of clinical developments—the belief that treatment with zidovudine (also known as azidothymidine, or AZT) could delay the onset of symptomatic AIDS and the recognition of the importance of primary prophylaxis against *Pneumocystis carinii* pneumonia—the medical significance of identifying those with early HIV disease had become clear. Consequently, the clinical and political context—involving a wide range of constituencies—of the debate about testing underwent a fundamental change (Bayer, Levine, and Wolf 1986). Gay organizations began to urge homosexual and bisexual men to have their antibody status determined under confidential or anonymous conditions. Physicians pressed for AIDS to be incorporated into the medical mainstream and for the HIV-antibody test to be treated like other blood tests—that is, given with the presumed consent of the patient.

Pressure to shift the paradigm of testing away from the exacting standard of informed consent was especially pronounced in the case of pregnant women and newborns (Bayer 1995). Diagnostic progress was to make it possible to determine whether HIV-positive newborns were truly infected soon after birth, and the improved prospects of clinical management were to make such determinations for infected infants appear all the more critical. So it is not surprising that pediatricians became increasingly impatient with the strict regimen of explicit and specific consent that surrounded the testing of newborns for HIV (Hegearty and Abrams 1992)—all the more so because routine and unconsented testing of newborns for inborn errors of metabolism such as phenylketonuria was mandated in virtually every state and had provoked little ethical objection.

In 1994 a research study discovered that the administration of zidovudine during pregnancy could reduce the rate of maternal–fetal HIV transmission by two-thirds (to about 8%) (Connor et al. 1994). In the aftermath of that finding, pressure mounted to ensure that infected women were identified early in pregnancy. In 1996 the American Medical Association's House of Delegates passed a resolution calling for mandatory testing of pregnant women (Shelton 1996). Even the Institute of Medicine (1999), which early in the epidemic had opposed testing policies that abrogated the privacy rights of pregnant women, was by the end of the 1990s to endorse routine testing on the basis of an informed right of refusal, a much less exacting standard than specific informed consent.

The retreat from the exacting standard of specific informed consent with pretest counseling has taken the form of efforts to integrate HIV testing into clinical practice where standards of presumed consent prevail. In 2006, frustrated by the fact that more than 25% of Americans with HIV infection were unaware of their status and that almost 40 percent of those with newly diagnosed AIDS discovered that they were infected less than a year before diagnosis, the CDC proposed that HIV screening be routinely offered in all health care settings. Importantly, the CDC urged that the standards of consent be significantly altered. Rather than the "opt-in" approach where individuals had to assert that they agreed to be tested, the CDC proposed that consent be presumed with the possibility of "opting out." For some this move presented an effort to make it easier to say "yes." For others it was an attempt to make it more difficult to say "no." Hence it was a burdening of the consent process.

At a global level a debate driven by the importance of identifying those with HIV infection also occurred. It too confronted the question of pretest counseling and the standards of consent that ought to apply.

In May 2007 the Joint United Nations Programme on HIV/AIDS (UNAIDS) and the WHO issued new guidelines on HIV testing. Prepared to meet the demands of the AIDS pandemic and the prospects of extending the benefits of antiretroviral therapy to regions where such treatment had been all but out of reach, the new guidance was the product of an extended period of sometimes acrimonious controversy both within the two United Nations (UN) agencies and globally. Those pressing for change had argued that a paradigm of testing that had emerged at a time when little could be done for those infected with HIV was inappropriate in the current moment. Those who viewed with skepticism, if not hostility, the claims that current practice and stringent ethical standards had become an impediment to effectively confronting the challenge of AIDS saw in the proposed changes a threat to the bedrock ethical principles of informed consent (Bayer and Edington 2009).

REPORTING OF HIV CASES

A course similar to that which occurred with testing characterized the debate surrounding case reporting for HIV infection. Given the profound stigma that surrounded AIDS in the epidemic's first years, and the extent to which individuals with or at risk for HIV feared the social consequences of having their diagnoses made public, it is not surprising that confidentiality of AIDS-related information assumed great salience. From the pragmatic perspective of public health officials, it was crucial to preserve confidentiality as a way of ensuring that those at risk would come forward for testing and counseling (Institute of Medicine 1986). Others objected on grounds of principle. Privacy was a value that should not be set aside lightly.

However central were the claims of privacy and the duty to protect confidentiality, they were not absolutes. One of the conventionally accepted limits to those claims occurred when individuals with infectious diseases were reported by name to confidential public health registries. It was thus not surprising that despite concerns about privacy, little opposition existed in the epidemic's first years to making AIDS cases reportable by name (Bayer 1989). The acceptance of AIDS case reporting requirements was facilitated by the well-established record of state health departments in protecting such records from unwarranted disclosure.

With the inception of HIV testing, however, debate emerged about whether the names of all infected persons, regardless of whether they had received an AIDS diagnosis, should be reported. Activists who accepted AIDS case reporting opposed HIV reporting because of heightened concerns about privacy, confidentiality, and discrimination. For them the potential public health benefits of reporting were too limited and the burden on those who would be the subject of reporting too great to justify an abrogation of privacy.

While many public health officials, especially those who came from states with large AIDS caseloads, opposed HIV reporting because of its potential effect on the willingness of people to seek testing and counseling, some public health officials did become strong advocates of such reporting. In their arguments in favor of such reporting, they sought to underscore the extent to which the public health benefits of HIV reporting would be similar to those that followed from more broadly conceived reporting requirements, such as those that applied to syphilis, tuberculosis, and AIDS itself (Vernon 1986).

As therapeutic advances began to emerge in the late 1980s, and as the logic of distinguishing between HIV and AIDS became increasingly difficult to sustain, fissures began to appear in the relatively broad and solid alliance against named HIV reporting. At the end of November 1990, the CDC declared its support for HIV reporting, which it asserted could "enhance the ability of local, state and national agencies to project the level of required resources" for care and prevention services (CDC 1990, 861). The House of Delegates of the American Medical Association also endorsed the reporting of names (Bayer 1999).

Central to the argument for HIV name reporting was the assertion that AIDS case reporting captured an epidemic that was as much as a decade old and that an accurate picture of the incidence and prevalence of HIV infection—especially in light of the impact of treatment—required a surveillance system based on HIV case reporting. At the end of 1999, in the face of lingering opposition from most AIDS activists, the CDC finally proposed that all states put in place an HIV reporting system. And while it left open the possibility of reliance on unique identifiers that met strict performance criteria, it was clear that the use of names was viewed as preferable (CDC 1999). Remarkably, of those states that adopted HIV case surveillance after the publication of the CDC's recommendations, virtually all adopted coded systems.

Since 2008 all states have required reporting to name-based confidential health department systems. More recently, innovative attempts and use required reporting of HIV, viral loads, and CD4 counts (a marker of immune status) to identify individuals who had never entered treatment, whose treatment has been interrupted, who had dropped out of treatment, or whose treatment appeared to be inadequate reflect a willingness to use surveillance data for clinical ends that would have been unthinkable on technical and ethical grounds in the recent past (Fairchild and Bayer 2011).

In Europe the situation was quite different until most recently. The unique constellation of social, psychological, and political factors surrounding the AIDS epidemic and especially concerns about stigma and of driving those most at risk away from contact with the health care system led many nations to avoid name reporting for HIV. Because of concerns about privacy and confidentiality, most European countries have not conducted name-based notification. In 2006, 28 nations in the WHO's European Region used coded identifiers for HIV case reports. In 11 countries, so great were the concerns about potential breaches of privacy that the codes contained no name-related elements. Only 12 nations used full names for HIV notification, 10 of which were in Eastern Europe or the former Soviet Union. The exceptions were Iceland and Israel.

PARTNER NOTIFICATION

In the controversy over partner notification the limits of privacy were also encountered. What emerged as a source of contention in the first decade of the epidemic was the extent to which the protection of identifiable third parties who had been or were currently placed at risk for HIV by already infected individuals provided a warrant for public health interventions. This was not a new issue; it had been confronted in the context of psychiatry in the so-called *Tarasoff* doctrine (from the mid-1970s court case, *Tarasoff v. Regents of the University of California*), which held that physicians who knew that their patients were about to inflict serious harm on other identifiable individuals had a duty to act to warn or protect. While opinions differed about the wisdom of such efforts, there was little principled objection to breaching confidentiality under such circumstances.

Thus in the mid- to late 1980s, when many AIDS activists argued that the principle of confidentiality had to be inviolable, and when public health officials were loath to endorse legislative mandates requiring third-party notification, many ethicists suggested that protection of unsuspecting sexual partners took precedence over privacy. In 1988 the American Medical Association's House of Delegates embraced the duty to warn.

Some states sought to meet the challenge of endangered third parties by enacting statutes that secured a "privilege to disclose." Under such laws physicians could, if they chose, breach confidentiality to warn unsuspecting individuals but would not be held liable if they failed to do so.

The depth of antagonism to public health interventions in matters of sexual intimacy was further demonstrated by the deep suspicion of contact tracing programs, under which public health officials would notify those who had been placed at risk without divulging the identity of the individual who had imposed the risk. Such efforts were typically voluntary and relied on the willingness of index patients to provide the names of their contacts.

Despite the four decades of experience with contact tracing, efforts to undertake such public health interventions in the context of AIDS met with fierce resistance in the first years of the epidemic. Opposition by gay leaders and civil liberties groups had a profound impact on the response of public health officials, especially in states with relatively large numbers of AIDS cases, where contact tracing efforts remained all but moribund (Bayer 1989). In part the opposition was fueled by the fact that throughout most of the 1980s, no therapy could be offered to asymptomatic infected individuals. Thus, the role of contact tracing in the context of HIV infection differed radically from its role in the context of other sexually transmitted diseases. In the latter case, effective treatments could be offered to notified partners. Once cured, such individuals would no longer pose a threat of transmission. In the case of HIV, nothing could be offered other than information about possible exposure.

Public health officials saw in such information an opportunity to target efforts to foster behavioral changes among individuals still engaging in high-risk behavior—behavior that could place both the individual contacted and future partners at risk; for such officials, this was reason enough to undertake the process. For opponents of contact tracing, the very effort to reach out to such individuals represented a profound intrusion on privacy with little or no compensating benefit. The task of behavioral change, they asserted, could be achieved more effectively and efficiently through community-based HIV prevention efforts (Bayer and Toomey 1992).

Early misapprehensions about the extent to which public health officials typically relied on overt coercion in the process of contact tracing, and the degree to which confidentiality might be compromised, had by the end of the 1980s all but vanished. With such concerns allayed, many gay leaders had come to recognize that partner notification, in fact, could be a "useful tool" in efforts to control AIDS (Schram 1988). The debate began to shift to one centered on relative efficacy (American Public Health Association 1988). That dispute was informed by questions that had already surfaced about the usefulness of contact tracing in the control of syphilis in populations where individuals had large numbers of sexual partners, many of whom were anonymous (Andrus et al. 1990).

PUBLIC HEALTH AND CLINICAL RESEARCH

The HIV epidemic provided the circumstances for the emergence of a broad and potent political movement that sought to reshape radically the conditions under which research was undertaken. Brought into question were the role of the randomized clinical trial, the importance of placebo controls, the centrality of academic research institutions, the dominance of scientists over subjects, the sharp distinction between research and therapy, and the protectionist ethos of *The Belmont Report* (the landmark formulation of research ethics issued in 1978 and published in 1979 by the National Commission for the Protection of Human Subjects of Biomedical and Behavioral Research). Although scholars concerned with the methodological demands of sound research and ethicists committed to the protection of research subjects played a crucial role in the ensuing discussions, both as defenders of the received wisdom and as critics, the debate was largely driven by the articulate demands of those most threatened by AIDS (Epstein 1996). Most prominent were groups such as the People with AIDS Coalition and ACT UP, organizations made up primarily of white, gay men. They were joined by community-based physicians who identified closely with the plight of their patients.

What was so stunning—disconcertingly so to some, exciting to others—was the rhythm of challenge and response. Rather than the careful exchange of academic arguments, there was the mobilization of disruptive and effective political protest. Most remarkable was the core demand. As Carol Levine noted in 1988, "The shortage of proven therapeutic alternatives for AIDS and the belief that trials are, in and of themselves, beneficial have led to the claim that people have a right *to be* research subjects. This is the exact opposite of the tradition started with Nuremberg—that people have a right *not to be* research subjects" (172). That striking reversal resulted in a rejection of the model of research conducted at remote academic centers, with restrictive (protective) standards of access and strict adherence to the "gold standard" of the randomized clinical trial.

Having blurred the distinction between research and treatment—expressed forcefully through the slogan "A Drug Trial Is Health Care Too"—those insistent on radical reform sought to open wide the points of entry to new "therapeutic" agents both within and outside of clinical trials; they demanded that the paternalistic ethical warrant for the protection of the vulnerable from research be replaced by an ethical regime informed by respect for the autonomous choice of potential subjects who could weigh, for themselves, the potential risks and benefits of new treatments for HIV infection. Moreover, the revisionists demanded a basic reconceptualization of the relationship between researchers and subjects. In place of protocols imposed from above, they proposed a more egalitarian and democratic model in which negotiation would replace a scientific authority. Indeed, research "subjects" were now thought of as "participants." Furthermore, the role of the carefully controlled clinical trial as providing protection against the wide-scale use of drugs whose safety and efficacy had not been proven no longer commanded unquestioned respect (Bayer 1990).

The new perspective did not go without challenge, of course. Some were concerned that the proposed regime would make all but impossible the conduct of research so crucial to the needs of those with HIV/AIDS ("Parallel Track" 1989), while others feared that desperate individuals would, in the absence of the now discredited (paternalistic) ethos, be subject to deception (Annas 1989).

The AIDS-inspired challenge to the ethics of research was not restricted to issues within the United States. Just as the protective regime surrounding research in the United States was a product of a history of abuse, efforts to enunciate ethical standards for the conduct of research in third world nations was shaped by a history of exploitation, a history characterized by investigations on the poor designed to serve the interests of the privileged. Central to those efforts was the belief that the ethical principles first encountered in industrialized nations had direct bearing on the norms that should govern research in very different settings (IJsselmuiden and Faden 1996). Such universalism took as a given the need to assume that insights regarding cultural differences not serve as the basis for moral relativism.

Just as individual informed consent was the first principle of the ethics of research in advanced industrial nations, it was at the heart of the codes designed to guide research in the poorest nations. To preclude exploitation, international consensus also existed on the extent to which it was critical that research be responsive to the health needs and priorities of the community in which it is to be carried out (Council for International Organizations of Medical Sciences [CIOMS] 1993). What would remain a matter of uncertainty, however, was whether the needs of the poorest and the requirement of responsiveness could justify research that would be unacceptable in the richest nations—whether the principle of universalism could accommodate research in Burundi that would be prohibited in Brooklyn.

That was the issue that would animate a furious international debate occasioned by the 1994 finding that AZT administered to infected women in the second and third trimesters and to their infants for six weeks could reduce by two-thirds the rate of mother-to-child HIV transmission (Connor et al. 1994). Although superficially a conflict over a technical matter involving research design—the role of placebos—the dispute touched on the deepest questions of what ethical conduct meant in a world characterized by great inequalities and profound inequities.

Given the burden of pediatric AIDS in Africa and Asia, it was a matter of some urgency that trials begin to determine whether radically cheaper alternatives to the standard regimen could achieve at least some measure of reduced maternal–fetal HIV transmission. In June 1994 a special consultation of the WHO considered the challenge and called for the launching of studies to achieve that goal. The consultation made clear its conclusion that placebo-controlled trials—trials in which a comparison is made between an inert substance and the potentially active agent—"offer the best option for obtaining rapid and scientifically valid results."

There was no question that a placebo-controlled trial would have been considered unethical in the United States or any other advanced industrial nation. No trial that denied access to the effective standard, or to an intervention thought to hold the promise of being at least as effective as, if not more effective than, the prevailing standard of care, would have satisfied the requirements of ethical review. The question posed by the furious controversy that unfolded was whether it was ethical to conduct such a trial in a poor country. In 1997 the *New England Journal of Medicine* gave its answer unambiguously: "Only when there is no known effective treatment is it ethical to compare a potential new treatment with a placebo. When effective treatment exists, a placebo may not be used. Instead, subjects in the control group of the study must receive the best known treatment" (Angell 1997, 847).

Given this premise, the *Journal* rejected as irrelevant the fact that health care available in most third world countries provided nothing like health care available in industrialized countries. Citing for authority the Declaration of Helsinki—the international code of research ethics adapted by the World Medical Association in 1964—the editorial noted that control groups had to be provided with the best current therapy, not simply that which was available locally. "The shift in wording between 'best' and 'local' may be slight, but the implications are profound. Acceptance of this ethical relativism could result in widespread exploitation of vulnerable Third World populations for research programs that could not be carried out in the sponsor country" (Angell 1997, 848).

Those who rejected the *Journal*'s viewpoint made clear that placebo-controlled trials were dictated by the urgency of the situation. Only placebo-controlled trials could provide "definitive," "clear," "firm" answers about which interventions worked, thus allowing governments to make "[a] sound judgment about the appropriateness and financial feasibility of providing the intervention" (Varmus and Satcher 1997, 1004). The failure to employ a placebo would have made it difficult to clearly determine whether the affordable but less effective intervention was better than no intervention at all. In short, they concluded that placebos were crucial to policy makers required to make relatively costly decisions under conditions marked by profound poverty and scarce public health resources (Varmus and Satcher 1997).

Paralleling the debates over maternal–fetal transmission of HIV were those that surfaced over the ethics of AIDS vaccine trials. In this case the focus was on those research participants who might become infected with HIV during a trial. On the one hand there were those who argued that such individuals be provided with optimal care—the retroviral therapy available in the developed countries. On the other hand there were those who asserted that care should reflect that which was consistent with what was available in the host nation (Bayer 2000). So divisive was this controversy that UNAIDS (2000) could not come to an agreement on the appropriate ethical norm and indeed had to settle for a procedural rather than substantive solution, a solution that focused on how to reach acceptable agreement rather than one that put forth a standard to guide such deliberations.

Thus were the issues joined. These controversies ultimately provoked an international effort to consider ethical standards of research in the third world. The World Medical Association undertook a series of consultations on the revision of the Declaration of Helsinki; the CIOMS did so as well. Finally, within the United States, which funded much of the international research that had been subject to scrutiny, the National Bioethics Advisory Commission took up the issue of studies in poor nations.

Whereas those who saw in any effort to craft "flexible" standards that reflected the uniquely pressing context of international poverty and inequality the treacherous embrace of moral relativism, their opponents persisted in arguing that a failure to consider the context of investigation was a failure of moral understanding. Principles could be universal; their application could not be rigid (Singer and Benatar 2001; Benatar and Singer 2000).

Finally, we turn to the question of epidemiological research. Like other matters involving scientific investigation the global AIDS epidemic had an enormous impact on international discussions, although it must be emphasized that broader concerns about morbidity and mortality were involved.

EPIDEMIOLOGICAL RESEARCH

Epidemiologists and ethicists began to discuss whether the principle of informed consent extended to the use of records and whether the insistence on individual consent of large numbers of individuals, many of whom would be difficult or impossible to locate, would render epidemiological research virtually *impossible*. "The clash between the privacy rights of persons and the need for access to and disclosure of personal health-related information," noted one observer, "is the most frequent ethical dilemma to confront epidemiologists."

In 1991 the CIOMS addressed the issues imposed by the use of existing clinical records as part of its broader analysis of the ethical issues posed by epidemiological studies. It acknowledged that prior efforts to provide ethical guidance for biomedical research were focused on "patients and individual subjects" and were not sufficient for studies involving "groups" of people. Thus, while emphasizing the importance of the principles of research ethics first propounded in *The Belmont Report*, it recognized that their application in the epidemiological context would require flexibility.

Most important, the CIOMS epidemiological guidelines, like those from nations that had addressed these issues earlier, noted that individual informed consent was not always practical in epidemiological studies. While asserting that individuals and their representatives should "normally" be told that their medical records or stored tissue samples might be used for future epidemiological studies, CIOMS acknowledged that such notification might not have always been undertaken. In the end, it was the duty of researchers who sought to undertake such records-based studies "to explain to an ethical review committee how the study would be ethical in [the absence of consent]: it may be impractical to locate subjects whose records are to be examined" (CIOMS 1991).

In lieu of individual consent, CIOMS suggested that the agreement of a representative of the community or group in which the proposed study would be conducted could be important. It recognized, however, that the identification and selection of such representatives might pose difficulties, especially if the "group" under study was, in fact, created by the investigators.

In 2009, after an extended process of consultation, CIOMS proposed revised guidelines for epidemiological research. In a fundamental way, they confirmed the analysis issued two decades earlier about the conditions under which epidemiological studies could be conducted in the absence of individual informed consent. Furthermore, they reemphasized the critically important role of community consultation in such instances (CIOMS 2009).

SECURING ACCESS TO CARE

In the first years of the epidemic there was little that medicine could offer those with HIV. Indeed, that was the context within which AIDS activists struggled to increase access to experimental trials. As the prospects for clinical intervention improved, first with the use of prophylactic treatment to prevent *Pneumocystis carinii* pneumonia and other opportunistic infections and then with AZT, the first widely prescribed antiretroviral agent, it was inevitable that the inequities of the US health care system would be encountered.

Some who needed treatment had private insurance, although they frequently faced efforts on the part of their insurers to deny them coverage for their HIV-related conditions; those who were poor or who became impoverished because of their disease could qualify for Medicaid, but many remained unprotected (Green and Arno 1990). To meet the needs of the latter group, special programs were developed. The federal government, through the Ryan White Comprehensive AIDS Resources Emergency Act of 1990, directed significant sums to localities to provide medical services. Among the initiatives under the act was the AIDS Drug Assistance Program (ADAP), designed to pay for AIDS-related medicines. Like the End Stage Renal Disease Program that ensured access to dialysis and transplantation regardless of the ability to pay, these AIDS programs left untouched the basic patterns of medical inequality.

When protease inhibitors emerged in the mid-1990s and combination antiretroviral therapy became the standard of care, the system was strained to the limits. Medication costs alone for those receiving care could range from $10,000 to $15,000 per year (Deeks et al. 1997). A review of dramatically improved therapeutic prospects added the caveat that the new achievements were important "at least for those socioeconomically privileged" (Richman 1996, 1887). ADAP experienced persistent shortfalls in funding. When that was the case, it was necessary to resort to a host of rationing strategies (Henry J. Kaiser Family Foundation 1998). At one point, nearly half of the ADAPs limited access to protease inhibitors (Carton 1996).

The remarkable advances in therapeutics have provided a critical element in the argument that the exceptionalism of the epidemic's early years is no longer appropriate. It is therefore a remarkable paradox that the very same achievements have set the stage for challenging the exceptionalist programs that seek to ensure—however inadequately—access to those same treatments. These expressions of disquiet must be understood, at least in part, as a reflection of concern that the American AIDS epidemic may no longer be seen as immediately threatening, that the unique services for those with HIV would be vulnerable unless they were embedded in a broader system of a just health care system.

On an international plane the prospect of effective antiretroviral treatment would pose challenges vaster by many orders of magnitude. What justification was there for a system of pricing that made the cost of drugs beyond the reach of the desperate? Could markets ever respond to need where effective demand was nil? Could the monopoly confirmed by patent rights be compatible with a response dictated by claims of the dying? Was the treaty on intellectual property rights, incorporated into the World Trade Organization's international regime, a barrier to survival in context of the AIDS epidemic? What moral obligation did the wealthiest nations have to the poorest to provide the resources necessary to purchase the new lifesaving agents and build the medical infrastructure necessary for their appropriate administration? Was there any reason to believe that a global community that permitted millions to die each year from treatable and preventable diseases such as tuberculosis and malaria would respond differently in the face of AIDS?

AIDS activists ultimately seized on this issue and began an international campaign to confront the pharmaceutical industry. What might have seemed an utterly quixotic undertaking would ultimately, however, take on worldwide dimensions linking protesters in the United States, France, and South Africa (Berkman 2001); institutional proponents of global health such as the WHO; and a sympathetic public. By the end of the 1990s the pharmaceutical industry was placed on the defensive, perceived as protecting narrow self-interests when the lives of millions were at stake. Against the claims that high prices were necessary to fuel the engine of research, and that patent protections were crucial to spurring investments in drug investigations, those who sought to turn the terms of discourse asserted that urgency demanded that the barriers to drug access tumble.

Ultimately, under pressure from generic drug manufacturers, prices began to fall, and pharmaceutical firms began to accept the notion of differential or equity pricing.

As prices began to fall, it became ever more apparent that even if drugs were to be provided at cost, even if the principle of equity pricing were to guide sales, even if nations pursued the option of compulsory licensing and parallel imports, the cost of providing antiretroviral therapy was simply beyond the reach of the poorest and most HIV-burdened nations. And even if drugs could be paid for, the necessity of a medical infrastructure that could offer and monitor the use of drugs in a way that was attentive to the needs of individual patients and the risks to public health from drug resistance would require huge investments. This was the context within which a remarkable movement would take shape to create a massive funding effort to respond to the threat of AIDS.

The moral urgency of AIDS treatment was amplified by UN Secretary-General Kofi Annan, who called for a global trust fund that would spend $7 billion to $10 billion a year over an extended period to face the threat to the world's poorest people. Most striking was his assertion that the care that had for so long eluded men, women, and children in the less-developed nations was a matter of moral right. Everyone who was infected should have access to medicine and medical care. That was a moral imperative. What was the unfortunate had become the unfair; inequality had become inequity (Bayer 2002).

Around the start of the twenty-first century it was inconceivable that antiretroviral treatment would be available in resource-constrained settings. Whatever the limits, and they are all too obvious, through the US for President's Emergency Plan for AIDS Relief (PEPFAR) program and UN's Global Fund to Fight AIDS, Tuberculosis and Malaria, what some had thought impossible has become possible and there is growing evidence at a country level of increases in life expectancy and recent discoveries that the use of antiretroviral medications by those who are infected can radically reduce their capacity to transmit HIV, treatment as prevention and that the use of such drugs by those who are not infected can provide protection from the acquisition of HIV infection (PrEP, or pre-exposure prophylaxis) will have a fundamental impact in linking the worlds of treatment and prevention. Those discoveries will pose significant ethical challenges about who is treated and at what course of their illness (Granich et al. 2009).

CONCLUSION

This discussion began with an analysis of ethical and policy issues that emerged in the United States as it confronted the AIDS epidemic. These issues were commonly addressed in other economically advanced nations bounded by the liberal tradition, even when the resolution of the controversies that surfaced took on divergent forms.

No ethical analysis of the challenges posed by AIDS will ever again be sufficient if it is restricted to the challenges faced in wealthy developed nations. Indeed, increasingly the analysis will need to be driven by the complexities of an epidemic in the world's poorest nations. Older concerns rooted in a focus on the need to protect the privacy rights of individuals will inevitably be overshadowed by new concerns about global equity.

SEE ALSO *AIDS: II. Health Care and Research Issues; Confidentiality; Epidemics; Health Care Resources, Allocation of; Homosexuality, Religious Perspectives; Human Dignity; Human Rights; Humanitarian Relief; Life, Quality of: I. Quality of Life in Clinical Decisions; Pandemics; Reductionism; Relativism, Cultural and Ethical; Rights*

BIBLIOGRAPHY

American Public Health Association (APHA). 1988. *Contact Tracing and Partner Notification.* Washington, DC: Author.

Andrus, Jon K.; David W. Fleming; Douglas R. Harger; et al. 1990. "Partner Notification: Can It Control Syphilis?" *Annals of Internal Medicine* 112 (7): 539–43.

Angell, Marcia. 1997. "The Ethics of Clinical Research in the Third World." *New England Journal of Medicine* 337 (12): 847–49.

Annas, George J. 1989. "Faith (Healing), Hope, and Charity at the FDA: The Politics of AIDS Drug Trials." *Villanova Law Review* 34 (5): 771–97.

Bayer, Ronald. 1989. *Private Acts, Social Consequences: AIDS and the Politics of Public Health.* New Brunswick, NJ: Rutgers University Press.

Bayer, Ronald. 1990. "Beyond the Burdens of Protection: AIDS and the Ethics of Research." *Evaluation Review* 14 (5): 443–46.

Bayer, Ronald. 1991. "Public Health Policy and the AIDS Epidemic: An End to HIV Exceptionalism?" *New England Journal of Medicine* 324 (21): 1500–1504.

Bayer, Ronald. 1995. "Women's Rights, Babies' Interests: Ethics, Politics, and Science in the Debate of Newborn HIV Screening." In *HIV Infection in Women*, edited by Howard L. Minkoff, Jack A. DeHovitz, and Ann Duerr. New York: Raven Press.

Bayer, Ronald. 1999. "Clinical Progress and the Future of HIV Exceptionalism." *Archives of Internal Medicine* 159 (10): 1042–48.

Bayer, Ronald. 2000. "Ethical Challenges of HIV Vaccine Trials in Less Developed Nations: Conflict and Consensus in the International Arena." *AIDS* 14 (8): 1051–57.

Bayer, Ronald. 2002. "From the Bowels of an Epidemic: AIDS, Human Rights, and International Equity." *Macalester International* 11:201–32.

Bayer, Ronald, and Claire Edington. 2009. "HIV Testing, Human Rights, and Global AIDS Policy: Exceptionalism and Its Discontents." *Journal of Health Policy, Politics and Law* 34 (3): 301–23.

Bayer, Ronald; Carol Levine; and Susan M. Wolf. 1986. "HIV Antibody Screening: An Ethical Framework for Evaluation Proposed Programs." *Journal of the American Medical Association* 256 (13): 1768–74.

Bayer, Ronald, and Gerald M. Oppenheimer. 2013. "Routine HIV Testing, Public Health, and the USPSTF—An End to the Debate." *New England Journal of Medicine* 368:881–84.

Bayer, Ronald, and Kathleen E. Toomey. 1992. "HIV Prevention and the Two Faces of Partner Notification." *American Journal of Public Health* 82 (8): 1158–64.

Benatar, Solomon R., and Peter A. Singer. 2000. "A New Look at International Research Ethics." *British Medical Journal* 321 (7264): 824–26.

Berkman, Allan. 2001. "Confronting Global AIDS: Prevention and Treatment." *American Journal of Public Health* 91 (9): 1348–49.

Carton, Barbara. 1996. "Life after Death: New AIDS Drugs Bring Hope to Provincetown, but Unexpected Woes." *Wall Street Journal,* October 3, A1.

Centers for Disease Control and Prevention. 1990. "Current Trends Update: Public Health Surveillance for HIV Infection: United States, 1989 and 1990." *Morbidity and Mortality Weekly Report* 39 (47): 853, 859–61.

Centers for Disease Control and Prevention. 1999. "Guidelines for National Human Immunodeficiency Virus Case Surveillance, Including Monitoring for Human Immunodeficiency Virus Infection and Acquired Immunodeficiency Syndrome." *Morbidity and Mortality Weekly Report* 48 (13): 1–28.

Connor, Edward M.; Rhoda S. Sperling; Richard Gelber; et al. 1994. "Reduction in Maternal–Infant Transmission of HIV Type 1 with Zidovudine Treatment." *New England Journal of Medicine* 331 (18): 1173–80.

Council for International Organizations of Medical Sciences (CIOMS). 1991. "International Guidelines for Ethical Review of Epidemiological Studies." *Journal of Law, Medicine and Health Care* 19 (3–4): 47–58.

Council for International Organizations of Medical Sciences. 2009. *International Ethical Guidelines for Epidemiological Studies.* Geneva: Author.

Council for International Organizations of Medical Sciences in collaboration with the World Health Organization (WHO). 1993. *International Ethical Guidelines for Biomedical Research Involving Human Subjects.* Geneva: Author.

De Cock, Kevin M.; Charles F. Gilks; Ying-Ru Lo; et al. 2009. "Can Antiretroviral Therapy Eliminate HIV Transmission?" *Lancet* 373 (9657): 7–9.

De Cock, Kevin M., and Anne M. Johnson. 1998. "From Exceptionalism to Normalization: A Reappraisal of Attitudes and Practice around HIV Testing." *British Medical Journal* 316:290–93.

Deeks, Steven G.; Mark Smith; Mark Holodniy; et al. 1997. "HIV-1 Protease Inhibitors: A Review for Clinicians." *Journal of the American Medical Association* 277 (2): 145–53.

Epstein, Stephen. 1996. *Impure Science: AIDS, Activism, and the Politics of Knowledge.* Berkeley: University of California Press.

Fairchild, Amy L, and Ronald Bayer. 2011. "HIV Surveillance and the Barrier between Public Health and Clinical Medicine: Will the Walls Come Tumbling Down?" *New England Journal of Medicine* 365 (8): 685–87.

Fairchild, Amy L.; Ronald Bayer; and James Colgrove; with Daniel Wolfe. 2007. *Searching Eyes: Privacy, the State, and Disease Surveillance in America.* Berkeley: University of California Press.

Granich, Reuben M.; Charles F. Gilks; C. Dye; et al. 2009. "Universal Voluntary HIV Testing with Immediate Antiretroviral Therapy as a Strategy for Elimination of HIV Transmission: A Mathematical Model." *Lancet* 373 (9657): 48–57.

Green, Jesse, and Peter S. Arno. 1990. "The 'Medicaidization' of AIDS: Trends in the Financing of HIV-Related Medical Care." *Journal of the American Medical Association* 264 (10): 1261–66.

Grodin, Michael A. 1992. "Historical Origins of the Nuremberg Code." In *The Nazi Doctors and the Nuremberg Code: Human Rights in Human Experimentation,* edited by George J. Annas and Michael A. Grodin, 121–48. New York: Oxford University Press.

Hegearty, Margaret, and Elaine Abrams. 1992. "Caring for HIV-Infected Women and Children." *New England Journal of Medicine* 326 (13): 887–88.

Henry J. Kaiser Family Foundation. 1998. "National ADAP Monitoring Project: Interim Technical Report." Menlo Park, CA: Author.

IJsselmuiden, Carel B., and Ruth R. Faden. 1996. "Medical Research and the Principle of Respect for Persons in Non-Western Cultures." In *The Ethics of Research Involving Human Subjects: Facing the Twenty-First Century,* edited by Harold Y. Vanderpool. Frederick, MD: University Publishing Group.

Institute of Medicine. 1986. *Confronting AIDS: Directions for Public Health, Health Care, and Research.* Washington, DC: National Academy Press.

Institute of Medicine, Committee on Perinatal Transmission of HIV, and U.S. National Research Council, Board on Children, Youth, and Families. 1999. *Reducing the Odds: Preventing Perinatal Transmission of HIV in the United States,* edited by Michael A. Stoto, Donna A. Almario, and Marie C. McCormick. Washington, DC: National Academy Press.

Joint United Nations Programme on HIV/AIDS (UNAIDS). 2000. *Ethical Considerations in HIV Preventive Vaccine Research: UNAIDS Guidance Document.* Geneva: Author.

Levine, Carol. 1988. "Has AIDS Changed the Ethics of Human Subjects Research?" *Journal of Law, Medicine and Health Care* 16 (3–4): 167–73.

McNeill, William H. 1976. *Plagues and Peoples.* Garden City, NY: Anchor Press.

National Bioethics Advisory Commission. 2001. *Ethical and Policy Issues in International Research: Clinical Trials in Developing Countries.* Vol. 1. Rockville, MD: Author.

National Commission for the Protection of Human Subjects of Biomedical and Behavioral Research. 1978. *The Belmont Report: Ethical Principles and Guidelines for the Protection of Human Subjects of Research.* Washington, DC: DHEW and US Government Printing Office.

Oppenheimer, Gerald M.; Ronald Bayer; and James Colgrove. 2002. "Health and Human Rights: Old Wine in New Bottles?" *Journal of Law, Medicine and Ethics* 30 (4): 522–32.

"Parallel Track System Defended." 1989. *CDC AIDS Weekly,* December 11.

Rennie, Stuart, and Frieda Behets. 2006. "Desperately Seeking Targets: The Ethics of Routine HIV Testing in Low-Income

Countries." *Bulletin of the World Health Organization* 84 (1): 52–57.

Rennie, Stuart; Abigail Norris Turner; Bavon Mupenda; et al. 2009. "Conducting Unlinked Anonymous HIV Surveillance in Developing Countries: Ethical, Epidemiological and Public Health Concerns." *PLoS Medicine* 6 (1): 30–34.

Richman, David D. 1996. "HIV Therapeutics." *Science* 272 (5270): 1886–88.

Rothman, David J. 1991. *Strangers at the Bedside: A History of How Law and Bioethics Transformed Medical Decision Making.* New York: Basic Books.

Schram, Neil. 1988. "Partner Notification Can Be Useful Tool against AIDS Spread." *Los Angeles Times*, July 28. http://articles.latimes.com/1988-07-28/local/me-9498_1_partner-notification

Shelton, Deborah L. 1996. "Delegates Push Mandatory HIV Testing for Pregnant Women: American Medical Association House of Delegates Vote: Annual Meeting News." *American Medical News* 31:1.

Singer, Peter A., and Solomon R. Benatar. 2001. "Beyond Helsinki: A Vision for Global Health Ethics." *British Medical Journal* 322 (7289): 747–48.

Tarasoff v. Regents of the University of California. 1974. 118 Cal. Rptr. 129 (Cal. Sup. Ct. 1974).

Varmus, Harold, and David Satcher. 1997. "Ethical Complexities of Conducting Research in Developing Countries." *New England Journal of Medicine* 337 (14): 1003–05.

Vernon, Thomas. 1986. "Remarks." In *AIDS: Impact on Public Policy*, edited by Robert Hummell, W. Leavy, R. Rampola, et al. New York: Plenum Press.

World Health Organization (WHO). 1994. "Recommendations from the Meeting on Mother to Infant Transmission of HIV, Geneva, Switzerland, June 23–25." Geneva.

World Health Organization (WHO). 2004. "Ethical Issues to Be Considered in Second Generation Surveillance." Accessed June 15, 2013. http://www.who.int/hiv/pub/surveillance/sgs_ethical/en/index.html

World Health Organization (WHO) and UNAIDS. 2007. "Guidance on Provider-Initiated HIV Testing and Counseling in Health Facilities." Accessed June 15, 2013. http://www.who.int/hiv/pub/guidelines/9789241595568_en.pdf

World Medical Association. 2000. *Declaration of Helskini: Ethical Principles for Medical Research Involving Human Subjects: Principle 22.* Accessed June 15, 2013. http://www.wma.net/en/30publications/10policies/b3/

Ronald Bayer (1995, 2004, 2014)
Center for the History and Ethics of Public Health, Mailman School of Public Health, Columbia University

II. HEALTH CARE AND RESEARCH ISSUES

The early ethical debates regarding the AIDS epidemic were largely driven by the concerns of the politically active, primarily white, homosexual or bisexual men in the United States in whom the disease was first identified. Because of severe discrimination against HIV/AIDS patients, early activists argued for special confidentiality protections for HIV information. Because infection at that time was almost always fatal, patients also demanded access to experimental treatments, which offered the only chance of survival. From the 1980s through the first decade of twenty-first century, however, the epidemic changed, as did many of the ethical issues.

The global impact of HIV/AIDS in the twenty-first century dominates ethical and policy debates. In 2010 an estimated 34 million people worldwide were living with HIV, with approximately 2.7 million new infections and 1.8 million deaths. These figures are lower than 2001 estimates because of increased use of antiretroviral treatments, particularly in resource-poor countries, which have been disproportionately affected by HIV/AIDS. More than 95 percent of new infections occur in developing countries. AIDS is the leading cause of death in sub-Saharan Africa and the fourth-leading cause of death worldwide. Although Africa has been particularly hard-hit by the AIDS epidemic with about 70 percent of the world's HIV-infected persons and new infections, there have been significant increases since 2001 in people living with HIV in eastern Europe and Asia. Failure of governments to acknowledge the threat of HIV has exacerbated the epidemic.

In the United States HIV/AIDS has been a serious public health problem. Spread primarily through sexual activity and injection drug use, the epidemic increasingly affects poor people of color. In 2012 approximately 1.1 million people in the United States were infected with HIV, with approximately 50,000 new diagnoses annually. But as a result of the introduction of highly active antiretroviral therapy (HAART) and prevention and education efforts, the number of AIDS deaths in the United States has fallen dramatically.

This entry discusses ethical issues regarding HIV testing, confidentiality of HIV information, HIV infection in women and children, end-of-life issues for HIV-infected patients, and access to health care for HIV disease. This entry also discusses clinical research issues with particular attention to international HIV research and HIV vaccine research.

HEALTH CARE ISSUES

Despite treatment advances and better understanding of the disease, fear and social stigma create barriers to seeking HIV testing or care. In the United States special procedures, protections, and programs were developed to encourage testing and to provide care.

Transmission and Prevention. HIV is transmitted by direct contact with bodily fluids that contain the virus.

The major modes of transmission are sexual contact and injection drug use (through sharing needles and drug paraphernalia). HIV also can be transmitted from mother to infant during pregnancy or through breast-feeding. Prevention measures, such as safer-sex education, use of condoms, needle exchange, and methadone maintenance, have proved effective at preventing HIV transmission.

Nevertheless, these prevention efforts often meet with strong resistance. Some critics object that providing condoms and discussing safer-sex techniques inappropriately encourage sexual behaviors outside of heterosexual marriage. Similarly, some opponents object that providing clean needles fosters illegal and harmful injection drug use. From a population perspective, however, such preventive measures reduce the incidence of a serious and, if untreated, often fatal illness. Empirical studies do not demonstrate an increase in high-risk behaviors related to these preventive interventions.

HIV Testing. Because of the sensitivity surrounding HIV, testing for the disease historically has been treated differently from most other medical tests. The 2006 US Centers for Disease Control and Prevention (CDC) recommendations seek to change this.

Special Procedures for HIV Testing (Historic). Because the physical risks are minimal, in the United States blood tests typically do not require extensive informed-consent discussions, and consent often is implied rather than explicit. Early in the AIDS epidemic, however, HIV testing was different from other blood tests because it presented serious psychosocial risks, such as familial rejection; employment discrimination; or loss of health care, insurance, and housing. Moreover, because there was no proven treatment at that time, the benefits of early diagnosis were uncertain. In recognition of these circumstances and to encourage voluntary testing, special procedures for obtaining consent for an HIV test (including pretest counseling and specific, often written, informed consent) and for protecting the confidentiality of HIV test results also were enacted. Nevertheless, states may permit HIV testing without informed consent under limited circumstances. For example, many states permit testing without patient permission after emergency response workers or health care workers are exposed to their blood or other fluids. The patient's permission must be requested, but it is not required. In addition, some states permit testing without consent of prisoners and persons accused of sex crimes. Many states require HIV testing of newborns under some circumstances, which indirectly reveals maternal HIV status.

Move to Routine Testing. In 2006 the US government, through the CDC, recommended HIV testing of all Americans ages thirteen to sixty-four as part of routine medical care. The CDC recommended testing on an opt-out basis, that is, that patients be notified that they would be tested for HIV unless they refuse testing. The CDC also recommended against specific written consent. The rationale for the proposed change was to increase the number of people who know their HIV status. Evidence shows that those who do not know their status account for some 20,000 new HIV infections annually and that knowledge of HIV status lowers the risk of transmission. While there are strong public health reasons for routine testing, there are some concerns about removing the protections afforded by pretest counseling and specific-consent requirements, including eliminating opportunities for HIV education.

Availability of Anonymous Testing. Because of the stigma and potential psychosocial risks associated with HIV testing and to encourage voluntary testing, most states offer anonymous HIV testing. At anonymous test sites, individuals are not required to provide any identifying information. Upon testing, they are given a unique code to use to obtain results. People identified as HIV positive at these sites are not reported to public health officials.

Conventional versus Rapid Testing. Effective interventions cannot be implemented without timely test results. Conventional HIV test results typically are not available for one to two weeks because initial positive tests must be confirmed with more sophisticated and accurate tests. In the United States such testing is used to avoid mistakenly informing people that they are infected with HIV based on a falsely positive test. However, this approach can be problematic when there is time urgency, such as when women of unknown HIV status first seek medical care when they are in labor or when people are unlikely to return for results, such as in clinics for sexually transmitted diseases.

Rapid HIV tests that provide results shortly after testing are available. Rapid testing carries an increased risk of false-positive tests, although this risk is lessened in settings that serve a population with a high HIV prevalence and by using more than one rapid test for each person tested. The US Food and Drug Administration (FDA) approved a rapid home HIV test in 2012. There are concerns with home testing because people are not connected directly to information and counseling to interpret results and the risk of false positives appears to be higher. However, the benefits of obtaining HIV test results quickly are considered to outweigh these risks.

Confidentiality. Although medical information generally is considered confidential, additional requirements apply to HIV-related information.

Protections. In the United States physicians and health care organizations have ethical and legal obligations to preserve the confidentiality of all medical information. Because of the sensitivity of HIV-related information, many states have adopted laws that provide additional protection to HIV-related medical information. For example, many states require specific authorization from patients to disclose HIV-related information to third parties. Such protections are particularly important where stigma associated with HIV infection is high. Although the US Supreme Court determined that HIV infection can be a disability under the Americans with Disabilities Act of 1990 (*Bragdon v. Abbott* 1998), HIV-infected individuals still experience negative effects. For example, the US Equal Employment Opportunity Commission reports that people living with HIV continue to experience significant discrimination in employment. In addition, the United States has eliminated its restrictions on travel by people living with HIV, but some countries continue to limit such travel.

Exceptions. There are many exceptions to the legal and ethical rules of HIV-related confidentiality. First, health care providers in the United States must report HIV infections and AIDS cases to public health authorities. The public health benefits of this reporting outweigh the duty to maintain confidentiality. Reporting of AIDS cases has always included disclosing the patient's name and other identifying information. Initially, HIV reports did not include names because of confidentiality concerns in light of the delay between infection and illness, but every state now requires name-based reporting. Although name-based reporting was viewed as controversial, the practice became accepted given the benefits of early HIV diagnosis for prevention in the age of HAART and of obtaining accurate epidemiological information about HIV infection for better planning and funding of HIV-related programs.

Second, public health officials commonly carry out partner notification. Although notification is typically conducted confidentially, it may inadvertently reveal the source patient's identity. In addition, health care providers may be permitted to inform an infected patient's sexual or drug-sharing partner of the patient's HIV infection. Such a breach of confidentiality is justified on the grounds that it is the only means of preventing serious harm to an identifiable person and that the breach of confidentiality is minimized.

Third, US policy recommends that an expert panel review the cases of any HIV-infected health care workers who perform invasive procedures that might lead to transmission of HIV/AIDS to decide whether that HIV-infected health care worker should be permitted to continue to perform such procedures or if doing so would constitute too great a risk to the patients. Additionally, the panel should decide if it is necessary to inform the health care worker's patients of any risk of infection, so that the patients can make an informed decision about whether they wish to continue in the health care worker's care. There is wide variation in state law, and not all states require disclosure of HIV infection.

HIV Infection in Women and Children. Worldwide, mother-to-child transmission is a major public health crisis. In parts of Africa 45 percent of pregnant women are HIV infected. Without treatment, their children contract HIV in 25 to 45 percent of cases, resulting in some 540,000 perinatal cases annually. In the United States HAART has significantly reduced mother-to-child HIV transmission; by 2007, there were fewer than 200 perinatal HIV cases annually.

United States. To take advantage of the proven effectiveness of HAART for preventing perinatal HIV transmission, women must know that they are HIV positive. US policy recommends routine HIV testing of all pregnant women unless a woman specifically refuses to be tested. However, state law may still require specific informed consent.

Developing World. When HAART first became available in 1996, the high costs, complex regimens, lack of prenatal care, and baby delivery outside the hospital limited access to it in developing countries. However, the use of HAART has expanded globally as regimens have become simpler to administer and more cost-effective. Studies have confirmed the cost-effectiveness of prenatal HAART in preventing mother-to-child transmission despite its cost, compared with overall per capita health expenditures in resource-poor countries. Many national governments have risen to the challenge of improving access to HAART with some notable successes but not without controversy. For example, the prenatal use of nevirapine, while it is simple and inexpensive, has resulted in nevirapine resistance and toxicity in some women.

Mother-to-child transmission may also occur through breast-feeding. Studies have shown that bottle-feeding instead of breast-feeding lowers the risk of transmission. Nevertheless, bottle-feeding is not a feasible option in many countries because of lack of access to clean water and the high cost of formula. Some women may resist bottle-feeding even when it is safe, because breast-feeding is the norm in many developing countries and may play an important symbolic role in conveying social status to mothers. In such cultures failure to breast-feed may indirectly reveal HIV status, which could subject women to the risk of physical harm or loss of housing and support, particularly when there is a history of domestic violence. Women need to know the steps they can take to reduce the risk of HIV transmission to their infants, so that they can assess the risks and benefits in light of their own circumstances and make informed decisions.

End-of-Life Issues. Early in the US epidemic, before HAART was available, HIV infection often quickly progressed to a terminal illness. As a result of complications from their disease, AIDS patients in many cases were unable to make medical decisions for their care, but there was uncertainty regarding who should serve as a patient's surrogate decision maker. In the absence of a patient's written advance directive, the law and physicians typically look to family members. But many homosexual men with AIDS were estranged from their families and often would have preferred to give decision-making authority to committed partners or friends with whom they had discussed their wishes. Because the availability of HAART has prolonged survival, end-of-life care in HIV infection has become a less-prominent issue in the United States.

Although access to antiretroviral therapy has increased significantly in the early twenty-first century, in the developing world palliative care, which focuses on relief of suffering, is still sometimes the only tenable goal. The World Health Organization (WHO) has recommended palliative care throughout the lifetime of an HIV patient as part of an integrated system in developing countries, even where HAART is available. However, severe resource constraints and lack of infrastructure make it difficult to provide even palliative measures. Under these circumstances, care may be limited to psychosocial and spiritual support and helping patients make plans for such practical issues as burial or child custody and support.

Access to Health Care for HIV Disease. Access to health care for HIV disease remains an important issue both domestically and internationally.

United States. In the United States the average annual health care cost for an HIV-infected individual is more than $20,000, primarily for HAART, and the annual cost for those with AIDS can be more. Access to health care in the United States may be provided through private insurance coverage or public programs.

HIV-infected individuals may face several difficulties with private health care insurance. Most individuals in the United States with health care coverage receive it through their employers, who may seek to control the soaring cost of health insurance by limiting coverage for HIV infection. A federal appeals court case affirmed employers' "freedom to amend or eliminate employee benefits" in health insurance, including benefits for any particular illness, even if all other medical conditions are covered (*McGann v. H & H Music Company* 1991). Another federal appeals court decision concluded that such limits do not violate the Americans with Disabilities Act (*Doe v. Mutual of Omaha Insurance Company* 2000). Those who do not receive health care coverage through their employers or who lose coverage when they are unable to work because of their disease may find it difficult to obtain private coverage because, if it is available at all, it is very expensive or provides limited benefits. The 2010 Affordable Care Act (ACA, commonly referred to as "Obamacare") addresses some of these challenges, for example, by expanding public programs, providing subsidies for some people who could not otherwise afford insurance, and eliminating annual and lifetime coverage limits and preexisting condition exclusions. The Supreme Court ruled that Congress had the constitutional authority to enact the ACA (*National Federation of Independent Business v. Sebelius* 2012), but its future remains uncertain because some politicians have pledged to repeal it. The House of Representatives has voted multiple times since 2010 to do so. Moreover, provisions take effect at different times, with many not going into effect until 2014.

About half of HIV-infected adults and 90 percent of HIV-infected children receiving medical care are covered through various publicly funded sources. First, patients may be insured through Medicaid. Historically, to qualify for Medicaid patients must be categorically eligible, typically because of AIDS or HIV-related disability, and meet (low) income requirements. The ACA expands Medicaid coverage, beginning in 2014, by eliminating the categorical eligibility requirement and determining eligibility solely on low income. Given the disproportionate impact of HIV/AIDS on the poor, this could greatly expand the number of people living with HIV/AIDS who have health insurance. However, as ACA remains under political attack, some states have indicated that they will not accept the expansion.

Second, state AIDS Drug-Assistance Programs (ADAPs), which are funded through the federal Ryan White Comprehensive AIDS Resources Emergency (CARE) Act of 1990, make HIV medications available to low-income and uninsured persons. Because each state receives different funding and determines eligibility and benefits packages, Medicaid coverage and access to medications vary widely from state to state. However, unlike Medicaid, ADAPs are not entitlement programs (programs in which all those who meet the eligibility criteria may receive the benefits) but are funded through annual appropriations, which may vary from year to year.

Finally, the CARE Act provides funding for HIV/AIDS services that are not covered by Medicaid or by state or local government funds. Although the majority of the

CARE Act funds are used for medical care (including the ADAPs), they also pay for HIV/AIDS-related support services, including counseling, emergency housing assistance, training for clinicians who treat HIV-infected patients, and developing programs to improve treatment. States and local governments receive CARE Act funds based in part on the prevalence of HIV/AIDS in their populations.

The reliance on Medicaid and other public funding causes several problems. Because of low reimbursement levels, many physicians do not accept Medicaid patients. As a result, emergency departments and public hospitals bear a greater burden of care. In addition, because of large budget deficits, many states and counties are finding it increasingly difficult to pay for such care. Some ACA provisions may alleviate these problems, although there are fears they may exacerbate them.

Specific funding that provides for HIV care but not for other fatal illnesses whose treatments are expensive, such as cancer, raises issues about equitable allocation of resources. AIDS activists exerted considerable political pressure to obtain this funding and to continue the programs supported by it. There are public policy reasons for making special funding available for HIV care. HIV is an infectious disease. Providing care and access to HAART slows the progress of the disease, which may decrease transmissibility and therefore help control the spread of the epidemic. Because the overall cost of antiretroviral therapy is less than that of caring for a patient with AIDS, it may be more cost-effective for the government to provide HAART to delay progression to AIDS.

Developing World. There have been many efforts to make HIV medications more available to the developing world by pressuring pharmaceutical manufacturers to lower prices, permitting production of generic versions of effective therapies, and providing funds for drug purchases. Even though the annual cost of antiretroviral therapy has been reduced to between $500 and $1,350 per patient for the developing world, this cost is beyond the means of many developing nations. In 2001 the secretary-general of the United Nations (UN), Kofi Annan, proposed a $7 billion to $10 billion fund to combat AIDS globally. Although many of the eight countries with the world's largest economies (G8 countries) contributed to the fund, the UN Global Fund is not expected to reach its goal until 2013 and needs more than originally contemplated just to continue to pay for existing programs. The United States has committed billions to treat HIV-infected individuals in resource-poor countries and to prevent new infections through the Global Fund and through programs funded by the President's Emergency Plan for AIDS Relief (PEPFAR) program created by President George W. Bush. Despite the pledge of 193 UN member states to provide universal access to HIV treatment, a 2010 report on the pledged goals indicates that universal access has not been achieved and that the number of new infections each year is still greater than the number of HIV patients who are gaining access to care.

The obligation of developed nations to address the AIDS epidemic in the developing world can be justified on several grounds. First, compassion may motivate developed nations to help alleviate the suffering caused by the AIDS epidemic. Second, to the extent that good health and health care are basic human rights, nations that are able should contribute resources to guarantee these rights. Third, because the wealth (and health) disparities between the developed and the developing nations are largely a legacy of colonialism, developed nations have a duty to address those problems to which they contributed. Finally, it is in the self-interest of developed nations to assist the developing world. If the AIDS epidemic is not controlled in the developing world, the resulting economic and political instability will threaten the security of all nations.

Even if antiretroviral therapy can be made affordable, there are challenges in providing treatment in developing countries that have little health care infrastructure. Because failure to adhere to the treatment regimen may lead to drug resistance, it is important to train host-country personnel to provide and monitor treatments and to develop treatment protocols that can be implemented effectively using existing infrastructure, such as once-a-day regimens and strategies for monitoring care when intensive laboratory testing is not available. Directly observed therapy (DOT), a treatment strategy that began as a means to treat tuberculosis, is being used in some developing countries to ensure effective delivery and to monitor HIV and related diseases. DOT-HAART requires community health workers to accompany HIV patients to their treatments on a daily basis to ensure greater compliance and thus greater success in treating the disease. This method has proved to be effective in many of the poorest countries, such as Haiti, where the prevalence of HIV is high.

CLINICAL RESEARCH ISSUES

Activists and the scope of the HIV epidemic forced society and scientists to reconsider fundamental questions about clinical trials of promising new therapies (Lo 2001).

What Is the Goal of the Clinical Trial? To most scientists and to the FDA, the goal of clinical trials is to determine the safety and effectiveness of new drugs. Historically, clinical research has been considered dangerous for subjects. The HIV epidemic, however, caused many patients to consider clinical trials beneficial rather than risky because they offer access to promising new treatments, closer medical follow-up, and more sophisticated laboratory monitoring than does standard care.

Who Should Participate in Clinical Trials? Historically, women, children, and people of color have been underrepresented in clinical trials. Usually, children are restricted from clinical trials to protect them from the risks of unproven therapies. Unlike adults, children cannot give informed consent. The rationale for excluding women of childbearing age, particularly women who are pregnant, is to protect their developing and future children from possible long-term side effects of unproven drugs, but restricting women and children from clinical trials also harms them. Unless they participate in clinical trials, the effectiveness and safety of therapies cannot be rigorously established. For example, trials of the effect of zidovudine (also known as azidothymidine or AZT) on mother-to-child transmission provided important information that has dramatically reduced rates of perinatal HIV transmission. Without the participation of pregnant women in clinical trials, the effectiveness of antiretroviral therapy in preventing mother-to-child transmission of HIV would not be established. Additionally, there would be no evidence basis for enhanced public health measures and increased funding to prevent mother-to-child transmission. Similarly, the increased inclusion of minorities in trials has provided information on the efficacy and adverse effects in these populations. Moreover, it is problematic to take away women's decision making about research participation simply because they are pregnant.

International Research. Because of the great wealth disparities between developed and developing nations and a history of exploitation, research conducted in the developing world has been the subject of controversy. There are concerns that research is conducted in developing countries solely because costs are lower and the local ethical requirements are not as onerous as those in the sponsoring nation. Moreover, there are concerns that people will participate in research regardless of the level of risk because participation represents the only opportunity to receive medical care. Nevertheless, HIV-related research in developing countries often is publicly funded and designed to assess efficacy of affordable treatment regimens or behavioral interventions rather than privately sponsored trials of new drugs that are unlikely to become available to the host country. Government involvement and sponsorship may result in research to address health policy issues that are more relevant to the host countries.

Controversy over Perinatal Trials. Placebo-controlled trials testing interventions to lessen rates of perinatal HIV transmission conducted by US researchers in Africa and Asia sparked extensive debate. Relying on the World Medical Association's (WMA) (1996, para. II.3) Declaration of Helsinki (first adopted in 1964), which states that "in any medical study, every patient—including those of a control group, if any—should be assured the best proven diagnostic and therapeutic methods," some critics argued that the placebo-controlled trials were unethical because zidovudine was a treatment proved to be effective even though it generally was not available in the countries in which the trials were taking place. Others argued that such placebo-controlled trials can be ethically justified because they provide information that responds to local needs. A developing country needs to know whether a simpler, cheaper therapeutic treatment is superior to what is currently available in the country (generally no therapy) rather than whether a simpler, cheaper treatment is comparable to the best proven treatment, which the country cannot afford.

Appropriate Comparison Group. The controversy over the perinatal HIV transmission trials influenced the larger debate regarding international research, particularly because the WMA revised the Declaration of Helsinki in 2000. The revision reads: "The benefits, risks, burdens and effectiveness of a new method should be tested against those of the best current prophylactic, diagnostic, and therapeutic methods. This does not exclude the use of placebo, or no treatment, in studies where no proven prophylactic, diagnostic or therapeutic methods exists" (WMA 2000, para. 29). Recognizing that it may be ethically permissible to compare an inexpensive, simple regimen to a current practice of no therapy in developing countries when the regimen used in developed countries is not feasible to employ, the WMA (2001, para. 29) issued a clarification after the 2000 revision: "A placebo-controlled trial may be ethically acceptable, even if proven therapy is available … where for compelling and scientifically sound methodological reasons its use is necessary to determine the efficacy or safety of a prophylactic, diagnostic or therapeutic method." However, improved access to therapies globally should limit the use of this exception, which remains in the text.

Posttrial Access to Treatment. There is general agreement that clinical research in a developing country should not go forward unless there is a realistic chance that its inhabitants will gain access to the treatment after the trial. For example, HIV vaccine trials would be permissible in a developing country only if the successful vaccine would be available in the host country. There is, however, disagreement regarding how far researchers' obligations extend toward ensuring access and to whom the obligation is owed (i.e., trial participants only or others in the community or nation), especially because researchers are not in control of government policy and funding for clinical care. There is a growing consensus that researchers should make good faith efforts to ensure that therapies are available after completing a trial, recognizing that successful results in a well-designed clinical trial may lead to availability of resources to provide a new therapy even though such resources were not available before the trial commenced.

Ancillary Care. There also is growing consensus that researchers conducting research in the developing world have obligations to provide ancillary care, "defined as health care that research participants need but that is not necessary to ensure the safety or scientific validity of the research [or] to redress injuries caused by research participation" (Merritt 2011, 312). This duty stems in part from the researcher-participant relationship, which requires the researcher to maximize benefits and minimize harms to the participant and places the researcher in a unique position to address these needs. However, there is disagreement regarding the extent of the researchers' obligations. While justice may demand some alleviation of problems that have arisen from historic inequities and exploitation, it would be unfair to expect the researcher to take responsibility for all problems created by others and could make it impossible to conduct the research.

Informed Consent. US regulations, the Declaration of Helsinki, and other international ethics guidelines all require individual consent for research participation. However, US informed consent requirements may present challenges for research in developing countries. Informed consent is often not the norm for clinical care in many developing nations. People may therefore be uncomfortable or even scared when asked to provide consent. In addition, it may be difficult to persuade people to appreciate the risks of research participation when most assume that doctors will recommend only treatments that are known to work. Women may be used to deferring decisions to husbands, fathers, or other family members. In some communities it may not be possible to approach individuals without the community leader's permission. Although assent from the authority figure may be needed to approach individuals in some cases, voluntary consent must be obtained from each participant. Finally, in some communities documenting consent may be difficult because of illiteracy or because people fear that a signed document may be used against them. In such cases, it may be necessary to seek approval of the institutional review board to modify the documentation requirements to accommodate these conditions.

Vulnerable Participants. Those infected with HIV may be medically vulnerable from their infection. In addition, homosexuals, injection drug users, minorities, and women, who for various reasons may be at higher risk of HIV infection, are more likely to be socially and economically vulnerable because of historical attitudes and discrimination. This may be particularly true in the international setting, and the degree of vulnerability for these groups may vary from country to country. Accordingly, investigators conducting HIV-related research must pay particular attention to vulnerability and take steps to protect potentially vulnerable research participants.

Special Issues in HIV Vaccine Research. HIV vaccine trials present special ethical concerns. First, HIV vaccine trials must go forward with less preclinical evidence of efficacy than other interventions because a good animal model does not exist, HIV is highly variable and undergoes rapid mutation, and there is little information about how to build protection against HIV. For these reasons, large numbers of participants are necessary for even a single study. Nevertheless, because of the enormous suffering caused by HIV, such trials are ethically appropriate if there are credible scientific reasons to believe that the candidate vaccine will be effective.

Second, vaccine trial participants may mistakenly believe that they will receive protection from the vaccine and therefore may increasingly engage in risky behaviors. However, unlike most vaccines, HIV vaccines are unlikely to confer full immunity. While researchers need outcomes (i.e., evidence of seroconversion, or positive HIV test results in persons who previously tested negative for HIV) to evaluate the efficacy of the vaccine candidate, they also have an obligation to protect research participants. Accordingly, researchers must provide high-quality risk-reduction counseling and emphasize uncertainty about the effectiveness of the candidate vaccine to all participants even though the clinical trial would be undermined if such counseling were totally effective. To avoid this potential conflict, it may be necessary to have separate staff for the counseling and the research aspects of the trial. Similar issues arise in studies of temporary prevention interventions, such as preexposure prophylaxis that uses chemicals to block infection exposure by exposure rather than conferring long-term immunity as vaccines do.

Finally, HIV vaccine trials pose unique risks to participants. Participants may be prevented from taking part in future vaccine trials, and subsequently developed vaccines may be less effective for them. Because participants may react positively to certain HIV antibody tests, they may be excluded from certain professions and activities, even if their seroconversion status does not represent a true infection. Subjects may also face stigmatization from family or friends to whom they disclose information. Mere participation in some trials may identify the subject as someone at high risk of contracting HIV. Because of the high stakes if confidentiality is breached, researchers should take extra steps to protect the confidentiality of the information they collect in HIV vaccine trials. In some cases, the intervention may cause physical harm to participants. For example, a large-scale vaccine trial was stopped early after finding that the vaccine candidate increased the risk of HIV infection. Studies of the use of microbicides, which could increase women's control over prevention, similarly have been stopped for increased risk of infection.

Overall, the potential benefits of well-designed vaccine trials and research into other prevention methods outweigh the risks, providing needed data about effective prevention methods. Certain studies, for example, led the FDA to approve one HIV medication, Truvada™ (which combines emtricitabline and tenofovir), for preexposure prophylaxis.

In summary, the HIV epidemic has raised new ethical and policy dilemmas and has forced reconsideration of established guidelines and policies that apply to a much broader range of issues. In the future, controversies will likely continue to focus on addressing the global impact of HIV/AIDS and what justice requires in health care access and research.

This is a revised version of the entry first written by Bernard Lo in 1995 and updated by Bernard Lo and Leslie E. Wolf in 2004.

SEE ALSO *Access to Health Care; Children: III. Health Care and Research Issues; Confidentiality; Epidemics; Health Care Resources, Allocation of; Homosexuality, Religious Perspectives; Human Dignity; Life, Quality of: II. Quality of Life in Health Care Allocation; Research Policy; Rights*

BIBLIOGRAPHY

Angell, Marcia. 1997. "The Ethics of Clinical Research in the Third World." *New England Journal of Medicine* 337 (12): 847–49.

Bayer, Ronald. 1991. "Public Health Policy and the AIDS Epidemic: An End to HIV Exceptionalism?" *New England Journal of Medicine* 324 (21): 1500–1504.

Bozzette, Samuel A.; Sandra H. Berry; Naihua Duan; et al. 1998. "The Care of HIV-Infected Adults in the United States." *New England Journal of Medicine* 339 (26): 1897–1904.

Bragdon v. Abbott. 1998. 524 U.S. 624.

Centers for Disease Control and Prevention. 2001a. "HIV and AIDS: United States, 1981–2000." *Morbidity and Mortality Weekly Report* 50 (21): 430–34.

Centers for Disease Control and Prevention. 2001b. "Revised Guidelines for HIV Counseling, Testing, and Referral." *Morbidity and Mortality Weekly Report* 50 (RR19): 1–58.

Centers for Disease Control and Prevention. 2001c. "Revised Recommendations for HIV Screening of Pregnant Women." *Morbidity and Mortality Weekly Report* 50 (RR19): 59–86.

Centers for Disease Control and Prevention. 2006. "Revised Recommendations for HIV Testing of Adults, Adolescents, and Pregnant Women in Health-Care Settings." *Morbidity and Mortality Weekly Report* 55 (RR-14): 1–17.

Centers for Disease Control and Prevention. 2011. "Diagnoses of HIV Infection and AIDS in the United States and Dependent Areas." *HIV Surveillance Report* 21:1–79.

Chesney, Margaret A.; Peter Lurie; and Thomas J. Coates. 1995. "Strategies for Addressing the Social and Behavioral Challenges of Prophylactic HIV Vaccine Trials." *Journal of Acquired Immune Deficiency Syndromes and Human Retrovirology* 9 (1): 30–35.

De Cock, Kevin M., and Robert S. Janssen. 2002. "An Unequal Epidemic in an Unequal World." *Journal of the American Medical Association* 288 (2): 236–38.

Doe v. Mutual of Omaha Insurance Company. 2000. 179 F.3d 557 (7th Cir. 1999), cert. denied 528 U.S. 1106.

Farmer, Paul; Fernet Léandre; Joia S. Mukherjee; et al. 2001. "Community-Based Approaches to HIV Treatment in Resource-Poor Settings." *Lancet* 358 (9279): 404–9.

Ferriman, Annabel. 2001. "Doctors Demand Immediate Access to Antiretroviral Drugs in Africa." *British Medical Journal* 322 (7293): 1012.

Global HIV Prevention Working Group. 2002. "Global Mobilization for HIV Prevention: A Blueprint for Action." Accessed December 14, 2012. http://www.globalhiv prevention.org/pdfs/hivprevreport_final.pdf

Gostin, Lawrence O. 2000. "A Proposed National Policy on Health Care Workers Living with HIV/AIDS and Other Blood-Borne Pathogens." *Journal of the American Medical Association* 284 (15): 1965–70.

Gostin, Lawrence O.; John W. Ward; and A. Cornelius Baker. 1997. "National HIV Case Reporting for the United States: A Defining Moment in the History of the Epidemic." *New England Journal of Medicine* 337 (16): 1162–67.

Guay, Laura A.; Philippa Musoke; Thomas Fleming; et al. 1999. "Intrapartum and Neonatal Single-Dose Nevirapine Compared with Zidovudine for Prevention of Mother-to-Child Transmission of HIV-1 in Kampala, Uganda: HIVNET 012 Randomised Trial." *Lancet* 354 (9181): 795–802.

Henry J. Kaiser Family Foundation. 2012a. "HIV/AIDS Policy: The HIV/AIDS Epidemic in the United States." Accessed December 14, 2012. http://www.kff.org/hivaids/upload/3029-13.pdf

Henry J. Kaiser Family Foundation. 2012b. "The U.S. President's Emergency Plan for AIDS Relief (PEPFAR)." U.S. Global Health Policy. Accessed December 14, 2012. http://www.kff .org/globalhealth/upload/8002-04.pdf

Joint United Nations Programme on HIV/AIDS (UNAIDS). 2000. *Ethical Considerations in HIV Preventive Vaccine Research: UNAIDS Guidance Document.* Geneva: Author. http://www unaids.org/publications/documents/vaccines/

Joint United Nations Programme on HIV/AIDS (UNAIDS). 2001a. *AIDS Epidemic Update, December 2001.* Geneva: Author. Accessed December 12, 2012. http://www.unaids.org/ en/media/unaids/contentassets/dataimport/publications/ irc-pub06/epiupdate01_en.pdf

Joint United Nations Programme on HIV/AIDS (UNAIDS). 2001b. *Children and Young People in a World of AIDS.* http://data.unaids.org/publications/irc-pub02/jc656-child_aids_en.pdf

Kallings, Lars, and Stefano Vella. 2001. "Access to HIV/AIDS Care and Treatment in the South of the World." *AIDS* 15 (7): IAS1–3.

Langan, Michael, and Chris Collins. 1998. *Paving the Road to an HIV Vaccine: Employing Tools of Public Policy to Overcome Scientific, Economic, Social, and Ethical Obstacles.* San Francisco: Center for AIDS Prevention Studies, AIDS Research Institute, University of California.

Levine, Carol; Nancy N. Dubler; and Robert J. Levine. 1991. "Building a New Consensus: Ethical Principles and Policies for Clinical Research on HIV/AIDS." *IRB: A Review of Human Subjects Research* 13 (1): 1–17.

Levine, Robert J. 1999. "The Need to Revise the Declaration of Helsinki." *New England Journal of Medicine* 341 (7): 531–34.

Lo, Bernard. 2000. "Confidentiality." In *Resolving Ethical Dilemmas: A Guide for Clinicians.* 2nd ed. Philadelphia: Lippincott, Williams, and Wilkins.

Lo, Bernard. 2001. "Addressing Ethical Issues." In *Designing Clinical Research,* 2nd ed., edited by Stephen Hulley, Steven R. Cummings, Warren S. Browner, et al. Philadelphia: Lippincott, Williams, and Wilkins.

Lo, Bernard, and Robert Steinbrook. 1992. "Health Care Workers Infected with the Human Immunodeficiency Virus: The Next Steps." *Journal of the American Medical Association* 267 (8): 1100–1105.

Lurie, Peter, and Sidney M. Wolfe. 1997. "Unethical Trials of Interventions to Reduce Perinatal Transmission of the Human Immunodeficiency Virus in Developing Countries." *New England Journal of Medicine* 337 (12): 853–56.

McDonough, John E. 2012. "The Road Ahead for the Affordable Care Act." *New England Journal of Medicine* 367 (3): 199–201.

McGann v. H & H Music Company. 1991. 946 F.2d 401 (5th Cir.).

Merritt, Maria W. 2011. "Health Researchers' Ancillary Care Obligations in Low-Resource Settings: How Can We Tell What Is Morally Required?" *Kennedy Institute of Ethics Journal* 21 (4): 311–47.

Montaner, Julio S. G.; Robert Hogg; Evan Wood; et al. 2006. "The Case for Expanding Access to Highly Active Antiretroviral Therapy to Curb the Growth of the HIV Epidemic." *Lancet* 368 (9534): 531–36.

National Federation of Independent Business v. Sebelius. 2012. 132 S.Ct. 2566.

Nduati, Ruth; Grace John; Dorothy Mbori-Ngacha; et al. 2000. "Effect of Breastfeeding and Formula Feeding on Transmission of HIV-1: A Randomized Clinical Trial." *Journal of the American Medical Association* 283 (9): 1167–74.

Steinbrook, Robert. 1998. "Caring for People with Human Immunodeficiency Virus Infection." *New England Journal of Medicine* 339 (26): 1926–28.

Steinbrook, Robert. 2002. "Beyond Barcelona: The Global Response to HIV." *New England Journal of Medicine* 347 (8): 553–54.

Stoto, Michael A.; Donna A. Almario; and Marie C. McCormick, eds. 1999. *Reducing the Odds: Preventing Perinatal Transmission of HIV in the United States.* Washington, DC: National Academy Press.

United Nations Department of Economic and Social Affairs. 2010. *The Millennium Development Goals Report 2010.* Accessed December 12, 2012. http://www.unfpa.org/public/home/publications/pid/6090

US National Bioethics Advisory Commission. 2001a. *Ethical and Policy Issues in Research Involving Human Participants.* Rockville, MD: Author.

US National Bioethics Advisory Commission. 2001b. *Report and Recommendations of the National Bioethics Advisory Commission.* Vol. 1 of *Ethical and Policy Issues in International Research: Clinical Trials in Developing Countries.* Bethesda, MD: Author.

Varmus, Harold, and David Satcher. 1997. "Ethical Complexities of Conducting Research in Developing Countries." *New England Journal of Medicine* 337 (12): 1003–5.

Wolf, Leslie E., and Bernard Lo. 1999. "What about the Ethics?" *Western Journal of Medicine* 171 (5–6): 365–66.

Wolf, Leslie E.; Bernard Lo; Karen P. Beckerman; et al. 2001. "When Parents Reject Interventions to Reduce Perinatal Transmission of HIV." *Archives of Pediatrics and Adolescent Medicine* 155:927–33.

World Health Organization. 2002. "Integrated Management of Adolescent and Adult Illness (IMAI) Modules." 3 by 5 Initiative. Accessed December 12, 2012. http://www.who.int/3by5/publications/documents/imai/en/

World Medical Association. 1996. *Declaration of Helsinki: Ethical Principles for Medical Research Involving Human Subjects.* Ferney-Voltaire, France: Author.

World Medical Association. 2000. *Declaration of Helsinki: Ethical Principles for Medical Research Involving Human Subjects.* Ferney-Voltaire, France: Author.

World Medical Association. 2001. *Declaration of Helsinki: Note of Clarification on Placebo-Controlled Trials.* Ferney-Voltaire, France: Author.

Leslie E. Wolf
Professor of Law, Georgia State University College of Law

Rachel L. Hulkower
Georgia State University College of Law

ALCOHOL AND OTHER DRUGS IN A PUBLIC HEALTH CONTEXT

Psychoactive drugs are substances that alter the mental state of humans after ingestion. There are a wide variety of such substances, both naturally occurring and synthesized, including tobacco, alcoholic beverages, coffee, tea, chocolate, and some spices, as well as substances that are legally available only through medical channels, such as benzodiazepines, cannabinoids, opiates, and cocaine. Such substances often have other use values along with their psychoactive properties. Users may like the taste or the image of themselves that the use of those substances conveys. Substance use may be a medium of sociability (Partanen 1991) or part of a religious ritual. Some substances have other useful properties; alcohol, for example, is a source of calories and is used as a solvent in tinctures.

Psychoactive drugs differ in their metabolic pathways and mechanisms of action in the human body, the strength of their effects, and the states of mind and feelings they induce. Yet the effects of drug use also are highly dependent on the pattern of use and on the set and setting—that is, the expectations of the user and of others who are present and the context of use (Zinberg 1984). Although the psychoactive effect of tobacco may not register in the consciousness of a habituated cigarette smoker, in other circumstances the effect of tobacco use may be so strong that the user is rendered unconscious, as early Spanish observers reported in describing tobacco use among native South Americans (Robicsek 1978).

Psychoactive substances frequently are valued by potential consumers well above the cost of production. On the one hand, this means that taxes on alcohol, tobacco, and other drugs have long been an important fiscal resource for the state. On the other hand, it means that there are substantial incentives for an illicit market to emerge in places where the sale of drugs is forbidden or stringently restricted.

A consideration of drugs in a public health context may start with an examination of general cultural patternings and understandings of drug use. This entry continues by discussing the major approaches to limiting harm from drug use. The entry concludes with a characterization of the major directions in the development of drug policies in the United States and other industrialized countries.

GENERAL CULTURAL FRAMINGS OF DRUG ABUSE

Three social patternings of psychoactive drug use can be distinguished as prototypical: medicinal use, customary regular use, and intermittent use. In many traditional societies some drugs or formulations have been confined to medicinal use—that is, use under the supervision of a healer to alleviate mental or physical illness or distress. For several centuries after the technique for distilling alcoholic spirits had diffused from the Arab world to Europe, for instance, spirits-based drinks were regarded primarily as medicines (Wasson 1984). This way of framing drug use has been routinized in the modern state through a prescription system, with physicians writing the prescriptions and pharmacists filling them. Drugs included in the prescription system usually are forbidden for nonmedicinal use (Babor et al. 2010).

When a drug becomes a regular accompaniment of everyday life, its psychoactivity often is muted and even unnoticed, as is often the case for a habitual cigarette smoker. Similarly, in southern European wine cultures wine is often differentiated from intoxicating "alcohol"; wine drinkers are expected to maintain their original comportment after drinking. This may be called a pattern of *banalized use*: A potentially powerful psychoactive agent is domesticated into a mundane article of daily life that is available relatively freely in the consumer market.

Intermittent use—for instance, on sacred occasions, at festivals, or only on weekends—minimizes the buildup of tolerance to a drug. It is in the context of those patterns that the greatest attention is likely to be paid to a drug's psychoactive properties. The drug may be understood by both the user and others as having taken control of the user's behavior and thus to explain otherwise unexpected behavior, whether bad or good (see the "disinhibition hypothesis" in Pernanen 1976; see also Room 2001b). As in nineteenth-century Scottish author Robert Louis Stevenson's fable of Jekyll and Hyde, normal self-control is expected to return when the effects of the drug wear off. In light of the power attributed to the substance, access to it may be limited: in traditional societies by sumptuary rules keyed to social differentiations and in industrial societies by other forms of market restriction.

In industrial societies a fourth pattern of use is commonly recognized for certain drugs: addicted or dependent use that is marked by regular use, often of large doses. Because the pattern of use of a particular drug is not defined in the society as banalized, addiction is defined as an individual failing rather than a social pattern. Although attention is paid to physical factors that sustain regular use, such as use to relieve withdrawal symptoms, most formulations of addiction focus on psychological aspects, including an apparent commitment to drug use to the exclusion of other activities and despite default in performing major social roles. An addiction concept thus also focuses on the loss of normal self-control, but the emphasis is not so much on the immediate effects of the drug as it is on a repeated or continuing pattern of an apparent inability to control or refrain from use despite the adverse consequences.

ADDICTION AS A MODERN GOVERNING IMAGE

The concept of addiction as an affliction of habituated drug users first arose in its modern form for alcohol as heavy drinking lost its banalized status in the United States and some other countries under the influence of the temperance movement of the nineteenth century (Levine 1978; Valverde 1998). Habitual drunkenness had been viewed since the Middle Ages as a subclass of gluttony; now abstinence from alcohol was singled out as a separate virtue and an important sign of the key virtue in a democracy of autonomous citizens: self-control. Along with other mental disorders, *chronic inebriety*, as habitual drunkenness became termed, was reinterpreted as a disease suitable for medical intervention, although without losing all of its negative moral loading.

In nineteenth-century formulations addictiveness was seen as an inherent property of alcohol no matter who used it, and that perception justified efforts to prohibit its sale. By the late nineteenth century such addiction concepts were being applied also to opiates and other drugs, and this formulation has remained the governing image (Room 2001a) for those drugs to the present day. But as temperance became unpopular with the repeal of national alcohol prohibitions in the United States in 1933 and in several other countries in the same period (Schrad 2010), for alcohol the concept was reformulated to be a property of the individual "alcoholic," who was mysteriously unable to drink like a normal drinker. This "disease concept of alcoholism" received its classic scholarly formulation by E. M. Jellinek (1952), although that author later (1960) retreated to a broader formulation of alcohol problems.

In popular thinking and often in official definitions, addiction has remained a property of the drug for illicit drugs but of the person for alcohol (Christie and Bruun 1969). The inherent addictiveness attributed to illicit drugs is the primary rationale for their prohibition (Room 2006a). The extent of the anathema imposed in US cultural politics by labeling a substance as addictive can be gauged from the unanimous testimony of cigarette company executives to the US Congress in 1994 that they did not believe that cigarettes are addictive despite the evidence of their own corporate research (Hilts 1994).

In the late twentieth and early twenty-first centuries, philosophers and cultural analysts have begun to question and rethink the meaning of addiction concepts (Fingarette 1988; Keane 2002) and consider the implications for drug policy (Husak 1992). In a related initiative, economists have begun propounding and testing theories of *rational addiction* (Elster and Skog 1999). More recently, there have been arguments against a neurobiological framing, emphasizing the role of environment in addiction (Levy 2013). As the addiction concept has been applied to more and more behaviors (Potenza 2006; Avena, Rada, and Hoebel 2008; Saïet 2011), its cultural power as a mysterious explanation of behavior may be weakening.

APPROACHES TO LIMITING THE PROBLEMS FROM DRUG USE

Most human societies have known of and used psychoactive drugs, and most also have made efforts to limit the use of one or more drugs, customarily if not legislatively. Historically, the main aim of those restrictions was to diminish threats to the social order or to increase the labor supply. Public health concerns sometimes were expressed in attempts to justify restrictions—for instance, in the early seventeenth-century efforts of James I of England to stem tobacco smoking (Austin 1979)—but such concerns were rarely decisive. The restrictions on the spirits market adopted in Britain as a response to the extreme alcoholization of eighteenth-century London (depicted in the English painter and engraver William Hogarth's famous print of *Gin Lane*) are an early example of limits substantially motivated by concern about public health (Warner 2002; Dillon 2003). Only since the 1970s have public health concerns become a major element in discussions of drug policies, although those concerns often are subordinated in the case of legal drugs to fiscal and economic considerations and in the case of illicit drugs to moral and lifestyle issues.

Health hazards from psychoactive drugs occur in two main ways: in connection with particular occasions of use and in connection with the patterning of use over time. Thus, an overdose from barbiturates, a traffic casualty from drunk driving, and an HIV infection from sharing a needle to inject heroin are all consequences associated with a particular occasion of use, whereas lung cancer from tobacco smoking, liver cirrhosis from alcohol use, and (by definition) addiction all reflect a history of heavy use. As is discussed below, measures to prevent event-related problems often differ from and even conflict with measures to prevent cumulative, condition-related problems. For alcohol the ethical situation with regard to public health measures is complicated by the possibility of a protective effect of drinking on heart disease that must be balanced against the undoubted negative health effects (Rehm, Sempos, and Trevisan 2003; Room 2006b).

Efforts to limit problems from drug use can be seen as oriented toward controlling whether a drug is used at all; influencing the amount, context, and pattern of use; or preventing harmful consequences of use (Bruun 1971; Moore and Gerstein 1981).

Prohibiting Use to All or Some. Efforts to impose a general prohibition on the use of a drug for all the members of a society have a lengthy history, although those efforts frequently have failed (Austin 1979). Perhaps the most sustained effort has been the prohibition on alcoholic beverages in Islamic societies (Michalak and Trocki 2006). In general, religious taboos on drug use have tended to have more lasting effects than have state prohibitions. Prohibiting the sale or use of a drug that some might choose to use and enjoy involves a degree of intervention in the marketplace and in private behavior that is unusual in modern democratic states. If there are people who use a drug without problems, the prohibition on their use of that drug must be justified as benefiting others who would have or would cause problems if they used it. In societies with a strong tradition of individual liberties and consumer sovereignty, discomfort with the use of this line of argument to support prohibition commonly is resolved by presumptions that users sooner or later will become addicted and that users without problems do not really exist.

A common form of prohibition of use in village and tribal societies has been sumptuary rules restricting use to particular status groups, most commonly the most powerful segments of the society. Depending on the culture, a variety of arguments are offered for the inability of lower-status groups to handle drug use appropriately. Because psychoactive drugs offer visions of an alternative reality (Stauffer 1971) and may be associated with disinhibition, dominant groups may fear challenges to their power if subordinates have access to drugs (Morgan 1983). The universalist ethic of modern states has made explicit sumptuary restrictions untenable, with the substantial exception of prohibitions on use by children. Yet provisions that the names of habitual drunkards be posted and that those listed be refused service of alcoholic drinks, mostly abandoned or disused since the 1960s, appear to be making a comeback (Room 2012).

A third form of modified prohibition of use that is often employed in modern societies is limitation to medicinal use. The individual's supply of such medications is controlled by state-licensed professionals who are backed up by a state system of market controls. National controls on psychopharmaceuticals are backed up by an unusual and elaborate international control structure (Bruun, Pan, and Rexed 1975; Babor, Caulkins, Edwards, et al. 2010). In principle, the prescribing and use of these drugs are limited to therapeutic purposes. For psychoactive drugs, which commonly are prescribed to relieve negative affective states or mental distress, the definition of therapeutic use is often quite wide, and a substantial proportion of the resources of the health system in industrial societies is absorbed in superintending the provision of psychoactive drugs.

Except for methadone or other opioids as a remedy for heroin addiction and nicotine as a remedy for tobacco smoking, it generally is considered illegitimate to prescribe a drug to help a person maintain a habitual pattern of use without withdrawal or other distress. Use for pleasure or for the sake of the psychoactive experience is considered nontherapeutic, and so the functions of drugs that are considered psychopharmaceuticals are always described in terms of the relief of distress rather than the provision of pleasure. To some extent the medical prescription system in a modern state serves as a covert form of control by status differentiation, according to the prejudices of the prescriber; for instance, older and more respectable adults find it easier than do the younger and more disreputable to obtain a prescription for a psychopharmaceutical (Babor, Caulkins, Edwards, et al. 2010).

Influencing the Pattern of Use. An enormous variety of formal and informal strategies have been used to influence the amount, pattern, and context of the use of drugs. Among the potential aims of those strategies is the public health goal of reducing the prevalence of hazardous use.

Controlling Availability. One class of such strategies attempts to reduce drug-related problems by controlling the market in drugs by means of taxes, general restrictions on availability, or user-specific restrictions (Room 2000; Babor, Caetano, Casswell, et al. 2010). Public health considerations are one reason among several that governments tax legally available drugs such as alcohol and tobacco. Such taxes often constitute a substantial portion of the price paid by the consumer. Raising taxes does diminish levels of use among heavier as well as lighter users, although demand usually diminishes proportionately less than the increase in price; that is, demand is relatively inelastic. Thus, short of levels that create an opening for a substantial illicit market, raising taxes on drugs tends both to have positive public health effects and to increase government revenues.

Governments often also control the conditions of availability, particularly for alcohol. Through a system of retail licenses or a government monopoly of sales, limits are placed on the hours and conditions of sale. Changes in those limits sometimes have been found to affect patterns of consumption and of alcohol-related problems (Babor, Caetano, Casswell, et al. 2010). But with the strengthening of the ideology of consumer sovereignty—legal goods should be readily available, with purchases limited only by the consumer's means—controls on availability tend to have been loosened in the contemporary period (Mäkelä et al. 1981).

A generally stronger and more direct effect on hazardous alcohol consumption has been found to result from measures that ration or restrict the availability of alcohol for specific purchasers (Babor, Caetano, Casswell et al. 2010). A general ration limit for all purchasers restricts heavy consumption or at least raises the effective price, but such measures strongly conflict with the ideology of consumer sovereignty and are thus politically impracticable nearly everywhere. As was noted above, proscriptions or limits on sales to named heavy users also fell out of favor because they were considered infringements on individual liberty, but such tactics are being revived, for instance in the United Kingdom and Australia (Room 2012).

Controlling the Circumstances of Use. Another class of strategies aims to deter drinking or drug use in particularly hazardous circumstances, usually through the use of criminal sanctions. The prototypical situation is driving after drinking. Because alcohol consumption impairs the ability to drive a vehicle, most countries treat driving with a blood-alcohol level above a set limit as a criminal offense, and the enforcement of those laws often absorbs a substantial proportion of the criminal justice system's resources. Popular movements as well as policy makers have expended much energy, particularly in the United States and other Anglophone and Scandinavian countries, in seeking a redefinition of drunk driving as a serious crime rather than a "folk crime" (Gusfield 1981). This type of situational limit or prohibition has been extended to other skill-related tasks and also has been applied to driving after using other psychoactive drugs, particularly illicit drugs. A related development has sought to eliminate illicit drug use in working populations and alcohol use in the workplace by means of random urine testing of workers, with job loss as the sanction (Zimmer and Jacobs 1992).

The ethics of this measure, which was pushed strongly by the US government in the 1980s, are controversial, particularly because the tests detect illicit drug use that has not necessarily affected work performance (Macdonald and Roman 1994). Random blood-alcohol tests of drivers to deter drinking before driving also have proved controversial: they are effective, well accepted, and widely applied in Australia (Homel 1990; Peek-Asa 1999) and northern Europe; legally permissible but not intensively applied in the United States; and in some countries viewed as too much of an infringement on individual liberty and privacy.

Education and Persuasion about Use. A third class of strategies seeks to educate people or persuade them not to engage in hazardous drug use. Because such strategies are seen as the least coercive, at least for those beyond school age, they are used very widely and commonly despite the frequent lack of clear evidence on their effectiveness (Paglia and Room 1999; Babor, Caetano, Casswell, et al. 2010; Babor, Caulkins, Edwards, et al. 2010). Education of schoolchildren about the hazards of drug use is very widespread, indeed nearly ubiquitous, in the United States. Most countries also have made at least a token effort at public information campaigns about the hazards of tobacco smoking, and poster and slogan campaigns against drinking before driving and illicit drug use are also widespread. Other public information campaigns on alcohol have promoted limits on drinking (e.g., suggestions of safe levels in Britain and Australia) or campaigned against drinking in various hazardous circumstances.

Often these public information campaigns have competed for attention in a media environment saturated with advertising from tobacco or alcohol companies on behalf of use. From the 1980s onward, there have been increasing restrictions on tobacco and, to a lesser extent, alcohol advertising, such as through bans advertisements on electronic media and via mandated warning labels in advertisements or on product packages. While US court decisions have limited such restrictions for alcohol as impermissible restrictions on the freedom of "commercial speech," tobacco advertising has been effectively restricted. Attempts by global producers to counter such restrictions as contrary to free-trade agreements have been more successful for alcohol than for tobacco (O'Brien 2013).

Reducing the Harm from Use. The strategies considered above are directed primarily at influencing the fact or pattern of use. They thus fall into the category of either supply reduction or demand reduction, to use terminology commonly applied to the use of illicit drugs. Since the late 1980s substantial attention has been directed toward a third option: harm reduction, or strategies that reduce the problems associated with drug use without necessarily reducing drug use (O'Hare et al. 1992; Heather et al. 1993). Attention to this class of strategies has a somewhat longer history for alcohol (Room 2004). Usually these strategies focus on the physical or social environment of drug use, seeking physical, temporal, or cultural insulation of the drug use from harm. Thus, needle exchanges are intended to remove the risk of HIV infection from injection drug use, and seat belts and air bags insulate drivers who drink and those around them from the possibility of becoming casualties.

The debate over harm reduction strategies for illicit drugs has raised classic ethical issues for public health. Some argue that insulating the behavior from harm will encourage and thus increase the prevalence of the undesirable behavior.

A further consideration is the effectiveness of the insulation provided. Thus, efforts to provide a safer tobacco cigarette largely have been undercut by compensatory changes in puffing and inhaling by smokers. At an empirical level it seems that insulating drug use from harm does not necessarily increase the prevalence of drug use (Yoast et al. 2001). Even if it did, an old public health tradition that is epitomized by the operation of venereal disease clinics would argue that reducing the immediate risk of harm has a higher ethical priority than affecting the prevalence of disapproved behaviors.

THE POLITICAL REALITY IN THE MID-2010s: LOPSIDED POLICIES AND SIGNS OF CHANGE

The United States and many other countries have experienced recurring "moral panics" from the 1960s on concerning illicit drug use and have invested substantial resources in efforts to prevent such use. These resources have been invested largely in two areas: a particular preventive strategy—interdicting the illicit market—and the provision of treatment. The first strategy has received the greatest investment of government resources. On a global level, the attempt to eliminate or at least reduce the illicit market has failed (Room and Reuter 2012).

At the level of individual countries, there are ebbs and flows in drug use. There was a substantial decrease in illicit drug use in North America in the late 1980s and early 1990s, but that was followed by a rise in the 1990s. In the early twenty-first century, the rates of current illicit drug use in the population were fairly stable, although cannabis use rose between 2007 and 2011 (SAMHSA 2012). Governments often are blamed or credited for these shifts up and down, but such trends may have more to do with cyclical patterns in youth fashions and social mores. The illicit market remains strong, and drug-related imprisonments are a primary reason that the United States has the highest rate of incarceration among industrial societies.

Meanwhile, the highest rates of health and social harm come from legal drugs. The contribution in 2010 of different risk factors to the total burden of disease globally is estimated at 6.3 percent for tobacco, 3.9 percent for alcohol, and 0.8 percent for all illicit drugs (Lim et al. 2012). In terms of a collective judgment by psychopharmacologists of the intrinsic harmfulness of twenty psychoactive substances, alcohol ranked highest and tobacco sixth (Nutt, King, and Phillips 2010). But the wide gulf in thinking established in the mid-twentieth century (Courtwright 2005) between illicit drugs, on the one hand, and alcohol and tobacco, on the other, has continued at the policy level, both nationally and globally. Alcohol and tobacco have therefore received a much lower policy priority, and government policy making, particularly regarding alcohol, often subordinates public health considerations to economic concerns.

A substantial emphasis on the treatment of addiction has accompanied the emphasis on attacking markets in illicit drugs. In this mixed policy environment, however, the role of treatment has been highly differentiated by the type of drug. To a large extent tobacco smoking has continued to be defined as a health problem rather than a social problem, with the emphasis on the health consequences of smoking rather than the physical dependence of smokers on tobacco. Thus, there has been very little public provision of treatment for smoking addiction; most of those who have quit have done it by themselves or by using nicotine substitutes. At the same time, public health advocates have had increasing success in many industrialized countries in tightening tobacco controls, eliminating smoking in the workplace and in indoor public spaces. In these circumstances, the rates of cigarette and other tobacco smoking have declined substantially since the 1960s. Tobacco producers have thus increasingly concentrated on low- and middle-income countries. It is estimated that between 1970 and 2000 tobacco consumption rose by 3.1 percent annually in developing countries while falling by 0.2 percent per year in developed countries (FAO 2003).

The goals for an illicit drug treatment system have often been highly ambitious. In theory, in the mid-1970s and again in the late 1980s, the United States aspired to provide treatment to every unincarcerated addict. Drug treatment provision substantially increased in the latter part of the twentieth century in many other countries as well (Klingemann and Hunt 1998). Quite explicitly, treatment for illicit drug use has been seen in the United States as a form of social control, and a high degree of coercion has been taken for granted (IOM 1990). On occasion, US drug strategies have argued for the provision of treatment as a means to encourage courts to be tougher on those who choose not to accept it (Strategy Council on Drug Abuse 1973), and drug treatment agencies have argued routinely for maintaining jail sentences for drug use in order to force users into treatment as an alternative.

In the case of alcohol there also has been substantial growth in treatment provision in the United States and elsewhere (Klingemann, Takala, and Hunt 1992). In English-speaking and northern European countries, where systems of alcohol regulation were substantially loosened in the second half of the twentieth century, the growth of alcohol treatment provision, it has been argued, accompanied and served as a "cultural alibi" for the dismantling of the alcohol control structure (Mäkelä et al. 1981). Although there is an increasing contradiction between the demands for sobriety in a technological environment and the increased market availability of alcohol, managing that contradiction is seen as a character test for the individual consumer, with treatment for alcoholism provided for those deemed to have failed the test (Room 2011).

By 2013 there were signs of change in policies. Tobacco was the furthest advanced on a new course, with the signing of the Framework Convention on Tobacco Use in 2003, and subsequent steps in implementing it, setting an international climate for strengthened regulation of tobacco. Change in alcohol policy was the least advanced. The World Health Assembly adopted a global strategy to reduce the harmful use of alcohol in 2010, but the World Health Organization had scant resources for action on the strategy, and political support was generally weak for strengthened public health measures. For illicit drugs—the drugs controlled by United Nations drug treaties—there had been little change in the international system, but it was increasingly subject to criticism and defection. With a variety of motivations, including an unwillingness to continue suffering the casualties of the so-called war on drugs on their territory, a number of Latin American countries were moving toward change at the domestic level. A 2013 report by the Organization of American States carried Latin American questioning of the system to a new level (OAS 2013). Perhaps most significantly, given the strong role the United States has played in the international drug prohibition system, there was, by 2013, majority support among US adults for legalizing cannabis sales, and two US states—Colorado and Washington—voted in 2012 to set up a regulated legal domestic market in cannabis. While the outcome of these steps remained uncertain, they were in themselves substantial signs of change.

SEE ALSO *Addiction and Dependence; Public Health: I. History; Smoking*

BIBLIOGRAPHY

Austin, Gregory A. 1979. *Perspectives on the History of Psychoactive Substance Use.* National Institute on Drug Abuse Research Issues 24. Washington, DC: US Government Printing Office.

Avena, Nicole M.; Pedro Rada; and Bartley G. Hoebel. 2008. "Evidence for Sugar Addiction: Behavioral and Neurochemical Effects of Intermittent, Excessive Sugar Intake." *Neuroscience and Biobehavioral Reviews* 32 (1): 20–39.

Babor, Thomas; Raul Caetano; Sally Casswell; et al. 2010. *Alcohol—No Ordinary Commodity: Research and Public Policy.* 2nd ed. Oxford: Oxford University Press.

Babor, Thomas; Jonathan Caulkins; Griffith Edwards; et al. 2010. *Drug Policy and the Public Good.* Oxford: Oxford University Press.

Bruun, Kettil. 1971. "Finland: The Non-medical Approach." In *Alcoholism and Drug Abuse: Proceedings of the 29th International Congress on Alcoholism and Drug Dependence, Sydney, Australia, February, 1970,* edited by L. G. Kiloh and D. S. Bell, 545–59. Chatswood, Australia: Butterworths.

Bruun, Kettil; Lynn Pan; and Ingemar Rexed. 1975. *The Gentlemen's Club: International Control of Drugs and Alcohol.* Chicago: University of Chicago Press.

Christie, Nils, and Kettil Bruun. 1969. "Alcohol Problems: The Conceptual Framework." In *Proceedings of the 28th International Congress on Alcohol and Alcoholism,* vol. 2, *Lectures in Plenary Sessions,* edited by Mark Keller and Timothy G. Coffey, 65–73. Highland Park, NJ: Hillhouse Press.

Courtwright, David T. 2005. "Mr. ATOD's Wild Ride: What Do Alcohol, Tobacco, and Other Drugs Have in Common?" *Social History of Alcohol and Drugs* 20 (1): 105–24.

Dillon, Patrick. 2003. *Gin: The Much-Lamented Death of Madam Geneva; The Eighteenth-Century Gin Craze.* Boston: Justin, Charles.

Elster, Jon, and Ole-Jørgen Skog, eds. 1999. *Getting Hooked: Rationality and Addiction.* Cambridge, UK: Cambridge University Press.

FAO (Food and Agriculture Organization of the United Nations). 2003. *Projections of Tobacco Production, Consumption, and Trade to the Year 2010.* Rome: Author.

Fingarette, Herbert. 1988. *Heavy Drinking: The Myth of Alcoholism as a Disease.* Berkeley: University of California Press.

Gusfield, Joseph R. 1981. *The Culture of Public Problems: Drinking-Driving and the Symbolic Order.* Chicago: University of Chicago Press.

Heather, Nick; Alex Wodak; Ethan Nadelmann; and P. A. O'Hare, eds. 1993. *Psychoactive Drugs and Harm Reduction: From Faith to Science.* London: Whurr.

Hilts, Philip J. 1994. "Embattled Tobacco: One Maker's Struggle" (three-part series of articles). *New York Times,* June 16, 17, and 18.

Homel, Ross. 1990. "Random Breath Testing and Random Stopping Programs in Australia." In *Drinking and Driving: Advances in Research and Prevention,* edited by R. Jean Wilson and Robert E. Mann, 159–204. New York: Guilford Press.

Husak, Douglas N. 1992. *Drugs and Rights.* Cambridge, UK: Cambridge University Press.

IOM (Institute of Medicine). Committee for the Substance Abuse Coverage Study. 1990. *Treating Drug Problems,* vol. 1, *A Study of the Evolution, Effectiveness, and Financing of Public and Private Drug Treatment Systems.* Edited by Dean R. Gerstein and Henrick J. Harwood. Washington, DC: National Academy Press.

Jellinek, E. M. 1952. "Phases of Alcohol Addiction." *Quarterly Journal of Studies on Alcohol* 13 (4): 673–84.

Jellinek, E. M. 1960. *The Disease Concept of Alcoholism.* New Haven, CT: Hillhouse Press.

Keane, Helen. 2002. *What's Wrong with Addiction?* Melbourne: Melbourne University Press.

Klingemann, Harald, and Geoffrey Hunt, eds. 1998. *Drug Treatment Systems in an International Perspective: Drugs, Demons, and Delinquents.* Thousand Oaks, CA: Sage.

Klingemann, Harald; Jukka-Pekka Takala; and Geoffrey Hunt, eds. 1992. *Cure, Care, or Control: Alcoholism Treatment in Sixteen Countries.* Albany: State University of New York Press.

Levine, Harry Gene. 1978. "The Discovery of Addiction: Changing Concepts of Habitual Drunkenness in American History." *Journal of Studies on Alcohol* 39 (1): 143–74.

Levy, Neil. 2013. "Addiction Is Not a Brain Disease (and It Matters)." *Frontiers in Psychiatry* 4:24. Accessed August 14, 2013. doi:10.3389/fpsyt.2013.00024.

Lim, Stephen S.; Theo Vos; Abraham D. Flaxman; et al. 2012. "A Comparative Risk Assessment of Burden of Disease and Injury Attributable to 67 Risk Factors and Risk Factor Clusters in 21 Regions, 1990–2010: A Systematic Analysis for the Global Burden of Disease Study 2010." *Lancet* 380 (9859): 2224–60.

Macdonald, Scott, and Paul Roman, eds. 1994. *Drug Testing in the Workplace.* Research Advances in Alcohol and Drug Problems 11. New York: Plenum Press.

Mäkelä, Klaus; Robin Room; Eric Single; et al., eds. 1981. *Alcohol, Society, and the State,* vol. 1, *A Comparative Study of Alcohol Control.* Toronto: Addiction Research Foundation.

Michalak, Laurence, and Karen Trocki. 2006. "Alcohol and Islam: An Overview." *Contemporary Drug Problems* 33 (4): 523–62.

Moore, Mark H., and Dean R. Gerstein, eds. 1981. *Alcohol and Public Policy: Beyond the Shadow of Prohibition.* Washington, DC: National Academy Press.

Morgan, Patricia. 1983. "Alcohol, Disinhibition, and Domination: A Conceptual Analysis." In *Alcohol and Disinhibition: Nature and Meaning of the Link,* edited by Robin Room and Gary Collins, 405–20. National Institute on Alcohol Abuse and Alcoholism Research Monograph 12. Washington, DC: US Government Printing Office.

Nutt, David J.; Leslie A. King; and Lawrence D. Phillips. 2010. "Drug Harms in the UK: A Multicriteria Decision Analysis." *Lancet* 376 (9752): 1588–65.

OAS (Organization of American States). General Secretariat. 2013. *The Drug Problem in the Americas.* Washington, DC: Author.

O'Brien, Paula. 2013. "Australia's Double Standard on Thailand's Alcohol Warning Labels." *Drug and Alcohol Review* 32 (1): 5–10.

O'Hare, P. A.; Russell Newcombe; Alan Matthews; et al., eds. 1992. *The Reduction of Drug-Related Harm.* London: Routledge.

Paglia, Angela, and Robin Room. 1999. "Preventing Substance Use Problems among Youth: A Literature Review and Recommendations." *Journal of Primary Prevention* 20 (1): 3–50.

Partanen, Juha. 1991. *Sociability and Intoxication: Alcohol and Drinking in Kenya, Africa, and the Modern World.* Finnish Foundation for Alcohol Studies (series) 39. Helsinki: Finnish Foundation for Alcohol Studies.

Peek-Asa, Corinne. 1999. "Effect of Random Alcohol Screening in Reducing Motor Vehicle Crash Injuries." *American Journal of Preventive Medicine* 16 (1), supp. 1, 57–67.

Pernanen, Kai. 1976. "Alcohol and Crimes of Violence." In *The Biology of Alcoholism,* edited by Benjamin Kissin and Henri Begleiter, vol. 4, *Social Aspects of Alcoholism,* 351–444. New York: Plenum Press.

Potenza, Marc N. 2006. "Should Addictive Disorders Include Non-substance-Related Conditions?" *Addiction* 101 (supp. s1): 142–51.

Rehm, J.; C. T. Sempos; and M. Trevisan 2003. "Average Volume of Alcohol Consumption, Patterns of Drinking, and Risk of Coronary Heart Disease: A Review." *European Journal of Cardiovascular Risk* 10 (1): 15–20.

Robicsek, Francis. 1978. *The Smoking Gods: Tobacco in Maya Art, History, and Religion.* Norman: University of Oklahoma Press.

Room, Robin. 1975. "Minimizing Alcohol Problems." In *Proceedings of the Fourth Annual Alcoholism Conference of the National Institute on Alcohol Abuse and Alcoholism: Research, Treatment, and Prevention, Washington, D.C., June 12–14, 1974,* edited by Morris E. Chafetz, 379–93. Department of Health, Education, and Welfare publication no. (ADM) 76-284. Washington, DC: US Government Printing Office.

Room, Robin. 2000. "Control Systems for Psychoactive Substances." In *Nicotine and Public Health,* edited by Roberta Ferrence, John Slade, Robin Room, and Marilyn Pope, 37–61. Washington, DC: American Public Health Association.

Room, Robin. 2001a. "Governing Images in Public Discourse about Problematic Drinking." In *International Handbook of Alcohol Dependence and Problems,* edited by Nick Heather, Timothy J. Peters, and Tim Stockwell, 33–45. Chichester, UK: Wiley.

Room, Robin. 2001b. "Intoxication and Bad Behaviour: Understanding Cultural Differences in the Link." *Social Science and Medicine* 53 (2): 189–98.

Room, Robin. 2004. "Alcohol and Harm Reduction, Then and Now." *Critical Public Health* 14 (4): 329–44.

Room, Robin. 2006a. "Addiction Concepts and International Control." *Social History of Alcohol and Drugs* 21 (2): 276–89.

Room, Robin. 2006b. "Looking towards Policy in Thinking about Alcohol and the Heart." In *Understanding Choice, Explaining Behaviour: Essays in Honour of Ole-Jørgen Skog,* edited by Jon Elster, Olav Gjelsvik, Aanund Hylland, and Karl Moene, 249–58. Oslo: Unipub forlag/Oslo Academic Press.

Room, Robin. 2011. "Addiction and Personal Responsibility as Solutions to the Contradictions of Neoliberal Consumerism." *Critical Public Health* 21 (2): 141–51.

Room, Robin. 2012. "Individualized Control of Drinkers: Back to the Future?" *Contemporary Drug Problems* 39 (2): 311–43.

Room, Robin, and Peter Reuter. 2012. "How Well Do International Drug Conventions Protect Public Health?" *Lancet* 379 (9810): 84–91.

Saïet, Mathilde. 2011. *Les Addictions* [The addictions]. Paris: Presses Universitaires de France.

SAMHSA (Substance Abuse and Mental Health Services Administration). 2012. *Results from the 2011 National Survey on Drug Use and Health: Summary of National Findings.* Rockville, MD: Author.

Schrad, Mark Lawrence. 2010. *The Political Power of Bad Ideas: Networks, Institutions, and the Global Prohibition Wave.* Oxford: Oxford University Press.

Stauffer, Robert B. 1971. *The Role of Drugs in Political Change.* New York: General Learning Press.

Strategy Council on Drug Abuse. 1973. *Federal Strategy for Drug Abuse and Drug Traffic Prevention.* Washington, DC: US Government Printing Office.

Valverde, Mariana. 1998. *Diseases of the Will: Alcohol and the Dilemmas of Freedom.* Cambridge, UK: Cambridge University Press.

Warner, Jessica. 2002. *Craze: Gin and Debauchery in an Age of Reason; Consisting of a Tragicomedy in Three Acts in which High and Low Are Brought Together, Much to Their Mutual Discomfort.* New York: Four Walls Eight Windows.

Wasson, R. Gordon. 1984. "Distilled Alcohol Dissemination." *Drinking and Drug Practices Surveyor* 19:6.

Yoast, Richard; Michael A. Williams; Scott D. Deitchman; and Hunter C. Champion. 2001. "Report of the Council on Scientific Affairs: Methadone Maintenance and Needle-Exchange Programs to Reduce the Medical and Public Health Consequences of Drug Abuse." *Journal of Addictive Diseases* 20 (2): 15–40.

Zimmer, Lynn, and James B. Jacobs. 1992. "The Business of Drug Testing: Technological Innovation and Social Control." *Contemporary Drug Problems* 19 (1): 1–26.

Zinberg, Norman E. 1984. *Drug, Set, and Setting: The Basis for Controlled Intoxicant Use*. New Haven, CT: Yale University Press.

Robin Room (1995, 2004, 2014)
Director, Center for Alcohol Policy Research, Turning Point
Professor, Melbourne School of Population and Global Health, University of Melbourne

ALTERNATIVE THERAPIES

This entry consists of the following:

I. SOCIAL HISTORY
Robert C. Fuller and Justin Stein
II. ETHICAL AND LEGAL ISSUES
James F. Drane

I. SOCIAL HISTORY

Healing is a profoundly cultural activity. The very act of labeling a disease and prescribing treatment expresses a healer's commitment to a particular set of assumptions about the nature and structure of reality. These assumptions not only help specify the agents thought to cause disease but also contain implicit understandings of what health optimally or normatively enables humans to do. Because rival medical systems typically subscribe to differing philosophical and cultural outlooks, the notion of orthodoxy pertains to medicine as surely as it does to religion or politics. What makes a therapy "orthodox" is its adherence to a belief system that, for intellectual and sociological reasons, informs the practice of the dominant members of a culture's medical delivery system. A therapy is therefore "unorthodox" to the extent that its diagnoses and treatments are not deemed legitimate by the dominant belief system.

The philosophical and professional differences that separate orthodox and unorthodox therapies give rise to complex ethical questions. How, for example, are we to understand medical "legitimacy" when this notion is the product of ever-changing philosophical, cultural, and social factors? What does it mean for a medical treatment to be unethical? Must it in some way bring about negative results, or is it unethical even if it is merely a harmless fraud—such as vitamin placebo treatment? What constitutes a therapeutic benefit? Is it solely determined by improvement in a person's physical well-being, or does it also include consideration of a person's mental or spiritual well-being?

First, the sheer diversity of alternative therapies hampers attempts to generalize about the kinds of ethical issues that unorthodox treatments present. There is an almost bewildering array of alternative therapies, ranging from chiropractic, osteopathy, and acupuncture to shiatsu, herbal medicine, and religious faith healing. Further complicating this task is the fact that these alternative therapies find themselves labeled unorthodox for quite different reasons. Some, for example, are practiced by healers committed to an alternative belief system or worldview that grants reality to causal forces that differ greatly from those specified by medical orthodoxy. Such is the case with Ayurveda and Chinese medicine, which describe fluids in patients' bodies that have no direct correlates in biomedicine. It is also true for religious therapies such as "faith healing" traditions and New Age medical systems that invoke overtly metaphysical explanations of the causes of physical illness and depict human health in terms of adherence to specific spiritual or moral outlooks on life.

Second, healing systems may become unorthodox when they employ therapies that, though they are predicated upon the consensus worldview, have not yet been validated or confirmed as efficacious by orthodox medical standards. Many of the treatments suggested for combating cancer or acquired immunodeficiency syndrome (AIDS) are considered unorthodox for this reason. Third, healers find themselves outside the medical mainstream when they provide services that are typically ignored or deemed of secondary importance by a culture's dominant medical practitioners. This has been the case, for example, with dentists in the nineteenth century, podiatrists in the early twentieth century, and midwives throughout most of modern history.

The case of midwifery is instructive. While it was never as widespread in the United States as in other parts of the world, midwives provided the only obstetrical assistance available to many women until early in the twentieth century. As obstetrics became a recognized medical specialty, primarily under the control of male physicians, hospitals equipped with surgical facilities supplanted the home as the normal site for giving birth. Increasingly the last resort of those who could not afford hospital births, midwifery generally fell into disrepute. Midwifery, then, became an "unorthodox" form of medical care not because it employed an alternative worldview or because it could not be validated as a treatment but because the dominant providers of medical services decided that the home and the assistance of other women at childbirth were not of primary importance. Interestingly, midwifery has witnessed a modest resurgence as part of a general cultural trend toward "natural" medicine and woman-centered health care. From 1980 to 2010, births attended by certified nurse-midwives went from just over 3 percent to about 8 percent of total births and 12 percent of all vaginal births (Declercq 2012). These numbers are roughly the same in Western Europe, with the exception of the Netherlands, where roughly one-third of all births are home births monitored by midwives and where midwives monitor almost 70 percent of hospital births (DeVries 2001).

What alternative therapies have in common is economic, legal, and cultural disenfranchisement from the socially empowered institution of scientific medicine. Any attempt to reflect upon the ethical questions raised by these "alternative" approaches to healing requires sensitivity to the historical and philosophical roots of this disenfranchisement. "Regular" physicians coalesced into state and local medical societies during the nineteenth century, securing an institutional power base for what was to become medical orthodoxy in the United States. This emerging corps of physicians shared a more or less common approach to medical practice, and they were eventually able to "institutionalize" this approach through the influence they exerted over licensure laws enacted by state and federal governments, the accreditation of medical schools, and access to technologically equipped hospitals.

The American Medical Association (AMA) (founded in 1847 but lacking strong organization and sufficient membership until the early twentieth century) eventually succeeded in organizing and promoting the interests of the nation's dominant medical practitioners. The AMA encouraged state and federal agencies to enact stricter licensing regulations and to restrict hospital access to graduates of AMA-accredited medical schools. These efforts undoubtedly furthered the cause of scientific medicine and surely protected the public from potentially harmful forms of quackery. They also, however, forced to the margins of the medical marketplace those whose approaches to healing utilized a nonscientific worldview or whose medical services did not fit with dominant approaches to medical care.

Medical orthodoxy aligned itself with the worldview spawned by the Western scientific tradition. Its approach to therapeutic intervention has been firmly rooted in the evolving body of information that has emerged from advances in physiology, chemistry, and pharmacology. Accompanying this reliance upon the Western scientific tradition has been an implicit endorsement of a secularist and rationalist ontology (i.e., a worldview skeptical of claims concerning the supernatural or other unquantifiable influences). What has given scientific medicine its "public" character is its insistence that theories concerning the etiology and treatment of disease specify causal forces that are physical, as opposed to spiritual or metaphysical. Its theories and strategies for therapeutic intervention are thus more susceptible to empirical verification, and disputes can at least potentially be resolved by an appeal to observable and quantifiable sets of data. This is also why scientific medicine found itself more amenable than many of its alternative counterparts to the economic and legal institutions of modern Western governments. Rejecting the "private" claims to truth made in religious arguments, Western democracies have required that all civic discourse be advanced according to rationalistic and public grounds of argumentation.

To the extent that scientific medicine's academic and experimental foundations facilitate such "public" argumentation, it has largely merited its enfranchisement within the legal and economic institutions that make judgments about the allocation of medical resources. Any consideration of the ethical status of these judgments and their effect upon the practice of alternative medical systems in the modern West must take into account the important role that such rational and public discourse has had in the development of Western culture.

EARLY CHALLENGES TO REGULAR MEDICINE

The Thomsonian System. One of the first challenges to the orthodoxy of "regular physicians" occurred in the early 1800s. Samuel Thomson (1769–1843) was a poor New Hampshire farmer whose mother and wife had suffered from the bleedings and mercurial drugs forced upon them by regular physicians. Thomson believed that better treatments must be available, and he began studying the therapeutic value of herbs. He soon developed his own system of botanical medicine predicated upon the assumption that there is only one cause of disease, cold, and one cure, heat. Thomson believed that by restoring heat to his patients' systems, he could cure any ailment. Using botanics such as cayenne pepper, supplemented with steam baths, Thomson sought cures without the incessant bloodletting or mercurial drugs utilized by the era's orthodox physicians.

The Thomsonian system reached the height of its popularity in the 1820s and 1830s. Some estimate that its methods were employed to varying degrees by as many as a million Americans. One obvious reason for its appeal was that its treatments were generally more benign than the aggressive arsenal of bloodletting, alcohol, opium, mercury, arsenic, and strychnine that many regular physicians used to stimulate their patients' systems. Perhaps more important, Thomsonianism could be studied relatively inexpensively (although the official price for the right to use his methods was a substantial $20) and practiced by family members. During the early days of medical professionalization in the United States, Thomsonianism strengthened the role of parents and especially mothers in caring for family members.

Thomsonianism also fit nicely with the period's moral and religious climate, which urged individuals to take responsibility for their own moral and spiritual regeneration. It endeavored "to make every man his own physician" and encouraged individuals to take responsibility for restoring their rightful relationship to the divinely decreed laws of nature. Of lasting significance is the fact that Thomsonianism was the first system to take on the issue of licensing of medical practitioners and to assert the public's right to free choice of healers. Thomsonians led the successful campaign to repeal medical licensing legislation in the mid-1800s and drew public attention to the somewhat predatory tactics with which orthodox physicians sought to restrict the right of would-be healers to practice whatever system they wanted.

Homeopathy. A second form of sectarian medicine, homeopathy, emerged more or less concurrently with the public's gradual loss of enthusiasm for the Thomsonian system. The homeopathic system of medicine was the creation of the German physician Christian Friedrich Samuel Hahnemann (1755–1843), who grew increasingly critical of the indiscriminate prescription of drugs by contemporary physicians. He coined the term *allopathic* to refer to orthodox medicine's alleged overreliance upon invasive therapeutic treatments (e.g., bloodletting, surgery, or the administration of strong pharmacological agents). In contrast to allopathic medicine, Hahnemann enunciated a medical theory that he thought relied more upon the body's natural powers to bring about recovery. The first principle of homeopathic medicine is "like cured by like." By this Hahnemann meant that physicians should treat symptoms by prescribing drugs that produce similar symptoms in a healthy individual. The second fundamental principle of homeopathic medicine is the doctrine of infinitesimals. It was Hahnemann's conviction that the greatest therapeutic benefit was to be achieved by administering diluted doses of a drug, sometimes only 1/1,000,000 of a gram.

Homeopathy spread quite rapidly in the United States. It was introduced by Hans Gram (1786–1840), who opened an office in New York after studying the homeopathic system in Europe. By 1835 a homeopathic college had been formed, and in 1844 the American Institute of Homeopathy was organized. Throughout the second half of the nineteenth century, 10 to 12 percent of the country's medical schools and medical school graduates were adherents of homeopathy. In contrast to Thomsonianism, which was practiced by nonprofessionals, homeopathic practitioners were educated professionals who often came from the ranks of regular physicians. Moreover, while those who received Thomsonian treatment tended to be rural and poor, homeopathy thrived among the urban upper and middle classes. This latter fact led to direct economic competition with the regular system and proved an important catalyst in the formation and success of the AMA as economic motives joined with scientific ones to rally regular physicians in opposition to their now "irregular" competitors.

As the most popular of the century's alternative systems, homeopathy raised a number of important ethical questions. For example, could allopathic physicians consult "unscientific" practitioners? (The AMA's original code of ethics included a consultation clause that prohibited such interactions.) Or should homeopathic physicians be allowed to practice in publicly supported hospitals or in the military? Even in the late twentieth century there was debate about whether pharmacies should be required to stock homeopathic medicines.

Hydropathy and Dietary Regimens. In the mid-1840s another alternative therapy, hydropathy (water cure), began to attract a following in the United States. Based on the theories of Vincenz Priessnitz (1799–1851) of Austria, hydropathy was based on enhancing the body's inherent vitality and purity. Priessnitz believed that pure water could be used to flush out bodily impurities and stimulate the body's inherent tendencies toward health. Water-cure treatments emphasized drinking large amounts of water and applying water externally through baths, showers, or wrapping wet sheets around the body. Most American adherents of water cure advocated an eclectic approach to health based on the curative powers of fresh air, diet, sleep, exercise, and proper clothing. The philosophy of water cure also had a decidedly moral tone.

Hydropathy equated disregard of the laws of healthful living with defiance of God's will. Systematic efforts to promote healthful living were not only the means to physical well-being but also the key to the spiritual renovation of Earth. The hydropathic cause naturally attracted many of the period's moral and religious reformers. William Alcott, Lucy Stone, Amelia Bloomer, Susan B. Anthony, and Horace Greeley visited major hydropathic retreat centers, where they circulated reformist agendas ranging from vegetarianism to utopian socialism. Critical of the alleged superiority of "official" medical authorities, advocates of hydropathy had a natural affinity with the feminist thought of the time. Hydropathy looked to nature, not credentialed male physicians, as the ultimate source of healing; in so doing, it provided a vehicle for those seeking to redress what they thought were faulty notions of social and political authority.

Another nineteenth-century forebear of contemporary alternative therapy in the United States was Sylvester Graham (1794–1851), who combined conservative religious beliefs with zealous concern for health reform. An ordained Presbyterian minister and itinerant evangelist, Graham believed that human physical, moral, and spiritual well-being required scrupulous adherence to the natural order established by God. Graham admonished his followers that avoiding alcohol and the overstimulation of the sexual organs could help them maintain moral and physical health. His advice for a healthful diet included a coarse bread, which was later produced in the form of a cracker that (in modified forms) still carries his name. Graham's dietary principles, widely circulated throughout the nineteenth century, served the cause of keeping the soul's "bodily temple" free from impurities.

Ellen White (1827–1915) occasionally visited a hydropathic resort in Dansville, New York, where she became a convert to Graham's dietary gospel. White thereafter had a series of mystical visions in which God revealed to her that he expected humans to follow the divinely given laws governing health and diet as faithfully as his moral laws. The Seventh-day Adventist denomination founded by White has since then adopted Grahamite principles and a vegetarian diet as essential parts of purifying themselves in expectation of the Second Coming of Christ. Seventh-day Adventists, one of the largest religious groups to originate in the United States, combine their evangelical religious faith with a strong emphasis on healthy dietary practices. This emphasis upon a healthful diet does not in and of itself constitute an alternative medical practice. Their dietary concerns are, however, closely connected with their belief in the efficacy of petitionary prayer. Furthermore, the Adventist church opened health sanitariums, including the renowned Battle Creek Sanitarium overseen by John Harvey Kellogg (1852–1943) of breakfast cereal fame. These sanitariums stressed hydrotherapy and nutrition but have since developed into a system of hundreds of biomedical hospitals and clinics around the world.

THE RISE OF MENTAL HEALING PRACTICES

Mesmerism. The introduction of Franz Anton Mesmer's "science of animal magnetism," commonly known as mesmerism, in the 1830s and 1840s popularized a belief in the power of the unconscious mind to draw upon an invisible healing energy. Mesmer (1734–1815), a Viennese physician, believed that he had detected the existence of an almost ethereal fluid that permeates the universe. This fluid, called animal magnetism, flows continuously into and is evenly distributed throughout a healthy human body. If for any reason an individual's supply of animal magnetism is thrown out of equilibrium, one or more bodily organs will begin to falter. Mesmer proclaimed, "There is only one illness and one healing." The science of animal magnetism revolved around the identification of techniques for restoring a patient's inner receptivity to this mysterious, life-giving energy.

Mesmer held magnets in his hands and repeatedly passed them over the heads and bodies of his patients in an effort to induce the flow of animal magnetism into their systems. His followers later dispensed with the magnets, finding that oral suggestions from the healer could induce patients into a trance, ostensibly heightening their receptivity to the influx of this metaphysical healing agent. Mesmerized patients claimed to feel prickly sensations running up and down their bodies, which they attributed to the influx and movement of animal magnetism. Awaking from their sleeplike trance, they reported feeling refreshed, invigorated, and healed of such disorders as arthritis, nervousness, digestive problems, liver ailments, stammering, insomnia, and the abuse of coffee, tea, or alcohol. Some patients even claimed that the mesmerizing process enabled them to open up the mind's latent powers for telepathy, clairvoyance, and precognition. These claims contributed as much or even more to mesmerism's growing popularity than its reputation for healing.

A good many of those drawn to mesmerism were middle- and upper-class individuals who styled themselves progressive thinkers and were interested in uniting science and religion in a single philosophical account of human nature. Mesmerism struck them as an important step in this direction. The phenomena surrounding mesmeric trances were thought to provide empirical proof that each human is inwardly connected with higher, metaphysical planes of reality. Adherents of mesmerism believed that under certain conditions of psychological receptivity, humans are able to open themselves to an influx of energy or guidance from these higher realms. American mesmerists borrowed terminology from transcendentalism, spiritualism, and Theosophy to provide their middle-class reading audience with a new vocabulary for understanding the interconnection of their physical, mental, and spiritual natures.

Mind Cure and Christian Science. A popular philosophy known as the mind cure, or New Thought movement, grew out of the mesmerists' healing practices. Mind-cure writers in the United States published books and pamphlets describing how thought controls the extent to which we are able to become inwardly receptive to spiritual energies. From Phineas P. Quimby and Warren Felt Evans in the 1800s to Norman Vincent Peale, Norman Cousins, and Bernie Siegel in the 1900s, to Rhonda Byrne in the early twenty-first century, Americans have displayed a remarkable enthusiasm for this "power of positive thinking" literature. The mind-cure movement gave rise to a novel form of religious piety based on the belief that the deeper powers of our minds control our access to a metaphysical power that can instantly help us to achieve peace of mind, improved health, and a never-ceasing flow of energy. The holistic health movement of the late twentieth century relied heavily upon this cluster of metaphysical ideas.

Mesmerism was also instrumental in the formation of Christian Science. In 1862 Mary Baker Eddy, in great physical and emotional distress, arrived on the doorstep of the famous mesmerist healer Phineas P. Quimby.

Quimby's treatments gradually cured her of her ailments; they also gave her a new outlook on life, based upon the principle that our thoughts determine whether we are inwardly open to or closed off from the creative activity of a spiritual energy (animal magnetism). Soon after Quimby's death, Eddy transformed his mesmerist teachings into the foundational principles of Christian Science. Her principal text, *Science and Health with Key to the Scriptures* (1875), reveals her intention to shift the science of mental healing away from the categories of mesmerism to those that bear more resemblance to Christian scripture, albeit her own unique interpretation of it.

The basic theological postulate of Christian Science is that God creates all that is and all that God creates is good. Sickness, pain, and evil are not creations of God, and therefore they do not truly exist. They are simply the delusions produced in an erring, mortal mind that has lost a firm hold on the belief that only those things created by God have true existence. For Christian Scientists the universe is spiritual. What we call matter (e.g., bacteria, viruses, and so on) consequently does not really exist and therefore has no causal power. Christian Science healers, known as practitioners, help individuals to overcome their faulty thinking and to elevate their mental attitudes above the delusions of the senses. Healing occurs as the individual learns to function on a metaphysical rather than a physical plane. Healings are understood not as miracles or faith healings but as the lawful consequence of exchanging false conceptions for true ones, which center solely on the higher laws of God's spiritual presence.

Both Christian Science and the "holistic" philosophies that emerged from the mind-cure tradition teach that our thoughts control the degree to which we avail ourselves of the higher spiritual source from which health proceeds. As a consequence, illness or disease is understood as something the sufferer has brought upon himself or herself through failure to sustain a "correct" mental posture toward life. Any ethical analysis of these forms of alternative therapy must take seriously their built-in skepticism about whether a medical system really needs to attend to material causes of illness (bacteria, viruses, and others). The issue is not as acute for holistic healing practices that do not deny that there are physical and material causes of illness but simply maintain that mental and spiritual factors are entailed in the etiology of most illnesses and must be taken into account in any comprehensive medical system. Although they insist that a patient's mental outlook often is a significant factor in the creation and cure of illness, they generally do not espouse a medical theory that puts all the "blame" for illness or "credit" for recovery upon the patient.

Christian Science, by contrast, goes much further in challenging the empirical and rational foundations of Western science. By denying the ontological reality of matter, and hence the causal power of viruses or bacteria, Christian Science is clearly at philosophical loggerheads with both medical orthodoxy and the legal systems of most Western, democratic nations. Although the courts allow Christian Scientists and others to avoid immunization, concern over the medical well-being of children has prompted judicial action to limit Christian Scientists' right to prevent minors from being denied medical treatment. In 1990 the US courts decided that two Christian Science parents were guilty of child neglect when their sole reliance on Christian Science methods was deemed responsible for their child's death Such cases draw attention to the important ethical distinction between "private" religious belief and actions that have consequences in the "public" domain regulated by the legal system.

CHIROPRACTIC AND OSTEOPATHIC MEDICINE

Osteopathic and chiropractic medicine provide interesting examples of the fate of alternative philosophical, religious, and ethical interpretations of healing in an age dominated by scientific medicine. Osteopathic medicine emerged from the healing philosophy of Andrew Taylor Still (1828–1917). A former spiritualist and mesmeric healer, Still developed techniques for manipulating vertebrae along the spine in ways that he thought removed obstructions to the free flow of "the life-giving current" that promotes health throughout the body. Still explained the healing principles of osteopathy (a term derived from two Greek words meaning "suffering of the bones") in overtly metaphysical terms that described the origin and nature of "the life-giving current" ultimately responsible for human well-being. His followers largely discarded the occult-sounding dimensions of Still's philosophy and instead insisted that osteopathic medical education be grounded in anatomy and scientific physiology. Thus, although osteopaths originally relied only upon manual manipulations of the spine as a means of restoring health, they soon added surgery and eventually drug therapy to their medical practice.

By the 1950s, so few differences existed in the training or practice of osteopaths and medical doctors that their two national organizations agreed to cease the rivalry that had existed for several decades and to cooperate in such matters as access to hospitals, residency programs, and professional recognition. Having jettisoned the alternative worldview of its founder, osteopathy no longer bore any overt signs of unorthodoxy and finally found itself within the medical mainstream. Interestingly, during the 1960s many osteopaths were concerned about being absorbed into allopathic medicine and gave renewed focus to osteopathy's philosophical origins. Their commitment to osteopathy's historical concern with enhancing the body's natural powers for recuperation made them champions of holistic medicine long before the term *holistic* became commonplace among alternative healers. As of 2012, there were over 82,500 osteopathic physicians in the United States, with the number estimated to top 100,000 by the end of the decade (American Osteopathic Association 2012, 2).

The case of chiropractic medicine is more complex. Chiropractic medicine originated in the work of Daniel David Palmer (1845–1913), a mesmerism-inspired magnetic healer in Iowa. Palmer, who knew of Still's osteopathic techniques, theorized that dislocations of the spine are able to block the free flow of the life force, which he called Innate (his nomenclature for animal magnetism). Palmer and his son, B. J. Palmer, explained that Innate Intelligence is a part of the Divine Intelligence that fills the universe, bringing full physical health whenever it flows freely through the human body. Chiropractic medicine represents the Palmers' art and science of adjusting the spine in ways that remove obstructions to the free flow of Innate Intelligence within the body.

Over the years, chiropractic physicians began playing down the movement's metaphysical origins and emphasized its scientific approach to the treatment of musculoskeletal disorders. In this way, they minimized their theoretical unorthodoxy and identified an area of medical practice largely ignored by most medical doctors. Chiropractic physicians' sustained attention to this void in the "orthodox" medical system has earned them a viable niche in the medical marketplace. In 1990 more than 19,000 chiropractic physicians in the United States were treating more than 3 million patients annually; a survey by the National Institutes of Health estimated that by 2006 osteopathic and chiropractic physicians were treating over 18.7 million Americans through manipulative treatments (Barnes, Bloom, and Nahin 2008, 10). Even though most medical insurance companies have come to recognize the medical functions performed by chiropractic medicine, medical doctors are still largely wary of chiropractic medicine because it has failed to elucidate an empirically validated theory that would substantiate its therapeutic claims. This professional tension provides a fascinating example of a continuing theme in the history of alternative medicine: the clash between orthodox medicine's rationalism (its insistence on an acceptable scientific explanation for all methods) and alternative medicine's pragmatism (discovery of therapies that produce results regardless of whether they are "proved" with rational theories).

ALTERNATIVE MEDICAL SYSTEMS

Around the world, a wide variety of therapies exist alongside those based on medical science. An estimated 80 percent of the world considers "alternative medicine" their primary health care option, while biomedical care is unavailable or is prohibitively expensive. Within the United States, variations of pow-wow, an eclectic tradition using charms, prayers, and rituals to prevent and cure disease, continue to be practiced by Pennsylvania Dutch; *curanderismo* still flourishes among Mexican-American communities in the American Southwest; and immigration from the Caribbean has rekindled African-American folk medicine practices. The continued presence of such "ethnomedical" treatments may represent attempts to preserve cultural identity, economic disenfranchisement from the nation's more expensive conventional medical system, or the revival of genuine medical pluralism. The contemporary medical landscape is not, however, one that ensures even ground for all competing systems. The very notion of "conventional" versus "alternative" reveals enduring discrepancies in legal status, institutional funding, and access to insurance coverage. Furthermore, conflicts between multinational pharmaceutical corporations and indigenous peoples and their advocates over the intellectual property rights to medicinal plants point to an ideological chasm between biomedicine and ethnomedicine. In any case, both legal and economic attitudes toward alternative therapies must be philosophically and culturally nuanced.

Immigration from Asia has increased the presence of Ayurveda and Chinese medicine in the West, and, in the case of the United States, use of these therapies dramatically increased immediately following the immigration reforms of 1965. The National Institutes of Health's National Center for Complementary and Alternative Medicine (NCCAM) classifies these as *alternative medical systems* or *whole medical systems* because they are "complete systems of theory or practice that have evolved over time … apart from conventional or Western medicine." NCCAM distinguishes such systems, which also include homeopathy and naturopathy, from *biologically based therapies*, such as supplements and diets; *manipulative therapies*, such as chiropractic and osteopathic manipulation; *mind-body therapies*, such as meditation and breathing exercises; and *energy-healing therapies*, such as Reiki and therapeutic touch. The fact that the "alternative medical system" of Chinese medicine includes therapies from the other four categories (e.g., herbs, massage, and internal and external qigong) demonstrates the arbitrariness of this delineation. Orthodox medicine's relationship with these systems lies somewhere between its acceptance of osteopathy and its continued mistrust of chiropractic: therapies like acupuncture are considered efficacious, although practitioners' explanations of how it works are still largely rejected.

Ayurveda. The best known of India's indigenous medical systems, Ayurveda is founded on ancient (c. 500 B.C.E.–600 C.E.) Sanskrit texts that emerged from the heterogeneous religious traditions of Brahmanism, Buddhism, and Jainism and circulated in translation across premodern Eurasia, from Italy to China. These texts outline Ayurvedic physiology, etiology, and diagnosis as well as surgical techniques and the preparation and dispensation of plant- and mineral-based medicines. Despite some similarities to biomedical procedures, Ayurvedic practices operate under different models of the body than biomedicine's aggregate of anatomical structures and physiological systems. Ayurveda describes the body as a series of seven layers (*dhatu*), animated by a vital energy (*ojas*) and circulating three fluids (*doshas*): wind (*vata*), bile (*pitta*), and phlegm (*kapha*). While one or two of these fluids dominates each individual's constitution, good health relies on a balance of the three, and Ayurveda tends to stress prevention over cure.

Even though biomedicine has achieved orthodoxy in postcolonial India, receiving the majority of state funding, indigenous practices like Ayurveda continue to thrive, partly through their adoption of the discursive, institutional, and technological practices of scientific medicine. In the West, however, where interest in Asian medical systems grew dramatically at the end of the twentieth century, it is precisely Ayurveda's difference from biomedicine that makes it attractive to medical consumers.

Traditional Chinese Medicine. Since the second half of the nineteenth century, waves of migration have brought Chinese medical practices, including herbalism, acupuncture, massage, cupping and moxibustion, to the Americas, Australia, and Europe. Like Ayurveda, Chinese medical discourse describes the body as a microcosm of the universe, through which courses a series of channels that carry the fluid called *qi* (or chi). Blockages, excesses, deficiencies, and imbalances of *qi* are considered to be the root of disease, and these are treated through diet, herbs, acupuncture, and other therapies. Several types of imbalances can occur, the most important being those between heat and cold; damp and dryness; and the "five phases" (*wuxing*) of wood, fire, earth, air, and water, which each correspond to one of five viscera.

There have been many competing schools of thought and practice in Chinese medical history, but massive standardization efforts in twentieth-century China resulted in what is called Traditional Chinese Medicine (TCM). This standardization is the result of professional unification by practitioners in the face of competition by Western biomedicine in the first half of the century as well as the state control of education and health care after the establishment the People's Republic in 1949. While other Chinese practices, such as *taijiquan* (or tai chi) and qigong, have also received international attention for their health benefits since the second half of the twentieth century, the NCCAM classifies them as "mind-body therapies" rather than part of the "alternative medical system" of Chinese medicine.

HOLISTIC MEDICINE

During the last few decades of the twentieth century, the holistic healing movement led a surge of popular interest in therapies based on an explicitly religious, or quasi-religious, interpretation of the healing process. The precise meaning of the term *holistic medicine* varies among healing systems. Among its meanings are emphasis upon "natural" therapies, patient education and responsibility, prevention, and treating patients as "whole" people. Also common to holistic healing is the basic assumption that, as one handbook put it, "every human being is a unique, wholistic, interdependent relationship of body, mind, emotions, and spirit" (Belknap, Blau, and Grossman 1975, 18). The term *spirit*, alongside *body*, *mind*, and *emotions*, carries holistic healing beyond psychosomatic medical models; it also represents commitment to a belief in the interpenetration of physical and nonphysical spheres of causality. Even holistic healing's exhortations concerning reliance on the body's own regenerative and reparative processes are typically laden with references to opening individuals up to the inflow of a divine healing energy. Persons who call themselves holistic health practitioners typically operate according to a worldview that is incompatible with the naturalistic framework of the modern Western scientific heritage.

One example of such a holistically oriented healing movement and its methods is Alcoholics Anonymous (AA) and its twelve-step program, which has influenced many other self-regenerative therapies. Founded in the 1930s, AA has well over 1 million members, with about 35,000 groups meeting weekly in over ninety countries. The principal founder of the movement, Bill Wilson, was an alcoholic who became aware of his inability to overcome his addiction. A mystical experience of "a great white light" (Kurtz 1979, 19) convinced him that a loving presence surrounds us and is capable of healing our broken inner lives. Wilson maintained that we need only cease relying upon our own willpower and surrender to this Higher Power. Wilson was wary of institutional religion's moralism. From psychologists such as William James and Carl Jung, he pieced together a spirituality based upon opening the unconscious mind to a higher metaphysical reality. AA counsels its members that "in order to recover, they must acquire an immediate and overwhelming 'God-consciousness' followed at once by a vast change in feeling and outlook" (Alcoholics Anonymous 1955, 569). AA's mystical, nonscriptural approach to personal regeneration sets its doctrines apart from most of the United States' religious establishment; its denunciation of both material and psychological/attitudinal factors in favor of an overtly spiritual view of healing sets its practices apart from the American medical and psychological establishments. But its open-minded and eclectic sense of the presence of spiritual forces in the determination of human well-being made it one of the most powerful mediators of wholeness in twentieth-century America.

The various religious and healing groups that constitute the New Age movement also endorse a holistic approach to health and medicine; they envision every human being as a unique combination of body, mind, emotions, and spirit. Central to New Age piety is the conviction that each person exists simultaneously on both the physical and the metaphysical (i.e., the astral and etheric) planes of reality. Many New Age therapies seek to channel healing energies from higher metaphysical planes into the physical body. Energy healing, for example, maintains that illness in the physical body is frequently caused by a disruption or disharmony of energies in the part of the body that extends into the metaphysical plane, called the *etheric body* or the *subtle body*. Healing consequently requires techniques to achieve harmony between the physical and metaphysical bodies.

Crystals are thought to have unique properties that enable them to serve as receptors and capacitors of energies from the metaphysical planes. Used properly, crystals are assumed to be capable of transmitting these energies in ways that bring the individual's physical, moral, and spiritual natures back into harmony. To this extent, New Age adherents do not reject the efficacy of established medical science (though they do condemn what they perceive to be an overreliance on drugs and invasive surgical techniques) so much as its secularist, materialistic worldview, which fails to take into account our spiritual potentials. Healing, for New Agers, is a by-product of the more fundamental goal of expanding their spiritual awareness. Many Westerners' attraction to Asian practices, including yoga, tai chi, and Reiki, is bound up with agendas left over from such nineteenth-century movements as mesmerism, spiritualism, and Theosophy. Even acupuncture is embraced by many Americans not only for its obvious physical benefits but also for its connections with Eastern mystical philosophies.

THE CHALLENGE TO BIOETHICS

Persons with life-threatening diseases who have not been helped by conventional treatments understandably become interested in pursuing alternative therapeutic strategies. The highly publicized debate in the late 1970s over the effectiveness of laetrile for retarding cancer drew attention to the potential risks of the regulation of medicine by the US Food and Drug Administration. At stake was the unresolved issue of whether a drug should be restricted only when it is known to cause harm or only when laboratory testing has failed to reveal measurable physical benefits. This debate continued in the 1980s and 1990s over various treatments for AIDS. Persons given a bleak prognosis by medical doctors sought immediate access to experimental drugs that had just entered the slow and laborious regulatory processes mandated by US federal law. Although much has been done to try to speed up the evaluation of experimental treatments for AIDS and other prevalent diseases such as cancer, there is always a subset of the population that finds itself barred from access to innovative scientific treatment.

The central ethical question raised by alternative therapies is whether genuine medical treatment can be distinguished from various forms of quackery. Except for isolated instances in which individuals engage in deliberate medical fraud, quackery is difficult to identify or prove. Any reliable definition of therapeutic benefit requires being able to define the factors "known" to affect human well-being and what optimal health consists of. The practitioners of many forms of alternative medicine criticize the assumptions they believe underlie contemporary medical science. They argue that alternative therapies better understand human well-being and are cognizant of mental, moral, and spiritual factors that go well beyond the physiological considerations on which scientific medicine relies. To those who say that their practices or those who utilize them are "irrational," they respond that every therapy is rational insofar as its methods of treatment are logically entailed by its fundamental premises or its assumptions about the nature of disease.

Establishing criteria with which to mediate between competing medical systems is complicated by the fact that the plausibility of the beliefs or assumptions that underlie them are every bit as dependent on sociological factors as on intellectual "proofs." What we consider valid evidence, whom we consider expert authorities, and how we should go about separating relevant from irrelevant information turn not on objective, rational criteria but on the ways we were socialized into one belief system or another. Who, then, is in a position to decide what is an "irrational" medical choice? With what degree of confidence or philosophical integrity can orthodox physicians seek to dissuade persons from seeking alternative treatments? Do persons have a right to what seems, to adherents of "accepted" forms of Western medicine, to be an utterly ineffective therapy simply because it conforms to their personal belief system?

Alternative therapies may reasonably be expected to demonstrate their benefits to patients and to substantiate the claim that their distinctive healing practices directly cause these therapeutic results. Medical ethics is concerned with protecting persons from intended or inadvertent harm. Well-intentioned tolerance of alternative therapies should not preclude their undergoing rigorous scrutiny. Governmental agencies, health care facilities, and insurance companies are forced to allocate limited resources and to ensure the welfare of the general public. They must be prepared to make reasonable assessments of alternative medical systems that are based on belief systems at considerable variance with modern Western science. Because quackery poses an inherent threat to both personal and public well-being, those who make ethical and policy-related judgments must exercise caution and strive for the unrelenting application of "public" (openly demonstrable and subject to empirical scrutiny) standards of evidence. Perhaps the most important consideration in assessing scientifically unvalidated therapies is that contemporary medicine differs from its predecessors not because we have become more rational but because we have learned to use the controlled trial to determine the relative merits of competing treatments.

Medical systems that are labeled alternative because their concerns or treatments are at the periphery of mainstream medicine are reminders that dominant professional groups tend over time to employ predatory tactics to ensure their continued supremacy and keep potential competitors at a distance. These "medically peripheral" systems alert us to the fact that medical science has philosophical and institutional blinders that may close off, rather than open, innovative approaches to human health. The presence of alternative health professionals in the wider system of health care helps safeguard against the kinds of complacency and narrowness of vision that frequently creep into economically entrenched professions. By providing a range of services that address both curative and preventive issues typically neglected by biomedical physicians, many of these alternative therapies potentially contribute to a comprehensive understanding of human health and well-being.

The twenty-first century is perhaps no closer to adjudicating the scientific, economic, and ethical controversies surrounding alternative medicines than previous eras. In 1991 US Senator Tom Harkin spearheaded the effort to create a special division of the National Institutes of Health dedicated to the research of promising unconventional therapies. The Office for Alternative Medicine was initially launched with a budget of $2 million and, by 2010, had grown into NCCAM with an annual budget of about $120 million. The center's use of the descriptive phrase "complementary medicine" seemingly endorses the view that alternative medicines might be used in combination with conventional medical treatments, as is also implied with other phrases such as "integrative medicine." The creation of NCCAM coincided with the United Kingdom's decision to fund homeopathic hospitals under the National Health Service. Governmental support for these alternative medicines predictably generated considerable criticism from physicians, scientists, and public policy analysts. Critics note that the use of public funds to research and promote complementary and alternative medicine (CAM) gives the misleading impression that these treatments have been clinically validated in addition to diverting research funds from the most scientifically promising treatments (Bausell 2007; Ernst 2008; Singh and Ernst 2008). Debates about whether NCCAM is driven more by scientific method or ideological agendas reflect the continuing public dilemma about how to assess the clinical and economic merits of alternative medicine.

SEE ALSO *America, Bioethics in: I. United States; Bioethics: VIII. Sociology of; Health and Disease: III. Anthropological Perspectives; Medicine, Anthropology of; Medicine, Philosophy of*

BIBLIOGRAPHY

Alcoholics Anonymous. 1955. *Alcoholics Anonymous*. 2nd ed. New York: Author.

American Osteopathic Association. 2012. *Osteopathic Medical Profession Report*. Chicago: Author.

Astin, J. A. 1998. "Why Patients Use Alternative Medicine: Results of a National Study." *Journal of American Medical Association* 279 (19): 1548–53.

Barnes, Linda L., and Susan S. Sered, eds. 2005. *Religion and Healing in America*. New York: Oxford University Press.

Barnes, Patricia M.; Barbara Bloom; and Richard L. Nahin. 2008. "Complementary and Alternative Medicine Use among Adults and Children: United States, 2007." *National Health Statistics Report* 10 (12): 1–23.

Bausell, R. Barker. 2007. *Snake Oil Science: The Truth about Complementary and Alternative Medicine*. New York: Oxford University Press.

Belknap, Mary; Robert Blau; and Rosaline Grossman, eds. 1975. *Case Studies and Methods in Humanistic Medicine*. San Francisco: Institute for the Study of Humanistic Medicine.

Bivens, Roberta. 2007. *Alternative Medicine? A History*. New York: Oxford University Press.

Bynum, William Frederick, and Roy Porter, eds. 1987. *Medical Fringe and Medical Orthodoxy, 1750–1850*. Wolfeboro, NH: Croom Helm.

Callahan, Daniel, ed. 2002. *The Role of Complementary and Alternative Medicine: Accommodating Pluralism*. Washington, DC: Georgetown University Press.

Cayleff, Susan E. 1987. *Wash and Be Healed: The Water-Cure Movement and Women's Health*. Philadelphia: Temple University Press.

Declercq, Eugene. 2012. "Trends in Midwife-Attended Births in the United States, 1989–2009." *Journal of Midwifery and Women's Health* 57 (4): 321–26.

DeVries, Raymond; Sirpa Wrede; Edwin van Teijlingen; and Cecilia Benoit. 2001. *Birth by Design: Pregnancy, Maternity Care, and Midwifery in North America and Europe*. New York: Routledge.

Eisenberg, David M.; Roger B. Davis; Susan L. Ettner; et al. 1998. "Trends in Alternative Medicine Use in the United States, 1990–1997: Results of a Follow-Up National Survey." *Journal of the American Medical Association* 280 (18): 1569–75.

Ernst, Edzard, ed. 2008. *Healing, Hype, or Harm? A Critical Analysis of Complementary or Alternative Medicine.* Exeter, UK: Societas.

Frohock, Fred M. 1992. *Healing Powers: Alternative Medicine, Spiritual Communities and the State.* Chicago: University of Chicago Press.

Fuller, Robert C. 1989. *Alternative Medicine and American Religious Life.* New York: Oxford University Press.

Gevitz, Norman. 1982. *The D.O.s: Osteopathic Medicine in America.* Baltimore: Johns Hopkins University Press.

Gevitz, Norman, ed. 1988. *Other Healers: Unorthodox Medicine in America.* Baltimore: Johns Hopkins University Press.

Goldstein, Michael S. 1999. *Alternative Health Care: Medicine, Miracle, or Mirage?* Philadelphia: Temple University Press.

Gordon, Rena J.; Barbara Cable Nienstedt; and Wilbert M. Gesler, eds. 1998. *Alternative Therapies: Expanding Options in Health Care.* New York: Springer.

Harrington, Anne. 2008. *The Cure Within: A History of Mind-Body Medicine.* New York: Norton.

Hodgson v. Minnesota. 1990. 497 U.S. 417 (1990).

Hufford, David. 1988. "Contemporary Folk Medicine." In *Other Healers: Unorthodox Medicine in America,* edited by Norman Gevitz, 228–64. Baltimore: Johns Hopkins University Press.

Inglis, Brian. 1965. *The Case for Unorthodox Medicine.* New York: G. P. Putnam.

Johnston, Robert D., ed. 2004. *The Politics of Healing: Histories of Alternative Medicine in Twentieth-Century North America.* New York: Routledge.

Kaufman, Martin. 1971. *Homeopathy in America: The Rise and Fall of a Medical Heresy.* Baltimore: Johns Hopkins University Press.

Kurtz, Ernest. 1979. *Not-God: A History of Alcoholics Anonymous.* Center City, MN: Hazelden Press.

National Center for Complementary and Alternative Medicine. 2008. "What Is Complementary and Alternative Medicine?" Accessed April 7, 2013. http://nccam.nih.gov/health/whatiscam

Numbers, Ronald L. 1976. *Prophetess of Health: A Study of Ellen G. White.* New York: Harper and Row.

Porter, Roy. 1989. *Health for Sale: Quackery in England, 1660–1850.* Manchester, UK: Manchester University Press.

Raboteau, Albert J. 1986. "The Afro-American Traditions." In *Caring and Curing: Health and Medicine in the Western Religious Traditions,* edited by Ronald L. Numbers and Darrel W. Amundsen, 539–62. New York: Macmillan.

Ramsey, Matthew. 1999. "Alternative Medicine in Modern France." *Medical History* 43 (3): 286–322.

Singh, Simon, and Edward Ernst. 2008. *Trick or Treatment: The Undeniable Facts about Alternative Medicine.* New York: Norton.

Whorton, James C. 1982. *Crusaders for Fitness: The History of American Health Reformers.* Princeton, NJ: Princeton University Press.

Young, James Harvey. 1967. *The Medical Messiahs: A Social History of Health Quackery in Twentieth-Century America.* Princeton, NJ: Princeton University Press.

Robert C. Fuller (1995, 2014)
Professor of Religious Studies, Bradley University

Justin Stein (2014)
Doctoral Candidate, Department for the Study of Religion, University of Toronto

II. ETHICAL AND LEGAL ISSUES

Alternative medicine covers a dizzyingly heterogeneous group of medical theories and practices that are not part of mainline conventional medicine. Alternatives range from the different forms of folk medicine to more scientific systems such as homeopathy, chiropractic, acupuncture, and naturopathy. Also included under the term *alternative* are hypnotherapy; herbalism; iridology; the traditional medicines of India, China, Japan, the Philippines, and indigenous peoples; yoga; diet; meditation; music therapy; massage therapy; and reflexology. Certain shared negative elements justify lumping together such diverse medical theories and practices. These include marginal social standing or fringe status in advanced cultures; exclusion from mainline professional journals; little public funding for research; exemption from mainline licensing requirements; and conflict (but sometimes cooperation) with mainline medicine. The essential ethical and legal considerations raised by alternative medicines are scientific objectivity, veracity, and beneficence and nonmaleficence. Because false claims of healing efficacy can cause direct and indirect harms to patients, such claims violate the essential ethical obligation of all medical practice, whether alternative or conventional—that is, to help and not to harm. On the other hand, there is an ethical issue that supports many alternative medicines: the frequent failures of mainline conventional scientific medicine to connect personally with the patient, to establish and then continue a personal relationship, and to pay primary attention to the patient rather than to technologies. Into the ethical vacuum in mainline medicine, created by the loss of personal relationship with patients, step many different forms of alternative and unconventional medicines.

THE MEANING OF *ALTERNATIVE* AND *CONVENTIONAL*

Once the Flexner Report (*Medical Education in the United States and Canada: A Report to the Carnegie Foundation for the Advancement of Teaching*) commissioned by the American Medical Association (AMA) was published in 1910 in order to improve medical education in the United States and bring quality controls to medical curricula,

Johns Hopkins Medical School became the standard for education in science-based mainline medicine. Then other medical schools and other forms of medical practice became "alternatives" to the new standard. One of the characteristics of many alternative medicines was maintaining health rather than fighting disease. Most alternatives held the belief that personal experience is as reliable as scientific data in determining effectiveness of interventions.

Alternative implies an available choice or an opportunity to choose a way of treating a condition that is different from or complementary to the treatments of orthodox, regular, mainline, conventional medicine. These descriptive terms refer to a medical theory, based on modern science, that began to emerge in the Renaissance. The medical innovators were persons such as Andreas Vesalius (1514–1564) and Paracelsus (1493–1541). Then came scientifically validated medical discoveries and procedures from Germany in the late 1800s, which blossomed in the twentieth century in the United States. If alternative medicine is characterized by an enormous variety of different medical theories and practices with little in common with each other either conceptually or culturally, conventional medicine has the appearance of a single powerful system based on one narrowly conceived scientific biology and focused primarily on organic pathologies. Besides being scientific and physical, mainline conventional medicine is also rationalistic. It is a system that relies on hard data from a hypothesis, observation, controlled experimentation, logical argument, and a somewhat narrow view of causality. Alternative and conventional medicines actually contribute to defining each other by contrast and opposition.

What today are classified as either *conventional* or *alternative* medicine were not always so designated. Formerly alternative medical theories and practices have over time moved into conventional mainline standing; an example is the use of antioxidant vitamins and other dietary remedies for both disease prevention and therapy (Rimm et al. 1993; Steinberg 1993). Likewise, formerly conventional medicines today are in the alternative category, for example, most nineteenth-century therapies such as baths, massage, and purgatives. Between the Renaissance beginnings of modern scientific orthodoxy and its dominance in the twentieth century, mainline medicine was practiced by relatively few university-trained physicians. Most sick people during these centuries got by on prayer or remedies developed under older theories. Even university physicians used bleedings and purgings, sweating, and vomiting in addition to a few new tested medications such as quinine and digitalis. Not much separated early scientific orthodoxy from nonscientific alternative practice when it came to medical interventions. All this changed in the nineteenth and twentieth centuries. University-educated physicians established their own medical associations, adopted updated ethical standards, reformed their educational systems, proved that microorganisms cause infectious disease, developed vaccines to control some infections, employed technologies to improve both diagnosis and therapy, and finally gained legal status for their practice, along with monopolistic control of health care institutions. The line between a unified, socially supported, conventional medicine on one side and alternative medical practices on the other became much more clearly drawn in the twentieth century.

Differences between conventional and alternative medicines now are accentuated by a continuing polemic. The term *alternative* is used by many conventional physicians as synonymous with quackery, falsehood, uselessness, and dishonesty. *Alternative* is frequently used to mean foreign or antiquated, or to emphasize different cultural origins. In literature favoring alternative therapies, conventional medicine is often synonymous with toxic and addictive drugs, high costs, aggressive procedures, impersonalness, unnecessary surgeries, economic monopoly, and iatrogenic or physician-induced illness. For their part, mainline critics of alternative medicines create the impression that alternatives are products of prescientific cultures, whereas conventional medicine is purely scientific and transcends historical and cultural influence.

What constitutes disease and illness, however, as well as how they are understood and treated by any medical system, is necessarily historical and cultural. Contemporary culture's medical-industrial complex, for example, has as much influence on mainline medicine as the military-industrial complex has on modern warfare. Indeed, the historical and cultural content of both conventional and alternative medicines is an important consideration whenever legal and ethical issues are addressed. What is ethically right cannot be simply reduced to what is culturally dominant. Cultural dominance does not equate with ethical correctness. Minority status or identification with another culture does not mean moral incorrectness. Only when cultural and historical factors are identified on both sides can ethical and legal questions about medicine be effectively addressed. Then dialogue can be substituted for hostile discourse, and common ethical standards can be developed for both types of practice. This is especially important today because many medical practices that once were defined as alternative and excluded from mainline medical facilities have gained a new acceptance. Now certain alternative practices are being made available in mainline hospitals.

The interaction between conventional mainline medicine and alternative medicines is increasing. Histories of alternative medicines are now available that explain their background beliefs about the body and illness and how they came to be promoted in Europe and the United States (Bivins 2008). Centuries before Edward Jenner discovered that exposure to mild forms of cowpox conferred immunity to smallpox, Asian healers engaged in a form of this same type medical theory and practice. Acupuncture has not yet become totally integrated into mainline practice, but like other alternative treatments from different cultures, it can be objectively or scientifically evaluated based on measured results from clinical interventions. Many medical schools now offer some instruction in alternative medicine. The fact that testing of all types of clinical interventions is now possible opens a gate for many alternative medicines that previously were scorned and ignored to enter the evidence-based orthodox medical world.

The fact that there is movement toward accepting alternative therapies of proven effectiveness means that the segregating line between alternative and conventional medicines is not impassable. More alternative practices have become complementary practices: that is, what was alternative medicine is now called complementary and alternative medicine (CAM). Attitudes of mainline physicians toward alternative practices are changing, if only slowly and selectively.

MAINLINE CONVENTIONAL MEDICINE

Allopathy (M.D.). One mainline medicine today is referred to as *allopathy*, a term that sets it apart from *homeopathy*. Allopathy is a system that counteracts disease by the use of remedies that produce effects different from those produced by the disease (*contraria contrariis curantur*). Allopathic medicine by definition combats, counteracts, and aggressively opposes specific disease entities. Today's conventional allopathic medicine has its own history and is the product of strong cultural influences. The allopathic approach, originating with the Hippocratics, was reinforced in the nineteenth century by opposition to a homeopathic alternative. Another important historical influence was a high school teacher from Kentucky, Abraham Flexner (1866–1959), whose book on US medical practices laid the foundations of what today has come to be orthodox, conventional, mainline medical practice.

The Flexner Report, published in 1910, not only took a critical view of medical education and practices in North America but also held up a model of medicine grounded in hard laboratory science and universal laws. For Flexner, the best medicine targeted diseased objects rather than patient complaints and, like engineering, was founded on hard science. Under Flexner's influence, nineteenth-century German medicine came to be orthodox medicine in the United States, and the medical school at Johns Hopkins University became the model for the way orthodox medicine should be taught and practiced. Doctors William Welch (1850–1934), William Osler (1847–1919), William S. Halsted (1852–1922), and Howard Kelly (1858–1943) at Johns Hopkins became the architects of the new orthodoxy, and all four physicians were themselves products of German medical training (Ackerknecht 1982). Because Flexner applied the imagery of war to medical practice, orthodox medicine became an aggressive science. Engineering and military science shaped mainline medical attitudes and procedures, while contemporary biology, histology, embryology, anatomy, physiology, pathology, and bacteriology provided the substance of mainline medical understanding. For Flexner, all other approaches were considered unscientific and unethical.

What came to be accepted over several centuries as modern science melded with mainline orthodox medicine, which now enjoys great power and prestige around the world. Mainline allopathic medicine, alone of the classic professions (law, medicine, ministry), wrapped itself in the mantle of hard science. Alternative medicines are alternative because they lack that mantle. If alternative medicine is ethically suspect, it is because hard science became the ethical as well as the epistemological standard in the twentieth century and remains so today. Being unscientific or deficiently scientific amounts to being irresponsible in medicine. All alternative medicines are not the same in this regard, but in general, alternative medicine's moral weakness can be traced to either absent or deficient science.

Some alternative medicines claim to use "a different science." They adopt the stance that mainline science is just another cultural variable or another historical belief system. Some defenders of alternative medicine argue that one cultural variable or belief system is as good as another. No objective rational ground exists, they claim, to prefer one medical system to another, or to assign to one a greater social and ethical standing. Radical advocates for alternative medicine make their argument for equal legal and ethical status based on the fact that mainline science is itself cultural and historical. Patients, they insist, should be totally free to make their own choices about treatment. Their argument is strengthened by calling attention to the theoretical flaws in modern science and to the corrupting influence of powerful financial interests (e.g., large pharmaceutical firms) on scientific research and even on scientific literature.

Karl Popper's work *The Logic of Scientific Discovery* (1939 German edition; 1959 English edition) on the concepts of verifiability and falsifiability weakened some claims about what is proved in science. He argued that the best science can do is demonstrate what is false, not prove what is true. Later, Popper's claims about falsifiability were themselves shown to be flawed. Then Thomas Kuhn

(*The Structure of Scientific Revolution*, 1962) showed how what he called a *paradigm* defines what counts as admissible evidence in science, and how these paradigms change. These classic works show that the foundations on which mainline medical orthodoxy bases its claims to ethical and social superiority are influenced by cultural historical factors.

Modern science and scientific proof claims may have rational and conceptual flaws, but all flaws are not equal. Despite the flawed epistemological foundations of science and the limitations of mathematics, they still can be used to build bridges that work and spacecrafts that arrive at their destinations. Modern medical science, too, has real explanatory power. This rigor of scientific explanation is often absent from alternative medicines. Mainline scientific research is much more credible than unscientific and unsubstantiated claims. Admittedly, alternative medicines lack the government funding to carry out the most sound research, which is expensive, but many alternative medicines ignore research and lack rigorous standards for subjecting therapeutic claims to critical review. When a medical practice is ethical and earns preferential legal status because it bases its claims on publicly confirmable evidence, then that medicine warrants the ethical and legal priority that it enjoys.

Osteopathy (D.O.). One medical practice that has moved from alternative status to integration with mainline conventional medicine is osteopathy. Osteopathic medicine in the United States brings together mainline medical practice with components of what once were considered alternative practices. Mainline physicians (M.D.s) now practice alongside osteopathic physicians (D.O.s). Osteopathic education now combines conventional medical education with osteopathic practices such as manipulation, physical therapy, and education about healthful body posture and positioning. The medical education of an osteopathic physician is similar to that of a mainline physician, except for some added practices and a more holistic background theory. D.O.s now prescribe drugs and perform surgery. Some D.O.s today belong both to the AMA and the American Osteopathic Association.

In osteopathy there is focus on the neuromusculoskeletal system because the structure of the body and body function are related. Medical problems in one part of the body affect other parts as well. Realignment of one part of the body can improve health and function in other parts. Manipulative techniques have been developed to bring about this realignment.

Osteopathy embraces a holistic perspective that supports a continuum between health and illness. Mainline conventional medicine focuses on specific body parts and particular causes of illness, and then attacks the causes of pathology. Osteopathy, in contrast, emphasizes the interactiveness of all parts of the body and the body's natural healing power. It focuses on the whole patient and the whole system (body, mind, and soul). Osteopathy has moved from alternative to mainline medical status in the United States, but in other countries it remains separate and complementary. Outside the United States, osteopaths mainly use spinal manipulation and are often confused with chiropractors. In the United States osteopaths treat many conditions, the same as mainline doctors do. If certain ailments were to be assigned to osteopaths, they might be conditions such as back pain, ankle injury, tennis elbow, and knee and joint injuries.

Osteopathic medical practice developed in the United States during the latter half of the nineteenth century. Andrew Still (1828–1917), its founder, was a creative, committed, hard-working M.D. physician. He developed a system of manipulation and spinal reflexes for the treatment of many different conditions and in 1874 created a new medical theory that he called osteopathy. Later, a school of osteopathic medicine was established and then a small hospital. Still authored many articles and several books. His osteopathic medicine is naturalistic, vitalistic, holistic. The body functions as a unit rather than a group of parts; diseased organs will alter the musculoskeletal system, and manipulation of this system can cure organ disease.

Still's vision was influenced by different philosophical theories circulating in the United States during the last decades of the nineteenth century. He was certainly influenced by Herbert Spencer, who in turn influenced Charles Darwin. The relationship between structure and function, and a holistic view of human nature, can be traced to these sources.

What began during the late nineteenth and early twentieth centuries as an alternative view has become integrated with mainline conventional medicine. In all fifty states an osteopathic license is equivalent to an M.D. degree. Arriving at this point was not easy. The AMA opposed this integration, trying to maintain its status as the only mainline medicine. Osteopaths first gained approval as military physicians during the Vietnam War. Now they serve in the military and the government and in religious and community health organizations.

At the twenty-nine osteopathic medical schools in the United States, the curriculum is the same as at allopathic schools, except that manipulation is added. With official approval and equivalence to mainline medicine, osteopathy has become less distinctive and more similar to mainline medicine in both theory and practice. The original medical theory and practices of Still have not disappeared, but they are less prominent in the medical practices of most of the 104,000 osteopathic physicians (American Osteopathic Association 2013). Many of Still's original insights have been confirmed by mainline science and have become part of mainline medicine.

Osteopathy has become part of mainline medicine, and mainline medicine has been influenced by osteopathy. This situation may be repeated with other medical theories and practices that today are still classified as alternative. Adding the term *complementary* to *alternative* (in CAM) is a step toward integration. In line for such integration are acupuncture, chiropractic, homeopathy, and naturopathy. Some medical theories and practices based on different physical or mental or spiritual perspectives of human life will remain separate from mainline scientific medicine. But it is possible that other different medical perspectives and approaches will someday be synthesized into one scientific holistic mainline medical theory and practice.

COMPLEMENTARY AND ALTERNATIVE MEDICINES

Homeopathy. Homeopathy is the creation of an eighteenth-century German physician, Christian Friedrich Samuel Hahnemann (1755–1843). Hahnemann was trained in the mainline medicine of his day, which made extensive use of practices such as bleeding and purging. He renounced these practices and was motivated by the traditional ethical commitment to "do no harm." Hahnemann's medical theory is summed up in the phrase *similes similibus curantur*, or "like cures like." According to this theory, small amounts of whatever could induce the patient's symptoms could cure the disease that is producing the symptoms. Over and against this theory is the opposite theory of mainline conventional medicine, *contraria contrariis curantur*; that is, cure occurs when a pathology is attacked by opposite influences. Conventional medicine does, however, recognize the effectiveness of the "law of similar" as expressed in vaccinations and allergy treatments. By administering trace amounts of a disease component or cause (e.g., a virus), antibodies are produced and immunity is created.

The term *homeopathy* was coined by Hahnemann using the Greek word *homeo* (the same), or *homoios* (similar), to describe his medical theory. This theory led to the production of its own pharmacological agents, using extremely diluted amounts of the symptom-causing agents. The agents can be plant, mineral, or animal substances. These agents are believed to have a healing effect even after multiple dilutions. A single homeopathic agent is given for a particular condition or set of complaints, and each agent is diluted many times until it becomes more powerful:

> Homeopathic remedies actually become stronger as they are diluted, as long as this dilution is accompanied by succussion (a carefully prescribed vigorous shaking of the mixture in a special manner). The final product is so diluted, in fact, that in many cases not a single molecule of the original substance would be expected to survive in the final product, which is important since many homeopathic remedies start out with toxic intent (e.g., the active ingredient in poison oak or the protective discharge emanating from the cuttlefish). The remaining substance is believed to possess the "memory" of what it started out as, but without its original toxicity. (Bausell 2007, 14–15)

Hahnemann's medicine came to the United States in 1828 and quickly spread. By the beginning of the twentieth century there were 15,000 homeopathic physicians and twenty-two homeopathic medical schools in the United States (Masiello 1999). These numbers declined sharply once contemporary hard scientific medicine was established at Johns Hopkins and then spread throughout the nation. Homeopathic remedies later gained legal status and became available as safe, even though their efficacy was not scientifically established. Gradually, clinical trials have been conducted and some remedies were proven effective. The results of these trials, however, are questioned by many mainline physicians.

Homeopathy today is complementary to mainline medicine, and pressures come from some homeopathic organizations to remove its alternative status and integrate it into conventional mainline medicine. But not all organizations agree. In 2010 the US Food and Drug Administration (FDA) issued warning letters regarding homeopathic swine flu remedies. Yet the National Center for Complementary and Alternative Medicine (NCCAM) at the National Institutes of Health (NIH), in a publication on homeopathy for public use, under the title *Side Effects and Risks*, stated the following: "A 2007 systematic review found that highly dilute homeopathic remedies, taken under the supervision of trained professionals, are generally safe and unlikely to cause severe adverse reactions" (NCCAM 2013). Proponents claim that homeopathic treatments are especially helpful for diseases such as diabetes, arthritis, asthma, epilepsy, skin conditions, allergies, and mental and emotional disorders. Homeopathy is practiced in the United States, Europe, India, Mexico, Argentina, Brazil, and elsewhere. As more of the limits of mainline scientific medicine are revealed, the uses of homeopathy become more likely to be legally and ethically approved.

Chiropractic. This CAM has roots in ancient Egypt and other early civilizations. It is based on hands-on manipulation of the back and adjustments of the spinal cord. The word *chiropractic* comes from the Greek words meaning "hand" and "done by." Contemporary chiropractic in the United States originated in Davenport,

Iowa, in 1895, with Daniel David Palmer's teachings that all illness originates in a dislocated spine and misaligned nervous system. Even ailments such as allergies, asthma, morning sickness, menstrual problems, insomnia, otitis media, bladder infections, depression, and addictions are believed to originate in dislocated spines and misaligned nervous systems.

Chiropractic adjustments are provided at office visits. A first visit is usually for acute symptoms. Second-level or repeated chiropractic adjustments are for maintenance, and third-level or periodic visits are to prevent new dislocations and misalignments that are believed to be the sources of different illnesses.

The first graduates of Palmer's College of Chiropractic in Iowa were physicians, and chiropractic retains a complementary relationship with mainline conventional medicine. Mainline physicians send patients to chiropractors, and chiropractors send patients for conventional care. Legally, the US Supreme Court upheld the right of mainline physicians to form partnerships or engage in group practice with alternative health care providers, thereby making chiropractic and mainline practice legally complementary.

Chiropractic practitioners call themselves doctors and complain about being excluded from mainline medical institutions. Osteopathic physicians are now considered mainline, and they receive training similar to chiropractors. The present integration of osteopathy with mainline medicine provides encouragement that chiropractors will achieve the same status at some point.

Chiropractic is probably the best-known alternative medicine in the United States. The effectiveness of manual manipulations is supported by scientific studies, but it is difficult for studies of hands-on chiropractic manipulation to eliminate a placebo effect and to satisfy double-blind requirements. One double-blind scientific study of the effectiveness of chiropractic versus conventional treatment conducted in 1990 by Dr. T. W. Meade and colleagues strongly favored chiropractic. Conventional physicians attacked the study's science, arguing that the statistics were unreliable because the study's method was not rigorous. The response to Meade and colleagues was extensive. The critical responders questioned the study's methodology and the effectiveness of chiropractic over traditional hospital treatments. The supporters were impressed both by the study and the results that favored chiropractic over mainline medical treatment. They insisted that the study be given serious consideration. The authors of the article replied to all respondents, answering questions, defining their methodology, and strengthening their conclusions ("Low Back Pain" 1990).

Most chiropractors are uncomfortable about requiring that any claim of effectiveness must satisfy a double-blind requirement, because doing so would throw doubt upon many of their own scientific studies of effectiveness, which are statistical but not double-blind. Some chiropractic medical schools have their own research institutes and are continuously involved in effectiveness and outcome studies. Despite extensive use of chiropractic in certain parts of the United States, serious dialogue and cooperation with mainline practitioners is still limited.

Naturopathy. The term *naturopathy* was used by Dr. John Schell of New York City to describe a healing method that he developed in 1895. The method first flourished, then declined, like many other medical practices in competition with mainline scientific medicine. Naturopathy never achieved the same political and professional support enjoyed by some other alternative medical systems. Today there are several naturopathic colleges that have been accredited by the profession. Bastyr University in Seattle, Washington, is its major academic center. Other schools that provide naturopathic medical education in North America are the following: Bastyr University, California; National College of Natural Medicine, Oregon; National University of Health Sciences, Illinois; Southwest College of Naturopathic Medicine, Arizona; University of Bridgeport, Connecticut; Canadian College of Naturopathic Medicine, Ontario; Boucher Institute of Naturopathic Medicine, British Columbia. Students study anatomy, physiology, basic science, and then applied practice. Naturopath practitioners usually make use of manipulation, massage, herbal remedies, acupuncture, and Eastern medicines.

In naturopathic theory, the practitioner treats the underlying causes of illness by energizing the body's "life force." As far back as Hippocrates, nature was seen as having healing powers. Practitioners are licensed legally in many states but still are not covered by most health insurances. Ethically, the issue is whether this medical system is subjecting its therapeutic claims and practices to objective scientific standards of efficacy.

Naturopathy falls under CAM because naturopath physicians use mainline research on natural therapies such as nutrition and botanicals, which also complement conventional medical therapies. They refer patients to mainline physicians and vice versa. There is a teamlike relationship with some mainline physicians.

As was the case with many other alternative medicines, there was a decline in the use of naturopathy following the successes of mainline research in the twentieth century and the flow of new medicines and technologies following government investment. Before the post World War II enormous government investment in mainline medicine, there were a number of naturopathic medical schools and thousands of practitioners using naturopathic therapies. In the 1970s, when many of the problems, limitations, and costs of mainline medicine emerged, naturopathy and many other alternative medical approaches experienced a resurgence. One of the hallmarks of naturopathic medicine is the greater amount of time that naturopaths spend with their patients.

Not only are patients increasingly using alternatives such as naturopathy, but also more and more cooperation exists between naturopathic and mainline physicians. The NIH has established an agency to test alternative medicines and therapies. States are developing naturopathic licensing laws. The locations that currently have licensing laws for naturopathic physicians are Alaska, Arizona, California, Colorado, Connecticut, District of Columbia, Hawaii, Idaho, Kansas, Maine, Minnesota, Montana, New Hampshire, North Dakota, Oregon, Utah, Vermont, Washington, and the US territories Puerto Rico and Virgin Islands (American Association of Naturopathic Physicians 2013).

Accredited university education programs, professional licensing, and commitment to scientific research all reflect the complementary status of naturopathy. An increasing number of patients are using naturopathic physicians for primary health care. There are 4,300 practicing naturopathic physicians, and their patients run into the millions (American Association of Naturopathic Physicians 2013).

Acupuncture. Many conventional mainline medical clinics and hospitals now offer acupuncture. There is an American Academy of Medical Acupuncture to which hundreds of physicians belong, where education and training are offered. Standards of practice have been set for the use of acupuncture in medical practice.

Acupuncture is used mainly for chronic pain relief but also for smoking cessation and conditions such as asthma, arthritis, and substance abuse. Different ethnic groups (e.g., Koreans, Chinese) disagree about the correct locations of acupuncture points. One common moral criticism of acupuncture is that many conventional physicians use it simply as a way to charge patients and insurance companies.

Acupuncture is grounded on a theory of "chee" or "chi" (or "qi"): a flow of energy or life force and a release of the body's natural opiate-like pain-relieving substances. The long thin needles inserted into the skin aid in maintaining or increasing the flow of energy. Although this background theory does not have confirmation from mainline medical science, the therapeutic effect of acupuncture has been confirmed by mainline groups such as the NIH.

> Promising results have emerged, showing efficacy of acupuncture in adult postoperative and chemotherapy nausea and vomiting and in postoperative dental pain. There are other situations such as addiction, stroke rehabilitation, headache, menstrual cramps, tennis elbow, fibromyalgia, myofascial pain, osteoarthritis, low back pain, carpal tunnel syndrome, and asthma, in which acupuncture may be useful as an adjunct treatment or an acceptable alternative or be included in a comprehensive management program. Further research is likely to uncover additional areas where acupuncture interventions will be useful. (NIH 1997)

The NIH panel's consensus statement recommends integrating acupuncture into standard medical practice and urges Medicare, Medicaid, and private insurance companies to begin paying for acupuncture treatments.

Biophysicists have been able to prove that electrical currents do flow along the ancient Chinese pathways, and that acupuncture points exist along the measurable lines. Efficacy tests involving thousands of patients carried out at respected universities have confirmed the efficacy of acupuncture for different conditions. Acupuncture has also been approved for pain conditions at military clinics and hospitals.

As the complementary use of acupuncture increases in mainline medicine, new acupuncture techniques have been developed, such as replacing needles with laser beams, light waves, or sound waves. Another variation called "cupping" uses glass, metal, wood, or bamboo cups of different sizes. The cups are warmed and placed top down on acupoints or areas of the skin. The cups draw blood to the cup location, and this influences the flow of energy (chee). Many other variations exist.

Thousands of acupuncturists in the United States have been licensed, registered, or certified, including more than 3,000 mainline physicians (M.D.s and D.O.s) (American Association of Acupuncture 2013). Certain official organizations do the certifications and set the standards, including the National Certification Commission for Acupuncture and Oriental Medicine (NCCAOM). Acupuncture remains in the category of CAM because although it is increasingly used in mainline medicine, it has not been recognized as mainline scientific medicine. It differs from mainline medicine in its theory that changes in the whole organism make specific symptoms disappear; in mainline conventional theory, directly targeted symptoms cause changes in the whole organism. Like mainline medicine, however, acupuncture operates on physiological processes of the organism, and it is overseen by official commissions.

ALTERNATIVE MEDICINES AND THERAPIES

Hypnosis, Hypnotherapy, and Biofeedback. The word *hypnosis* refers to a technique introduced by Franz Anton Mesmer (1734–1815), a German physician, and then later developed by a British ophthalmologist, James Braid (1795–1860). It was Braid who changed the name of the technique from *mesmerism* to *hypnosis* (from Hypnos, the Greek god of sleep). The technique guides a patient into an altered state of consciousness, a deep relaxation or trance-like state. It is used to treat stress, anxiety, addictions, panic attacks, and many other psychological and physical problems. The power of suggestion is used to bring about an altered mental and emotional state that in turn will have an effect on one's physical state. Sigmund Freud (1856–1939), the father of contemporary psychiatry, used hypnosis in his practice in the nineteenth century.

It was not until 1955 that hypnotherapy was officially recognized as a medical treatment by the British Medical Association, and three years later by the AMA. Soon after, the American Institute of Hypnotherapy was established, with a membership made up of physicians, psychiatrists, psychologists, dentists, and other health professionals. Although it is not yet supported by hard scientific evaluations, the technique is taught in many psychiatric residency programs and used by many practitioners. The induced deep relaxation is beneficial for many different pathologies.

Biofeedback is a recording of different body functions that picks up signals from physical bodily activities. If a person is under stress, the signals will show how the body is handling the stress. The recordings help a person to learn how to use relaxation techniques to alter the signals. Biofeedback helps the person to reduce stress, reduce anxiety, and alter other states that create the signals. It helps persons to be attentive to certain physical causes and then to modify their effects.

Hypnosis, guided imagery, hypnotherapy, and biofeedback are all forms of visualization therapy often used in orthodox treatment centers. Practitioners may be mainline physicians, psychologists, social workers, or nurses. The conditions addressed include everything from mental and emotional illness to immunological disorders, childhood hyperactivity, cancer, and senility. On the theoretical level, practitioners and advocates work to demonstrate just how the mind controls the brain and the immune system. The effect of biofeedback on the psyche (e.g., stress reduction) and physiology (e.g., temperature, heart rate, blood pressure) is well documented.

Whether visualization techniques will be considered an alternative therapy or an extension of conventional medicine, in the sense that they broaden conventional medicine's physical base to include the psyche, will depend on whether they can generate satisfactory scientific proof of effectiveness. Advocates of mainline medicine such as Norman Cousins, Bernie Siegel, and Andrew Weil call for a wider theoretical base for mainline practices, one that includes a place for the mind's influence on bodily healing (Cousins 1979; Weil 1983; Siegel 1986).

Meditation, Massage, and Relaxation. Mainline conventional physicians recognize the benefits that come from psychiatry as well as from practices such as meditation, massage, and relaxation for helping patients with illnesses related to stress and anxiety. It is when these techniques alone are used for certain physical pathologies that they qualify as alternative medicines. The fact that personal beliefs play a role in mainline medical practice as well as mainline research is clear from placebo-effect evidence.

The biological sciences of orthodox medicine are materialistic (i.e., grounded in physical realities and quantifiable data) and are ill-equipped to handle many of the problems listed as disease categories in psychiatry's diagnostic manual (cf. the American Psychiatric Association's *Diagnostic and Statistical Manual of Mental Disorders*). A narrowly focused conventional psychiatry relies on chemical therapies and restricts practice to drug prescriptions and medication reviews. Beyond this narrow range of orthodoxy, psychological and social theories have added a broad assortment of nonchemical approaches to conventional practice—from classical psychoanalysis to cognitive, behavioral, and group treatments, to visualization therapies.

Diet and Nutrition. The role of good diet in health preservation has long been recognized in mainline conventional medicine. Certain diets are part of standard treatment for pathologies such as heart disease and diabetes. Certain vitamins are also part of mainline conventional medicine. Dieticians work in mainline hospitals and are used as consultants by conventional physicians. Only when dietary interventions alone are used by alternative practitioners, and when certain dietary supplements are promoted by them, does diet and nutrition fall into the category of alternative medicine.

Energy Medicine, Reflexology, and Reiki. Electrical power is commonly used in diagnostic and therapeutic medical procedures. Electroencephalograms (EEGs), electrocardiograms (ECGs), and magnetic resonance imaging (MRI) are all examples of electrical energy used for diagnostic purposes. Energy is also used for healing in procedures such as therapeutic touch, reflexology, and reiki. In therapeutic practices, the energy is directed, modulated, balanced, and interfaced with other therapeutic modalities. According to proponents of these therapies, the energy is transferred from one human being to another in order to create a therapeutic effect. In lesser degrees there is a transfer of energy that goes on continuously from one person to another. When the energy transfer is joined to a therapeutic intention, its healing power is increased.

Electrical therapy, light therapy, electroacupuncture, and sound therapy are all examples of energy medicine. Electric pain therapy involves placing electrodes at or near where pain is felt, then running an electric current into the electrodes in order to relieve the pain. Transcutaneous electrical nerve stimulation (TENS) is thought to stimulate the body's natural pain killers (endorphins) and to prevent the brain from perceiving painful brain sensations. This energy medicine is used in the treatment of arthritis, sciatica, neuralgia, shingles, chronic back pain, dental pain, musculoskeletal pain, cancer, angina, menstrual pain, migraine, carpal tunnel, and nerve damage pain.

Herbal Medicine. Human beings lived for many thousands of years in small hunter-gatherer groups. During this longest period of human existence, medicines came in the form of plants. Forests were abundant and rich in plant life. People passed down information from generation to generation about the therapeutic effects of certain plants. Much of this information continued to be passed down to populations in later civilizations, some with advanced testing capabilities. Mainline scientific medicine used some traditional information about herbal remedies and tested traditional claims about the benefits of herbal medicines. Herbal remedies in teas and tablets continue to be used. They retain alternative status because most of their therapeutic claims have not been subjected to hard scientific testing. Folk healers and herbalists qualify as alternative healers. Herbal remedies can be marketed without FDA approval, and therapeutic claims are often exaggerated by promoters.

Iridology. Iridology is a diagnostic method developed by a homeopathic physician in Hungary more than 100 years ago. It is based on examination of the iris and what it reveals about the presence of disease in different parts of the body. Dr. Ignaz von Peczely (1826–1911) noticed a black mark on the eye of an owl with a broken leg, then later he saw a similar mark on the iris of a person with a similar break. From then on he focused on the iris as an indicator of pathology in other parts of the body. This theory had ancient roots in Egypt and China and in the ancient medicine of Greece (e.g., Hippocrates). The diagnostic method required no special technologies (only a light and a magnifying glass) and no invasions of other body parts or disruptions of other body functions. This alternative medicine's diagnostic method could not replace the diagnostic methods of mainline medicine, however, and its alternative status was fixed.

Music Therapy. Music therapy is the employment of music to bring about change in the psychological, physical, mental, or social functioning in a patient. The practitioners who use music in this way are music therapists. The focus of music therapy is on the process rather than on determining how it works or why it works.

Yoga. The word *yoga* comes from Sanskrit and means yoke, union, to join. There are many creators of different types of yoga. Some types are more like religions and involve primarily spiritual exercises such as meditation. Others are more like physical medicinal practices, usually with some meditation.

Yoga as alternative medicine makes claims of deliverance from pain and sorrow, remedy of heart disease, psychiatric disorders, AIDS, and the power to achieve a full life. Yoga with physical focus is often integrated with mainstream fitness programs. Different types of yoga blend the physical and spiritual dimensions of the tradition, which traces its roots to 3000 B.C.E.

Many spiritual forms of yoga are geared toward achieving moral objectives such as compassion, humility, courage, truthfulness, love, non-covetousness, and strength to cope with fears. These yoga forms have clear psychiatric and psychological objectives. More physical forms provide alternative therapies for stress relief, pain relief, and relaxation. They often employ different tools such as bells and blocks. Yoga, even in its physical forms, is still a long way from mainline scientific medicine, but it is more and more frequently approved by mainline practitioners.

Because of the vast variety of different styles of yoga, there is also a vast variety of legal and ethical evaluations available. A book by William Broad (*The Science of Yoga*, 2012) explores the different styles and tries to evaluate in scientific terms both the different claims made and the evidence available to support the claims. He makes the point that not all yoga is beneficial or safe. He also weighs the reliability of the journals in which the yoga studies were published.

Broad traces yoga's history and finds that what today in the United States is an activity of mainly upper-middle-class Americans was historically in India the practice of vagabonds who promoted their body movements to win money and sex. A 2012 sex scandal involving the founder of Anusara Yoga, reconnects with that ancient tradition. Yoga's new face radiates with health, fitness, and even with some science. Many of the practices of contemporary yoga in the United States are modern inventions. Alongside the health benefit claims, however, there are also many yoga injuries. Yoga can produce painful impairments such as torn Achilles tendons, nerve damage, back injuries, and even strokes. Overall, though, it seems to do more good than harm. After centuries of practice it is understandable that its record includes both positive benefits and negative effects. Any approach to broader medical acceptability will have to involve, among other things, more controlled and systematic training for yoga teachers.

ORTHODOX PUBLIC HEALTH AND ALTERNATIVE PRACTICES

No medicine has been more orthodox since the nineteenth century than public health medicine. When microscopic technologies aided the discovery of bacterial causes of infectious diseases, public health physicians became energetic in the application of laboratory science on behalf of societal health. Public health physicians were laboratory science's strongest advocates. They insisted upon strict quantitative standards of proof for what they considered ethical medical practice. Only what could be shown quantitatively to be effective (e.g., vaccines) commanded their respect and endorsement. Laboratory science alone was the basis for medical respectability. They used the state power associated with public health (health laws and their enforcement) to support a narrow, positivistic foundation for conventional medicine. Medicine for them was narrowly focused on microbes, and they tended to leave aside broader social and cultural issues. We know, however, that an adequate science does not ignore sociocultural influences on behaviors that spread disease.

Contemporary public health practice requires "cultural competence," that is, an understanding of the culture of the people to whom public health policies are applied. Ethnic ways, which include particular attitudes and practices related to health and disease, have to be taken into consideration in order to provide the most effective public health services. Cooperation between mainline physicians and alternative practitioners will make the difference between compliance and noncompliance, especially in minority populations. What is true in public health also applies in private practice.

The World Health Organization (WHO) has strongly advocated cooperation between conventional physicians and alternative practitioners because neither one is likely to disappear. In the European Union and the United States, over 100 million citizens use alternative medicines (WHO 2001; Bausell 2007). In the Netherlands, a survey of 293 conventional physicians showed that many believe in the efficacy of certain alternative practices such as manual therapy, yoga, acupuncture, hot baths, and homeopathy (Knipschild 1990). In Germany, a distinction is made between scientifically supported alternatives such as naturopathy and unscientifically based alternatives; the former are covered by some insurance policies and the state plan pays a subsidy to patients using them (German Health Insurance Program 2013). In Norway, conventional physicians and alternative practitioners have moved toward ever closer cooperation (Rankin-Box 1992).

Because the use of alternative treatments continues to increase both in the United States and in Europe, new studies of alternative approaches have been initiated. The NIH established the NCCAM to test the safety and efficacy of alternative therapies and to keep the public informed of research results. Congress mandated the creation of this project and required that the NIH spend part of its annual budget on it. An oversight committee includes both conventional physicians and alternative practice advocates, who have agreed that alternative practices will be evaluated with the same methods and standards as conventional therapies (outcome research, relative efficiency, double-blind studies where possible). This is an important development because ethical considerations of alternative practices have to start from reliable information about their effectiveness. This project has added an ethical component because the projects funded require cooperation and collaboration between alternative and conventional practitioners wherever possible.

ETHICAL STANDARDS AND ALTERNATIVE PRACTICE

Alternative medicine is governed by ethical obligations derived from the principles that medical practitioners of all varieties publicly profess and from what societies have always required of them: to heal, to relieve pain, to restore function, and to comfort and accompany the dying when patients are beyond treatment. In the Hippocratic tradition these basic ethical standards were encapsulated in the imperative "to help and not to harm." Twenty-first-century medical ethics references these same basic ethical obligations using the principles of beneficence and nonmaleficence.

Alternative or mainline medical interventions that harm patients without providing offsetting benefits are unethical. Alternative treatments that are harmless may not violate either individual or social ethical standards—especially if patients have strong faith in them or if the illnesses for which they are used are self-limiting and conventional treatments are expensive, have serious side effects, or have proven ineffective. When diseases being treated are more serious, however, harmlessness is not enough to satisfy individual and social ethical standards. If harmless alternative remedies prevent patients from seeking an effective treatment available from conventional medicine, then alternative practitioners are actually preventing patients from being helped, and just social policies would require that such practices be curtailed. Although alternative remedies are often adjuvant and complementary to mainline remedies, it remains important to respect the social and professional ethical requirement that treatments actually provide benefit to patients. Patient benefit is a complicated concept that sometimes involves unquantifiable quality of life considerations, but patient benefit cannot be permitted to slip beyond empirical proof entirely. Societies have to make laws that use rigorous empirical standards for approval of treatment modalities. Anecdotal evidence of therapy effectiveness or claims of effectiveness dependent upon depth of commitment to an alternative belief system are not enough to satisfy basic individual and social medical ethical standards.

Modern medical-ethical standards add yet another basic obligation derived from patient rights—that is, that the patient has the right to consent to treatment or to refuse consent. Alternative practitioners, like conventional doctors, are ethically obligated to provide patients with information relevant to their decisions and to protect them from coercion, fraud, or manipulation. If patients are not competent, informed consent or refusal must be provided by surrogates—either family members or, in their absence, a guardian. Even decisions by competent patients must meet professional standards, therefore an irrational choice or insistence upon a treatment that is futile or economically devastating should not be respected. The modern principle of patient autonomy must be balanced with the ageless principle of beneficence/nonmaleficence, which protects patients against irrational or incompetent decisions that involve harm without offsetting benefit. Care must be exercised, however, in judging possibly irrational decisions, so as not to confuse them with decisions based on value systems different from those of the treating physician or practitioner. Patients have their own values, and these cannot be set aside because they differ from what a scientifically focused specialist may think is best for a patient. True patient benefit requires consideration of both personal and scientific interests.

A competent adult may refuse an effective but burdensome conventional treatment and choose instead an unproven or ineffective alternative therapy. Similar choices that are made on behalf of children or incompetent adults without advance directives, however, are neither ethically nor legally respectable. Justice and autonomy, and beneficence and nonmaleficence, are broad and abstract ethical standards. Agreement about these standards in their abstract form is possible even in pluralistic and heterogeneous societies. But principles can come into conflict with one another. Respect for patient autonomy may mean not providing patient benefit or violating principles of justice and equality. When such conflict occurs, ethics at a more pragmatic level of discourse is required; that is, concrete norms and rules are required that attempt to facilitate compromise or to bring about a balance between conflicting principles. Working out the relationship between mainline conventional medicine and alternative practices involves just this form of concrete ethics. Appeal to abstract principles only, in a situation of conflict between conventional and alternative medicine, can turn an ethics discussion into an exchange of slogans. One important test of an ethics that addresses the relationship between alternative and conventional medicine is whether it encourages a needed dialogue between different practitioners and whether it can generate concrete norms and public policies to handle interaction between the two traditions (Eisenberg et al. 1993).

Ethics has been intimately associated with mainline medicine since its beginning in Hippocratic times. Hippocratic physicians were distinguished from other healers not only by their emphasis on a type of science but also by their commitment to patient benefit rather than to the selfish goals of healers. Medicine of any variety derives its ethics from obligations generated by a doctor-patient relationship in which a healer commits himself or herself to help someone in need, by cure or pain relief or function restoration. Unselfishness and altruism are at the core of medicine's professional ethics. Truthfulness traditionally was not part of medical ethics, but it has been added in order to fulfill the obligations associated with patient autonomy. This essential and structural medical ethics is applicable to both alternative and conventional medicine.

Mainline medicine obliges physicians to conform to high ethical standards, but mainline medicine has been weak in policing deviant members and in sanctioning ethical failures. Alternative practitioners are not as well organized as conventional physicians, and some lack the strong ethical emphasis of the mainline tradition. Both types of practitioners face a daunting challenge: developing and maintaining the character traits of true professionals, without which concrete moral rules and abstract ethical principles become ineffective in an economic culture that encourages profit making more than altruism.

SEE ALSO *Autonomy; Beneficence; Emotions; Health Care Professionals, Legal Regulation of; Medicine, Philosophy of; Public Health: II. Law*

BIBLIOGRAPHY

Ackerknecht, Erwin H. 1982. *A Short History of Medicine*. Rev. ed. Baltimore, MD: Johns Hopkins University Press.

American Association of Acupuncture. 2013. Accessed September 19, 2013. http://www.Aaaomonline.Org

American Association of Naturopathic Physicians. 2013. Accessed September 19, 2013. http://www.naturopathic.org

American Cancer Society. 2002. *American Cancer Society's Complementary and Alternative Cancer Methods Handbook.* Atlanta, GA: Author.

American Institute of Homeopathy. 2013. Accessed September 19, 2013. http://www.osteopathic.org/Pages/default.aspx

American Osteopathic Association. 2013. "About the AOA." Accessed September 19, 2013. http://www.osteopathic.org/inside-aoa/about/Pages/default.aspx

American Pharmacists Association. 1994. *Code of Ethics for Pharmacists.* Accessed September 19, 2013. http://www.pharmacist.com/code-ethics

American Psychiatric Association. 2013. *Diagnostic and Statistical Manual of Mental Disorders.* 5th ed. (DSM-5). Washington, DC.

Bausell, R. Barker. 2007. *Snake Oil Science: The Truth about Complementary and Alternative Medicine.* New York: Oxford University Press.

Bivins, Roberta. 2008. *Alternative Medicine? A History.* New York: Oxford University Press.

Broad, William. 2012. *The Science of Yoga.* New York: Simon and Schuster.

Callahan, Daniel, ed. 2002. *The Role of Complementary and Alternative Medicine: Accommodating Pluralism.* Washington, DC: Georgetown University Press.

Clouser, K. Danner, and David J. Hufford. 1993. "Nonorthodox Healing Systems and Their Claims." *Journal of Medicine and Philosophy* 18 (2): 101–6.

Clouser, K. Danner; David J. Hufford; and B. B. O'Connor. 1996. "Informed Consent and Alternative Medicine." *Alternative Therapies in Health and Medicine* 2 (2): 76–78.

Cohen, Michael H., and David M. Eisenberg. 2002. "Potential Physician Malpractice Liability Associated with Complementary and Integrative Medical Therapies." *Annals of Internal Medicine* 136 (8): 596–603.

Cousins, Norman. 1979. *Anatomy of an Illness.* New York: Norton.

Davidoff, F. 1998. "Weighing the Alternatives: Lessons from the Paradoxes of Alternative Medicine." *Annals of Internal Medicine* 129 (12): 1068–70.

Eisenberg, David M. 1997. "Advising Patients Who Seek Alternative Medical Therapies." *Annals of Internal Medicine* 127 (1): 61–69.

Eisenberg, David M.; Ronald C. Kessler; Cindy Foster; et al. 1993. "Unconventional Medicine in the United States: Prevalence, Costs and Patterns of Use." *New England Journal of Medicine* 328 (4): 246–52.

Ernst, Edzard, and Michael H. Cohen. 2001. "Informed Consent in Complementary and Alternative Medicine." *Archives of Internal Medicine* 161 (19): 2288–92.

Ernst, Edzard; Michael H. Cohen; and Julie Stone. 2004. "Ethical Problems Arising in Evidence Based Complementary and Alternative Medicine." *Journal of Medical Ethics* 30:156–59.

FDA (Food and Drug Administration). 2010. Accessed September 19, 2013. http://www.fda.gov/ICECI/EnforcementActions/WarningLetters/ucm215236.htm

Flexner, Abraham. 1910. *Medical Education in the United States and Canada: A Report to the Carnegie Foundation for the Advancement of Teaching.* Birmingham, AL: Classics of Medicine Library.

Fuller, Robert C. 1992. "The Turn to Alternative Medicine." *Second Opinion* 18:11–31.

German Health Insurance Program. 2013. Accessed September 19, 2013. http://www.howtogermany.com/pages/healthinsurance.html

Gevitz, Norman C., ed. 1988. *Other Healers: Unorthodox Medicine in America.* Baltimore, MD: Johns Hopkins University Press.

Holtz, Carol. 2008. *Global Health Care: Issues and Policies.* Sudbury, MA: Jones and Bartlett.

International Hahnemannean Association (IHA). Accessed September 19, 2013. http://www.wholehealthnow.com/homeopathy_pro/iha.html

Kaptchuk, Ted J., and Franklin G. Miller. 2005. "Viewpoint: What Is the Best and Most Ethical Model for the Relationship between Mainstream and Alternative Medicine: Opposition, Integration, or Pluralism?" *Academic Medicine* 80 (3): 286–90.

Knipschild, Paul. 1990. "Belief in the Efficacy of Alternative Medicine among General Practitioners in the Netherlands." *Social Science Medicine* 31 (5): 625–26.

Kottow, Michael H. 1992. "Classical Medicine v. Alternative Medical Practice." *Journal of Medical Ethics* 19 (1): 51.

Kuhn, Thomas. 1996 [1962]. *The Structure of Scientific Revolution.* Chicago: University of Chicago Press.

Larson, Christine A. 2007. *Alternative Medicine.* Westport, CT: Greenwood.

"Low Back Pain: Comparison of Chiropractic and Hospital Outpatient Treatment" (letters). 1990. *British Medical Journal* 300 (6740): 1647–50. (Other doctors who supported Dr. Meade were Dr. J. C. T. Fairbank, Dr. R. M. Ellis, and Dr. A. O. Frank.)

Lynöe, Niels. 1992. "Ethical and Professional Aspects of the Practice of Alternative Medicine." *Scandinavian Journal of Public Health* 20 (4): 217–25.

Masiello, Domenick. 1999. "Homeopathy." In *The Illustrated Encyclopedia of Body-Mind Disciplines,* edited by Nancy Allison, 10–14. New York: Rosen.

Mayo Clinic. 2010. *Mayo Clinic Book of Alternative Medicine.* 2nd ed. New York: Time Inc. Home Entertainment Books.

Meade, T. W.; Sandra Dyer; Wendy Browne; et al. 1990. "Low Back Pain of Mechanical Origin: Randomised Comparison of Chiropractic and Hospital Outpatient Treatment." *British Medical Journal* 300 (6737): 1431–37.

Murray, Raymond H., and Arthur J. Rubel. 1992. "Physicians and Healers—Unwitting Partners in Health Care." *New England Journal of Medicine* 326 (1): 61–64.

National Center for Complementary and Alternative Medicine (NCCAM). 2013. "Homeopathy: An Introduction." Accessed September 19, 2013. http://www.pharmacist.com/code-ethics

National Institutes of Health (NIH). 1997. "Acupuncture: NIH Consensus Statement." November 3–5, 15 (5): 1–34.

Popper, Karl R. 1959. *The Logic of Scientific Discovery.* New York: Basic Books.

Rankin-Box, Denise. 1992. "European Developments in Complementary Medicine." *British Journal of Nursing* 1 (2): 103–5.

Rimm, Eric B.; Meir J. Stampfer; Alberto Ascherio; et al. 1993. "Vitamin E Consumption and the Risk of Coronary Heart Disease in Men." *New England Journal of Medicine* 328 (20): 1450–56.

Schneiderman, L. J. 2000. "Alternative Medicine or Alternatives to Medicine? A Physician's Perspective." *Cambridge Quarterly of Healthcare Ethics* 9 (1): 83–97.

Siegel, Bernie S. 1986. *Love, Medicine, and Miracles: Lessons Learned about Self-Healing from a Surgeon's Experience with Exceptional Patients*. New York: Harper and Row.

Steinberg, Daniel. 1993. "Antioxidant Vitamins and Coronary Heart Disease." *New England Journal of Medicine* 328 (20): 1487–89.

Still, Andrew. 2010. *The Philosophy and Mechanical Principles of Osteopathy*. Whitefish, MT: Kessinger.

Stone, Julie. 2002. *An Ethical Framework for Complementary and Alternative Therapists*. New York: Routledge.

Studdert, Daniel M.; David M. Eisenberg; Frances H. Miller; et al. 1998. "Medical Malpractice Implications of Alternative Medicine." *Journal of the American Medical Association* 280 (18): 1610–15.

Sugarman, Jeremy, and Larry Burk. 1998. "Physicians' Ethical Obligations regarding Alternative Medicine." *Journal of the American Medical Association* 280 (18): 1623–25.

Thorne, Sally, and Allan Best. 2002. "Ethical Dimensions in the Borderland between Conventional and Complementary/Alternative Medicine." *Journal of Alternative and Complementary Medicine* 8 (6): 907–15.

Weil, Andrew. 1983. *Health and Healing: Understanding Conventional and Alternative Medicine*. Boston: Houghton Mifflin.

Weintraub, Michael I. 1999. "Legal Implications of Practicing Alternative Medicine." *Journal of the American Medical Association* 281 (18): 1698–99.

World Health Organization (WHO). 2001. *Legal Status of Traditional Medicine and Complementary/Alternative Medicine: A Worldwide Review*. Geneva: WHO.

James F. Drane (1995, 2014)
James F. Drane Bioethics Institute, Edinboro University of Pennsylvania

AMERICA, BIOETHICS IN

This entry consists of the following:

I. UNITED STATES

THE UNITED STATES IN THE TWENTY-FIRST CENTURY

Bioethics originated in the late 1960s in the United States. Its roots are in the traditional medical ethics of Anglo-American medicine; in the cultural setting of American health care; and in certain social, religious, and moral perceptions that had emerged in the American ethos. As the 1970s opened a number of scholars were attempting to analyze issues in medical ethics using the perspectives and methodologies of the two disciplines traditionally concerned with ethics, philosophy and theology. As these scholars began to publish and discuss their work, a distinct field of study called bioethics came into being. The word *bioethics* was coined by Van Rensselaer Potter (1971) and first applied to the ethics of population and environment. It soon became the rubric for a diverse collection of considerations about the ethical issues inherent in health care and the biological sciences (Callahan 1973).

The term, although considered unsatisfactory even by some of those who employed it, was canonized by the inauguration of the *Encyclopedia of Bioethics* project in 1972 and by the publication of the first edition, edited by Warren T. Reich, in 1978 (Post 2004 [1978]). Scholars in the contemporary bioethics field now come from many disciplines, such as theology, philosophy, the social sciences, and law. As now understood, bioethics concentrates on the specific set of issues and employs the range of analytic methodologies as set out in texts such as *Principles of Biomedical Ethics* (Beauchamp and Childress 2001) for the more theoretical questions and in *Clinical Ethics* (Jonsen, Siegler, and Winslade 2001) for the more practical questions. The field has professors, students, texts, journals, learned societies, and research centers. By 2013 more than a dozen graduate programs offered higher degrees to students trained in the topics and methods of the field.

This entry delineates the background for the development of bioethics and then discusses the events, issues, and concepts that stimulated its growth during the latter half of the twentieth century and its continued evolution into the twenty-first century.

THE DEVELOPMENT OF US MEDICINE

Bioethics comprehends much more than medicine and medical science. Nevertheless, the development of bioethics can best be understood against the background of the development of medicine in the United States from 1900. The twentieth century saw enormous growth in American medicine—in scientific understanding, the amount of money devoted to medical care, the number of persons with access to care, the number of personnel and specialties, the complexity of institutional systems, and the invention of diagnostic and therapeutic technologies. Three principal lines of development contribute to the interest in ethical questions: (1) the changing role of the hospital; (2) the ascendance of science and technology; and (3) the trend toward specialization (Jonsen 1998; Garrett, Jotterand, and Ralston 2013).

Beginning in the late nineteenth century hospitals were founded at an increasing rate and eventually became the principal sites of medical care in the United States. As medical diagnosis and treatment increasingly involved elaborate techniques and devices, it was seen as more efficient and economical to centralize care in hospitals. Physicians could allocate their time more conveniently, and nurses, technicians, and medical specialists could coordinate their work more effectively. Communities sought to establish hospitals as a matter of pride; cities needed hospitals for indigent patients. The passage in 1946 of the Hill-Burton Act, which provided federal support for local hospital construction, and the tendency of newly popular health insurance to reimburse hospital care rather than office or home care accelerated the evolution of the hospital in the United States (Rosenberg 1987; Stevens 1989).

With seminal discoveries in bacteriology, pathology, and physiology during the nineteenth century, medicine became increasingly scientific. This scientific medicine was integrated into medical practice after the extensive reorganization of medical schools in the decades around 1900—a period marked by the vigorous efforts of the American Medical Association (AMA) to reform medical education and to improve the standards of medical practice. Medical school reform was greatly stimulated by Abraham Flexner's report, *Medical Education in the United States and Canada* (1910), sponsored by the Carnegie Foundation for the Advancement of Teaching. This report insisted on two years of scientific study prior to clinical teaching. Experimentation involving human subjects, both patients and health volunteers, became more widespread as the National Institutes of Health sponsored clinical research centers after World War II. Medical school faculties began to consist of many research physicians supported by federal grants. The twentieth century brought a "new" medicine, one profoundly shaped by the biological sciences. Diagnosis and treatment took on forms dictated by the scientific knowledge generated in the laboratory, tested in clinics, and assessed by statistical methods.

The fascination of scientific knowledge and techniques drew many physicians into narrower fields of concentration. The vastly increased body of general medical knowledge became too much for individual physicians to master; deeper knowledge of specific problems required focused study. Moreover it became possible for physicians to build careers by performing procedures aimed at defined medical problems. Thus scientific medicine fostered the growth of specialties. Specialty boards, organized to test and certify competence in the particular fields of medicine, were established for a variety of specialties and subspecialties, beginning in the United States with the Board of Ophthalmology in 1917 (Stevens 1971). The social and economic status of physicians improved significantly during the first half of the twentieth century, and with assured incomes from insurance reimbursement, American physicians gradually moved from middle- to upper-class status, which distinguished them in attitudes, lifestyles, and places of residence from many of their patients (Starr 1982).

In general the three developments described above set the scene for the ethical concerns that began to surface in the United States in the 1960s. The concentration of specialized medical care in hospitals encouraged an impersonal, organizational approach to medical care. Although social, behavioral, environmental, and personal aspects of illness were not totally neglected, scientific medicine focused on the biological and physical aspects; complaints that physicians had lost the ability to care for the "whole patient" were increasingly heard. As scientific knowledge increased, teaching in the sciences tended to crowd other concerns from the basic medical curriculum. Specialization narrowed attention to particular organ systems and diseases, and patients were shuttled among a variety of specialists rather than cared for by the family doctor. Leading medical educators felt obliged to continually stress the more comprehensive view of medicine, but educational, economic, and professional pressures constantly obscured these calls. By the 1960s physicians, formerly close and familiar to their patients, had become, in David J. Rothman's (1991) words, "strangers at the bedside." As Rothman notes, this alienation was an important impetus for the emergence of bioethics.

SOCIAL, CULTURAL, AND POLITICAL TRENDS

In addition to these directions within medicine, cultural and social movements involved the public in the ethics of medical care to an unprecedented extent. By emphasizing new discoveries, dramatic incidents, and "human interest" stories, the mass media stimulated public interest in medicine while also highlighting growing tensions between complex medical technology and its humane use. Although growing urbanization and the consequent uneven distribution of population heightened existing obstacles to health care, a higher standard of living and increased educational achievement for many led to greater patient sophistication. During the 1950s and 1960s federal government support of biomedical research grew, thrusting research into the realm of public policy.

The introduction of employment-based insurance in the 1930s dramatically improved people's ability to purchase health care. The passage of Medicare and Medicaid in 1965 augmented this ability for the poor and the elderly. However, health care in the United States, while technically superb, became increasingly costly; because of its cost and organization, large numbers of Americans became excluded from adequate care. By the late 1980s this situation had evolved into a social and political crisis, and the costs of both medical care and medical insurance continued to rise through the twenty-first century. The passage of the Patient Protection and Affordable Care Act in 2010 marked the first significant political step on the national scale toward incorporating most Americans in health insurance plans.

Several movements of the late twentieth century began to influence the health care system. The steadily building influence of consumerism, which began with concern about adulteration of food in the early decades of the twentieth century, led to militant demands for consumers' rights in the 1970s. Also in that decade the patients' rights movement, a segment of a larger movement for civil rights, and the women's movement heightened sensitivity to the unmet health care needs of people of color and women. The issues of birth control and abortion, central to feminist concerns, divided the public on the role of health professionals in family and population policies. Raw practitioners from a culturally broader population and many new allied health professions and technical specialties were added to health care. The peace movements of the 1960s and 1970s and growing ecological movements drew attention to burgeoning international health problems arising from war, environmental hazards, and pollution (Leaf 1989; McCally and Cassel 1990). These concerns challenged the adequacy of medicine in maintaining the overall health and well-being of the world population. Physicians for Social Responsibility was founded in 1971 on the premise that it was physicians' duty to address the health risks of nuclear armaments, a matter of pressing concern during the Cold War. Although threats to the global biological environment emerged as major research and political concerns in the 1970s, the study of ethical issues in these areas remained rather separate from the study of ethical issues in medicine and health sciences (Geiger 1971; Jonsen and Jameton 1977; Cassel and Jameton 1982).

These sociocultural and political trends, together with the direction of the biological and medical sciences, were the background for the bioethics movement that began in the 1960s. Bioethics as it is known in the early twenty-first century had its roots in general public concerns over issues of individual rights, social justice, and environmental quality that marked American culture in that era. Before examining the bioethics movement itself, it is advisable to examine the ideas, activities, and interests that were its precursors.

TRADITIONAL MEDICAL ETHICS

The effort to establish a unified medical profession during the nineteenth century and the accompanying internecine strife among physicians of various doctrinal allegiances profoundly influenced the nature and content of medical ethics at the opening of the twentieth century. Although ethicists invoked strains of the Hippocratic, medieval, and Enlightenment traditions, the dominant themes were the ideals of respectability and professional collegiality and the etiquette of professional relationships that promoted those ideals. At the beginning of the twentieth century this goal of a unified profession was within reach. The AMA, through the strenuous efforts of its chief spokesperson, Joseph McCormack, represented the profession as dedicated to orthodox scientific medicine, the advancement of medical education, the elimination of quackery, and the promotion of public health, particularly through support of pure food and drug legislation (Burrow 1977; Baker et al. 1999; Jonsen 2000).

One crucial mandate of professional ethics was firmly in place in the early twentieth century: ethical physicians did not consult with or refer patients to unorthodox practitioners, such as homeopaths and naturopaths. Before the turn of the century and for several decades afterward, the poor quality of medical education and the inadequacy of licensing laws allowed many ill-trained or even untrained persons to advertise as "medical practitioners." A vast number of bogus medicines and devices were promoted as cures for any and all disorders. Many voices favored freedom to choose one's practitioner, claiming that the "scientific" practitioners and drugs offered nothing better than what their untutored and untested competitors advised. Others, particularly the more educated practitioners, set out to discredit quacks, nostrums, and patent medicines.

This concern stimulated the debate among physicians over cooperation between physicians and "irregular" practitioners. Many regular physicians refused to treat patients who had received prior treatment from irregulars; medical society codes of ethics barred irregular practitioners from society membership, hospital admitting privileges, and joint practice with regular practitioners (Gevitz 1988). Prior to World War I (1914–1918) the AMA led a fight that finally persuaded state legislatures and Congress to pass legislation controlling the practice of medicine and the sale of drugs. Midwives were among the targets of the campaign against quackery. Despite better health outcomes by many midwives at the turn of the century, the campaign for "scientific" practice won public support and drove midwifery out of obstetrical care until their return in the 1980s (Leavitt 1986). Thus in this period medical ethics appeared to be exclusively concerned with restricting practice to "orthodox" physicians. Although self-interested motives can be imputed to organized medicine, many physicians repudiated the "freedom of choice" argument out of the sincere concern that medicine, as stated in the Hippocratic oath, "at least do no harm" (Burrow 1977). Still, as many commentators have noted, medical ethics in this matter served the ends of medical monopoly (Berlant 1975).

A second important question about consultation and referral was vigorously debated: whether referring physicians were entitled to a fee or "kickback" for having sent a patient to a specialist or consultant. This practice was particularly common in surgery. Some surgeons solicited patients through general practitioners, who in turn found it lucrative to refer patients who sometimes did not require surgery. The abuses of fee splitting scandalized the public and many professionals. The American College of Surgeons, founded in 1915, required its fellows to take an oath that explicitly repudiated fee splitting. Although branded by all professional organizations as unethical, this practice continued in a covert way for many years (Davis 1960).

The Patient-Physician Relationship. Perhaps the most agitated debate in traditional medical ethics during the first half of the twentieth century was over the integrity of the patient-physician relationship. Private practice was the predominant mode of medical care: physicians practiced alone (solo practitioners) or in partnership, charged patients for each consultation (fee-for-service), and sought to develop their own followings of patients. Some contract practice, in which a physician undertook to provide unlimited service to a designated population for an agreed amount, had long existed. Plantations in the American South had used this method for the medical care of slaves. Fraternal organizations formed by immigrant populations had insured their members in this way, and in the West the railroad and lumber industries contracted with physicians to care for their workers. In these plans a group of physicians would be employed by the organization or would join together to offer services. Many in the organized profession, however, objected to contract practice, condemning it as cut-rate medicine, as inferior to private practice in the quality of care and personal relationship, and as allowing a third party to dictate conditions of care to the possible detriment of the patient.

The same objections met the forms of group practice that evolved from contract practice in the first half of the twentieth century. Bitter battles raged over these issues; many medical societies excluded physicians who were involved in these "schemes." A series of antitrust decisions by the US Supreme Court, beginning in the 1940s and continuing into the 1970s, gradually cleared the way for the development of a variety of corporate practice forms, such as health maintenance organizations, that a few decades before would have been considered unethical forms of medical practice.

The Debate over Payment. Another closely related ethical issue was the debate over payment for medical care. Traditional ethics had required physicians to charge their patients fairly and to provide free or discounted services to those who could not pay. The emergence of free public clinics and hospitals in the late nineteenth century threatened that ethic. Many physicians claimed that even patients who could pay sought free care, draining physicians' practices and making it impossible for them to provide charitable services: they needed a steady income from paying patients to be able to afford to provide such services. Thus at the turn of the century extensive public use of free clinics was debated as an ethical question. Some argued that it was conducive to continued pauperization; others claimed that forcing poor people to pay for needed medical care was immoral. Some practitioners opposed free clinics because they viewed them as unfair competition by medical schools, which they saw as using free clinics to obtain patients for medical education.

At the same time the organized profession realized that the costs of care were beyond many persons' ability to pay and that physicians' incomes were low. Initial support was given to proposals emanating from organized labor for government-supported compulsory health insurance. By 1916 a broad coalition of organized medicine, labor, and social reformers had almost achieved the passage of national health insurance. World War I intervened, and the coalition was weakened: many viewed national health insurance as a "Germanic" proposal (Germany had long had such a program) or "socialistic." Organized medicine from then on firmly opposed almost all forms of government health insurance. Again it was proclaimed that because this would interpose government between doctor and patient, such programs would be unethical. This opposition persisted down to the passage of Medicaid and Medicare in 1965 (Marmor 1970; Fein 1986). These claims continued to be heard in the political debates over health care in the first two decades of the twenty-first century.

The AMA Code. The AMA revised its 1847 code of ethics in 1903, 1912, 1947, 1957, and 1980. The revisions, successively more succinct, reflected an increased sense of professionalism and ideals about the scientific excellence of the practitioner. At the same time the professional ethics expressed in official codes and in the positions taken by organized medicine on social questions reflected an interest in maintaining the status quo of the profession and the practice of medicine as it had been evolving in the late nineteenth and early twentieth centuries. With few exceptions, such as increased tolerance for group practice, the 1957 revision of the AMA code, which consists of a condensation into ten principles of medical ethics, bears little evidence of the major social changes that had begun to affect medical care in the United States. In 1985 the AMA Judicial Council, charged with enforcement of the code of ethics, changed its name to the Council on Ethical and Judicial Affairs. It now issues regular statements on issues of current ethical import, such as euthanasia, the obligation to care for patients with AIDS, and financial conflict of interest. Many major medical organizations, such as the American College of Physicians and the American Academy of Pediatrics, have formed ethics committees with a similar purpose. Although commentaries and informal codes on the conduct of nurses can be found as far back as the founding of the profession by Florence Nightingale (1820–1910), the American Nurses Association did not adopt an official code of ethics for nurses until 1950.

Thus during the first half of the twentieth century medical ethics consisted of professionally devised propositions to enhance the unity and monopoly of the profession. Professional self-interest sometimes hid behind ethical claims that were often to the detriment of the public. At the same time the profession, in encouraging improved medical education and advocating public health and safety measures, lived up to its more noble traditions (Jonsen 1990).

THE INFLUENCE OF THEOLOGICAL AND PHILOSOPHICAL ETHICS

The medical profession in the United States imbibed an ethic from the Judeo-Christian culture of the nation. The ethical physician was expected to be respectful of religion and to be a "good Christian gentleman" (Burns 1977). The dominant Protestant culture offered some admonitions about health and medicine, with denominations expressing opinions on abortion, contraception, and euthanasia. In the nineteenth century physicians of strong Protestant faith urged the enactment of strict laws against abortion, but the scholarly ethics of Protestant denominations did not elaborate on this or other issues (Mohr 1978).

Roman Catholic moral theology, by contrast, had a long tradition of concern with moral questions in medicine. Since the seventeenth century principles of Scholastic philosophy and theology had been applied to such issues as abortion, sterilization, and the duties of physicians and patients. Acute analyses had been made of the duty to sustain life and the circumstances under which the death of a patient could be permitted. This tradition was conveyed to students in the Catholic medical schools that were founded in the nineteenth century. Charles Coppens, Society of Jesus, lectured in the Medical Department of Creighton University, in Omaha, Nebraska, at the turn of the century. His 1905 book, *Moral Principles and Medical Practice: The Basis of Medical Jurisprudence*, treated abortion, sexual behavior, and the duties of physicians in light of philosophical and theological principles. His work represented "the emergence of medical ethics as a medical school subject, especially at religiously affiliated schools" (Burns 1980, 282). During the 1940s and 1950s this tradition was carried on in the extensive writings of the theologians Edwin Healy, Gerald Kelly, Charles McFadden, Francis Connell, and Patrick Finney. In 1949 the Catholic Hospital Association issued *Ethical and Religious Directives for Catholic Health Facilities* (revised in 1954 and 1971), which obliged all physicians and health professionals working in Catholic institutions to follow Catholic moral tenets with regard to a number of specific medical procedures (US Catholic Conference, Department of Health Affairs [1949]).

Catholic reflection on medical moral issues continues in the *Linacre Quarterly*, published by the Catholic Medical Association since 1934. Charles Curran, Richard McCormick, Edmund D. Pellegrino, Lisa Cahill, and Margaret Farley have been important voices in the Catholic dialogue. The Catholic tradition, in its doctrine of natural law, has affirmed that moral questions can be analyzed from a philosophical viewpoint without explicit reference to revealed theological truths. Thus common ground can be found with those who do not share the Catholic faith. This somewhat nonsectarian approach has allowed Catholic analysis of problems to have a significant influence on the intellectual development of secular bioethics.

Groundbreaking and Influential Works. In 1950 Willard Sperry, the dean of Harvard Divinity School, published lectures given at Massachusetts General Hospital and the University of Michigan Medical School under the title *The Ethical Basis of Medical Practice*. As the era of medical technology was opening, he offered thoughtful, humane, literary, but unsystematic commentary on such problems as truth telling, prolongation of life, and euthanasia. In 1954 the Episcopal theologian Joseph F. Fletcher published the groundbreaking study *Morals and Medicine*. Fletcher's work was the first to emphasize the patient's rights as the center of an ethics of medicine and to argue "the ethical case for our human rights … to use contraceptives, to seek insemination anonymously from a donor, to be sterilized and to receive a merciful death from a medically competent euthanasist" (Fletcher 1954, 25). He strongly asserted the patient's right to be told the truth about his or her diagnosis and prognosis. Fletcher's book is the pioneering work of the new medical ethics.

Sixteen years later the Methodist theologian Paul Ramsey produced the foundational work of bioethics, *Patient as Person* (1970b). Ramsey, a professor of religion at Princeton University, took the unusual step of spending a year in intense dialogue with physicians, scientists, and students at Georgetown Medical School and immersing himself in the clinical activities of the University Hospital. *Patient as Person*, first delivered as the Beecher Lectures at Yale University in 1969, examines questions, such as organ transplantation, experimentation with human subjects, and the use of life-supporting technologies, that had not been on the agenda of previous commentators on the moral aspects of medicine. Although he spoke from a very different theological ground than did Fletcher, Ramsey also placed the freedom and rights of the patient at the center of his ethic but subsumed patients and physicians within the scope of a theologically defined covenant. The distinctive features of modern bioethics begin to appear in Fletcher and Ramsey: attention to the effects of new technologies, affirmation of the centrality of the patient as free and responsible agent, and the invocation of the concepts and method of moral analysis from the classical disciplines of theology and philosophy.

Despite the theological tone and language of Ramsey's work, its cogent analyses of issues such as consent were widely influential. At about the same time James Gustafson (1970) of Yale Divinity School produced thoughtful essays on the implications of medical and scientific advances. Many Protestant theologians followed the paths laid down by these pioneers. In 1987 in Chicago the Park Ridge Center for the Study of Health, Faith, and Ethics was founded under the auspices of the Lutheran Hospital Association to foster religious reflection on the issues of bioethics. The center published a fine series of volumes describing the teachings about medicine and morality of major Christian denominations and other world religions (Marty 1983; Vaux 1984).

The Jewish faith has an ancient tradition of reflection on questions of life, death, health, and medical care. Issues in medical ethics, such as allocation of scarce resources, risk-benefit evaluation, quality of life, abortion, contraception, and indications of death, are discussed in great detail in Talmudic literature. The doctoral thesis of Immanuel Jakobovits, published in 1959 as *Jewish Medical Ethics*, drew these teachings together and brought them into contact with modern scientific advances. In so doing Jakobovits gave a distinct identity to a field of study that had not been previously singled out in Jewish scholarship. Talmudic scholars, such as Moshe Tendler, David Bleich, David Feldman, Elliot Dorff, and Laurie Zoloth, and the physician Fred Rosner have continued this effort. The first course in Jewish medical ethics was taught by Tendler at Yeshiva University in 1956, and the Institute for Jewish Medical Ethics was established in San Francisco in the early 1980s.

Moral, Academic, and Legal Philosophy. Moral philosophy came rather late to the analysis of medical-moral questions. Although the first AMA Code of Ethics was strongly influenced by the English physician Thomas Percival (1740–1804), who was familiar with the philosophers of the Scottish Enlightenment, American philosophers had paid scant attention to these questions. In 1927 Chauncey D. Leake noted in his edition of *Percival's Medical Ethics* (Percival 1927 [1803]) that all of the classic codes represented "medical etiquette" or the tenets of professional courtesy rather than medical ethics. "It is interesting," Leake wrote, "that writers on medical ethics have seldom availed themselves of the philosophical analyses of the principles of ethical theory made by recognized ethical scholars" (Percival 1927 [1803], 3). In words that predict the bioethics movement of the 1960s, Leake called for a medical ethics that would bring the systems of moral philosophy to bear on the problems of medical practice. He undertook to do this in a dialogue with the philosopher Patrick Romanell (Leake and Romanell 1950). Three decades later moral philosophers began to show interest in the ethics of health care.

Academic philosophy did not find it easy to approach the practical problems posed by evolving science and medicine. In the 1950s philosophical ethics was struggling with the theoretical challenges of naturalism, relativism, utilitarianism, Marxism, linguistic analysis, and positivism; hardly any attention was paid to the analysis of actual moral problems. This began to change in the 1960s, as students vociferously questioned their professors about the moral legitimacy of the Vietnam War and racial discrimination. Interest in practical philosophy slowly appeared within academic philosophy, and the journal *Philosophy and Public Affairs* appeared in 1971. The questions of life and death raised by new technologies also began to intrigue some philosophers. In 1969 Nicholas Rescher wrote an early article on the allocation of "exotic medical lifesaving therapy," such as dialysis and transplantation. Medical ethics began to be taught as an undergraduate philosophy course for which textbooks were produced (Gorovitz et al. 1973; Gorovitz et al. 1976). Daniel Callahan, trained in the analytic philosophy tradition at Harvard University, realized the ethical dimensions of the new medicine and in 1979 founded, with the psychiatrist Willard Gaylin, the Institute of Society, Ethics, and the Life Sciences, later renamed the Hastings Center. Philosophers such as Baruch Brody, K. Danner Clouser, Samuel Gorovitz, Ruth Macklin, Tom L. Beauchamp, Stephen Toulmin, and Martha Nussbaum made significant contributions to the methods and substantive analysis of biomedical problems. Indeed as

Toulmin (1982) claimed, "medicine saved the life of ethics," imparting an intellectual vitality and moral urgency to a field that had turned away from the moral concerns of personal and social life.

Legal scholars were also prominent in the early years of bioethics. William Curran and Paul A. Freund of Harvard University and Jay Katz of Yale University contributed to the important symposium on experimentation with human subjects sponsored by the American Academy of Arts and Sciences in 1966. Katz subsequently published major work in this area (Freund 1970; Katz, Capron, and Glass 1972). The Catholic legal scholar John Noonan wrote perceptively on abortion and contraception. As the issues surrounding death and dying became prominent, particularly with the 1975 Karen Ann Quinlan case—in which the parents of a young woman in an apparently permanent coma who could be maintained alive indefinitely on a respirator sought the removal of life support—lawyers became deeply involved, because law has always taken a serious interest in the determination of the causes of human death. Similarly the evolution of the doctrine of informed consent has been strongly influenced by jurisprudence and judicial opinion. It is difficult to distinguish between the lawyer and the bioethicist in such figures as George J. Annas, John Robertson, Alexander M. Capron, and William J. Winslade. Indeed in a 1993 book Annas (1993, 2) asserted that "American law, not philosophy or medicine, is primarily responsible for the agenda, development and current state of American bioethics."

Many physicians and scientists have become adept at bioethics. As the field developed, however, the majority of its practitioners came from theology and philosophy; relatively few physicians have devoted themselves to scholarly productivity. Notable exceptions are Pellegrino, Mark Siegler, Howard Brody, Eric Cassell, and Joseph Fins. Their contributions exhibit the sense and sensitivity of the practicing physician.

ETHICS EDUCATION IN MEDICINE

Although medical jurisprudence, the study of the relationship between medical practice and the law, had been taught in American medical schools during the nineteenth century, no course on medical ethics as such is known to have been offered until the late 1920s except in Catholic medical schools. The curriculum of the first known course in a secular medical school, offered by Park White at Washington University School of Medicine, Saint Louis, in 1924, included discussion of group practice, consultations, relations with other practitioners, quackery, eugenics, euthanasia, and birth control (Burns 1980). In 1926 the AMA recommended that medical ethics be made part of the medical curriculum. By 1931 it was reported that 43 percent of the sixty-seven American medical schools offered a course in medical ethics, most of these courses in the required curriculum. Approximately the same level was maintained through the 1950s, although course time was stretched to cover other subjects, such as medical sociology and economics, and it is unclear what topics were covered as medical ethics. During this era Richard Clarke Cabot, who was both professor of medicine and professor of social ethics at Harvard University, was a dominant figure. He stressed the importance of personal integrity and honesty in the physician, as had the earlier professional ethics, but he placed this within the evolving framework of scientific medicine: integrity must be manifested in clinical competence, the primary ethical obligation of the practitioner (Burns 1977).

As the century progressed and the social and psychological sciences spread in collegiate education, discussion of the art of character development became increasingly overlaid with psychological and psychiatric analysis of the physician's character. Indeed in the 1940s and 1950s the Freudian model of psychological dynamics and of the doctor-patient relationship became prominent in the analyses of the virtues of physicians (Binger 1945). Meanwhile the increasing mid-century confidence in the social sciences tended to displace ethics terminology with concepts of "professional development," "human engineering," and so forth, sometimes even denigrating the admonitions of traditional morality as no more than "taboos." Ethics was often seen as so colored by religion that its teaching was bound to be covert indoctrination. In the secular climate of that time, any formal acknowledgment of ethics was suspect. Even the National Endowment for the Humanities, which eventually became a strong supporter of bioethics, originally excluded ethics from the list of the humanities whose study it would fund. Thus ethics was rarely taught in higher education and even more rarely in medical education. This hiatus in the teaching of medical ethics during the 1950s may be seen as a prelude to the bioethics movement, in which neglected ethical questions forced their way back into the consciousness of the profession and the public alike.

The first national conference on the teaching of medical ethics was held in 1972 under the sponsorship of the Institute of Society, Ethics, and the Life Sciences and Columbia University College of Physicians and Surgeons. By this time, out of 114 medical schools, only 3 required an ethics course, and only 33 offered ethics as an elective (Veatch, Gaylin, and Morgan 1973). The Society for Health and Human Values, formed in 1969, and its attendant Institute on Human Values in Medicine encouraged medical ethics teaching. In the decade that followed the number of schools providing organized teaching of ethics increased, and faculty members, often philosophers and theologians, were appointed. The content of the course shifted from the traditional topics, such as truth telling, confidentiality, care of indigent patients, care of the dying, and relations among practitioners, to the newer problems raised by technology and the social setting of modern medical care. In 1987 ninety-five American medical schools reported that they required a course in medical ethics, and the Association of American Medical Colleges strongly urged the inclusion of ethics in the curriculum (Bickel 1987).

NURSING ETHICS

Although medical students received little formal instruction in ethics, nursing schools had developed a strong tradition of ethics teaching. Several major works on ethics were published by nurses at the start of the twentieth century, notably *Nursing Ethics* (1901) by Isabel Hampton Robb. Although her text is marked by a stern and self-sacrificing message to nurses, it includes sensitive discussion of many aspects of nurse-patient and nurse-physician relations. Textbooks on nursing ethics published in the first two decades of the century went through many editions before fading from popularity in the 1940s and 1950s. Notable among the authors were Charlotte Aikens (1916) and Thomas Verner Moore (1935), whose books made extensive use of case studies. In 1931 the religious educator Paul M. Limbert published a defense of nursing ethics courses. They were needed, he argued, to make ethical concerns explicit and to assist student nurses in interpreting their clinical experiences in such a way as to foster good professional character. As in the medical ethics of that era, the emphasis was on the character development of the nurse rather than on principle-centered or patient-centered ethics.

An important theme for nursing ethics has always been the impact of the feelings and character—the "humanness"—of the practitioner on the care and cure of the patient. As new technologies developed with increasing efficacy, practitioners felt the need to redefine their role in relationship to those technologies. Andrew Jameton (1984) introduced an important concept, "moral distress," to designate the ethical problem that nurses face: because of their subordinate position within the hospital power structure, they are unable to manage ethical problems that they see in patient care.

At the beginning of the twentieth century nursing was predominantly a home-based practice; by the end of the century it had become predominantly institution based. This redefinition of the nursing role stimulated recurring issues in the early nursing literature. For instance, whether a nurse should do housework, such as washing diapers or tending the fire in the grate, was a significant issue until the 1950s. How the nurse should react to the errors of quacks and regular physicians continued to be a prominent issue. In all such cases texts resolved the questions in terms of dedication to the welfare of patients. Indeed nursing ethics took an early stand against dangerous practitioners, whether nurses or physicians. Since the late twentieth century nurses have taken an increasing role in institutional quality control.

Like physicians, nurses struggled with the problem of "irregular" practitioners. The nursing ethics literature of the first years of the century represented the "untrained nurse" as ethically as well as technically incompetent. The emergence of the licensed practical nurse in the 1930s and the increasing number of nursing aides during the century challenged professional nursing, and the ethics of relationships among members of these occupations has been delicate. In the 1970s the American Nurses Association took a stand that a bachelor's degree was necessary for professional nursing, calling into question the standing of nurses whose sole training was in hospitals. In the 1980s nursing was again challenged by an AMA call for the creation of a "registered care technician" to perform some of the technical functions of nurses.

The ethics of the relationship of nurse to physician is still debated in the nursing ethics literature in the early twenty-first century. It is commonly asserted that power and gender relationships are central to the ethics of nursing. Notable among commentators on the ethics of nursing are Mila Aroskar, Martin Benjamin, Joy Curtis, Anne Davis, Marsha Fowler, Sara T. Fry, Sally Gadow, Amy Haddad, Jameton, Christine Mitchell, James Myskens, and Michael Yeo. Their work carries the themes of nursing ethics into the broader stream of bioethics. The bioethics movement has also touched the many other professions involved in the care of patients: dentists, occupational therapists, pharmacists, physical therapists, physician assistants, medical technicians, and social workers.

ETHICAL ISSUES IN THE EMERGING BIOMEDICAL TECHNOLOGIES

In the years after World War II (1939–1945) the rapid advances of biomedical science were translated into clinical interventions that could save and sustain life in ways never before possible. These technological advances brought not only the benefits of improved health and prolonged life but also a range of puzzling moral questions (Jonsen 1998). One of the first of these technologies to raise explicit ethical concerns was the 1961 invention by Belding Scribner at the University of Washington of a technique for chronic hemodialysis of persons with end-stage renal disease. Because the first artificial kidney center in Seattle had limited machines and trained personnel, it could serve only a tiny portion of the estimated 15,000 to 20,000 Americans in need of such lifesaving care. A committee consisting of seven lay members and two physician-advisers was chosen to select patients who would be admitted to treatment. Those who were not admitted would die. The committee relied on social criteria, such as productive livelihood and respectable citizenship, for selecting candidates from among the many medically eligible patients. When this practice was publicized in the press, public and scholarly opinion strongly criticized the use of social values in life-and-death decisions (Fox and Swazey 1974).

Philosophers and theologians took note of the issue and engaged in debate over it (Rescher 1969; Childress 1970; Ramsey 1970b). The crisis of rationing the scarce resource of dialysis was resolved in 1972 by an amendment to the Social Security Act providing payment for about 90 percent of the high cost of dialysis. This led to further discussion comparing the plight of other persons in high-cost disease categories, such as hemophilia, with that of kidney patients. In justice, the argument ran, various other groups ought to receive similar public aid. This early example of the ethical dilemmas posed by the new technology exemplified some of the themes that would become central to bioethics: the admittance of lay opinion into decisions formerly reserved to physicians, the appearance of philosophical and theological analyses of the issue, the recognition of questions of fairness in application of medical resources, and the profound implications of life-and-death decisions. Indeed the questions Who should live? Who should die? Who should decide?, reflected in the title of the journalist Shana Alexander's (1962) article on the Seattle dialysis committee, became the theme of bioethics (Jonsen 2005).

The first heart transplantations were done in South Africa in 1968, and similar operations were attempted shortly thereafter in the United States. Optimistic claims by medical innovators fostered public enthusiasm, which turned to disillusionment when, after three years, the very poor survival rate resulted in a virtual moratorium on heart transplants (Fox and Swazey 1974). As heart and kidney transplantation became more effective, ethical issues surrounding organ donorship arose. To encourage cadaver donorship, the Uniform Anatomical Gift Act was proposed by the US National Conference of Commissioners on Uniform State Laws in 1968 and subsequently adopted by all states (Katz, Capron, and Glass 1972). Because of high costs and the scarcity of organs, transplantation forcefully raised questions whether the gains of new technology could justify the costs. At the same time the determination of how death was declared, traditionally done by noting the cessation of cardiorespiratory functions, began to be questioned. These criteria seemed obsolete under conditions of artificial respiratory support and did not allow for removal of organs for transplantation. A vigorous debate ensued about the ethical and legal implications of shifting to clinical criteria that would focus on cessation of brain, rather than cardiac, activity. In 1968 a committee at Harvard Medical School formulated a statement defining brain death and establishing it as a criterion for declaring death. Brain death criteria were accepted and legalized slowly, beginning in Kansas in 1970. Still, considerable confusion required further refinement of the concept, leading eventually to the recommendation in 1981 by the President's Commission for the Study of Ethical Problems in Medicine and Biomedical and Behavioral Research of a uniform statute for the determination of death, which was adopted by most states as the Uniform Determination of Death Act.

During this same period artificial implants to assist or replace damaged hearts were being developed. Denton Cooley in Houston, Texas, unsuccessfully attempted to implant an artificial heart in 1969. In anticipation of the time when such a device might be ready for use in humans, the National Heart and Lung Institute (now the National Heart, Lung, and Blood Institute) in 1971 established a panel to study the possible ethical, social, economic, legal, medical, and psychiatric consequences of its development. This was the first effort by the federal government to explore the ethical implications of new medical technologies (Jonsen 1973). The first actual US implantation of an artificial heart—in Barney Clark in Salt Lake City in 1982—aroused considerable debate about the appropriateness of this device (Shaw 1984).

ETHICS OF RESEARCH WITH HUMAN SUBJECTS

By the mid-1960s issues of research ethics had begun to ferment among scientists (Ladimer and Newman 1963). The Nuremberg trials in 1947 revealed the horrors of the Nazi concentration camps, where cruel and lethal medical experiments had been performed on prisoners. Several articles on the ethics of human experimentation had appeared in American medical literature, but these issues were not widely discussed, perhaps because many believed that nothing so horrible could happen in the United States (Alexander 1949; Annas and Grodin 1992). During World War II, however, the intense efforts to improve the capabilities of military medicine occasionally spurred researchers to design experiments in which persons were treated dangerously and without their consent. In the postwar years biomedical research was fueled by large infusions of funds from the newly expanded National Institutes of Health, and research projects were sponsored in hospitals throughout the country. As the volume and intensity of research increased, questionable practices appeared and were tolerated as the price to be paid in the war against disease. Concern about the effects of nuclear radiation prompted researchers to expose unknowing patients (Faden 1996). Informed consent of research subjects was rarely obtained, and oversight by anyone other than the researcher was unusual. In 1962 a number of children were born with serious congenital defects due to their mothers' ingestion of thalidomide, an unapproved drug. This tragedy stimulated congressional hearings at which the ethics of human experimentation, then largely uncontrolled, was aired. Subsequently, amendments to the federal Food, Drug, and Cosmetic Act in 1964 required full and free consent of all subjects of drug trials.

In a 1966 article Henry K. Beecher, professor of anesthesia at Harvard University, brought problems in the ethics of experimentation to the attention of the medical community. He detailed twenty-two medical experiments performed by respected investigators that he branded as unethical because of lack of consent or inappropriate assessment of risks in relation to benefits. In 1966 (with revisions in 1968) the US Public Health Service formulated guidelines for protection of the rights and welfare of human subjects in all federally supported research. In 1971 these guidelines became regulations of the Department of Health, Education, and Welfare, requiring research institutions to set up medical and lay panels to review all federally funded experimentation to ensure that subjects are informed and freely consent to the research procedure and to determine that the scientific benefits justify the risks of the research (Levine 1986).

A number of scandals in research ethics brought public attention to the need for regulation. At Willowbrook State Hospital in New York, a series of studies on hepatitis were conducted from 1965 to 1971 that involved infecting mentally retarded children with hepatitis virus. At the Jewish Chronic Disease Hospital in Brooklyn in 1963, live cancer cells were injected into senile patients without their knowledge or consent. In 1971 a study begun in the 1930s in Tuskegee, Alabama, came to public attention: a number of poor African American farmers diagnosed with syphilis had been left untreated to ascertain the "natural history" of the untreated disease (Jones 1981). In response to these and several other scandals, the US Congress established the National Commission for the Protection of Human Subjects of Biomedical and Behavioral Research (1974–1977) to make recommendations for federal policy on the broad problems of human subjects in research and the special problems posed by research with fetuses, children, prisoners, and other dependent or vulnerable persons. These recommendations were codified in federal regulations and are now widely enforced in research institutions.

The scholarship of bioethics was significantly advanced by the work of this commission. Several scholars in ethics sat on the commission, and many philosophers, theologians, lawyers, and sociologists were asked to contribute to its deliberations, thereby stimulating thought about the issues and making public careful analyses of the problems and principles. The commission's *Belmont Report* (1978), stating the principles of research with human subjects, first enunciated the triad of bioethical principles: autonomy, beneficence, and justice. Federal regulations codified the commission's recommendations, and for the next several decades clinical research, scrutinized for ethical probity by institutional review boards, proceeded without incident. In the late 1990s, however, several deaths of research subjects and widespread evidence of inadequate review of research led to a revival of concern. The ethics of research returned to the agenda of bioethics.

ETHICS OF DEATH AND DYING

It became increasingly common during the twentieth century for people to die in a hospital, often under conditions of dehumanizing technology. This reawakened age-old discussions of death, dying, and euthanasia, now in light of the new technical potential of modern medicine. Although there had been several unsuccessful attempts to make euthanasia legal in the early years of the century, death and dying had become a taboo subject in medicine. Elisabeth Kübler-Ross's sensitive interviews with dying patients, captured in her 1969 book *On Death and Dying*, did much to awaken interest in the psychology of dying.

In 1976 California passed novel legislation about termination of life support. The Natural Death Act authorized patients to sign a legal document directing physicians to remove or to withhold life-support devices under carefully defined circumstances. Many states followed California by enacting legal forms of "advance directives" or "durable powers of attorney" (because they allow the signer to designate someone to make decisions on his or her behalf) to guide physicians in following the wishes of their dying patients. In 1976 a New Jersey Supreme Court decision allowed the parents of Quinlan to have their daughter removed from the respirator (New Jersey Superior Court 1975). Subsequent judicial decisions in many states and one US Supreme Court decision—*Cruzan v. Director, Missouri Department of Health* (1990)—have elucidated the conditions under which life support might be forgone. Many of these decisions have been influenced by the bioethical debates over active and passive euthanasia.

In the 1990s the debate over legalization of active euthanasia was renewed, spurred by the public perpetration of euthanasia by the physician Jack Kevorkian (1928–2011) and by the advocacy of the Hemlock Society, which promoted legislation that would authorize physicians to provide "aid in dying" at the request of terminal patients. In that decade several states held initiatives to legalize this practice, with Oregon voters the first to approve it. Since 1994 citizens of that state have been permitted to seek, under stringent conditions, the aid of a physician to end their lives. Washington State and Montana have followed. This and other efforts to make euthanasia legal have prompted important judicial decisions, even in the US Supreme Court (*Vacco v. Quill* [1997] and *Washington v. Glucksberg* [1997]) (Hillyard and Dombrink 2001). These questions about the nature of appropriate care for the terminally ill and many other ethical questions are made more urgent by the increase in the numbers of elderly people in the United States. Since the beginning of the twentieth century the number of Americans over the age of sixty-five has tripled in proportion to the general population (Jecker 1991).

BIOETHICS COMMISSIONS

In 1978 the US Congress set up a successor to the National Commission for the Protection of Human Subjects. Its broader mandate was reflected in its title, the President's Commission for the Study of Ethical Problems in Medicine and Biomedical and Behavioral Research (1978–1983). The definition of death, genetic screening, access to health care, and the use of life-sustaining technologies were among its reports (President's Commission for the Study of Ethical Problems in Medicine and Biomedical and Behavioral Research 1981, 1983a, 1983b, 1983c). Like its predecessor, it called on scholars from many disciplines to contribute to its deliberations, and its reports make up a veritable canon of bioethics. Its recommendations on the definition of death were enacted into law in 1981 as the Uniform Determination of Death Act.

Subsequent administrations authorized bioethical commissions. Presidents Bill Clinton, George W. Bush, and Barack Obama established advisory and investigative bodies by executive order. Each of these bodies was given a broad mandate to study ethical issues arising in the biomedical sciences, although several were given specific instructions to explore the growing field of stem cell research, cloning, and genomics. The remarkable expansion of molecular genetics posed new and unique issues about human identity, privacy, and indeed human nature itself. Federal studies of the late twentieth and early twenty-first centuries concentrated on these questions and their public policy relevance.

President Obama continued this line of inquiry. He directed his Presidential Commission for the Study of Bioethical Issues to study ethical issues raised by "synthetic biology," the creation of life in the laboratory. In *New Directions: The Ethics of Synthetic Biology and Emerging Technologies* (2010), the commission noted that these efforts are still in their earliest stages and suggested that federal oversight maintain "prudent vigilance" while encouraging creativity and innovation from the private sector. In addition the commission prepared a report on whole genome sequencing for disease management and the privacy implications of these advances. In a mandate recalling the topic that had initiated federal bioethics investigations thirty years before, President Obama ordered an inquiry into alleged US Public Health Service abuse of research studies on Guatemalan citizens in the 1950s. Chair Amy Guttman was asked to convene an international panel to examine global human subjects research and to ensure that current federal and international standards for human subjects research were sufficiently rigorous.

These government commissions and counsels, while having mixed influence, have shown that bioethics is more than an academic field: it is a public enterprise. Made up of participants from a variety of professional and public backgrounds—scientists, lawyers, clergy, scholars from various disciplines, and citizens at large—they represent a wide array of views about ethical issues. Few participants were experts in academic ethics, although the bodies were supported by persons trained in ethics and advised by many scholars familiar with ethics and related disciplines. The unique contribution of these bodies, with their mandates to study particular issues, was the focus on immediate practical problems and the production of recommendations that can be translated into public policy. Moral philosophy had never seen such concentrated attention to matters that were not simply to be thought about but to be acted on.

As bioethics was developing, there was also popular, political, and scholarly debate over the nature of health care itself. Popular and academic works investigated the conceptions of health employed in medicine and the efficacy of medical services offered (Illich 1976). They explored the nature and authority of the health professions and raised questions about ethical responsibilities of health professionals whose attitudes are shaped by economic and social forces (Freidson 1988 [1970]). The proper role of health professionals has been questioned in many contexts, including the right of health professionals to strike and the extent to which they bear responsibility for patients' lives, for behavioral factors affecting health, and for social and political factors causing disease. The helplessness of individuals in the face of a massive medical establishment led to a patients' rights movement. The American Hospital Association (1992 [1973]) published "A Patient's Bill of Rights" in 1973 with the suggestion that it be adopted by all hospitals. (In 2003 the American Hospital Association replaced "A Patient's Bill of Rights" with *The Patient Care Partnership*.) In 1975 the book *The Rights of Patients*, by the bioethicist Annas, provided the bioethical grounding for those rights. As demanded by the unique nature of medicine directed toward the protection of the community as a whole, a distinct bioethics of public health slowly emerged (Beauchamp and Steinbock 1999). The appearance of the HIV/AIDS epidemic in the 1980s impelled many bioethicists to explore this perspective (Jonsen and Stryker 1993; Feldman and Bayer 1999).

REPRODUCTIVE ETHICS

During the first part of the twentieth century birth control was an important issue in the feminist movement. Not until the late 1960s were restrictions on the use and teaching of birth control removed in most states. The feminist movement, especially through Margaret Sanger (1879–1966), also sponsored and encouraged research on new birth control methods that led to hormonal contraceptives (the Pill) (Gordon 1976). In the 1960s abortion became a center of debate. The discussion began with the American Law Institute's model statute permitting abortion for medical and psychological conditions as well as after rape and for fetal defect. The public debate evolved into a rigid polarity between those viewing the issue in terms of a woman's right to control her body and those viewing it in terms of the fetus's right to life. The US Supreme Court in *Roe v. Wade* (1973) chose a position protecting a woman's decision to have an abortion in the first trimester of pregnancy with increasing possibility for legal restrictions during the second and third trimesters. Abortion, because of its intriguing questions about personhood, stimulated considerable professional, philosophical, and theological reflection (Callahan 1970; Grisez 1970; Kamm 1992). That reflection in the 1990s and into the next decade ceded to vigorous, sometimes violent political activism.

In the 1960s advances in genetics and reproductive technology caused much speculation about the social consequences of such possible innovations as cloning, in vitro fertilization, and extrauterine gestation. The concern over cloning human beings was vigorously debated in the 1960s, when the question was still speculative (Ramsey 1970a). It resumed in 1996 after the successful cloning of a sheep, called Dolly, by two Scottish researchers (MacKinnon 2000). Interest in the potential and the dangers of genetic manipulation was heightened by the development of recombinant DNA technology in the mid-1970s. Amniocentesis (a test to diagnose certain fetal disorders during early pregnancy) and improvements in taking genetic histories made possible the development of genetic counseling as a profession in the late 1960s with attendant ethical questions (Hilton et al. 1973). Many questions considered speculative in the 1980s came close to realization by the early twenty-first century. The American College of Obstetricians and Gynecologists and the American Fertility Society set up the National Advisory Board on Ethics and Reproduction, which sat from 1991 to 1998 (Cohen 1996).

The federally sponsored project to map the entire human genome has become a focus for the study of the ethical questions involved in genetic diagnosis, treatment, and social policy. The Ethical, Legal, and Social Implications Research Program has sponsored a wide variety of scholarly and institutional activities in the ethics of genetics (Juengst and Watson 1991; Cooke-Deegan 1994). Scientific interest in the therapeutic value of embryonic stem cells stirred up an ethical storm (Green 2001). In 2001 President George W. Bush said in a public address that "embryonic stem cell research is at the leading edge of a series of moral hazards" and announced that he would appoint a council to monitor stem cell research and investigate other bioethical questions. The President's Council on Bioethics was established in 2002 and was headed by a distinguished bioethicist, Leon Kass. Certain forms of stem cell research were allowed to proceed under stringent oversight. The promise of genetic therapy, bright at the opening of the twenty-first century, has dimmed as a variety of trials have produced meager results.

PSYCHIATRIC ETHICS AND NEUROETHICS

In the bioethics field and in public debate, there were persistent questions about the biological basis of personality, achievement, and social behavior. In the early part of the twentieth century the eugenics movement fostered many state laws requiring or allowing sterilization of persons with mental retardation or illness. Debate over sterilization arose again around 1970, when protection of women and minority groups against pressure for sterilization became an issue. The role of genetics in behavior continued to be debated with the development of sociobiology and studies on IQ and heredity. There was disagreement over the goals of genetic counseling as well as over whether genetic factors in behavior could or should be identified. Screening of populations for genetically determined conditions was much debated (President's Commission for the Study of Ethical Problems in Medicine and Biomedical and Behavioral Research 1983c; Holtzman 1989). Surgical interventions to treat behavioral disorders (psychosurgery) were introduced in the mid-twentieth century. The crude operation, prefrontal lobotomy, was widely used for decades after its introduction in 1935 to treat an ill-defined range of "insanity," from depression to violence. With improvements in surgical techniques in the 1960s, new types of brain surgery were attempted for more specific conditions, such as obsessive-compulsive disorders. The use of psychosurgery on prisoners became a public issue (Valenstein 1974). The National Commission for the Protection of Human Subjects issued a report on this practice, recommending its use only in strictly controlled experimental applications.

Although psychosurgery is the most physically invasive mode of treatment for behavioral problems, all levels of psychiatric treatment were subject to ethical inquiry. The warrant and nature of involuntary commitment to mental hospitals has long been a source of contention (Rothman 1980). Commitment laws in many US states were modified in the 1960s to increase protection of individuals from arbitrary commitment, although at the same time the policy of deinstitutionalization thrust many mental patients into a world for which they were unprepared. The right of hospitalized mental patients to receive treatment was established in the United States initially by the Supreme Court decision in *Wyatt v. Stickney* (1972). The use of drugs in treating psychiatric disorders became an issue after chlorpromazine and related major tranquilizers became widely available in the 1950s, reducing the need for hospitalization. The conventional medical view of behavioral problems as disease came under attack from radical psychiatrists, such as Thomas S. Szasz (1961). Goals and values in psychotherapy came to the fore in discussions about treating patients who manifested "antisocial" behavior. During the first decade of the twenty-first century the detection of potential terrorists, assassins, and mass shooters posed ethical questions about preemptive restrictions and surveillance, challenging traditional libertarian values.

In the last decades of the twentieth century the new field of neuroscience took shape using remarkable imaging techniques to capture the activity of the brain at the very moment that persons are acting, thinking, imagining, and even intending to act. Mapping brain activity in response to various stimuli quickly inspired commentators to raise the ancient questions about free will and personal responsibility and enhancement of cognitive and affective life. The initiation of a national effort to map brain activity, announced by President Obama in 2013, is likely to stimulate a vast array of bioethical questions about consciousness, personal identity, and responsibility. Neuroscience may be the richest and most challenging area for contemporary bioethics (Marcus 2002).

HIV/AIDS

In 1981 a previously unknown disorder of the immune system appeared, at first in men known to engage in homosexual activities. This disorder, named acquired immunodeficiency syndrome (AIDS), was quickly traced to a blood-borne retroviral infection. The resulting disease was relatively slow to appear but, given the therapeutic possibilities then available, was inevitably fatal. It spread in epidemic fashion among gay men and among those who shared needles while taking drugs intravenously. Fear of the disease and widespread homophobia led to discriminatory actions against those infected. Old ethical questions about restricting the freedom of persons suspected of having a communicable disease were revived. Public health needs appeared to conflict with personal rights. The duty of health care professionals to treat infected persons was vigorously debated, as was the right of infected care providers to practice. Bioethics, by now adept at the discussion of practical ethics, made a major contribution to these debates (Bayer 1989; Juengst and Koenig 1989).

HEALTH CARE REFORM

The problem of just allocation of health care was recognized in the earliest days of bioethics. At that time, however, it was largely defined in terms of selection of patients for rare and expensive technologies, such as dialysis. In the early 1980s the fact that some 35 million Americans were not covered by any health insurance became a pressing public matter (President's Commission for the Study of Ethical Problems in Medicine and Biomedical and Behavioral Research 1983b; Churchill 1987; Dougherty 1988). Ethical questions about the justice of such a system were raised as health policy experts began to note the rapid inflation in health care costs. Lack of access to care competed with cost containment in public debate and political maneuvering. These problems became central to the concerns of many bioethicists, who began to produce acute analyses of the issues of justice in the health care system and its financial base. These ethicists raised and examined the politically unpalatable issue of rationing of health care resources (Daniels 1985; Callahan 1988; Menzel 1990; Morreim 1991). Two major political initiatives to enact comprehensive health insurance for all Americans—the first during the Clinton administration, which ended in stalemate, and the second under President Obama, which ended in the 2010 passage of a new health care law—raised major ethical questions about justice. Although bioethicists contributed to these debates, their ideas were largely submerged by the torrent of political and economic arguments.

BIOETHICS AS ACADEMIC DISCIPLINE

Bioethicists show considerable interest in the theoretical definition of the field and its methodologies. In 1974 Albert R. Jonsen and André E. Hellegers published an essay delineating bioethics as a mélange of traditional professional ethics, philosophical ethics, and theological ethics. Robert M. Veatch, however, was the first to attempt a full exposition of the theoretical underpinnings of bioethics. His 1981 book, *A Theory of Medical Ethics*, set the field firmly on the ethical considerations relative to autonomy of the patient. H. Tristram Engelhardt Jr. (1996 [1986]) followed in 1986 with *The Foundations of Bioethics*, an even more strongly stated thesis about autonomy as the basis of the discipline. Nevertheless, some have asserted that bioethics, though it had its origins in the strong affirmation of autonomy for patients, may have moved too far in this direction and thereby neglected other aspects of health care, such as benevolence, community, and social justice (Daniels 1985; Pellegrino and Thomasma 1988).

The study of bioethics, together with other fields in applied ethics, has inspired much debate about the methods appropriate to studying practical ethics in general. Many of these nascent methods have lent a richer, more detailed texture to ethical discussion than is permitted by principle- and theory-based ethics. The long-abandoned casuistry that employs rhetorical and analogical reasoning to examine cases is being viewed in the early twenty-first century with renewed and critical interest (Jonsen and Toulmin 1988; Arras 1991; Sugarman and Sulmasy 2001). Mathematical decision analysis has been used to study values through systematically related cases (Smith and Wigton 1987). Stories, real and fictional, are used as texts open to moral interpretation according to the methods of hermeneutics (Brody 1987; Hunter 1991), and phenomenology seeks to capture the ethical subtleties of clinical encounters (Zaner 1988; Carson 1990). Echoing the language of ethics from the nineteenth century but with much greater attention to depth and detail, interest in virtue- and character-based ethics is vigorous (Shelp 1985; Drane 1988).

Clinical Ethics. In the 1970s, as faculty members were appointed to teach ethics in medical schools, it became common for the ethicist to accompany physicians on teaching rounds. This led to the participation of ethicists in consultations about cases that presented particularly difficult ethical decisions. This practice came to be called clinical ethics. In 1977 the ethicist John C. Fletcher was appointed assistant for bioethics to the director of the Clinical Center at the National Institutes of Health with responsibility for ethics consultation. Because philosophy itself provides little guidance about how to assist in actual decision making, various methods that, like classical casuistry, attempted to disclose the ethical dimensions of particular situations were devised to apply principles to practice. Clinical ethics spread from university hospitals to community hospitals; many individuals, physicians and philosophers alike, now act as clinical ethics consultants. The *Journal of Clinical Ethics* was initiated in 1991. As might be expected, some dispute surrounds the idea and practice of ethics consultation because it seems to imply that some persons are "ethical experts," a notion rather foreign to a morally pluralistic culture (Fletcher, Quist, and Jonsen 1989). In 2010 the American Society for Bioethics and the Humanities published the second edition of its criteria for clinical ethics consultation. A number of training programs provide an introduction to the skill of clinical consultation.

Clinical ethics, deeply engaged in practical decision making about patient care, has inspired empirical study of ethics in health care. This in turn has fostered cooperation between the social sciences and normative philosophical ethics. Termed the *contextual approach* by some authors, it calls attention to significant social and cultural features of life that affect ethical expression and debate (Weisz 1990; Thomasma 1984). Some researchers have used in-depth ethnographic techniques, such as participant observations and interviews, to study the context of clinical settings; others are employing epidemiological methods to ascertain frequency of behaviors, such as resuscitation. The empirical social sciences and philosophy have begun to converse with each other on the common ground of bioethics (Bosk 1979; Guellemin and Holmstrom 1986).

Feminine and feminist issues have become an intrinsic part of humanist and social science disciplines. Although early bioethics was dominated by male scholars, women, such as Renée C. Fox, Loretta Kopelman, Karen Lebacqz, Macklin, Ruth Purtilo, Cahill, and Nussbaum, have made significant contributions to theoretical and practical bioethics, and feminist ethics has attracted much attention. Feminist bioethics offers social criticism of the treatment of women as patients and as physicians, discusses the interrelationship between gender and power, provides fresh analyses of issues of traditional concern to women (such as pregnancy, birth, and reproductive choices), and emphasizes important theoretical concepts—such as caring, community, and responsibility—neglected by male scholars (Holmes and Purdy 1992; Sherwin 1992).

Events and Organizations for the Study of Bioethics. As the field of bioethics was beginning to form, conferences and symposia were an important source for developing literature, teaching, and publicity. Some of the more important early conferences were the Joseph P. Kennedy Jr. Foundation's International Conference on Abortion, held in 1967 in Washington, DC; a New York Academy of Sciences conference, "New Dimensions in Legal and Ethical Concepts for Human Research," held in 1969; a National Academy of Sciences Institute of Medicine conference, "Health Care and Changing Values," held in 1973; a series of transdisciplinary symposia on philosophy and medicine, the first of which was held in Galveston, Texas, in 1974 (Engelhardt and Spicker 1975); and the 1975 conference "Experiments and Research with Humans: Values in Conflict" sponsored by the National Academy of Sciences. In the 1990s such conferences, on a wide variety of topics, were announced at a dizzying pace.

Several privately funded institutes were devoted primarily to the study of bioethics. The Institute of Religion, established in 1954 at the Texas Medical Center in Houston, began to devote attention to bioethical issues in the late 1960s. The Society for Health and Human Values evolved in 1969 from a smaller interdisciplinary group that had formed the Committee on Health and Human Values in 1963 with support from the ecumenical United Ministries in Higher Education. In 1998 the Society for Health and Human Values, the Society for Bioethics Consultation, and the American Association of Bioethics united to form the American Society for Bioethics and Humanities, which by 2002 had enrolled 1,500 members drawn from bioethics, medicine, nursing, law, religion, and the social sciences. The Hastings Center, founded by Daniel Callahan and Willard Gaylin in 1969 as the Institute of Society, Ethics, and the Life Sciences, investigates social, legal, and ethical aspects of the health sciences. Located in Garrison, New York, it conducts a program for visiting fellows and associates; publishes the most widely read of the ethics journals, *Hastings Center Report* and *IRB: A Review of Human Subjects Research*; organizes study groups on special topics; and conducts courses for health professionals and others. In 2013 the Hastings Center had 195 fellows and almost 12,000 members.

For several years in the 1970s the Joseph P. Kennedy Jr. Foundation funded the Interfaculty Program in Medical Ethics, which joined Harvard University's Medical School, School of Public Health, and Divinity School to train scholars in this new field. After this program came to an end, the Kennedy Foundation then founded the Joseph and Rose Kennedy Institute for the Study of Human Reproduction and Bioethics, led by Hellegers and now known as the Kennedy Institute of Ethics, at Georgetown University. This program has supported research by permanent and visiting scholars, courses and workshops in bioethics, and cooperative and consulting programs with private and governmental institutions. Starting in 1972 the institute sponsored Reich's project for the preparation of the *Encyclopedia of Bioethics*, a landmark in US bioethical studies. Its National Resource Center prepares the computer-based bibliography of bioethical literature for the National Library of Medicine's website PubMed, which was published annually from 1975 to 2009 in book form as *Bibliography of Bioethics*. The Kennedy Institute originated the *Journal of Philosophy and Medicine*, which in the early twenty-first century is published independently, and produces the *Kennedy Institute of Ethics Journal.*

As bioethics flowered, many ethical issues were being debated as matters of public policy. Some bioethicists found themselves working as public employees to aid in policy formation, and others served as members of and consultants to advisory bodies, such as the National Commission for the Protection of Human Subjects of Biomedical and Behavioral Research; the President's Commission for the Study of Ethical Problems in Medicine and Biomedical and Behavioral Research; the now defunct Ethics Advisory Board of the Department of Health and Human Services; and state bodies, such as New York's Task Force on Life and the Law and New Jersey's Bioethics Commission. Ten of the eighty-two "special government employees" working with the 1993 Task Force on Reform of Health Care were identifiable as bioethicists. Beyond these official bodies, several thousand physicians, nurses, clergy, and laypersons sit on the hospital ethics committees that have since the 1980s become part of most medical centers in the United States. Grassroots bioethics activities, such as the Oregon Health Decisions Project, strive to involve laypersons in making decisions about the ethics of health care allocation policy. The environmental movement has also raised many questions about human interaction in the biosphere. Though not yet a formal part of bioethics, these questions, particularly as they affect human health, are bound to enter into it. Bioethics has become, to some extent, a philosophy for the people.

Although bioethics in the United States was charged in the past with a failure to reflect the concerns of people of color, work began to appear that increasingly reflected diverse viewpoints, including collections of narratives of the African American experience with disease and health care (White 1990; Secundy and Nixon 1992). The Center for Bioethics was inaugurated at Tuskegee University at the time of President Bill Clinton's formal apology to African Americans for the Tuskegee syphilis experiments; this center concentrates on ethnic issues in bioethics. Some authors have discussed the tensions between expressed philosophical ideals and systematic patterns of discrimination, such as abuses of birth control, sterilization, and selection of subjects for research (Dula 1991; Flack and Pellegrino 1992). Bioethics has slowly recognized global issues, such as poverty and hunger, and the social systems that underlie them as major bioethical topics (Singer 2010). US bioethics has become more international and less ethnocentric in its concerns. American bioethicists have visited many nations, and bioethicists from around the world have spent time in American programs, stimulating cross-cultural comparisons and analyses (Fox and Swazey 1984; Harding 1987; Sagoff 1991; Macklin 1999), and American scholars are active in the International Association for Bioethics.

Since its beginnings the bioethics movement has demonstrated extraordinary vitality in the United States. Its work effected significant changes in the practices of health care. Its first historian, Rothman, wrote only a few years after its origins: "The record since 1966, I believe, makes a convincing case for a fundamental transformation in the substance as well as the style of medical decision making" (1991, 251). That transformation consists largely in the flow of lay opinion and judgment into the formerly closed world of medical decision and policy, in both clinical and research settings, and into the restricted world of academic ethics. Many central concepts of bioethics have become embedded in common thought about medicine and science.

By the 1990s bioethics was firmly established as a field of study in academic settings. This status gives it a prestige and institutional base that it had previously lacked but may also imperil its vitality and independence. Although initially seen by some as a fad, bioethics is linked with social and personal issues deeply rooted in the culture of the United States during the twentieth century.

The impact of technology on human life, the distribution of increasingly scarce health resources in an otherwise affluent society, the role of government in the pursuit of health by individuals and populations, and the voice of the consumer-patient in decisions about medical care—all these issues are central to the concerns of bioethics. Inevitably ethical issues in the life sciences also embrace the larger social problems of environment and population. It is likely that the diffuse field of bioethics will take shape as it increasingly finds its place in the education of future health professionals, as it becomes part of the attempt by schools and consumer organizations to increase personal responsibility for health and environment, and as it attends to the formulation of public policy about social life in the biosphere.

SEE ALSO *Bioethics Commissions, History of*

BIBLIOGRAPHY

Aikens, Charlotte. 1916. *Studies in Ethics for Nurses*. Philadelphia: Saunders.

Alexander, Leo. 1949. "Medical Science under Dictatorship." *New England Journal of Medicine* 241 (2): 39–47.

Alexander, Shana. 1962. "They Decide Who Lives, Who Dies." *Life*, November 9, 102–25.

American Hospital Association. 1992 [1973]. "A Patient's Bill of Rights." http://www.carroll.edu/msmillie/bioethics/patbillofrights.htm

American Hospital Association. 2003. *The Patient Care Partnership*. Chicago: Author. http://www.aha.org/content/00-10/pcp_english_030730.pdf

Annas, George J. 1975. *The Rights of Patients*. Carbondale: Southern Illinois University Press.

Annas, George J., and Michael A. Grodin. 1992. *The Nazi Doctors and the Nuremberg Code: Human Rights in Human Experimentation*. New York: Oxford University Press.

Arras, John D. 1991. "Getting Down to Cases: The Revival of Casuistry in Bioethics." *Journal of Medicine and Philosophy* 16 (1): 29–51.

Baker, Robert; Arthur Caplan; Linda Emanuel; et al. 1999. *The American Medical Ethics Revolution: How the AMA's Code of Ethics Changes Its Relationship to Practitioners, Patients, and the Public*. Baltimore, MD: Johns Hopkins University Press.

Bayer, Ronald. 1989. *Private Acts and Social Consequences: AIDS and the Politics of Public Health*. New York: Free Press.

Beauchamp, Dan, and Bonnie Steinbock. 1999. *New Ethics for the Public's Health*. New York: Oxford University Press.

Beauchamp, Tom L., and James F. Childress. 2001. *Principles of Biomedical Ethics*. 5th ed. New York: Oxford University Press.

Beecher, Henry K. 1966. "Ethics and Clinical Research." *New England Journal of Medicine* 274 (24): 1354–60.

Berlant, Jeffrey L. 1975. *Profession and Monopoly: A Study of Medicine in the United States and Great Britain*. Berkeley: University of California Press.

Bickel, Janet. 1987. "Human Values Teaching Programs in the Clinical Education of Medical Students." *Journal of Medical Education* 62 (5): 369–78.

Binger, Carl A. L. 1945. *The Doctor's Job*. New York: Norton.

Bosk, Charles L. 1979. *Forgive and Remember: Managing Medical Failure*. Chicago: University of Chicago Press.

Brody, Howard. 1987. *Stories of Sickness*. New Haven, CT: Yale University Press.

Burns, Chester R. 1977. "Richard Clarke Cabot (1868–1939) and Reformation in American Medical Ethics." *Bulletin of the History of Medicine* 51 (3): 353–68.

Burns, Chester R. 1980. "Medical Ethics and Jurisprudence." In *The Education of American Physicians: Historical Essays*, edited by Ronald L. Numbers, 273–89. Berkeley: University of California Press.

Burrow, James G. 1963. *AMA: Voice of American Medicine*. Baltimore, MD: Johns Hopkins University Press.

Burrow, James G. 1977. *Organized Medicine in the Progressive Era: The Move toward Monopoly*. Baltimore, MD: Johns Hopkins University Press.

Callahan, Daniel. 1970. *Abortion: Law, Choice, and Morality*. New York: Macmillan.

Callahan, Daniel. 1973. "Bioethics as a Discipline." *Hastings Center Studies* 1 (1): 66–73.

Callahan, Daniel. 1988. *Setting Limits: Medical Goals in an Aging Society*. New York: Simon and Schuster.

Carson, Ronald A. 1990. "Interpretive Bioethics: The Way of Discernment." *Theoretical Medicine* 11 (1): 51–59.

Cassel, Christine K., and Andrew Jameton. 1982. "Medical Responsibility and Thermonuclear War." *Annals of Internal Medicine* 97 (3): 426–32.

Childress, James F. 1970. "Who Shall Live When Not All Can Live?" *Soundings* 53: 39–55.

Churchill, Larry R. 1987. *Rationing Health Care in America: Perceptions and Principles of Justice*. Notre Dame, IN: University of Notre Dame Press.

Cohen, Cynthia B., ed. 1996. *New Ways of Making Babies: The Case of Egg Donation*. Bloomington: Indiana University Press.

Cooke-Deegan, Robert. 1994. *The Gene Wars: Science, Politics, and the Human Genome*. New York: Norton.

Coppens, Charles. 1905. *Moral Principles and Medical Practice: The Basis of Medical Jurisprudence*. 4th rev. ed. New York: Benziger.

Daniels, Norman. 1985. *Just Health Care*. New York: Cambridge University Press.

Davis, Loyal Edward. 1960. *Fellowship of Surgeons: A History of the American College of Surgeons*. Springfield, IL: Charles Thomas.

Dougherty, Charles J. 1988. *American Health Care: Realities, Rights, and Reforms*. New York: Oxford University Press.

Drane, James F. 1988. *Becoming a Good Doctor: The Place of Virtue and Character in Medical Ethics*. Kansas City, MO: Sheed and Ward.

Dula, Annette. 1991. "Toward an African-American Perspective on Bioethics." *Journal of Health Care for the Poor and Underserved* 2 (2): 259–69.

Engelhardt, H. Tristram, Jr. 1996 [1986]. *The Foundations of Bioethics.* 2nd ed. New York: Oxford University Press.

Engelhardt, H. Tristram, Jr., and Stuart F. Spicker, eds. 1975. *Evaluation and Explanation in the Biomedical Sciences: Proceedings of the First Trans-Disciplinary Symposium on Philosophy and Medicine, Held at Galveston, May 9–11, 1974.* Dordrecht, Netherlands: Reidel.

Faden, Ruth, ed. 1996. *The Human Radiation Experiments: Final Report of the President's Advisory Committee.* New York: Oxford University Press.

Fein, Rashi. 1986. *Medical Care, Medical Costs: The Search for a Health Insurance Policy.* Cambridge, MA: Harvard University Press.

Feldman, Eric, and Ronald Bayer. 1999. *Blood Feuds: AIDS, Blood, and the Politics of Medical Disaster.* New York: Oxford University Press.

Flack, Harley E., and Edmund D. Pellegrino, eds. 1992. *African-American Perspectives in Biomedical Ethics.* Washington, DC: Georgetown University Press.

Fletcher, John C.; Norman Quist; and Albert R. Jonsen, eds. 1989. *Ethics Consultation in Health Care.* Ann Arbor, MI: Health Administration Press.

Fletcher, Joseph F. 1954. *Morals and Medicine.* Princeton, NJ: Princeton University Press.

Flexner, Abraham. 1910. *Medical Education in the United States and Canada.* New York: Carnegie Foundation for the Advancement of Teaching.

Fox, Renée C., and Judith F. Swazey. 1974. *The Courage to Fail: A Social View of Organ Transplants and Dialysis.* Chicago: University of Chicago Press.

Fox, Renée C., and Judith F. Swazey. 1984. "Medical Morality Is Not Bioethics: Medical Ethics in China and the United States." *Perspectives in Biology and Medicine* 27 (3): 336–60.

Freidson, Eliot. 1988 [1970]. *The Profession of Medicine: A Study of the Sociology of Applied Knowledge.* Chicago: University of Chicago Press.

Freund, Paul A., ed. 1970. *Experimentation with Human Subjects.* New York: George Braziller.

Garrett, Jeremy R.; Fabrice Jotterand; and D. Christopher Ralston, eds. 2013. *The Development of Bioethics in the United States.* New York: Springer Science and Business Media.

Geiger, H. Jack. 1971. "Hidden Professional Roles: The Physician as Reactionary, Reformer, Revolutionary." *Social Policy* 1 (6): 24–33.

Gevitz, Norman, ed. 1988. *Other Healers: Unorthodox Medicine in America.* Baltimore, MD: Johns Hopkins University Press.

Gilligan, Carol. 1982. *In a Different Voice: Psychological Theory and Women's Development.* Cambridge, MA: Harvard University Press.

Gordon, Linda W. 1976. *Woman's Body, Woman's Rights: A Social History of Birth Control in America.* New York: Grossman.

Gorovitz, Samuel; Andrew L. Jameton; Ruth Macklin; et al., eds. 1976. *Moral Problems in Medicine.* Englewood Cliffs, NJ: Prentice-Hall.

Gorovitz, Samuel; Ruth Macklin; Andrew Jameton; et al. 1973. *Teaching Medical Ethics: A Report on One Approach.* Cleveland, OH: Case Western Reserve University, Department of Philosophy and School of Medicine.

Green, Ronald M. 2001. *The Human Embryo Research Debates: Bioethics in the Vortex of Controversy.* Oxford: Oxford University Press.

Grisez, Germain G. 1970. *Abortion: The Myths, the Realities, and the Arguments.* New York: Corpus.

Guellemin, Jeanne Harley, and Lynda Lytle Holmstrom. 1986. *Mixed Blessings: Intensive Care for Newborns.* New York: Oxford University Press.

Gustafson, James. 1970. "Basic Ethical Issues in the Bio-Medical Field." *Soundings* 53:430–55.

Harding, Sandra. 1987. "The Curious Coincidence of Feminine and African Moralities: Challenges for Feminist Theory." In *Women and Moral Theory,* edited by Eva Feder Kittay and Diana T. Meyers, 296–315. Totowa, NJ: Rowman and Littlefield.

Harvard Medical School, Ad Hoc Committee of the Harvard Medical School to Examine the Definition of Brain Death. 1968. "A Definition of Irreversible Coma." *Journal of the American Medical Association* 205 (6): 337–40.

Hillyard, Daniel, and John Dombrink. 2001. *Dying Right: The Death with Dignity Movement.* London: Routledge.

Hilton, Bruce; Daniel Callahan; Maureen Harris; et al., eds. 1973. *Ethical Issues in Human Genetics: Genetic Counseling and the Use of Genetic Knowledge.* New York: Plenum.

Holmes, Helen Bequaert, and Laura Martha Purdy, eds. 1992. *Feminist Perspectives in Medical Ethics.* Bloomington: Indiana University Press.

Holtzman, Neil A. 1989. *Proceed with Caution: Predicting Genetic Risks in the Recombinant DNA Era.* Baltimore, MD: Johns Hopkins University Press.

Hunter, Kathryn Montgomery. 1991. *Doctors' Stories: The Narrative Structure of Medical Knowledge.* Princeton, NJ: Princeton University Press.

Illich, Ivan. 1976. *Medical Nemesis: The Expropriation of Health.* New York: Pantheon.

Jakobovits, Immanuel. 1959. *Jewish Medical Ethics: A Comparative and Historical Study of the Jewish Religious Attitude to Medicine and Its Practice.* New York: Bloch.

Jameton, Andrew. 1984. *Nursing Practice: The Ethical Issues.* Englewood Cliffs, NJ: Prentice-Hall.

Jecker, Nancy S., ed. 1991. *Aging and Ethics: Philosophical Problems in Gerontology.* Clifton, NJ: Humana.

Jones, James H. 1981. *Bad Blood: The Tuskegee Syphilis Experiment.* New York: Free Press.

Jonsen, Albert R. 1973. "The Totally Implantable Artificial Heart." *Hastings Center Report* 3 (6): 1–4.

Jonsen, Albert R. 1990. *The New Medicine and the Old Ethics.* Cambridge, MA: Harvard University Press.

Jonsen, Albert R. 1998. *The Birth of Bioethics.* New York: Oxford University Press.

Jonsen, Albert R. 2000. *A Short History of Medical Ethics.* New York: Oxford University Press.

Jonsen, Albert R. 2005. *Bioethics beyond the Headlines: Who Lives? Who Dies? Who Decides?* Lanham, MD: Rowman and Littlefield.

Jonsen, Albert R., and André E. Hellegers. 1974. "Conceptual Foundations for an Ethics of Medical Care." In *Ethics of Health Care: Papers of the Conference on Health Care and Changing Values, November 27–29, 1973*, edited by Laurence R. Tancredi, 3–20. Washington, DC: National Academy of Sciences.

Jonsen, Albert R., and Andrew Jameton. 1977. "Social and Political Responsibilities of Physicians." *Journal of Medicine and Philosophy* 2 (4): 376–400.

Jonsen, Albert R.; Mark Siegler; and William J. Winslade. 2001. *Clinical Ethics: A Practical Approach to Ethical Decisions in Clinical Medicine*. 5th ed. New York: Macmillan.

Jonsen, Albert R., and Jeff Stryker, eds. 1993. *The Social Impact of AIDS in the United States*. Panel on Monitoring the Social Impact of the AIDS Epidemic: Committee on AIDS Research and the Behavioral, Social, and Statistical Sciences; Commission on Behavioral and Social Sciences and Education; National Research Council. Washington, DC: National Academies Press.

Jonsen, Albert R., and Stephen E. Toulmin. 1988. *The Abuse of Casuistry: A History of Moral Reasoning*. Berkeley: University of California Press.

Juengst, Eric, and Barbara Koenig, eds. 1989. *The Meaning of AIDS: Implications for Medical Science, Clinical Practice, and Public Health Policy*. New York: Praeger.

Juengst, Eric, and James Watson. 1991. "Human Genome Research and the Responsible Use of New Genetic Knowledge." *International Journal of Bioethics* 2:99–102.

Kamm, Frances. 1992. *Creation and Abortion: A Study in Moral and Legal Philosophy*. New York: Oxford University Press.

Katz, Jay; Alexander M. Capron; and Eleanor Swift Glass, eds. 1972. *Experimentation with Human Beings: The Authority of the Investigator, Subject, Professions, and State in the Human Experimentation Process*. New York: Russell Sage Foundation.

Kübler-Ross, Elisabeth. 1969. *On Death and Dying*. New York: Macmillan.

Ladimer, Irving, and Roger W. Newman, eds. 1963. *Clinical Investigation in Medicine: Legal, Ethical, and Moral Aspects*. Boston: Law-Medicine Research Institute, Boston University.

Leaf, Alexander. 1989. "Potential Health Effects of Global Climatic and Environmental Changes." *New England Journal of Medicine* 321 (23): 1577–83.

Leake, Chauncey D., and Patrick Romanell. 1950. *Can We Agree? A Scientist and a Philosopher Argue about Ethics*. Austin: University of Texas Press.

Leavitt, Judith W. 1986. *Brought to Bed: Childbearing in America, 1750–1950*. New York: Oxford University Press.

Levine, Robert. 1986. *Ethics and Regulation of Clinical Research*. 2nd ed. Baltimore, MD: Urban and Schwarzenberg.

Limbert, Paul M. 1931. "Are Courses in the Ethics of Nursing Worthwhile?" *Trained Nurse and Hospital Review* 87 (4): 472–76.

MacKinnon, Barbara, ed. 2000. *Human Cloning: Science, Ethics, and Public Policy*. Urbana: University of Illinois Press.

Macklin, Ruth. 1999. *Against Relativism: Cultural Diversity and the Search for Ethical Universals in Medicine*. New York: Oxford University Press.

Marcus, Steven J., ed. 2002. *Neuroethics: Mapping the Field*. New York: Dana.

Marmor, Theodore R. 1970. *The Politics of Medicare*. London: Routledge and Kegan Paul.

Marty, Martin E. 1983. *Health and Medicine in the Lutheran Tradition: Being Well*. New York: Crossroad.

McCally, Michael, and Christine K. Cassel. 1990. "Medical Responsibility and Global Environmental Change." *Annals of Internal Medicine* 113 (6): 467–73.

Menzel, Paul T. 1990. *Strong Medicine: The Ethical Rationing of Health Care*. New York: Oxford University Press.

Mohr, James C. 1978. *Abortion in America: The Origins and Evolution of National Policy, 1800–1900*. New York: Oxford University Press.

Moore, Thomas Verner. 1935. *Principles of Ethics*. Philadelphia: Lippincott.

Morreim, Haavi. 1991. *Balancing Act: The New Medical Ethics of Medicine's New Economics*. Dordrecht, Netherlands: Kluwer Academic.

National Academy of Sciences. 1975. *Experiments and Research with Humans: Values in Conflict*. Washington, DC: Author.

National Commission for the Protection of Human Subjects of Biomedical and Behavioral Research. 1978. *The Belmont Report: Ethical Principles and Guidelines for the Protection of Human Subjects of Research*. Washington, DC: DHEW and US Government Printing Office.

National Heart and Lung Institute, Artificial Heart Assessment Panel. 1973. *The Totally Implantable Artificial Heart: Economic, Ethical, Legal, Medical, Psychiatric, and Social Implications*. Bethesda, MD: National Institutes of Health.

New Jersey Superior Court. 1975. *In the Matter of Karen Quinlan: The Complete Legal Briefs, Court Proceedings, and Decisions in the Superior Court of New Jersey*. Arlington, VA: University Publications of America.

Pellegrino, Edmund D., and David C. Thomasma. 1988. *For the Patient's Good: The Restoration of Beneficence in Health Care*. New York: Oxford University Press.

Percival, Thomas. 1927 [1803]. *Percival's Medical Ethics*. Edited by Chauncey D. Leake. Baltimore, MD: Williams and Wilkins.

Post, Stephen G., ed. 2004 [1978]. *Encyclopedia of Bioethics*. 5 vols. New York: Macmillan Reference USA.

Potter, Van Rensselaer. 1971. *Bioethics: Bridge to the Future*. Englewood Cliffs, NJ: Prentice-Hall.

President's Commission for the Study of Bioethical Issues. 2010. *New Directions: The Ethics of Synthetic Biology and Emerging Technologies*. http://bioethics.gov/sites/default/files/PCSBI-Synthetic-Biology-Report-12.16.10.pdf

President's Commission for the Study of Ethical Problems in Medicine and Biomedical and Behavioral Research. 1981. *Defining Death: A Report on the Medical, Legal, and Ethical Issues in the Determination of Death*. Washington, DC: US Government Printing Office. http://bioethics.georgetown.edu/pcbe/reports/past_commissions/defining_death.pdf

President's Commission for the Study of Ethical Problems in Medicine and Biomedical and Behavioral Research. 1983a. *Deciding to Forego* [sic] *Life-Sustaining Treatment: A Report on the Ethical, Medical, and Legal Issues in Treatment Decisions.* Washington, DC: US Government Printing Office. http://bioethics.georgetown.edu/pcbe/reports/past_commissions/deciding_to_forego_tx.pdf

President's Commission for the Study of Ethical Problems in Medicine and Biomedical and Behavioral Research. 1983b. *Screening and Counseling for Genetic Conditions: A Report on the Ethical, Social, and Legal Implications of Genetic Screening, Counseling, and Education Programs.* Washington, DC: US Government Printing Office. http://bioethics.georgetown.edu/pcbe/reports/past_commissions/geneticscreening.pdf

President's Commission for the Study of Ethical Problems in Medicine and Biomedical and Behavioral Research. 1983c. *Securing Access to Health Care: A Report on the Ethical Implications of Differences in the Availability of Health Services.* Washington, DC: US Government Printing Office. http://bioethics.georgetown.edu/pcbe/reports/past_commissions/securing_access.pdf

President's Council on Bioethics. 2002. *Human Cloning and Human Dignity: An Ethical Inquiry.* Washington, DC: Government Printing Office. http://bioethics.georgetown.edu/pcbe/reports/cloningreport/

Ramsey, Paul. 1970a. *Fabricated Man: The Ethics of Genetic Control.* New Haven, CT: Yale University Press.

Ramsey, Paul. 1970b. *Patient as Person: Explorations in Medical Ethics.* New Haven, CT: Yale University Press.

Rescher, Nicholas. 1969. "The Allocation of Exotic Medical Lifesaving Therapy." *Ethics* 79 (3): 173–86.

Robb, Isabel Hampton. 1901. *Nursing Ethics: For Hospital and Private Use.* Cleveland, OH: Savage.

Rosenberg, Charles E. 1987. *The Care of Strangers: The Rise of America's Hospital System.* New York: Basic Books.

Rothman, David J. 1980. *Conscience and Convenience: The Asylum and Its Alternatives in Progressive America.* Boston: Little, Brown.

Rothman, David J. 1991. *Strangers at the Bedside: A History of How Law and Bioethics Transformed Medical Decision Making.* New York: Basic Books.

Sagoff, Mark. 1991. "Zuckerman's Dilemma: A Plea for Environmental Ethics." *Hastings Center Report* 21 (5): 32–40.

Secundy, Marian Gray, and Lois LaCavita Nixon, eds. 1992. *Trials, Tribulations, and Celebrations: African-American Perspectives on Health, Illness, Aging, and Loss.* Yarmouth, ME: Intercultural.

Shaw, Margery W., ed. 1984. *After Barney Clark: Reflections on the Utah Artificial Heart Program.* Austin: University of Texas Press.

Shelp, Earl E., ed. 1985. *Virtue and Medicine: Explorations in the Character of Medicine.* Dordrecht, Netherlands: Reidel.

Sherwin, Susan. 1992. *No Longer Patient: Feminist Ethics and Health Care.* Philadelphia: Temple University Press.

Singer, Peter. 2010. *The Life You Can Save: How to Do Your Part to End World Poverty.* New York: Random House.

Smith, David G., and Robert S. Wigton. 1987. "Modeling Decisions to Use Tube Feeding in Seriously Ill Patients." *Archives of Internal Medicine* 147 (7): 1242–45.

Sperry, Willard. 1950. *The Ethical Basis of Medical Practice.* New York: Hoeber.

Starr, Paul. 1982. *The Social Transformation of American Medicine.* New York: Basic Books.

Stevens, Rosemary. 1971. *American Medicine and the Public.* New Haven, CT: Yale University Press.

Stevens, Rosemary. 1989. *In Sickness and in Wealth: American Hospitals in the Twentieth Century.* New York: Basic Books.

Sugarman, Jeremy, and Daniel Sulmasy. 2001. *Methods in Medical Ethics.* Washington, DC: Georgetown University Press.

Szasz, Thomas S. 1961. *The Myth of Mental Illness: Foundations of a Theory of Personal Conduct.* New York: Harper and Row.

Thomasma, David C. 1984. "The Context as a Moral Rule in Medical Ethics." *Journal of Bioethics* 5 (1): 63–79.

Toulmin, Stephen. 1982. "How Medicine Saved the Life of Ethics." *Perspectives in Biology and Medicine* 25 (4): 736–50.

US Catholic Conference, Department of Health Affairs. 1971 [1949]. *Ethical and Religious Directives for Catholic Health Facilities.* Washington, DC: Author.

Valenstein, Elliot S. 1974. *Brain Control: A Critical Examination of Brain Stimulation and Psychosurgery.* New York: Wiley.

Vaux, Kenneth L. 1984. *Health and Medicine in the Reformed Tradition: Promise, Providence, and Care.* New York: Crossroad.

Vawter, Dorothy E.; Warren Kearney; Karen G. Gervais; et al. 1990. *The Use of Human Fetal Tissue: Scientific, Ethical, and Policy Concerns.* Minneapolis: University of Minnesota, Center for Biomedical Ethics.

Veatch, Robert M. 1981. *A Theory of Medical Ethics.* New York: Basic Books.

Veatch, Robert M.; Willard Gaylin; and Councilman Morgan, eds. 1973. *The Teaching of Medical Ethics: Proceedings of a Conference Sponsored by the Institute of Society, Ethics, and the Life Sciences and Columbia University College of Physicians and Surgeons, June 1–3, 1972.* Hastings-on-Hudson, NY: Institute of Society, Ethics, and the Life Sciences.

Walters, LeRoy, ed. 1975–2009. *Bibliography of Bioethics.* Washington, DC: Georgetown University, Kennedy Institute of Ethics.

Weisz, George, ed. 1990. *Social Science Perspectives on Medical Ethics.* Philadelphia: University of Pennsylvania Press.

White, Evelyn C., ed. 1990. *The Black Women's Health Book: Speaking for Ourselves.* Seattle: Seal.

Zaner, Richard M. 1988. *Ethics and the Clinical Encounter.* Englewood Cliffs, NJ: Prentice-Hall.

Andrew Jameton (1995, 2004)
Professor, College of Public Health, University of Nebraska Medical Center

Albert R. Jonsen (1995, 2004, 2014)
Senior Ethics Scholar, Program in Medicine and Human Values, California Pacific Medical Center, San Francisco

II. CANADA

Two aspects of Canadian society are particularly determinative of the Canadian approach to bioethics: (1) the country's universally accessible, publicly funded health care system and (2) the interplay between jurisprudence, legislation, and ethics. While a multitude of bioethical issues have occupied Canadians since the 1960s, the thought and actions of Canadians and Canadian bioethicists have been intensively mobilized around issues at the beginning of life (abortion and assisted human reproduction), issues at the end of life (cessation of treatment, unilateral decision making, physician-assisted suicide, and voluntary euthanasia), research ethics (use of placebos, conflict of interest), and public health ethics (pandemic planning).

The history of bioethics in Canada can be divided into two time periods: from 1800 to the 1960s and from the 1960s to the present. In the first period medical ethics predominated, although nursing ethics and theological ethics were also important. In the second period all of these spheres of interest were incorporated into the field of bioethics (understood as applied ethics in the life sciences—primarily in the areas of health care and biology).

1800s–1960s

Canada was proclaimed a nation in 1867. This is also the year in which the Canadian Medical Association (CMA) was formed as an organization to protect the interests of licensed practitioners. At its first annual meeting in 1868, the CMA adopted the Code of Ethics of the Canadian Medical Association, which was closely modeled on the American Medical Association's code of ethics. Since 1868 there have been no less than twenty updates to the CMA Code of Ethics. The most recent version was published in 2004 (Canadian Medical Association 2004) and was reviewed in March 2012 (at which time it was deemed "still relevant"). The code focuses on decision making, consent, privacy, confidentiality, research, and physician responsibilities. It outlines fundamental responsibilities: responsibilities to the patient, responsibilities to society, responsibilities to the profession, and responsibilities to oneself.

The Canadian Nurses Association (CNA) was established in 1908. In 1954 the CNA adopted the code of ethics of the International Council of Nurses (first published in 1953). In 1980 the CNA established its own code, published as the *CNA Code of Ethics: An Ethical Basis for Nursing in Canada.* This code has been revised on several occasions, most recently in 2008. It is now titled the *Code of Ethics for Registered Nurses.* The code identifies seven primary nursing values: providing safe, compassionate, competent, and ethical care; promoting health and well-being; promoting and respecting informed decision making; preserving dignity; maintaining privacy and confidentiality; promoting justice; and being accountable.

The Roman Catholic Church has played an important role in health care in Canada since colonial times. The Catholic Hospital Association of the United States and Canada (CHAUSC), founded in 1915, adopted a code of ethics in 1921 that dealt primarily with surgical issues in obstetrics and gynecology. This document was updated in 1935, and in 1949 it was revised and published as *Ethical and Religious Directives for Catholic Hospitals.* In 1939 the Catholic Hospital Council of Canada declared its independence from the CHAUSC and later renamed itself the Catholic Hospital Association of Canada. It adopted its own moral code in 1955. Now named the Catholic Health Alliance of Canada (since 2009), this organization in 1990 updated and renamed its moral code the *Health Ethics Guide.* The most recent version of this guide was published in 2012. This document addresses issues related to social services and organizational ethics, with particular attention to the communal nature of health care, the dignity of the human person, human reproduction, organ and tissue donation and transplantation, care of the dying person, research on human subjects, and governance and administration.

In the early days the medical ethics literature was primarily authored by physicians and focused narrowly on physician behavior. The most renowned Canadian physician of this period, influential in Canada and abroad, was Sir William Osler (1849–1919). The chief virtues of the individual physician are variously referred to in his writings as equanimity (*aequanimitas*), imperturbability, and detachment. His stated ideal for the medical profession was that of "noblesse oblige" (Osler 1985).

Not until the 1940s did a significant number of Canadian publications in medical ethics begin to appear, most of them written by Catholic theologians (e.g., LaRochelle and Fink 1943). Some Catholic schools of medicine (e.g., the University of Ottawa) and nursing (e.g., the University of Montreal) made faculty appointments in medical ethics, and the professors who took these posts contributed to the growing body of Catholic literature in this field (e.g., Paquin 1954). Comparable work by philosophers and health professionals was noticeable by its absence.

1960s–2010s

In the mid-1960s the field of medical ethics underwent a radical transformation propelled in part by advances in medical technology and in American bioethics. By the end of the 1970s the field displayed all the features of what has become known as bioethics. In Canada the major actors in the development of bioethics have been professional health associations, governmental organizations, academic institutions, and academics.

The major professional health associations expanded their ethics activities during this period. In the 1970s the CMA remandated its Committee on Ethics to develop policies and guidelines to deal with a wide range of bioethical issues. In 1989 the CMA established a Department of Ethics and Legal Affairs. This later became the Office of Ethics and is now (since 2008) the Office of Ethics, Professionalism, and International Affairs. The Royal College of Physicians and Surgeons of Canada created a Biomedical Ethics Committee in 1977 to develop bioethical curricula for specialists in training, and the College of Family Physicians of Canada followed suit in 1991. The CNA established an ad hoc ethics committee that met regularly from 1985 to 1997 to revise its code of ethics. In the spring of 1997 this committee was given permanent standing. As well, during this period there was a proliferation of codes of ethics among a number of professional health associations.

There are four federal agencies with significant ethics portfolios. The Canadian Institutes of Health Research (CIHR) is Canada's major health research funding agency. It has an Ethics Office to assist with its legislated mandate to promote, assist, and undertake research that meets the highest international scientific standards of excellence and ethics; to foster the discussion of ethical issues and the application of ethical principles to health research; and to monitor, analyze, and evaluate issues, including ethical issues, pertaining to health and health research. This broad mandate is also supported by the CIHR Standing Committee on Ethics. The Public Health Agency of Canada has a Public Health Law and Ethics Program (PHLEP) with three interrelated streams: public health law, public health ethics, and research ethics. The Interagency Advisory Panel on Research Ethics (PRE) is the federal organization responsible for the development, interpretation, and implementation of the *Tri-Council Policy Statement: Ethical Conduct for Research Involving Humans* (Canadian Institutes of Health Research, Natural Sciences and Engineering Research Council of Canada, and Social Sciences and Humanities Research Council of Canada 2010), now in its second edition (TCPS2). And finally, there is the Health Canada and Public Health Agency of Canada's Research Ethics Board, which is responsible for the ethics review of research proposals received by either of these organizations.

Academic institutions have experienced tremendous growth in the area of bioethics since the 1960s. Courses in this field have proliferated in philosophy and religious studies departments, where they are often the most heavily subscribed offerings at the undergraduate level (e.g., Baylis et al. 2011; Boetzkes and Waluchow 2012). Bioethics instruction is now offered in every Canadian medical school at the basic degree level and is expanding into residency training programs. As well, nursing (Storch, Rodney, and Starzomski 2012), health administration, and dentistry programs have formalized ethics teaching, and in many universities instruction in the ethical aspects of animal experimentation is required for biology, zoology, and psychology students. Many law schools also include courses that wholly or in part deal with bioethics and the law.

Academic research and writing in bioethics has been fostered by the creation of centers, institutes, and professional associations. The Center for Bioethics of the Clinical Research Institute of Montreal, established in 1976, was the first such organization in Canada. It was followed three years later by the Westminster Institute for Ethics and Human Values based in London, Ontario. Both of these organizations are now defunct. In 2012 there were twenty-five academic bioethics centers in Canada, most of them university based. A national association, the Canadian Bioethics Society, was established in 1988. Another major influence on research and writing in bioethics has been targeted funding for ethics research in social science– and humanities-related disciplines. For example, Genome Canada has dedicated funding for Genomics and Its Ethical, Economic, Environmental, Legal, and Social Aspects (GE^3LS) research. There are both stand-alone ethics projects and integrated ethics projects (i.e., where ethics researchers are embedded in scientific or clinical research protocols). This has exponentially increased the number of ethics publications on genetics and genomics.

THE CANADIAN HEALTH CARE SYSTEM

The Canadian health care system is not a single system but rather a network of ten provincial and three territorial health care systems. The coherence of this network derives from the Canada Health Act (1984) and a series of accords between the federal, provincial, and territorial governments. The federal government provides funds to the provinces and territories for health care; the latter governments in return agree to incorporate the essential features of the national health insurance program into their health care systems.

The Canadian health insurance system, as defined in the Hospital Insurance and Diagnostic Services Act (1957) and reaffirmed in the Canada Health Act (1984), is founded on a Canadian values system. The principal features of this program (public administration, comprehensiveness, universality, portability, and accessibility) derive from Canadians' commitment to the principle of equality. Equality before the health care system, as Robert G. Evans has phrased it, is as strong a principle in Canada as equality before the law (Evans 1988). The basis of this principle is that all Canadians should have access to a similar level of care regardless of their ability to pay for it.

There have been challenges to the principle of universal access to hospital and medical services. The practice of user fees and extra billing by doctors, which is prohibited by the Canada Health Act, represents one such challenge. Extra billing would allow doctors to bill patients for charges exceeding what the national health insurance plan paid doctors for a medical service. For a short time in the mid- to late 1980s, extra billing occurred in seven provinces. In response to this violation of the Canada Health Act, the federal government stopped transfer payments to these provinces, thereby providing the provincial governments with an incentive to enforce the principles of the Canada Health Act.

The way a country organizes its health care system as a whole is not just an issue of economics and administration. It is also an issue of public ethics and is deeply rooted in the conflict between powerful interest groups and the requirements of justice (as interpreted by a society's governing ethos). The Canadian ethos of universal access with equal terms and conditions for all is being challenged by new questions of fairness. For example, the current Canadian Medicare program pays for physician and hospital services but not drugs (unless these are administered in a hospital). For many patients, good health depends on access to expensive medications, and since these are not covered by provincial and territorial health care systems, Canadians who need expensive medications are at risk of incurring significant debt or, worse, doing without their medications. This explains frequent calls on the federal government to expand the Canada Health Act to include prescription drug costs.

In 2002 there was renewed debate about the future of the health care system in Canada, with particular focus on two issues: (1) public administration (whether there should be a single insurer/funder model or a multipayer system) and (2) delivery of goods and services (whether this should be public, private nonprofit, or private for-profit). Two reports looked at the sustainability of the universally accessible, publicly funded health care system, with particular attention to the question of whether Canada should move to a two-tier system by allowing the use of private hospitals and private insurance. The first of these reports, *The Health of Canadians: The Federal Role* (Standing Senate Committee on Social Affairs, Science, and Technology 2002), looked at the state of the health care system in Canada and the federal role in that system. The report is widely known as the Kirby Report in reference to Senator Michael Kirby, who chaired the committee. It recommends restructuring the hospital and doctor system to improve efficiency and effectiveness, and it endorses an increased role for private health care corporations.

The second report, *Building on Values: The Future of Health Care in Canada* (Commission on the Future of Health Care in Canada 2002), is widely known as the Romanow Report after the commission chair, Roy Romanow. The report examines four strategies for continuing to ensure access to high quality of care regardless of ability to pay: (1) more public investment (paid for by raising taxes or diverting resources from other programs); (2) more user pay (through charging fees as an incentive to deter abuse); (3) increasing private choice (either for-profit or nonprofit); or (4) completely reorganizing the health care delivery system. A commitment to health care as a social good and service, not an economic commodity only available to those who can pay, informs the analysis.

A direct, successful attack on the public financing of health care is the 2005 case *Chaoulli v. Québec (Attorney General)*. A patient, Mr. Zeliotis was frustrated with the wait times he experienced in accessing health services. Together he and Dr. Jacques Chaoulli (a physician who wanted to establish a private medical practice) challenged Québec's provincial legislation prohibiting citizens from purchasing health insurance for private access to services otherwise available in the public system. The Supreme Court of Canada decided that the ban on private insurance was not necessary to protect Canadian Medicare and that it should be possible for Québecers to purchase private insurance when wait times in the public system were unreasonable. In response to this decision, the province of Québec pledged to reduce wait times and, when there were unreasonable delays, to provide the service at a private clinic or out of province at public expense, thereby seeking to stave off any potential rush to buy private insurance for the private delivery of health care. This case was decided on the basis of Québec's Charter of Human Rights and Freedoms (Québec Charter). The ban on private insurance was deemed a violation of the right to personal security guaranteed in the Québec Charter. It is unclear what would happen in other provinces were a similar legal challenge to be mounted, as the Canadian Charter of Rights and Freedoms (Canadian Charter) (Government of Canada 1982) is not as broad as the Québec Charter.

In Canada, the Constitution Act (1867) was amended in 1982 through the introduction of the Canadian Charter, which obliges government actors not to violate rights and freedoms considered fundamental. Such rights and freedoms include the right to life, liberty, and security of the person; the right to the equal protection and equal benefit of the law without discrimination; freedom of conscience and religion; and freedom of thought, belief, opinion, and expression. The section of the Canadian Charter that guarantees security of the person is section 7, and this section contains a limitations clause: "7. Everyone has the right to life, liberty and security of the person and the right not to be deprived thereof *except in accordance with the principles of fundamental justice*" (Government of Canada 1982; emphasis added). As of 2010 it is estimated that close to 30 percent of Canada's health care system is financed privately (e.g., assisted human reproduction, cosmetic surgery, pharmaceuticals, dental care) (Flood and Thomas 2010).

KEY ISSUES IN CANADA

Issues at the Beginning of Life. Between the 1960s and the 1990s the issue of abortion dominated the public-policy debate in Canadian bioethics. The debate was ignited in the late 1960s, when the federal government proposed changes to the Criminal Code that would relax restrictions on divorce, homosexual acts between consenting adults, the distribution of contraceptives, and abortion. The last issue was the most contentious and engendered widespread public discussion and lobbying of members of Parliament. The abortion law in effect since 1869 prohibited termination of pregnancy under any circumstances, and criminal sanctions could be brought against the pregnant woman and anyone who would perform the abortion. In 1969 a new abortion law was adopted that retained the criminal sanctions against both the woman seeking an abortion and anyone who would perform the act but legalized termination of pregnancy if the following conditions were met: (1) the abortion had to be performed by a qualified medical practitioner in an accredited or approved hospital; (2) it had to be approved by a therapeutic abortion committee of the hospital; and (3) the continuation of the pregnancy would or would be likely to endanger the life or health of the woman seeking the abortion.

Following this liberalization of the abortion law, there were many complaints of unequal access to abortion services as well as accusations from antiabortion groups that the law was being applied too loosely. Since the federal government refused to revise the law, both proponents and opponents of abortion decided to challenge the law in the courts.

In 1970 Dr. Henry Morgentaler established an abortion clinic in Montréal in clear opposition to the law. After his third jury acquittal in 1976 on charges of performing an illegal abortion, the Québec government announced that it would no longer prosecute Morgentaler and thereby allowed his clinic to operate, despite vigorous protests from antiabortion forces. In 1983 Morgentaler set up an abortion clinic in Toronto and was promptly arrested and charged, along with two colleagues. A jury once again acquitted him. This decision was appealed, and in 1985 the Ontario Court of Appeal overturned the decision of the jury and ordered a new trial. Morgentaler appealed this ruling to the Supreme Court of Canada. On January 28, 1988, the Supreme Court, in a 5–2 decision, overturned the Court of Appeal decision and restored the original jury acquittal. The Supreme Court also declared the 1969 abortion law unconstitutional, because it violated the Canadian Charter (*R. v. Morgentaler* 1988).

Between 1988 and 1991 the federal government made several attempts to pass a new abortion law, but none were successful. A bill introduced in 1989 would have recriminalized abortion except when performed by a doctor "of the opinion that, if the abortion were not induced, the health or life of the female person would be likely to be threatened" (Bill C-43 1989). This bill was defeated in the Senate January 31, 1991. Health was defined as including physical, mental, and psychological well-being. The bill was approved by the House of Commons in May 1990 by a narrow margin (140–131), and it was then sent to the Senate. In January 1991 a vote was taken, but the Senate was deadlocked. Under Canada's Senate rules, a tie is considered a defeat. As a result, Canada is in the unusual circumstance of having no criminal restrictions on abortion.

New reproductive technologies have also generated considerable public-policy activity in Canada and have been the subject of several public inquiries, including a federal Royal Commission on New Reproductive Technologies. The Royal Commission (1993) issued its final report, *Proceed with Care*, in 1993. The report recommended federal oversight of assisted human reproduction. In 1996 Bill C-47, the Human Reproductive and Genetic Technologies Act, was introduced in the House of Commons. This bill did not complete the legislative process before an election was called. Years later, in May 2002, Bill C-56, the Assisted Human Reproduction Act, was introduced. While Parliament was prorogued before this bill could complete the legislative process, Bill C-56 did not share the same fate as the earlier bill. It was reinstated as Bill C-13.

Significantly, the general purpose of Bill C-13 found favor with the Canadian bioethics community, which applauded the government for introducing legislation to promote the safety and well-being of those who use and those who are born of assisted human reproduction. Support for the legislation was communicated in an open letter to the government distributed in Parliament. Never before or since have members of the Canadian bioethics community taken this kind of initiative on a matter of bioethical import. On March 24, 2004 (more than ten years after the Royal Commission issued its final report), the Assisted Human Reproduction Act received royal assent.

Shortly thereafter the Québec government challenged the constitutionality of the legislation. The Québec Court of Appeal held that several sections of the act were indeed unconstitutional. In turn the federal government appealed this decision to the Supreme Court of Canada. On December 22, 2010, the Supreme Court rendered its decision. The prohibitions listed in the act (such as the prohibitions of human cloning, creating in vitro embryos for research purposes, manipulating embryos to increase the probability of a particular sex, and payment for surrogacy or for the purchase of gametes) were deemed to be a valid exercise of the federal government's criminal law powers. However, most of the legislation dealing with controlled activities (which would have seen the introduction of a federal licensing system overseen by Assisted Human Reproduction Canada) was found to be unconstitutional (Reference re Assisted Human Reproduction Act 2010). As a consequence of this decision, it became clear that the regulation of much of assisted human reproduction is a provincial responsibility. By 2013, only the Québec government had seriously taken on this responsibility.

Meanwhile, another assisted human reproduction law case was winding its way through the courts. This class-action lawsuit was initiated by Olivia Pratten on behalf of donor-conceived individuals to bring an end to donor anonymity. Pratten was conceived using donor sperm, and she argued that donor-conceived individuals have a right to know the identities of their biological parents. In May 2011, the British Columbia Supreme Court ruled in favor of Pratten. In November 2012, the British Columbia Court of Appeal ruled against Pratten. Pratten then sought leave to appeal to the Supreme Court of Canada; leave was denied (*Olivia Pratten v. Attorney General of British Columbia* 2013).

Issues at the End of Life. An ethical and legal consensus has emerged in Canada in support of the view that competent adults should not be treated against their will, even when treatment refusal may result in death. Further, in cases involving incompetent patients it is agreed that, pursuant to legally valid advance directives, physicians can withhold or discontinue treatments that do little more than prolong a patient's dying and suffering. However, there continues to be debate about unilateral decision making by physicians, physician-assisted suicide, and voluntary euthanasia (Baylis 2000; Downie 2004; College of Physicians and Surgeons of Manitoba 2007; Sumner 2011), as illustrated in the legal cases summarized below.

In 1992 the Superior Court of Québec affirmed that the request of a competent patient to discontinue life-supporting treatment should be honored (*Nancy B. v. Hôtel-Dieu de Québec*). Nancy B., a twenty-five-year-old woman, was permanently dependent on a respirator due to Guillain-Barré syndrome. After two years, while lucid and without clinical depression, she asked that the respirator be stopped, knowing that this would lead to her death. The court held that discontinuing treatment would not constitute criminal negligence or homicide. This case has been cited approvingly by the Supreme Court of Canada.

A year later, in 1993, Sue Rodriguez—a competent woman suffering from amyotrophic lateral sclerosis who wanted to commit assisted suicide—brought a challenge to the prohibition against assisted suicide found in the Criminal Code. The Supreme Court of Canada upheld the prohibition by a 5–4 margin based on its application of the Canadian Charter to the facts of the case (*Rodriguez v. British Columbia [Attorney General]*). Despite this decision, Rodriguez ultimately died as a result of physician-assisted suicide, and no one was prosecuted in connection with her death.

Also in 1993 Robert Latimer was charged with first-degree murder in the death of his twelve-year-old daughter, Tracy Latimer. Latimer had placed his severely handicapped daughter (a quadriplegic child with the intellectual capacity of a three-month-old) in the cab of his truck and, with the intent of alleviating her suffering, asphyxiated her with carbon monoxide. In 1994 Latimer was convicted of second-degree murder and given the mandatory sentence of life imprisonment without eligibility for parole for ten years. He successfully appealed his conviction to the Supreme Court of Canada, and a new trial was ordered. In 1997 Latimer was tried on a charge of second-degree murder, was again convicted, but was now sentenced to two years less a day (instead of the mandatory sentence of at least ten years in prison). Latimer again appealed his conviction, and the Crown appealed the sentence. The Court of Appeal dismissed Latimer's appeal, allowed the Crown's appeal, and imposed the mandatory minimum sentence. Latimer then appealed to the Supreme Court, and in 2001 it upheld the conviction and the life sentence with no possibility of parole for ten years (*R. v. Latimer*).

Another important Canadian case is that of Hassan Rasouli. Following surgery to remove a benign brain tumor, Rasouli developed bacterial meningitis resulting in severe brain damage. Having determined that the patient was in a permanent vegetative state, his physicians sought to withdraw interventions they deemed to be of no medical value to the patient (mechanical ventilator, and artificial nutrition and hydration) and to provide palliative care. His wife and legal substitute decision maker, Ms. Salasel, objected to the proposed plan. The physicians involved in Rasouli's care insisted that they did not require her consent to withdraw life-sustaining treatment. Because of specific definitions of "treatment" and "plan of treatment" in the relevant legislation (which include "the withholding or withdrawal of treatment"), the Supreme Court of Ontario found in favor of Rasouli and concluded that the proposal to withdraw treatment must be referred to the Consent and Capacity Board and that the physicians were not permitted to withdraw treatment and transfer Rasouli to palliative care. The case was dismissed by the Court of Appeal for Ontario (*Rasouli v. Sunnybrook Health Sciences Centre* 2011) and then appealed to the Supreme Court of Canada. The Supreme Court of Canada heard oral arguments in December 2012, and a decision was expected in 2013.

These cases show that the courts in Canada will respect the wishes of competent adults to refuse potentially life-sustaining treatment; will reject the wishes of competent patients to actively bring about their own deaths through physician-assisted suicide; will not tolerate deliberate actions to bring about the death of another person, even when the motive is to alleviate suffering; and will not endorse unilateral decision making by physicians to limit or cease treatment.

By and large these court decisions are consistent with contemporary bioethics literature in Canada. Many suspect, however, that change is in the offing (in both the literature and the law). In 2011 the Royal Society of Canada Expert Panel released its final report, *End-of-Life Decision Making*, in which it recommended revisions to the Criminal Code to permit assisted suicide and voluntary euthanasia in limited circumstances. At more or less the same time, the Parliamentary Committee on Palliative and Compassionate Care (2011) released its report, *Not to Be Forgotten: Care of Vulnerable Canadians*, advocating for improved quality end-of-life care. In March 2012 the Québec Assembly Select Committee on Dying with Dignity published its final report, recommending improved palliative care and endorsing medical aid in dying. The report recommends that persons who meet all of the following criteria be eligible for medical aid in dying: be a Québec resident; be an adult able to consent to treatment; be able to make a free and informed decision to request medical aid in dying; have a serious and incurable disease; have no chance of improvement; and be experiencing constant and unbearable physical or psychological suffering (recommendation 13).

In 2012 a case similar to the 1993 Rodriguez case went before the British Columbia Supreme Court (*Carter v. Canada [Attorney General]*). The plaintiffs, relying on the Canadian Charter, challenged the Criminal Code provisions prohibiting physician-assisted suicide. The British Columbia Supreme Court found in favor of the plaintiffs. Subsequently the British Columbia Court of Appeal heard the case in March 2013). The expectation is that whatever decision the Court of Appeal renders, leave to appeal to the Supreme Court of Canada will be sought.

Research Ethics. In Canada, unlike in some other countries, guidelines play a significant role in the governance of research involving humans. The first such guidelines were promulgated by the Medical Research Council of Canada in 1978 and were later revised in 1987. Some years later, in the wake of a number of research-related controversies, a Tri-Council Working Group involving all three federal research-funding agencies—the Medical Research Council of Canada (as it was then), the Natural Sciences and Engineering Research Council of Canada (NSERC), and the Social Sciences and Humanities Research Council of Canada (SSHRC)—was convened to develop a common set of ethics guidelines that would govern virtually all publicly funded research involving humans in Canada (an international first). In 1998 the *Tri-Council Policy Statement on Research Involving Humans* (TCPS) was adopted. These guidelines outline the expectations regarding ethics review and set out the rules for researchers and institutions that receive research funds from these agencies. The TCPS is the responsibility of the Interagency Advisory Panel on Research Ethics (PRE)—an organization that reports to the three federal funding agencies: the Canadian Institutes of Health Research (CIHR), which replaced the Medical Research Council in 2000, the NSERC, and the SSHRC.

In 2002, in the absence of specific guidelines for research involving human stem cells, the CIHR issued guidelines for CIHR-funded stem cell research titled (following a series of revisions) *Updated Guidelines for Human Pluripotent Stem Cell Research* (Canadian Institutes of Health Research 2010). In 2007 additional research ethics guidelines were issued to promote ethical and culturally competent research involving aboriginal people: *CIHR Guidelines for Health Research Involving Aboriginal People* (Canadian Institutes of Health Research 2007). In December 2010 the second edition of the TCPS (TCPS2) was released. The guidelines for research involving aboriginal people were incorporated into chapter 9 of the TCPS2, while the stem cell guidelines were only incorporated by reference (meaning the stem cell guidelines remained a stand-alone document under the purview of the CIHR). In 2013, recognizing the wisdom of having one comprehensive set of research ethics guidelines, the PRE elected to revise the TCPS2 to fully incorporate the stem cell guidelines, thereby ensuring that there would only be one national research ethics oversight organization.

A contentious issue in Canadian research ethics is conflict of interest. For years there have been repeated calls for the federal research granting agencies to step away from the governance of research ethics because of structural conflict of interest (i.e., they have a mandate to promote research and a mandate to regulate research and, most importantly in doing so, to protect research participants). This recommendation was made most forcefully in the 2008 final report of the Experts Committee for Human Research Participant Protection in Canada (2008), titled *Moving Ahead: Final Report.* Specifically, the Experts Committee recommended that a new organization, the Canadian Council for the Protection of Human Research Participants, be created to oversee research ethics programs and that the council be responsible for developing research ethics policies, education standards, and an accreditation program. While there has been some work on the recommendations regarding policy, education, and accreditation, there has been no action on the recommendation to establish an independent national council.

In addition to concerns about structural conflict of interest, there have been concerns about competing interests in the context of university-industry partnerships. The *Report of the Committee of Inquiry on the Case Involving Dr. Nancy Olivieri, the Hospital for Sick Children, the University of Toronto, and Apotex Inc.* (Thompson, Baird, and Downie 2001) addresses the issue of academic freedom for researchers and emphasizes its importance in relation to the obligation to promote the public interest. The central issue in this case was the right of research participants to be informed of research risks identified during the course of a clinical trial and the obligation of the researcher to disclose such risks in the face of objections from the industry sponsor.

Another important national research ethics report is the *Final Report of the National Placebo Working Committee on the Appropriate Use of Placebos on Clinical Trials in Canada* (National Placebo Working Committee 2004). This report concludes that clinicians both within and outside clinical research have a fiduciary obligation to patients and that the concept of clinical equipoise can be used to test whether a clinician-researcher's fiduciary obligation is met in a specific protocol. This view informs Canadian policy on placebo-controlled clinical trials in TCPS2 and explains the limits on the use of placebos with control groups. Canadians have made important contributions to the literature on clinical equipoise, placebo-controlled trials, and therapeutic misconception (Freedman, Glass, and Weijer 1996a, 1996b; Kimmelman 2007).

Public Health Ethics. A number of public health threats, starting in 2000, prompted renewed interest in public health ethics in Canada with a focus on infectious disease control. In May 2000 there was an outbreak of *E. coli* in Walkerton, Ontario. In April 2001 there was an outbreak of *Cryptosporidium parvum* in North Battleford, Saskatchewan. In 2003 there was the severe acute respiratory syndrome (SARS) epidemic in the Greater Toronto area followed by the pending threat of a global pandemic.

The Public Health Agency of Canada (PHAC) was created in September 2004, and the Public Health Agency of Canada Act received royal assent in December 2006. Though created in response to crises in infectious disease, the PHAC's mandate is much broader. It is to "promote health; prevent and control chronic diseases and injuries; prevent and control infectious diseases; prepare for and respond to public health emergencies; and strengthen public health capacity in a manner consistent with a shared understanding of the determinants of health and of the common factors that maintain health or lead to disease and injury" (Public Health Agency of Canada 2011). Within the PHAC there is a Public Health Law and Ethics Program.

In 2005 the University of Toronto Joint Centre for Bioethics Pandemic Influenza Working Group published *Stand on Guard for Thee: Ethical Considerations in Preparedness Planning for Pandemic Influenza.* This document was widely consulted and influenced a number of policy documents, including the World Health Organization's 2007 report *Ethical Considerations in Developing a Public Health Response to Pandemic Influenza.* The Canadian document addressed ethical, legal, and social issues related to influenza response, with particular attention to "health workers' duty to provide care during a communicable disease outbreak; restricting liberty in the interest of public health by measures such as quarantine; priority setting, including the allocation of scarce resources, such as vaccines and antiviral medicines; and global governance implications, such as travel advisories" (World Health Organization 2007). This report built on prior work by Ross Upshur (2002) to develop a public health ethics framework.

Reaching beyond pandemic planning to public health ethics, in 2008 Françoise Baylis, Nuala Kenny, and Susan Sherwin (2008, 196) proposed a framework for relational public health ethics that aims to "embrace the full spectrum of public health responsibilities from poverty, to sanitation, to pollution, to infectious disease, to epidemics and pandemic threats, to global warming, to bioterrorism." Their work has been well received in government circles.

UNIQUE FEATURES OF CANADIAN BIOETHICS

It has been said that Canadians are but Americans with good health care. This jest points to an important feature of Canadian bioethics. The commitment to publicly funded health care and the multicultural nature of Canadian society make for different starting assumptions in contemporary bioethics discussions. Another unique feature of bioethics in Canada is the role of the Canadian Charter.

In addition Canada's prominence in feminist bioethics is noteworthy. Feminist bioethics is especially concerned with systematic oppression on the basis of gender, race, class, ethnicity, disability, sexual orientation, and so on. Canadian scholars have made important contributions to the theoretical and applied literature in feminist ethics. Canadians are regular contributors to the *International Journal of Feminist Approaches to Bioethics* (*IJFAB*). Moreover year after year Canadians have been elected to the Board of the International Network of Feminist Approaches to Bioethics, including Susan Sherwin, Françoise Baylis, Carolyn McLeod, Carolyn Ells, and Kirstin Borgerson. Another area of strength is mental health ethics and neuroethics. Prolific contributors to the relevant literature include Walter Glannon, Judy Illes, and Eric Racine.

More generally bioethics in Canada is now widely recognized as an established multidisciplinary field. It has made, and continues to make, important contributions to public policy (both nationally and internationally), with particular attention to issues of social justice. Indeed a Canadian, Michèle Stanton-Jean, was president of the United Nations Educational, Scientific and Cultural Organization (UNESCO) International Bioethics Committee from 2002 to 2005, during which time the Universal Declaration on Bioethics and Human Rights was developed (adopted in 2005).

This is a twice-revised version of the entry that was first written by John R. Williams and David J. Roy in 1995.

BIBLIOGRAPHY

Baylis, Françoise. 2000. "Expert Testimony by Persons Trained in Ethical Reasoning: The Case of Andrew Sawatzky." *Journal of Law, Medicine and Ethics* 28 (3): 224–31.

Baylis, Françoise; Barry Hoffmaster; Susan Sherwin; and Kirstin Borgerson, eds. 2011. *Health Care Ethics in Canada.* 3rd ed. Toronto: Nelson.

Baylis, Françoise; Nuala Kenny; and Susan Sherwin. 2008. "A Relational Account of Public Health Ethics." *Public Health Ethics* 1 (3): 196–209.

Boetzkes Gedge, Elisabeth, and Wilfrid Waluchow, eds. 2012. *Readings in Health Care Ethics.* 2nd ed. Peterborough, ON: Broadview.

Canadian Institutes of Health Research. 2007. *CIHR Guidelines for Health Research Involving Aboriginal People.* http://www.cihr-irsc.gc.ca/e/29134.html

Canadian Institutes of Health Research. 2010. *Updated Guidelines for Human Pluripotent Stem Cell Research.* http://www.cihr-irsc.gc.ca/e/42071.html

Canadian Institutes of Health Research, Natural Sciences and Engineering Research Council of Canada, and Social Sciences and Humanities Research Council of Canada. 2010. *Tri-Council Policy Statement: Ethical Conduct for Research Involving Humans.* http://www.pre.ethics.gc.ca/pdf/eng/tcps2/TCPS_2_FINAL_Web.pdf

Canadian Medical Association. 2004. *CMA Code of Ethics.* http://policybase.cma.ca/dbtw-wpd/PolicyPDF/PD04-06.pdf

Canadian Nurses Association. 2008. *Code of Ethics for Registered Nurses.* http://www2.cna-aiic.ca/CNA/documents/pdf/publications/Code_of_Ethics_2008_e.pdf

Carter v. Canada (Attorney General). 2012. BCSC 886 (CanLII).

Catholic Health Alliance of Canada. 2012. *Health Ethics Guide.* 3rd ed. http://www.chac.ca/resources/ethics/ethicsguide_e.php

Chaoulli v. Québec (Attorney General). 2005. SCC 35 (CanLII), [2005] 1 SCR 791.

College of Physicians and Surgeons of Manitoba. 2007. *Withholding and Withdrawing Life-Sustaining Treatment.* Statement no. 1602. http://cpsm.mb.ca/cjj39alckF30a/wp-content/uploads/st1602.pdf

Commission on the Future of Health Care in Canada. 2002. *Building on Values: The Future of Health Care in Canada.* http://publications.gc.ca/collections/Collection/CP32-85-2002E.pdf

Downie, Jocelyn. 2004. *Dying Justice: A Case for Decriminalizing Euthanasia and Assisted Suicide in Canada.* Toronto: University of Toronto Press.

Downie, Jocelyn, and Jennifer Llewellyn, eds. 2011. *Being Relational: Reflections on Relational Theory and Health Law.* Vancouver: UBC Press.

Evans, Robert G. 1988. "'We'll Take Care of It for You': Health Care in the Canadian Community." *Daedalus* 117 (4): 155–89.

Experts Committee for Human Research Participant Protection in Canada. 2008. Moving Ahead: Final Report. Ottawa. http://noveltechethics.ca/files/files/Policy/Research_Ethics/Moving_Ahead.pdf

Flood, Colleen, and Bryan Thomas. 2010. "Blurring of the Public/Private Divide: The Canadian Chapter." *European Journal of Health Law* 173 (3): 257–78.

Freedman, Benjamin; Kathleen Glass; and Charles Weijer. 1996a. "Placebo Orthodoxy in Clinical Research, I: Empirical and Methodological Myths." *Journal of Law, Medicine and Ethics* 24 (3): 243–51.

Freedman, Benjamin; Kathleen Glass; and Charles Weijer. 1996b. "Placebo Orthodoxy in Clinical Research, II: Ethical, Legal, and Regulatory Myths." *Journal of Law, Medicine and Ethics* 24 (3): 252–59.

Glannon, Walter. 2007a. *Bioethics and the Brain.* New York: Oxford University Press.

Glannon, Walter, ed. 2007b. *Defining Right and Wrong in Brain Science: Essential Readings in Neuroethics.* New York: Dana.

Glannon, Walter. 2011. *Brain, Body, and Mind: Neuroethics with a Human Face.* New York: Oxford University Press.

Government of Canada. 1989. Bill C-43, An Act Respecting Abortion, 2nd Sess., 34th Parl.

Government of Canada. 1982. Constitutions Act, 1982 c,11 (U.K.) Schedule B Canadian Charter of Rights and Freedoms. http://laws-lois.justice.gc.ca/eng/Const/page-15.html

Illes, Judy. 2006. *Neuroethics: Defining the Issues in Theory, Practice, and Policy.* Oxford: Oxford University Press.

Illes, Judy, and Barbara Sahakian, eds. 2011. *The Oxford Handbook of Neuroethics.* Oxford: Oxford University Press.

Kimmelman, Jonathan. 2007. "The Therapeutic Misconception at 25: Treatment, Research, and Confusion." *Hastings Center Report* 37 (6): 36–42.

LaRochelle, Stanislas, and C. T. Fink. 1943. *Handbook of Medical Ethics for Nurses, Physicians, and Priests*. 2nd ed. Translated by M. E. Poupore. Westminster, MD: Newman Book Shop.

Nancy B. v. Hôtel-Dieu de Québec. 1992. 69 CCC (3d) 450 (Qc Sup Ct).

National Placebo Working Committee. 2004. *Final Report of the National Placebo Working Committee on the Appropriate Use of Placebos on Clinical Trials in Canada*. http://www.cihr-irsc.gc.ca/e/25139.html#toc1

Olivia Pratten v. Attorney General of British Columbia, et al. 2013. CanLII 30404 (SCC).

Osler, William. 1985. *The Collected Essays of Sir William Osler*. Vol. 1, *The Philosophical Essays*. Edited by John P. McGovern and Charles G. Roland. Birmingham, AL: Classics of Medicine Library.

Paquin, Jules. 1954. *Morale et Médecine*. Montreal: Comité des Hôpitaux du Québec.

Parliamentary Committee on Palliative and Compassionate Care. 2011. *Not to Be Forgotten: Care of Vulnerable Canadians*. http://pcpcc-cpspsc.com/wp-content/uploads/2011/11/ReportEN.pdf

Public Health Agency of Canada. 2011. "Mandate." http://www.phac-aspc.gc.ca/about_apropos/what-eng.php

Québec Assembly, Select Committee on Dying with Dignity. 2012. *Dying with Dignity*. http://www.dyingwithdignity.ca/database/files/library/Quebec_death_with_dignity_report.pdf

R. v. Latimer. 2001. SCC 1 CanLII [2001] 1 SCR 3.

R. v. Morgentaler. 1988. CanLII 90 (SCC), [1988] 1 SCR 30.

Racine, Eric. 2010. *Pragmatic Neuroethics: Improving Treatment and Understanding of the Mind-Brain*. Cambridge, MA: MIT Press.

Rasouli v. Sunnybrook Health Sciences Centre. 2011. ONCA 482 (Can LII).

Reference re Assisted Human Reproduction Act. 2010. SCC 61 (CanLII), [2010] 3 SCR 457.

Rodriguez v. British Columbia (Attorney General). 1993. Can LII 75 (SCC), [1993] 3 SCR 519.

Royal Commission on New Reproductive Technologies. 1993. *Proceed with Care: The Final Report of the Royal Commission on New Reproductive Technologies*. Vol. 1. Ottawa: Minister of Supply and Services Canada.

Royal Society of Canada Expert Panel. 2011. *End-of-Life Decision Making*. http://rsc-src.ca/sites/default/files/pdf/RSCEndofLifeReport2011_EN_Formatted_FINAL.pdf

Sherwin, Susan. 1992. *No Longer Patient: Feminist Ethics and Health Care*. Philadelphia: Temple University Press.

Standing Senate Committee on Social Affairs, Science, and Technology. 2002. *The Health of Canadians: The Federal Role; Final Report*. Vol. 6, *Recommendations for Reform*. http://www.parl.gc.ca/Content/SEN/Committee/372/soci/rep/repoct02vol6-e.htm

Storch, Janet; Patricia Rodney; and Rosalie Starzomski, eds. 2012. *Toward a Moral Horizon: Nursing Ethics for Leadership and Practice*. 2nd ed. Toronto: Pearson Education Canada.

Sumner, L. Wayne. 2011. *Assisted Death: A Study in Ethics and Law*. Oxford: Oxford University Press.

Thompson, Jon; Patricia Baird; and Jocelyn Downie. 2001. *Report of the Committee of Inquiry on the Case Involving Dr. Nancy Olivieri, the Hospital for Sick Children, the University of Toronto, and Apotex Inc.* Toronto: CAUT.

University of Toronto Joint Centre for Bioethics, Pandemic Influenza Working Group. 2005. *Stand on Guard for Thee: Ethical Considerations in Preparedness Planning for Pandemic Influenza*. http://www.jointcentreforbioethics.ca/publications/documents/stand_on_guard.pdf

Upshur, Ross. 2002. "Principles for the Justification of Public Health Intervention." *Canadian Journal of Public Health* 93 (2): 101–3.

World Health Organization. 2007. *Ethical Considerations in Developing a Public Health Response to Pandemic Influenza*. http://www.who.int/csr/resources/publications/WHO_CDS_EPR_GIP_2007_2c.pdf

Françoise Baylis (2004, 2014)
Professor and Canada Research Chair in Bioethics and Philosophy, Novel Tech Ethics, Faculty of Medicine, Dalhousie University

III. LATIN AMERICA

This entry presents a historical panorama of biomedical ethics in Latin America, the name given to a linguistic and cultural community encompassing South America, Central America, Mexico, and part of the Caribbean. From political, economic, and social points of view, the Latin American nations are quite different, although at present they have underdevelopment in common.

Since bioethics as a discipline flourished first in the United States, it is useful to compare medical ethics in North America, with its predominantly Anglo and northern European culture, and in Latin America, pointing out the differences between the two traditions within the Western culture.

First, the Latin American tradition of medical ethics is described; next, the incipient bioethics movement in Latin America is considered; then the major bioethical problems of the region are noted; and finally, the challenge to Latin American bioethics is discussed.

THE LATIN AMERICAN TRADITION OF MEDICAL ETHICS

When Spain and Portugal established colonies in the Americas, they brought with them the profound influence of the Roman Catholic Church, heir to that Western culture whose roots are Greek philosophy, Judaism, and Roman law. The Catholic tradition has in fact defined Latin American ethics and the Latin American ethos. First, Catholic moral theology built a system of medical ethics based on (1) natural-law theory as the basis of morality; (2) the principle of the sanctity of human life as a moral criterion; and (3) the commandment of love, or the virtue of charity, as the golden rule. Second, through their pastoral role and religious authority, priests reinforced the paternalistic medical ethos of the Hippocratic tradition. The paternalistic model of medical responsibility centered on the principle of beneficence (that benefit must be produced and harm avoided); the principle of autonomy is not taken into account. Beneficent paternalism has dominated the relationships between doctor and patient, and between medicine and society, in Latin America up to the present day.

As the cultures of northern and southern Europe evolved in the Americas, the differences between the two were accentuated. Modernity did not have the same secular, liberal, and pluralistic cast in Latin America as it did in North America. In Latin America, morality was not detached from metaphysics and religion; it did not establish a new basis in scientific and political rationalism, nor did it set itself up as critical and autonomous over against the natural and supernatural order of the medieval epoch.

Beginning in the eighteenth century, it is possible to contrast two ethics: the classical tradition of virtue, represented by the Mediterranean peoples (particularly the Italians and Spaniards), and the tradition in which principles are central, dominant in the English- and German-speaking countries (McIntyre 1984). In Latin America, the political paternalism of the *ancien régime* and the medical paternalism of the Hippocratic tradition go together; the result is a paternalistic model on both the individual-clinical and the social policy levels.

The ethics and ethos of Latin American medicine are expressed in professional codes of ethics and in health policy and legislation. The forebear of all these normative institutions was the *protomédicato*. Originating in the Roman Empire, the *protomédicato* was a tribunal of royal physicians (*protomédicos*) that granted professional licenses and acted as a judicial and legislative body in health matters. In the thirteenth century, Castile was one of the first kingdoms to establish legal regulations for medical practice and public health; examples of this were found in the School of Salerno and the laws of Frederick II in Sicily (Mainetti, 1989). The *protomédicato* was transplanted from Spain to the Americas, where it endured until the period of independence (early nineteenth century), at which point medical instruction, practice, and policy began to be modernized.

In the twentieth century, professional associations and medical colleges in various countries began to formulate their own codes of ethics, in accordance with the deontological tradition that regulates the relationships of doctors among themselves, with the public, and with the state. One of the first such codes was drawn up in 1918 by Luis Razetti, a leading Venezuelan physician who specialized in medical deontology, under the influence of the French—an influence that was at that time very perceptible in Latin American society in general and in the medical culture in particular. This same code was later adopted in Colombia (1919) and in Peru (1920); it provided a basic model for other Latin American codes, which are essentially traditional guides for professional courtesy or etiquette, the relationships of physicians among themselves, with the patient, and with the state (León 1973).

The medical codes promulgated in many Latin American countries are influenced by a variety of factors, among them biomedical progress, malpractice legislation, and the political changes throughout the region after decades of military rule. Brazil's Federal Code of Medical Ethics (1988), for example, incorporates concern about new problems like AIDS and reformulates the rule of medical confidentiality. The Medical College of Chile has been very active since 1984, demonstrating its sensitivity to—among other issues—the participation of Chilean physicians in torture during the years of authoritarian rule that ended in 1984 (Mainetti 1990).

The state's responsibility for health care has constitutional status in Latin American countries (Pan American Health Organization 1989). The right to health care is included among social and economic rights. The first nation to incorporate the right to health care in its constitution was Chile, in 1925, followed by Bolivia, Cuba, Guatemala, Guyana, Haiti, Honduras, Mexico, Nicaragua, Paraguay, Peru, Uruguay, and Venezuela. The responsibility of the state for health planning is legislated by many Latin American countries, which provide for universal access to essential medical services and a national health care system that is either free or based on co-payments, but with limited coverage. In Latin American government, health policy generally demonstrates a significant gap between principle and practice: between justice, which theoretically endorses the equal right to health care, and actual practice in societies that, owing to their social and economic development, are not able to guarantee that this and other rights will be respected.

Codes of ethics and health legislation are based on a moral view that is both dogmatic (codified and legalistic, in contrast with philosophic, analytic, and critical) and authoritarian (based on professional authority, which is partly religious and partly governmental, rather than civic or democratic). The Latin American tradition of medical ethics can be defined as naturalistic, paternalistic, dogmatic, and authoritarian. The new Latin American medical ethics, represented by bioethics, has developed in contrast with this older tradition.

THE BIOETHICS MOVEMENT IN LATIN AMERICA

The bioethics revolution that has occurred in the industrialized nations has arisen both from the scientific and technological progress of biomedicine and from the liberal and pluralistic character of those nations. By contrast, in the developing Latin American countries bioethical interests correspond more to those of a low-technology society and a tradition of confessional morality (Mainetti 1988). Bioethics, based on the principles of beneficence, autonomy, and justice, may be seen as civic morality to which the parties to an increasingly conflictual relationship—physician, patient, and society—appeal. Or bioethics may be seen as medical culture, expressed in the "introduction of the moral subject into medicine," the promotion of the rational, free agent in the therapeutic relationship. It is fair to say, however, that bioethics has barely arrived in Latin America in either guise.

Latin American bioethics evolved over a period of thirty years, in three decade-long stages, commencing in the 1970s: reception, assimilation, and re-creation. Public and academic interest in bioethical topics appeared in the 1980s with the proliferation of new medical technologies, such as those used in intensive care units, transplants, and assisted reproduction, and with the appearance of democratic governments in the region. On the one hand, legal intervention in medical cases increased, due perhaps to the distances created between the professional and the patient by specialization. Malpractice and a patient's rights movement in Latin America imitated the early history of US bioethics. On the other hand, there was an academic rehabilitation of practical, moral, and political philosophy as they could be applied to medicine. This development was in keeping with the kind of ideological pluralism and consensus formation that has characterized bioethics as a discipline in the United States.

The academic and professional development of bioethics in Latin America has been a process of incorporating the US model in stages. As the twentieth century neared its end, the institutionalization of the discipline as expressed in the creation of research centers, professorships at universities, ethics committees at hospitals, and national commissions on bioethics could not be said to be significant. Nor had the three main functions of bioethical studies been carried out. These are the educational function (deontology and legal medicine still stand for ethics at medical schools); the consultative function (clinical and health care ethics are not practiced in hospitals and other health care facilities); and the political function (groups of experts have not formed to advise public institutions on biomedical norms). Bioethics is also just beginning to capture the attention of the public and the media.

Among the groups active on the Latin American bioethics scene, two deserve mention: the Instituto de Humanidades Médicas y Centro de Bioética of the Fundación Mainetti (Institute for the Medical Humanities and Center for Bioethics of the Mainetti Foundation) in La Plata, Argentina, and the Instituto Colombiano de Estudios Bioéticos (Colombian Institute for Bioethical Studies) in Bogotá, Colombia. The former, established in 1972, combines the European and Anglo-American traditions of medical humanism, serving as a model and resource center for other countries in the region, particularly through its Escuela Latinoamericana de Bioética (Latin American School of Bioethics, ELABE), directed by Juan Carlos Tealdi. The latter, founded in 1985 by Fernando Sánchez Torres, former dean of the National University of Colombia, together with the ASCOFAME (Colombian Association of Medical Faculties) with its Center for Medical Ethics, directed by Alfonso Llano Escobar, S.J., and the Colombian School of Medicine and its Health Care Ethics Committee, also lead in the process of renovating medical ethics in the region.

Other academic and professional associations have emerged in Latin American countries in recent years for the purpose of developing programs of bioethical studies: the Department of Bioethics of the Catholic University of Uruguay; the Sindicato Médico of Uruguay, a very important professional organization that appointed a bioethics commission; the Department of Bioethics of the Chilean Catholic University; and the Chilean Medical College, mentioned above. These associations work actively on deontological questions, and the Brazilian Association of Medical Ethics Teachers emphasizes bioethical issues.

The bioethics enterprise also can be evaluated by the number of people interested in the discipline; by courses, conferences, and other scientific activities; and by the publication of books and articles. The classic 1973 Latin American text on medical ethics, by Augusto León, was followed by several bioethics texts (Mainetti 1988; Varga 1988; Velez and Alfonso 1989). According to a 1990 report issued by the Pan American Health Organization, conditions in Latin America were expected to encourage the development of programs to integrate medical ethics into the health system. This integration could occur along a broad spectrum ranging from legislation and public policies to academic curricula, and should include the revision of the ethics codes of established medical associations. To this end, the Latin American School of Bioethics has been coordinating a regional program of hospital ethics committees since 1989 (Tealdi and Mainetti 1990). The growth of interest in bioethics justified a Latin American bioethics association to unite isolated efforts, and thus to offer a concerted response to the needs of the region. Meeting in La Plata, Argentina, in December 1991, representatives from several Latin American nations founded the Federaciòn

Latinoamericana de Instituciones Bioéticas (FELAIBE; Latin American Federatíon of Bioethics Institutions).

In 1990 the Pan American Health Organization (PAHO) commissioned James Drane of the United States to produce a decisive report that reviewed the development of bioethics in Latin America and proposed several steps for the further regional development of the discipline (Drane and Fuenzalida 1991). That same year, PAHO published a special issue on bioethics, edited by Susan Scholle Connor and Hernán Fuenzalida-Puelma, formally introducing bioethics in Latin America. This was the first collection in which early authors in the field addressed diverse topics and set out different perspectives on the discipline. Finally, PAHO, a pioneer among international health organizations, created the Regional Program on Bioethics (1994) with headquarters in Santiago de Chile, but whose activities are decentralized in order to serve all the member countries of PAHO. This program—a comprehensive policy in bioethics and its associated disciplines—entered a new stage under the outstanding scholar Fernando Lolas Stepke's leadership (Programa Regional de Bioética 2000).

Bioethics has become a field of new challenges in Latin America. A seeming uniformity hides a rich, heterogeneous set of activities. Not only European and Christian influences but also indigenous intellectual traditions are very important in the development of Latin American bioethics. It does not have its own philosophy, as Anglo-American bioethics is perceived to have, but it does have its own literature or narrative. The particular historical setting, cultural ethos, and social reality of Latin America could infuse new life into the global bioethics community. In this sense, a symptom of the new times is the fact that the Second Congress of the International Association of Bioethics took place in Buenos Aires, Argentina, in 1994, and the Sixth Congress was held in Brasilia, Brazil, in 2002. A "new Brazilian bioethics" or "hard bioethics," inspired by Brazil's contradictory social reality, began to flourish at the turn of the twentieth century, and explores alternative perspectives to traditional bioethical currents (Garrafa 2000).

Bioethics first arrived in Latin America as a foreigner, and later underwent a transcultural shaping. Transplanted to a new habitat, bioethics took on its own distinctive character and voices and has become a strong intellectual and political enterprise (Lolas Stepke 1994, 1998).

In comparison to the North American style of bioethics, Latin American bioethics takes a more theoretical and philosophical approach. As a search for a *critical, radical,* and *global* bioethics, Latin American bioethics represents a global, "post-bioethical" age (Drane 1998; Spinsanti 1995). Although Latin American bioethics is far from being a unified theoretical system or a single coherent perspective, it represents the *ethica spes* of the new millennium.

MAJOR TOPICS IN LATIN AMERICAN BIOETHICS

Latin American countries share a concern about a number of problems with implications for both law and policy. A common sociocultural and public-health situation defines the Latin American biomedical ethos. Ethnomedical ethics ought to be an essential topic because the health and disease conceptions, practices, and values, as well as the needs, of the native (precolonial) Latin American peoples are not properly understood by academic medicine and the health policy of the dominant culture. These peoples still await the fulfillment of the World Health Organization's proclamation calling for the integration of their healing arts into modern medicine. Among the most pressing bioethical issues facing Latin America are the following.

Reproductive Ethics. Both the prevention of human reproduction (contraception, sterilization, and abortion) and assisted human reproduction (reproductive technologies) are central issues for Latin American population policy. This policy is clearly linked to health and to religious, secular, and geopolitical factors. Underdevelopment and overpopulation form a vicious circle that distances societies more and more from the goal of sustainable development. The Catholic Church does not tolerate what it calls "artificial" control of fertility and condemns abortion, which is legally prohibited in most Latin American countries. To date neither public debate nor legislative reform has occurred, although the widespread and frequent practice of clandestine abortion effectively expresses Latin American governments' laissez-faire policies. The ethical complexity of assisted reproduction provokes polemics about the status of the embryo without leading to a declared war between "Catholics" and "secularists, " but this area requires legal regulation.

The Ethics of Death and Dying. In Latin America, death is not as medicalized nor is the medical profession as tormented about it as is the case in the First World. The technological assault on dying, the new *danse macabre* in the intensive care unit, does not offer the same sort of spectacle in Latin America as it does in the United States. Nevertheless, the contemporary "art of dying" is a challenge in Latin America, too, even if living wills, do-not-resuscitate orders (DNRs), the ethical principles of critical care medicine, and the pro-euthanasia movement have yet to become major issues. Palliative medicine, the hospice movement, and campaigns for death with dignity are the modern Latin American versions of *ars moriendi.* At the beginning of life, pediatrics ethics committees are improving regulations regarding the treatment of premature and disabled newborns. At the end of life, legislation authorizing removal and transplantation of organs has advanced markedly in many Latin American countries (Fuenzalida-Puelma 1990).

Research Ethics. Biomedical research in Latin America lacks both a legislative framework and an effective set of controls. Much research also lacks scientific validity and, motivated more by monetary interest than by interest in knowledge, overlooks patient's rights such as consent and confidentiality. Developing countries must create the scientific and financial conditions for research itself; they must also attract projects that involve international cooperation while avoiding the risks such cooperation often brings with it, including economic and human exploitation. Oversight committees are needed so that international standards, with criteria appropriate to the cultural modalities of each community, may be applied. US standards of consent, for instance, cannot be implemented easily in the social conditions of developing countries (Levine 1982). Questions that must be considered in the future include research priorities, allocation of resources for research, and access to new, experimental drugs. This last issue, which has an especially high profile because of the global AIDS crisis, now involves not only the right of patients to protection from possible ill effects but also their right to have access to such drugs, which may prolong or save their lives.

Health Care Ethics. Health status in Latin America must be seen within a larger picture of underdevelopment, poverty, hunger, and economic crisis aggravated by the foreign debt of the region. Two global short-term goals set by the World Health Organization have not yet been reached in Latin America: Infant mortality has not been brought below 5 percent, and life expectancy has not risen beyond sixty-five years. Health care expenditures in Latin America did not exceed 5 percent of the gross national product in the 1970s and 1980s, compared with 10 percent for the so-called developed countries.

Although there is a plethora of medical students and an oversupply of physicians, approximately 75 percent of the population of Latin America does not receive medical attention. This dramatizes the gap between the proclaimed right to health care and the conditions necessary to exercise it. Primary care—including family planning, maternal and child care, immunization, health counseling and education, campaigns against tuberculosis, and treatment of infectious diseases—should be the goal of health policy in all developing nations. Health care policy must be focused on health as an indicator of development, oriented to the basic needs of the majority of the population, and designed to promote medical care based on criteria of equity, integration, participation, and efficiency (Pan American Health Organization 1989).

Between 80 and 90 percent of the resources allocated to health care in Latin America is spent on secondary and tertiary care. "Bioethics in the time of cholera," to paraphrase the novelist Gabriel García Márquez—medical ethics faced with plagues like cholera and AIDS—sums up the challenge to health care ethics in Latin America.

Environmental Ethics. The environmental problems of Latin America are in part peculiar to the region and in part similar to those in western Europe and the United States. Overpopulated cities like Mexico City, Caracas, and São Paulo are more polluted than their European counterparts, and the Latin American urban crisis ranges from street cleaning to disposing of radioactive wastes from nuclear power plants.

In agricultural areas, the indiscriminate use of biocides contaminates crops and reduces the fertility of the soil. The extinction of animal and plant species produces imbalances in the ecosystem. Of worldwide importance is the devastation of the Amazon rainforest, the largest jungle in the world. An ecological reserve with an influence on world climate, the area has been deforested by 10 percent. It faces the prospect of destruction within half a century, for reasons not unrelated to the sizable foreign debt owed by Brazil.

Governments and publics in Latin America are just beginning to become conscious of the importance of the environment to human and animal health; to national, regional, and world economies; to the preservation of nature and of life itself. Some countries have environmental protection legislation, projects to protect or preserve natural resources, and active ecology movements. Bioethics, however, has yet to raise its voice in civic and public arenas with regard to environmental ethics (that is, ecological rights), a new type of third-generation human rights, and policies of sustainable development (Pan American Health Organization 1987).

THE CHALLENGE OF BIOETHICS FOR LATIN AMERICA

Because of its humanistic medical tradition and the social conditions of developing countries, Latin America can offer a distinctive bioethics perspective. There are two dimensions to this perspective. First, a discipline established along European lines of the general philosophy or theory of medicine, with three main branches (medical anthropology, epistemology, and axiology), may be better equipped to transform academic, scientific medicine into a new humanistic biomedical paradigm (Mainetti 1988). Such an approach would guard against the accusations often lodged against bioethics in the United States and Europe: that the discourse of bioethics only appears to humanize medicine while obscuring the real dehumanization of the system. For example, the bioethical discourse on autonomy may hide the depersonalization of medical care and its risks of iatrogenesis, exploitation of the body, and alienation of health. In response to the development of biomedicine in a technological era, bioethics may be able to play a more critical role, one that is less complacent or optimistic about progress.

Second, the Latin American reality of "bioethics in the time of cholera" requires an orientation toward social ethics, with an accent on the common welfare, the good society, and justice rather than on individual rights and personal virtues (the modern and classical traditions of morality, respectively). A macroethics of health or public health may be proposed as an alternative to the Anglo-American tradition of micro or clinical ethics. Greater emphasis can be placed on the social importance of medicine; as far as medical ethics is concerned, the great need in the developing countries is fairness in the allocation of resources and the distribution of health services. Latin America has not lost hope that it might be the continent of justice.

Several decades after its birth, bioethics in the United States is moving toward new intellectual models. This movement shows up in the revisionist-foundationalist debate within the discipline; the application of ethics to other discourses, including the political arena; the rediscovery of ethics of virtue; the return to what is experiential; and the cross-cultural and international dialogue. The bioethics revolution in North America and Europe—summarized in a high-technology *bios* and individualized ethos—must be complemented in Latin America by a humanistic *bios* and a communitarian ethos.

A promising outlook is emerging as the bioethics traditions and problematics of the two Americas move closer to one another. Perhaps in the context of the new world order and the beginning of the twenty-first century, bioethics—the bridge toward the future of humanity—will also be a bridge of inter-American cooperation and integration.

BIBLIOGRAPHY

Brazil. 1988. *Federal Code of Medical Ethics.*

Drane, James F. 1996. "Bioethical Perspectives from Ibero-America." *Journal of Medicine and Philosophy* 21 (6): 557–69.

Drane, James F. 1998. "Universal Medical Ethics." *Quirón* 29 (2): 53–64.

Drane, James F. 1999. "Commentary" (to José A. Mainetti's "Complejo Bioético: Pigmalión, Narciso y Knock"). *Acta psiquiátrica y psicológica de América latina* 45 (2): 109–21.

Drane, James F., and Hernán Fuenzalida. 1991. "Medical Ethics in Latin America: A New Interest and Commitment." *Kennedy Institute of Ethics Journal* 1 (4): 325–38.

Escobar Triana, Jaime. 1996. "Humanistic and Social Education for Physicians: The Experience of the Colombian School of Medicine." *Journal of Medicine and Philosophy* 21 (6): 651–57.

Figueroa, Patricio R., and Hernán Fuenzalida. 1996. "Bioethics in Ibero-America and the Caribbean." *Journal of Medicine and Philosophy* 21 (6): 611–27.

Fuenzalida-Puelma, Hernán. 1990. "Organ Transplantation: The Latin American Legislative Response." *Bulletin of the Pan American Health Organization* 24 (4): 425–45.

Garrafa, Volnei. 2000. "A Bioethical Radiography of Brazil." *Acta Bioethica* 6 (1): 163–81.

León, Augusto. 1973. *Ética en Medicina.* Barcelona: Científico-Médica.

Levine, Robert J. 1982. "Validity of Consent Procedures in Technologically Developing Countries." In *Human Experimentation and Medical Ethics*, edited by Zbigniew Bankowski and Norman Howard-Jones. Geneva: Council for International Organizations of Medical Sciences.

Lolas Stepke, Fernando. 1994. "El discurso bioético: Una anécdota personal." *Quirón* 25 (4): 28–30.

Lolas Stepke, Fernando. 1998. *Bioética.* Santiago de Chile: Editorial Universitaria, S.A.

Lolas Stepke, Fernando. 2000a. "Bioethics and the Culture of Life: A Contribution to Peace." *Bioética Informa* VI (19): 8–11.

Lolas Stepke, Fernando. 2000b. *Bioética y Antropología Médica.* Santiago de Chile: Mediterraneo.

Macklin, Ruth, and Florencia Luna. 1996. "Bioethics in Argentina: A Country Report." *Bioethics* 10 (2): 140–53.

Mainetti, José Alberto. 1988. "Bioethical Problems in the Developing Word: A View from Latin America." *Unitas* 60 (June): 238–48.

Mainetti, José Alberto. 1989. *Ética médica: Introducción histórica.* La Plata, Argentina: Quirón.

Mainetti, José Alberto. 1990. "Bioethics: A New Health Philosophy." *Bulletin of the Pan American Health Organization* 24 (4): 578–81.

Mainetti, José Alberto. 1996. "In Search of Bioethics: A Personal Postscript." *Journal of Medicine and Philosophy* 21 (6): 671–79.

McIntyre, Alistair C. 1984. *After Virtue: A Study in Moral Theory,* 2nd ed. Notre Dame, IN: University of Notre Dame Press.

Pan American Health Organization. 1987. *Informe anual del director.* Washington, DC: Guerra de Macedo, Carlyle (Director).

Pan American Health Organization. 1989. *El derecho a la salud en las Américas: Estudio constitucional comparado.* Washington, DC: Author.

Programa Regional de Bioética OPS/OMS. 2000. "Instituciones y Centros especializados en Bioética en América Latina y el Caribe." Santiago de Chile: Author.

Razzetti, Luis. 1963. *Deontología médica,* Volume 1: *Obras completas.* Caracas: Ministerio de Sanidad y Asistencia Social.

Scholle Connors, S., and Hernán L. Fuenzalida-Puelma. 1991. *Bioethics. Sigues and Perspectivas.* Scientific Publications No. 527 of the Panamerican Health Organization.

Spinsanti, Sandro. 1995. "José Alberto Mainetti: Simboli dell' antichitá classica in America Latina." In *La bioetica: Biografie per una disciplina.* Milano: Franco Angeli.

Tealdi, Juan Carlos, and Mainetti, José Alberto. 1990. "Hospital Ethics Committees." *Bulletin of the Pan American Health Organization* 24 (4): 410–18.

Varga, Andrew C. 1988. *Bioética: Principales problemas*, translated by Alfonso Llano Escobar as *The Main Issues of Bioethics*. Bogotá: Ediciones Paulinas.

Velez, Correa, and Alfonso, Luis. 1989. *Etica médica: Interrogantes acera de la medicina, la vida y la muerte*. Medellín, Colombia: Corporación para Investigaciones Biológicas.

José Alberto Mainetti (1995, 2004)
Instituto de Bioética y Humanidades Médicas de la Fundación Mainetti, Centro Oncologico de Excelencia
Translated by Mary M. Solberg

III. LATIN AMERICA [ADDENDUM]

In the 2000s, bioethics became widely acknowledged as a field throughout Latin America. A number of programs have since developed: educational ones with a regional flavor, enhanced through distance learning, such as the degree offered by the Facultad Latinoamericana de Ciencias Sociales (FLACSO) that grants an accredited diploma—an online specialization and a master's program conceived in Argentina that extends to the region as a whole—as well as onsite programs offering PhDs from different universities (e.g., El Bosque University, Colombia). Substantial improvements have also occurred in research ethics education. In 2000 the Fogarty International Center (National Institutes of Health) launched an international program on the topic, strengthening different bioethics departments in the region (those at the University of Chile, "Ethics of Research in Latin American Countries," and at FLACSO, "A Training Program in Research Ethics in the Americas"). Since the inception of this initiative, research ethics has gone from being a largely foreign concept and an unfamiliar practice to an integral and growing feature of the health care sector (Saenz et al. n.d.). UNESCO also began working in the region offering courses as well as an electronic journal.

Several theoretical analyses have developed. One of which is the scope of "conscientious objection" (Vazquez 2007, 2008; Diniz 2012) following its use by the Catholic Church as a resource to hinder reproductive policies. In addition, new analyses in research ethics have been presented, such as the layered notion of the concept of vulnerability (Luna 2009), standards in research (Luna 2001), or proposals concerning fair benefits or obligations to research participants (Mastroleo 2007; Bergel 2012). Finally, specific situations have also influenced discussions. Consider, for example, violence—such as that occurring in Mexico—or domestic violence (Bardales Mendoza 2012; de la Garza 2012), corruption (Luna 1999), or the inequalities and imbalances perceived in the region (Luna 2005; Arosteguy 2012; Viera Charro 2012). These have been reflected in a number of Latin American concerns and analyses (Luna 1999; Bardales Mendoza 2012; de la Garza 2012).

The 2000s have also been a period of numerous changes in public policies and laws. While some progressive ideas have arisen, other contradictions and loyalties to the Catholic Church still prevail. In a progressive and inclusive spirit, Argentina was the first country in the region to legislate marriage equality, allowing persons of the same sex to marry (InfoLEG Información Legislative 2010) in 2010; in 2012 the opportunity to undergo sex-change surgery covered by the public health care system was passed. In addition, in 2007, following heated debates, abortion laws were enacted in Mexico City, and in 2012 Uruguay (Poder Legislativo 2012) allowed abortion to be performed within the first twelve weeks of pregnancy. This was carried out in a region where countries like Honduras, Chile, Dominican Republic, Salvador, and Nicaragua (GIRE n.d.) still enforce absolute restrictions. The only other countries with permissive laws are Cuba and Guyana. Regarding assisted reproduction, the region witnessed the prohibition of these techniques in Costa Rica and a case was argued against this country before the Inter-American Court of Human Rights (Luna 2008). While this emblematic case was under discussion, a law ruling the free provision of assisted reproduction in public hospitals was approved in a province of Argentina (Law 14.208). Surprisingly, this was done without establishing the status of embryos—a taboo in some countries, where embryos are valued more than women. In this contradictory line, the new project to reform Argentina's Civil Code accepts postmortem insemination and surrogacy (highly controversial practices) and includes one article to grant a different status to ex uterus embryos while, quite inconsistently, still considering in uterus embryos "persons."

Despite the recognition and wide acceptance of bioethics in academia, commissions, and ethics committees, Latin American laws reflect a regionally complex and contradictory reality. They also reveal the obstacles to reproductive rights and the lack of a true valorization of women.

BIBLIOGRAPHY

Arosteguy, Julieta. 2012. "Pensar la salud en Latinoamérica: pobreza, desigualdad, justicia y los determinantes sociales de la salud." In *Cuestiones de Bioética en y desde Latinoamérica*, edited by María Casado and Florencia Luna, 83–98. Navarra, Spain: Aranzadi.

Bardales Mendoza, Olga. 2012. "Violencia familiar y sexual: desafíos actuales para la investigación en Latinoamérica." In *Cuestiones de Bioética en y desde Latinoamérica*, edited by María Casado and Florencia Luna, 439–52. Navarra, Spain: Aranzadi.

Bergel, Salvador. 2012. "El derecho de acceso a los medicamentos: su reconocimiento y las barreras puestas a su ejercicio." In *Cuestiones de Bioética en y desde Latinoamérica,* edited by María Casado and Florencia Luna, 333–48. Navarra, Spain: Aranzadi.

Debora, Diniz. 2012. "Objeción de conciencia y aborto: derechos y deberes de los médicos respecto de la salud pública en Brasil." In *Cuestiones de Bioética en y desde Latinoamérica,* edited by María Casado and Florencia Luna, 145–56. Navarra, Spain: Aranzadi.

Garza, Victoriano de la. 2012. "Bioética en contextos de violencia extrema: vivir y morir en Juárez." In *Cuestiones de Bioética en y desde Latinoamérica,* edited by María Casado and Florencia Luna, 65–82. Navarra, Spain: Aranzadi.

GIRE. n.d. "Informe sobre la situación de la accesibilidad al aborto no punible en América Latina y el Caribe." Accessed March 1, 2013. http://www.gire.org.mx/index.php?option=com_content&view=article&id=568&Itemid=1161&lang=es

InfoLEG Información Legislative. 2010. "Civil marriage." Accessed March 1, 2013. http://www.infoleg.gov.ar/infolegInternet/anexos/165000-169999/169608/norma.htm

Law 14.208 of the Province of Buenos Aires. Accessed March 1, 2013. http://www.gob.gba.gov.ar/legislacion/legislacion/l-14208.html

Luna, Florencia. 1999. "Corruption and Research." *Bioethics* 13 (3/4): 262–72.

Luna, Florencia. 2001. "Is 'Best Proven' a Useless Criterion?" *Bioethics* 15 (4): 273–88.

Luna, Florencia. 2005. "Poverty and Inequality: Challenges for the IAB." *Bioethics* 19 (5/6): 431–59.

Luna, Florencia. 2008. *Reproducción Asistida, Género y Derechos Humanos en Latinoamérica.* San José, Costa Rica: Instituto Interamericano de Derechos Humanos.

Luna, Florencia. 2009. "Elucidating the Concept of Vulnerability: Layers not Labels." *International Journal of Feminist Approaches of Bioethics* 2 (1): 121–39.

Mastroleo, Ignacio. 2007. "Justicia global e investigación biomédica: la obligación post investigación hacia la comunidad anfitriona." *Perspectivas Bioéticas* 23: 76–92.

Poder Legislativo. 2012. Accessed March 1, 2013. http://www.mysu.org.uy/IMG/pdf/ley_promulgada_por_el_poder_ejecutivo-2.pdf

Saenz, C., et al. n.d. "Twelve Years of Fogarty-Funded Bioethics Training in Latin America and the Caribbean: Achievements and Challenges." Unpublished manuscript.

Vazquez, Rodolfo. 2007. *Laicidad una asignatura pendiente.* Coyoacán, Mexico: Fontamara Ediciones.

Vazquez, Rodolfo. 2008. "Laicidad, religión y deliberación pública." *Perspectiva Bioéticas* 13 (24–25): 44–58.

Viera Cherro, Mariana. 2012. "Inequidades múltiples y persistentes en el campo de la reproducción asistida." *Revista de Antropología Social* 21:251–71.

Florencia Luna
Independent Researcher, Consejo Nacional de Investigaciones Científicas y Técnicas (CONICET)
Director of Bioethics Program, Facultad Latinoamericana de Ciencias Sociales (FLACSO)

ANIMAL RESEARCH

This entry consists of the following:

I. HISTORICAL ASPECTS

Ethical discussion of animal experimentation is as old as experimentation itself. Its history encompasses the development of experimentation and changing views about animals that led to the emergence of ethical debates. Culture, religion, philosophy, and politics shaped the ways science developed as well as the development of ethical critiques of it. Animal experimentation is often identified with vivisection—the cutting open of living animals to observe their inner structure and function—but that constitutes only a portion of its practice. Other forms of experimentation include the administration of drugs or diseases, dietary manipulation, and alteration of environment. The purpose of such experimenting was to discover the structure and function of the human and animal body. The improvement of medical practice was an ultimate goal, but knowledge of the body for its own sake was equally important.

EXPERIMENTATION FROM THE GREEKS TO HARVEY

Ancient Greek philosophers such as Aristotle (384–322 B.C.E.) observed and manipulated numerous animals, establishing that mammals in particular resembled humans to the extent that they could act as stand-ins. For much of antiquity dissecting the human body was not allowed. Aristotle did not vivisect animals but others did, particularly the Alexandrian physicians Herophilus (c. 335–c. 280 B.C.E.) and Erasistratus (fl. c. 250 B.C.E.). The Roman physician Galen (129–c. 199 C.E.) followed the Alexandrians in systematically vivisecting animals to examine function. He tied off the ureters to show they channeled urine from the kidneys to the bladder, and he cut the spinal cord in different places to demonstrate the connections between nerves and various body parts. Galen revealed the inner workings of the animal body, and his treatise *De anatomicis administrationibus* (*On Anatomical Procedures* [1956]) explained how it could be done. Galen's concept of the human body, based entirely on his work with animals, remained the model until the sixteenth century.

Scientific inquiry declined along with the Roman Empire's decline. Although Greek and Arab scholars preserved ancient texts, experimental practices did not revive until the late Middle Ages and the development of universities in western Europe. Dead animals were dissected in some Italian medical schools in the twelfth century and dead humans by the early fourteenth. But the questioning of ancient ideas about the body that led to a revival of experimentation (not merely demonstration) began only around 1500. The key text in this revival was *De humani corporis fabrica* (1543; *On the Fabric of the Human Body*) by the Flemish anatomist Andreas Vesalius (1514–1564). Following many of Galen's methods from *On Anatomical Procedures*, Vesalius employed human dissection and animal vivisection to revise the dominant Galenic ideas about the human body, which had been based entirely on animal dissection and vivisection. Over the next century, physicians continued the experimental reevaluation of ancient ideas.

HARVEY AND THE NEW SCIENCE

The English physician William Harvey (1578–1657) overturned the central concept of Galen's physiology with his experimental proof of the circulation of the blood throughout the body. Galen believed blood was formed in the liver and did not circulate but was absorbed by the tissues. Harvey experimented on dozens of different animals, including using vivisection and performing such procedures as ligation of the aorta and vena cava. His *De Motu Cordis* (1628; *The Circulation of the Blood* [1990]) initiated a widespread experimental program across Europe that dismantled the edifice of ancient physiology at the same time that the works of Nicolaus Copernicus and Galileo Galilei dismantled ancient ideas about astronomy and physics, respectively. By 1685, Daniel Le Clerc and Jean-Jacques Manget, the authors of the collection *Bibliotheca Anatomica* (*Anatomical Library*), had declared that more had been learned about the body in the previous fifty years than in all past times. Researchers vivisected animals and otherwise experimented with them to investigate respiration, glandular secretion, nervous function, digestion, and blood pressure, among other functions.

Nonetheless, experimentation did not become the dominant approach to understanding the human and animal body until after 1800. Important experimental work continued in the eighteenth century, such as the 1752 work of the Swiss biologist Albrecht von Haller (1708–1777) on irritability and sensibility. But vitalist physicians, who believed that the functions of life were spontaneous and unrepeatable, rejected experimentation. Many relied on the dissection of dead animals and humans to deduce function from structure.

The 1789 revolution in France led to reforms of its medical and veterinary schools and an increased emphasis on experimenting over theorizing. The surgeon and anatomist Xavier Bichat (1771–1802) established criteria for experimenting with animals, and his student François Magendie (1783–1855) brought the experimental method back to the forefront of physiology. Magendie experimented on live animals to look at the nervous system, digestion, and the way poisons work, claiming he could make physiology as certain a science as Isaac Newton's physics.

THE EMERGENCE OF EXPERIMENTAL PHYSIOLOGY

Magendie's student Claude Bernard (1813–1878) added chemical analysis to animal experimentation but insisted on the uniqueness of life, in contrast to his contemporaries in the German states who aimed to reduce biology to chemistry and physics. Bernard narrowly defined the scope of experimental physiology to exclude questions about the nature of life (the concern of the vitalists), confining his research to explaining specific vital phenomena. In this he was extraordinarily successful, making many major discoveries on digestive and neuromuscular function. Bernard's *Introduction à l'étude de la médecine expérimentale* (1865; *Introduction to the Study of Experimental Medicine* [1957]) was a manifesto for a new science. He argued forcefully for the value of animal experimentation, including vivisection. In his view, it was unethical to perform harmful experiments on humans, but scientists had the right, "wholly and absolutely," to vivisect animals (102). Although various anesthetic agents including ether and chloroform began to appear in the 1840s, scientists did not consistently use anesthesia in animal experiments, fearing it would alter desired outcomes.

As physiology and other experimental medical sciences became distinct disciplines over the nineteenth century, institutional structures also changed. Researchers became professional scientists rather than physicians conducting research in their spare time. Universities in the German states took the lead in establishing state-supported institutions that encouraged cross-disciplinary research and emphasized medical applications, uniting the laboratory with the clinic in the research hospital. These universities competed with each other for the best students and researchers. The German model was widely imitated, including in the United States, where the medical school at Johns Hopkins University (founded in 1893) became the model for the reform of US medical education.

THE GERM THEORY AND THE NORMALIZATION OF ANIMAL RESEARCH

The germ theory of disease, the major medical (rather than physiological) discovery of the era, was as much a result of the diligent individual genius of men such as

Louis Pasteur (1822–1895) and Robert Koch (1843–1910) as of modern institutions of science. Like physiology, the discovery and application of the germ theory relied heavily on animal experiments. But the scale changed: where Bernard had used dozens of animals, Pasteur in France and Koch in Germany used hundreds, and Koch's student Paul Ehrlich (1854–1915) thousands. Physiological research relied on surgical vivisections, but the new bacteriology used animals as living test tubes to grow and test pathogens, vaccines, and antitoxins. Although dogs and pigs continued to be experimental subjects, rats, mice, guinea pigs, and rabbits became much more common in laboratories. Monkeys and other nonhuman primates, however, were rare.

The success of the germ theory was immediate and dramatic. Dozens of microbial diseases were identified between 1880 and 1910, and the development of vaccines and antitoxins radically changed the medical response to infectious disease. Childhood diseases such as diphtheria virtually disappeared within a generation, and the combination of anesthesia with antiseptic practices made surgery far more effective and safe. Success bred further success. Ehrlich sacrificed thousands of mice to discover arsphenamine (sold under the commercial name Salvarsan), the first specific cure for syphilis (1907), and many thousands more led to the discovery and testing of sulfanilamide (1935), penicillin (discovered in 1928 but not used in humans until 1940), and streptomycin (1943).

Unlike bacterial diseases, viral diseases such as polio were more species specific. Polio appeared to attack only primates, and Jonas Salk (1914–1995) and Albert Sabin (1906–1993) developed polio vaccines in the 1950s in monkeys. Monkeys and apes also became the preferred animals for psychological research; although Ivan Pavlov (1849–1936) tested conditioned reflex in dogs (1903), Harry Harlow (1905–1981) in the 1950s tested the nature of motherly love in monkeys.

As these examples indicate, by the twentieth century the experimental use of animals extended to every aspect of the life sciences. Basic physiological work faded as attention turned to disease and other medical research, including drug testing and psychological studies. The establishment of safety standards for food, drugs, and consumer products, beginning in the United States with the Pure Food and Drug Act of 1906, led to the extensive use of animals in product testing. Most recently, new uses for animals have emerged with experiments in cloning and xenotransplantation. But the very ubiquity of animals in science led some to question whether their use was ethical.

ETHICAL DEBATES FROM ANTIQUITY TO BENTHAM

The ethical debates on animal use in science are inextricably tied to broader issues of animal cognition and the human-animal relationship. Aristotle's disciple Theophrastus (c. 372–c. 287 B.C.E.) recognized that the physical analogies between animals and humans made human uses of animals ethically questionable. But he blunted the impact of this insight by arguing that human necessity could overrule ethical considerations. Others in antiquity made similar arguments, but the Christian view as enunciated by Augustine of Hippo (354–430 C.E.)—that animals lack a rational soul and are therefore outside humanity's moral realm—came to dominate in western Europe. When experimentation was revived during the Renaissance, Augustine's distinction between animal and human sanctioned the use of animals. But the medieval theologian Thomas Aquinas (c. 1224–1274) added an important caveat: if compassion was a quality of a good Christian, then humans should not be cruel, even to animals. Cruelty to animals would corrupt the soul and lead to cruel behavior toward humans.

Ethical attention to animal experiments emerged in the seventeenth century for two reasons: the enormous increase in animal research following the work of Harvey and the "beast-machine" doctrine developed by the French philosopher René Descartes (1596–1650). Descartes argued, like Augustine, that animals lacked a rational soul, using their lack of speech as proof. But he further claimed that therefore they were merely automata who lacked the mental capacity to experience pain. It is not clear whether Descartes believed animals feel no pain or only that they cannot cognitively perceive it. In any case, the "beast-machine" notion was received with broad skepticism and some active opposition. Few scientists believed animals could not feel pain, and even fewer used that concept to justify experimenting on them. Most experimenters acknowledged that their actions caused pain but believed it was justified for the greater human good. But some, including the English naturalist John Ray (1627–1705), went further: he wrote in 1693, "the torture of animals is no part of philosophy" (12).

This debate continued through the eighteenth century. The protagonist in a series of engravings titled "The Four Stages of Cruelty" by the English artist William Hogarth (1697–1764) began his career by torturing animals and ended it with murder; the German philosopher Immanuel Kant (1724–1804) had these images in mind when he argued in his *Lectures on Ethics* (1780) that cruelty to animals would damage human moral sensibility, echoing Thomas Aquinas. But, he added, humans have no moral obligations to animals. In the same year (but not published until nearly a decade later), the English political philosopher Jeremy Bentham (1748–1832) changed the terms of the debate: the question, he said, "is not, Can they *reason*? nor, Can they *talk*? but, Can they *suffer*?" (Bentham 1823 [1789], 142–43). According to his utilitarian philosophy, the goal of government and of ethics was to maximize happiness and minimize pain, and because animals could experience happiness, they were within humanity's moral realm.

THE RISE AND DECLINE OF NINETEENTH-CENTURY ANTIVIVISECTION

Early-nineteenth-century efforts toward animal protection did not follow Bentham's arguments but returned to the earlier connection between cruelty to animals and human sensibility. In the 1820s the British Parliament passed the first law forbidding cruelty to farm animals. The Society for the Prevention of Cruelty to Animals was founded around the same time ("Royal" was later added to the name when Queen Victoria became its patron, making its acronym RSPCA). Antivivisection sentiment was strong in Britain, even though few British scientists at this time employed vivisection; when François Magendie visited London in 1824, he was widely condemned in the press. Although the emphasis of critics was on vivisection, this term became shorthand for any experimentation on live animals. The development of anesthesia as well as opiate-based pain relief such as morphine (1804) made the infliction of pain a central issue.

By the 1860s a French society for animal protection existed, but the RSPCA did not hesitate to condemn French practices. In addition, an Englishwoman in Florence, Frances Power Cobbe (1822–1904), led a campaign against a local physiologist who experimented on animals. Cobbe, a journalist and feminist, became the leader of an antivivisection movement in Britain and agitated for antivivisection legislation as British scientists increasingly experimented with animals. The result, the Cruelty to Animals Act of 1876, was the first attempt by a national government to regulate animal experimentation. It required the licensing and inspection of experimenters and facilities. Anesthesia was required except in special circumstances. Scientists, however, were expected to regulate each other, a provision that Cobbe found unacceptable. She continued to press for the abolition of vivisection.

The successes of the new bacteriology made Cobbe's battle an uphill one. Opponents of vivisection often also opposed the germ theory, and the Socialist playwright George Bernard Shaw wittily attacked vivisection, the germ theory, vaccines, and the medical profession itself in the preface to his 1911 play *The Doctor's Dilemma*. Henry Bergh (1811–1888) had founded the American Society for the Prevention of Cruelty to Animals (ASPCA) in 1866, but several attempts to pass federal legislation regulating animal experimentation failed. US Senate hearings in 1896 and 1900 on proposals to regulate vivisection served to mobilize scientists, and the successes of the germ theory made antivivisectionists' arguments that experimentation was useless unconvincing. By the 1920s the antivivisection movement seemed moribund if not dead.

ANIMAL LIBERATION AND NEW REGULATIONS

The revelation after World War II (1939–1945) of Nazi experimentation on humans ironically worked against the regulation of animal experimentation. The Nuremburg Code of 1947 precluded research on human subjects for ends that could be attained by other means and required prior experiments on animals before human trials could take place. Increasingly funded by national governments, biological experimentation grew enormously after 1945 with little criticism on ethical grounds. But the intellectual and social turmoil of the 1960s reopened and transformed old debates. Increasing recognition of universal human rights led to a new consideration of the rights of animals, a concept that had first been argued by the English writer Henry S. Salt (1851–1939) in his *Animals' Rights: Considered in Relation to Social Progress* (1892). Salt's argument that all beings have the right to live their lives without interference gained particular resonance in the context of the liberation movements of the 1960s.

A founding document of the new movement, which encompassed antivivisection as part of a broader agenda, was Australian philosopher Peter Singer's 1975 book *Animal Liberation*. Singer returned to Bentham's utilitarian philosophy to argue that animals have equal interests with humans in maximizing their pleasure and minimizing their pain. He supported his ideas with numerous examples of animal exploitation, employing the term *speciesism* (coined by the animal activist Richard Ryder a few years earlier) as a parallel with *racism* and *sexism*. A few years later, in *The Case for Animal Rights* (1983), the American philosopher Tom Regan argued for animal rights from the basis of inherent rights.

The new movement rejected traditional animal welfare groups such as the RSPCA and ASPCA as accommodationist, and new groups such as the Animal Liberation Front (ALF), founded by British activist Ronnie Lee in 1976, and People for the Ethical Treatment of Animals (PETA), founded in 1980 by Ingrid Newkirk and Alex Pacheco, have employed a variety of tactics to bring attention to animal abuse in laboratories and elsewhere. ALF, the more radical group, has "liberated" lab animals, destroyed property, and threatened scientists. PETA has planted undercover operatives in labs and other animal facilities to reveal abuses.

In the United States, triggered in part by scandals over "puppy mills" that sold pets for research, Congress passed the Laboratory Animal Welfare Act in 1966 to regulate animal dealers and facilities. This act (later known as the Animal Welfare Act) has been amended several times, most recently in 2008; perhaps the most important revision was in 1985, when institutional animal care and use committees were required for institutions that used animals in research. These committees review all animal research at institutions that receive federal funding, using for their reviews the "three Rs" enunciated in *The Principles of Humane Experimental Technique* (1959) by W. M. S. Russell and R. L. Burch. The three Rs—replacement, reduction, and refinement—are supplemented by an extensive literature, including the National Research Council's *Guide for the Care and Use of Laboratory Animals*, first published in 1963. The 1985 revision was provoked in part by PETA's revelation of abuses of monkeys in a laboratory in Silver Springs, Maryland, in 1981. Animal research in the United States is overseen by several overlapping agencies; to give one example, the Animal Welfare Act excludes rats, mice, birds, and fish, but the National Institutes of Health, which fund much biomedical research, include rats and mice in their regulatory policies.

The 1980s saw the institution of laboratory welfare regulation in most European countries and many others around the world. The European Union adopted legislation in 1986 (revised in 2010) that required member nations to regulate animal research. The British act from 1876 was replaced in 1986. Regulations vary from country to country; in general, European laws are more stringent than those of the United States, and laws and regulations are constantly revised to reflect new techniques and changing sensibilities.

Since the 1980s, increased public consciousness of animal awareness and cognition has led to significant changes in animal use. The use of animals for product testing has declined precipitously, owing to public preference for so-called cruelty-free products. This label has no legal standing, however, and may disguise the fact that products or their components were tested on animals in the past but are not presently. The kinds of animals used in research have also changed. The overwhelming majority of research animals—something like 95 percent in the United States in 2010—are rats and mice. Specially bred mice and rats for research began to be marketed to scientists in the 1920s; now sophisticated genetic engineering can create custom animals for a variety of research projects.

In addition, the use of nonhuman primates in research has become increasingly controversial. Starting with the research of the primatologist Jane Goodall on chimpanzees in Africa, and including several experiments in teaching language to primates, knowledge about primate intelligence, social life, and complexity has greatly increased. Extending the insight of Theophrastus, the very similarities to humans that make nonhuman primates such good experimental subjects also make their use in science particularly problematic. In the mid-1990s Goodall, Singer, and others developed the Great Ape Project, which aimed to give chimpanzees, gorillas, and orangutans the status of "persons," which would give them the human rights to life, individual liberty, and freedom from torture. The Spanish parliament passed a nonbinding resolution in 2008 that recognized these principles. By 2013 the European Union was examining the feasibility of phasing out research on nonhuman primates. There is concern, however, that if Western countries abandon primate research, countries such as China, where regulation is much more lax, may take it over.

Although many millions of animals—primarily rats and mice—continue to be used for research around the world, there has been considerable growth in moral concern and regulatory legislation since the early 1970s. The historical trajectory of Western science, and its undeniable success in improving human and animal health and adding to the knowledge of the human and animal body, makes it unlikely that animal experimentation will disappear anytime soon. But it is much more highly regulated than in the past, and as values continue to change, so too will laws and practices.

SEE ALSO *Cloning: I. Scientific Background; Harm; Hinduism, Bioethics in; Jainism, Bioethics in; Moral Status; Pain and Suffering; Veterinary Ethics; Xenotransplantation*

BIBLIOGRAPHY

Bentham, Jeremy. 1823 [1789]. *An Introduction to the Principles of Morals and Legislation*. 2nd ed. London: W. Pickering and E. Wilson.

Bernard, Claude. 1957 [1865]. *Introduction to the Study of Experimental Medicine*. Translated by Henry Copley Greene. New York: Dover.

Coleman, William, and Frederic L. Holmes, eds. 1988. *The Investigative Enterprise: Experimental Physiology in Nineteenth-Century Medicine*. Berkeley: University of California Press.

European Commission. 2013. "Animals Used for Scientific Purposes." Last modified March 7. http://ec.europa.eu/environment/chemicals/lab_animals/home_en.htm

Finsen, Lawrence, and Susan Finsen. 1994. *The Animal Rights Movement in America: From Compassion to Respect*. New York: Twayne.

French, Richard D. 1975. *Antivivisection and Medical Science in Victorian Society*. Princeton, NJ: Princeton University Press.

Fye, W. Bruce. 1987. *The Development of American Physiology: Scientific Medicine in the Nineteenth Century*. Baltimore, MD: Johns Hopkins University Press.

Galen. 1956. *On Anatomical Procedures*. Translated by Charles Singer. London: Oxford University Press.

Great Ape Project. 2013. Accessed September 15, 2012. http://www.greatapeproject.org

Guerrini, Anita. 2003. *Experimenting with Humans and Animals: From Galen to Animal Rights*. Baltimore, MD: Johns Hopkins University Press.

Haller, Albrecht von. 1936 [1752]. *A Dissertation on the Sensible and Irritable Parts of Animals*. Translated by Owsei Temkin. Baltimore, MD: Johns Hopkins University Press.

Harvey, William. 1990 [1628]. *The Circulation of the Blood and Other Writings*. Translated by Kenneth J. Franklin. London: J. M. Dent.

Jasper, James M., and Dorothy Nelkin. 1992. *The Animal Rights Crusade: The Growth of a Moral Protest*. New York: Free Press.

Kant, Immanuel. 1997 [1780]. *Lectures on Ethics*. Edited by Peter Heath and J. B. Schneewind. Translated by Peter Heath. New York: Cambridge University Press.

Le Clerc, Daniel, and Jean-Jacques Manget. 1685. *Bibliotheca Anatomica*. Geneva: Chovet.

Lesch, John E. 1984. *Science and Medicine in France: The Emergence of Experimental Physiology, 1790–1855*. Cambridge, MA: Harvard University Press.

National Research Council. 2011. *Guide for the Care and Use of Laboratory Animals*. 8th ed. Washington, DC: National Academies Press.

Passmore, John. 1975. "The Treatment of Animals." *Journal of the History of Ideas* 36 (2): 195–218.

Rader, Karen A. 2004. *Making Mice: Standardizing Animals for American Biomedical Research, 1900–1955*. Princeton, NJ: Princeton University Press.

Ray, John. 1693. *Synopsis methodica animalium quadrupedum et serpentini generis*. London: S. Smith and B. Walford.

Regan, Tom. 2004. *The Case for Animal Rights*. Rev. ed. Berkeley: University of California Press.

Ritvo, Harriet. 1987. *The Animal Estate: The English and Other Creatures in the Victorian Age*. Cambridge, MA: Harvard University Press.

Rowan, Andrew N. 1984. *Of Mice, Models, and Men: A Critical Evaluation of Animal Research*. Albany: State University of New York Press.

Rudacille, Deborah. 2000. *The Scalpel and the Butterfly: The War between Animal Research and Animal Protection*. New York: Farrar, Straus, and Giroux.

Rupke, Nicolaas A., ed. 1987. *Vivisection in Historical Perspective*. London: Croom Helm.

Russell, W. M. S., and R. L. Burch. 1959. *The Principles of Humane Experimental Technique*. London: Methuen.

Salt, Henry S. 1892. *Animals' Rights: Considered in Relation to Social Progress*. London: Bell.

Shaw, George Bernard. 1911. "Preface on Doctors." In *The Doctor's Dilemma*, v–xcii. New York: Brentano's.

Singer, Peter. 1990. *Animal Liberation*. 2nd ed. New York: New York Review of Books.

Sorabji, Richard. 1993. *Animal Minds and Human Morals: The Origins of the Western Debate*. Ithaca, NY: Cornell University Press.

Turner, James. 1980. *Reckoning with the Beast: Animals, Pain, and Humanity in the Victorian Mind*. Baltimore, MD: Johns Hopkins University Press.

US Department of Agriculture. Animal and Plant Health Inspection Service. 2012. "Animal Welfare Act." Last modified August 15. http://www.aphis.usda.gov/animal_welfare/awa_info.shtml

US Food and Drug Administration. 2013. "Science and Research." Accessed March 16. http://www.fda.gov/ScienceResearch/

Vesalius, Andreas. 1543. *De humani corporis fabrica*. Basel, Switzerland: Joannes Oporinus.

Wise, Steven M. 2000. *Rattling the Cage: Toward Legal Rights for Animals*. Cambridge, MA: Perseus Books.

Anita Guerrini
Horning Professor in the Humanities and Professor of History, Oregon State University

II. PHILOSOPHICAL ISSUES

For several centuries the issue of animal use in research, testing, and education has generated intense debate. In the early twenty-first century a complex range of opinions are in play in philosophy, policy, and public discourse, and it is not apt or especially helpful to cast the debate as one between those who favor animal use and those who do not. As an ethical question, the use of animals is deeply linked to debates over genetic engineering, biotechnology, cloning, xenotransplantation, stem cell research, and clinical trials with humans. It is also bound up with changing scientific and technological understanding about preclinical research and study as well as growing demands for a human systems biology approach better suited to human medical needs. Finally, there is a strong push for the development and implementation of reliable and human-relevant methods, directly applicable to the human condition, for the testing of pharmaceuticals and other products. These trends and a changing social consensus promise to transform both ethical discussion and the practical use of animals in the future.

The topic of animal use encompasses two distinct questions. Does such use yield useful knowledge that could not be gained from other sources, and is it morally acceptable for humans to use animals in ways that can cause them harm? The two questions are certainly related. If it were the case that nothing useful and distinctive is learned from animal use, it would be quite difficult to justify it on any basis. At the same time the fact that humans can learn useful things from research on animals would not by itself show that animal use is justified or—if it can be justified at all—under what conditions it would be justified. As explained in more detail below, further ethical discussion would be required to decide that question.

Ethical problems related to research on nonhuman animals are grounded in the assertion that animals have conscious experiences and that their lives can go well or badly. Central to this issue is the belief that nonhuman animals can experience pain and other unpleasant or distressing mental states. The French philosopher René Descartes (1596–1650) denied this (Regan and Singer 1989 [1976]), as have one or two contemporary philosophers (Carruthers 1992). On the whole, however, popular opinion and the overwhelming majority of contemporary scientists and philosophers agree that animals, especially vertebrate animals, can suffer (Smith and Boyd 1991; DeGrazia 1996, 2002). To take a contrary view, one must refute not just the everyday observations that people make about their animal companions but also the increasing body of empirical evidence, both physiological and behavioral, suggesting close parallels between animal experience and human experience (Dawkins 1980, 1993; Griffin 1992; Rollin 1998 [1989]). Such parallels are supported by the known similarities among the nervous systems of all vertebrate animals and by the common evolutionary origin of animals and humans (Rachels 1990).

NATURE AND EXTENT OF ANIMAL EXPERIMENTATION

Animal use in biomedical laboratories involves three broad classifications: (1) research, (2) product development and safety testing, and (3) education and training. Each area of use can take multiple forms. Research may be applied toward the diagnosis, understanding, treatment, or prevention of an existing medical problem, as in the development and testing of therapies and preventive vaccines. It may be "fundamental" or "basic," aiming at greater understanding about how the body works, without necessarily addressing a specific medical problem. Product development and safety testing encompasses assessments of the safety and effectiveness of drugs, consumer products, and other substances. Education and training involves classroom dissection and vivisection as well as animal use in teaching of or learning about biomedical techniques, such as surgery. These three categories of research, testing, and education can also overlap with one another.

Animal experimentation takes place at universities, medical centers, corporate testing facilities, and contract laboratories. In the United States it is frequently funded by the federal government, primarily the National Institutes of Health (NIH), which had a 2012 research budget of $32 billion. Approximately 40 percent of NIH-funded research involves experimentation on nonhuman animals (Monastersky 2008). Private foundations and charities also finance animal experiments.

Some governments provide detailed information on the experiments carried out each year, but many do not, making it difficult to arrive at a reliable estimate of the number of animals used in research, testing, and education. One 2005 estimate put worldwide use between 58.3 million and 115.3 million (Taylor et al. 2008), whereas another placed the range at 50.0 million to 100.0 million (Nuffield Council on Bioethics 2005). Animal use worldwide reached its height in the 1970s, and several analysts place the overall number in the early twenty-first century at approximately half of what it was in that decade (Van Zutphen 1998; Nuffield Council on Bioethics 2005; Rowan 2011).

Animal use appears to be increasing again, however, in part a result of the expanded breeding and use of genetically modified animals of many different strains. In the United Kingdom the 2000 annual report for the Animals (Scientific Procedures) Act showed that 2.71 million procedures had been performed, a significant decrease from the 1970s, when the figure topped an estimated 6.50 million. By 2010 the number of procedures in the United Kingdom was rising and at 3.7 million was 3 percent more than in 2009 and 1.0 million more than the number of procedures conducted in 2001 (the year that marked the lowest number of procedures since that statistical measure took hold in 1987). An increase in genetically altered animals was a factor, but the 2010 annual report also showed a 23 percent increase in the number of procedures involving birds and a 10 percent increase in procedures involving nonhuman primates, mostly Old World monkeys (Balls 2011). Overall, during the period from 1995 to 2005 the number of animals used for breeding and research rose by 11 percent (Festing 2008), mostly because of an increase in breeding "procedures."

In the United States official figures do not include purpose-bred rats, mice, and birds, the species most commonly used, or reptiles, amphibians, and fish, but a 1986 report from the US Congress's Office of Technology Assessment estimated that 17 million to 22 million animals were used annually. US government statistics put the number of regulated animals used in 2010 at 1,134,693 (Taylor et al. 2008; US Department of Agriculture Animal and Plant Health Inspection Service 2011). An upward adjustment by the authors of this article to account for the fact that the statistics do not include mice, rats, fish, birds, and amphibians (based on these species comprising an estimated 93.2 percent of the European Union figure for 2005) produces an estimate of about 17 million used per year. This figure, however, is likely a low estimate. In 2004, acknowledging the rising trend in production and use of transgenic animals, a laboratory animal veterinarian posited that as many as 100 million rodents alone were being used in US laboratories (Carbone 2004). Given the trends in breeding, maintenance of breeding colonies, and use, the real figure almost certainly lies somewhere in between these estimates.

The collection of data concerning the numbers of animals used in research and related information, such as the purposes of use and the severity of the procedures involved, is a practical challenge. Yet it seems necessary to the goals of increasing transparency; reducing pain, suffering, and distress; and assessing opportunities to secure further advances in the reduction, refinement, and replacement of animals used in research as well as with respect to improved husbandry, quality of care, and living standards for animals.

INSTITUTIONAL GUIDELINES AND CODES

Since the 1980s the networks for ethically informed decision making concerning animal use in laboratories have improved. Many countries have national, legally enforceable guidelines for the protection of animals in research, and a growing number require experiments to be approved by ethics committees. Among the more advanced approaches, in Australia the ethics committees must include a lay member and a person from an animal welfare organization, and in Sweden the ethics committees consist of six scientists and six lay members, including representatives from animal organizations, and are chaired by a judge.

Both the European Union and the Council of Europe have their own codes, which, like the most frequently cited international code, the International Guiding Principles for Biomedical Research Involving Animals developed by the Council for International Organizations of Medical Sciences (1985) (CIOMS), date from the mid-1980s. In the United States institutional animal care and use committees (IACUCs) are part of a system enacted following passage of the 1985 amendments to the Animal Welfare Act. The committee members are supposed to include individuals representing a broader community interest. They periodically review the institution's animal care and use programs and regularly review research proposals.

Most analysts looking at animal care committees cite such problems as insufficient training, competency, and expertise; weak guidelines; and inadequate protocol review or peer oversight. The committees are not mentioned in the relevant national legislation in all cases, and there is inconsistent interpretation and implementation of the laws. In some committees members only advise, whereas in others they approve, modify, or reject proposals. Ethical consideration focuses largely on practical matters, such as the appropriateness of the pain reliever used and its dose, as distinct from any sophisticated grappling with the costs and benefits of a given research protocol.

A 2005 audit report by the US Department of Agriculture Office of Inspector General, Western Region, revealed problems with IACUCs, including insufficient monitoring of animal care, protocols, and alternative research methods; unsatisfactory or no follow-up on the correction of deficiencies; and inaccurate annual reporting. IACUCs also had high rates of turnover, failed to properly train their members, and conducted only sporadic reviews. The report noted that the number of research facilities cited for violations had steadily increased in recent years.

A National Science Foundation study published in *Science* in July 2001 concluded that IACUC reviews of animal experiments were of limited reliability. The three-year study found that animal use committees unfamiliar with the university and personnel involved do not make the same approval decisions as those that know the university and personnel, often asking for more information rather than approving studies (Plous and Herzog 2001).

Some degree of regulation seems to have become necessary to securing public consent for the continued use of animals, in part as a result of the perceived need for accountability and transparency in all areas of public life but also because of the erosion of faith in value- or bias-free science (Rollin 2006b). In prior decades, when the activities of researchers were much less regulated, allegations persisted concerning mistreatment of animals, lack of awareness or recognition of their capacity to suffer, and insufficient reflection on the likely benefits or probability of success of experiments. Without question, more could be done to promote the discussion of ethics and to create a culture of care within institutions, and there is room for improvement, but animal care committees represent a rudimentary framework for such exchanges and activities.

THE PUBLIC POLICY ARENA

The use of animals in research, testing, and education has been the subject of government regulation somewhere in the world since 1876, the year Great Britain passed its Cruelty to Animals Act. In the twenty-first century the use of animals in most Organisation for Economic Co-operation and Development (OECD) countries is subject to an extensive and ever more sophisticated regime of regulation. For moral and technical reasons, there is a great deal of momentum in support of new approaches, generally favoring the development of nonanimal methods on account of their aptness, accuracy, speed, and economy.

The discussion of nonanimal methods is grounded in the three Rs (reduction, refinement, and replacement), a concept outlined by W. M. S. Russell and R. L. Burch in *The Principles of Humane Experimental Technique* (1959). This breakthrough conceptual framework undergirds legislative, administrative, and regulatory approaches in dozens of countries. A number of academic and government centers are devoted to alternatives to animal use, and nine World Congresses on Alternatives and Animal Use in the Life Sciences (1993–2014) have helped further interest and action concerning nonanimal methodologies in scientific research.

Even as the codification of the three Rs into law, policy, guidelines, and public discussion continues, advocates and regulators are engaged in continuing reflection and exchange on their meaning, their application, and their expansion to include new developments in animal use. Russell and Burch placed emphasis on reducing animal pain and distress, and this focus remains important. The three Rs, however, may not accommodate all situations in the twenty-first century. There are many factors that can affect animal welfare from species to species, including breeding, transportation, feeding, housing, handling, and quality of life, and many challenges associated with research involving genetically modified animals and animals bred as models of particular diseases. There have been special pleas raised for certain species asking that they simply not be used. The three Rs framework is elastic enough to accommodate some of these developments, and its potential is not exhausted. But it may be that other approaches will be needed over time (Nuffield Council on Bioethics 2005; Schuppli and Fraser 2005).

There are many signs of the significant progress that has resulted from the confluence of public pressure, a growing appreciation of the advantages of nonanimal methods, and dissatisfaction with the status quo in the form of government reports, blue-ribbon committees, increasing numbers of validated and accepted alternatives on the AltTox (2013) website and elsewhere, and other manifestations. Tremendous advances have occurred in some areas. In the United States the 2007 National Research Council report titled *Toxicity Testing in the 21st Century* proposed a bold new vision concerning the assessment of biological and chemical compounds, one that would phase out animal use via a gradual reshaping of government regulation, budgeting priorities, and other levers (see also Stephens 2010).

Another bellwether was the Institute of Medicine and the National Research Council's 2011 report *Chimpanzees in Biomedical and Behavioral Research*. While the Institute of Medicine and National Research Council committee took up only the question of the scientific necessity for chimpanzee use in biomedical and behavioral research, it signaled its view that such an assessment inevitably raises ethical issues. The chimpanzee's genetic proximity to humans makes it "a uniquely valuable species for certain types of research" but also demands "a greater justification for conducting research using this model" (Institute of Medicine and National Research Council 2011, 2). The final report includes a summary of basic ethical principles that might distinguish the use of the chimpanzee from the use of other species, concluding that "the use of chimpanzees should face the most stringent requirements for justification" (Institute of Medicine and National Research Council 2011, 15).

PAIN AND DISTRESS

Pain and distress have long been of special concern in the realm of ethics and animal use. In the early twenty-first century the positive influences of law, research, and ethical discussion have led to genuine improvement, and campaigners, policy makers, and others are rightly focused on more serious treatment of associated issues (Rollin 2006a, 2006b). In 2011 twelve countries employed classification systems relating to pain and suffering: Australia, Canada, Finland, Germany, Great Britain, the Republic of Ireland, the Netherlands, New Zealand, Poland, Sweden, Switzerland, and the United States. Many codes regulating animal experimentation instruct committees to assume that procedures that would cause pain in humans also will cause pain in vertebrate animals unless there is evidence to the contrary. The regulatory framework in Great Britain requires that any research on vertebrate animals (and the common octopus) that may cause pain, suffering, distress, or lasting harm must be licensed.

In the United States prior to 1963 regulation was solely the responsibility of individual investigators. Only with the 1963 publication of the *Guide for Laboratory Animal Facilities and Care* (later renamed the *Guide for the Care and Use of Laboratory Animals* [National Research Council 2011]) and the passage of the Laboratory Animal Welfare Act of 1966 did a regulatory framework emerge. The act was amended in 1970 to add reporting requirements and in 1985 to add provisions to minimize pain and distress, to focus on psychological health and well-being, and to promote the search for alternatives to painful procedures (Carbone 2004).

A 2010 study by Leah M. Gomez, Kathleen M. Conlee, and Martin L. Stephens revealed numerous instances of animal pain, suffering, and death when research institutions failed to follow minimum legal standards. The authors examined reports submitted to the NIH's Office of Laboratory Animal Welfare by ninety-one research facilities that collectively receive hundreds of millions of dollars in federal funding. Their analysis was based on 124 noncompliance reports over a three-month period, and there were at least 1,000 animals affected, including monkeys, rabbits, guinea pigs, hamsters, mice, and rats. The most common problems involved animal care and management, such as not providing pain relief following surgery, improper killing of animals, and failure to provide adequate food and water, in one case leading to death. In many instances, investigators performed animal studies that involved painful procedures without proper approval.

A 2009 National Research Council report called for more research to determine when laboratory animals are suffering and how to relieve that pain (see also Marris 2009). Nevertheless it is plain that animals do suffer pain and distress in use, and opinion surveys suggest that public approval of experiments is lower the more pain and distress there is perceived to be. One major humane organization has called for a phaseout of significant pain and distress by 2020 (Plous 1996a, 1996b; Aldous, Coghlan, and Copley 1999; Stephens and Conlee 2004).

To achieve such an outcome, regulatory systems must address the question of pain more seriously and above all promulgate methods for its assessment, whether they involve retrospective reviews of the suffering involved or other measures. The scientific community will also need to address the challenges associated with genetically modified animals, who frequently manifest unexpected effects and associated suffering along with the predictable symptoms of the conditions they are being used to model.

IN DEFENSE OF ANIMAL EXPERIMENTATION

If experiments being carried out in the early twenty-first century inflict substantial suffering on animals, how can this practice be defended? The primary reason given for using animals in research is to ensure scientific progress in basic and applied biological and medical science. Defenders of the practice emphasize the use of animals in medical experimentation, particularly in areas such as diabetes and hypertension research, where the use of animals is claimed to have led to important medical breakthroughs (Paton 1984; US Congress, Office of Technology Assessment 1986). They assert that statistics on the large numbers of animals used can be misleading, because a great deal of animal experimentation is of a relatively harmless nature—for example, running a rat through a maze with a reward of food as encouragement for good performance rather than an electric shock as punishment for poor performance. They argue that animal experimentation is the primary way to advance basic knowledge of human anatomy and physiology and that it offers the best hope of finding cures for diseases such as cancer and AIDS. They may argue that some animal experimentation is carried out to find ways to treat diseases that affect animals. Sometimes too it is said that the goal of increasing scientific knowledge provides sufficient justification for whatever suffering might be inflicted in the process of advancing toward that goal.

Behind such arguments lie a variety of philosophical positions. For instance, it may be said that, as related in Genesis 1:26, God has given human beings "dominion" over the other animals, to use them as humans please. Combined with other theological notions, such as the idea that humans, alone of all animals, have immortal souls, this idea has been influential throughout the Christian world. But it can be turned the other way. As long ago as 1713 the English poet Alexander Pope argued against cruel experiments on the grounds that dominion requires humans to play the role of the good shepherd, caring for our flock (Turner 1992 [1964]). More recently a number of Christians have suggested that the gift of dominion should be interpreted as one of "stewardship," which makes us responsible for the care of the nonhuman creation (Attfield 1991 [1983]). It remains unclear, however, precisely what follows from this reinterpretation. Does it imply that humans are not entitled to use animals in harmful experiments or only that there must be a strong reason for doing so?

It also has been said by writers as diverse as the Italian philosopher and theologian Thomas Aquinas (c. 1224–1274) and the German philosopher Immanuel Kant (1724–1804) that animals are not "ends in themselves" and have no rights (Regan and Singer 1989 [1976]). In support of this idea it is alleged that the status of a being who is an "end in itself" or has rights belongs only to a being who is rational, is capable of autonomous action, or is a moral agent. This position attempts to equate the universe of moral agents—those to whom moral judgments or prescriptions can sensibly be addressed—with the universe of moral patients—those about whom it matters, morally, what people do. One possible justification for this equation would be a social contract model of ethics. Humans have a moral obligation to respect the rights or interests only of those who can reciprocate respect for their rights or interests (Gauthier 1986; Carruthers 1992). This position, however, does not provide any grounds for distinguishing between nonhuman animals, on the one hand, and infants and the profoundly intellectually disabled, on the other. It may be true that many people care more about members of their own species and hence wish to give infants and the intellectually disabled "courtesy status" as members of the moral community. But what if they do not? A social contract theory of morality, then, offers no footing for insisting on equal consideration for the interests of those human beings. Indeed some philosophers think that the best understanding of the social contract model includes animals as well as humans (Rowlands 2009).

A second justification claims that all human beings form a moral community not because of an implicit contract but because of people's natural feelings for members of the human species. Those feelings, it is argued, resemble the natural affection of parents for their own children, which people take as a basis for the special moral obligation they think parents have to give preference to the interests of their own children over the greater interests of the children of strangers. The natural ties between members of a species should, the argument continues, serve as the basis for holding that humans have a greater obligation to other humans than they do to members of other species (Midgley 1984; Gray 1991a, 1991b).

If this argument were valid, it is not clear how much experimentation on animals it would justify, because people do not think that parents are justified in causing serious harm to the children of strangers to benefit their own children. But is this argument valid? Understandably those who use these arguments are silent about the obvious case that lies between the family and the species: preference for the interests of the members of one's own ethnic group or race over the greater interests of members of other ethnic groups or races. It would seem that if the argument works for both the narrower circle of the family and the wider sphere of the species, it also should work for the middle case. If one rejects the extension from families to ethnic groups, the further extension to the whole of the human species looks very dubious (Singer 1991).

A utilitarian defense of contemporary use might be based on the idea that the benefits produced outweigh the harm done to animals (Paton 1984; US Congress, Office of Technology Assessment 1986). Prominent among the claimed benefits is a considerable extension of the human life span. The first question raised by this defense is how much animal experimentation has helped extend human longevity. In polemical debates dramatic claims are often made, but the consensus among those who have studied trends in human health from a historical point of view is that almost all of the increase in human longevity that has occurred since the early twentieth century has been the result of improved sanitation, diet, and living conditions rather than to medical research of any kind, whether on animals or not (McKeown 1979; McKinlay, McKinlay, and Beaglehole 1989).

It is possible to accept this verdict but to maintain that medical research, including research on animals, has benefited humans; increasing longevity may be a poor measure of research value, because it does not address reductions in morbidity and human suffering. Defenders of the value of animal research often point as well to the development of coronary artery bypass graft surgery as an achievement facilitated by research on animals. The contribution of this surgery to the prolongation of life is not clear, but the surgery is more effective than conventional medication in relieving angina, a painful condition that results from coronary artery disease (US Congress, Office of Technology Assessment 1986). Thus it may contribute to a better quality of life rather than to a greater quantity of life.

A second point in considering a genuinely utilitarian defense of early twenty-first-century practice in animal research is that the classical utilitarian tradition has steadfastly required people to take all suffering—that of humans and that of nonhuman animals—into consideration. The leading nineteenth-century utilitarians—Jeremy Bentham (1948 [1789]), John Stuart Mill (1963–1991), and Henry Sidgwick (1966 [1874])—were unwavering on this point. Modern utilitarians who cast their views in terms of the satisfaction of preferences rather than in terms of pleasure and pain are equally comprehensive in the scope of their theories (Hare 1981; Singer 2011 [1979]). This makes it more difficult to claim that a genuinely utilitarian approach favors animal experimentation in general or as an institution. Nevertheless some individual experiments—those that do not involve any or very much suffering for the animals and promise major benefits for humans or animals—may be defensible on utilitarian grounds (Singer 2006).

Some seek to justify what researchers do to animals by appealing to a human-centered version of utilitarianism. In the extreme version of this view the conscious experiences of beings who are not members of the human species do not matter at all. In the more moderate version those experiences do matter, but they do not matter as much as the similar experiences of members of the human species. Both positions frankly endorse an ethic that is limited to or biased toward the human species. Once such an ethic is accepted of course, the justification for animal experimentation becomes much easier. The difficulty of this position lies in defending such a speciesist ethic.

Finally, defenders of early twenty-first-century practice often accuse their opponents of a lack of consistency in objecting to the deaths of animals in laboratories while continuing to participate in the practice of rearing and killing animals for food. The rise of the animal rights movement has made this accusation less effective, because a great percentage of those actively involved in that movement have been vegetarians or vegans as well as opponents of animal experimentation. In any case, the issue of whether animal experimentation is justified cannot be resolved by reference to the character of some individuals who object to animal experimentation.

OBJECTIONS TO ANIMAL EXPERIMENTATION

Critics of experimenting on animals tend to fall into two groups: abolitionists and reformers. Abolitionists usually rely on the principle that the end does not justify the means. To inflict pain and death on an innocent being is, they maintain, always wrong. They point out that people do not think that the possibility of advancing scientific knowledge justifies taking healthy human beings and inflicting painful deaths on them; similarly, they say, the infliction of suffering on animals cannot be justified by reference to future benefits either for humans or for other animals (Ryder 1983 [1975]; Regan 2004 [1983]).

A weakness of the abolitionist position is that when the end is sufficiently important, most people think that otherwise unacceptable means are justifiable if there is no other way of achieving the end. People do not approve of telling lies, but most people accept the idea that politicians should tell lies to mislead the enemy when their country is fighting a war that they believe is right. Similarly if the prospects of finding a cure for cancer depended on a single experiment, most people probably would think that the experiment should be carried out.

In response to objections along these lines, some abolitionists argue that although a single experiment, taken in isolation, may appear justifiable, the benefits of such experiments do not outweigh the suffering inflicted by the institution of animal experimentation as a whole. One also must take into account, these abolitionists would say, two other factors. First, a large (if uncertain) proportion of experimentation is worthless; second, even if no pain or distress is caused by the experiments, experimental animals typically have been raised in conditions that constitute severe deprivation for beings of their species. The common laboratory rat, for instance, is a highly intelligent animal with a strong urge to explore new surroundings. Rats also like to get into small, dark spaces, yet in most laboratories they are kept in barren plastic container bins with a bit of sawdust or other absorbent at the bottom. Such treatment indicates the lack of consideration for the interests of animals that prevails in the world of animal experimentation, and abolitionists doubt that this will ever change as long as people regard laboratory animals primarily as tools for research.

Since the early 1970s some of those arguing from an ecofeminist or a feminist ethic of care perspective have also argued for abolition, but others have taken the reformist side. This ethical approach, based on a unified sensibility that addresses the interconnecting dominations of women, animals, and nonsentient nature and making the point that there is no reason animals' difference cannot be grounds for caring and for relationships characterized by ethically significant attitudes, such as respect, gratitude, compassion, and fellow or sisterly feeling, is sufficiently broad to encompass both reformist and abolitionist views (Slicer 2007 [1991]; Gruen 2011 [2001]).

Reformers believe that a changed practice of experimenting on animals could be defensible. They demand that any benefits that are believed to be likely to arise from the experimentation should be sufficiently probable and sufficiently great to offset the costs to the animal subjects; they urge that every experiment should come under close and impartial scrutiny to determine whether this is the case.

Reformers point out that since the 1980s and 1990s several countries have developed legally obligatory systems of review based on an institutional ethics committee's review of proposals to carry out experiments on animals but that experimenters usually are well represented on such committees, whereas animal welfare advocates either are not represented or are heavily outnumbered by experimenters. An impartial committee that weighed the cost to the animal in the same way that people would weigh a comparable cost to a human would, the reformers maintain, approve at most a small fraction of the experiments performed in the early twenty-first century. In other countries, such as the United States, institutional ethics committees exist but are not legally required for corporations or other institutions that do not receive federal funds, and their coverage of animal experimentation is incomplete. Moreover in the United States these committees do not always have the authority to prevent experimenters from going ahead with painful experiments if the experimenters assert that alleviating the animals' pain would interfere with the purpose of the experiment (US Congress, Office of Technology Assessment 1986; Dresser 1988; Smith and Boyd 1991; Gavaghan 1992; Orlans 1993).

Among opponents of early twenty-first-century forms of animal experimentation, the line between reformers and abolitionists is not clear-cut, because questions of long-term goals and short-term strategy intervene. A threefold division might be more appropriate. In the first category one could place those whose long-term goals do not extend beyond better regulation and control of animal experiments to eliminate the most painful and trivial experiments. In the next category would be those who have the long-term goal of abolishing all or virtually all animal experiments but who consider this an ideal rather than a realistic objective for the immediate future (Stephens 2012). This group therefore seeks reforms in the interim period, and its short-term goals do not differ significantly from those of the members of the first category. The third category consists of those who aim at abolition and are not interested in advocating anything less.

Although members of these three categories disagree sharply among themselves, they all agree that the early twenty-first-century situation is not acceptable. They also agree on promoting the use of alternatives to animal experimentation, and many believe that alternative methods would be developed more rapidly if they received more substantial government support (Ryder 1983 [1975]; Rowan 1984; Balls 1992).

The ethical stance of those in the first category, who seek only limited reforms, is often of a relatively conventional type. They can be thought of as following an "animal welfare" line rather than accepting an ethic of "animal rights" or "animal liberation." They accept the idea that animals may be used for human purposes but want safeguards to ensure that the purposes are serious ones and that no more suffering occurs than is necessary for the purpose to be realized. Those who take an animal rights or animal liberation stance want to narrow the ethical gulf that separates humans from other animals in regard to conventional morality. They thus raise a philosophically deep question with implications that go beyond experimentation, extending to the treatment of animals in general.

THE MORAL STATUS OF ANIMALS

In examining the case for early twenty-first-century practices, this entry examined some attempts to justify in ethical terms the sharp distinction that is made between the treatment of members of the human species and the treatment of members of other species. The problems noted bedevil all attempts to make the boundary of the human species coincide with the boundary of human moral obligations. Although it is said frequently that humans are superior to other animals in such respects as rationality, self-awareness, the ability to communicate with others, and a sense of justice, human infants and humans with severe intellectual disabilities fall below many nonhuman animals on any objective test of abilities that could mark humans as superior to other animals. Yet surely these less capable human beings are also "ends in themselves," and it would not be legitimate to experiment on them in the ways people experiment on animals. For a contrary view that accepts the moral possibility of harmful experimentation on both nonhuman animals and humans at a similar mental level, see Raymond G. Frey's 1983 article "Vivisection, Morals, and Medicine."

Richard D. Ryder, Peter Singer, Tom Regan, and other thinkers claim that respect for the interests of those humans and comparative neglect of the interests of members of other species with equal or superior capacities constitutes speciesism, a prejudice in favor of "one's own kind" that is analogous to and no more justifiable than racism. This argument has been seen by many people as the most difficult for defenders of animal experimentation to counter, so much so that a leading philosopher has referred to it as a "won argument" (McGinn 1991).

Certainly the view that species is in itself a reason for giving more weight to the interests of one being than to the interests of another is more often assumed than explicitly defended. Some writers who have claimed to be defending speciesism have in fact been defending a very different position: that the morally relevant differences between species—such as differences in mental capacities—entitle people to give more weight to the interests of the members of the species with the superior mental capacities (Cohen 1986; Leahy 1991). If this argument were successful, it would not justify speciesism, because the claim would not be that species in itself is a reason for giving more weight to the interests of one being than to those of another. The real reason would be the difference in mental capacities, which happens to coincide with the difference in species. But in view of the overlap in mental capacities between some members of the species *Homo sapiens* and some members of other species, it is difficult to see how this argument can be used to defend early twenty-first-century practices. In other contexts people insist on treating beings as moral individuals rather than lumping them together as members of a group; it is precisely those who practice racism and sexism who treat all members of a group in the same way (for instance, assuming that women cannot perform heavy physical labor as well as men can) without recognizing individual variation.

Defenders of animal experimentation sometimes have portrayed the animal rights position in an extreme form, for example, as implying that it is as wrong to kill a mosquito as it is to kill a normal human adult. This is, however, a caricature. Animal advocates do not claim that all animals have the same interests, only that interests are not to be given less consideration solely on the grounds of species. Thus it is compatible with the animal liberation view to say that the interests of beings with different mental capacities vary and that these variations are morally significant (DeGrazia 1996, 2002). If people are forced to choose between saving the life of a being who understands the meaning of death and wants to go on living and saving the life of a being who is not capable of having desires for the future because that being's mental capacities do not enable it to grasp that it is a "self," a mental entity existing over time, it is entirely justifiable to choose in favor of the being who wants to go on living. This is a choice that is based on mental capacity and not on species membership, as one can see by considering that the former being may be a chimpanzee and the latter being a human with profound brain damage (Singer 1990 [1975]).

There have been those who attempted to sweep aside such issues by denying that animal experimentation raises a moral issue at all. Unfortunately these individuals do not attempt to explain why, to take only one example, the clear proposal of utilitarian writers—that pain as such is evil regardless of the species of the being that suffers it—is devoid of meaning. It may be difficult to compare the suffering of a human and that of, say, a rabbit, but sometimes rough comparisons can be made. It seems undeniable that to put into the eye of a rabbit a chemical that causes the eye to blister or become ulcerated is to do more harm to the rabbit than people would do to any number of human beings by denying them the possibility of using a new type of shampoo that could be marketed only if the chemical was tested in this way. When such rough comparisons can be made, the mere fact that rabbits are "lower animals" is no reason to give less weight to their suffering.

Seen in this light, the argument that restricting experiments on animals interferes with scientific freedom and medical progress appears less conclusive. People do not grant scientists the freedom to experiment at will on humans, although such experiments would do more to advance knowledge of human physiology and be more likely to find cures for diseases such as AIDS than would animal experiments. It would seem therefore to be incumbent on the defenders of experiments on animals to show that there is a relevant difference between all humans and other animals that justifies experiments on the latter but not on the former. Success at this task, however, still eludes defenders of animal experimentation.

CONCLUSION

For many decades the debate over animal use in research, testing, and education has been highly polarized, and especially in the United States, public exchanges between those who support such use and those who do not have usually resulted in more heat than light. Since the late 1980s, however, thoughtful discussion of the status of animals within philosophy, public policy circles, and popular discourse has transformed the landscape of animal use in research, testing, and education. Government agencies, research groups, and corporations in the early twenty-first century spend $200 million annually worldwide on developing alternative toxicity tests that do not involve animals, and the conversation about not using certain species, such as primates, has reached a serious level.

Most biomedical research does not involve animals, although many nevertheless consider it important to a full program of research. Animals do suffer pain in such use, however, and a regulatory system that is meaningful and effective, emphasizing alternatives to animal use and the highest possible care for those animals used, must become a priority for ethical reasons above all.

There is certainly room for additional moral debate, but such debate on its own cannot resolve the question of whether animal use in research, testing, and education is justified. This makes support for methods that reduce conflict and animal suffering and the validation and implementation of such methods a moral imperative. Doubts continue to grow about the extrapolation of information from animal studies to human health and safety issues and whether fundamental biological differences between species and indeed strains of animals can be eliminated by manipulating animal models (Bhogal 2010). In some areas the transformative revolution in biology and biotechnology will help enable the replacement of animals in toxicity and other testing, and growing social disapproval may well lead to a future in which the use of species more highly placed on the phylogenic scale, such as primates, becomes anathema. It is also possible that the point will be reached at which a social consensus favors the elimination of studies that are not likely to have an impact on important human health problems and settles on the fundamental principle that animals may be used for research only if there is no other way of obtaining the results anticipated from an experiment. At the same time societal expectations and the imperatives of continuing progress in the effort to secure human safety, health, and well-being remain powerful drivers in the evolution of animal use in research, testing, and education as well as in the ensuing ethical discussion of such use, and they will do so for the foreseeable future.

SEE ALSO *Animal Welfare and Rights: I. Ethical Perspectives on the Treatment and Status of Animals; Conscience, Rights of; Moral Status; Nazi Legacy and Bioethics; Research Policy: II. Risk and Vulnerable Groups; Veterinary Ethics; Xenotransplantation*

BIBLIOGRAPHY

Aldous, Peter; Andy Coghlan; and Jon Copley. 1999. "Let the People Speak." *New Scientist*, May 22, 26–31.

AltTox.org. 2013. "Non-animal Methods for Toxicity Testing." Accessed March 1, 2013. http://alttox.org

Altweb: The Global Clearinghouse for Information on Alternatives to Animal Testing. 2013. Johns Hopkins Bloomberg School of Public Health. Accessed March 1, 2013. http://altweb.jhsph.edu

Animal Ethics Infolink. 2013. New South Wales Department of Primary Industries and Animal Research Review Panel. Accessed March 1, 2013. http://www.animalethics.org.au

Association of Medical Research Charities. 2013. Accessed August 14, 2013. http://www.amrc.org.uk/news-policy—debate_animal-research

Attfield, Robin. 1991 [1983]. *The Ethics of Environmental Concern*. 2nd ed. Athens: University of Georgia Press.

Baird, Robert M., and Stuart E. Rosenbaum, eds. 1991. *Animal Experimentation: The Moral Issues*. Buffalo, NY: Prometheus.

Balls, Michael. 1992. "Time to Reform Toxic Tests." *New Scientist*, May 2, 31–33.

Balls, Michael. 2011. "The Three Rs and Animal Experimentation: Documented Signs of Advancement or of Stagnation." *Alternatives to Laboratory Animals* 39 (4): 299–301.

Bayne, Kathryn A. L.; Molly Greene; and Ernest D. Prentice, eds. 1995. *Current Issues and New Frontiers in Animal Research*. Greenbelt, MD: Scientists Center for Animal Welfare.

BBC. 2013. "Experimenting on Animals." Accessed March 1, 2013. http://www.bbc.co.uk/ethics/animals/using/experiments_1.shtml

Beauchamp, Tom L.; F. Barbara Orlans; Rebecca Dresser; et al. 2008. *The Human Use of Animals: Case Studies in Ethical Choice*. 2nd ed. Oxford: Oxford University Press.

Bentham, Jeremy. 1948 [1789]. *An Introduction to the Principles of Morals and Legislation*. New York: Hafner.

Bhogal, Nirmala. 2010. "A Time to Replace Animal Models? A Clinical Perspective; Reflections on the Keynote Address." *Alternatives to Laboratory Animals* 38 (supp. 1): iii–v.

Boyd Group. 2013. Accessed August 14, 2013. http://www.boyd-group.demon.co.uk

British Union for the Abolition of Vivisection. 2013. Accessed March 1, 2013. http://www.buav.org

Canadian Council on Animal Care. 2013. "CCAC Training Module on Ethics in Animal Experimentation." Accessed March 1, 2013. http://ccac.ca/en_/education/niaut/stream/cs-ethics

Carbone, Larry. 2004. *What Animals Want: Expertise and Advocacy in Laboratory Animal Welfare Policy*. Oxford: Oxford University Press.

Carruthers, Peter. 1992. *The Animals Issue: Moral Theory in Practice*. Cambridge, UK: Cambridge University Press.

Cohen, Carl. 1986. "The Case for the Use of Animals in Biomedical Research." *New England Journal of Medicine* 315 (14): 865–70.

Council for International Organizations of Medical Sciences. 1985. "International Guiding Principles for Biomedical Research Involving Animals (1985)." http://cioms.ch/publications/guidelines/1985_texts_of_guidelines.htm

Dawkins, Marian Stamp. 1980. *Animal Suffering: The Science of Animal Welfare*. London: Chapman and Hall.

Dawkins, Marian Stamp. 1993. *Through Our Eyes Only? The Search for Animal Consciousness*. Oxford: Freeman.

DeGrazia, David. 1996. *Taking Animals Seriously: Mental Life and Moral Status*. Cambridge, UK: Cambridge University Press.

DeGrazia, David. 2002. *Animal Rights: A Very Short Introduction*. Oxford: Oxford University Press.

Dresser, Rebecca. 1988. "Standards for Animal Research: Looking at the Middle." *Journal of Medicine and Philosophy* 13 (2): 123–43.

European Commission. 2013. "Legislation for the Protection of Animals Used for Scientific Purposes." http://ec.europa.eu/environment/chemicals/lab_animals/legislation_en.htm

Festing, Simon. 2008. "Animal Experimentation: The Need for Deliberation and Challenge." *Alternatives to Laboratory Animals* 36 (1): 1–4.

Frey, Raymond G. 1983. "Vivisection, Morals, and Medicine." *Journal of Medical Ethics* 9 (2): 94–97.

Fund for the Replacement of Animals in Medical Experiments. 2013. Accessed March 1, 2013. http://www.frame.org.uk

Gauthier, David. 1986. *Morals by Agreement*. Oxford: Clarendon.

Gavaghan, Helen. 1992. "Animal Experiments the American Way." *New Scientist*, May 16, 32–36.

Glock, John P.; Tony DiPascuale; and F. Barbara Orlans, eds. 2002. *Applied Ethics in Animal Research: Philosophy, Regulation, and Laboratory Applications*. West Lafayette, IN: Purdue University Press. http://docs.lib.purdue.edu/press_ebooks/16/

Gomez, Leah M.; Kathleen M. Conlee; and Martin L. Stephens. 2010. "Noncompliance with Public Health Service (PHS) Policy on Humane Care and Use of Laboratory Animals: An Exploratory Analysis." *Journal of Applied Animal Welfare Science* 13 (2): 123–36.

Gray, Jeffrey A. 1991a. "On Speciesism and Racism: Reply to Singer and Ryder." *Psychologist* 4 (5): 202–3.

Gray, Jeffrey A. 1991b. "On the Morality of Speciesism." *Psychologist* 4 (5): 196–98.

Griffin, Donald R. 1992. *Animal Minds*. Chicago: University of Chicago Press.

Gruen, Lori. 2011 (2001). *Ethics and Animals: An Introduction*. Cambridge, UK: Cambridge University Press.

Hare, Richard M. 1981. *Moral Thinking: Its Levels, Method, and Point*. Oxford: Clarendon.

Institute of Medicine and National Research Council. 2011. *Chimpanzees in Biomedical and Behavioral Research: Assessing the Necessity*. Washington, DC: National Academies Press.

Kraus, A. Lanny, and David Renquist, eds. 2000. *Bioethics and the Use of Laboratory Animals: Ethics in Theory and Practice*. Chester, NH: American College of Laboratory Animal Medicine.

LaFollette, Hugh, and Niall Shanks. 1996. *Brute Science: Dilemmas of Animal Experimentation*. London: Routledge.

Leahy, Michael P. T. 1991. *Against Liberation: Putting Animals in Perspective*. London: Routledge.

Marris, Emma. 2009. "More Pain Studies Needed." *Nature* 458 (7237): 394–95.

McGinn, Colin. 1991. "Eating Animals Is Wrong." *London Review of Books* 13 (2): 14–16.

McKeown, Thomas. 1979. *The Role of Medicine: Dream, Mirage, or Nemesis?* Oxford: Blackwell.

McKinlay, John B.; Sonia M. McKinlay; and Robert Beaglehole. 1989. "Trends in Death and Disease and the Contribution of Medical Measures." In *Handbook of Medical Sociology*, 4th ed., edited by Howard E. Freeman and Sol Levine, 14–45. Englewood Cliffs, NJ: Prentice Hall.

Midgley, Mary. 1984. *Animals and Why They Matter*. Athens: University of Georgia Press.

Mill, John Stuart. 1963–1991. *Collected Works*. 33 vols. Edited by John M. Robson and Jack Stillinger. Toronto: University of Toronto Press.

Monastersky, Richard. 2008. "Protesters Fail to Slow Animal Research." *Chronicle of Higher Education*, April 18.

National Institutes of Health. 2013. Office of Laboratory Animal Welfare. Accessed March 1, 2013. http://grants.nih.gov/grants/olaw/olaw.htm

National Research Council. 2007. *Toxicity Testing in the 21st Century: A Vision and a Strategy*. Washington, DC: National Academies Press.

National Research Council. 2009. *Recognition and Alleviation of Pain in Laboratory Animals*. Washington, DC: National Academies Press.

National Research Council. 2011. *Guide for the Care and Use of Laboratory Animals*. 8th ed. Washington, DC: National Academies Press.

Nuffield Council on Bioethics. 2005. *The Ethics of Research Involving Animals*. London: Author.

O'Donoghue, Philip N., ed. 1998. *The Ethics of Animal Experimentation: Proceedings of the EBRA/FELASA European Congress*. London: European Biomedical Research Association.

Orlans, F. Barbara. 1993. *In the Name of Science: Issues in Responsible Animal Experimentation*. Oxford: Oxford University Press.

Paton, William. 1984. *Man and Mouse: Animals in Medical Research*. Oxford: Oxford University Press.

Paul, Ellen Frankel, and Jeffrey Paul, eds. 2001. *Why Animal Experimentation Matters: The Use of Animals in Medical Research*. New Brunswick, NJ: Transaction.

Plous, Scott. 1996a. "Attitudes toward the Use of Animals in Psychological Research and Education: Results from a National Survey of Psychologists." *American Psychologist* 51 (11): 1167–80.

Plous, Scott. 1996b. "Attitudes toward the Use of Animals in Psychological Research and Education: Results from a National Survey of Psychology Majors." *Psychological Science* 7 (6): 352–58.

Plous, Scott, and Harold Herzog. 2001. "Reliability of Protocol Reviews for Animal Research." *Science* 293 (5530): 608–9.

Rachels, James. 1990. *Created from Animals: The Moral Implications of Darwinism*. Oxford: Oxford University Press.

Regan, Tom. 2004 [1983]. *The Case for Animal Rights*. Rev. ed. Berkeley: University of California Press.

Regan, Tom, and Peter Singer, eds. 1989 [1976]. *Animal Rights and Human Obligations*. 2nd ed. Englewood Cliffs, NJ: Prentice Hall.

Rollin, Bernard E. 1998 [1989]. *The Unheeded Cry: Animal Consciousness, Animal Pain, and Science*. Rev. ed. Ames: Iowa State University Press.

Rollin, Bernard E. 2006a. "The Regulation of Animal Research and the Emergence of Animal Ethics: A Conceptual History." *Theoretical Medicine and Bioethics* 27 (4): 285–304.

Rollin, Bernard E. 2006b. *Science and Ethics*. Cambridge, UK: Cambridge University Press.

Rowan, Andrew N. 1984. *Of Mice, Models, and Men: A Critical Evaluation of Animal Research*. Albany: State University of New York Press.

Rowan, Andrew N. 2011. "Avoiding Animal Testing." *Scientist*, December 1. http://www.the-scientist.com/?articles.view/articleNo/31401/title/Avoiding-Animal-Testing/

Rowlands, Mark. 2009. *Animal Rights: Moral Theory and Practice*. 2nd ed. Houndmills, UK: Palgrave MacMillan.

Russell, W. M. S., and R. L. Burch. 1959. *The Principles of Humane Experimental Technique*. London: Methuen.

Ryder, Richard D. 1983 [1975]. *Victims of Science: The Use of Animals in Research*. 2nd ed. London: National Anti-Vivisection Society.

Schuppli, Catherine A., and David Fraser. 2005. "The Interpretation and Application of the Three Rs by Animal Ethics Committee Members." *Alternatives to Laboratory Animals* 33 (5): 487–500.

Sidgwick, Henry. 1966 [1874]. *The Methods of Ethics*. New York: Dover.

Singer, Peter. 1990 [1975]. *Animal Liberation*. 2nd ed. New York: New York Review of Books.

Singer, Peter. 1991. "Speciesism, Morality, and Biology: A Response to Jeffrey Gray." *Psychologist* 4 (5): 199–200.

Singer, Peter. 2006. "Setting Limits on Animal Testing." *Sunday Times* (London), December 3.

Singer, Peter. 2011 [1979]. *Practical Ethics*. 3rd ed. Cambridge, UK: Cambridge University Press.

Slicer, Deborah. 2007 [1991]. "Your Daughter or Your Dog? A Feminist Assessment of the Animal Research Issue." In *The Feminist Care Tradition in Animal Ethics: A Reader*, edited by Josephine Donovan and Carol J. Adams, 105–24. New York: Columbia University Press.

Smith, Jane A., and Kenneth M. Boyd, eds. 1991. *Lives in the Balance: The Ethics of Using Animals in Biomedical Research: The Report of a Working Party of the Institute of Medical Ethics*. Oxford: Oxford University Press.

Stephens, Martin L. 2010. "An Animal Protection Perspective on 21st Century Toxicology." *Journal of Toxicology and Environmental Health B, Critical Reviews* 13 (2–4): 291–98.

Stephens, Martin L. 2012. "Pursuing Medawar's Challenge for Full Replacement." *ALTEX Proceedings: 8th World Congress, Montreal, 2011* 1 (1): 23–26.

Stephens, Martin L., and Kathleen M. Conlee. 2004. "The HSUS's Pain and Distress Initiative: Overview and Update." *Alternatives to Laboratory Animals* 32 (supp. 1): 423–27.

Taylor, Katy; Nicky Gordon; Gill Langley; and Wendy Higgins. 2008. "Estimates for Worldwide Laboratory Animal Use in 2005." *Alternatives to Laboratory Animals* 36 (3): 327–42.

Turner, Ernest S. 1992 [1964]. *All Heaven in a Rage*. Fontwell, UK: Centaur.

Understanding Animal Research. 2013. Accessed March 1, 2013. http://www.understandinganimalresearch.org.uk

US Congress, Office of Technology Assessment. 1986. *Alternatives to Animal Use in Research, Testing, and Education*. Washington, DC: US Government Printing Office.

US Department of Agriculture Animal and Plant Health Inspection Service. 2011. "Annual Report Animal Usage by Fiscal Year: 2010." http://www.aphis.usda.gov/animal_welfare/efoia/downloads/2010_Animals_Used_In_Research.pdf

US Department of Agriculture Office of Inspector General, Western Region. 2005. "Audit Report: APHIS Animal Care Program Inspection and Enforcement Activities." http://www.usda.gov/oig/webdocs/33002-03-SF.pdf

Van Zutphen, L. F. M. 1998. "Refinement, the Cinderella of the 3Rs." In *The Ethics of Animal Experimentation: Proceedings of the EBRA/FELASA European Congress*, edited by Philip N. O'Donoghue, 143–50. London: European Biomedical Research Association.

Peter Singer (1995, 2004)
IRA W. Decamp Professor of Bioethics, University Center for Human Values, Princeton University
Laureate Professor, School of Historical and Philosophical Studies, University of Melbourne

Bernard Unti (2014)
Senior Policy Adviser, Humane Society of the United States

III. LAW AND POLICY

This entry describes the laws and policies of the United States governing the care and use of animals in research, education, and testing; the history of these policies and laws since 1966; the issues addressed by these laws; and the lawsuits that have followed publication of regulations implementing these laws. Two federal laws govern the use of animals: the Health Research Extension Act of 1985 and the Animal Welfare Act, as amended. While all states have laws governing the care of animals, research usage is often exempted. Twenty states have simple facility licensure, and a few have only very general regulations governing research usage of animals. In reality, nearly all states defer to federal law in this area. A National Institutes of Health (NIH) document, *Public Health Service Policy on Humane Care and Use of Laboratory Animals*, which was revised in 2002, implements the Health Research Extension Act for all activities involving animals conducted or supported by the Public Health Service (PHS), while regulations implementing the Animal Welfare Act are in the *Code of Federal Regulations*, Title 9, Chapter 1, Subchapter A, Parts 1, 2, and 3 (known as animal welfare regulations). The PHS includes twelve health agencies within the US Department of Health and Human Services (HHS).

HISTORY OF PUBLIC HEALTH SERVICE POLICY

As Robert Whitney notes in his 1987 article "Animal Care and Use Committees: History and Current National Policies in the United States," regulations have been promulgated by the PHS since 1935, originally through one of its constituents, the National Institutes of Health. NIH guidelines have provided direction and recommendations for caring for and using laboratory animals at NIH. Subsequently, a committee of laboratory scientists assembled by the Institute of Laboratory Animal Resources of the National Research Council (NRC) wrote the *Guide for the Care and Use of Laboratory Animals* (NRC guide). First published in 1963 and updated many times since, this work has become the standard guide in the field. The first policy based upon the 1963 NRC guide came from NIH in 1971. The PHS published its first policy on animal care in 1973, with revisions in 1973, 1979, 1986, 1996, and 2002. Each successive revision increased the specificity and level of responsibility of animal-care committees in the supervision of animal use.

At the outset of NIH policymaking in animal care and use in 1971, all institutions and organizations using warm-blooded animals for the purpose of research or other projects supported by NIH were required to give assurances that facilities for animals met "acceptable standards for the care, use, and treatment of such animals." This assurance could be met either by gaining accreditation through a professional laboratory-accrediting body (such as the Association for Assessment and Accreditation of Laboratory Animal Care International [AAALAC]) or by establishing a committee to evaluate the care and housing of animals used for NIH-sponsored activities. Institutions were also obligated to follow pertinent sections of the animal welfare regulations. In 1973, the NIH policy was replaced by the first of the PHS policies. Like the NIH policy preceding it, the first PHS policy required institutions either to be fully accredited or to have a standing institutional committee with a minimum of three members, including a veterinarian for those institutions using a "significant" number of animals. These committees were required to conduct periodic facility inspections, with the review of applications and proposals involving the use of animals considered optional.

The 1979 revision to the PHS policy required all institutions using animals, regardless of numbers used and accreditation status, to have a standing committee whose responsibility was oversight of the institution's animal-care program. In addition to the establishment of a committee of at least five members, including one veterinarian, the institution was obligated to establish a mechanism to review its facilities for warm-blooded animals for adherence to the principles contained in the NRC guide. The PHS policy recommended that AAALAC accreditation was the best means of satisfying this obligation, although periodic committee review of facilities and animals' care would suffice. Absent from the 1979 PHS policy was the requirement for review of individual proposals or projects, although review was encouraged. In 1986, however, the PHS policy was revised again, this time requiring the animal-care committees of institutions to take responsibility for specific organizational and supervisory duties in an effort to strengthen the system of institutional assurance.

HISTORY OF ANIMAL WELFARE REGULATIONS

A 1966 *Life* magazine feature titled "Concentration Camps for Dogs," along with other works published around this time, dramatized poor care and treatment of animals by some dealers who sold animals for biomedical research. This disclosure and the ensuing public outcry resulted in the introduction of twenty-nine bills in the US Congress relating to the regulation of animal research. The bill that eventually became law was the Laboratory Animal Welfare Act of 1966 (LAWA; in 1970, after passage of the first amendments, the name was shortened to the Animal Welfare Act, or AWA). This act was limited to regulation of the sale and transportation of animals by dealers and the holding of animals by certain research facilities. Although the bill was passed, it was a compromise between far-reaching legislation and none at all; it did not apply to actual research usage of animals. The regulations implementing the LAWA specified that the housing facility provide shelter and protection from temperature extremes, that food and water be provided at least daily, and that cages be of a certain size and cleaned daily. These regulations also specified cage sizes and frequency of feeding and watering during transportation. Passage of amendments in 1970, 1976, 1985, and 1990 and of a law calling for the PHS policy extended federal regulations into areas covering the appropriate use and humane treatment of laboratory animals. The 1966 law regulated dogs, cats, hamsters, guinea pigs, rabbits, and nonhuman primates. The 1970 amendment broadened it to include all warm-blooded animals, but regulations excluded birds, rats, and mice.

The 1970 amendments broadened the US Department of Agriculture's (USDA) administrative responsibility to cover animal care throughout an animal's stay in research facilities, including the period during which research was being conducted. The 1976 amendments brought transportation carriers under the purview of the act, leading to more stringent standards for shipment of animals. The 1985 version of the AWA invested the USDA with responsibility for issuing and enforcing regulations regarding humane care, handling, and treatment of animals. Animals covered under the AWA include warm-blooded animals—such as dogs, cats, monkeys, guinea pigs, hamsters, rabbits, marine mammals, and normally wild animals—being used for research, testing, experimentation, exhibition purposes, or as a pet. Excluded from coverage are birds, rats, mice, and horses and other farm animals intended for use as food or fiber, or for use in improving animal nutrition, breeding or management. The 1990 changes to the act added college-student work with animals to the list of areas over which a research institution has oversight responsibility.

PUBLIC HEALTH SERVICE POLICY

PHS policy requires that each awardee institution provide a written assurance setting forth how that institution will comply with regulations. This assurance then forms the basis for the care and use of animals in research, education, and testing at that institution and is the basis for judging the adequacy of the institution's compliance with the policy. PHS policy calls for the establishment of a program for animal care and use, using the NRC guide as a basis for developing the program. Also required is the creation of an institutional animal care and use committee (IACUC), appointed by the chief executive officer of the institution. This committee must have at least five members, including at least one veterinarian experienced in laboratory animal science, one scientist, one layperson, and one person unaffiliated with the institution. PHS policy then charges this committee with oversight responsibility for: semi-annual review of the program of animal care and use; semi-annual inspection of facilities; review of research protocols, or proposals for the use of animals; investigation of all concerns raised by anyone regarding the humane use of animals at the institution; recommendations for personnel training; and suspension of activities deemed improper.

An institution's program for the care and use of laboratory animals encompasses institutional policies, laboratory-animal husbandry procedures, and veterinary care practices. Institutional policies address such personnel provisions as veterinary qualifications, procedures for safely handling hazardous agents, occupational health and personal hygiene, including appropriate clothing and practices, and the prohibition of smoking and eating in animal rooms; special considerations are also addressed through policies, such as those concerning prolonged physical restraint of animals and multiple surgeries on a single animal. Laboratory animal husbandry procedures include housing systems (size of cages and provision for social interaction among animals where appropriate); temperature, humidity, ventilation, lighting control, and cage and room sanitation schedules; and methods of animal identification and of clinical record keeping. Veterinary care practices include preventive medicine strategies; methods for detecting and treating diseases; giving investigators advice about appropriate anesthesia, analgesia, and surgical and postoperative care; and methods of euthanasia.

Facility inspection covers not only visiting the physical plant but also assessing the health of the animals and reviewing portions of the institutional program for animal care. The physical plant should be properly constructed to house the species being used and to permit sterile surgery to be performed, if necessary.

PHS policy sets forth several criteria to be followed by the IACUC in reviewing protocols. These criteria go beyond mere care and housing guidelines. The care and use of animals in proposed research must be consistent with the NRC guide, unless acceptable scientific justification is provided for any deviation. The investigator must explain the rationale for using animals at all in the proposed research as well as the appropriateness of the species to be used, the number of animals, and their proposed use. PHS policy stipulates requirements for the use of sedatives, analgesics, and anesthetics if the proposed procedure might cause more than slight pain or distress; it also requires prompt euthanasia at the end of (or, when appropriate, during) a procedure for "animals that would otherwise suffer severe or chronic pain or distress that cannot be relieved" and imposes methods of euthanasia consistent with American Veterinary Medical Association (AVMA) guidelines. All personnel involved in the use of animals in research must be appropriately trained and qualified in the procedures to be employed in the experiment.

Each IACUC must have procedures for investigating concerns raised about the care and use of animals at the institution. In addition, the IACUC must ensure that the institution has a training program for both animal-care staff (people actually caring for the animals) and research staff; videotapes and training handbooks may be used to satisfy this requirement. The final charge—the power to suspend an improperly conducted activity—must come from an official of the institution such as the chief executive officer or the vice president. Without this official support, the IACUC cannot fulfill its duty to ensure compliance with PHS policy.

Several features of PHS policy are of special importance. While its legal force is restricted to awardee institutions, its scope includes all live vertebrates. It was the first US law to call for a consideration of animal welfare during a procedure and to call for the establishment of a committee to review protocols for the appropriateness of design, the importance of knowledge sought (as set forth in the "U.S. Government Principles for the Utilization and Care of Vertebrate Animals Used in Testing, Research, and Training," published in both the PHS policy and the NRC guide), and the competency of personnel. Thus, through PHS policy, committees have been created to review the use of animals in research, much like the committees that review the participation of humans in research.

ANIMAL WELFARE REGULATIONS

Animal welfare regulations (AWRs) pertaining to the care and use of laboratory animals were extensively modified and rewritten following the 1985 amendments of the Animal Welfare Act to include provisions for an IACUC, for protocol review, and for more social interaction among the same species and between animals and their caretakers. These regulations are similar to PHS policy provisions because the secretary of the USDA was directed to consult with the secretary of the HHS concerning the writing of regulations. In the AWRs, an IACUC committee with only slight differences from PHS policy is required (e.g., three members instead of five as a minimum, including an unaffiliated member and a veterinarian). The duties of the committee are very similar to the duties specified by PHS policy; instructions for reviewing protocols, however, are more detailed than those included in PHS policy. The AWRs require the investigator to search for alternatives to any procedure that may cause more than slight pain or distress and to assure that the proposed activity does not unnecessarily duplicate previous work. Several aspects of a personnel-training program are specified. In contrast to PHS policy, which requires institutions to develop an animal care and use program based upon the NRC guide, the AWRs have an extensive set of standards specifying the humane handling, care, treatment, and transport of various species of animals. The standards section of the regulations detail facility and operating standards, animal health and husbandry standards, and transportation standards for each regulated species. In addition, detailed specifications are given for marking dogs, cats, and other animals for the purpose of identification. In most, but not all, cases, the standards of the AWRs are the same as those of the PHS policy and, thus, are similar to the guidelines given in the NRC guide.

The AWA calls for the USDA to issue regulations in several areas. These regulations, which have engendered considerable public debate as well as the filing of a lawsuit, require exercise of dogs and the provision of a physical environment adequate to promote the psychological wellbeing of nonhuman primates. After considerable debate, the final regulations combined performance-based standards (standards that specify the desired outcome and leave the details of achieving that outcome to the regulated party) with design or engineering standards (standards that specify in measurable and objective terms how a particular outcome is to be achieved). It is the choice of performance-based standards that is especially controversial because plaintiffs in a lawsuit alleged that they allow too much latitude for compliance by the regulated parties. It is generally true, however, that humane care and use of animals can be achieved under a variety of circumstances, making it difficult to use detailed engineering standards or specifications. For example, the regulations call for dry floors for most mammals. This can be accomplished by mopping the floor until dry, by wet-vacuuming the floor, by sloping the floor and letting water run off before placing an animal on the surface, and so on. Thus, there are a number of ways of achieving the desired goal, and it is the outcome itself that is specified rather than the steps needed to reach it. Critics of performance standards state that the goal often is not well described, leaving too much discretion to the regulated parties.

Another controversial aspect of the AWRs is that the regulatory definition of *animal* excludes birds, rats, and mice that have been bred for use in research; hence, these animals are not protected under the AWRs. The exclusion is a major one because more than 85 percent of animals used in research, education, and testing are rats, mice, and birds. The reason for the exclusion is to limit the scope and cost of annual USDA inspections; there are barely enough inspectors to review facilities and procedures involving larger vertebrate animals, whose use is thought to require more sensitivity and therefore more intense scrutiny. Adding rats, mice, and birds to the mandatory inspection list would exceed the capacity of the USDA, both because of the increased numbers of animals to be inspected and because there would be an increase in the number of registered research facilities requiring inspection. (A number of institutions use only rats and/or mice and therefore are not subject to inspection.) Because PHS policy defines *animal* as any vertebrate (with no exclusions), rats, mice, and birds are covered by PHS policy. As Orlans notes in her 2000 article "The Injustice of Excluding Laboratory Rats, Mice, and Birds from the Animal Welfare Act," in institutions not covered by PHS policy (e.g., industry and colleges not receiving PHS funds), the use of rats and mice remains largely unregulated, a glaring oversight unique to the United States.

PROTOCOL REVIEW: CONSIDERATION OF PAIN AND DISTRESS AND NUMBERS OF ANIMALS USED

Because both PHS policy and the AWRs explicitly require minimization of pain and distress of animals during research, there have been examinations of the implications and possible effectiveness of the IACUC consideration of these issues during protocol review (Dresser 1988; Brody 1989). Both regulations attempt to incorporate cost-benefit considerations, utilitarian theory, and some elements of a modified rights-based philosophy (Dresser 1988). The success of PHS policy and the AWRs depends fundamentally on the recognition that animals can experience pain and distress that can be alleviated (NRC 1992). The USDA requires an annual report from all registered institutions that lists the numbers of animals used in research and testing, classified by the degree of pain and distress: (1) minimal, transient or no pain or distress; (2) pain and distress relieved by anesthetics, analgesics, or tranquilizers; and (3) pain and distress not treated. A detailed statement on category 3 procedures is required, including scientific justification for withholding drugs. Another classification scheme, developed by the Scientists Center for Animal Welfare, lists six categories instead of three (Orlans 1987). Many IACUCs use some classification scheme for pain and distress, reducing the number of animals used in research that fall into the higher categories of pain and distress by applying the "three Rs" (replacement, reduction, and refinement) of William M. S. Russell and Rex L. Burch, authors of a book first published in 1959 called *The Principles of Humane Experimental Technique.*

Some observers feel that IACUC review does not adequately reduce the number of animals used in research or the pain and distress of these animals. In a 1989 article, Mimi Brody suggested new legislation that would implement two oversight levels—first, a local committee; second, a national committee—to review uses of animals with "high ethical cost." Gary L. Francione argued in a 1990 article that open IACUC meetings, publicly announced and attended by interested members of the community, would improve the quality of protocol review. The two-committee approach has the disadvantage of delaying approval of certain types of research and has the potential for becoming excessively bureaucratic. The open-meetings approach presumes that the general public could comprehend the scientific details of the described procedures and would be able to judge the ethical and social justifications for the proposed procedure.

LAWSUITS CONCERNING THE ANIMAL WELFARE REGULATIONS

As mentioned earlier, the definition of animals in the AWRs excludes birds, rats, and mice specifically bred for use in research. After parts one and two of the AWRs became final in 1989, the Animal Legal Defense Fund (ALDF) and the Humane Society of the United States (HSUS) filed a rule-making petition with the USDA to amend the regulations to include rats, mice, and birds in the definition of animals. After the USDA denied the petition in 1990, the ALDF and the HSUS brought suit in federal court, seeking a declaratory judgment and an injunction preventing the USDA from excluding coverage of rats, mice, and birds. In 1992 the ALDF and the HSUS were granted summary judgment, and the USDA was ordered to reconsider its denial of plaintiffs' petition in light of the court's opinion holding the exclusion of rats, mice, and birds to be arbitrary and capricious (*Animal Legal Defense Fund v. Madigan*, 1992). The USDA appealed, and on May 20, 1994, the court of appeals vacated the district court's decision and directed the lower court to dismiss, holding that none of the petitioners had demonstrated both constitutional standing to sue and a statutory right to judicial review under the Administrative Procedure Act—leaving regulations, and presumably practice, to stand unchanged (*Animal Legal Defense Fund v. Espy*, 1994). In 1998, however, the Alternatives Research and Development Foundation filed a new suit to force the inclusion of rats, mice, and birds under AWA. The USDA settled the case (*Alternatives Research and Development Foundation v. Glickman*) in 2000, agreeing to inclusions. But the Farm Security and Rural Investment Act of 2002 blocked the settlement. This amendment permanently denied rats, mice, and birds legal protection under AWA.

The USDA regulations concerning requirements for exercise of dogs and for a physical environment adequate to promote the psychological well-being of nonhuman primates were published in February 1991. The ALDF and others sued, alleging that these regulations did not comply with the 1985 amendments of the AWA because they did not provide minimum standards for exercise of dogs and for adequate cage size and environmental enrichment for nonhuman primates as required by Congress. The district court granted plaintiffs' motion for summary judgment in February 1993 (*Animal Legal Defense Fund v. Secretary of Agriculture*, 1993). It was unclear at the time of this decision whether the federal government would appeal the decision, so the National Association for Biomedical Research (NABR) moved to intervene in the case to ensure an appeal. Although the NABR motion was originally denied, the denial was reversed by the court of appeals. The federal government subsequently decided to pursue an appeal, and the consolidated appeal was argued in May 1994. Two months later, the court of appeals vacated the district court's decision and directed the lower court to dismiss, concluding that the ALDF and the other appellees lacked standing to challenge USDA regulations (for the same reasons cited in the ALDF/ HSUS case), again leaving policy unchanged.

CONCLUSION

Federal laws and policies regarding the use of animals in research, education, and testing have progressed rapidly from the first enunciation of principles for the care of laboratory animals in the early days of NIH and the first animal welfare laws passed in 1966. Early policy had limited effects on the use of animals because of the generally careful practice standards already in place as well as the lack of enforcement of the new policy. Several US programs and institutions had their funding suspended in the early 1980s, with increased USDA inspections and subsequent violations at numerous institutions in the years that followed, all of which serve as a warning that all animal-care policies must be followed (Rozmiarek 1987). The evolution of policies for animal care and use shows a trend toward increased responsibility for and supervision by IACUCs, with greater emphasis on the level of assurances institutions must give, on IACUC membership, on the process of protocol review, and on the committee's power in matters involving activities using animals. This has resulted in more scrutiny of the care and use of animals in scientific research. The regulations in effect are comprehensive and, if followed, result in excellent care for animals. The penalties for not adhering to the regulations are great enough to encourage compliance and will assure that the privilege of using animals in research is carried out in a humane and careful manner.

BIBLIOGRAPHY

Alternatives Research and Development Foundation v. Glickman. 2000. 101 F.Supp.2d 7 (D.D.C. 2000).

American Veterinary Medical Association (AVMA). Panel on Euthanasia. 2001. "2000 Report of the AVMA Panel on Euthanasia." *Journal of the American Veterinary Medical Association* 218 (5): 669–96.

Animal Legal Defense Fund v. Espy. 1994. 23 F.3d 496 (C.A.D.C. 1994).

Animal Legal Defense Fund v. Madigan. 1992. 781 F.Supp. 797 (D.D.C. 1992).

Animal Legal Defense Fund v. Secretary of Agriculture. 1993. 813 F.Supp. 882 (D.D.C. 1993).

Animal Welfare Act, as Amended. US Code 7 secs. 2131–56.

Brody, Mimi. 1989. "Animal Research: A Call for Legislative Reform Requiring Ethical Merit Review." *Harvard Environmental Law Review* 13 (2): 423–84.

Dresser, Rebecca. 1988. "Assessing Harm and Justification in Animal Research: Federal Policy Opens the Laboratory Door." *Rutgers Law Review* 40 (3): 723–95.

Francione, Gary L. 1990. "Access to Animal Care Committees." *Rutgers Law Review* 43 (1): 1–14.

Health Research Extension Act of 1985. 1985. Public Law 99-158, U.S. Statutes at Large 99 (1985).

Laboratory Animal Welfare Act of 1966. US Code 7 secs. 2131–56.

National Institutes of Health. Office of Laboratory Animal Welfare. 2002. *Public Health Service Policy on Humane Use of Laboratory Animals.* Rev. ed. Rockville, MD: National Institutes of Health.

National Research Council (NRC). Commission on Life Sciences. Institute of Laboratory Animal Resources. 1996. *Guide for the Care and Use of Laboratory Animals.* Rev. ed. Washington, DC: National Academy Press.

National Research Council (NRC). Commission on Life Sciences. Institute of Laboratory Animal Resources. Committee on Educational Programs in Laboratory Animal Science. 1991. *Education and Training in the Care and Use of Laboratory Animals: A Guide for Developing Institutional Programs.* Washington, DC: National Academy Press.

National Research Council (NRC). Commission on Life Sciences. Institute of Laboratory Animal Resources. Committee on Pain and Distress in Laboratory Animals. 1992. *Recognition and Alleviation of Pain and Distress in Laboratory Animals.* Washington, DC: National Academy Press.

Orlans, F. Barbara. 1987. Research Protocol Review for Animal Welfare. *Investigative Radiology* 22 (3): 253–58.

Orlans, F. Barbara. 1993. *In the Name of Science: Issues in Responsible Animal Experimentation.* New York: Oxford University Press.

Orlans, F. Barbara. 2000. "The Injustice of Excluding Laboratory Rats, Mice, and Birds from the Animal Welfare Act." *Kennedy Institute of Ethics Journal* 10 (3): 229–38.

Rozmiarek, Harry. 1987. "Current and Future Policies Regarding Laboratory Animal Welfare." *Investigative Radiology* 22 (2): 175–79.

Russell, William M. S., and Rex L. Burch. 1992 [1959]. *The Principles of Humane Experimental Technique.* Potters Bar, UK: Universities Federation for Animal Welfare.

Silva, M. 1966. "Concentration Camps for Dogs." *Life*, February 4, 22–29.

Southwick, Ron. 2002. "Researchers Face More Federal Scrutiny on Animal Experimentation." *Chronicle of Higher Education,* June 28, 23.

Whitney, Robert A., Jr. 1987. "Animal Care and Use Committees: History and Current National Policies in the United States." *Laboratory Animal Science* 37 (suppl.): 18–21.

Jeffrey Kahn (1995, 2004)
Robert Henry Levi and Ryda Hecht Levi Professor of Bioethics and Public Policy, Berman Institute of Bioethics, Johns Hopkins University

Susan Parry (2004)
Hennepin Technical College

Ralph Dell (1995)
Professor of Pediatrics, College of Physicians & Surgeons, Columbia University
Chair, Health Sciences Institutional Animal Care and Use Committee

III. LAW AND POLICY [ADDENDUM]

The most dramatic development in US animal research policy involves a reduction in the amount and types of research on chimpanzees that the National Institutes of Health (NIH) will fund. In early 2011 the NIH asked the Institute of Medicine (IOM) to examine the continued US funding of biomedical research on chimps. In December of that year a committee of the IOM and the National Research Council of the National Academies published *Chimpanzees in Biomedical and Behavioral Research: Assessing the Necessity*. The report concluded that most current use of chimps in biomedical research was unnecessary and recommended that use of chimpanzees in biomedical research be limited to cases in which no other suitable research model was available, the research in question could not ethically be performed on human beings, and forgoing research on chimpanzees would significantly slow or prevent advancements that could prevent, control or treat life-threatening or debilitating conditions (Institute of Medicine and National Research Council of the National Academies 2011). In June 2013 the NIH implemented the IOM recommendations, effectively reducing the number of federally funded chimpanzee research subjects in the US from over 1,000 to approximately 50. Most continuing chimp research involves hepatitis (National Institutes of Health 2013).

A less dramatic but more far-reaching development was the publication in 2011 of the first update in fourteen years of the *Guide to the Care and Use of Laboratory Animals* (National Resource Council of the National Academies 2011). The eighth edition of the guide has been adopted by the NIH as its standard for animal care. The new guide is nearly twice as long as its predecessor and contains many more mandatory statements (as opposed to mere recommendations). Many of these pertain to standards relating to the housing of laboratory animals, including recommendations about enhancement techniques; others are broader statements about the goals and structure of an animal care and use program and the newly introduced concept of "animal biosecurity"—measures used to protect animals from infection.

In the autumn of 2011 the Association for Assessment and Accreditation of Laboratory Animal Care International (2013) (AAALAC) began recognizing the revised guide as one of three primary standards it would use to evaluate animal care and use programs, the other two being the Federation of Animal Science Societies' *Guide for the Care and Use of Agricultural Animals in Science and Teaching* (2010) and the European Convention for the Protection of Vertebrate Animals Used for Experimental and Other Scientific Purposes (Council of Europe 2005). Where the standards differ (as in certain kinds of research on agricultural animals), the AAALAC relies on the collective professional judgment of veterinarians, Institutional Animal Care and Use Committee (IACUC) members, and principal investigators to determine which of the standards is most appropriately met given the nature of the research in question.

SEE ALSO *Animal Welfare and Rights: VII. Policies and Organizations; Law and Morality; Research Policy: I. General Background; Xenotransplantation*

BIBLIOGRAPHY

Association for Assessment and Accreditation of Laboratory Animal Care International. 2013. *AAALAC Now Using Three Primary Standards.* Accessed August 11, 2013. http://www.aaalac.org/about/guidelines.cfm

Council of Europe. 2005. "European Convention for the Protection of Vertebrate Animals Used for Experimental and Other Scientific Purposes." http://conventions.coe.int/treaty/en/treaties/html/123.htm

Federation of Animal Science Societies. 2010. *Guide for the Care and Use of Agricultural Animals in Research and Teaching.* 3rd ed. Champaign, IL: Author.

Institute of Medicine and National Research Council of the National Academies. 2011. *Chimpanzees in Biomedical and Behavioral Research: Assessing the Necessity.* Washington, DC: National Academies Press.

National Institutes of Health. 2013. "NIH to Reduce Significantly the Use of Chimpanzees in Research." News and Events. June 26, 2013. http://www.nih.gov/news/health/jun2013/od-26.htm

National Resource Council of the National Academies. 2011. *Guide for the Care and Use of Laboratory Animals.* 8th ed. Washington, DC: National Academies Press.

Stephen R. Latham
Director, Interdisciplinary Center for Bioethics, Yale University

ANIMAL WELFARE AND RIGHTS

This entry consists of the following:

I. ETHICAL PERSPECTIVES ON THE TREATMENT AND STATUS OF ANIMALS

Normative ethical theory may be conceived as the systematic inquiry into the moral limits on human freedom. Philosophers and theologians throughout history and across cultures have offered different, often contradictory, answers to the central question of ethics thus conceived. Some have argued, for example, that the only justified limits on human freedom are those grounded in the rational self-interest of the agent, whereas others have maintained that the foundations of morality, and thus the basis of morally justified limitations on human freedom, are logically distinct from self-interest, though not from the dictates of reason. Still others have alleged that the foundations of morality have nothing to do with either reason or self-interest.

In view of the variety and conflicting nature of answers to the central question of normative ethics, it is hardly surprising that ethical theories sometimes offer strikingly different accounts of the moral status of those nonhuman animals we humans raise or hunt for food and clothing, use as beasts of burden, train to entertain us, and use as models for purposes of biomedical research. No philosopher or theologian has gone so far as to say that, from the moral point of view, there are no justified limits on what we may do to these animals. Even René Descartes, much celebrated for his theory that nonhuman animals are automata and thus incapable of feeling either pain or pleasure (Descartes, "Animals Are Machines," in Regan and Singer 1976, 1989), is said to have treated his dog humanely. At a certain minimal level, then, all normative ethical theories speak with one voice. But at other levels, the differences are both real and deep.

DIRECT AND INDIRECT DUTIES

These differences emerge clearly when we consider how competing theories answer two distinct but related questions. The first asks, What are the grounds for morally limiting human freedom when it comes to human interactions with nonhuman animals? The second asks, How extensive are these moral limits on human freedom? The former inquires as to why human freedom should be limited at all when our actions affect other animals; the latter challenges us to investigate how much our freedom should be limited. Of the two questions, the first is the more basic, for the reasons given in support of views about how much our freedom should be limited ultimately are based on views about why our freedom should be limited in the first place.

Two opposed possibilities present themselves as answers to the first, more basic question. One possibility holds that it is because of how animals themselves are affected or treated by human agents that we should limit our freedom. Viewed from this perspective, nonhuman animals are entitled to a certain kind of consideration or treatment. Because such views stress the idea that something is owed or is due directly to these animals, it is common to refer to them as "direct duty" views.

The second possibility locates the ground of moral constraint in some basis other than the animals. Viewed from this perspective, humans owe nothing to other animals, nor do these animals deserve any sort of treatment or consideration. Rather, human freedom should be limited because, for example, human cruelty to other animals will cause humans to treat one another cruelly. Because such views deny that we have duties directly to other animals, while recognizing that other factors should limit our freedom in our dealings with them, they are commonly referred to as "indirect duty" views.

All normative ethical theories, as they address the moral status of nonhuman animals, fall into one or the other of these two classes. That is, either they affirm that we have direct duties to nonhuman animals, or they deny that we have direct duties. Some of the major theoretical options within each class, as these have been developed by ethicists within the history of Western thought, will be considered in what follows.

ABOLITION, REFORM, AND STATUS QUO

As noted earlier, a second important question asks how much our freedom should be limited in our dealings with other animals. Three sorts of options may be distinguished: abolitionist, reformist, and status quo. An abolitionist position argues on behalf of ending human practices that routinely utilize nonhuman animals (for example, as a source of food or as models in scientific research). A reformist position accepts these institutions in principle but seeks in various ways to improve them in practice (for example, by enlarging the cages for animals used in research). A status quo position, unlike the abolitionist position, accepts these institutions in principle and, unlike the reformist position, does not recognize the need to improve them. Representative examples of each outlook and their logical relationship to competing normative ethical theories will be explained below.

Although the heated, sometimes acrimonious, debate among partisans of abolition, reform, and the status quo captures the attention of the media, far less attention has been devoted to the critical assessment of the competing ethical philosophies, whether of the direct or indirect duty variety. This by itself suggests the degree to which the public debate over "animal rights," broadly conceived, has assumed the greater part of what is most in need of informed, critical reflection. For clearly, whether we should favor the goals of supporters of abolition, reform, or the status quo in practice depends on determining the most adequate account of how we should treat nonhuman animals in theory. It is to a consideration of some of the major options in ethical theory that this entry now turns.

PERFECTIONISM

Aristotle (384–322 B.C.E.) presents the broad outlines of a moral theory that goes by the name "perfectionism." The cornerstone of this theory has a high degree of initial plausibility. Justice, it is claimed, consists in giving to individuals what they are due, and those individuals whose character is morally better (more "perfect") than the character of others prima facie deserve more of what is good in life than do other, less good people. Aristotle's accounts of what makes people morally better and of "the good of man" have helped shape much of Western moral theory. Concerning the latter first, Aristotle accepts the commonplace notion that the good we humans seek is happiness, but he argues that the true happiness we seek is not wealth, fame, or even pleasure in abundance but, rather, the possession and exercise of those virtues (those "excellences") that are uniquely human. Thus happiness, in his view, is characterized as "an activity of the soul in accordance with virtue." Those are happiest who optimally express their humanity in how they live and, in doing so, take pleasure in being the human beings they are.

As for the moral virtues (prudence, justice, courage, and temperance), Aristotle characterizes each as a mean between the extremes of excess and deficiency. A courageous person, for example, is neither foolhardy (an excess) nor cowardly (a deficiency); a courageous person has the right mix of the willingness to take risks and the fear of doing so. Among the intellectual virtues, a detached, contemplative wisdom, wherein one knows eternal truths and in this way shares in that knowledge possessed by the gods, is the highest. In the case of both the moral and the intellectual virtues, finally, the human capacity to reason plays a decisive role. For man is, in Aristotle's view, unique in being "a rational animal," and "the good of man" consists in actualizing, to the fullest extent possible, those unique potentialities that define what it is to be human. Thus, since those are happiest who optimally express their humanity in how they live, those are happiest who exercise their reason optimally.

Because it prescribes the distribution of what is good in life on the basis of one's possessing the favored virtues and, thus, on the basis of degrees of human perfection, perfectionism can—and in Aristotle's hands, does—sanction or require radically inegalitarian treatment of different individuals. In the case of nonhuman animals in particular, perfectionism provides no direct protection. Despite his teaching, in sharp contrast to Descartes's, that these animals share many of the same psychological capacities possessed by humans—including, for example, sensation and desire—Aristotle confidently denies that they share the capacity to reason. Moreover, because in his view the "lesser" exists to serve the interests or purposes of the "greater," Aristotle maintains that nonhuman animals exist for the purpose of advancing the good of human beings. He writes: "Other animals exist for the sake of man, the tame for use and food, the wild, if not all, at least the greater part of them, for food, and for the provision of clothing and various instruments" (Aristotle, "Animals and Slavery," in Regan and Singer 1976, 110; 1989, 5). There is no implication here that Aristotle's teachings permit the wanton infliction of pain on nonhuman animals for no good reason. What is clear is that because he recognizes no greater purpose for nonhuman animals than to serve the interests of human beings, Aristotle can recognize only indirect duties in their case. Finally, whereas controversial practices involving human utilization of nonhuman animals, such as factory farming and animal-to-human organ transplants, were unknown in his day, all the available evidence seems to indicate that Aristotle was well disposed to the status quo with respect to the relevant practices current while he was alive.

It is not only nonhuman animals, however, that exist for the sake of those who are more perfect. In general, women do not measure up to Aristotle's standards of "the good of man." "The male is by nature superior, and the female inferior," he writes, "and the one rules, and the other is ruled; this principle, of necessity, extends to all mankind" (ibid.). Moreover, some humans, whether male or female, lack the ability to grasp through reason those truths understood by the more virtuous among us; of such individuals Aristotle writes that they are "slave[s] by nature" (ibid.). And so it is that Aristotle affirms the obvious parallel, given the form perfectionism takes in his hands, between the moral status of human slaves and nonhuman animals: "The use made of slaves and of tame animals is not very different; for both with their bodies minister to the needs of life" (ibid.). Those humans who, because of their superior rationality, are morally more perfect are entitled to make use of those, whether human or not, who lack the virtues defining human perfection.

Few today will publicly embrace Aristotle's perfectionism. Not only does his view of women offend emancipated gender egalitarianism, but the comfortable elitism and classism that enable him to pronounce some humans "slaves by nature" will find no home among the most basic precepts of contemporary moral, political, and legal thought. The practical implications for humans of the fundamental principle of Aristotelian perfectionism—that those who are lacking in reason exist to serve the interests of those who are most virtuous—is morally offensive. It is one thing to affirm that those people who are more perfect than others prima facie deserve more of what is good in life; it is quite another to maintain that those who are less perfected exist for the sole purpose of ministering to the more virtuous. Moreover, since we cannot rationally defend the exploitation of some humans on the grounds that "by nature" they lack the potential to acquire the virtues possessed by those who exploit them, we cannot rationally defend human exploitation of nonhuman animals by offering an analogous defense—cannot, that is, rationally defend such exploitation by claiming that nonhuman animals "by nature" lack the potential to acquire uniquely human virtues.

DESPOTISM AND STEWARDSHIP

An alternative to Aristotle's philosophy is rooted in the biblical teaching that the God of Judaism and Christianity gives human beings dominion over nature in general and other animals in particular. As so often happens, however, there is more than one way to interpret the biblical message. Two ways in which human dominion can be understood—despotism and stewardship—will be sketched here.

Despotism teaches that nature in general and the other animals in particular are created by God for the sake of humans, and thus are ordained by the divine creator to serve such myriad human purposes as a source of food and clothing. Nothing within the natural order, save humans, has value in and of itself; what value the natural world possesses is entirely dependent on the extent to which it serves human interests. In this sense, human interests *are* the measure of all things, at least all things of value. Various biblical passages are cited to confirm the despotic reading, for example, "Then God said, 'Let us make man in our image, after our likeness; and let them have dominion over the fish of the sea, and over the birds of the air, and over the cattle … and over all the earth'" (Gen. 1:26).

Seen in this light, despotism's appeal to what God has ordained provides a reason for human supremacy over nonhuman animals that Aristotle's appeal to what is guaranteed "by nature" seems to lack, and it is a small step from acceptance of the despotic interpretation of human dominion to the conclusion that we owe nothing to nonhuman animals. Thus we find Saint Thomas Aquinas (c. 1225–1274), for example, urging in words barely distinguishable from those of Aristotle except for their reference to God that it is by "Divine ordinance that the life of animals and plants is preserved not for themselves but for man" (Thomas Aquinas, "On Killing Living Things and the Duty to Love Irrational Creatures," in Regan and Singer 1976, 119; 1989, 11). Mindful, moreover, that some biblical passages prohibit cruelty to nonhuman animals, Aquinas firmly places himself within the indirect duty tradition when he maintains that the import of such prohibitions is, for example, "to remove man's thoughts from being cruel to other men, and lest through being cruel to animals one become cruel to human beings" (Thomas Aquinas, "Differences between Rational and Other Creatures," in Regan and Singer 1976, 59; 1989, 9).

To the extent that Saint Thomas's philosophy is rooted in the scripture of the Christian tradition, those who stand outside this tradition are unlikely to be persuaded that God established in nature what nature was incapable of establishing by itself. Even granting biblical underpinnings to one's ethic, moreover, questions arise concerning the accuracy of the despotic interpretation of human dominion. Although the Hebrew concept of *rada*, translated as "having dominion," often is interpreted to mean human despotism over the nonhuman world—an idea that, according to some early critics (White 1967; McHarg 1969), is the root cause of today's environmental crisis—a significantly different interpretation has been proposed by more recent thinkers (Barr 1974; Linzey 1987; McDaniel 1989; Callicott 1993).

For *rada* can be understood as the idea of human responsibility toward and care for a created order that is good independent of the human presence. According to this latter interpretation, commonly referred to as stewardship, humans are given the task of being as loving within the natural order as God was in creating the natural order in the first place. Humans, that is, are to be the loving caretakers of an independently good creation. Because, viewed from the stewardship perspective, the natural world in general, and those nonhuman animals with whom we share it in particular, are good apart from human interests, our duties with regard to these animals emerge as direct duties owed to them rather than indirect duties owed either to other humans or to their creator.

Although when thus interpreted all of creation is seen as having a kind of value that is independent of human interests, the value of nonhuman animals arguably is especially noteworthy. One might note, first, that these animals were created on the same day—the sixth—as were humans (Gen. 1:24–27); that in the original state of perfection, in Eden, humans did not eat other animals (Gen. 1:29); and that, in God's covenant with Noah after the flood (Gen. 9:8–12), animals (but not plants) are included. Using these images, one can argue that the choice we face today is *either* to continue to move further from the sort of relationship with the animals God hoped would prevail when the world was created *or* to make daily efforts to recapture that relationship—to journey back to Eden, as it were. Given this latter reading, the practical consequences of a stewardship interpretation of dominion would depart significantly from those favored by the status quo position, just as the goals one would hope to achieve would differ from those advanced by reformists. For if our righteous relationship with the other animals, in our capacities as their caretakers and protectors, is one of nonutilization (they are not to be eaten, not to be worn, etc.), then the stewardship interpretation of human dominion would seem to support an abolitionist ideal.

However these matters are to be settled, the biblical grounding of morality characteristic of both despotism and stewardship places these moral perspectives outside the mainstream of normative ethical theory, at least from the Enlightenment forward, where rigorous, imaginative attempts have been made to ground ethics independently of belief in God and the moral authority of the Bible. One such attempt is contractarianism.

CONTRACTARIANISM

Among the most influential nontheological political and moral theories, contractarianism has a legacy that reaches at least as far back as Thomas Hobbes (1588–1679) and, among our contemporaries, includes such notable philosophers as John Rawls (1971) and Jan Narveson (1988). Like other theorists united by a common outlook, contractarians often disagree on many of the most fundamental points. It will not be possible to do justice to the rich fabric of disagreement that characterizes proponents of the theories under review.

As its name suggests, contractarianism conceives of morality as a kind of contract into which people (the "contractors") enter voluntarily. For contractarians, morality emerges as a set of mutually agreed upon and enforceable constraints on human freedom, constraints that each party to the contract rationally believes to be in his or her own self-interest. There is, then, according to contractarian theory, nothing that by its nature is morally right or wrong, just or unjust; rather, acts or institutions become right or wrong, just or unjust, as a result of the agreements reached by rational, self-interested contractors. In this sense, all of morality is conventional, and none is natural. Morality is created, not discovered, by human beings.

Both the self-interest that motivates and the rationality that guides the contractors are significant. We are not to imagine that people, as they deliberate about what limits on their freedom they will accept, are motivated by a natural sympathy for the misfortune of others or that they are willing altruistically to accept personal loss so that others might gain. Each contractor is motivated exclusively by his or her self-interest. The conception of individual self-interest each contractor has, moreover, is neither whimsical nor uninformed. Each person asks the same basic question: From the point of view of what is best for me, rationally considered, what limitations on my freedom would I be willing to accept? Morality, understood as rational, enforceable constraints on human freedom, arises when all the contractors jointly agree on the same constraints, not out of sympathy for others or because of altruistic motivations, but because each judges the outcome to be in his or her personal self-interest.

Two fundamentally opposed forms of contractarianism may be distinguished. The first permits the contractors to enter into their contractual deliberations equipped with the knowledge of who they are and what they want out of life, given their individual interests, talents, and hopes. This is the form of contractarianism favored by Hobbes and Narveson, for example. The second, favored by Rawls, requires that the contractors imagine that they lack such detailed knowledge of their individual psychology and circumstances, and instead deliberate about the terms of the contract from behind what Rawls calls "a veil of ignorance." Why Rawls would have recourse to this imaginative point of view will be explained momentarily. First, however, the implications of Hobbesian contractarianism for the treatment of nonhuman animals deserve attention.

Judged on the basis of the interests of these animals, the implications are not particularly salutary. In view of their inability to express these interests and to negotiate with others, nonhuman animals obviously are not to be counted among the potential contractors. Moreover, even while it is true that some things are in the interests of pigs and wolves, for example, the idea that these animals can have an informed understanding of what is in their rational self-interest has no clear meaning. Not surprisingly, therefore, what protection these animals are provided by Hobbesian contractarianism necessarily depends on what interests the human contractarians happen to have in them.

Narveson, for one, cheerfully indicates that this need not be very much (Narveson, "A Defense of Meat Eating," in Regan and Singer 1989). Because many contractors have a special place in their hearts for companion animals ("pets"), these animals will be treated reasonably well, not because they are entitled to such treatment but because we owe it to their human friends not to upset them (these humans) gratuitously. In the case of most other nonhuman animals, however, including those slaughtered for food or used in research, Narveson finds no good reason to cease and desist. Clearly, then, given Hobbesian contractarianism, all our duties with respect to other animals are indirect duties owed to those human beings who help forge the contract. And just as clearly, considered from a political perspective, one finds little within this version of contractarianism that could mount an abolitionist or a far-reaching reformist approach to how other animals are treated; what one finds instead is a theory well disposed to the status quo while remaining open to modest reforms.

Critics of Hobbesian contractarianism have raised various objections (Regan 1983). One concerns the possibility of arbitrary discrimination between people—for example, discrimination based on race. If we imagine that a large majority of potential contractors (say, 95%) are white, and the remainder black, then it is not obviously irrational for those who make up the majority to exclude members of the minority from negotiating the contract; perhaps the majority might even agree to keep the minority in bondage, as chattel slaves, the better to advance the rational self-interests of those individuals constituting the majority. That such an arrangement would be unjust seems too obvious to need a supporting argument. And (for Hobbesian contractarianism) there's the rub. For since what is just and unjust is created by the agreements reached by the contractors, there is, within this form of contractarianism, no theoretical grounding for the evident injustice involved in excluding the minority from participating. The theory, that is, not only fails to illuminate why such discrimination is unjust, but it also seems to deprive us of the means even to raise this objection. If a moral theory is so fundamentally flawed when it comes to how human beings, given their differences in skin pigmentation, should be treated, it is unclear how it can be any nearer the truth when it comes to how nonhuman beings, given their species differences, should be treated.

Rawls's introduction of the veil of ignorance, mentioned earlier, can be interpreted as his attempt to preserve the spirit of Hobbesian contractarianism while departing importantly from the letter. Rawls invites would-be contractors to imagine themselves in what he calls the "original position," in which, because they deliberate from behind the veil of ignorance, they do not know when they will be born or where, whether they will be rich or poor, of exceptional intelligence or below average, male or female, Caucasian or non-Caucasian. The question now to be asked, by each of the contractors, is what limits on human freedom each would accept, in the face of such profound ignorance concerning such details.

The full scope of Rawls's answer need not concern us. Only two points are of particular importance here. The first concerns how Rawlsian contractarianism improves on Hobbesian contractarianism when it addresses the issue of discrimination based on race. Hobbesian contractors, as noted above, can have a self-interested reason for accepting such discrimination, given that they know they belong to a racial majority. Rawlsian contractors, in contrast, lack such a reason since, for all they know, they might be one of the minority. In this respect, Rawlsian contractarianism seems to represent a notable improvement over Hobbesian contractarianism.

Despite its apparent strengths in response to issues involving arbitrary discrimination, Rawls's account of the moral status of nonhuman animals seems to fail to live up to its own standards (VanDeVeer 1979). Although the imaginary contractors behind the veil of ignorance are denied detailed knowledge about their individual interests and circumstances, and thus do not know whether, say, they will be male or female, black or white, Rawls does permit them to know that they will be born as human beings. To allow knowledge of this detail, however, seems to prejudice the case against nonhuman animals from the start. Granted, rational, self-interested contractors, making choices from behind the veil of ignorance, will negotiate direct duties to human beings and indirect ones to nonhumans, if they know they will be born human. But this only shows that these contractors will discriminate against these animals if they are provided with an arbitrary reason for doing so. In short, neither Hobbesian nor Rawlsian contractarianism seems to offer a reasonable basis on which to ground the only duties each recognizes in the case of nonhuman animals: indirect duties.

KANTIANISM

A final example of an indirect duty view is provided by the great Prussian philosopher Immanuel Kant (1724–1804). In some respects Kant's moral philosophy regarding the treatment of nonhuman animals is an amalgam of Aristotle's and, stripped of its appeals to God, Aquinas's. In concert with both, Kant emphasizes rationality as the defining characteristic of being human and, echoing Saint Thomas, objects to cruelty to animals because of the deleterious effect this has on how humans are treated. "He who is cruel to animals," Kant writes, "becomes hard also in his dealings with men," whereas "tender feelings towards dumb animals develop humane feelings towards mankind" (Kant, "Duties in Regard to Animals," in Regan and Singer 1976, 123; 1989, 24).

Despite these historical echoes, Kant's moral philosophy is in many ways highly original. Of particular note is his thesis that humanity exists as an "end in itself." Kant does not attempt to prove this thesis by appeal to some more basic principle; rather, it is set forth as a postulate in his system. In this capacity it places humans and other rational, autonomous beings in a unique moral category that distinguishes them, as "persons," from everything else that exists. Like Aristotle and Aquinas before him, Kant views the rest of the natural order as existing to serve human interests. In particular, animals, in his words, exist "merely as a means to an end. That end is man" (ibid.). Thus, whereas in Kant's view we are morally free to use other animals as we wish, subject only to the injunction to avoid cruelty, we are not morally free to treat human beings in a comparable fashion. Because humans exist as ends in themselves, we are never to treat them merely as means, Kant argues, which is what we would be doing if we treated them as we treat other animals (for example, if we raised humans as a food source). An abolitionist, a radical reformist, Kant is not. Provided only that we are not cruel in our treatment of nonhuman animals, we do nothing wrong when we treat them as we do.

A common objection against Kant's position is the argument from marginal cases (Regan 1983; for criticism of this argument, see Narveson 1977). All humans, Kant implies, exist as ends in themselves. To restrict this supreme moral value to humans among terrestrial creatures is not arbitrary, Kant believes, because humans, unlike the other animals, are unique in being rational and autonomous. However, not all humans are rational and autonomous. Those who are mentally enfeebled or deranged, for example, lack these capacities. Are these humans nevertheless ends in themselves? If Kant's answer is affirmative, then it is not the presence of rationality and autonomy that ground this supreme moral value; if, however, Kant's answer is negative, then it follows that these "marginal" human beings do not exist as ends in themselves, in which case it would seem that they, no less than other animals, may be treated as mere means. Because one assumes that this latter consequence would be seen by Kant to be morally grotesque, it seems fair to assume that he would want to avoid it; but he can do so, it seems, only by accepting the view that individuals who are neither rational nor autonomous nevertheless exist as ends in themselves, a view that undermines his confident assertion that nonhuman animals, deficient in reason and autonomy, exist "merely as means to an end," the end being "man."

UTILITARIANISM

The pioneering work of the nineteenth-century utilitarians Jeremy Bentham (1748–1832) and John Stuart Mill (1806–1873) represents a significant departure from the Aristotelian legacy we find in Kant's moral theory. Bentham, referring to nonhuman animals, writes, "The question is not, Can they *reason?* nor, Can they *talk?* but, Can they *suffer?*" (Bentham, "A Utilitarian View," in Regan and Singer 1976, 130; 1989, 26). The possession of sentience (the capacity to experience pleasure and pain), not the possession of rationality, autonomy, or linguistic competence, entitles any individual to direct moral consideration; and it is the possession of this particular capacity, in Bentham's and Mill's view, that creates in humans the direct duty not to cause nonhuman animals to suffer needlessly. We owe it to these animals themselves, not to those humans who might be affected by what we do, to take their (the nonhuman animals') pleasures and pains into account and, having done so, to ensure that we never make them suffer without good reason.

Both Bentham and Mill give a utilitarian interpretation of what such a good reason might be. Utilitarianism, roughly speaking, is the view that our duty is to perform that act that will bring about the best consequences for all those affected by the outcome. For value hedonists like Bentham and Mill, who recognize only one intrinsic good, pleasure, and only one intrinsic evil, pain, the best consequences will be those that include the greatest possible balance of pleasure over pain. A good reason for permitting animal suffering, then, is that such suffering is a necessary price to pay in bringing about the best consequences, all considered. How much of the spirit of reform, abolition, or the status quo happens to characterize individual utilitarians depends on how much animal suffering is judged to be necessary. Bentham opposes hunting, fishing, and the baiting of animals for sport, for example, whereas Mill's name is to be found among the earliest contributors to England's Royal Society for the Prevention of Cruelty to Animals. But neither Bentham nor Mill aligns himself with the cause of antivivisection, and both are lifelong meat eaters. So reformers they are, but abolitionists they are not. Even so, in their time, and given the broader social context in which they lived, they were seen by many of their contemporaries as radicals, if not extremists.

The degree to which utilitarians can differ over important practical matters is illustrated in our time by Peter Singer and R. G. Frey. Singer is justly famous for his seminal 1975 book, *Animal Liberation*. Frey has written two books (1980, 1983) and many essays devoted to the issues under review. The two philosophers, although agreeing on some of the most fundamental points in ethical theory, disagree on many of the most important consequences each believes follow from the application of utilitarianism, including how nonhuman animals should be treated. For example, in *Animal Liberation* Singer advocates vegetarianism, on moral grounds; Frey disagrees, appealing to the same grounds in his *Rights, Killing, and Suffering: Moral Vegetarianism and Applied Ethics* (1983). It will be useful to explain how such profound disagreements can arise between partisans of the same moral philosophy.

By its very nature, utilitarianism is a forward-looking moral theory. The consequences of our actions, and the consequences alone, determine the morality of what we do. As such, utilitarians will reach opposing judgments about what is right and wrong if they have opposing views of what the consequences of a given act will be. In the case of vegetarianism in particular, utilitarians like Singer believe that, taking everyone's interests into account, and counting equal interests equally, the consequences that flow from abstaining from animal flesh will be better than if people continue to include animal flesh in their diets; Frey, however, believes that the consequences of a vegetarian diet are not sufficiently better so as to impose an obligation on us to become vegetarians. It is, then, factual disagreements over what the future might hold that underlie the type of moral disagreement separating Singer and Frey on the issue of vegetarianism.

Some critics of utilitarianism (e.g., Clark 1977) argue that the apparently unresolvable impasse created by Singer's and Frey's application of utilitarian theory to the particular case of vegetarianism illustrates a major weakness in utilitarian theory in general. Because so much—indeed, because everything—depends on our ability to know what will happen in the future, and in view of the limitations of human knowledge in this regard, utilitarianism, these critics maintain, reduces moral judgment to guesswork about what might or might not occur.

Despite this problem, utilitarianism may seem to be a congenial theory for those who utilize nonhuman animals in animal model research. The most common justification of such research consists in appealing to the improvements in human health and longevity to which this research allegedly has led; and although researchers may recognize the need to look for alternatives to the animal model, lest these animals be used unnecessarily, it seems clear that the moral justification they offer is utilitarian. (For dissenting voices regarding the human benefits of such research, from the perspective of the history of medicine, see McKinlay and McKinlay 1977; for epistemological concerns, see LaFollette and Shanks 1993.) Part of the enduring greatness of *Animal Liberation* lies in Singer's relentless documentation of how much of this research prima facie fails to meet the utilitarian standard favored by researchers themselves. No less important is the way Singer exposes a prejudice that he, following Richard Ryder (1975), denominates "speciesism," and that he characterizes as "an attitude of bias in favor of the interests of members of one's own species and against those of other species" (Singer 1990, 6). Research scientists, Singer believes, frequently offer at best half a utilitarian justification of their work: Human interests are considered; those of nonhuman animals are not. To be consistent, the interests of both must be counted, and counted equitably. It is Singer's considered judgment that few researchers are consistent in this regard.

Frey, too, examines the lack of moral consistency among researchers ("Vivisection, Morals, and Medicine," in Regan and Singer 1989). Given any reasonable view about the richness and variety of psychological life, it is unquestionably true, Frey believes, that the psychological life of nonhuman primates, or even that of a cat or a dog, is richer and more varied than the psychological life of some human beings (a child born with only the stem of the brain, for example). Thus, if the moral defense of animal model research is supposed to lie in the good results allegedly produced by using these animals, then a similar defense for utilizing marginal humans is at hand. To be consistent in their utilitarianism, therefore, Frey believes that researchers should be willing to conduct their studies on marginal humans—a finding researchers are unlikely to welcome. Frey is unperturbed, insisting that researchers cannot have it both ways, using utilitarian modes of thinking when they believe it justifies their practice of using other than human animals in their studies, only to discard utilitarianism when its implications for the selection of marginal humans as research subjects are made manifest.

Whatever form utilitarianism takes, one of the principal objections its advocates face centers on questions of justice (Lyons 1965). What limits, if any, can utilitarianism recognize on how future good is to be obtained? The theory seems to imply that good ends justify whatever means are necessary to achieve them, including means that are flagrantly unjust. Classic examples include situations in which the judicial execution of the innocent is sanctioned on the grounds that others will be deterred from committing similar offenses. Here, critics concede, good consequences are brought into being, but the means used to secure them are reprehensible because they are unjust.

Utilitarians have replies to this and similar lines of criticism that go beyond the scope of the present entry (Brandt 1979). Suffice it to say that among those philosophers who are not utilitarians, many dissociate themselves from utilitarianism because they believe that respect for the rights of the individual is a principle that should not be compromised in the name of achieving some greater good for others. Not surprisingly, perhaps, a position of this kind, one that prohibits the use of nonhuman animals in the name of advancing the general human welfare, has been advanced (Regan 1983). Though not the only possible theory of animal rights (see, e.g., Rollin 1981, 1989), this particular theory (the "rights view") can be seen as an attempt to blend certain features of utilitarianism and Kant's theory.

THE RIGHTS VIEW

Kant, it will be recalled, recognizes only indirect duties to nonhuman animals; we humans are not to be cruel to animals, for example, not because we treat them wrongly by our cruel treatment but because cruelty to animals can lead people to be cruel to one another. By contrast, utilitarians from Bentham to Singer recognize direct duties to nonhuman animals; they believe that there are certain things we owe to these animals, apart from how humans will be affected. On this divisive issue the rights view sides with utilitarians against Kantians: Nonhuman animals are of direct moral significance; we have direct duties in their case.

In a second respect, however, the rights view sides with Kantians against utilitarians. Utilitarians believe that duty is determined by the comparative value of consequences; the right thing to do is what causes the best results. Kant and his followers take a decidedly different view: What is right does not depend on the value of consequences, it depends on the appropriate, respectful treatment of the individual—in particular, whether humans are treated as ends, not merely as means. In this regard, the rights view is cut from Kantian, not utilitarian, cloth. What is right depends not on the value of consequences but on the appropriate, respectful treatment of the individual, including individual nonhuman animals. Thus, the fundamental principle of the rights view (the respect principle) is Kantian in spirit: We are always to treat individuals who exist as ends in themselves (those who have "inherent value") with respect, which means, in part, that we are never to treat them merely as means.

One problem the rights view faces concerns which nonhuman animals possess value of this kind. Like other line-drawing issues ("Exactly how tall do you have to be to be tall?" "Exactly how old do you have to be to be old?"), this one has no precise resolution, in part because the criterion for drawing the line is imprecise. The criterion the rights view proposes is that of being the subject of a life, a criterion that specifies a set of psychological capacities (the capacities to desire, remember, act intentionally, and feel emotions, for example) as jointly sufficient. At least some nonhuman animals (e.g., mammals and birds) arguably possess these capacities, thus are subjects of a life, and thus, given the rights view, are to be treated as ends in themselves. (For criticism, see Frey 1980.)

Such a view, for obvious reasons, has massive political, social, and moral implications concerning how these animals ought to be treated. From an animal rights perspective of this kind, the abolition of human exploitation of these animals, whether on the farm, at the lab, or in the wild—not merely the reform of these practices, and certainly not approval of the status quo—is what duty requires.

Line-drawing issues aside, the rights view faces daunting challenges from other quarters. One concerns the idea of inherent value. Some critics (e.g., Sapontzis 1987) allege that the idea is "mystifying," meaning that it lacks any clear meaning. Advocates of animal rights reply that the notion of inherent value is no less "mystifying" than Kant's idea of end in itself. As applied to human beings, Kant's idea of end in itself attempts to articulate the cherished belief that the value or worth of a human being is not reducible to instrumental value—not reducible, that is, to how useful a human being happens to be in forwarding the interests or purposes of other human beings. Neither John Doe nor Jane Doe, in Kant's view, exists as a mere resource relative to what other people want for themselves, and to treat the Does as if their value—their worth or dignity—consists merely in their resource or instrumental value for others is morally wrong. All that the rights view alleges, then, is that to be consistent, the same moral judgment must be made in those cases where nonhuman animals that are subjects of a life are treated in a similar fashion.

Another set of challenges alleges that the philosophy of animal rights, if acted upon, would lead to catastrophic consequences, either to human interests in particular or to the community of life in general. Concerning the former challenge, some critics argue that human health and longevity would be seriously harmed if, as the philosophy of animal rights requires, nonhuman animals ceased to be used as models of human disease (see C. R. Gallistel, "The Case for Unrestricted Research Using Animals," in Regan and Singer 1989; and Cohen 1986). Several responses seem apposite.

First, given the massive allocation of public monies that fund such research, it needs to be asked whether abandoning reliance on the whole-animal model really is contrary to what is in the collective best interests of human beings. Some (e.g., Sharpe 1988) argue that customary reliance on this well-entrenched scientific methodology retards the development of alternative methodologies that would be more useful in understanding and curing major human diseases; in addition, these critics insist that humans would benefit more if the dominant focus of biomedical research were shifted away from curing disease to preventing it, a goal that is more efficiently advanced, these critics allege, by methodologies other than the use of the whole-animal model.

Second, recall one of the fundamental objections raised against utilitarianism: just as one does not justify the violation of a human being's rights because doing so will benefit others, so one does not justify the violation of the rights of nonhuman animals on similar grounds. More generally, some gains others might obtain may be ill-gotten, and they are ill-gotten if the price of obtaining them involves the violation of another's rights. Thus, even if it is true that humans stand to lose some benefits if animal model research is abandoned, this by itself does not constitute a telling moral objection to the abolitionist implications of the philosophy of animal rights, assuming that these animals, like humans, have the right to be treated as ends in themselves.

Concerning the second line of criticism—the one alleging that acting on the philosophy of animal rights would have catastrophic implications for the community of life in general—the principal objection may be summarized as follows. Predatory animals obviously live off the death and flesh of their prey. Because prey animals have the right to be treated with respect, according to the rights view, critics (e.g., Callicott 1980; Sagoff 1984) allege that it follows that we should intervene to stop predatory animals in their natural depredations. However, if we were to do this, there would be no check on the balance that exists in nature between predators and prey; instead, the population of prey animals would explode, and this would have the effect of irreparably damaging the balance and sustainability of life forms within the larger life community.

Advocates of the philosophy of animal rights have a number of possible replies to the predation problem, the principal one of which is the following. Situations can and do arise where the right thing to do is to come to the assistance of another, whether the potential victim is a human or a nonhuman animal. However, in these situations the potential victim not only is at risk of serious injury but also is less than capable of mounting a defense. Thus, an elderly woman who is attacked by a psychotic killer, or a puppy who is being tormented by children, merits our intervention. But the predator–prey relationship seems to bear little resemblance to such cases. Most prey animals, most of the time, are perfectly capable of eluding their predators without anyone's assistance. Thus it would seem to be human arrogance, not informed responsibility, that would lead humans to believe that because animals in the wild have rights, we are duty bound to "police" nature. From an animal rights perspective, we have no general duty to intervene in predator–prey relations; that being so, the catastrophic environmental costs alleged to be implied by acting on the rights view seem to be more in the nature of fiction than of fact. (For a different response to the predation problem, see Sapontzis 1987.)

DEEP ECOLOGY

Despite the significant differences separating the philosophy of animal rights and other, more traditional moral theories, such as Kant's, there are important similarities. For example, like Kant's theory, the philosophy of animal rights recognizes the noninstrumental value of the individual; and animal rights philosophy, as is true not only of Kant's theory but of utilitarianism as well, articulates an abstract, universal, and impartial fundamental moral principle—abstract because the respect principle enjoins us to treat others with respect, without regard to time, or place, or circumstance; universal because the respect principle applies to everyone capable of making moral decisions; and impartial because this principle does not favor some individuals (e.g., family members or companion animals) over others. Some contemporary moral philosophers find this approach to ethics archaic; among these critics, some of those who classify themselves as deep ecologists (see, in particular, Devall and Sessions 1985) command a growing audience. (For a more systematic and in some ways different version of deep ecology, see Naess 1989. For importantly different approaches to environmental ethics, see Callicott 1980; Taylor 1986; Rolston 1988.)

Both traditional moral theories and the philosophy of animal rights are doubly to be faulted, according to Devall and Sessions (1985)—first, because these moral outlooks offer an overly intellectualized account of the moral life, and second, because they perpetuate the myth of the moral preeminence of the individual. Considering this latter charge first, Devall and Sessions argue that the concept of the isolated, atomistic individual, which arises out of the anthropocentric traditions of Western philosophy, is false to the facts of all life's embeddedness in the larger life community. People are not independent bits of mind existing by themselves; they are enmeshed in networks of relationships that bind them both to their evolutionary past and to their ecological present. Expressed another way, humans do not stand "above" or "apart from" nature; they stand "within" nature. And the natural world does not exist "for us," as a storehouse of renewable human resources (a view that is symptomatic of a "shallow" view of humanity's relationship to nature); we are inseparable from the natural environment (a view that indicates a "deeper" understanding of what it means to be human).

Thus, acceptance of the illusory concept of the isolated individual, existing outside the natural order, has done, and continues to do, incalculable damage to those who seek self-understanding. So long as we carry out this quest with a fundamentally flawed preconception of our place in the larger scheme of things, the longer we search, the less we will understand. As for the charge that traditional moral theories overintellectualize the moral life,

Devall and Sessions argue that the moral life should be viewed as primarily experiential, not inferential, a life that is characterized by our coming to experience certain values in the concrete particularities of day-to-day life, rather than by apprehending abstract, universal, impartial moral principles by means of our rational powers.

Among those values to be found in the concrete particularities of day-to-day life, some involve other animals; and although deep ecologists have not written extensively on some of the most pressing practical issues, the general disdain these thinkers display toward reductionist science and industrial societies' technological domination of the natural world suggests that they would be strong reformists, at a minimum, in response to such practices as factory farming and animal model research. In the case of sport and recreational hunting, however, Devall and Sessions not only find nothing wrong, they applaud the practice. In pursuit of their prey, hunters tap into natural means whereby, through the act of killing, they can obtain greater self-understanding. Viewed in this light, Devall and Sessions seem to understand our duties with respect to animals as indirect duties limited by the overarching quest for self-knowledge. Although, therefore, deep ecologists like Sessions and Devall can be counted upon to add their voices to those of reformists and abolitionists in some cases, they emerge as defenders of the status quo in others.

ECOFEMINISM

Ecofeminists, not just advocates of the rights view, are among those contemporary moral philosophers who differ significantly with deep ecologists. Like other isms, ecofeminism is not a monolithic position (see Adams 1990; Diamond and Orenstein 1990; Warren 1990; Gaard 1993); instead, it represents a number of defining tendencies, including in particular a principled stance that puts its advocates on the side of those who historically have been victims of oppression. For obvious reasons, women are pictured as among the oppressed, but the scope of ecofeminism's concern is not limited to women. The same ideology that sanctions oppression based on gender, ecofeminists maintain, also sanctions oppression based on race, class, and physical abilities, for example; moreover, beyond the boundaries of our species, this same ideology, ecofeminists believe, sanctions the oppression of nature in general and of nonhuman animals in particular.

In a number of fundamental ways, ecofeminism's diagnosis of the ideology of oppression resembles deep ecology's diagnosis of the deficiencies of traditional moral theory. As is true of the latter, ecofeminism challenges the myth of the isolated individual, existing apart from the world, and instead affirms the interconnectedness of all life. Moreover, no less than deep ecologists, ecofeminists abjure the overintellectualization of the moral life characteristic of traditional moral theories, with their abstract, universal, and impartial fundamental principles. But whereas deep ecologists locate the fundamental cause of moral theory gone awry in anthropocentrism (human-centeredness), ecofeminists argue that it is androcentrism (male-centeredness) that is the real cause.

Nowhere is this difference clearer than in the case of sport or recreational hunting. Devall and Sessions (1985) celebrate the value of this practice as a means of bonding ever more closely with the natural world, of discovering "self in Self"; ecofeminists, by contrast, detect in the hunt the vestiges of patriarchy—the male's need to dominate and subdue (Kheel 1991). More fundamentally, deep ecologists seem to continue to view the natural world instrumentally, as a means to greater self-awareness and self-knowledge. In this respect, and despite appearances to the contrary, deep ecology does not represent a "paradigm shift" away from the anthropocentric worldview it aspires to replace.

Ecofeminists believe they offer a deeper account of the moral life than do deep ecologists, one that goes to the very foundations of Western moral theorizing. The idea of "the rights of the individual" is diagnosed as a symptom of patriarchal thought, rooted in the (male) myth of the isolated individual. Morally, a "paradigm shift" occurs when, in place of assertions of rights, we freely, lovingly choose to take care of and assume responsibility for those who are victims of oppression, both within and beyond the extended human family, other animals included. Writing for the growing number of ecofeminists, Josephine Donovan states:

> Natural rights and utilitarianism present impressive and useful arguments for the ethical treatment of animals. Yet, it is also possible—indeed, necessary—to ground that ethic in an emotional and spiritual conversation with nonhuman life forms. Out of a woman's relational culture of caring and attentive love [there] emerges the basis for a feminist ethic for the treatment of animals. We should not kill, eat, torture, and exploit animals because they do not want to be so treated, and we know that. If we listen, we can hear them. ("Animal Rights and Feminist Theory," in Gaard 1993, 185)

Thus, whereas the grounds for practical action offered by ecofeminists differ fundamentally from those favored by the rights view, and despite the foundational gulf that separates these two theories, both philosophies arguably have the same abolitionist practical implications.

CONCLUSION

The "animal rights debate," broadly conceived, is more than a contest of wills representing professional, economic, and ethical concerns; it is also a divisive, enduring topic in normative ethical theory (Vance 1992). Until comparatively recently, discussions of the moral status of nonhuman animals had all but disappeared from the work of moral philosophers. (For a historical overview, see Ryder 1989.) Beginning in the 1970s (Godlovitch, Godlovitch, and Harris 1972; Singer 1975; Linzey 1976; Clark 1977), however, we have witnessed a historically unprecedented outpouring of philosophical and theological interest in exploring the moral ties that bind humans to other animals, and there is every indication that this interest will intensify in the coming decades. The moral theories of philosophers are not the stuff of politics; still, the contributions philosophers make can help shape the political debate by clarifying the major theoretical options available to an informed public.

Principal among these options are those that have been canvassed here: perfectionism, despotism and stewardship, contractarianism, Kantianism, utilitarianism, the rights view, deep ecology, and ecofeminism. Doubtless other options will evolve as the discussion continues (Garner 1994). Among these options, two in particular—utilitarianism and the rights view—have offered the most systematic accounts of those duties owed directly to nonhuman animals. It will be instructive, before concluding, to highlight some of the important practical differences, particularly as these pertain to animal model research, that flow from these competing philosophies.

Because utilitarianism is committed to reducing the total amount of suffering in the world, its proponents must be prepared to recognize the moral legitimacy of some research on nonhuman animals. Even Peter Singer, contemporary utilitarianism's most forceful critic of such research, has conceded this possibility (Singer 1993). Moreover, utilitarians must be similarly well disposed to the activities of animal care and use committees (Singer has served as a member of such a committee), provided that these committees conscientiously work to eliminate unnecessary animal suffering. Legislative attempts to improve the well-being of animals, whether in laboratories or on the farm, find support among utilitarians. Viewed in these respects, utilitarianism offers a philosophical basis for those who would reform the ways in which nonhuman animals are utilized by humans; what it does not offer is a categorical condemnation of this utilization. For this reason utilitarianism is congenial to those individuals and groups working to advance animal welfare—who accept, that is, the morality of human utilization of nonhuman animals in principle but who seek to improve it, by making it more humane, in practice.

The rights view has a different perspective on such matters (Regan, Francione, and Newkirk 1992). This philosophy is opposed to human utilization of nonhuman animals in principle and seeks to end it in practice. Its practical implications are abolitionist, not reformist. Because those nonhuman animals who exist as ends in themselves are never to be treated merely as means, it is wrong to experiment on them in the name of advancing the well-being of others. Moreover, to the extent that animal care and use committees and reformist legislation help perpetuate social acceptance of human exploitation of these animals, whether on the farm or in the laboratory, advocates of the rights view will—or, to be consistent, should—withhold their support. What animal rights advocates *can* consistently support are incremental steps that put an end to certain practices within the larger context of animal exploitation—for example, legislation that would prohibit the use of nonhuman animals in cosmetic testing and in drug addiction experiments, and the creation of policies that end compulsory vivisection and dissection in the classroom (Francione and Charlton 1992). When, as can often happen, utilitarians deem such practices unjustified because they cause gratuitous animal suffering, these two conflicting normative ethical philosophies—utilitarianism and the rights view—can speak with one voice. And when this happens, their potential political power is greater than the sum of its parts.

No one can predict which of the tendencies examined above—reform, abolition, or the status quo—will prevail in the coming years. Some positions (e.g., the rights view and ecofeminism) call for fundamental social change; others (e.g., Aristotelian perfectionism and Kant's view) call for much less. To the extent that people act because of their beliefs, the future of how humans treat other animals depends on what we humans believe the latter to be and how we think they should be treated. Because what we should do in practice depends on understanding what we ought to do in principle, our ability to give an appropriate response to the practical issues constituting the animal rights debate, broadly conceived—from whether we ought to be vegetarians to whether we should continue to use nonhuman animals in biomedical research—depends on our ability to make an informed, rational choice among normative ethical theories. In this respect, while a fair consideration of such theories may not be the end-all, it can make some claim to being at least part of the begin-all of a commitment to seek understanding and truth in these troubled waters.

BIBLIOGRAPHY

Adams, Carol J. 1990. *The Sexual Politics of Meat: A Feminist-Vegetarian Critical Theory*. New York: Continuum.

Barr, James. 1974. "Man and Nature: The Ecological Controversy over the Old Testament." In *Ecology and Religion in History*, edited by D. Spring and E. Spring, 58–72. New York: Harper and Row.

Beauchamp, Tom L. 1997. "Opposing Views on Animal Experimentation: Do Animals Have Rights?" *Ethics and Behavior* 7 (2): 113–21.

Brandt, R. B. 1979. *A Theory of the Good and the Right.* Oxford: Clarendon Press.

Callicott, J. Baird. 1980. "Animal Liberation: A Triangular Affair." *Environmental Ethics* 2 (4): 311–28. Reprinted in *In Defense of the Land Ethic: Essays in Environmental Philosophy,* 15–38. Albany: State University of New York Press, 1989.

Callicott, J. Baird. 1993. "The Search for an Environmental Ethic." In *Matters of Life and Death: New Introductory Essays in Moral Philosophy,* 3rd ed., by Tom L. Beauchamp et al., edited by Tom Regan, 322–82. New York: McGraw-Hill.

Cavalieri, Paola. 2001. *The Animal Question: Why Non-Human Animals Deserve Human Rights.* Translated by Catherine Woollard. New York: Oxford University Press.

Clark, Stephen R. L. 1977. *The Moral Status of Animals.* Oxford: Clarendon Press.

Cohen, Carl. 1986. "The Case for the Use of Animals in Biomedical Research." *New England Journal of Medicine* 315 (14): 865–70.

DeGrazia, David. 1996. *Taking Animals Seriously: Mental Life and Moral Status.* Cambridge, UK: Cambridge University Press.

Devall, Bill, and George Sessions. 1985. *Deep Ecology: Living as if Nature Mattered.* Salt Lake City, UT: Gibbs Smith.

Diamond, Irene, and Gloria Fenman Orenstein, eds. 1990. *Reweaving the World: The Emergence of Ecofeminism.* San Francisco: Sierra Club.

Francione, Gary L., and Anna E. Charlton. 1992. *Vivisection and Dissection in the Classroom: A Guide to Conscientious Objection.* Jenkintown, PA: American Anti-Vivisection Society.

Frey, R. G. 1980. *Interests and Rights: The Case against Animals.* Oxford: Clarendon Press.

Frey, R. G. 1983. *Rights, Killing, and Suffering: Moral Vegetarianism and Applied Ethics.* Oxford: Basil Blackwell.

Frey, R. G. 1997. "Moral Community and Animal Research in Medicine." *Ethics and Behavior* 7 (2): 123–36.

Gaard, Greta C., ed. 1993. *Ecofeminism: Women, Animals, Nature.* Philadelphia: Temple University Press.

Garner, Richard. 1994. *Beyond Morality.* Philadelphia: Temple University Press.

Godlovitch, Stanley; Roslind Godlovitch; and John Harris. 1972. *Animals, Men, and Morals: An Enquiry into the Maltreatment of Non-Humans.* New York: Taplinger.

Kheel, Marti. 1991. "Ecofeminism and Deep Ecology: Reflections on Identity and Difference." *Trumpeter* 8 (2): 62–72.

LaFollette, Hugh, and Niall Shanks. 1993. "Animal Models in Biomedical Research: Some Epistemological Worries." *Public Affairs Quarterly* 7 (2): 113–30.

Linzey, Andrew. 1976. *Animal Rights: A Christian Assessment of Man's Treatment of Animals.* London: SCM Press.

Linzey, Andrew. 1987. *Christianity and the Rights of Animals.* New York: Crossroad.

Linzey, Andrew, and Tom Regan, eds. 1988. *Animals and Christianity: A Book of Readings.* New York: Crossroads.

Lyons, David. 1965. *Forms and Limits of Utilitarianism.* Oxford: Clarendon Press.

Magel, Charles R. 1981. *A Bibliography on Animal Rights and Related Matters.* Washington, DC: University Press of America.

Magel, Charles R. 1989. *Keyguide to Information Sources in Animal Rights.* Jefferson, NC: McFarland.

McDaniel, Jay B. 1989. *Of God and Pelicans: A Theology of Reverence for Life.* Louisville, KY: John Knox.

McHarg, Ian L. 1969. *Design with Nature.* Garden City, NY: Natural History Press.

McKinlay, John B., and S. McKinlay. 1977. *Health and Society.* London: Milbank.

Midgley, Mary. 1983. *Animals and Why They Matter.* Harmondsworth, UK: Penguin.

Naess, Arne. 1989. *Ecology, Community, and Lifestyle: Outline of an Ecosophy.* Edited and translated by David Rothenberg. Cambridge, UK: Cambridge University Press.

Narveson, Jan. 1977. "Animal Rights." *Canadian Journal of Philosophy* 7 (1): 161–78.

Narveson, Jan. 1988. *The Libertarian Idea.* Philadelphia: Temple University Press.

Orlans, Barbara F.; Tom L. Beauchamp; Rebecca Dresser; et al. 1998. *The Human Use of Animals: Case Studies in Ethical Choice.* New York: Oxford University Press.

Rachels, James. 1990. *Created from Animals: The Moral Implications of Darwinism.* Oxford: Oxford University Press.

Rawls, John. 1971. *A Theory of Justice.* Cambridge, MA: Belknap Press of Harvard University Press.

Regan, Tom. 1983. *The Case for Animal Rights.* Berkeley: University of California Press.

Regan, Tom, ed. 1986. *Animal Sacrifices: Religious Perspectives on the Use of Animals in Science.* Philadelphia: Temple University Press.

Regan, Tom. 1997. "The Rights of Humans and Other Animals." *Ethics and Behavior* 7 (2): 103–11.

Regan, Tom. 2001. *Defending Animal Rights.* Urbana: University of Illinois Press.

Regan, Tom; Gary Francione; and Ingrid Newkirk. 1992. "A Movement's Means Create Its Ends." *Animals' Agenda* 12 (1): 40–43.

Regan, Tom, and Peter Singer, eds. 1976. *Animal Rights and Human Obligations.* Englewood Cliffs, NJ: Prentice-Hall.

Regan, Tom, and Peter Singer, eds. 1989. *Animal Rights and Human Obligations.* 2nd ed. Englewood Cliffs, NJ: Prentice-Hall.

Rollin, Bernard E. 1981. *Animal Rights and Human Morality.* Buffalo, NY: Prometheus.

Rollin, Bernard E. 1989. *The Unheeded Cry: Animal Consciousness, Animal Pain, and Science.* New York: Oxford University Press.

Rolston, Holmes, III. 1988. *Environmental Ethics: Duties to and Values in the National World.* Philadelphia: Temple University Press.

Rowlands, Mark. 2002. *Animals Like Us.* New York: Verso Books.

Ryder, Richard D. 1975. *Victims of Science: The Use of Animals in Research.* London: Davis-Poynter.

Ryder, Richard D. 1989. *Animal Revolution: Changing Attitudes towards Speciesism.* Oxford: Basil Blackwell.

Sagoff, Mark. 1984. "Animal Liberation and Environmental Ethics: Bad Marriage, Quick Divorce." *Osgoode Hall Law Journal* 22 (2): 297–307.

Sapontzis, Steve F. 1987. *Morals, Reason, and Animals.* Philadelphia: Temple University Press.

Sharpe, Robert. 1988. *The Cruel Deception: The Use of Animals in Medical Research.* Wellingborough, UK: Thorsons.

Singer, Peter. 1975. *Animal Liberation: A New Ethics for Our Treatment of Animals.* New York: New York Review.

Singer, Peter. 1990. *Animal Liberation.* 2nd ed. New York: New York Review of Books.

Singer, Peter. 1993. "Animals and the Value of Life." In *Matters of Life and Death: New Introductory Essays in Moral Philosophy,* 3rd ed., by Tom Beauchamp et al., edited by Tom Regan, 280–321. New York: McGraw-Hill.

Singer, Peter. 2002. *Animal Liberation.* 3rd ed. Chicago: Ecco Press.

Taylor, Paul W. 1986. *Respect for Nature: A Theory of Environmental Ethics.* Princeton, NJ: Princeton University Press.

Vance, Richard P. 1992. "An Introduction to the Philosophical Presuppositions of the Animal Liberation/Rights Movement." *Journal of the American Medical Association* 288 (13): 1715–19.

VanDeVeer, Donald. 1979. "Of Beasts, Persons, and the Original Position." *Monist* 62 (3): 368–77.

Warren, Karen J. 1990. "The Power and the Promise of Ecological Feminism." *Environmental Ethics* 12 (2): 125–46.

Warren, Mary Anne. 1998. *Moral Status: Obligations to Persons and Other Living Things.* Issues in Biomedical Ethics. New York: Oxford University Press.

White, Lynn, Jr. 1967. "The Historical Roots of Our Ecological Crisis." *Science* 155 (3767): 1203–7.

Tom Regan (1995)
Professor Emeritus of Philosophy, North Carolina State University

I. ETHICAL PERSPECTIVES ON THE TREATMENT AND STATUS OF ANIMALS [ADDENDUM]

Ethical concerns about nonhuman animals arise from the recognition that many animals, such as mammals, birds, and vertebrates generally, as well as some invertebrate species, are conscious and sentient, that is, capable of negative and positive sensations. Further mental states attributed to many animals include beliefs, desires, reasoning, memory, expectations for the future, rich and varied negative and positive emotions, social engagement, self-awareness, and a psychological unity that enables identity over time.

A growing body of research in cognitive ethology, the branch of scientific research focused on animal minds, is providing increasingly stronger reasons—beyond common sense, observations, and arguments from analogy to human behavior, physiology, and evolution—to believe that many animals are, like human beings, minded, psychologically complex beings whose lives can go better and worse for them and thus are capable of being harmed (Armstrong and Botzler 2008). Little scientific research supports an opposing view that all animals are mindless, incapable of suffering or experiencing negative emotions, or are otherwise incapable of being harmed or made worse off.

In light of this understanding of animals' cognitive and emotional lives, most contemporary ethicists who address these issues argue that there are some direct moral duties owed to conscious, sentient animals, although they disagree on the extent and seriousness of these obligations. And there are debates about what difference the cognitive sophistication of the species might make to our obligations concerning individuals of that species: for example, might a prima facie obligation to not harm be stronger concerning chimpanzees, less toward chickens, and even less for fish? Answers here depend on our scientific understanding of the mental lives of the species, as well as our moral theorizing.

Moral arguments in favor of either the abolition or major reform of animal-harming industries and practices have been developed out of nearly every major ethical theory or tradition: Aristotelian ethics; virtue ethics; natural law; Christian, Jewish, and other religious ethics; Kantian ethics; Rawlsian or ideal contractarianisms or contractualisms; utilitarianism and other consequentialisms; rights-based theories; and more (Taylor 2009; Beauchamp and Frey 2011). Many of these ethicists appeal to our considered moral judgments about human beings, especially those who are vulnerable or mentally challenged, and argue that there is no relevant difference between humans and animals that justifies protecting human beings but not also many animals (Dombrowski 1997).

Much work on animal ethics in the 1970s and 1980s focused on Peter Singer's arguments that animals' interests deserve equal consideration to comparable human interests and that the denial of this is an unjustified prejudice, *speciesism,* which is analogous to sexism and racism. There was also considerable focus on Tom Regan's arguments that animals possess moral rights to respectful treatment comparable in strength and seriousness to the moral rights possessed by nonrational human beings. These arguments remain controversial, and critics have offered reasons why animals' interests do not deserve equal considerations to similar human interests, and why animals lack moral rights.

One response to these critics, beyond attempts to demonstrate that that their criticisms fail, is that we can accept these criticisms but still have adequate theoretical resources to explain why many harmful uses of animals are wrong. Some ethicists have argued that we can accept, either sincerely or for the sake of argument, that speciesism—not giving animals' interests serious weight because they are not of our species—is a justified prejudice, that animals' interests should not be given equal consideration to humans' comparable interests, and that animals lack moral rights, but argue that most, if not all, harmful uses of animals are wrong nevertheless (Garrett 2012). These thinkers appeal to common, less controversial, moral presumptions against unnecessary harms, or harms unnecessary for greater goods, or causing harms to innocents, arguing that these principles apply to many uses of animals and justifying evaluating them as wrong.

Insofar as many critics of the main early contemporary theoretical defenses of animals accept these common presumptions, their critics argue that their positions, contrary to their stated goals to undermine arguments in defense of animals, seem to justify the judgment that many harmful uses of animals are wrong, even if animals lack rights and even if their interests shouldn't be given equal consideration to humans' interests (Garrett 2012). That is, the notion that animal interests should be given some consideration may be a sufficient basis to condemn many uses and much harmful treatment of animals. Some philosophers also argue that theoretical positions that justify harmful animal use typically fail to adequately justify moral protections for vulnerable human beings, citing this as a sufficient reason to reject these theoretical positions (Taylor 2009).

A growing body of discussion and research exists concerning the practical uses and treatment of animals, including the ethics of using animals for food, animal research, biotechnology, education, training, zoos, aquariums, circuses, rodeos, and as companion animals. Discussion and research continue also on the ethics of ecosystem management and the treatment of wildlife, such as hunting and fishing, including dolphin hunting and whaling, and our obligations toward rare and exotic species (Armstrong and Botzler 2008).

Regarding the use of animals for food, it is difficult to find a philosophical ethicist who defends the status quo concerning standard methods of animal agriculture known as "factory farming" and slaughter insofar as such methods cause unnecessary and unjustified pain, suffering, and other harms to animals (Sapontzis 2004; Beauchamp and Frey 2011). Indirect concerns about animals arise from environmental concerns about animal agriculture, because it is a major polluter and producer of greenhouse gases, as well as from antibiotic overuse in animal agriculture, which may lessen or eliminate antibiotics' effectiveness in human medicine (Taylor 2009).

Some critics of factory farming propose an agrarian alternative where animals are raised on a smaller scale in ways that show greater concern for their welfare: these animals experience less pain and perhaps no suffering. These views, however, must explain why killing animals to satisfy nonvital human interests is permissible if killing these animals harms them by depriving them of their valuable futures or the chance to satisfy any of their interests. Some philosophers argue that beings who lack a sense of the future or cannot conceive of themselves in the future or have no explicit interests in or plans for the future are either not harmed by death or lack a right to life, and so killing them painlessly is not wrong (Beauchamp and Frey 2011). These theories are controversial, however, especially concerning their implications for human beings who lack a sense of the future. Their applications to animals, of course, depend on developing scientific understanding of animals' minds: which animal species, if any, have a sense of the future strong enough to grant them a right to life on these theories? Especially relevant here is recent research on fish: although they are arguably conscious, do they have a moment-to-moment existence, or do they have memories and anticipations of the future and thus a sense of themselves over time? (Braithwaithe 2010).

Instead of arguing for the reform of animal agriculture, others argue for its abolition: as we can meet our dietary needs on vegan or vegetarian diets, the serious harms to animals who are raised and killed to be eaten are morally unjustified because these harms are inflicted, critics argue, not for any good reason, but only for our pleasure, convenience, tradition, financial gain, and other reasons insufficient to justify the harms done to animals (Sapontzis 2004).

Concerning animal experimentation and research, greater scientific rigor has been applied to attempting to quantify and measure benefits and harms, allowing evidence-based answers to questions concerning the human benefits from animal research. Systematic reviews to identify the human clinical utility of animal experiments have suggested that data gained from animal experiments have little value to human medicine, and citation analyses show that data from animal studies are not likely to be cited in human medicine (Knight 2011). The common assumption that animal models are reliably predictive of human responses is perhaps not evidence-based. Insofar as common moral defenses of animal experimentation accept this assumption, the relevant science suggests that these arguments are deficient.

Animal researchers have promised to engage the public on the scientific and moral merits of their work and some progress has occurred in these areas. However, activist protest of animal research has often contributed to researchers focusing on evaluating activist tactics instead of engaging the moral question of why harmful experimentation on animals is morally permissible, when analogous experimentation on human beings, especially vulnerable humans, would be judged as clearly wrong.

Finally, concerns about the ethical treatment of animals have given rise to the growing field of animal law (Sunstein and Nussbaum 2004). Some philosophers have begun to bring issues in animal ethics to political theory. The success of integrating animals into the field of philosophy and ethics has contributed to the development of animal studies, the study of animals through any relevant academic discipline. And there is a growing literature on how to best teach animal issues in many fields and at all levels of education (DeMello 2010).

SEE ALSO *Animal Research: II. Philosophical Issues; Endangered Species and Biodiversity; Environmental Ethics: I. Overview; Pain and Suffering; Veterinary Ethics*

BIBLIOGRAPHY

Armstrong, Susan J., and Richard G. Botzler, eds. 2008. *The Animal Ethics Reader*. 2nd ed. New York: Routledge.

Beauchamp, Tom L., and R. G. Frey, eds. 2011. *The Oxford Handbook of Animal Ethics*. Oxford: Oxford University Press.

Braithwaite, Victoria. 2010. *Do Fish Feel Pain?* Oxford: Oxford University Press.

DeMello, Margo, ed. 2010. *Teaching the Animal: Human-Animal Studies across the Disciplines*. New York: Lantern Books.

Dombrowski, Daniel A. 1997. *Babies and Beasts: The Argument from Marginal Cases*. Urbana: University of Illinois Press.

Garrett, Jeremy R., ed. 2012. *The Ethics of Animal Research: Exploring the Controversy*. Cambridge, MA: MIT Press.

Knight, Andrew. 2011. *The Costs and Benefits of Animal Experiments*. New York: Palgrave Macmillan.

Sapontzis, Steven, ed. 2004. *Food for Thought: The Debate over Eating Meat*. Amherst, NY: Prometheus Books.

Sunstein, Cass R., and Martha C. Nussbaum, eds. 2004. *Animal Rights: Current Debates and New Directions*. Oxford: Oxford University Press.

Taylor, Angus. 2009. *Animals and Ethics: An Overview of the Philosophical Debate*. 3rd ed. Peterborough, ON: Broadview Press.

Nathan Nobis
Assistant Professor of Philosophy, Morehouse College

II. VEGETARIANISM

Vegetarianism is traditionally defined as the practice of abstaining from eating animal flesh. Modern vegetarian societies, such as the Vegetarian Society of the United Kingdom, define the practice as abstaining from flesh, fish, and fowl, with or without the addition of dairy produce and eggs. Those who wholly or occasionally abstain from "red meat" but eat fish or poultry or both are described as "demi-" or "semi-" vegetarians. Veganism, or "pure" vegetarianism, is the practice of abstaining as completely as possible from all products and by-products of the slaughterhouse, including products derived from treatment deemed exploitative to animals. Vegans do not consume dairy produce or eggs and also exclude products such as honey on the ground that animals are used or killed in producing such types of human nourishment. Many vegetarians do not wear slaughterhouse by-products such as leather, and vegans avoid wearing any animal products, such as leather and wool.

HEALTH VEGETARIANS

As late as the 1950s, the unwritten consensus among health specialists and dieticians was that animal protein in some form is essential to maintaining adequate human health. While this position has not been completely reversed, medical advice from official studies increasingly recommends low-animal-fat diets, some of which eschew animal protein completely. Studies suggest that vegetarians have lower rates of diet-related cancer (Chang-Claude et al. 1992), especially colon and rectal cancer (Phillips 1975; Willett et al. 1990) and prostate cancer (Giovannucci et al. 1993). Vegetarians experience lower mortality rates from coronary heart disease than nonvegetarians, possibly owing to their lower serum cholesterol levels (Burr and Butland 1988). One study has shown that the mortality rate from cardiovascular disease among vegetarians is less than half that of the general population (Chang-Claude et al. 1992; see also Snowdon et al. 1984). Vegetarians suffer less from hypertension (Armstrong et al. 1977; Rouse et al. 1983), obesity (Thorogood et al. 1989), and diabetes (Snowdon and Phillips 1985).

Interpretation of these and other studies has become a source of controversy, with advocates for each side citing evidence in their favor (Frey 1983; Robbins 1987). Increasingly, however, health specialists seem to favor vegetarian diets on medical grounds alone. According to present knowledge, a balanced vegetarian diet poses no health problems and offers some indisputable advantages.

"GREEN" VEGETARIANS

Green political parties in Europe (i.e., those parties committed to programs that give priority to ecological sustainability) increasingly advocate a vegetarian diet or at least reduced meat consumption for environmental reasons. For example, the policy of the Green Party of the United Kingdom "encourage[s] a reduction in consumption of animal produce and promote[s] the development and use of foods which are more healthy and humane" (Green Party 1993, 15). They offer two arguments. The first is that if enough Westerners become vegetarians, worldwide food distribution will become more equitable. It is calculated that "if we all had a vegetarian diet and shared our food equally, the biosphere could support around six billion people; if 15 percent of our calories came from animal products (and again food were shared equally), the figure would come down to four billion people; if 25 percent of our calories came from animal products, then it would fall to three billion; and if 35 percent of our calories came from animal products, as in North America today, then it would fall to 2.5 billion" (Myers 1990; Tickell 1992, 67). The second argument is that the present system of intensive farming, while it is cost-efficient, will prove inefficient in the long run in terms of energy and environmental costs (Porritt 1984). Hence, Greens argue that the "expanding livestock industry contributes to … the destruction and pollution of the planet" by being "energy intensive rather than labour intensive" and contributes to "world starvation" (Green Party 1993, 15).

Assessing these arguments is problematic. While intensive farming is energy inefficient and environmentally damaging—apart from concerns it raises about animal welfare—any measurement of food resources must take into account not only the quantity of food available but also the way in which complex systems of supply and demand militate against egalitarian food distribution. Again, while animal farming is not always an efficient use of food resources, it is not clear that the political will exists to adopt alternative economic policies. Those who are sympathetic to vegetarianism on environmental grounds believe that widespread vegetarianism can and will affect worldwide trade. Despite the evident increase in the number of vegetarians in the West, it is as yet unclear whether and how much such minorities will have lasting economic impact.

In response to the "Green" argument in favor of vegetarianism, some environmental ethicists, while sympathetic to the view that modern industrial agriculture is environmentally damaging, hold that because nature is a predatory system, it is natural for humans as well as animals to consume sentient life-forms. Frederick Ferré argues that "from the broadest biotic perspective, life is cannibalistic upon itself; an ecological ethic must begin with the affirmation of the nutrient cycle" (1986, 392; see also Birch and Cobb 1981). This view is reinforced by Holmes Rolston III, who states that "humans in their eating habits follow nature; they can and ought to do so." Rolston's argument is dependent upon a distinction between nature and culture: "Humans, then, can model their dietary habits on their ecosystems, but they cannot and should not model their interpersonal justice or charity on ecosystems" (1988, 81).

Both arguments presuppose to some degree that what should be must be modeled on what is. Only faintly, if at all, do ethical considerations fundamentally apply to the human act of killing sentient animals even when it is unnecessary. Ferré and Rolston do not sufficiently consider that what is "given in nature" is as much a social construct as what may be presupposed in "human nature." No perception of nature is value-free. What we judge to be "given in nature" often turns out to be what we ourselves judge on other criteria should be the case. In sum, there is no ecological shortcut to avoiding the question of whether the human killing of sentient animals is a moral issue. Because not all ethicists, especially theological ethicists, are convinced that the natural order exists as God intended, arguments based on what is "natural" leave open metaphysical questions about the justice of what is (Linzey 1987, 1994; Clark 1993).

ETHICAL VEGETARIANS

Of three main arguments for vegetarianism on ethical grounds, the first is based on the value of animal life. Even if we grant animal life secondary or even minimal value, it is difficult to see how human taste preference alone can justify killing. In general, killing for food when it is not required for human health or survival fails the test of moral necessity. Consuming flesh when we could do otherwise is "empty gluttony" (Clark 1977, 183). Some philosophers have contended that it is not justifiable to kill animals even painlessly, asserting that it is logically inconsistent to care whether animals suffer without also valuing animal life itself (Godlovitch 1971).

Other philosophers perceive gradations of value. Ferré, for example, argues against the assertion that all beings with inherent value possess that value equally. "There is no reason to suppose that the quality and intensity of the mental life—and with it its value for itself—of an oyster is on a par with that of a pheasant; but there is likewise no reason to suppose that the quality and intensity of the mental life of the pheasant is on a par with that of a human child" (1986, 396). Ferré further states that "there is no 'line.…' All living beings have some degree of inherent value … but different organisms call for different forms of respect" (397–98). But even if such gradations are admitted, the case of mammals, as distinct from plants, calls for greater ethical justification. We still need to know how the killing of animals—which are sentient beings with inherent value superior to that of plants—without strict necessity is compatible with appropriate "respect" for their lives. The logic of Ferré's position is inclusive. Even the killing of plants requires strong ethical justification.

The second argument derives from considerations of animal welfare. If animals should be spared unnecessary suffering, then eating meat should be avoided, because the rearing, transport, and slaughter of farm animals invariably—and in some cases, necessarily—involves suffering, sometimes of a severe and prolonged kind (Singer 1976; Frey 1983). This argument gains credibility in light of modern farming methods and the recognized fallibility of slaughtering techniques (Harrison 1964; Mason and Singer 1980; Johnson 1991).

Ferré accepts that many modern farming practices are cruel but reasons that "moderate" meat eating is justifiable if "nearly painless methods" of slaughter are adhered to (1986, 400). If such a goal were to be achieved, fundamental changes would be required at all levels of livestock management. Minimally, slaughtering techniques would have to be indisputably humane (i.e., rendering the animal instantaneously unconscious), slaughterhouses would have to be regularly inspected, and regulations would need to be enforced by law. Animals would need to be killed as close as possible to their point of origin to avoid suffering in transit. Handling of animals on farms would have to be subject to a new range of welfare criteria. Conscientious meat eaters could justify eating meat only in specific circumstances when all such conditions have been met. The failure to secure humane farm management and slaughter renders "moderate" meat eating ethically problematic. While in theory this second argument justifies only provisional vegetarianism in most, perhaps all, circumstances as a protest against animal abuse, it is difficult to envisage a time when conditions will universally prevail so as to preclude animal suffering in agriculture.

The third argument appeals to notions of animal rights. Sentient beings, or beings that can be classed as "subjects of a life," have a right to live that is equal to, or analogous with, human beings' right to live. Vegetarianism, according to the rights view, is obligatory in principle and entails the end of commercial animal agriculture in practice. However, even this animal right not to be harmed is viewed as "a prima facie, not an absolute right" (Regan 1983, 330).

The precise implications of this argument are not always clear. Do animals have in each and every case an equal right with humans to life? To what extent may individual rights be overridden in particular crisis situations? Commercial nonanimal agriculture also depends to some degree upon the control of competing species. Some animal rightists defend a stricter definition of avoidability or necessity than others. For example, some would concede that meat eating may be justified in those limited situations where alternative resources are inadequate (Linzey 1987).

Discussion has sometimes centered on the cultural survival of the Inuit peoples, for example, and the question of whether their cultural rights should override the rights of the animals they hunt for food and clothing. Some animal rightists would accept the legitimacy of a limited human preference approach in such circumstances. George Woodcock maintains that there is not "a single responsible person in the animal rights movement who would object to the Indian or Inuit, where he can, following a partly subsistence life of hunting for food" (1989, 5). Other animal rightists, however, would question whether cultural considerations should be paramount when considering the exploitation of animals. Both "moderate" and "strong" animal rights positions would, however, concur with Woodcock's judgment that both indigenous peoples, as well as fur-bearing animals, "have always been the victims of the fur trade" (5). The rights position may be described as the strong welfare position, more uncompromising in its insistence upon the correctness of not harming animals as a prima facie duty. The rights view may not always require absolute (as distinct from obligatory) vegetarianism, but it would contend that vegetarianism should be the ethical and social norm.

RELIGIOUS VEGETARIANS

Two primary motifs, ascetic and mystical, have informed ethico-religious awareness on this subject. Vegetarianism has an established place in some Indian religious traditions, especially Jainism and, to some degree, Buddhism and Hinduism. The ascetic motif, particularly within Jainism, is based on the doctrines of nonviolence and nonpossessiveness. The goals of the spiritual life are, among other things, renunciation of aggressive and possessive urges and following the path of purification (Jaini 1979).

While Christianity has not formally endorsed vegetarianism, some strands of Christian tradition have affirmed that abstaining from meat can have value as a spiritual discipline. Some religious orders—for example, the Benedictines—eschewed meat as part of their ascetic regime (Sorrell 1988). Self-denial as part of striving toward moral perfection has sometimes formed the basis for vegetarian lifestyles (Tolstoy 1961). Ascetic practices may involve a vegetarian diet as a conscientious ecological response to wasteful consumerism and affluence (Lappé 1982).

Allied to asceticism has been a mystical appreciation of other creatures as valuable beyond human calculations of utility, because of their divine creation. The origins of this outlook are clear in the early and medieval periods (Sorrell 1988). Only in modern times has this viewpoint received systematic expression in notions of reverence for life or in life-centered ethics (Schweitzer 1961; McDaniel 1989; Linzey 1994). Historical Christianity has not fostered these insights, mainly because of its continuing anthropocentric theology. However, theological affirmations that animals are humans' fellow creatures, whose life or spirit belongs to God—and that they are therefore worthy of respect—undergird an ethical impulse to minimize injury and harm to them. Because of the rights of their creator, animals can be said to bear "theos-rights," or God-rights (Linzey 1987, 68).

The modern vegetarian movement—in the sense of organized societies specifically founded to advance ethical or religious vegetarianism—can be traced to the emergence of humanitarian sensibility from the nineteenth century onward. The Bible Christian Church, founded in 1809 by an Anglican priest, William Cowherd, made vegetarianism compulsory among its members and heralded the later growth of specifically vegetarian societies in the United Kingdom and the United States. The Bible Christian Church found its inspiration in what was understood to be a biblical command, recorded in Genesis 1:29, to be herbivores. Later commands to eat flesh (for example, in Genesis 9:3) were understood as permission given to humankind only after the Fall and the Flood. (For a discussion of Judaism and vegetarianism, see Schwartz 1988.)

The Bible is, however, ambivalent about meat eating. While carnivorousness may be construed as a divine concession to human sinfulness (Baker 1975), almost all biblical writers accepted the practice as ethically justifiable. Moreover, Jesus Christ was not a "pure" vegetarian; the Gospel accounts record that he ate fish. There were various sects advocating vegetarianism in early Jewish and Christian circles, but none of their practices became normative within Judaism or Christianity (Beckwith 1988). Carnivorousness has seldom been theologically challenged within mainstream religious traditions, and only in modern times has ethical vegetarianism emerged as a serious option. Some modern-day Jewish vegetarians (see, e.g., Kook 1979) maintain that abstaining from meat is one step toward realizing the biblical vision of universal peace as described by such prophets as Isaiah (11:6f). Some Christian theologians hold that contemporary vegetarianism constitutes a more Christlike response to the evil of animal exploitation (Linzey 1994).

The best defense of meat eating is based not only on a denial that animals have rights (Frey 1980, 1983; Leahy 1991; Carruthers 1992) but also on a denial that they have any moral status. According to this view, the gastronomic pleasures humans experience by consuming flesh far outweigh the value of animal life and suffering. "By comparison with animals, our lives are of an incomparably greater texture and richness, and when we say of a dying man that he has led a rich, full life we allude to something incomparably beyond to what we would allude, were we to say the same of a dying chicken, cat or chimpanzee" (Frey 1983, 110).

It is difficult to see how such a position can be sustained without putting at risk the moral status of some classes of humans, for example, the mentally handicapped, the comatose, or newborns. Furthermore, it follows from the denial of animal status that a species superior to humans—as some humans now regard themselves in relation to animals—would not be morally obligated to respect human lives and suffering. The hope that "our aliens' nobility will match the quality of their imagined mentality" (Ferré 1986, 406) and that therefore they will spare us unnecessary suffering and death sadly cannot be deduced from humans' own moral record in relation to sentient nonhumans.

What has given contemporary secular and theological arguments for vegetarianism their strength and cogency is the realization that meat is not generally essential for human health and well-being. Consuming meat may have been necessary at certain times in the past; it may sometimes be necessary in the present. But eating a balanced vegetarian diet carries with it no medical or nutritional handicap. And, more important, it respects the ethical injunction to avoid killing sentient beings whenever possible.

BIBLIOGRAPHY

Adams, Carol J. 1990. *The Sexual Politics of Meat: A Feminist-Vegetarian Critical Theory.* New York: Continuum.

Armstrong, Bruce K.; Anthony J. Van Merwyck; and Harvey Coates. 1977. "Blood Pressure in Seventh-day Adventist Vegetarians." *American Journal of Epidemiology* 105 (5): 444–49.

Baker, John Austin. 1975. "Biblical Attitudes to Nature." In *Man and Nature,* edited by Hugh Montefiore, 87–109. London: Collins.

Beckwith, Roger T. 1988. "The Vegetarianism of the Therapeutae, and the Motives for Vegetarianism in Early Jewish and Christian Circles." *Revue de Qumrân* 13 (49–52): 407–10.

Birch, Charles, and John B. Cobb Jr. 1981. *The Liberation of Life: From the Cell to the Community.* New York: Cambridge University Press.

Burr, Michael L., and Barbara K. Butland. 1988. "Heart Disease in British Vegetarians." *American Journal of Clinical Nutrition* 48 (3 suppl): 830–32.

Carruthers, Peter. 1992. *The Animals Issue: Moral Theory in Practice.* New York: Cambridge University Press.

Chang-Claude, Jenny; Rainer Frentzel-Beyme; and Ursula Eilber. 1992. "Mortality Pattern of German Vegetarians after 11 Years of Follow-up." *Epidemiology* 3 (5): 395–401.

Clark, Stephen R. L. 1977. *The Moral Status of Animals.* Oxford: Clarendon Press.

Clark, Stephen R. L. 1993. *How to Think about the Earth: Philosophical and Theological Models for Ecology.* London: Mowbray.

Ferré, Frederick. 1986. "Moderation, Morals and Meat." *Inquiry* 29 (1–4): 391–406.

Fiddes, Nick. 1991. *Meat: A Natural Symbol.* London: Routledge.

Fox, Michael W., and Nancy E. Wiswall. 1989. *The Hidden Costs of Beef.* Washington, DC: Humane Society of the United States.

Frey, Raymond G. 1980. *Interests and Rights: The Case against Animals.* Oxford, UK: Clarendon Press.

Frey, Raymond G. 1983. *Rights, Killing and Suffering: Moral Vegetarianism and Applied Ethics.* Oxford, UK: Basil Blackwell.

Giovannucci, Edward; Eric B. Rimm; Graham A. Colditz; et al. 1993. "A Prospective Study of Dietary Fat and Risk of Prostate Cancer." *Journal of the National Cancer Institute* 85 (19): 1571–79.

Godlovitch, Roslind. 1971. "Animals and Morals." In *Animals, Men, and Morals: An Enquiry into the Maltreatment of the Non-Human*, edited by Stanley Godlovitch, Roslind Godlovitch, and John Harris, 156–72. London: Victor Gollancz.

Green Party. 1993. "Animal Rights." In *Green Party Manifesto for a Sustainable Society,* 15–16. London: Author.

Harrison, Ruth. 1964. *Animal Machines: The New Factory Farming Industry.* London: Vincent Stuart.

Jaini, Padmanabh S. 1979. *The Jaina Path of Purification.* Berkeley: University of California Press.

Johnson, Andrew. 1991. *Factory Farming.* Oxford, UK: Basil Blackwell.

Kook, Abraham Isaac. 1979. "Fragments of Light: A View as to the Reasons for the Commandments." In *The Lights of Penitence, The Moral Principles, Lights of Holiness, Essays, Letters, and Poems*, translated by Ben Zion Bokser, 303–23. London: SPCK.

Lappé, Frances Moore. 1982. *Diet for a Small Planet*, 2nd rev. ed. New York: Ballantine.

Leahy, Michael. 1991. *Against Liberation: Putting Animals in Perspective.* London: Routledge.

Linzey, Andrew. 1976. *Animal Rights: A Christian Assessment of Man's Treatment of Animals.* London: S. C. M. Press.

Linzey, Andrew. 1987. *Christianity and the Rights of Animals.* London: SPCK.

Linzey, Andrew. 1994. *Animal Theology.* London: S. C. M. Press.

Mason, Jim, and Peter Singer. 1980. *Animal Factories.* New York: Crown.

McDaniel, Jay B. 1989. *Of God and Pelicans: A Theology of Reverence for Life.* Louisville, KY: Westminster/John Knox Press.

Myers, Norman. 1990. "Mass Extinctions: What Can the Past Tell Us about the Present and the Future?" *Palaeogeography, Palaeoclimatology, Palaeoecology* 82 (1–2): 175–85.

Phillips, Roland L. 1975. "Role of Life-style and Dietary Habits in Risk of Cancer among Seventh-day Adventists." *Cancer Research* 35 (11. pt. 2): 3513–22.

Porritt, Jonathon. 1984. *Seeing Green: The Politics of Ecology Explained.* Oxford, UK: Basil Blackwell.

Regan, Tom. 1983. *The Case for Animal Rights.* London: Routledge and Kegan Paul.

Robbins, John. 1987. *Diet for a New America: How Your Food Choices Affect Your Health, Your Happiness, and the Future of Life on Earth,* 2nd rev. ed. Walpole, NH: Stillpoint.

Rolston, Holmes, III. 1988. *Environmental Ethics: Duties to and Values in the Natural World.* Philadelphia: Temple University Press.

Rouse, Ian L.; Bruce K. Armstrong; and Lawrence J. Beilin. 1983. "The Relationship of Blood Pressure to Diet and Lifestyle in Two Religious Populations." *Journal of Hypertension* 1 (1): 65–71.

Schwartz, Richard H. 1988. *Judaism and Vegetarianism.* Marblehead, MA: Micah.

Schweitzer, Albert. 1961. *Civilization and Ethics*, 2nd ed. Translated by C. T. Campion. London: Unwin.

Singer, Peter. 1976. *Animal Liberation: A New Ethics for Our Treatment of Animals.* London: Jonathan Cape.

Snowdon, David A., and Roland L. Phillips. 1985. "Does a Vegetarian Diet Reduce the Occurrence of Diabetes?" *American Journal of Public Health* 75 (5): 507–12.

Snowdon, David A.; Roland L. Phillips; and Gary E. Fraser. 1984. "Meat Consumption and Fatal Ischemic Heart Disease." *Preventive Medicine* 13 (5): 490–500.

Sorrell, Roger D. 1988. *St. Francis of Assisi and Nature: Tradition and Innovation in Western Christian Attitudes toward the Environment.* New York: Oxford University Press.

Thorogood, Margaret; Klim McPherson; and Jim Mann. 1989. "Relationship of Body Mass Index, Weight and Height to Plasma Lipid Levels in People with Different Diets in Britain." *Community Medicine* 11 (3): 230–33.

Tickell, Crispin. 1992. "The Quality of Life: What Quality? Whose Life?" *Environmental Values* 1 (1): 65–76.

Tolstoy, Leo. 1961. "The First Step." In *Recollections and Essays,* 4th ed. Translated by Aylmer Maude, 123–34. London: Oxford University Press.

Willett, Walter C.; Meir J. Stampfer; Graham A. Colditz; et al. 1990. "Relation of Meat, Fat and Fiber Intake to the Risk of Colon Cancer in a Prospective Study among Women." *New England Journal of Medicine* 323 (24): 1664–72.

Woodcock, George. 1989. "A Briefing on the Fur Trade and Aboriginal Cultures." In *Skinned,* by George Woodcock et al., 1–5. Nottingham, UK: Lynx.

Andrew Linzey (1995)
Faculty of Theology and Religion, University of Oxford

II. VEGETARIANISM [ADDENDUM]

THE RISE OF VEGANISM

From the early nineteenth century there have been individuals in Great Britain and America who have avoided the use of animals for food. Founded in 1838 by the self-styled "sacred socialist" and mystic James Pierrepont Greaves, the Alcott House Concordium, in Ham Common, Surrey, was a utopian community based on the principles of simple living, celibacy, and a predominantly raw food vegan diet. Members followed a fully vegan lifestyle that excluded the use of animals in farming and for food and the use of animal products for clothing. The Concordists were responsible for calling a meeting to form a society of vegetarians in 1847 and, along with the Bible Christians of Salford, played a significant role in the founding and first year of the Vegetarian Society in Great Britain.

There were always members of the Vegetarian Society who followed a simple vegetarian diet that excluded eggs and dairy products, but interest in the nondairy diet grew in the early decades of the twentieth century. Some members of the British Vegetarian Society suggested the formation of a nondairy section, but this idea was rejected by the members as divisive. However, the nondairy vegetarians ultimately created a new organization, the Vegan Society, in November 1944 with a membership of twenty-five. Founding member Donald Watson suggested the name of the new society by taking the beginning and end of *vegetarian*. In the first issue of *Vegan News*, Watson writes of vegetarianism as being "a half-way house between meat-eating and a truly humane and civilised diet" (*Vegan News* 1944, 1). Watson compares the exploitation of animals to society's former dependence on slavery and considers that a "great impediment to man's moral development may be that he is a parasite of lower forms of animal life" (*Vegan News* 1944, 1). Veganism, particularly in the United Kingdom, has always had a strongly ethical basis linked to concerns for animal welfare and animal rights. Increasingly vegans espouse concerns for environmental stability, including concerns for global food security. The term *dietary vegan* is sometimes used to describe vegans who do not adhere to the vegan lifestyle regarding animal-free clothing, cosmetics, and toiletries but who are vegan in their dietary practices. This is usually the case where the vegan is interested in perceived health benefits of veganism rather than animal welfare or animal rights issues.

There is a paucity of historical data for the levels of veganism in society. Surveys that considered vegetarianism, such as the British Realeat Vegetarian Surveys of the 1980s and 1990s, did not ask about veganism; for this reason, it is not possible to chart the levels of veganism in this period in the same way as those of vegetarianism. And although British World War II rationing records confirm that the number of vegetarians in 1945 was 100,000, we do not know how many of them were vegan. The UK Department of Health and Food Standards Agency (FSA) National Diet and Nutrition Survey of 2012 gave the level of vegans at less than 1 percent based on a survey of 1,582 children (1.5–18 years old) and 1,491 adults (Vegetarian Society 2012). The same survey put the level of vegetarians (i.e., those eating eggs or dairy products in addition to vegan foods) at 2 percent of UK adults and children. The same study was conducted in 2010 and 2011, and the figures for vegetarianism and veganism remained stable throughout that period at 2 percent and less than 1 percent, respectively (Bates et al. 2013). The FSA figure for 2012 includes children under the age of sixteen; because veganism rates are low in this age group, the study reflects a lower percentage of the population than if the figure were given as a percentage of the adult population.

These sample sizes are small for minority groups. Moreover veganism is not evenly distributed throughout the population but appears in concentrations in London and the southeast of England. As a result the UK Vegan Society estimates that there are approximately 150,000 vegans in the country. In the United States a survey by Public Policy Polling (2013) found that 13 percent of the people surveyed considered themselves to be either vegetarians (6 percent) or vegans (7 percent). A Gallup poll of 2012, however, put the figure for self-declared vegetarians at 5 percent and for vegans at 2 percent. With a sampling error margin of up to 4 percent, these results have to be treated with caution. Since 2000 veganism has been increasingly associated in the media with high-profile figures and celebrities, such as former US president Bill Clinton; actors Woody Harrelson, Joaquin Phoenix, and Alicia Silverstone; singers Bryan Adams, k.d. lang, and Moby; athlete Carl Lewis; and poet and Vegan Society patron Benjamin Zephaniah. As a result veganism's profile is increasingly entering the mainstream in a way similar to vegetarianism in the 1980s.

VEGETARIANISM AND THE ENVIRONMENT

A concern for environmental ethics can be traced back at least to Plato, but there has been a steady growth in interest in the environment since the 1960s because of awareness of the effects of population and economic growth and the concomitant growth in industry and intensive farming methods. Vegetarians have long made the case that theirs is a diet that can make the best use of land and water resources and that eating plants directly rather than "cycling" them through animals would produce far more food for humankind and best serve a growing population. The United Nations estimates that 3 billion people could live on the grain fed to farm animals (United Nations Environment Programme 2009, 27). At the end of the twentieth century greenhouse gas (GHG) emissions became a concern; in this context vegetarians felt their diet had a positive impact on the environment. A United Nations Food and Agriculture Organization review noted that the livestock sector is a significant source of worldwide GHG emissions (Steinfeld et al. 2006). Livestock contribute both directly from enteric fermentation and manure management and indirectly from feed production and the conversion of forests to pasture for livestock use: "Based on a life cycle assessment (LCA) approach, it was estimated that the sector emits about 7.1 Gt of CO^2-eq, or about 18 percent of total global anthropogenic GHG emissions" (Gerber, Henderson, and Makkar 2013, 1).

It has been estimated that livestock farming is responsible for more GHG emissions than the world's transport system, which is calculated at 13.5 percent (Steinfeld et al. 2006). Vegetarian and vegan organizations argue that a vegetarian diet can lessen reliance on animal agriculture, make more efficient use of water and land resources, limit the effects of deforestation and soil erosion caused by cattle, and slow down the rate of GHG emissions. The UK Vegan Society promotes not just a plant-based (vegan) diet but also vegan-organic and stock-free farming, which uses green manures, crop rotation, and composting as low-cost alternatives to animal manures. The society claims that stock-free farming would have benefits to farmers in the United Kingdom and the developing world by freeing them from the burden of fluctuating animal feed costs and the worry of such animal diseases as bird flu and bovine spongiform encephalopathy (commonly called mad cow disease) and in the developing world would reduce the risk of conflict over scarce water and land resources.

SEE ALSO *Ecological Bioethics; Harm; Hinduism, Bioethics in; Jainism, Bioethics in; Moral Status*

BIBLIOGRAPHY

Bates, Beverly; Alison Lennox; Ann Prentice; et al. 2013. "National Diet and Nutrition Survey: Headline Results from Years 1, 2, and 3 (Combined) of the Rolling Programme (2008/2009–2010/11)." Accessed September 18, 2013. https://www.gov.uk/government/uploads/system/uploads/attachment_data/file/207708/NDNS-Y3-report_All-TEXT-docs-combined.pdf

Gallup. 2012. "In U.S., 5% Consider Themselves Vegetarians." July 26. Accessed November 2, 2013. http://www.gallup.com/poll/156215/consider-themselves-vegetarians.aspx

Gerber, Pierre J.; Benjamin Henderson; and Harinder P. S. Makkar, eds. 2013. *Mitigation of Greenhouse Gas Emissions in Livestock Production*. Rome: Food and Agriculture Organization of the United Nations. Accessed November 2, 2013. http://www.fao.org/docrep/018/i3288e/i3288e.pdf

Ginsberg, Caryn, and Alissa Ostrowski. 2013. "The Market for Vegetarian Foods." Accessed June 18, 2013. http://www.vrg.org/nutshell/market1.htm

Leneman, Leah. 1999. "No Animal Food: The Road to Veganism in Britain, 1909–1944." *Society and Animals* 7 (3): 219–28. http://tier-im-fokus.ch/wp-content/uploads/2009/09/leneman99.pdf

Marcus, Erik. 2001. *Vegan: The New Ethics of Eating*. Ithaca, NY: McBooks.

Public Policy Polling. 2013. "Food Issues Polarizing America." February 26. Accessed November 2, 2013. http://www.publicpolicypolling.com/main/2013/02/food-issues-polarizing-america.html

Steinfeld, Henning; Pierre Gerber; Tom Wassenaar; et al. 2006. *Livestock's Long Shadow: Environmental Issues and Options*. Rome: FAO. Accessed June 18, 2013. ftp://ftp.fao.org/docrep/fao/010/a0701e/a0701e00.pdf

Stepaniak, Joanne. 2000. *Being Vegan: Living with Conscience, Conviction, and Compassion*. Los Angeles: Lowell House.

United Nations Environment Programme. 2009. "The Environmental Food Crisis." Nairobi: Author. Accessed November 2, 2013. http://www.grida.no/publications/rr/food-crisis/

Vegan News. 1944. Accessed November 2, 2013. http://issuu.com/vegan_society/docs/the_vegan_news_1944#embed

Vegan Society. "Guide to Vegan Living." 2013. Accessed June 12, 2013. http://www.guidetoveganliving.org.uk/what-is-vegan-living/

Vegetarian Society. 2012. "UK Department of Health and Food Standards Agency (FSA) National Diet and Nutrition Survey." Accessed November 2, 2013. https://www.vegsoc.org/sslpage.aspx?pid=753

Vegetarian Society. 2013. "Fact Sheets: Statistics." Accessed June 17, 2013. https://www.vegsoc.org/sslpage.aspx?pid=750

Samantha Jane Calvert
University of Birmingham

III. WILDLIFE CONSERVATION AND MANAGEMENT

Wildlife management may be thought a contradiction in terms. The logic of "wild" precludes "managed." Wildlife lived for millions of years unmanaged by humans. Part of what humans value in wildlife is animals that can look out for themselves. Wildlife that is managed is not wild; it is managed life. So there is logical difficulty in the idea. There is also ethical difficulty. Perhaps humans are not responsible for wildlife; wild lives are on their own. But then again, human activities affect wildlife quite adversely. Have we no duty to care for it either because of what humans have at stake or because of what wildlife is in itself?

The main issues of wildlife management discussed in this entry include the contemporary crisis of conserving historically evolved wildlife populations on rapidly developing human landscapes; ownership, control, management, and stewardship responsibilities for wildlife; conservation of endangered wildlife species; fishes and fisheries as managed wildlife populations; wildlife as game for hunting and trapping, including hunting as a conservation strategy; "hands-on" versus "hands-off" management; rural and urban wildlife and feral animals. These are issues of management, but there are ethical questions at every point.

WILDLIFE AND HUMAN POPULATIONS: AN EMERGING CRISIS

There are more species on earth in the early twenty-first century than there have ever been in the 2.5-billion-year history of life. Estimates run from 5 to 30 million species; 10 million is a typical figure. Most of the vertebrate wildlife and birds are known; most unknowns are in the invertebrate animal, insect, and plant species. During evolutionary history, there was no wildlife management; wildlife conservation takes care of itself if no humans intervene. On statistical average, more species have been produced than have become extinct; diversity has gradually increased.

Some five catastrophic extinctions have been followed by rather swift respeciation of new replacement species. On landscapes that have grown colder or drier, species may become fewer. Some groups of species were more numerous in the past, such as dinosaurs in the Cretaceous period and birds in the Pleistocene. Nevertheless, diversity is at an all-time high. In one sense, all biology is conservation biology (biology that conserves life), whether or not humans are involved.

There are many more humans on earth in the early twenty-first century than ever, and the expansion of human habitat, coupled with pollution, hunting, and trade in wildlife, threatens populations of wild animals and their habitats. Humans now threaten the biological processes that have been creating and conserving life for billions of years. Hardly an American landscape has not been impoverished of its native fauna. The larger once-dominant animals, such as eagles, wolves, cougars, grizzly bears, wolverines, bison, otters, and crocodiles, are especially depleted. The New World depletion in both hemispheres results from Europeans entering two relatively empty continents several centuries ago and engaging in explosive development. In contrast, Amerindians had coexisted with wildlife for 10,000 to 15,000 years, though they too may have contributed to some extinctions.

Long-settled continents do not escape the problem. Humans have inhabited Africa since evolving there over 100,000 years ago, but only in the twentieth century, as contemporary nations grew rapidly, were African mega-fauna and avifauna seriously threatened. Bush meat hunting is now a multibillion-dollar trade in the tropics (Carey 1999; McNeil 1999). Wildlife in China, India, and Tibet, among the oldest settled areas in the world, though long affected by humans, continued for the most part to survive, but lately this wildlife has been greatly depleted. The crisis is as serious in the Old World as in the New.

The crisis, now potentially more urgent than at any time in the history of the planet, generates unprecedented responsibilities, because humans previously did not have a great effect on wildlife. Now there are unprecedented demands for trade-offs between human values and the welfare of wildlife and unprecedented implications because of the global and irreversible scale of threats to wildlife.

The challenge for wildlife conservation is to balance human and wildlife values. Fortunately, wildlife is valuable to humans and so far can be included among the human values. Humans wish to hunt and fish. They enjoy watching wildlife. Wildlife art is the most popular American art form. If backyard bird feeding is included, almost one in four Americans spends some time bird-watching. Animals are chosen as state animals; sports teams and automobiles are named for animals. Many animals serve useful roles in ecosystems; hawks catch mice, and birds control insect populations. Wildlife can indicate the health of an ecosystem. Unfortunately, many human values conflict with wildlife on landscapes, as shown by the massive depletion of wildlife. We also now know that many diseases of wildlife are transmitted to humans, evidenced by bird flu and fears of pandemics. Here human interests seem contrary to wildlife's flourishing. But even if wildlife were not valuable to humans, would we not have some responsibility for the values of wild things for what they are in themselves?

The Wildlife Society (1990), the principal professional organization of management and conservation, affirms that "wildlife, in its myriad forms, is basic to the maintenance of a human culture that provides quality living." The society seeks "to develop and promote sound stewardship of wildlife resources and of the environments upon which wildlife and humans depend; to undertake an active role in preventing human-induced environmental degradation; to increase awareness and appreciation of wildlife values." It also urges "ethical restraints in the use of living natural resources."

OWNERSHIP, CONTROL, MANAGEMENT, AND STEWARDSHIP RESPONSIBILITIES FOR WILDLIFE

According to a long legal tradition in the United Kingdom, Canada, the United States, and many other nations, individual persons do not own vertebrate wildlife. Animals and birds do not belong to the landowner on whose property they are found. They move around, with dens and nests in particular places, but the larger animals and the birds can range over hundreds or thousands of square miles. They sometimes live on public land, sometimes on different tracts of private land. Continental European nations, by contrast, sometimes hold that property owners own wildlife resident on their lands. The Michigan State University College of Law maintains the Animal Legal and Historical Center with information about past and present attitudes toward and laws pertaining to animals.

In the Anglo-American tradition, landowners have the right to control access to their property. They control who, for instance, may hunt there. But the state determines whether and how much game may be taken. Individuals can "take" wildlife—capture or kill it—at which point the animal enters into their possession. State control of wildlife was long understood as state ownership, but wildlife pays no more attention to state lines than to local property boundaries; indeed, migratory birds reside in various nations. The US government has often regulated wildlife, because much wildlife crosses state lines and much inhabits federal lands. In court decisions, the state ownership doctrine has been rejected as based on a flawed characterization of wildlife. That doctrine has been replaced by an expanding public trust doctrine that says that wildlife should be regulated like other natural resources considered commons, not so much owned as held in trust. Particular state ownership of wildlife has been subsumed under broader state and federal power to regulate all natural resources. Wildlife is a public good held in trust for the benefit of the people (Bean 1983).

The general idea is that, in the context of the public interest and stewardship, society as a whole has a responsibility for wildlife, a duty to the people concerning wildlife in which they have an interest that encourages individual persons to relate to wildlife, care for it, tolerate it, perhaps hunt it. Animal welfare was long subsumed under this rubric, because maintaining this public good required healthy wildlife populations. But animal welfare has increasingly become a concern in its own right, independent of human benefits. This is called the intrinsic value of wildlife, a value also held in trust. This concern becomes evident in protection of endangered species and in shifting attitudes toward hunting.

CONSERVATION OF ENDANGERED WILDLIFE SPECIES

The legal tradition arose with regard to individual animals, but protecting endangered species has increasingly figured in regulations covering both game and nongame species. State departments of "game and fish" have largely been renamed departments of "wildlife." Although hunting and fishing remain a large part of their assignments, their interest in threatened wildlife has dramatically increased. If the government can regulate individual animals, by the same logic it can regulate species. For example, in the fall of 1981, when black-footed ferrets were discovered on private ranches near Meeteetse, Wyoming, the ranchers were legally obligated to protect them. Furthermore, the federal government can designate critical habitat on private land.

Landowners ought not shoot the bald eagles that fly over their property or cut the trees in which they nest. In compliance with the Endangered Species Act of 1973, the Weyerhaeuser Company in the early 1980s set aside more than 900 acres, representing more than $9 million in unharvested timber, in Washington and Oregon to protect eighty bald eagle nesting sites. Lest it be supposed that the bald eagle, the national symbol, is a unique public good, to comply with the law Weyerhaeuser also set aside 155 acres in southern states to protect twenty-two colonies of the endangered red-cockaded woodpecker. These woodpeckers prefer to nest in prime timber, eighty-year-old pine forests. Loggers would rather cut these lands more often than that, but the law causes them to protect eagles and woodpeckers, species that, though on their land, do not belong to them but are a common good.

The Endangered Species Act of 1973 is the most far-reaching wildlife statute adopted by any nation. The US Fish and Wildlife Service is charged by the act to list both domestic and foreign wildlife species threatened with extinction. No government agency may undertake projects likely to jeopardize listed species (including disruption of habitat) at home or abroad except under authority of a high-level committee that has granted few exemptions. Persons cannot take listed wildlife species on either public or private lands. In evaluating whether to list a species, economic considerations may not be considered, a point of repeated contention but one that the US Congress has reaffirmed several times. Importing species on the worldwide list into the United States is illegal except under specific conditions.

This concern, enacted into legislation, reveals an increasing sense of duty toward wildlife that comes into focus when a species becomes endangered. Game managers who may once have thought their responsibility was to maintain an annual crop of game to shoot now see themselves as wildlife managers whose responsibility is to provide for a diverse native fauna both for the benefits such wildlife brings to humans and out of respect for what all species of wildlife, not just the game species, are in themselves.

FISH AND FISHERIES AS MANAGED WILDLIFE POPULATIONS

Analogous changes have taken place with regard to fishes. Once what one wanted was fish to catch, and fishing remains a popular recreation. But concern for all species of native fish is increasing.

The native fish fauna of North America has been tampered with possibly as extensively as, and certainly more rapidly than, the fish on any other continent. Managers have introduced "game" and eliminated "trash" fish. Humans have made dams and water developments for domestic, industrial, and agricultural uses. Humans have polluted, caused erosional sedimentation, and accidentally introduced parasites and diseases. Of the endangered fishes of the world, about 70 percent are in

North America, and 56 percent are receiving some degree of protection. The fish in the United States have been as disturbed as any other wildlife, more so in the West than in the East (Minckley and Deacon 1991). The Endangered Species Committee of the Desert Fishes Council identifies 164 fish in North American deserts as endangered, vulnerable, rare, or warranting various degrees of concern (Williams et al. 1985).

In the Pacific Northwest between 1930 and the late 1970s about 200 dams, including 19 major hydroelectric dams, were constructed in the Columbia Basin to provide water for irrigation, flood control, barging, and cheap electricity. The Columbia River was turned into a series of dams and reservoirs. These dams have decimated salmon by blocking and flooding salmon habitat; killing or stunning fish as they pass through dam turbines; and increasing migration times, predation, and stress. Many attempts to find a solution have largely failed, including fish ladders, barging salmon around the dams, spilling more water over dams in migration season, hatcheries, and severe reductions in commercial and sport fishing. Salmon have disappeared from about 40 percent of their historical breeding ranges in the US West, and many populations are depressed in areas where they were formerly abundant (National Research Council Committee on Protection and Management of Pacific Northwest Anadromous Salmonids 1996). Outlook for salmon is generally bleak despite sometimes aggressive efforts to facilitate their recovery.

Concern for fish has at times modified or stopped water development projects. On the Virgin River and its tributaries in Utah in 1980, for example, water authorities abandoned the Warner Valley project lest it jeopardize the woundfin and built the Quail Creek project instead. Water release from dams may be adjusted in time and volume for the benefit of endangered fish and bird species (Deacon 1988).

Endangered species legislation represents a change in what humans think they ought to manage. The shift is from maintaining game species to protecting native fishery populations. Wildlife managers especially show an increasing sense of duty to ensure the presence of fish as an integral part of the wildlife community, not just for human benefit but out of respect for what these fish are in themselves and for their roles in riparian ecosystems.

HUNTING AND TRAPPING: HUNTING AS A CONSERVATION STRATEGY

Wildlife management has traditionally meant game management. Hunting both for meat and for sport is an ancient practice. Humans evolved as omnivores. Meat has been important in human nutrition although it is quite possible for humans to be well nourished as vegetarians. The character of hunting has accentuated sport hunting in modern times; few hunters of the early twenty-first century are primarily meat hunters, although in most cases the carcass will be eaten. Most hunters have a code of ethics. They think it unethical to waste the meat. Hunters also seek a fair chase, a clean kill, minimal suffering, and respect for the animal, and hunters have long been among the most effective conservationists, at least of their hunted species and their habitats. Predators, especially wolves, were often eliminated as competitive hunters.

Since the mid-1960s a strong antihunting movement has emerged on the grounds that shooting animals for sport is unethical, even if the hunter's ethic is observed (Cartmill 1993; Regan 2004; Singer 1990). Yet hunters continue to defend the hunt (Evans 2005; Kowalsky 2010; Pauley 2003). Antihunters regard as morally wrong wildlife management for the purpose of maintaining hunting. But much funding for wildlife conservation comes from hunting and fishing licenses, and if these activities are curtailed, alternative funding sources will have to be found. Hunters argue that properly managed hunting can ensure conservation, because this activity makes wildlife valuable both to the hunter and to others who profit from the hunter's presence.

Such an argument is especially used for African wildlife. In Africa, although much hunting is legal, poaching has also been rampant, resulting in an international ban on skins, hides, horns, tusks, and other parts of various species. Wildlife managers may argue that whereas such bans may discourage poachers, they also discourage legal hunting, which can be quite profitable if such animal products are sold in markets. This makes wildlife worthless to native peoples, who can neither hunt for food nor sell wildlife products. Even the products from culled animals (shot to reduce excess populations) cannot be sold. Ivory has been a case in point. Most world ivory trade has been made illegal, but some authorities argue that the sale of legal ivory could greatly benefit elephant conservation.

Trapping has been a traditional use of wildlife, largely for pelts and hides made into mink coats, beaver hats, alligator-skin purses and shoes, and so on. Given available substitutes, many people object to this use of animals on the grounds that trapping involves cruelty. They argue that furs on fashion models simply flatter female vanities, somewhat as trophy animals mounted in sportmen's dens flatter male vanities. The leghold trap is especially objectionable to opponents of trapping. A counterargument is that a high value on animal skins with effective management can ensure conservation. Most of the world's crocodile species are endangered. But because crocodiles are dangerous and often frequent rivers where humans are present, only if they are of considerable value to local peoples are they likely to be tolerated and saved.

"HANDS-ON" VERSUS "HANDS-OFF" MANAGEMENT

Although there is a growing consensus that humans have an urgent responsibility actively to conserve wildlife, many argue that the less wildlife is managed the better. So far as wild animals are managed, their wildness is compromised—the paradox of wildlife management. The animals become artifacts, more like pets. This leads to a debate between "hands-on management," which favors active intervention, habitat enhancement, supplemental feeding, breeding, radio-collared monitoring, and so on, and "hands-off management," which favors as little management as possible consistent with animal welfare.

From a medical point of view, there is contention whether veterinarians ought to treat wildlife diseases. Like all physicians, veterinarians seek good health. Colorado veterinarians treated a lungworm disease in bighorn sheep successfully. By contrast, when an epidemic of pinkeye ravaged the bighorn sheep of Yellowstone Park in 1981–1982, authorities refused to let Wyoming veterinarians treat the disease. The welfare of the sheep, they said, required letting the disease take its course; disease-resistant sheep would survive, and the genetic fitness of the herd would improve. Whether the disease is introduced by humans is a factor. The *Chlamydia* parasite producing pinkeye was not thought to be introduced; some said that the lungworm was introduced from domestic sheep or that the sheep were weakened due to human disruptions, especially of their winter range. Although more than half the Yellowstone herd perished by starvation and injury following partial blindness, the herd recovered although not to its former numbers (Thorne 1987).

Many argue that hands-off management is ideal for animals that inhabit extensive ranges but that, because of development and human needs, insufficient habitat remains for hands-off management. With elephants in Africa, they say, only hands-on management is possible. Given the elephant's destructiveness and its tendency to migrate, herds must be fenced, water holes provided, herds culled, and so on. A balance between responsibilities to elephants and the needs of humans must be found. A controversial case in the United States involved supplemental feeding for grizzly bears in Yellowstone Park. After decades of supplemental feeding, park officials, preferring a wild bear over a managed bear, elected in 1971 to risk letting the endangered species survive on its own. The bears subsequently survived rather well.

RURAL WILDLIFE, URBAN WILDLIFE, FERAL ANIMALS

Although foxes, rabbits, thrushes, and eagles are wild, they often inhabit rural and semideveloped landscapes, such as parks. Indeed, nationwide most wildlife is not on wild lands but on landscapes that are hybrids of both nature and culture. Wildlife is often important to the human sense of place. No one since Rachel Carson coined the term wants a "silent spring" in the Shenandoah Valley, on Cape Cod, or in the Lake District. Salmon have such great cultural, economic, recreational, and symbolic significance in the Pacific Northwest that the Roman Catholic bishops there, in "The Columbia River Watershed: Caring for Creation and the Common Good," expressed their view of salmon as a sign not only of the ecological health of the river but also of the "spiritual vitality" of the people in the watershed (Roman Catholic Bishops of the Pacific Northwest and British Columbia 1999).

Some wildlife is urban and suburban. Robins and squirrels find their way into cities and suburbs, and even rabbits and foxes can be found there. These animals are mostly welcomed, but some—raccoons, coyotes, and deer, for example—can become pests, raiding trash cans, catching and eating pets, browsing garden plants. Hungry bears find their way into town. Such animals may have to be controlled, preferably by better trash cans or fences; perhaps they must be relocated or killed. Some wild animals live in zoos, safari parks, and research laboratories, if such animals can still be considered wild. These animals in large part come under the federal Animal Welfare Act of 1966 and related state laws and are overseen by institutional animal use and care committees. Zoos frequently claim to be important in conservation, but few actually are. Almost none of the hundreds of thousands of zoo animals will or could be released into the wild.

An early twenty-first-century perspective is that our obligations to animals include the need to consider these animals in their various contexts (Palmer 2010). One must and morally ought to treat wolves in the wilderness quite differently from warblers at the bird feeder and those warblers at the feeder differently from warblers in the wilderness. Salmon can no longer be wild, but they ought to be carefully managed (as in hatcheries or fish ladders) for a semblance of wildness. The central theme here is that obligations to wildlife and semiwildlife are graded in accordance with the degrees of habituation, domestication, capture, or behavioral modifications by humans.

Feral animals are those introduced by humans, not native to landscapes, that have managed to survive on their own. Management of such animals is disputed, especially of mustangs and burros in the western United States. Although not now living in their native ecosystems, such animals may have been living wild for centuries. Management policy is typically to eliminate them on the grounds that they are not authentic wildlife, although the US Congress has mandated preserving mustangs in some localities. Animal welfare advocates have protested eliminating the mustangs and burros. Other cases involve feral hogs and goats. On San Clemente Island off the coast of California, nearly 30,000 goats were eliminated in the 1980s, about half of them shot, the other half captured and relocated—with poor survival rates—to protect endangered species of plants and to prevent further degradation of the island ecosystem. The goats had been left there by the Spanish in earlier centuries. The argument here is that we have a greater responsibility to native wildlife and plants than to feral species.

SEE ALSO *Biodiversity Conservation; Ecological Bioethics; Environmental Ethics*

BIBLIOGRAPHY

Animal Legal and Historical Center, Michigan State University College of Law. http://www.animallaw.info

Bailey, James A. 1984. *Principles of Wildlife Management.* New York: John Wiley.

Bean, Michael J. 1983. *The Evolution of National Wildlife Law.* Rev. ed. New York: Praeger.

Carey, John. 1999. "Where Have All the Animals Gone?" *International Wildlife* 29 (6): 12–20.

Carson, Rachel. 1951. *Silent Spring.* Boston: Houghton Mifflin.

Cartmill, Matt. 1993. *A View to a Death in the Morning: Hunting and Nature through History.* Cambridge, MA: Harvard University Press.

Deacon, James E. 1988. "The Endangered Woundfin and Water Management in the Virgin River, Utah, Arizona, Nevada." *Fisheries* 13:18–24.

Endangered Species Act of 1973. 1973. Publ. L. no. 93–205, 87 Stat. 884.

Evans, Joseph Claude. 2005. *With Respect for Nature: Living as Part of the Natural World.* Albany: State University of New York Press.

Hargrove, Eugene C., ed. 1992. *The Animal Rights, Environmental Ethics Debate: The Environmental Perspective.* Albany: State University of New York Press.

Kowalsky, Nathan, ed. 2010. *Hunting: Philosophy for Everyone in Search of the Wild Life.* Malden, MA: Wiley-Blackwell.

McNeil, Donald G. 1999. "The Great Ape Massacre." *New York Times Magazine,* May 9, 54–57.

Minckley, W. L., and James E. Deacon, eds. 1991. *Battle against Extinction: Native Fish Management in the American West.* Tucson: University of Arizona Press.

National Research Council Committee on Protection and Management of Pacific Northwest Anadromous Salmonids. 1996. *Upstream: Salmon and Society in the Pacific Northwest.* Washington, DC: National Academies Press.

Palmer, Clare. 2010. *Animal Ethics in Context.* New York: Columbia University Press.

Pauley, John A. 2003. "The Value of Hunting." *Journal of Value Inquiry* 37 (2): 233–44.

Regan, Tom. 2004. *The Case for Animal Rights.* Berkeley: University of California Press.

Roman Catholic Bishops of the Pacific Northwest and British Columbia. 1999. "The Columbia River Watershed: Caring for Creation and the Common Good." Accessed November 2, 2013. http://www.thewscc.org/images/stories/Resources/Statements/colrvr-e.pdf

Singer, Peter. 1990. *Animal Liberation.* 2nd ed. New York: New York Review of Books.

Thorne, Tom. 1987. "Born Looking for a Place to Die." *Wyoming Wildlife* 51 (3): 10–19.

Wildlife Society. 1990. *Conservation Policies of the Wildlife Society.* Bethesda, MD: Wildlife Society.

Williams, Jack E.; David B. Bowman; James E. Brooks; et al. 1985. "Endangered Aquatic Ecosystems in North American Deserts with a List of Vanishing Fishes of the Region." *Journal of the Arizona-Nevada Academy of Science* 20:1–62.

Holmes Rolston III (1995, 2014)
University Distinguished Professor, Department of Philosophy, Colorado State University

IV. PET AND COMPANION ANIMALS

The term *companion animals* refers to those animals that human beings keep for purposes of control, companionship, and comfort. The word *pet,* which suggests the indulgent use of animals (Shell 1986), is being increasingly replaced by the term *companion animals.* However, the term *pet animal* seems indispensable in conveying the relationship of intimacy between some humans and selected domesticated species.

THE EMERGENCE OF PET KEEPING

The precise origins of pet keeping are obscure. There appear always to have been symbiotic relationships both between species and within species (see, for example, Kropotkin 1939), though some argue that "almost alone among animals, humans domesticate and dwell with other animals" (Clark 1982, 110). Keeping animals as companions may have been a by-product of both killing and domesticating them. Stephen Clark argues that "people who cared for their animals [kept for food] left more descendants than those who used them carelessly" and that "it 'paid' our ancestors to love what wasn't human" (1982, 111). Some animals were undoubtedly kept for their own value as sources of fascination or as mediators of unusual benefits. For example, cats, though they were domesticated for a much briefer time than other species, have frequently been associated with the supernatural, as agents of either benign or malign forces (Clutton-Brock 1993).

English society in the eighteenth and nineteenth centuries saw the emergence of widespread pet keeping, especially among the upper classes. Keith Thomas writes of how, as early as 1700, "symptoms of obsessive pet-keeping were in evidence," especially in the keeping of horses, cats, dogs, and birds (Thomas 1983, 117). These species were clearly "privileged" in comparison with food animals, which were still reared and killed with hideous cruelty. Although the "idea of a pedigree did not originate in the nineteenth century," Harriet Ritvo shows how the notion of purity of species through selective breeding became widespread among the middle and upper classes, for whom particular companion animals were themselves indicators of social class and good breeding (Ritvo 1986).

Since the nineteenth century, the phenomenon of pet keeping has increased not only among all English classes but also within continental European and US societies. Although reliable estimates of animal populations are difficult to obtain (partly because of nonexistent or unenforced licensing laws), one conservative estimate is that the total annual US turnover in owned dogs in 1991 was 7.71 million, 4 million of which were handled by animal shelters and 2.1 million of which were euthanized (Patronek and Glickman 1994). The current situation in the Western world of millions of animals being kept for purposes of companionship extends far beyond any reasonable interpretation of symbiosis and is historically without parallel.

Quite apart from the personal and psychological factors involved, one obvious reason accounts for this development. Pet owning has become an established part of consumer-oriented cultures in which animals are bought and sold like any other commodity. The pet industry itself, not to mention the allied supply (including veterinary) services, benefit directly or indirectly from the trade, management, and treatment of companion animals. In 1991, in the state of Washington alone, it is estimated that the number of dogs available from pet stores amounted to 11,442, and through breeders the number was 37,523 (Patronek and Glickman 1994).

THE BENEFITS OF PET KEEPING

The benefits of pet keeping may be classed under three broad headings: psychological benefits to humans, benefits to human society, and benefits to pet animals.

Psychological Benefits to Humans. It seems impossible to doubt that some human-animal bonds can contribute significantly to human flourishing. Relationships with pets seem to help prevent two sources of emotional disorder: deprivation and frustration. They enable nongenital physical contact, provide tactile comfort, improve self-esteem, enhance emotional security, boost personal prowess (as when a beautiful or socially appealing animal is owned), and engender loving relationships that are sometimes seemingly impossible with other humans (Ryder 1973; Levinson 1978; Fogle 1981; Serpell 1986).

Potential or actual benefits for pet owners specifically include lower blood pressure (Baun et al. 1984), lower heart rates (Wilson and Nettling 1987; Deshriver and Riddick 1990), reduced anxiety (Wilson 1991), and reduced depression (Bolin 1987). However, Cindy Wilson argues that although "much has been made over the potential benefits of a pet," it is also true that a large amount of such research "remains anecdotal, nongeneralizable, and scientifically flawed" and that a new methodology should be based on assessable "quality of life measurements" (1994, 4–8).

In the absence of large amounts of data based on objective evidence, interpretation of the psychological effects of pet keeping turns on whether interspecies relations are natural and commendable. Richard Ryder warns against the view that such interspecies relationships are "unnatural or cranky" (1973, 5); nonetheless, it is still questionable to what extent legitimate psychological needs are met through pet keeping and whether these needs can or should be met through relationships with members of our own species.

Benefits to Human Society. It has long been thought that pet keeping can help sensitize children, even train them in attitudes of care and respect (Rothschild 1986). One study goes so far as to claim that "companion animals are a vital part of the healthy emotional development of children" (Robin and ten Bensel 1991, 174). Studies have also suggested that relationships with pets can contribute to the psychological and social well-being of adult humans, especially elderly people who live alone (Connell and Lago 1991). Animal-assisted therapy is sometimes utilized for patients in psychiatric hospitals and for individuals with special needs, such as people with the human immunodeficiency virus or acquired immunodeficiency syndrome (Gorczyca 1991) and those suffering from chronic schizophrenia (Bauman et al. 1991).

Benefits to Pet Animals. The benefits of pet keeping to the animals themselves are difficult to quantify. Leaving aside the wider ethical question of whether animals should be domesticated at all, the impact on the individual pet depends on how well it is kept and to what degree its owners understand and meet its emotional and environmental needs. For example, although pet keeping can provide a stimulus to sensitize children, it can also conversely provide an opportunity for cruelty by abused or disturbed children or by children who lack parental supervision. Some commentators see something psychologically, even politically, perverse about indulging pet animals (see, for example, Shell 1986), and, as discussed later, it is not clear that such indulgence is always beneficial to the animals' welfare.

THE DISADVANTAGES OF PET KEEPING

Formidable ethical and welfare problems are associated with pet keeping (Carpenter et al. 1980). These issues may be classified under three headings: abuse, overpopulation, and commercial usage.

Abuse. Recorded acts of cruelty against pets appear to be increasing in both the United States and the United Kingdom. Whatever the benefits to both parties, living in proximity to animals substantially increases the risk of abuse. Apart from deliberate acts of cruelty, even sadism, unsuitable environmental conditions can cause unacceptably high levels of stress for animals. Few owners fully understand the complex psychological and physiological needs of the animals they keep. Cruelty sometimes arises through ignorance and misunderstanding rather than deliberate neglect, especially when the subjects are exotic animals. Abuse or neglect does occur despite the many and various pet-care programs available.

Overpopulation. Present high levels of pet populations inevitably mean death and sometimes suffering for other animals. In order to sustain high populations of such species as cats and dogs, for example, other species, such as whales, kangaroos, and horses, must be killed in order to feed them. Few pet animals of any size can be sustained without meat, though it appears that dogs can live well on an appropriately balanced vegetarian diet. The commercial production of pet food has also been criticized as a waste of resources. The average cost of feeding an eighty-pound dog has been estimated at $8,353 for its lifetime (Shell 1986).

High pet populations also raise other problems for humans. These include possible health hazards, nuisance, and social control. Dogs can communicate diseases such as *Toxocara canis*, which can cause blindness in children. Fortunately, such cases are rare, but an awareness of this hazard in the United Kingdom has led local councils to outlaw dogs from public parks, particularly children's parks. Animal organizations, such as the United Kingdom's Royal Society for the Prevention of Cruelty to Animals (1984), have argued the case for compulsory registration of dogs as a means of ensuring responsible ownership; so far, such schemes have operated only on a voluntary or local basis. In 1992, the Dangerous Dogs Act was introduced in the United Kingdom to deal with the threat posed by aggressive dogs after some distressing incidents in which children were attacked by uncontrolled dogs.

Commercial Usage. Because domestic animals have almost everywhere only the legal status of property (Sandys-Winsch 1984; Sweeney 1990), the breeding and sale of pets is subject to few legal constraints, save principally that direct and "unnecessary" cruelty must be avoided. The view that pets are merely human property has inevitably led, as with other consumer items, to the refashioning of pets. Nonveterinary mutilation of pets (e.g., tail docking, ear cropping, declawing, and removal of a dog's larynx to prevent barking) is not uncommon, though in the United Kingdom the British Veterinary Association refuses to authorize all nonveterinary procedures; performance of such procedures can lead to revocation of a veterinarian's license. The society likewise opposes all "selective breeding of animals which produces changes in bodily form and/or function," in addition to the commercial sale of puppies and kittens in pet shops (1984, 7–8).

Animal protectionists argue that the commercial trade in animals leads inevitably to overbreeding and the consequent abandonment and disposal of millions of unwanted animals. In the United Kingdom, the RSPCA estimates that it destroys on average about 1,000 unwanted dogs every week. In the United States, estimates vary from 2.1 million to 9.1 million per year for dogs alone (Patronek and Glickman 1994). Such a wide discrepancy in the figures indicates, among other things, the difficulty in collecting uniform data from the estimated 1,800 to 3,000 US animal shelters. Widespread euthanasia suggests a prima facie disregard for the worth of pet animals. (For a discussion of the ethical problems surrounding large-scale euthanasia, see Kay et al. 1988.)

IS PET KEEPING IMMORAL?

Despite the emergence of a strong animal-rights movement since the mid-1970s, the ethics of pet keeping is seldom questioned. The major works in animal ethics (Singer 1976; Clark 1977; Regan 1983; Rodd 1990) largely or entirely bypass this question, and only lone voices are raised in critical opposition (Linzey 1976; Bryant 1990). Animal rights philosophy has evolved without offering any critical analysis of the pet trade, though some argue that abuse of pet animals is a "human breach of contract" (Rollin 1992, 219). Because so many animal rights thinkers oppose a purely utilitarian justification for animal exploitation, this omission is surely anomalous.

Part of the reason may be that, historically speaking, sensibility to animal suffering seems to have arisen as a necessary corollary to the practice of keeping pets (Thomas 1983; Tester 1991). The physical inclusion of animals in the human community seems to have signified a moral inclusiveness also. It may be no accident that the first country to found a society for the prevention of cruelty to animals—England—was also the country renowned for its love of pet animals. Moreover, one cannot but be struck by the way in which anecdotes about animal behavior, especially that of pet animals, have formed the basis for a whole string of pioneering humanitarian books appealing for greater kindness to animals and a fundamental recognition of their rights (see, for example, Youatt 1839; Wood 1875; Nicholson 1879; Lessing 1991;Thomas 1993).

Yet questions must be asked about the ethical appropriateness of the psychological needs that pet animals apparently meet. Ryder accepts that some of these are "selfish" (1973, 8). One early critique argued that "we need to distinguish between a kind of love which respects animals for what they are and allows them to pursue their own lives according to their own natural instincts, and another selfish form of love which seeks to condition animal lives in accordance with our own human desires." Pet keeping, it is argued, represents a "false anthropomorphism" in which we seek to "humanise" animals and "regard them as extensions of our own egos" (Linzey 1976 68). This view was subsequently modified on the ground that "all loving is in practice a subtle blend of altruism and self-seeking," though "where the interests of animals are entirely subordinated to human emotional needs, we need to beware that we are not involved in a self-deceiving tyranny" (Linzey 1987, 137). According to this perspective, at least some forms of pet keeping are wrong because they are insufficiently symbiotic and fail to recognize the right of animals to their own natural life.

BIBLIOGRAPHY

Anderson, Robert S., ed. 1975. *Pet Animals and Society*. London: Baillière Tindall.

Bauman, Lawrence; Monte Posner; Karl Sachs; et al. 1991. "The Effects of Animal-assisted Therapy on Communications Patterns with Chronic Schizophrenics." In *Universal Kinship: The Bond between All Living Things*, edited by the Latham Foundation staff, 21–48. Saratoga, CA: R & E.

Baun, Mara M.; Nancy Bergstrom; Nancy F. Langston; et al. 1984. "Physiological Effects of Human/Companion Animal Bonding." *Nursing Research* 33 (3): 126–29.

Bolin, Sharon E. 1987. "The Effects of Companion Animals during Conjugal Bereavement." *Anthrozoös* 1 (1): 26–35.

Bryant, John. 1990. *Fettered Kingdoms: An Examination of a Changing Ethic*, rev. ed. Winchester, UK: Fox.

Carpenter, Edward; Angela Bates; Trevor Beeson; et al. 1980. *Animals and Ethics: Report of the Working Party*. London: Watkins.

Clark, Stephen R. L. 1977. *The Moral Status of Animals*. Oxford, UK: Clarendon Press.

Clark, Stephen R. L. 1982. *The Nature of the Beast: Are Animals Moral?* Oxford, UK: Oxford University Press.

Clutton-Brock, Juliet. 1993. *Cats, Ancient and Modern*. Cambridge, MA: Harvard University Press.

Connell, Cathleen M., and Daniel J. Lago. 1991. "Effects of Pets on the Well-being of the Elderly." In *Universal Kinship: The Bond between All Living Things*, edited by the Latham Foundation staff, 51–62. Saratoga, CA: R & E.

Davis, S. L., and P. R. Cheeke. 1998. "Do Domestic Animals Have Minds and the Ability to Think? A Provisional Sample of Opinions on the Question." *Journal of Animal Science* 76 (8): 2072–79.

Dawkins, Marian Stamp. 1993. *Through Our Eyes Only?: The Search for Animal Consciousness*. New York: W. H. Freeman.

Deshriver, Mary M., and Carol Cuttler Riddick. 1990. "Effects of Watching Aquariums on Elders' Stress." *Anthrozoös* 4 (1): 44–48.

Fogle, Bruce, ed. 1981. *Interrelations between People and Pets*. Springfield, IL: Charles C. Thomas.

Francione, Gary L. 1995. *Animals, Property, and the Law*. Philadelphia: Temple University Press.

Francione, Gary L. 2000. *Introduction to Animal Rights: Your Child or the Dog?* Philadelphia: Temple University Press.

Gorczyca, Ken. 1991. "Special Needs for the Pet Owner with AIDS/HIV." In *Universal Kinship: The Bond between All Living Things*, edited by the Latham Foundation staff, 13–20. Saratoga, CA: R & E.

Kay, William J.; Susan P. Cohen; Carole E. Fudin; et al., eds. 1988. *Euthanasia of the Companion Animal: The Impact on Pet Owners, Veterinarians, and Society*. Philadelphia: Charles Press.

Kropotkin, Petr Alekseevich. 1939. *Mutual Aid: A Factor of Evolution*. Harmondsworth, UK: Penguin.

Lessing, Doris. 1991. *Particularly Cats—and Rufus*, rev. ed. New York: Alfred A. Knopf.

Levinson, Boris M. 1978. "Pets and Personality Development." *Psychological Reports* 42 (3) pt. 2: 1031–38.

Linzey, Andrew. 1976. *Animal Rights: A Christian Assessment of Man's Treatment of Animals*. London: S. C. M. Press.

Linzey, Andrew. 1987. *Christianity and the Rights of Animals*. London: SPCK.

Linzey, Andrew. 1995. *Animal Theology*. London: S. C. M. Press.

Nicholson, Edward W. B. 1879. *The Rights of an Animal: A New Essay in Ethics*. London: C. Kegan Paul.

Patronek, Gary J., and Lawrence T. Glickman. 1994. "Development of a Model for Estimating the Size and Dynamics of the Pet Dog Population." *Anthrozoös* 7 (1): 25–41.

Patronek, Gary J., and Charlotte A. Lacroix. 2001. "Developing an Ethic for the Handling, Restraint, and Discipline of Companion Animals in Veterinary Practice." *Journal of the American Veterinary Medical Association* 218 (4): 514–17.

Regan, Tom. 1983. *The Case for Animal Rights*. Berkeley: University of California Press.

Ritvo, Harriet. 1986. "Pride and Pedigree: The Evolution of the Victorian Dog Fancy." *Victorian Studies* 29 (2): 227–53.

Ritvo, Harriet. 1994. "A Dog's Life." *New York Review of Books*, January 13.

Robin, Michael, and Robert ten Bensel. 1991. "Pets and the Socialization of Children." In *Universal Kinship: The Bond between All Living Things*, edited by the Latham Foundation staff, 173–96. Saratoga, CA: R & E.

Rodd, Rosemary. 1990. *Biology, Ethics, and Animals*. Oxford, UK: Clarendon Press.

Rollin, Bernard E. 1992. *Animal Rights and Human Morality*, rev. edition. Buffalo, NY: Prometheus Books.

Rothschild, Miriam. 1986. *Animals and Man*. New York: Oxford University Press.

Royal Society for the Prevention of Cruelty to Animals. 1984. *Policies on Animal Welfare*, rev. ed. Horsham, Sussex, UK: Author.

Ryder, Richard D. 1973. *Pets Are Good for People*. London: Pet Manufacturers' Association.

Sandys-Winsch, Godfrey. 1984. *Animal Law*, 2nd ed. London: Shaw and Sons.

Serpell, James. 1986. *In the Company of Animals: A Study of Human-Animal Relationships*. New York: Basil Blackwell.

Shell, Marc. 1986. "The Family Pet." *Representations* 15 (summer): 121–53.

Singer, Peter. 1976. *Animal Liberation: A New Ethics for Our Treatment of Animals*. London: Jonathan Cape.

Stallones, Lorann. 1994. "Pet Loss and Mental Health." *Anthrozoos* 7 (1): 43–54.

Sweeney, Noël. 1990. *Animals and Cruelty and Law*. Bristol, UK: Alibi Books.

Tester, Keith. 1991. *Animals and Society: The Humanity of Animal Rights*. London: Routledge.

Thomas, Elizabeth Marshall. 1993. *The Hidden Life of Dogs*. Boston: Houghton Mifflin.

Thomas, Keith. 1983. *Man and the Natural World: A History of the Modern Sensibility*. New York: Pantheon.

Wilson, Cindy C. 1991. "The Pet as an Anxiolytic Intervention." *Journal of Nervous and Mental Disease* 179 (8): 482–89.

Wilson, Cindy C. 1994. "A Conceptual Framework for Human-Animal Interaction Research: The Challenge Revisited." *Anthrozoös* 7 (1): 4–24.

Wilson, Cindy C., and F. Ellen Nettling. 1987. "New Directions: Challenges for Human-Animal Bond Research and the Elderly." *Journal of Applied Gerontology* 6 (2): 189–200.

Wood, John George. 1875. *Man and Beast: Here and Hereafter. Illustrated by More Than Three Hundred Original Anecdotes*. London: Daldy, Isbister.

Youatt, William. 1839. *The Obligation and Extent of Humanity to Brutes, Principally Considered with Reference to Domesticated Animals*. London: Longman, Orme, Brown, Green, and Longman.

Andrew Linzey (1995)
University of Oxford

IV. PET AND COMPANION ANIMALS [ADDENDUM]

The use of animals during the treatment of human patients can be traced back to the times of the ancient Egyptians, Greeks, and Romans (Shubert 2012). A dramatic increase in such animal-assisted interventions within medicine, social work, and related fields of health care, however, has occurred in recent years. Such interventions aim to improve the physical, emotional, cognitive, or social health and functioning of people who participate in them. Related programs may be classified into animal-assisted activities (AAAs), service animal programs (SAPs), and animal-assisted therapies (AATs) (Muñoz Lasa et al. 2011).

Of these programs, SAPs have the greatest prominence and lengthiest history. The animals used in these programs are intended to enhance the capabilities of humans disabled through impairment of sensory capacities, such as sight or hearing. Such animals are typically dogs, often highly trained through programs such as Guide Dogs for the Blind, which are run in several countries by various charities. They assist beneficiaries with everyday activities, thereby reducing their dependency on other people.

The use of animals may also be aimed at achieving specific medical or therapeutic benefits for patients, such as the alleviation of pain or depression or the lowering of blood pressure or stress levels. Horses, for example, have been used to facilitate the normalization of muscle tone and improved motor skills in children with cerebral palsy and in patients with lower limb spasticity (Muñoz Lasa et al. 2011).

AAAs provide motivational, educational, or recreational opportunities designed to enhance the quality of life, without the kind of specific treatment goals characteristic of AATs (Shubert 2012). Reported benefits of AAAs include enhancement of socialization, leisure, and recreational skills; reduction of stress, anxiety, and loneliness; and improvement in mood and general well-being (Muñoz Lasa et al. 2011). For elderly people or others who may lack adequate social contact, "animals allow people to escape from everyday reality, offer friendship and love and … also [a] sense of safety and needfulness," as M. Fejsáková and colleagues (2009, 62) have noted.

Considerable attention has focused on the potential human therapeutic or other benefits of such programs, particularly in the case of newer modalities, such as AATs and AAAs. In contrast, relatively little consideration has been afforded to the impacts experienced by the animals used. Sentient animals have their own intrinsic worth, independent of any instrumental value to humans. Or, put another way, their lives are morally significant in their own right. Each animal has its own set of interests, which it seeks to pursue by means of both individual and species-specific behaviors. When we frustrate those behaviors or inflict harms on animals, there are, of course, moral consequences. Unfortunately, animal-assisted interventions may potentially cause such harms, in several ways.

First, animals are frequently taken from their natural families and locales and then provided with limited, if any contact with their own kind. Instead, they receive the companionship of humans, who may not be entirely sound in body or mind. Human psychological or behavioral disorders may have consequences for animal companions. People who are overly anxious or needy for companionship, for example, may place their animal companions under stress, from which they have limited ability to escape. Where animals are transferred from patient to patient, they also have to endure changing homes and human companions, who are likely to have varying personal characteristics and levels of prior experience with animal guardianship. Lack of control over an animal's environment or social milieu can be a significant source of stress. As Fejsáková and colleagues (2009, 63) put it, "The majority of AAA/AAT animals are 'imprisoned' in systems in which they have little self-control over their social life and are unable to avoid … unwanted social environment[s]."

Such harms can become even more significant when nondomesticated species are used. Such species are more likely to have specialized dietary and other husbandry requirements; the risk is that such needs may not be met, resulting in detrimental effects on welfare. They are also less likely to cope well in artificial, captive environments and particularly stressful environments. They may also be considerably more difficult to train. Fejsáková and colleagues (2009) described the training of white-headed capuchin monkeys (*Cebus capucinus*) for use in an AAT program. Because of their potentially aggressive and unpredictable behavior, in the majority of cases these monkeys had to wear remote electric collars or harnesses and undergo castration and removal of their eyeteeth to control their behavior and safeguard patients.

Similarly, extreme measures may be required to allow the use of animals—whether domesticated or not—when patients are markedly immunocompromised, such as those suffering from AIDS or receiving high-dose steroid therapy. Owing to the risk of infections resulting from cat scratches, for example, feline companions of such patients may undergo onychectomy, or declawing surgery. This effectively amputates every toe at the first joint, resulting in avoidable risks associated with general anesthesia and of complications such as postoperative stump and phantom pain, hemorrhage, and infection and substantial reduction in self-defense capacity during encounters with other animals. Accordingly, onychectomy is extremely controversial within veterinary medicine (Atwood-Harvey 2005).

Clearly, the use of animal-assisted interventions can be more morally problematic than is apparent at first glance. Such problems may be exacerbated by inconsistency of standards for selection, training, and evaluation of both animals and therapists (Fejsáková et al. 2009). At a minimum, animal-assisted therapists should be intimately familiar with normal behavioral repertoires of the species in question and skilled at reading animal body language and detecting signs of stress, discomfort, fear, and fatigue. The wider adoption and harmonization of minimum standards would help ensure that therapists are adequately trained and experienced. Such standards should also be directed toward ensuring safe, stable, and physically and psychologically healthy environments for the animals used and also at identifying animals or species that cannot be used in such programs without incurring unacceptable risks to the health and welfare of the animals or their intended human companions.

Vegetarian companion animal diets also remain the subject of controversy. It is because of the ethical concerns of a growing population of vegetarian animal guardians about the farming and killing of animals raised for food and because of medical conditions such as allergies caused by beef, lamb, and other animal-derived dietary ingredients that vegetarian pet food brands were first developed. However, there is no scientific reason why a diet entirely comprising plant, mineral, and synthetically based ingredients cannot be formulated to meet all of the palatability, nutritional, and bioavailability needs of dogs, cats, humans, or indeed any other species for which they are intended. After all, each species requires particular dietary nutrients, not specific ingredients (Knight 2005). Indeed, an increasing number of such purely vegetarian diets are now commercially available for both dogs and cats.

SEE ALSO *Care: I. History of the Notion of Care; Environmental Ethics: I. Overview; Grief, Ethical Implications of; Moral Status*

BIBLIOGRAPHY

Atwood-Harvey Dana. 2005. "Death or Declaw: Dealing with Moral Ambiguity in a Veterinary Hospital." *Society and Animals* 13 (4): 315–42.

Fejsáková, M.; J. Kottferová; J. Mareková; et al. 2009. "Ethical Aspects Related to Involvement of Animals in Animal Assisted Therapy." *Folia Veterinaria* 53 (1): 62–64.

Knight Andrew. 2005. "In Defense of Vegetarian Cat Food." *Journal of the American Veterinary Medical Association* 226 (4): 512–13.

Muñoz Lasa, S.; G. Ferriero; E. Brigatti; et al. 2011. "Animal-assisted Interventions in Internal and Rehabilitation Medicine: A Review of the Recent Literature." *Panminerva Medica* 53 (2): 129–36.

Shubert Jan. 2012. "Therapy Dogs and Stress Management Assistance during Disasters." *U.S. Army Medical Department Journal* (April–June): 74–78.

Andrew Knight

Associate Professor of Welfare and Ethics, Ross University School of Veterinary Medicine, St. Kitts, West Indies

V. ZOOS AND ZOOLOGICAL PARKS

Humans have housed and maintained wild animals for public display for millennia. Egyptian priests kept menageries of live animals of religious significance at their temples, including lions, baboons, and ibises (Cherfas 1984; Croke 1997). In the twelfth century the Chinese emperor Wen-Wang constructed a 600-hectare Garden of Intelligence to house a large collection of animals. Like China, Greece valued the pursuit of knowledge and education, and as early as the fourth century most large city-states likely had their own animal collections. Montezuma, the great Aztec ruler, maintained an impressive menagerie at his palace at Tenochtitlan, reputedly employing as many as 300 keepers. The Romans captured and maintained wild animals primarily for entertainment. The Roman emperors made killing exotic animals a central part of the violent gladiatorial games in the Coliseum. Urban zoos began to emerge in Europe and North Africa in the sixteenth century. The first modern zoo dedicated to the scientific study of captive wildlife—the London Zoo—opened in 1828 (Blunt 1976). The Philadelphia Zoo—chartered in 1859 and opened in 1874—is generally recognized as the first American zoo (Croke 1997). The US Congress established the Smithsonian's National Zoo in 1887 for the purpose of breeding captive wildlife for conservation (Bechtel 2012). The New York Zoological Park or Bronx Zoo was created shortly thereafter in 1898. Zoos continued to evolve in the twentieth and early twenty-first centuries, adopting a broad mission that now includes research, education, conservation, and recreation (Hutchins, Smith, and Allard 2003).

Captive animal facilities, including zoos, aquariums, safari parks, and wildlife theme parks, continue to be very popular worldwide. Annual zoo visitation in the United States exceeds 100 million (Croke 1997), and visitation worldwide exceeds 600 million (International Union of Directors of Zoological Gardens and International Union for Conservation of Nature and Natural Resources and Species Survival Committee Captive Breeding Specialist Group 1993). There are approximately 1,000 professionally managed zoos and aquariums worldwide in addition to thousands of roadside menageries and petting zoos. It is important to note, however, that the quality of these facilities varies widely, with the best of zoological institutions being accredited by national associations, such as the Association of Zoos and Aquariums (AZA) in the United States (Barber et al. 2010). These institutions are further linked by the World Association of Zoos and Aquariums (WAZA). Many nations now also have legislation that regulates zoos and sets standards for their operation (Cooper 2003); however, developing countries have lagged behind in this regard. For the purposes of this discussion, the term *zoo* shall refer only to those zoos or aquariums that meet professional standards as defined by the AZA (Barber et al. 2010), standards that greatly exceed those required by the US Department of Agriculture's Animal and Plant Inspection Service for US licensed animal exhibitors. There is still considerable variation in quality even among AZA-accredited institutions.

Despite their popularity, zoos and aquariums have been criticized on ethical grounds. As the public has become more sensitive to animal welfare and conservation issues, animal protectionists have questioned whether the benefits of zoos outweigh their costs in terms of diminished animal welfare and the removal of animals from the wild, some of which are threatened or endangered (Jamieson 1985, 1995). In addition, with the recent rise of animal rights philosophy, some of the more radical fringes of the protectionist movement see no redeeming qualities of zoos at all, regardless of the professionalism of their care or the quality of their facilities (Regan 1995).

ETHICAL CONSIDERATIONS

Zoo critics have focused on four major ethical issues related to the keeping of wild animals in captivity.

Animal Acquisition. Conservationists have sometimes criticized zoos for their animal acquisition practices (Koontz 1995). In the 1990s, for example, controversy arose over the short-term loans of endangered giant pandas from China, which critics contended were a commercial activity (Croke 1997). However, an agreement was eventually worked out between the AZA, the US Fish and Wildlife Service, and the Chinese government for long-term loans that sent millions of dollars to China to aid in panda conservation. In addition US zoos seeking to acquire threatened or endangered species must now contribute financially to their conservation in nature to obtain an import permit (Shoemaker 2012). In 2012 the AZA presented its highest conservation award to the four zoos that pioneered the long-term lease of pandas and the associated conservation plans that were created to protect giant pandas in the wild.

Animal Care and Welfare. Animal rights and welfare proponents have criticized zoos for the quality of their facilities and for concerns about animal care and welfare (Regan 1995; Jensen and Tweedy-Holmes 2007). They claim that zoo animals exhibit aberrant, stereotypical behavior and that this is a reflection of their unnatural surroundings and boredom, resulting in stress, suffering, and early death. More recently this has played out over the keeping of elephants (Hancocks 2008), great apes (Cavalieri and Singer 1993), and large, far-ranging animals (Clubb and Mason 2003). Some accredited zoos still have small, sterile, or outdated enclosures; however, this is changing as zoos have modernized, moving toward larger, more naturalistic enclosures and appropriate, species-specific group sizes and compositions (Hutchins and Smith 2003). In addition zoos have also moved to implement environmental enrichment programs intended to facilitate natural behavior and reduce boredom (Shepherdson, Mellen, and Hutchins 1998). In general professionally managed zoos are paying more attention to welfare concerns (Maple, McManamon, and Stevens 1995; Margodt 2000; Thusty and Mellen 2012) and to ethical issues in general (Stevens and McCalister 2003; Kreger and Hutchins 2010). Furthermore all accredited zoos now have access to professional veterinary care and utilize many of the same technologies that are available in human hospitals (Kirkwood 2003). All national and regional associations have issued language supporting improvements in zoo animal welfare in their member institutions. Although zoos have not been as vocal about welfare, they spend most of their money on animal and veterinary care (Maple and Perdue 2013). With the Detroit and Brookfield Zoos establishing Centers for Animal Welfare, the zoo commitment to animal welfare is becoming more visible.

Disposition of Surplus Animals. Animal protectionists have long been concerned about the disposition of surplus animals, which may include aged animals no longer needed for exhibition and/or surplus offspring produced from breeding programs (Fox 1990; Jensen and Tweedy-Holmes 2007). In particular they have argued that some surplus exotic animals have gone into the pet trade, have been kept in substandard conditions, and/or have been used in canned hunts, all practices that diminish animal welfare. Some zoo administrators have argued that surplus animals should be culled (Lacy 1995), but others have questioned the ethics of controlling populations through culling when other alternatives, such as contraception and separation of the sexes, are available (Lindburg and Lindburg 1995). Modern zoos now carefully plan breeding of many species to limit surplus animal production (Asa and Porton 2005) and maintain genetic diversity (Ballou et al. 2010). In addition accrediting bodies, such as the AZA, have strict rules about animal disposition that seek to protect animals from transactions that compromise their welfare.

Entertainment. Animal protectionists have protested the use by zoos of animals in circus-like shows that use aversive conditioning to force animals to perform unnatural behaviors (e.g., bike-riding bears, hoop-jumping dolphins) or that portray animals with disrespect. Visitor safety is another aspect of this, as some performing animals are allowed close to the public, thus increasing the risk of injury or death. However, most progressive zoos no longer permit animal demonstrations performed solely for entertainment. Gone are the days of elephant and camel rides or young apes dressed in human clothing. Although some aquariums and zoos continue to feature performing marine mammals, this practice has also been criticized by animal activists. Developing the right balance between education and entertainment has been a source of contention even within the contemporary zoo community (Shifflett 2012), especially with the emergence of facilities like Disney's Animal Kingdom (Stevens, Ogden, and Sams 2007). The greatest controversy has been generated by theme parks and aquariums that feature performing dolphins and orcas.

Captivity and Individual Animal Rights. Animal rights proponents have criticized zoos based on the principle that all sentient animals have an inalienable right to life, freedom, avoidance of suffering, and avoidance of use as a means to an end, that is, solely for human benefit (Bostock 1993; Regan 1995). Animal rights proponents therefore believe that there is a moral presumption against capturing or holding wild animals in captivity (Jamieson 1985, 1995; Regan 1995). This is a value judgment that can be overcome if one considers the important justifications for modern zoos, particularly their roles in wildlife and habitat conservation, research, and education (Hutchins, Smith, and Allard 2003). Indeed animal rights philosophy itself—with its sole focus on the rights of individual animals versus the health of populations, species, and ecosystems—has been criticized as being anticonservation (Hutchins 2007). Zoos have successfully rescued species at risk of extinction (e.g., the California condor, the American bison, and the black-footed ferret), and there may be other situations in the future when zoos and wildlife agencies and organizations collaborate to save species. Wild tigers are at great risk of extinction, so captive tiger breeding programs in world zoos may become a critical strategy for conservation.

JUSTIFICATIONS OF ZOOS

Conservation. Animal advocates have long been critical of zoo contributions to species and habitat conservation, arguing that zoo breeding programs can do little to stem the massive tide of extinction washing over our planet (Fox 1990; Jamieson 1985, 1995). They have also criticized zoo breeding programs for promoting inbreeding and loss of natural behaviors. However, zoo-based conservation efforts advanced tremendously in the late twentieth and early twenty-first centuries and include captive breeding for reintroduction, field research, habitat restoration, in-country training, and fund-raising to support field (in situ) conservation (Hutchins and Conway 1995; Christie 2007; Zimmerman 2010). Collectively AZA zoos spent more than $130 million each year in 2007–12 supporting 4,000 scientific projects and conservation programs in over 100 countries worldwide. In addition their science-based captive breeding programs maximize the amount of genetic diversity maintained through planned breeding (Ballou et al. 2010), and based on the success of many reintroduction programs (e.g., black-footed ferrets), instinctive behaviors are maintained or can—at least in some cases—be reinforced through prerelease conditioning programs (Miller et al. 1998). Zoo education programs are a form of social marketing and should not be underestimated as a factor in promoting conservation values and citizen action.

Science. Animal activists have questioned both the quality and the usefulness of zoo-based research (Fox 1990; Jamieson 1985, 1995). In addition animal rights proponents do not condone any scientific research that harms or violates the rights of individual animals (Regan 1995). However, zoo-based scientists do not believe that research is inherently wrong. Indeed knowledge of basic animal biology and ecology is essential for conservation, thus making scientific research a necessity (Hutchins, Smith, and Allard 2003). Furthermore the scientific capability of the zoo community blossomed in the late twentieth and early twenty-first centuries, resulting in thousands of peer-reviewed publications on a wide variety of relevant topics, including field conservation, husbandry, reproductive biology, reintroduction, behavior, pathology and disease, and education (Maple and Bashaw 2010). Field biologists need the specialized knowledge and the collaboration of zoo professionals, especially zoo veterinarians, as they manage wild populations and prevent disease in nature. Animal health, welfare, and conservation are linked in the field.

Education. Public education is one of the primary stated missions of modern zoos (Hutchins and Smith 2003), but animal activists have attacked this justification for zoos as well, stating that zoos teach nothing about how animals live in nature and that they reinforce an attitude of human dominion over animals (Jamieson 1985, 1995; Fox 1990; Malamud 1998; Jensen and Tweedy-Holmes 2007). However, numerous studies affirm that both formal and informal education at zoos can be effective in promoting conservation messages to an urban public that is already divorced from nature (Anderson 2003; Reading and Miller 2007; Routman, Ogden, and Winsten 2010; Esson and Moss 2013). The results of these studies are not yet conclusive (Balmford et al. 2007), suggesting that further research on and development of zoo education programs is necessary. Robert Sommer acknowledged that zoos were the only institutions known for "hard architecture" (hospitals, prisons, zoos) that had significantly improved in the twenty-five years after publication of his iconic 1974 book *Tight Spaces*.

Recreation. Animal activists have frequently questioned the justification of keeping animals in captivity solely for entertainment or recreational purposes, arguing that such uses cannot overcome the moral presumption against captivity dictated by animal rights philosophy (Regan 1995). Urban dwellers certainly do need wholesome recreational activities that are focused on families, and zoos are, as discussed above, popular destinations. Conversely it would be difficult to justify the existence of zoos even from a purely animal welfare perspective solely on their entertainment and recreational value (Hutchins and Smith 2003). Zoos provide restoration and revitalization for urban-dwelling zoo visitors in the midst of botanically enriched, naturalistic, and immersive zoos and aquariums. Zoos also support the global effort to design a sustainable planet (Association of Zoos and Aquariums 2010).

CONCLUSION

Animal activists, especially animal rights proponents, have very different values from conservationists, whether zoo based or not (Hutchins 2007). Animal protectionists' core focus is on the rights and welfare of individual animals (Regan 1995), while conservationists are primarily concerned about the survival of populations, species, and ecosystems. The two values are not always compatible. As a result there will continue to be tension between zoo and animal rights proponents. The ethical arguments against zoos will become much weaker if zoos significantly improve their husbandry and exhibitry, making animal welfare a priority while at the same time expanding their contributions to conservation, science, and education (Hutchins, Smith, and Allard 2003).

SEE ALSO *Animal Research: I. Historical Aspects; Biodiversity Conservation; Ecological Bioethics; Endangered Species and Biodiversity; Environmental Ethics: I. Overview; Veterinary Ethics*

BIBLIOGRAPHY

Anderson, L. L. 2003. "Zoo Education: From Formal School Programmes to Exhibit Design and Interpretation." *International Zoo Yearbook* 38:75–81.

Asa, Cheryl S., and Ingrid J. Porton. 2005. *Wildlife Contraception: Issues, Methods, and Applications.* Baltimore, MD: Johns Hopkins University Press.

Association of Zoos and Aquariums. 2010. "AZA's Newest Initiative: Reducing Climate Impacts on Wildlife and Wildlife Habitats." *AZA Connect*, May, 22–23.

Ballou, Jonathan; Caroline Lees; Lisa J. Faust; et al. 2010. "Genetic and Demographic Management of Captive

Populations." In *Wild Mammals in Captivity*, 2nd ed., edited by Devra G. Kleiman, Katerina V. Thompson, and Charlotte Kirk, 219–52. Chicago: University of Chicago Press.

Balmford, Andrew; Nigel Leader-Williams; Georgina M. Mace; et al. 2007. "Message Received?: Quantifying the Impact of Informal Conservation Education on Adults Visiting UK Zoos." In *Zoos in the 21st Century: Catalysts for Conservation?*, edited by Alexandra Zimmerman, 120–36. Cambridge, UK: Cambridge University Press.

Barber, Joseph; Denny Lewis; Govindasamy Agoramoorthy; et al. 2010. "Setting Standards for Evaluation of Captive Facilities." In *Wild Mammals in Captivity*, 2nd ed., edited by Devra G. Kleiman, Katerina V. Thompson, and Charlotte Kirk, 22–34. Chicago: University of Chicago Press.

Bechtel, Stefan. 2012. *Mr. Hornaday's War: How a Peculiar Victorian Zookeeper Waged a Lonely Crusade for Wildlife That Changed the World.* Boston: Beacon.

Blunt, Wilfrid. 1976. *The Ark in the Park: The Zoo in the Nineteenth Century*. London: Hamish Hamilton.

Bostock, Stephen St. C. 1993. *Zoos and Animal Rights*. London: Routledge.

Cavalieri, Paola, and Peter Singer. 1993. *The Great Ape Project: Equality Beyond Humanity*. New York: St. Martin's.

Cherfas, Jeremy. 1984. *Zoo 2000: A Look behind the Bars*. London: British Broadcasting Corporation.

Christie, Sarah. 2007. "Zoo-Based Fund-Raising for In Situ Wildlife Conservation." In *Zoos in the 21st Century: Catalysts for Conservation?*, edited by Alexandra Zimmerman, 303–21. Cambridge, UK: Cambridge University Press.

Clubb, Ros, and Georgia Mason. 2003. "Captivity Effects on Wide-Ranging Carnivores." *Nature* 425:473–74.

Cooper, M. E. 2003. "Zoo Legislation." *International Zoo Yearbook* 38:81–93.

Croke, Vicki. 1997. *The Modern Ark*. New York: Scribner.

Esson, Maggie, and Andrew Moss. 2013. "The Risk of Delivering Disturbing Messages to Zoo Family Audiences." *Journal of Environmental Education* 44 (2): 79–96.

Fox, Michael W. 1990. *Inhumane Society*. New York: St. Martin's.

Hancocks, D. 2001. *A Different Nature: The Paradoxical World of Zoos and Their Uncertain Future*. Berkeley: University of California Press.

Hancocks, David. 2008. "Most Zoos Do Not Deserve Elephants." In *Elephants and Ethics: Toward a Morality of Coexistence*, edited by Christen Wemmer and Catherine A. Christen, 259–83. Baltimore, MD: Johns Hopkins University Press.

Hancocks, David. 2010. "The History and Principles of Zoo Exhibition." In *Wild Mammals in Captivity*, 2nd ed., edited by Devra G. Kleiman, Katerina V. Thompson, and Charlotte Kirk, 121–36. Chicago: University of Chicago Press.

Hutchins, Michael. 2003. "Zoo and Aquarium Animal Management and Conservation: Current Trends and Future Challenges." *International Zoo Yearbook* 38:14–28.

Hutchins, Michael. 2007. "The Animal Rights–Conservation Debate: Can Zoos and Aquariums Play a Role?" In *Zoos in the 21st Century: Catalysts for Conservation?*, edited by Alexandra Zimmerman, 92–109. Cambridge, UK: Cambridge University Press.

Hutchins, Michael, and William G. Conway. 1995. "Beyond Noah's Ark: The Evolving Role of Zoos and Aquariums in Field Conservation." *International Zoo Yearbook* 35:117–30.

Hutchins, Michael, and Brandie Smith. 2003. "Characteristics of a World-class Zoo or Aquarium in the 21st Century." *International Zoo Yearbook* 38:130–41.

Hutchins, Michael; Brandie Smith; and Ruth Allard. 2003. "In Defense of Zoos and Aquariums: The Ethical Basis for Keeping Wild Animals in Captivity." *Journal of the American Veterinary Medical Association* 223 (7): 958–66.

International Union of Directors of Zoological Gardens and International Union for Conservation of Nature and Natural Resources and Species Survival Committee Captive Breeding Specialist Group. 1993. *The World Zoo Conservation Strategy*. Brookfield, IL: Chicago Zoological Society.

Jamieson, Dale. 1985. "Against Zoos." In *In Defense of Animals*, edited by P. Singer, 108–17. Oxford: Basil Blackwell.

Jamieson, Dale. 1995. "Zoos Revisited." In *Ethics on the Ark: Zoos, Animal Welfare, and Wildlife Conservation*, edited by Bryan G. Norton 52–66. Washington, DC: Smithsonian Institution Press.

Jensen, Dale, and Karen Tweedy-Holmes. 2007. *Thought to Exist in the Wild: Awakening From the Nightmare of Zoos*. Santa Cruz, CA: No Voice Unheard.

Kirkwood, J. K. 2003. "Welfare, Husbandry, and Veterinary Care of Wild Animals in Captivity: Changes in Attitudes, Progress in Knowledge and Techniques." *International Zoo Yearbook* 38:124–30.

Koontz, Fred. 1995. "Wild Animal Acquisition Ethics for Zoo Biologists." In *Ethics on the Ark: Zoos, Animal Welfare, and Wildlife Conservation*, edited by Bryan G. Norton, 127–45. Washington, DC: Smithsonian Institution Press.

Kreger, Michael, and Michael Hutchins. 2010. "Ethics of Keeping Mammals in Zoos and Aquariums." In *Wild Mammals in Captivity*, 2nd ed., edited by Devra G. Kleiman, Katerina V. Thompson, and Charlotte Kirk, 3–10. Chicago: University of Chicago Press.

Lacy, Robert. 1995. "Culling Surplus Animals for Population Management." In *Ethics on the Ark: Zoos, Animal Welfare, and Wildlife Conservation*, edited by Bryan G. Norton, 187–94. Washington, DC: Smithsonian Institution Press.

Lindburg, Donald, and Linda Lindburg. 1995. "Success Breeds a Quandary: To Cull or Not to Cull?" In *Ethics on the Ark: Zoos, Animal Welfare, and Wildlife Conservation*, edited by Bryan G. Norton, 195–208. Washington, DC: Smithsonian Institution Press.

Malamud, Randy. 1998. *Reading Zoos: Representations of Animals and Captivity*. New York: New York University Press.

Maple, Terry L. 1995. "Towards a Responsible Zoo Agenda." In *Ethics on the Ark: Zoos, Animal Welfare, and Wildlife Conservation*, edited by Bryan G. Norton, 20–30. Washington, DC: Smithsonian Institution Press.

Maple, Terry L., and M. J. Bashaw. 2010. "Research Trends in Zoos." In *Wild Mammals in Captivity*, 2nd ed., edited by Devra G. Kleiman, Katerina V. Thompson, and Charlotte Kirk, 288–98. Chicago: University of Chicago Press.

Maple, Terry L., and Suma Mallavarapu. 2006. "Values, Advocacy, and Science: Toward an Empirical Philosophy for Zoo and Aquarium Leadership." In *Museum Philosophy for the Twenty-First Century*, edited by Hugh H. Genoways, 177–200. Lanham, MD: Rowman and Littlefield.

Maple, Terry L.; Rita McManamon; and Elizabeth Stevens. 1995. "Defining the Good Zoo: Animal Care, Maintenance, and Welfare." In *Ethics on the Ark: Zoos, Animal Welfare, and Wildlife Conservation*, edited by Bryan G. Norton, 219–34. Washington, DC: Smithsonian Institution Press.

Maple, Terry L., and Bonnie Perdue. 2013. *Zoo Animal Welfare.* New York: Springer.

Margodt, Koen. 2000. *The Welfare Ark.* Brussels: VUB University Press.

Miller, Brian; Dean Biggins; Astrid Vargas; et al. 1998. "The Captive Environment and Reintroduction: The Black-Footed Ferret as a Case Study with Comments on Other Taxa." In *Second Nature: Environmental Enrichment for Captive Animals*, edited by David J. Shepherdson, Jill D. Mellen, and Michael Hutchins, 97–112. Washington, DC: Smithsonian Institution Press.

Reading, Richard P., and Brian J. Miller. 2007. "Attitudes and Attitude Change among Zoo Visitors." In *Zoos in the 21st Century: Catalysts for Conservation?*, edited by Alexandra Zimmerman, 63–91. Cambridge, UK: Cambridge University Press.

Regan, Tom. 1995. "Are Zoos Morally Defensible?" In *Ethics on the Ark: Zoos, Animal Welfare, and Wildlife Conservation*, edited by Bryan G. Norton, 38–51. Washington, DC: Smithsonian Institution Press.

Routman, Emily; Jackie Ogden; and Keith Winsten. 2010. "Visitors, Conservation Learning, and the Design of Zoo and Aquarium Experiences." In *Wild Mammals in Captivity*, 2nd ed., edited by Devra G. Kleiman, Katerina V. Thompson, and Charlotte Kirk, 137–50. Chicago: University of Chicago Press.

Shepherdson, David; Jill Mellen; and Michael Hutchins, eds. 1998. *Second Nature: Environmental Enrichment for Captive Animals.* Washington, DC: Smithsonian Institution Press.

Shifflett, Tracey Lynn. 2012. "Dolphin Discovery: National Aquarium Makes Connections with New Dolphin Program." *AZA Connect*, June, 22–24.

Shoemaker, Alan. 2012. "Cash for Conservation: To Import Species, Zoos Export Funds to Support Wildlife." *Wildlife Professional* 5 (4): 42–43.

Sommer, Robert. 1974. *Tight Spaces: Hard Architecture and How to Humanize It.* Englewood Cliffs, NJ: Prentice-Hall.

Stevens, Beth; Jackie Ogden; and Kim Sams. 2007. "Creating a Culture of Conservation: A Case Study of a Backyard Approach." In *Zoos in the 21st Century: Catalysts for Conservation?*, edited by Alexandra Zimmerman, 110–19. Cambridge, UK: Cambridge University Press.

Stevens, P. M. C., and E. McCalister. 2003. "Ethics in Zoos." *International Zoo Yearbook* 38:94–101.

Thusty, M., and Jill Mellen. 2012. "Thinking about and Discussing Welfare of Zoo and Aquarium Animals." *AZA Connect*, May, 16–17.

Zimmerman, Alexandra. 2010. "The Role of Zoos in Contributing to *In Situ* Conservation." In *Wild Mammals in Captivity*, 2nd ed., edited by Devra G. Kleiman, Katerina V. Thompson, and Charlotte Kirk, 303–21. Chicago: University of Chicago Press.

Michael Hutchins
Executive Director/CEO, The Wildlife Society
Adjunct Associate Professor, Graduate Program in Sustainable Development and Conservation Biology, University of Maryland;
Affiliate Professor, Department of Environmental Science and Policy, George Mason University

Terry L. Maple
Director, Georgia Tech Center for Conservation & Behavior
Director Emeritus, Zoo Atlanta

VI. ANIMALS IN AGRICULTURE AND FACTORY FARMING

For almost all of human history, animal agriculture has involved human management of animals under living conditions for which the animals were biologically and evolutionarily adapted. Human intervention has consisted largely in ensuring the animals' health, nutrition, and reproduction by providing supplementary rations when forage was scarce, medical assistance, shelter from harsh elements, and so on. The symbiotic relationship between human and animal has been strongly reinforced by the cultural values of animal agricultural societies. In the early twenty-first century, for example, among ranchers in the American West, who are primarily traditional agriculturists and raise animals on open ranges, one finds a doctrine passed from generation to generation that we take care of the animals, and the animals take care of us.

FACTORY FARMING

Intensive agriculture, also known as confinement agriculture or factory farming, differs dramatically from traditional animal agriculture. The key notion behind confinement agriculture is the application of industrial methods to producing animals or animal products. This way of thinking about agriculture emerged in the middle of the twentieth century; before that, neither the technology nor the social conditions existed to make confinement agriculture possible. After World War II various technological developments and changing social conditions combined to alter radically the face of animal agriculture and to model farms on factories. At about the same time, departments of "animal husbandry" in agricultural universities began to change their names to departments of "animal science." Increasingly, agriculture became a business, not merely a way of life combined with a way of making a living.

The conditions that generated confinement or intensive agriculture are relatively clear. After World

War II increasing numbers of workers moved from rural agricultural regions into urban localities, where wages were higher and economic opportunities were perceived to be greater. At the same time, urban centers grew, encroaching onto traditional farmland, so that rising land prices and higher taxes militated against keeping that land for agricultural use. Inevitably the land was developed. Thus fewer and fewer people were directly involved in production agriculture.

With less land and fewer workers (by 1993, 1.7 percent of Americans were engaged in production agriculture), it was difficult to keep animals under far-ranging, open, extensive conditions. With fewer people caring for them, animals were brought into closer and closer confinement, both outdoors and indoors, so that effects of temperature, rain, snow, and so on could be minimized. Instead of depending on human labor, farmers began to rely on machinery to feed, clean, water, milk, collect eggs, and so forth. Animal agricultural operations became capital intensive rather than labor intensive.

Animals began to be crowded together in an attempt to get as many as possible into the expensive production unit. Laying hens, for example, are typically placed 5 to 6 and often more birds in a 12-by-18-inch cage, and up to 100,000 birds may be kept in one building. Broiler chickens are raised in huge open sheds at a density of approximately two birds per square foot. Beef cattle, traditionally raised on range grass, are moved for the latter portion of their lives into feedlots where they are fed grain diets, thus producing both increased weight gain and a lucrative outlet for US grain surplus. Hogs are increasingly raised in confinement buildings where they never see the light of day. Buildings holding 500 to 1,000 sows are not uncommon. Breeding sows, the source of the pigs processed into meat, may weigh over 600 pounds but are commonly kept in sow stalls or gestation crates whose recommended dimensions, according to the National Pork Producers, are 2 feet by 3 feet by 7 feet but in some cases are smaller. The sow is thus unable to stand up, turn around, and in some cases even lie flat without arching. (When kept under extensive conditions, sows will cover a mile a day foraging.) Most notoriously, veal calves are raised in small crates to restrict movement and keep their flesh tender and are also kept anemic or near anemic to keep the meat "white."

Thus animals are forced into environments for which they are not biologically suited. Because the operations are so expensive, producers are motivated to crowd as many animals as possible into the systems, owing to the small profit per animal. Thus even though it is well-known that chickens will lay more eggs if given more space, it is more profitable to crowd as many birds as possible into cages, yielding fewer eggs per bird but more eggs for the operation as a whole. Such methods would be impossible without recent technology. On June 29, 2010, the *New York Times* reported that

> the F.D.A. issued a "draft guidance" on the "judicious use" of medically important antimicrobial drugs in food-producing animals. The document suggested that the use of such drugs should be limited to treating or controlling infectious disease in animals or to prevent infections before an outbreak occurs. And in all of those cases, the drugs should be administered in consultation with a veterinarian whose oversight would likely restrain excessive use.

In the absence of antibiotics and vaccines, the spread of disease would decimate the animals in weeks. Without growth promoters, the animals could not be processed quickly enough to be profitable. Broiler chickens, for instance, now reach full growth in seven weeks, where once the same growth took more than four months. The rise of confinement agriculture has, according to its proponents, provided cheap and plentiful food. For example, the price of chicken has remained virtually the same for more than twenty years, even in the face of inflation. Advocates of intensive agriculture also argue that confinement provides animals with shelter from extremes of weather, protection from predators, and a consistent nutritional regimen.

HARMS OF CONFINEMENT

There are hidden costs offsetting these benefits, the most important of which is the cost to the animals. The animals being produced in confinement are still essentially the animals that were genetically adapted to extensive conditions. Their fundamental biological interests are systematically violated in confinement. Thus animals that are built to move about are unable to do so. Social animals may be deprived of companionship. Air laden with dust and ammonia in confinement chicken, egg, and swine barns is execrable; in some swine operations, workers must wear respirators. Diets designed to maximize growth may lead to metabolic disease for some of the animals, even though this loss is balanced by economic gain in the other animals. In chicken and swine barns, unnatural floor surfaces, such as wire and concrete slats, may lead to leg, foot, and joint problems. With the advent of confinement agriculture, there has arisen a class of diseases known as "production diseases" that result from the systems of production. Because intensive systems have a low profit margin, they are often understaffed, and care of sick or injured animals is impossible for workers whose other duties stretch them to their limit and who are usually ignorant of basic animal husbandry. Animal genetics and breeding are focused overwhelmingly on maximizing productivity at the expense of health, soundness, leg strength, maternal instinct, and sociability.

As a result of such systematic violation of their physical and psychological (animal scientists prefer the word *behavioral*) needs, animals suffer psychologically as well as physically. Many animals in confinement show chronic signs of long- and short-term stress, which can lead to both disease and behavioral problems. Cannibalism among chickens increases in the absence of either space to flee or small enough numbers to establish a pecking order. To prevent cannibalism, producers "debeak" chickens with a hot blade and without anesthesia, sometimes producing chronic pain by virtue of uncontrolled nerve growth following debeaking, which results in painful neuromas. Similarly, pigs are tail docked to prevent tail biting, a stress-induced result of confinement. Confined animals also show many bizarre, stereotypical behaviors that seem to result from the thwarting of natural inclinations and from boring, austere environments. Pigs and cattle are castrated without anesthesia or analgesia.

Confinement agriculture also exacts other social costs. In an industry requiring large amounts of capital, small operators cannot compete effectively, and large, well-capitalized corporations inevitably drive out small "family farmers." Young people cannot afford to enter agriculture.

Efficiency and productivity eclipse other values traditionally maintained in small farm communities, such as independence, self-sufficiency, and husbandry. Such environmental problems as waste disposal and water and energy consumption(factories use vast amounts of water and energy) also arise from intensive agriculture. Lack of pasturing of animals contributes to soil erosion when land no longer used for pasture is tilled for grain. Drug residues in animal products may pose human health problems, and widespread use of antibiotics essentially breeds for resistant pathogens by eliminating microbes susceptible to the drugs. *Salmonella* and *Campylobacter* bacterial contamination are significant problems in chickens, turkeys, and eggs, because they can cause severe enteric disease in humans who consume these products.

TOWARD REFORM

Agriculturists have recognized that the welfare of animals in confinement represents one of the three major challenges to agriculture in the twenty-first century, the other two being food safety and environmental concerns. When the British public became aware of factory farms in the 1960s as a result of Ruth Harrison's pioneering book *Animal Machines: The New Factory Farming Industry* (1964), the outcry generated a royal commission, the Brambell Committee, that was highly critical of confinement agriculture as violating the animals' natures. In the face of confinement agriculture, European society is moving toward legal protection for farm animals. Laws in Britain, Denmark, Germany, and Switzerland have restricted certain aspects of confinement agriculture. Sweden has essentially abolished such agriculture and guaranteed certain rights for farm animals in a law that has been called a "bill of rights" for farm animals, because it aims at protecting their fundamental interests. In the United States public attention was first directed toward animals in research, and certain basic protections for such animals have been legally encoded in two federal laws passed in 1985. Public attention is beginning to focus on the treatment of farm animals as well as on the environmental consequences of confinement agriculture, and articles in agricultural journals show that agriculture is starting to pay more attention to these concerns.

Until the late twentieth century US confinement agriculturists (in contrast to their counterparts in Europe and Canada) tended to deny that there were any problems of animal welfare intrinsically related to confinement agriculture and acknowledged only occasional "bad management." This was further exacerbated by widespread skepticism in the scientific community about the existence and knowability of animal consciousness, pain, and suffering. Since the early 1990s, however, there have been indications that at least some parts of the industry and government are engaging such issues as animal deprivation, boredom, and inability to move in confinement primarily by inaugurating research into improving animal welfare.

Beginning in the twenty-first century two major phenomena led US society to an awareness of farm issues. First was the Pew Commission on Industrial Farm Animal Production, chartered with funding from the Pew Charitable Trusts. Fifteen experts were assembled and worked for over two and half years to provide the first-ever critical evaluation of industrial animal agriculture in a variety of areas. The commission included a former secretary of agriculture; a former governor; and experts on public health, animal welfare, social justice, veterinary medicine, animal health, environmental despoliation, rural communities, nutrition, and agricultural economics. The issues examined by the commission included animal welfare, environmental damage caused by confined animal feeding operations (CAFOs), loss of sustainability, effects of CAFOs on human and animal health and disease, including physical and psychological effects on rural communities, loss of small farms, social justice, diminution of competition in agriculture, feeding of antibiotics to farm animals at low levels to promote growth (driving the resistance of pathogens to these drugs), and externalization of costs associated with animal-feeding operations. The commission report (Pew Commission on Industrial Farm Animal Production 2008) garnered positive editorial comments in more than 800 newspapers and prompted much new social concern about all aspects of confinement agriculture fueled by significant media coverage of food and animal agriculture issues.

The second momentous development stimulating increased societal attention to industrial animal agriculture was the work of the Humane Society of the United States (HSUS) under the leadership of Wayne Pacelle. HSUS galvanized public referenda in eight states to eliminate veal crates, sow stalls, and battery cages for egg-laying hens. All of the referenda passed by votes of approximately two to one. In Colorado the referendum was avoided when HSUS and the agricultural community working together passed joint legislation. Media coverage of these referenda significantly raised public awareness of welfare issues attendant on factory farming.

Dialogue conducted in 2007 between this author and senior executives of Smithfield Farms, the world's largest pork producer, led to Smithfield's announcement that it would phase out sow stalls by 2017. By the summer of 2012 Smithfield had moved a quarter of a million sows into open group housing. In 2011 the United Egg Producers, working with HSUS, jointly sponsored federal legislation aimed at replacing small, barren cages for laying hens with larger and enriched cages, taking cognizance of hen behavioral needs. In Europe momentum has gathered to eliminate castration of animals without anesthesia. The market for husbandry-based animal agricultural products has dramatically increased across Europe, and North America, Australia, and New Zealand.

It is unlikely that industrialized agriculture will ever revert to being fully or even largely extensive, but it is possible to make intensive agriculture much more "animal welfare friendly" and perhaps to change certain systems from full to partial confinement. For example, it is possible to raise swine profitably without keeping sows confined in small gestation crates for their entire lives. In addition, concern about sustainable agriculture may well result in a concerted social effort to return to less industrialized systems guided by husbandry. Confinement agricultural systems are being introduced into third world countries as a shortcut to rapid economic growth and as a way of adding animal products to the diets of people in these countries. This has generated a variety of ethical concerns, including fear of environmental despoliation, concern that successful indigenous agriculture will be lost, worries about importing European and North American health problems to these countries, and concern about proliferating animal suffering.

GROWING SOCIAL CONCERN

As the Pew Commission demonstrated, animal agriculture raises other animal-welfare issues beyond confinement. Although cattle ranching is extensive and in fact presupposes a good fit between animal and environment, management techniques, such as castration without anesthesia, hot-iron branding, and dehorning without anesthesia, produce pain and suffering in these animals. Transportation of agricultural animals over long distances, for example, to slaughter, is stressful and may cause disease and injury. Handling of farm animals by people ignorant of their behavior is a widespread problem that creates high levels of stress and significant injury. Slaughter of food animals raises the issue of whether these animals can be provided with a death free of pain, suffering, and fear. This problem is particularly acute in the area of Jewish and Muslim religious slaughter, where preslaughter stunning has been considered incompatible with religious demands. Genetic engineering of farm animals for traits that are desirable to producers for reasons of efficiency and productivity may well exact costs in welfare from the animals' perspectives. For example, swine and chickens engineered for greater size have suffered from a variety of diseases, including foot and leg problems. In one case, a cow engineered for double muscling was unable to stand on its own and required euthanasia. In the absence of full knowledge of the consequences of adding or deleting genes, unintended negative consequences occur. Alternatively, genetic engineering can also work to the benefit of farm animals, for example, by engineering for disease resistance.

Other branches of animal agriculture rear animals for uses other than food. Raising traditionally "wild" animals for various purposes has generated concerns about their well-being: pheasants for hunting, mink for fur, and deer for antler velvet (which is considered an aphrodisiac in parts of Asia) provide salient examples. Numerous welfare concerns have also been raised by the production of horses for human purposes, such as breakdown and injury in racehorses; injury in endurance horses (those used in long, grueling competitive rides over difficult terrain); heat, water deprivation, and poor air for urban carriage horses. Aquaculture may cause major stress and illness in farmed fish. Indeed, no branch of animal agriculture is being ignored by the growing social concern about farm animal welfare. Inspection and accreditation of animal production operations by independent auditors is a growing trend. Placing video cameras in such operations and streaming pictures online represents an emerging strategy aimed at reassuring the public about the well-being of animals raised in CAFOs.

SEE ALSO *Agriculture and Biotechnology; Animal Research; Ecological Bioethics; Endangered Species and Biodiversity; Enhancement Uses of Medical Technology; Environmental Health Ethics; Food; Veterinary Ethics*

BIBLIOGRAPHY

Benson, G. John, and Bernard E. Rollin, eds. 2004. *The Well- Being of Farm Animals: Challenges and Solutions.* Ames, IA: Blackwell.

Dawkins, Marian S. 1980. *Animal Suffering: The Science of Animal Welfare.* London: Chapman and Hall.

Dawkins, Marian S., and Roland Bonney, eds. 2008. *The Future of Animal Farming: Restoring the Ancient Contract.* Oxford: Blackwell.

Fox, Michael W. 1984. *Farm Animals: Husbandry, Behavior, and Veterinary Practice; Viewpoints of a Critic.* Baltimore: University Park Press.

Goodwin, Jeff L. 2001. "The Ethics of Livestock Shows: Past, Present, and Future." *Journal of the American Veterinary Medical Association* 219 (10): 1391–93.

Harrison, Ruth. 1964. *Animal Machines: The New Factory Farming Industry.* London: Vincent Stuart.

Hodges, John, and In K. Han, eds. 2000. *Livestock, Ethics, and Quality of Life.* New York: Oxford University Press.

Martin, Jerome, ed. 1991. *High Technology and Animal Welfare: Proceedings of the 1991 High Technology and Animal Welfare Symposium.* Edmonton: University of Alberta Press.

Mason, Jim, and Peter Singer. 1990. *Animal Factories.* Rev. ed. New York: Harmony Books.

Nolen, R. S. 2001. "Welfare on the Farm: Treating Pain and Distress in Food Animals." *Journal of the American Veterinary Medical Association* 219 (12): 1657.

Pew Commission on Industrial Farm Animal Production. 2008. "Putting Meat on the Table: Industrial Farm Animal Production in America." Accessed November 2, 2013. http://www.ncifap.org/_images/PCIFAPFin.pdf

Rollin, Bernard E. 1989. *The Unheeded Cry: Animal Consciousness, Animal Pain, and Science.* New York: Oxford University Press.

Rollin, Bernard E. 1990. "Animal Welfare, Animal Rights, and Agriculture." *Journal of Animal Science* 68:3456–61.

Rollin, Bernard E. 1993. *Social, Bioethical, and Researchable Issues Pertaining to Farm Animal Welfare.* Washington, DC: Government Printing Office.

Rollin, Bernard E. 1995. *Farm Animal Welfare.* Ames: Iowa State University Press.

Rollin, Bernard E. 2004. "Annual Meeting Keynote Address: Animal Agriculture and Emerging Social Ethics for Animals." *Journal of Animal Science* 82 (3): 955–64.

Rollin, Bernard E. 2006. *Animal Rights and Human Morality.* Buffalo, NY: Prometheus Books.

Rollin, Bernard E. 2011. *Putting the Horse before Descartes: My Life's Work for Animals.* Philadelphia: Temple University Press.

Sandøe, Peter; Birte L. Nielsen; Lars G. Christensen; et al. 1999. "Staying Good While Playing God: The Ethics of Breeding Farm Animals." *Animal Welfare* 8 (4): 313–28.

Theil, Deborah E. 2002. "A Resource for Veterinarians on Recognizing and Reporting Animal Abuse." *Canadian Veterinary Journal* 43 (2): 97–98.

Thompson, Paul B. 1998. *Agricultural Ethics: Research, Teaching, and Public Policy.* Ames: Iowa State University Press.

Bernard E. Rollin (1995, 2014)
University Distinguished Professor, Colorado State University

VII. POLICIES AND ORGANIZATIONS

Protections for nonhuman animals found in or near human communities around the world vary greatly. Further, even within the local communities in any one nation, protection levels and approaches can differ significantly. Protections may be based on specific laws enacted in an entire country or local jurisdiction, or protections may be anchored by contemporary social attitudes and practices not prescribed in any laws. Such nonlegal social customs, which may have their roots in traditional values, such as those prevailing in the communities of a specific religious tradition or some long-standing cultural practice or institution, essentially establish de facto public policy that can be just as effective in a community as formal public policy spelled out in specific laws and then enforced in full or in part by government officials.

Concerns for the welfare of nonhuman animals are expressed in both legal and nonlegal forms along a continuum from the truly robust to the exceptionally weak. Robust expressions of concern, often framed in terms of animal rights or animal welfare, provide fundamental, effective protections accomplished by establishment and enforcement of specific legal protections for an individual's most basic and important interests. An example of such a fundamental protection is the right to a life free from unnecessary harms and intentional deprivations, such that an individual has freedom to pursue species-specific behaviors within a healthy community of its own kind.

At the opposite end of the continuum, weak expressions of concern for animal welfare may involve making minor improvements in harsh conditions, for example, providing larger cages that permit each individual to turn around or stretch a wing, or some minor form of enrichment, such as a plastic toy, for animals confined indoors for their entire lives. Typically following such improvements the nonhuman animals remain in conditions and receive treatment that the ordinary person would not associate with far richer senses of the word *welfare* or notions such as a good life that prevail at the other, more robust end of the animal welfare continuum.

The weakest expressions of concern for animal welfare are commonly promoted by individuals and businesses that insist that there are no moral problems when humans use nonhuman animals as mere resources; this view has sometimes led to the issue of animal protection being framed as a question of "rights versus welfare." The dualism implicit in this framing can be unpacked, because, like *animal welfare*, the term *animal rights* means a variety of things depending on context. For an increasing number of people in industrialized societies around the world, animal rights does in fact mean law-specified protections explicitly called out for certain nonhuman animals. In industrialized societies, for example, the owned dogs, cats, and horses commonly called "companion animals" are most often the beneficiaries of such legal protections.

There is another, older sense of animal rights, however, that many other people around the world use for different forms of effective, fundamental animal protection. Such forms include the ancient, morals-driven values, often originating in religions, that recognize that humans may define *welfare* to include other animals living a normal life free of intentional harms caused by humans. Such morality-based protections, compassion, and respect for the freedom and life of certain animals were developed far earlier than legal protections and can still be found, although sometimes in attenuated form, in most cultures. Their hallmark is a serious concern for the well-being of individual nonhumans and freedom from harms, like captivity and pain, as well as the freedom to move around as part of their own community. In an important sense both the ancient, robust sense of animal welfare and the morals-based sense of animal rights (that is, morality-based, not merely law-based, protection) hold in every respect concern for the welfare of individual animals to be of great importance to any moral being.

The coexistence of these diverse, sometimes conflicting strong and weak forms of animal protection means that the dualism "rights versus welfare" can be misleading, because it relies on the weaker notion of welfare—that welfare exists through amelioration of some aspect of harms now being done to nonhuman animals. It remains silent, however, on key elements in the more robust idea of the welfare of nonhuman animals. This view, promoted by modern industries using nonhuman animals for profit, ignores the position that when freedoms are limited or altogether erased, there may be very little true welfare afforded the nonhuman animals. Thus the weaker sense of welfare not only preserves but also enhances human domination over nonhuman animals. Advocates of this weak sense of animal welfare characteristically maintain that conceding minor welfare improvements to captive animals in production-focused industries, laboratory research facilities, or even shelters for unwanted animals makes humans' domination of these animals ethically acceptable.

Such reasoning invokes some features of utilitarianism, such as the improved welfare brought about by the minor improvements that either increase happiness or decrease suffering. Importantly, though, essential features of the utilitarian tradition are ignored in such calculus, for there is little or no inquiry by which humans balance in a realistic way human-side benefits against the continuing harms to those nonhuman animals who remain in captivity, because even after the improvement they are still deemed mere resources. Instead advocates of the weak sense of animal welfare gloss over the minor nature of the improvements when balanced against the major harms that remain in place in factory farms, research facilities, zoos, and other forms of captivity that totally curtail the nonhuman animals' lives for human benefit.

The tensions inherent in purporting to care about the welfare of nonhuman animals who, though benefiting from minor improvements, still suffer prolonged and serious harms at the hands of humans, including isolation and death, are difficult to ignore. The ready acceptance of the "rights versus welfare" contrast reveals that humans often use different kinds of reasoning to justify the long-standing tradition of harming nonhuman animals for human profit. The philosopher Robert Nozick (1974), 39) used the phrase "utilitarianism for animals, Kantianism for people" to describe what he concluded was a "too minimal" position on the issue of animal protection.

An assessment of advocacy for animal welfare, animal welfare reform, and animal rights will likely depend, then, on whether the advocate advances the original, more robust sense of animal welfare that takes seriously the claim that animals matter in and of themselves or, alternatively, promotes the view that humans are deserving of benefits and privileges such that human interests justify continuing, serious harms to nonhuman animals even when the benefits (such as making a profit or providing nutrition for affluent humans who have many other alternatives) are relatively minor. Because improvements proposed under the weaker sense of animal welfare are often made in public policy venues, such as legislatures, debates on this topic are often intensely political in nature, even polarized, because reformers want change while those benefiting from current practices resist all but minor concessions. Opponents of "welfarist" approaches (that is, those approaches that advocate only minor improvements, not fundamental change) deride compromises putting in place minor concessions that leave intact human domination and cruel practices, because the results of such compromises are, such opponents assert, multiple—they include entrenchment of human privilege, a blunting of criticism of the continuing cruelty experienced by captive animals, and financial advantage for those who currently treat many nonhuman animals not as sentient beings but rather as mere resources to be handled much as a business would handle inanimate objects.

From an ethics standpoint, clarity about what is at stake whenever any form of animal welfare or improvement is proposed requires that a moral agent factor in what conditions and harms still prevail after the proposed changes are in place. A significant number of ethicists hold that a moral person should consider the vantage point of the nonhuman animal being discussed—for example, if given an option to choose his or her present form of confinement or a larger space, what would a particular nonhuman animal choose? Scientific approaches pioneered by Marian Stamp Dawkins (1985, 1993) and others make it possible to ask such questions. Further, while some argue that it is wrong to support minor welfare changes that leave major harms unaddressed, others believe that if one concludes that the animals themselves would prefer even a minor change, then taking the nonhuman animals' viewpoint seriously means that one should respect such a preference by supporting even those changes that ameliorate harmful conditions in only minor ways.

It often is the case, however, that there is little frank discussion of such problems, because contemporary political realities in many industrialized countries assume that continued use of certain animals, such as pigs, cattle, and chickens, for food and production are necessary for human thriving. This is why the dualism "rights versus welfare" tends to prevail in countries where private property rights are politically so popular that people and businesses can cite them as controlling and thereby subordinate the moral issues arising out of domination and harming of other living beings.

It is not only the business establishment of industrialized societies that continues to be a mainstay of this human-centered vision but also influential circles of law and legal education, mainline religious communities in general, and public policy circles and education programs. Many sectors of modern, consumer-oriented societies intentionally promote forms of industrialized food production or "factory farming" reliant on crowded indoor facilities, because these not only are considered morally acceptable but also are typically centerpieces of current public policy and law. The result is that many tens of billions of food and production animals are killed annually around the world, with this form of human-nonhuman interaction growing in both industrialized countries and the developing world (see Waldau 2011, 36). A common figure given for the United States alone in 2011–2012 is over 10 billion farmed animals killed annually. Foer (2009, 329) cites the researcher Noam Mohr's work with statistics available through the US Department of Agriculture that put the 2010 US figure for finfish at over 13 billion and for shellfish at over 40 billion (see also Farm Animal Rights Movement 2011).

Such practices have long been challenged through nonlegal means. As early as 1964 Ruth Harrison in *Animal Machines: The New Factory Farming Industry* described concentrated, highly mechanical production processes as going "to the degree where the animal is not allowed to live before it dies" (3). In a preface to this book written shortly before her death, Rachel Carson suggested that the moral implications of this newly industrialized practice "ought to shock the complacency out of any reader" (vii). While the efficiencies of the new processes produced profit and production benefits argued to justify the harming of the food animals themselves, this more efficient form of production comes with a startling range of evident problems on the human side. For example, the 2008 report of the Pew Commission on Industrial Farm Animal Production, titled *Putting Meat on the Table*, a project of the Pew Charitable Trusts and Johns Hopkins Bloomberg School of Public Health, concluded after examining the economic contribution of factory farming to local communities in the United States, "the *costs* to rural America have been *significant*." In addition the report reflects harms to family farms, "reduced civic participation rates, higher levels of stress, and other less tangible impacts" as well as "a substantial environmental problem for air quality, surface and subsurface water quality, and the health of workers, neighboring residents, and the general public." Comparably serious problems were cited in the 2006 report *Livestock's Long Shadow* from the Food and Agriculture Organization (FAO) of the United Nations.

Law-based public policy clearly permits such harms, as does the weaker sense of animal welfare. The more robust sense of animal welfare that operates much as do the moral and legal rights sense of animal rights provides a number of bases for challenging the harms that modern production processes cause both nonhumans and human communities. The Pew Commission (2008) report is blunt about the ethical dimensions of such production processes: "By most measures, confined animal production systems in common use today fall short of current ethical and societal standards." The reason for such a condemnation can be found in many best-selling texts, such as *The Omnivore's Dilemma* (2006) by Michael Pollan and *Dominion: The Power of Man, the Suffering of Animals, and the Call to Mercy* (2002) by Matthew Scully, the senior speechwriter of President George W. Bush. For example, after describing how the impoverished life and learned helplessness of pigs confined indoors in factory farms leads to infections, Pollan (2006, 218) explains, "Since treating sick pigs is not economically efficient, these underperforming production units are typically clubbed to death on the spot."

POLICIES FOR DOMESTIC AND FERAL CATS, DOGS, HORSES, AND OTHERS

Animal welfare's high-water mark in many industrialized countries can be found in policies and laws meant to protect those domestic animals commonly known as "companion animals" or "pets." Along with food animals, these animals are often lumped into the category "domesticated." But there are major differences for dogs, cats, horses, and a few others when they are owned animals, for owned animals of these species are often informally deemed "family members" in many modern societies (in fact in some industrialized nations more households have companion animals than have children). Because of the great connection that humans have to these animals, as evidenced by the "family member" designation, these nonhumans are treated differently than are those nonhuman animals that humans designate food animals. It remains the case that in some cultures dogs and cats are eaten, and when this is their fate, they do not enjoy the protections that are afforded the owned dogs, cats, birds, and other nonhumans we deem "companion animals."

This category of nonhuman animals is important for a number of reasons. It is, for example, the most important paradigm driving changes in animal protection laws of many countries. Humans widely advocate in the early twenty-first century for effective protections for their owned companion animals, such that more than a thousand legislative proposals are advanced every year in industrialized countries in an attempt to put effective protections into place. These animals receive not only more law-based protections in an increasing number of societies (though not yet specific legal rights as individuals) but also are the beneficiaries of a more robust sense of animal welfare and morals-based protections.

Yet whereas the number of owned companion animals worldwide is in the range of more than 100 million, there is at least an equal number of unowned, feral dogs and cats who, by and large, do not receive comparable protections. The number of feral dogs and cats, who are tolerated at times but also exterminated regularly, likely exceeds the number of owned dogs and cats worldwide. Further, even when owned, these animals are often relinquished to shelters and killed. Some reports indicate that the leading cause of death among cats and dogs in some industrialized countries is euthanasia, simply because shelters are overcrowded with unwanted animals.

As with dogs and cats, the tens of millions of owned horses can receive rather robust animal welfare protections in some situations, but when feral or unwanted by owners, they suffer notoriously harsh fates. In addition a great variety of birds have long been held captive by humans, and worldwide numbers reach well over 100 million (in China alone the number is estimated to be more than 70 million).

Given the number of feral dogs, cats, horses, and formerly captive birds and sundry other exotic animals set free by owners (such as snakes and mice), it is possible to recognize that urban, suburban, and even rural settings feature diverse animals that have escaped from human control. In addition there is a considerable body of work on "urban animals" other than humans (this category can include wildlife of course, but often the focus is primarily on those that have escaped from human control). All the living beings in these categories are given virtually no protection other than those afforded by social mores—in other words, official public policy and law protecting these living beings is practically nonexistent.

ANIMAL WELFARE ORGANIZATIONS WORLDWIDE

The number of animal protection organizations around the world is in the low tens of thousands. The World Animal Net Directory at the end of 2012 listed 17,000 organizations in 170 countries (World Animal Net 2013). While a small fraction of these organizations focuses on formal legal rights, most of them focus on protections for only a small number of nonhuman animals that fall under either a robust sense of animal welfare or a partial, more dilute form of animal protection reflecting the weaker sense of animal welfare described above. Whereas such organizations can be found in virtually any populated region of the world, they are most common in cities and suburbs throughout Europe, North America, Australia, and New Zealand. These continents also host the largest animal protections organizations in terms of members, fund-raising, and impact. Which organizations are the largest and most effective is, however, a matter of debate. A number of different organizations claim to be the "world's largest." For example, the Humane Society of the United States (2013) claimed in its "Annual Report 2012" to be "the world's largest animal protection organization" with "over 11 million members." On its website People for the Ethical Treatment of Animals (2013) describes itself as "the largest animal rights organization in the world, with more than 3 million members and supporters." Because environmental protection is a very important form of animal protection, any list of the organizations that protect nonhuman animals must include some of the world's largest environmental organizations, such as Conservation International and Greenpeace, alongside animal protection organizations with international reach, such as the World Society for the Protection of Animals International, International Fund for Animal Welfare, and Humane Society International (affiliated with the Humane Society of the United States).

Many large and small organizations can also be found in South America, Central America, South and East Asia, Africa, and the Middle East. The animals protected include not only companion animals but often working animals and local wildlife. Migrating animals and food animals too can receive welfare-based attention of one kind or another, but such concerns still remain undeveloped in the vast majority of human communities.

POLICIES AND ETHICS OF WILD ANIMALS ON PRIVATE PROPERTY

Public policy that addresses wild animals in one's home or on one's property is dealt with in a variety of ways, although the dominant theme is found in laws that permit landowners, in the vast majority of situations, to treat uninvited wild animals entering private property (for example, local raccoons, squirrels, and deer) as pests and invaders to be killed at the owner's whim. A noteworthy exception to such laws involves limited rights to kill members of an endangered species. The relevant ethical principles are diverse, because so much ethical analysis assumes without argument that humans are the privileged animals. But some ethical systems, such as the ancient concept known as ahimsa or nonviolence, do mandate that individual humans protect local wildlife on owned property as sentient creatures whose lives must be respected unless some sort of danger to the humans is a factor.

The distinct issue of keeping wild animals captive on private property (as opposed to keeping them in zoos or sanctuaries) revolves around the kind of animals so kept. If the animals are physically dangerous to other humans or their property (including the nonhuman animals owned by other people), then traditional law often provides that the owner of the dangerous animal has liability whenever harms are caused by the dangerous animal. If the animals being kept are members of an endangered species, then laws promulgated by national or regional governments very likely apply, as might also international treaties between two or more countries. If the animals involved pose the threat of disease transmission, then national or regional laws enacted to protect "public health" (with the "public" being humans or their owned animals) will apply and may result in the sick animals being killed for precautionary reasons.

The ethical standards that might be brought to bear on such practices are far more diverse. Some societies have traditionally held that any wild animal captured by an individual for either food or nonfood purposes belongs to that individual, but many modern ethical systems treat a number of nonhumans (typically the more complicated of our fellow mammals, though not, for example, much smaller animals that humans cannot recognize as individuals) as worthy of protection and respect. An obvious standard by which to measure the morality of acts depriving a wild animal of its freedom is to assess the seriousness of any harm done to the captured animal. Yet given the heavy concentration on human-centered standards in ethical traditions (evidenced, for example, by zoos' claim that captivity of any and all nonhuman animals can be morally justified in terms of humans' education), such a standard would be novel. Another standard measure used in ethics is a utilitarian balancing of the good consequences of an act over the bad, but it is notoriously difficult for any human to measure such consequences honestly from the vantage point of nonhuman animals' interests. It is true, however, that some nonhuman animals can be kept in captivity without the levels of extreme harm that captivity causes to large-brained, eminently social mammals, such as elephants, nonhuman great apes, dolphins, and whales. Finally, an ethics-sensitive individual might also focus on ecological risks caused by such practices. Wildlife depletion driven by consumer demand for exotics has become a serious problem (sometimes illegal trade in nonhuman animals is ranked as the third most serious international crime behind only illegal arms and illegal drugs). Further, the environmental consequences of invasive species are known to be extremely severe, and moral issues may arise whenever nonnative captive animals escape and then, after thriving, begin to threaten or even eliminate native forms of wildlife.

SEE ALSO *Agriculture and Biotechnology; Animal Research*

BIBLIOGRAPHY

Conservation International. 2013. Accessed August 14, 2013. http://www.conservation.org/Pages/default.aspx

Dawkins, Marian Stamp. 1985. "The Scientific Basis for Assessing Suffering in Animals." In *In Defence of Animals*, edited by Peter Singer, 27–40. New York: Basil Blackwell.

Dawkins, Marian Stamp. 1993. *Through Our Eyes Only? The Search for Animal Consciousness*. New York: Freeman.

DeMello, Margo, ed. 2010. *Teaching the Animal: Human-Animal Studies across the Disciplines*. New York: Lantern.

Farm Animal Rights Movement. 2011. "Report: Number of Animals Killed in US Increases in 2010." http://farmusa.org/statistics11.html

Foer, Jonathan Safran. 2009. *Eating Animals*. New York: Little, Brown.

Food and Agriculture Organization of the United Nations. 2006. *Livestock's Long Shadow: Environmental Issues and Options*. Rome: Author. Accessed November 2, 2013. http://www.fao.org/docrep/010/a0701e/a0701e00.HTM

Frasch, Pamela D.; Katherine M. Hessler; Sarah M. Kutil; and Sonia S. Waisman. 2011. *Animal Law in a Nutshell*. Saint Paul, MN: Thomson/West.

Greenpeace. 2013. Accessed August 14, 2013. http://www.greenpeace.org/usa/en/

Harrison, Ruth. 1964. *Animal Machines: The New Factory Farming Industry*. London: Stuart.

Humane Society International. 2013. Accessed August 14, 2013. http://www.hsi.org/

Humane Society of the United States. 2013. "Annual Report 2012." Accessed June 2, 2013. http://www.humanesociety.org/about/overview/financials/annual-report-2012.html

International Fund for Animal Welfare. 2013. Accessed August 14, 2013. http://www.ifaw.org/united-states

Irwin, Paul. 2003. "A Strategic Review of International Animal Protection." In *The State of the Animals II, 2003*, edited by Deborah Salem and Andrew Rowan, 1–8. Washington, DC: Humane Society.

Nierenberg, Danielle. 2005. *Happier Meals: Rethinking the Global Meat Industry*. Worldwatch Paper 171. Washington, DC: Worldwatch Institute.

Nozick, Robert. 1974. *Anarchy, State, and Utopia*. New York: Basic Books.

People for the Ethical Treatment of Animals. 2013. "About PETA: Our Mission Statement." Accessed June 2, 2013. http://www.peta.org/about/default.aspx

Pew Commission on Industrial Farm Animal Production. 2008. *Putting Meat on the Table: Industrial Farm Animal Production in America*. A Project of the Pew Charitable Trusts and Johns Hopkins Bloomberg School of Public Health. Baltimore, MD: Author. http://www.ncifap.org/_images/PCIFAPFin.pdf

Pollan, Michael. 2006. *The Omnivore's Dilemma: A Natural History of Four Meals*. New York: Penguin.

Scully, Matthew. 2002. *Dominion: The Power of Man, the Suffering of Animals, and the Call to Mercy*. New York: St. Martin's.

Trent, Neil; Stephanie Edwards; Jennifer Felt; and Kelly O'Meara. 2005. "International Animal Law, with a Concentration on Latin America, Asia, and Africa." In *The State of the Animals III, 2005*, edited by Deborah Salem and Andrew Rowan, 65–77. Washington, DC: Humane Society.

Wagman, Bruce, and Matthew Liebman. 2011. *A Worldview of Animal Law*. Durham, NC: Carolina Academic.

Waldau, Paul. 2011. *Animal Rights*. New York: Oxford University Press.

Waldau, Paul. 2013. *Animal Studies: An Introduction*. New York: Oxford University Press.

World Animal Net. 2013. "World Animal Net Directory." Accessed June 2, 2013. http://www.worldanimal.net/directory

World Society for the Protection of Animals International. 2013. Accessed August 14, 2013. http://www.wspa.ca/

Paul Waldau

Associate Professor, Anthrozoology, Canisius College

ARTIFICIAL NUTRITION AND HYDRATION

INTRODUCTION

Artificial nutrition and hydration (ANH)—nonoral feedings delivered directly into the upper digestive tract via a nasoenteric or percutaneous tube—has become an essential component of multidisciplinary care in acutely ill or injured patients. Not surprisingly as a result of these experiences with acute illness, ANH has been proposed for patients with chronic illnesses who have lost the ability to take in adequate calories. However, the benefits of long-term ANH in many settings have not been defined in controlled clinical trials. Whereas observational studies using a case-control or cohort design have provided insight into this area and have shown benefit for, for example, patients with stroke-related swallowing problems and patients with head and neck cancer undergoing therapy, such is not the case for patients with other conditions, such as advanced dementia, terminal cancer, and catastrophic neurological injury. But it is the latter group that has generated the most controversy in decision making. Is providing food and water using alternative access to the gastrointestinal tract the same as providing it orally under all circumstances? This is the question that has provoked controversy and at times emotional rejoinders.

Background. Historically when long-term artificial feeding was considered, surgical gastrostomy provided enteral access. This method has been largely replaced by percutaneous endoscopic gastrostomy (PEG), which can be performed if necessary at the bedside. This technique does not require general anesthesia, has less associated morbidity, and can be performed for a fraction of the cost of that for surgical techniques. During this procedure the patient is sedated, and using local anesthesia, the abdominal wall is punctured. With the aid of an endoscope, a feeding tube is pulled through the abdominal wall and secured, and the anterior wall of the stomach is anchored to the abdominal wall. Radiological methods are similar and also minimally invasive. In the Medicare population alone, well over 100,000 PEGs are placed annually.

Divergent Views. There are two perspectives about the use of ANH in the context of chronic illness. One viewpoint favors enteral feeding in most situations in which the ability to eat and drink has been lost. After all, it is a comparatively simple and straightforward process, and the risk involved in providing access is relatively small. Many would argue that doing so is in fact an obligation—that food and water are basic human needs under all circumstances and that if it cannot be given orally, alternative access is necessary. They do not view ANH as medical or life-sustaining therapy. Moreover there is the concern that because food and water are often viewed as a good, withholding or withdrawing them will cause suffering akin to the traditionally held concepts of starvation.

An alternative and competing viewpoint is based on the belief that whereas the traditional position just described is at first glance justified by the clinical circumstances, it is one for which factual support is lacking. ANH is not the same as oral feeding. Further, there is evidence that in some clinical settings, particularly terminal conditions, including advanced dementia, ANH fails to provide benefit and may actually be harmful, adding to the burden of suffering medical providers are trying to minimize. This viewpoint also holds that ANH is medical treatment; it is initiated in the setting of illness, requires forced administration of nutrition and hydration, and is provided artificially via alternative access to the digestive system using specially designed equipment. It also requires assessment of risk and benefit as with any medical decision making. As such it is different from oral ingestion of food and water, which provide nurture and comfort.

WHAT IS KNOWN ABOUT ANH

Since the first report of PEG in infants in 1980, an extensive clinical experience has evolved. Because of the relative ease of placement with low complications, it soon became the default intervention for any circumstance in which ANH was being considered.

Clinical Experience. At the turn of the twenty-first century two articles appeared in mainstream medical journals that called attention to the use of ANH in patients with advanced dementia (Finucane, Christmas, and Travis 1999; Gillick 2000). Both independently concluded that the available evidence failed to support the use of ANH in these patients. The conclusion was the same regardless of which outcome variable was measured; risk for aspiration, malnutrition, pressure sores, infections, and functional status were not favorably affected. Moreover patients with advanced dementia did not live longer with ANH, and up to 50 percent of patients who were given PEGs to receive ANH were dead within a month of the procedure, reflecting the terminal nature of their illness at the time the decision to provide ANH was made. No reports have appeared to challenge this concept; moreover a *Cochrane Database of Systematic Reviews* evaluation of evidence-based health care drew similar conclusions (Sampson, Candy, and Jones 2009a). A simultaneously published commentary noted that enteral tube feeding in individuals with advanced dementia deprived them of the opportunity to interact with others and the basic enjoyment of tasting food while reducing dignity and autonomy and making personal care task-oriented (Sampson, Candy, and Jones 2009b).

These were not new concepts. The Alzheimer's Association has recognized at least since the mid-1990s that ANH is optional in patients with advanced dementia who are no longer taking food or fluid orally (Alzheimer's Association 2012). The association continues to note that ANH has failed to benefit these patients and that significant complications that add to the burden of suffering can ensue. The association likewise champions the concept of assisted oral feeding as an alternative way to provide comfort and nurture for such patients. A similar experience has been reported among patients with advanced or terminal cancer. Permanent vegetative state (PVS) is a very different condition from dementia and cancer but one for which the use of ANH is often debated. PVS is a condition in which patients with brain injury, often from trauma or anoxia, may exhibit wakefulness but otherwise have no detectable awareness. ANH is clearly life-sustaining in this setting. Brain injury this devastating is lethal, and it is only with artificial provision of nutrition and fluids and, in some cases, other supportive interventions that these patients continue to live.

Adverse Effects of ANH. Complications of ANH derive from the PEG tube itself as well as the feedings. When they materialize, they may actually exacerbate suffering for dying patients. Among these problems are placement and mechanical complications, wound infection, diarrhea with incontinence, aspiration, and fluid overload. Another problem in the context of dementia is the common need for restraints for patients with feeding tubes. Restraining patients can be humiliating and demeaning, their dementia notwithstanding. PVS patients do not experience pain and suffering, but indirect adverse effects, such as incontinence and requirement for diapers, may likewise jeopardize individual dignity.

Perceptions about Artificial Feeding. Perceptions about enteral tube feedings vary, but in general surveys of elderly patients show that the majority would not want artificial feeding were they to develop advanced dementia. These opinions were common in groups educated about both the procedures involved and the adverse effects, in particular the possible need for restraints. Surveys of physicians generally support not placing feeding tubes when elderly patients or patients at the end of their lives are no longer eating; in reality feeding tubes appear to be used more often than such surveys would predict. Surrogates opt for feeding tubes more often than the patients would, but these decisions likely rely on an incomplete knowledge base of benefits and adverse effects.

Not surprisingly withholding food and water also raises concerns about starvation and dehydration. At face value these are circumstances that cause pain and suffering. While the prospect of going without food or water may be untenable for healthy individuals, anecdotal reports in the medical literature consistently note that dying patients actually appear comfortable without food and water, and even euphoria has been described. Further, urine volumes fall, and respiratory and gastrointestinal secretions decrease, lessening cough, congestion, vomiting, and diarrhea. Robert M. McCann, William J. Hall, and Annmarie Groth-Juncker (1994) reported an experience with thirty-two dying cancer patients in a hospice-like setting. These patients were sufficiently aware to judge hunger and thirst and were offered food and water as desired. Nearly two-thirds experienced neither hunger nor thirst; one-third were hungry only initially. Oral feeding as desired or mouth lubrication effectively met needs when they occurred, and caregivers could focus on patient comfort. In patients with advanced dementia, discomfort scores, as measured by a validated instrument, actually declined when ANH was forgone (Pasman et al. 2005). While the physiological basis for these effects is incompletely understood, a patient's needs can be met in a dignified manner by assisted oral feeding as the individual might desire. There are no reports concerning PVS patients, but loss of sentience in this condition precludes pain and suffering.

Legal Issues in Nonoral Enteral Feeding. To the extent that death is predictable in a period of hours, days, or even weeks, the intellectual and emotional struggles discussed earlier are less intense. But with respect to patients with terminal disorders in whom the timing of death is less certain or PVS patients who might live for years with artificial feeding, this is less likely to be the case. As a result disagreement has spilled over into the legal system. Subsequent judgments have provided legal support for the following concepts:

1. Artificial feeding is medical treatment and can be viewed on a level with other life-sustaining interventions (mechanical ventilation, dialysis, antibiotics, and others).
2. Competent patients may refuse life-sustaining treatment. This is a right also afforded to incompetent patients, particularly when there has been prior indication of this desire. State interests do not trump these rights.
3. Withholding and withdrawing life-sustaining treatment, including artificial feeding, are equal under the law. There is no requirement to continue a treatment once started if the proportionality of benefits and burdens is unfavorable.
4. Withholding or withdrawing life-sustaining treatment in a patient with a terminal disease is neither killing nor euthanasia.

OBSTACLES AND CHALLENGES TO ETHICAL DECISION MAKING

As commentators continued to question why feeding tubes are still being placed in patients with advanced dementia and related conditions when ethicists, geriatricians, and neurologists support a palliative approach, the issue of ANH entered the public domain in 2005 with a highly publicized case of a PVS patient. Terri Schiavo had been kept alive with a feeding tube after suffering a devastating neurological injury from hypoxic injury complicating sudden cardiac arrest fifteen years earlier. When Schiavo's husband petitioned to have the tube removed, a conflict with Terri Schiavo's parents ensued, leading to a lengthy court and legislative battle, the latter reaching the level of the federal government. Ultimately the feeding tube was removed, and she died shortly thereafter. With this case the issue of tube feeding became fair game for public debate, the accrued data presented notwithstanding. It led many to question the appropriate use of ANH in all clinical settings, even though dying patients with cancer or dementia are very different from those with devastating neurological injury resulting in PVS. Prolife and disability activists cited the horrors of starvation and dehydration in individuals who were being viewed by others as "better dead than disabled."

With the intense interest in artificial feeding, new or amending legislation was proposed in several states that would restrict the rights of patients or families to withhold or withdraw ANH (Brody et al. 2011). Many of these laws blanketed all clinical circumstances, not just PVS, and would have applied equally to patients with advanced dementia and other terminal illnesses. Even before the Schiavo case, however, a number of states had laws that held refusal of ANH to a higher standard than existed for other life-sustaining treatments. Examples of such standards include the need for more stringent evidence of a patient's wishes than for other treatments, specific authorization on an advance directive, the existence of so-called qualifying medical conditions, or a requirement for a second specialty opinion. Conscience-clause legislation allows health care providers not to acquiesce to patient's wishes about treatments, including ANH, if it is contrary to their moral or religious beliefs. Such laws have also affected any individual's option to forgo or withdraw ANH.

Roman Catholic teaching has had an impact on this area as well, and church doctrine would appear to have changed over the years. In the 1950s alleviation of pain and suffering, not merely prolongation of life, was the goal of medical treatment. At the time tube feeding was considered extraordinary care and as such could be refused if viewed by patients or families as excessive or burdensome. In the early years of the twenty-first century, however, the position of the church on ANH has been more difficult to discern. Church doctrine has seemed to evolve to a more restrictive posture, suggesting that ANH is in fact ordinary care to be rendered under any circumstance. Moreover forgoing or withdrawing ANH is considered killing by omission, essentially euthanasia, which is clearly contrary to Roman Catholic belief. But it is viewed as ordinary care "in principle." Commentators have construed this position as creating room for interpretation on a case-by-case basis, permitting the forgoing or withdrawing of ANH when it would be excessively burdensome or when the patient is actively dying. Still, the picture remains somewhat confusing. Further, whereas the "in principle" caveat creates options for providers with individual patients, Roman Catholic institutions might also interpret these guidelines differently, such that the wishes of patients or families could be overridden or ignored in an effort to conform to what is viewed as the church's moral teaching.

However, the disconnect between the continued use of ANH, on the one hand, but the lack of supporting evidence coupled with risk for harm, on the other, is not entirely explained by the public passion, state laws, and uncertain changes in Roman Catholic doctrine just discussed. The circumstances that promote ANH in these settings are likely much more complicated. There are pressures and incentives to proceed with ANH that are independent of both the medical circumstances and, in many cases, patients' preferences. Not surprisingly family members given decision-making power may be unwilling to accept a terminal prognosis, particularly if they expect that the dying process would be more painful without ANH. "Doing everything" even if there is no expectation of benefit may absolve the guilt that families may experience in this setting. Because technology is available that is relatively easy to apply, it may seem almost intuitive that we should use it when a chronically ill or dying patient is no longer eating. The idea that nutritional deficiencies or other problems cannot be corrected in this setting or that artificial feeing can add to the burden of suffering may at first glance seem inconsequential. Moreover whereas there remains a knowledge gap for many providers, even those who are aware of the studies noted earlier find such discussions with patients and families cumbersome if not difficult; they require time that is already at a premium, and the default decision to simply proceed with ANH is far easier to implement.

There are also financial and regulatory incentives. For the surgeon or gastroenterologist and the facility, placing a gastrostomy tube to deliver ANH generates a charge. In nursing homes reimbursement is far greater for ANH than it is for assisted oral feeding, even though the latter is more costly by virtue of the time commitment required. Furthermore federal regulations for nursing homes promote the use of nutritional supplements by requiring that certain parameters of nutritional status, such as albumin levels, be attained to maintain their certification. These incentives, a motivation to avoid conflict with families and referring physicians, and concerns about litigation often drive the decision to implement ANH in the context of advanced dementia and other terminal conditions regardless of one's perspective about ordinary versus extraordinary care. Only by changing the incentives, argue some, are we likely to have a chance to align our practice patterns with the existing evidence about benefit and risk (Finucane, Christmas, and Leff 2007).

OBLIGATIONS AND OPTIONS IN ANH

Confronting the obstacles and challenges begins with individuals. Misconceptions and knowledge gaps abound concerning ANH, and acting preemptively before the circumstance arises that requires a quick decision will obviate the need for agonizing discussions and, in many cases, ill-fated decisions. Primary care physicians therefore need to have end-of-life discussions with patients and families sooner rather than later. This allows time to educate patients and families to ensure that knowledge and understanding are on a par, so that decision making may be shared. An important part of these discussions is the completion of an advance directive and the designation of a surrogate who understands the patient's perspective and will be an advocate if and when that individual is unable to speak on his or her own behalf.

It is important to understand that the dying process changes body needs. For example, families are often concerned that forgoing nutrition and hydration will actually cause suffering, projecting from their own experiences with hunger and thirst. Good counseling and discussion with physicians can alleviate that concern in most cases. Whereas both ANH and oral feeding offer physiological benefits, it is the latter that provides comfort and pleasure to the extent that one wants to eat. It also respects autonomy in that one is left in control of oral intake. Assisting in this process is a nurturing act and should be considered an obligation rather than an option, as permitted by the clinical situation.

All too often, though, these conversations take place at the hospital bedside when decisions about ANH are needed quickly. In this setting they are much more challenging and as a result less effective. This is a circumstance in which the palliative care service can play an important role. In one center establishing a requirement that every patient with chronic illness being considered for ANH have a palliative care consultation resulted in a significant reduction in the number of dying patients with advanced dementia who received this intervention (Monteleoni and Clack 2004). Many if not most major hospitals now have multidisciplinary palliative care teams with trained providers who have expertise and time to present and discuss appropriate kinds of care—not just ANH—that will also address the family's and the patient's needs. Such teams are adept at communicating the concept that a recommendation to withhold or withdraw a useless, burdensome treatment can be a more caring act than any other. Issues addressed are the patient's prognosis and how feeding is expected to either positively or negatively affect the medical condition (benefits and burdens), taking into account expected life span, the patient's comfort, and as applicable, any previously expressed wishes about use of life-sustaining treatment. A critical step is to define goals as one might with any treatment modality. With disagreements about management that involves ethical issues for some, the institutional ethics committee can be helpful in shedding light on the pertinent issues and improving communication among the involved parties. This is a valuable resource in resolving looming conflicts but also in providing support for providers and family in emotionally charged situations.

Beyond the bedside, more needs to be done at the regulatory level to recognize and support interventions that make sense. These goals are more difficult to achieve if only because they can become politicized. But reforming state laws, for example, to allow decisions about ANH to be made on the basis of medical treatment, just as any other decision is made, would be a step in the right direction. These are individual decisions, and laws that assume that all incapacitated patients would want ANH may be contradictory to patients' interests. Nursing home regulations that promote care that for some patients, such as those noted earlier, would be counter-productive need to be revised in accordance with these differing treatment goals. Care is not the same for all with chronic or terminal illnesses, and there should be, for example, reimbursement for patient-specific services, such as assisted oral feedings in the context of advanced dementia, just as there exists for taking care of enteral feedings in other patients.

SUMMARY AND CONCLUSION

The importance our society places on eating a meal understandably drives a desire to provide nutrition when this is no longer possible. Technology affords us a relatively easy means of artificially providing food and fluids when oral intake diminishes or ceases. Thus placing a feeding tube relieves providers of concerns about their possible liability in not treating, and family or surrogates are relieved of guilt for not feeding. Yet a tension exists. The idea of employing a seemingly simple way to provide food when a patient is not eating conflicts with the more ominous themes in the clinical settings considered herein of failing to benefit, adding to suffering, and using technology that may be dehumanizing and disrespectful. Howard Brody and colleagues (2011, 1056) have suggested that "we seem to have forgotten the difference between people who die because they stop taking in food and water, and people who stop taking in food and water because of the natural dying process."

A principle-based analysis would likewise argue that both beneficence and autonomy may be in jeopardy if artificial nutrition and hydration are initiated in patients with terminal illness. A physician is not obligated to provide treatment that he or she considers futile. While sometimes considered an affront to autonomy, an element of paternalism may contribute to effective medical decision making, although physicians may hesitate to exercise it. For many patients with advanced dementia, terminal cancer, and neurological devastation, artificial feeding is inappropriate. The ethical and legal basis for withholding this treatment discussed earlier is sound. Whereas our morally pluralistic society will always generate different views because of competing value systems, the differences may not be as great as they may seem. While respecting these views, the goal of ethically sound decision making can realistically be achieved in most cases in a manner satisfactory to all.

SEE ALSO *Aging and the Aged: II. Health Care for the Aging; Autonomy; Chronic Illness; Clinical Ethics: I. Development, Role, and Methodologies; Dementia; DNR (Do Not Resuscitate); Harm; Informed Consent: I. History of Informed Consent; Judaism, Bioethics in; Long-Term Care: I. Concepts and Policies; Surrogate Decision Making; Technology: I. History of Medical Technology*

BIBLIOGRAPHY

Alzheimer's Association. 2012. "End-of-Life Decisions: Honoring the Wishes of the Person with Alzheimer's Disease." http://www.alz.org/national/documents/brochure_endoflifedecisions.pdf

Baxter, J. D. "Air versus Water." 2010. *Annals of Internal Medicine* 153 (9): 616–17.

Brody, Howard; Laura D. Hermer; Larry D. Scott; et al. 2011. "Artificial Nutrition and Hydration: The Evolution of Ethics, Evidence, and Policy." *Journal of General Internal Medicine* 26 (9): 1053–58.

Casarett, D.; J. Kapo; and A. Caplan. 2005. "Appropriate Use of Artificial Nutrition and Hydration: Fundamental Principles and Recommendations." *New England Journal of Medicine* 353 (24): 2607–12.

Drane, James F. 2006. "Stopping Nutrition and Hydration Technologies: A Conflict between Traditional Catholic Ethics and Church Authority." *Christian Bioethics* 12 (1): 11–28.

Dugdale, Lydia S., and Autumn Alcott Ridenour. 2011. "Making Sense of the Roman Catholic Directive to Extend Life Indefinitely." *Hastings Center Report* 41 (2): 28–29.

Dy, S. M. 2006. "Enteral and Parenteral Nutrition in Terminally Ill Cancer Patients: A Review of the Literature." *American Journal of Hospice and Palliative Care* 23 (5): 369–77.

Finucane, Thomas E.; Colleen Christmas; and Bruce A. Leff. 2007. "Tube Feeding in Dementia: How Incentives

Undermine Health Care Quality and Patient Safety." *Journal of the American Medical Directors Association* 8 (4): 205–8.

Finucane, Thomas E.; Colleen Christmas; and Kathy Travis. 1999. "Tube Feeding in Patients with Advanced Dementia." *Journal of the American Medical Association* 282 (14): 1365–70.

Ganzini, L. 2006. "Artificial Nutrition and Hydration at the End of Life: Ethics and Evidence." *Palliative and Supportive Care* 4 (2): 135–43.

Garrow, Donald; Pam Pride; William Moran; et al. 2007. "Feeding Alternatives in Patients with Dementia: Examining the Evidence." *Clinical Gastroenterology and Hepatology* 5 (12): 1372–78.

Gillick, Muriel R. 2000. "Rethinking the Role of Tube Feeding in Patients with Advanced Dementia." *New England Journal of Medicine* 342 (3): 206–10.

Gillick, Muriel R., and Angelo E. Volandes. 2008. "The Standard of Caring: Why Do We Still Use Feeding Tubes in Patients with Advanced Dementia?" *Journal of the American Medical Directors Association* 9 (5): 364–67.

Janes, Simon E. J.; C. S. G. Price; and S. Khan. 2005. "Percutaneous Endoscopic Gastrostomy: 30-Day Mortality Trends and Risk Factors." *Journal of Postgraduate Medicine* 51 (1): 23–29.

Klein, S., and R. L. Koretz. 1994. "Nutrition Support in Patients with Cancer: What Do the Data Really Show?" *Nutrition in Clinical Practice* 9 (3): 91–100.

Lynn, Joanne. 1989. *By No Extraordinary Means: The Choice to Forgo Life-Sustaining Food and Water.* Bloomington: Indiana University Press.

McCann, Robert M.; William J. Hall; and Annmarie Groth-Juncker. 1994. "Comfort Care for Terminally Ill Patients: The Appropriate Use of Nutrition and Hydration." *Journal of the American Medical Association* 272 (16): 1263–66.

Monteleoni, C., and E. Clark. 2004. "Using Rapid-Cycle Quality Improvement Methodology to Reduce Feeding Tubes in Patients with Advanced Dementia: Before and after Study." *British Medical Journal* 329 (7464): 491–94.

Pasman, H. Roeline W.; Bregje D. Onwuteaka-Philipsen; Didi M. W. Kriegsman; et al. 2005. "Discomfort in Nursing Home Patients with Severe Dementia in Whom Artificial Nutrition and Hydration Is Forgone." *Archives of Internal Medicine* 165 (15): 1729–35.

Post, Stephen G. 2001. "Tube Feeding and Advanced Progressive Dementia." *Hastings Center Report* 31 (1): 36–42.

Rabaneck, Linda; Laurence B. McCullough; and Nelda P. Wray. 1997. "Ethically Justified, Clinically Comprehensive Guidelines for Percutaneous Endoscopic Gastrostomy Tube Placement." *Lancet* 349 (9056): 496–98.

Sampson, Elizabeth L.; Bridget Candy; and Louise Jones. 2009a. "Enteral Tube Feeding for Older People with Advanced Dementia." *Cochrane Database of Systematic Reviews* 15 (2): CD007209.

Sampson, Elizabeth L.; Bridget Candy; and Louise Jones. 2009b. "Enteral Tube Feeding for Older People with Advanced Dementia: Findings from a Cochrane Systematic Review." *International Journal of Palliative Nursing* 15 (8): 396–404.

Scott, Larry D. 2005. "The PEG 'Consult.'" *American Journal of Gastroenterology* 100 (4): 740–43.

Shega, Joseph W; Gavin W. Hougham; Carol B. Stocking; et al. 2003. "Barriers to Limiting the Practice of Feeding Tube Placement in Advanced Dementia." *Journal of Palliative Medicine* 6 (6): 885–93.

Sieger, Carol E.; Jason F. Arnold; and Judith C. Ahronheim. 2002. "Refusing Artificial Nutrition and Hydration: Does Statutory Law Send the Wrong Message?" *Journal of the American Geriatrics Society* 50 (3): 544–50.

Slomka, Jacquelyn. 1995. "What Do Apple Pie and Motherhood Have to Do with Feeding Tubes and Caring for the Patient?" *Archives of Internal Medicine* 155 (12): 1258–63.

Teno, Joan M.; Susan L. Mitchell; Sylvia K. Kuo; et al. 2011. "Decision-Making and Outcomes of Feeding Tube Insertions: A Five-State Study." *Journal of the American Geriatrics Society* 59 (5): 881–86.

Larry D. Scott (2004, 2014)
Professor, Division of Gastroenterology, Hepatology, and Nutrition, Department of Internal Medicine, University of Texas Medical School at Houston

ASIA

SEE *China, Bioethics in; Japan, Bioethics in; South Asia, Bioethics in; Southeast Asia, Bioethics in.*

AUSTRALIA AND NEW ZEALAND, BIOETHICS IN

Bioethics in Australia and New Zealand (Australasia) evolved slowly until the early 1980s, when major advances in reproductive technologies prompted widespread public discussion of bioethical issues surrounding human conception.

EARLY HISTORY

In the early decades of the twentieth century, ethical debates centered on issues of professionalism in the delivery of medical services, such as the permissibility of advertising by individual practitioners and the setting of standard fees to avoid "undercutting" by competitors. The branches of the British Medical Association (BMA) that had been set up in the colonial Australian states were federated in 1912, when a unified code of professional ethics, dealing mainly with the regulation of advertising and etiquette toward patients, was introduced (Egan 1988). After World War I, medical schools in Australasian universities began to include brief didactic instruction in the ethical obligations of physicians. There was also some public discussion of abortion, methods of birth control, and confidentiality in relation to patients with venereal disease.

A Labour government with a strong social welfare platform was elected in Australia in 1941. In the late 1940s this government attempted to introduce a national health service, which would have provided universal access to health care for the first time in Australia. However, a bitter debate developed with the BMA, the majority of whose members saw the government's plans as a threat to the autonomy of medical practitioners and as the first step toward the nationalization of medicine. After legal challenges, the plans for a national health program were defeated in 1949 (Gillespie 1991). Under the free-market policies of subsequent Liberal governments, access to publicly funded health care was available only to recipients of old-age and invalid pensions. This situation persisted until 1975, when the Labour government introduced Medibank, Australia's first national health care program, which provided access to government-subsidized health care for all. While the incoming Liberal/National coalition government gradually dismantled this program during the late 1970s, it was reinstated as Medicare in 1983 by the newly elected Labour government, and has continued to operate into the twenty-first century.

Ethical issues in reproduction became a major concern in Australasia in the early 1980s, following pioneering research on in vitro fertilization (IVF) carried out by a joint research team led by Carl Wood and Ian Johnston at the Monash University Queen Victoria Medical Centre and the Royal Women's Hospital in Melbourne during the 1970s. In 1983 this research led to the world's first live IVF births from frozen embryos and donated eggs, and the embryo research carried out by Monash University scientists in order to improve IVF and other assisted reproduction techniques sparked worldwide interest. These developments in reproductive technology stimulated much public discussion in Australia, particularly among Roman Catholics, who constitute just over a quarter of the population.

EUTHANASIA

Care for the terminally ill became another widely debated issue in Australia in the 1980s. Influenced by the growing public support for voluntary euthanasia, the state governments of South Australia and Victoria passed legislation (in 1983 and 1988, respectively) permitting patients to refuse medical treatment in certain circumstances, even where such treatment might prolong their lives. In 1995 the Northern Territory's single-chamber parliament passed the Rights of the Terminally Ill Act, making it the first jurisdiction in the world to legalize active voluntary euthanasia. This legislation permitted doctors to carry out voluntary euthanasia, under certain specified conditions, for terminally ill patients with unbearable suffering. The lives of several patients were lawfully ended under this act before it was overruled by the Euthanasia Laws Act, passed by the Australian federal parliament in 1997. Voluntary euthanasia and physician-assisted suicide remain illegal in Australia and New Zealand.

ETHICS CENTERS

Australasia's first research center in bioethics, the Monash University Centre for Human Bioethics, was established by the philosophy professor Peter Singer, together with colleagues in medicine, science, and the law, in 1980. A number of smaller research centers for bioethics were set up in Australasia during the next two decades, including Melbourne's St. Vincent's Bioethics Centre, Adelaide's Southern Cross Bioethics Institute (both of which took a Christian perspective on bioethics), Sydney's John Plunkett Centre for Ethics in Health Care, the Ethics Unit at Melbourne's Murdoch Children's Research Institute, and the University of Otago Bioethics Research Centre in Dunedin, New Zealand. Bioethics research is also pursued at the University of Sydney Centre for Values, Ethics and the Law in Medicine, founded in 1995; at the Children's Bioethics Centre in Melbourne's Royal Children's Hospital; and by several of the large groups of philosophers appointed to the Centre for Applied Philosophy and Public Ethics, which was established by Charles Sturt University in both Canberra and Melbourne in 2000. The interdisciplinary Australasian Bioethics Association was formed in 1990, and its inaugural conference was held in Melbourne in 1991. In 2009 this association was combined with the Australian and New Zealand Institute of Health Law and Ethics to form the Australasian Association of Bioethics and Health Law, which holds an annual conference in Australia or New Zealand.

With Helga Kuhse and others from the Monash Centre, Peter Singer has written extensively on ethical issues in assisted reproduction and on questions surrounding the care of terminally ill adults and infants. Other noteworthy contributors to bioethical debates include Australians Linda Barclay, Paul Biegler, Russell Blackford, Annette Braunack-Mayer, Max Charlesworth, Steve Clarke, Dean Cocking, Susan Dodds, Lynn Gillam, Stan van Hooft, Megan-Jane Johnstone, Jeanette Kenneteil Levy, Miles Little, Bebe Loff, Catriona Mackenzie, Rosalind McDougall, Catherine Mills, Wendy Rogers, Julian Savulescu, Michael Selgelid, Robert Sparrow, Merle Spriggs, Nicholas Tonti-Filippini, Bernadette Tobin, Dominic Wilkinson, Robert Young, and Deborah Zion; New Zealanders Nicholas Agar, Alastair Campbell, Grant Gillett, Gareth Jones, Andrew Moore, and Martin Wilkinson; feminist academics Renate Klein and Robyn Rowland; lawyers Don Chalmers, Michael Kirby, Margaret Otlowski, Ron Paterson, Loane Skene, Cameron Stewart, and Colin Thomson; and theologian Norman Ford. In

1989 the Monash Centre introduced Australasia's first master's program in bioethics, and this institution also publishes Australia's first peer-reviewed bioethics journal, *Monash Bioethics Review*. The University of Sydney Centre for Values, Ethics and the Law in Medicine has subsequently developed a bioethics master's program, and in 2004 launched a new interdisciplinary bioethics journal, the *Journal of Bioethical Inquiry*, continuing from the *New Zealand Bioethics Journal*, which had been edited at the University of Otago Bioethics Centre since 2000.

REPRODUCTIVE TECHNOLOGIES

In 1982 advances in infertility research in Victoria led the government of that state to appoint Louis Waller, a professor of law at Monash University and an Australian law reform commissioner, to chair a committee whose mandate was to consider the social, ethical, and legal issues arising from IVF. The three reports produced by this committee supported the use of IVF under certain regulations, prompting the Victorian Parliament in 1984 to enact the Infertility (Medical Procedures) Act, the world's first legislation to deal specifically with these new reproductive technologies (see Charlesworth 1989). Among other provisions, this legislation allowed IVF to be carried out at approved hospitals, for married couples who have already sought infertility treatment for at least twelve months prior to attempting IVF. This legislation was subsequently amended in 1997 to allow IVF access to couples in de facto relationships, and again in 2008 to allow same-sex couples and single women to lawfully access IVF.

At the federal level in Australia, the National Bioethics Consultative Committee (NBCC) was established in 1988 as an advisory committee on issues such as access to information about their origins for children conceived through IVF; artificial insemination by donor; surrogate motherhood; and embryo experimentation. In 1990 this committee issued a report that supported surrogacy arrangements and proposed draft legislation to regulate such arrangements. In light of the heated public controversy that ensued, however, the Australian government decided against implementing its recommendations nationally. Nevertheless, most Australian states have not outlawed IVF-assisted surrogacy in cases where the surrogate mother receives no fee, and in 1994 the Australian Capital Territory enacted legislation to regulate such surrogacy arrangements. In 1991 the NBCC was subsumed under the existing National Health and Medical Research Council (NH&MRC), which merged the functions of the NBCC and the Medical Research Ethics Committee to form the Australian Health Ethics Committee, which continues to operate. One area of much debate has been the question of access by children born from gamete donation to information about their genetic parents. In 2012 the Parliament of Victoria Law Reform Committee produced a pioneering report recommending that children born of anonymous gamete donation be given access to identifying information about their donors, even if the donors had been assured of anonymity at the time of the donation, and the federal government has indicated that it is likely to support similar access rights at a national level. In New Zealand, the National Ethics Committee on Assisted Human Reproduction was established in 1995 to provide advice to government and ethics committees on ethical issues in assisted reproduction, and in 2004 this committee was superseded by the Advisory Committee on Assisted Reproductive Technology.

The groundbreaking work of Australian researchers with human embryonic stem cells and biotechnology became the focus of much public discussion at the beginning of the present century. The cloning of human beings was outlawed in 2002, following the recommendations of a federal parliamentary standing committee, but research is permitted on stem cells that had been extracted from human embryos prior to early 2001. Also, stem cell researchers can apply to a federal licensing committee to undertake such research using excess IVF embryos or embryos created through somatic cell nuclear transfer cloning. A 2011 review of this legislation endorsed many of its provisions, while also recommending that scientists be allowed to create gametes from induced pluripotent stem cells, on the condition that any embryo created with such gametes is not implanted. There are also emerging ethical debates about the use of stem cells in translational research for clinical applications, particularly in regard to issues concerning safety, informed consent, and justice in access to such therapies.

RESEARCH ON HUMANS

Australasia's first recorded institutional ethics committee to review research on humans was set up at the Royal Victorian Eye and Ear Hospital in Melbourne in 1957 (McNeill 1993 and, at the instigation of the NH&MRC (which allocates government funding for medical research), Australian universities began, in the 1980s, to form ethics committees to oversee medical and other research undertaken at those institutions. Following wide community consultation and a 1996 federal government review of the relatively brief NH&MRC guidelines on human experimentation, the detailed and remarkably broad-ranging *National Statement on Ethical Conduct in Research Involving Humans*, was issued by the NH&MRC in 1999 as a guide for all human research ethics committees (HRECs) in Australia. A revised version of these guidelines, the *National Statement on Ethical Conduct in Human Research* was issued in 2007 by the

NH&MRC, along with the Australian Research Council and the Australian Vice-Chancellors' Committee. The 2007 *National Statement* places the ethical oversight of research within the broader concept of research governance and provides HRECs with more detailed guidance than the 1999 version, while also allowing somewhat greater flexibility in the ethical review process. The basic principles in the *National Statement* are research merit and integrity, justice, beneficence, and respect, which are developed in more detail through their application to a variety of different types of research (see also Dodds and Thomson 2006).

In New Zealand, the Medical Research Council (set up in 1937 by the government to supervise medical research) decided in 1968 that all research must adhere to the World Medical Association's Declaration of Helsinki, which stressed nonmaleficence and the need for informed consent by experimental subjects. In 1987 unprecedented public outrage followed revelations of an experiment involving clandestine selective nontreatment of women with cervical cancer, which was carried out at the National Women's Hospital in Auckland from 1966 to 1981. The New Zealand government immediately set up an inquiry into the experiment. This inquiry (known as the "Cartwright Inquiry," after its Chair, Judge Silvia Cartwright) resulted in the Human Rights Commission Act of 1977 being amended to add a statement of patients' rights to proper standards of care and adequate disclosures to enable genuinely informed consent. This amendment also provided for the appointment of a national health commissioner to encourage awareness of these rights by members of the medical profession (Campbell 1989; Manning 2009). Another outcome of this inquiry was that area health boards were required to establish their own research ethics committees. The first national *Standard for Hospital and Area Health Board Ethics Committees Established to Review Research and Treatment Protocols*, providing guidance to these committees, was published by the Department of Health in 1988 and the *Guidelines on Ethics in Health Research* was published in 2002 by the Health Research Council (successor to the Medical Research Council). Revised, more streamlined versions of these guidelines were published by the National Ethics Advisory Committee in 2012 as the *Ethical Guidelines for Intervention Studies* and the *Ethical Guidelines for Observational Studies: Observational Research, Audits, and Related Activities*.

PATIENTS' RIGHTS

During the 1990s there was considerable discussion in Australia about patients' legal rights to treatment information, prompted by the Australian High Court decision in *Rogers v. Whitaker* (1992), which gave legal recognition to a patient-centered standard of disclosure of medical information. Following this decision, the NH&MRC issued a booklet containing guidelines on providing information to patients.

Influenced by the increasing recognition of patients' rights, Australasian medical schools gradually wove the teaching of ethics into their curricula. For example, the University of New South Wales in Sydney and the University of Newcastle began teaching substantive courses in ethics to medical undergraduates in the 1970s, and the University of Adelaide's medical school introduced ethics into the undergraduate syllabus in the early 1980s. Following the recommendations of the National Inquiry into Medical Education—a committee of academics and health professionals set up by the federal minister for health, which heard submissions during 1987 and 1988—all other Australian medical schools have included clinical ethics as part of their undergraduate programs. Innovative methods of teaching medical ethics have been developed at various institutions, including an experiential approach at the Australian National University, as a way of helping medical graduates to act with professional integrity in the face of various obstacles in clinical practice. These developments in bioethics education should help promote lively and informed discussions of medical ethics issues in Australasia as they arise in the future.

BIBLIOGRAPHY

Armit, Henry William. 1924. "Medical Practice." *Medical Journal of Australia* (October 25): 413–21.

Campbell, Alastair A. 1989. "A Report from New Zealand: An 'Unfortunate Experiment.'" *Bioethics* 3 (1): 59–66.

Charlesworth, Max J. 1989. *Life, Death, Genes, and Ethics: Biotechnology and Bioethics*. Sydney: ABC Books.

Charlesworth, Max J. 1993. *Bioethics in a Liberal Society.* Cambridge, UK: Cambridge University Press.

Coney, Sandra. 1988. *The Unfortunate Experiment*. Harmondsworth, UK: Penguin.

Dodds, Susan, and Thomson, Colin. 2006. "Bioethics and Democracy: Competing Roles of National Bioethics Organisations" *Bioethics* 20:326–38.

Egan, Bryan. 1988. "Nobler Than Missionaries: Australian Medical Culture c. 1880–c. 1930." Ph.D. diss., Monash University, Melbourne.

Ford, Norman. 1988. *When Did I Begin?: Conception of the Human Individual in History, Philosophy, and Science.* Cambridge, UK: Cambridge University Press.

Gillespie, James A. 1991. *The Price of Health: Australian Governments and Medical Politics, 1910–1960.* Cambridge, UK: Cambridge University Press.

Kasimba, Pascal, and Peter Singer. 1989. "Australian Commissions and Committees on Issues in Bioethics." *Journal of Medicine and Philosophy* 14:403–24.

Kuhse, Helga, and Peter Singer. 1985. *Should the Baby Live?: The Problem of Handicapped Infants.* Oxford, UK: Oxford University Press.

Kuhse, Helga, and Peter Singer, eds. 2009. *A Companion to Bioethics.* 2nd ed. Malden, MA: Wiley-Blackwell.

Manning, Joanna, ed. 2009. *The Cartwright Papers: Essays on the Cervical Cancer Inquiry 1987–88.* Wellington: Bridget Williams Books.

McNeill, Paul M. 1993. *The Ethics and Politics of Human Experimentation.* Cambridge, UK: Cambridge University Press.

Rowland, Robyn. 1987. "Making Women Visible in the Embryo Experimentation Debate." *Bioethics* 1:179–88.

Singer, Peter; Helga Kuhse; Stephen Buckle; et al., eds. 1990. *Embryo Experimentation.* Cambridge, UK: Cambridge University Press.

Singer, Peter, and Deane Wells. 1984. *Making Babies: The New Science and Ethics of Conception.* Oxford, UK: Oxford University Press.

Justin Oakley (1995, 2004, 2014)
Associate Professor and Deputy Director, Centre for Human Bioethics, Monash University

AUTHENTICITY

Authenticity is an important ethical concept. It is also a potentially confusing one because of the variety of ways it has been used throughout its history. Artifacts such as paintings or dollar bills can be described as authentic or inauthentic. In such cases, the attribution of authenticity suggests, as indicated by the *Oxford English Dictionary* (*OED*), that something is "what it professes in origin or authorship … genuine" ("Authenticity" 2012). But more important for a discussion of the concept within bioethics, people and their choices, actions, and lives are also assessed in terms of their authenticity. The term is then susceptible of a wider range of possible meanings (even though it can still be used in a similar sense to that relevant to inanimate objects), which this entry will attempt to spell out. Despite this plurality of meanings, however, authenticity is typically assumed to be a desirable thing. In the health care context, for instance, it is deemed of crucial importance that a patient's decision, say to refuse treatment, should be authentic; if there are grounds for thinking that it is not, this may be taken to mean that it is permissible to override it. Authenticity is also usually viewed as a significant consideration in the private conduct of one's life. As Charles Taylor (1992), among others, has pointed out, many people in Western society—especially since the 1960s—are committed to the moral ideal of living an authentic life, a life that is uniquely their own. This use of the concept has, for example, become salient in the debate on the ethics of human enhancement.

A BRIEF HISTORY OF THE CONCEPT

As traditionally conceived, authenticity fundamentally involves the idea of being true to oneself. This idea, however, can itself be understood in different ways. One major sense, connected to the *OED*'s definition of *authenticity* given above, has to do with sincerity: being true to oneself, on this construal, means accurately representing who one is, including one's beliefs and feelings, to others. This is the sense already found in the famous lines spoken by Polonius in Shakespeare's *Hamlet*, in which the character advises his son, Laertes:

> This above all: to thine own self be true,
> And it must follow, as the night the day,
> Thou canst not then be false to any man.
>
> (*HAMLET*, ACT 1, SCENE 3)

In his classic work *Sincerity and Authenticity* (1972), Lionel Trilling precisely argues that sincerity really came to prominence as a value in Western society at about the time *Hamlet* was written, the late sixteenth century. Although this value has retained its importance through the following centuries, it is only once being true to oneself starts mattering beyond the fundamentally public virtue of sincerity that the moral ideal of authenticity is truly born. Taylor traces this development of the ideal in *The Ethics of Authenticity* (1992), through Jean-Jacques Rousseau and in particular Johann Gottfried von Herder and the romantic movement. For the romantics, we should be true to ourselves not simply for the sake of presenting our true colors to others but also, more importantly, because of the intrinsic value of expressing and realizing our fundamental, inner nature. For one thing, this means realizing our best capacities, resulting, for instance, in the creation of great works of art. But an even more pressing reason for living authentically is, on this view, that this true self or inner nature is the ultimate source of knowledge for us about how we ought to live, about what a good life means for each of us as the individual she or he is. As Taylor (1992, 29) puts it, "There is a certain way of being human that is *my* way. I am called upon to live my life in this way, and not in imitation of anyone else's" (emphasis in original).

In the twentieth century, however, the romantic tenet of a true self in accordance with which one ought to shape one's life came under attack from existentialist philosophers, with whose thought the term *authenticity* is perhaps most closely associated. This criticism is most evident in the work of Jean-Paul Sartre. Sartre (1980 [1946], 28) adamantly rejected the idea that we have anything like a true self, a rejection most radically expressed in his early work *Existentialism and Humanism*, where he famously maintained that "man is nothing but that which he makes of himself." To believe, as the romantics did, that features one has not chosen can even partly define who one is represents, for Sartre, just an instance of bad faith, the very opposite of authenticity. Authenticity for Sartre means avoiding bad faith by facing up to the fact that we are fundamentally free to write the story of our life and thus are fundamentally responsible for the kind of person we become; there is no pregiven self laying down in advance the path we ought to follow.

TWO CONTRASTING APPROACHES TO AUTHENTICITY IN ANALYTIC PHILOSOPHY

The contrast between the romantic view of authenticity and the Sartrean one is reflected in the more general contrast drawn by some authors (such as Erik Parens [2004] and Neil Levy [2011]) between accounts of authenticity that emphasize self-discovery and those that focus on self-creation. The main analyses of authenticity stressing self-creation that have been proposed after Sartre tend to acknowledge more explicitly the limits that constrain our ability to shape ourselves as we wish. They do, however, still reject the idea of a pregiven self providing guidance as to how to live authentically—unless such a self is identified with our highest-priority values and commitments. Authenticity, according to the self-creation approach, involves living our life in accordance with these. No further constraints are placed on the authenticity of our choices and actions: for instance, someone could in principle make an authentic decision to radically change his or her physical appearance and psychological makeup provided that he or she did so in keeping with his or her core values and commitments. This approach thus treats authenticity as closely related to—if not identical with—the notion of autonomy, understood broadly as self-governance in the light of one's highest-priority values. In *The Importance of What We Care About* (1988), Harry G. Frankfurt can be read as providing an analysis of authenticity as autonomy: on this account, acting authentically means acting on the basis of desires that one wholeheartedly endorses. The notion of wholeheartedness implies the absence of ambivalence in one's second-order endorsement of those first-order desires as well as the absence of any inconsistency between one's second-order attitudes. David DeGrazia's (2005) account of authenticity in his book *Human Identity and Bioethics* is in many ways similar to Frankfurt's, though DeGrazia views autonomy as a necessary but not sufficient condition of authenticity. Honesty, in the sense of accurate presentation (both to others and oneself) of who one is, is required as well (DeGrazia 2005, 108–12).

Detailed, systematic expositions of the self-discovery approach to authenticity are more difficult to come by in analytic philosophy. Nevertheless, supporters of that approach can be said to share the following two ideas. First, each of us does have something like a true self, a set of traits (not limited to our values and commitments) that, taken together, define who we fundamentally are and do so whether or not we happen to endorse them. Second, authenticity entails living in accordance with such a true self, that is to say, expressing it, when appropriate, in our behavior (rather than hiding or repressing it) or preserving it even when we might be tempted to change it, for instance, because it would promote some of our interests. Taylor's *Ethics of Authenticity* (1992) can be taken to provide one of the most comprehensive outlines of the self-discovery model (though in some of his other works, it is less clear that Taylor Is willing to accept the idea of a true self that includes things beyond a person's values and commitments). Bernard A. O. Williams also expressed an affinity with that model. As he summed up to the journalist Stuart Jeffries (2002): "If there's one theme in all my work it's about authenticity and self-expression.… It's the idea that some things are in some real sense really you, or express what you [are] and others aren't." Among bioethicists, Carl Elliott (1998, 2003) and the President's Council on Bioethics (2003) have also endorsed a true-self approach to authenticity. They differ, however, in the exact way they understand the notion of a true or authentic self. Whereas the President's Council appears to identify it with an essence of some kind, Elliott does not.

In the light of those descriptions, the distinction between the self-discovery and self-creation approaches should not be interpreted too rigidly. Versions of the self-creation model less radical than Sartre's, such as DeGrazia's view, do make some space for the possibility of self-discovery. They do not rule out, for instance, that we might discover what our fundamental values and commitments are. Conversely, not all variants of the self-discovery approach posit an essential, unchangeable self. Some—perhaps the more plausible ones—do allow that we can to some degree deliberately shape who we authentically are, by working on ourselves to develop new traits and skills. Still, there remains an important difference between even the more moderate versions of each approach: DeGrazia, for instance, is keen to emphasize that only those of our features that we identify with and have made part of our own self-conception can define who we are fundamentally, that is, our identity as individuals.

It should finally be mentioned that the various accounts considered so far are primarily aimed at offering a criterion for the authenticity of our choices and actions rather than our psychological features, such as our emotions, desires, or moods. Authenticity in relation to such features has usually been discussed in a separate literature. Some authors, however, do use criteria that echo those described above. Kevin Mulligan (2009), for example, has argued that authentic emotions must escape rational and willful control, emphasizing, in the spirit of the self-discovery model, the need for spontaneity; other authors differ, stating instead that an authentic emotion must simply cohere with our autonomously formed values and beliefs (see Kraemer 2009 for a summary of that debate). Given that discussions about authenticity in bioethics are often concerned with the alteration of our psychological makeup (including our emotions or moods) for purposes of treatment or enhancement, such discussions might benefit from taking into account both of these bodies of literature on the concept of authenticity.

The following sections will consider the relevance of the concept of authenticity to three areas of debate in bioethics: end-of-life decision making, the technological enhancement of human beings, and the treatment of mental disorders.

AUTHENTICITY AND END-OF-LIFE DECISION MAKING

The issue of authenticity arises in the medical context when a person must decide whether or not to undergo some treatment to save his or her life. It also arises when someone seeks help with actively ending his or her life in countries—such as the Netherlands—where practices such as euthanasia and physician-assisted suicide are legal. The question then is whether the person's expressed wish (say, to end his or her life) is authentic or not. This wish may be directly expressed by the person at the present time, or it may have been formally expressed in the past through an advance directive, the latter being relevant when the person is now regarded as lacking decision-making capacity, for instance, as a result of a neurodegenerative disease. In either case, however, the concern about the authenticity of the person's request has to do with whether it accurately reflects his or her preferences and values. The relevant sense of authenticity at stake here is thus analogous to autonomy as conceived by Frankfurt or DeGrazia. It is considered important to ensure that someone's decision to end his or her life should be truly his or her own and that it should not have been distorted by false or incomplete information or by social pressures. If a person's choice is indeed judged authentic in this sense, the conclusion will usually be that it ought to be respected.

In such cases, considerations of authenticity are viewed as taking precedence even over the patient's best interests. Consider an adult who, on religious grounds, refuses a blood transfusion that would almost certainly save his or her life. Many would regard his or her decision as going against his or her own interests. Nevertheless, the consensus among doctors is that this decision should not be overridden if it is a genuine expression of the person's core values. Best interests can carry more weight in cases where a patient has lost capacity and no formal expression of his or her wishes regarding treatment is available. Even then, however, they need not be the decisive consideration. If the person deciding on behalf of the patient (the "surrogate") possesses sufficient knowledge of the latter's beliefs and values, he or she is supposed to try to determine what the patient would have chosen if he or she still had capacity. In other words, the decision he or she reaches should ideally be an authentic reflection of the patient's values and beliefs. Again, such a decision might not necessarily coincide with what most would regard as the patient's best interests.

The self-creation approach to authenticity seems of greater relevance than the self-discovery one to the question of whether a person's decision to refuse life-saving treatment (or his or her request to be helped to die) should be respected. Even if such a person possessed, for instance, great artistic gifts, few would argue that this would justify paternalistically overriding his or her refusal of treatment on the grounds that he or she should keep on living to give full expression to his or her authentic self. That said, such considerations might legitimately be appealed to in an attempt to persuade the person to change his or her mind. They might also appropriately figure in his or her own decision-making process: "Art still needs my contribution; I must go on." This suggests that although the self-creation model is more relevant to issues of public regulation, the self-discovery model might be more important for the personal question of how one ought to live.

AUTHENTICITY AND THE ENHANCEMENT DEBATE

The late twentieth and early twenty-first centuries have seen a growing interest in questions of authenticity within the debate on the technological enhancement of human beings—particularly "neuroenhancement," the process of intervening into a healthy person's brain, using procedures like psychoactive drugs or brain stimulation, to modify his or her mood, personality, or other psychological features in desired ways. A key impulse behind that debate was the publication in 1993 of the psychiatrist Peter Kramer's book *Listening to Prozac*. In it Kramer describes some patients who no longer meet the strict criteria for depressive (or any other) disorder yet are reportedly transformed by the use of the drug in ways many would judge desirable. Vulnerable, shy, and unconfident people become resilient, assertive, and socially savvy, with such benefits for their social and professional lives that some of them asked Kramer to allow them to remain on Prozac even when they were no longer considered at risk of relapsing into depression.

Kramer's account raises a general worry, shared by authors such as Elliott and the President's Council. Although this kind of neuroenhancement might seem to carry great benefits, does not it threaten the authenticity of the subject being enhanced?

This worry needs to be spelled out further. It is sometimes suggested that the enhanced individual will not be the same person as the initial one and that this is inherently problematic. However, as DeGrazia (2005, 231–32) has shown, this suggestion seems based on a failure to sufficiently distinguish between different senses of the phrase "being the same person" or of the idea of individual "identity." It seems implausible to think that the technological alteration of our personality or mood must produce a numerically distinct individual, with the implication that the original one has simply been destroyed. An alternative line of argument states instead that the qualitative changes to the person's identity produced by neuroenhancers are problematic from the perspective of authenticity. Yet why should they be regarded as such? One of the strongest arguments offered for that conclusion is Elliott's suggestion that mood brighteners such as Prozac might disconnect certain people from the appropriate sense of alienation they are experiencing in the face of a world that is amiss. His worry is that the drug might make the person feel better at the cost of silencing the voice of his or her authentic self, a voice that might not be pleasant yet is nevertheless a source of important insights about his or her life circumstances (see Elliott 1998).

Authors such as DeGrazia have responded to Elliott by arguing for a different understanding of the notions of authenticity and identity. Suppose that someone experiencing the feelings of alienation described by Elliott wants to get rid of them with the help of Prozac. To the extent that this person does not identify with his or her sense of alienation, this feature is not part of his or her identity on DeGrazia's view. Therefore removing it through pharmacological means does not threaten his or her authenticity. It will not betray anything like a true self. On the contrary, the person's decision to shape his or her psychology in this way can be fully authentic, provided that it is in line with his or her values and preferences and does not involve deception of any kind. This brings us back to the fundamental disagreement between the self-discovery and the self-creation approaches to authenticity.

Levy (2011) has proposed a way of resolving the conflict between these two approaches, using an analogy with people who choose to undergo sex reassignment surgery on the basis of their feeling that they are, for instance, really a woman trapped in a man's body. Such cases, Levy argues, illustrate the fact that enhancement technologies can actually help people become who they really are, allowing their authentic self (as the self-discovery model understands it) to shine through. He thinks that claim should be extended to the use of pharmaceuticals such as Prozac for enhancement purposes. He concludes that regardless of which approach to authenticity one subscribes to, the use of neuroenhancers can be seen as promoting our authenticity. The statements made by some of Kramer's patients, who claimed that they were "no longer themselves" without Prozac, do seem to lend support to that conclusion. Yet although Levy seems right that the self-discovery model does not warrant a systematic condemnation of enhancement use as inauthentic, it has nevertheless been argued that this model is in fact more conducive to worries about authenticity than the self-creation one (see Erler 2012). If so, the debate between the two camps is not at an end yet.

AUTHENTICITY AND MENTAL DISORDERS

A third context within bioethics in which the concept of authenticity has received much attention is the treatment of mental disorders. The issues here largely overlap with those raised in relation to the enhancement debate—unsurprisingly, since both discussions focus on interventions into the brain involving similar procedures (antidepressants such as Prozac, stimulants such as Ritalin), only for different purposes (treatment versus enhancement). Indeed these interventions were originally designed with the aim of treating psychological disorders, such as depression or attention deficit/hyperactivity disorder (ADHD), and their enhancement potential was discovered only accidentally. The issue of authenticity has been discussed in relation to various groups of people with mental disorders. Ilina Singh (2005) has studied children with ADHD; Ineke Bolt and Maartje Schermer (2009) have interviewed adults with the same condition. Tony Hope and colleagues (2011) have interviewed female patients with anorexia nervosa, and David A. Karp (2006) has related the experiences of people with depressive disorder.

In all of these contexts, a key question that arises, particularly for patients and their relatives, is whether medication that treats the disorder undermines the person's authenticity. The worry that it might do so is arguably less widely shared than the corresponding worry in relation to neuroenhancement, yet some patients (and, in the case of children with ADHD, their parents) do give voice to it. Others, by contrast, take the view that medication actually helps restore the authentic self that had been masked by pathology—a view with which many clinical practitioners would agree. Alternatives are to regard both the disordered and the "well" self as equally authentic or to simply reject the notion of an authentic self altogether. Patients who feel that medication takes away part of their identity by removing the disorder sometimes suggest that they are thereby being deprived of intrinsically valuable features, such as spontaneity or creativity in the case of ADHD. But the worry about losing part of oneself does not seem to systematically depend on the assumption that the relevant aspect of one's identity is valuable independent of its being part of oneself.

What do the philosophical perspectives on authenticity considered above imply in this sort of case? For advocates of the self-creation model, concerns about authenticity are appropriate only when a patient does not clearly endorse his or her motives for seeking treatment or the changes that the medication produces in him or her. If he or she does endorse them wholeheartedly or autonomously, his or her use of medication must count as fully authentic.

It is unclear whether supporters of a true-self analysis of authenticity will want to disagree here. This will depend on whether they are prepared to accept that mental disorder can be part of a person's authentic self. Although several of the authors mentioned earlier in this section agree that the self-discovery approach can help illuminate discussions of mental disorder and authenticity, they understandably tend to avoid taking a firm stand on the nature of the relation between the two. In favor of the view that mental disorder necessarily overshadows a person's authentic self, one might stress the common intuition that treating clinical depression through medication does not fundamentally change who the patient is but simply restores him or her.

However, as mentioned previously, this intuition is not universally accepted with respect to all forms of mental disorder. To this should be added that the way the concept of mental disorder is applied by the medical profession at any point in time does not stand beyond criticism. Some characteristics, such as homosexuality, were once viewed as disorders but are no longer so, and some that are still so classified in the 2013 version of the *Diagnostic and Statistical Manual of Mental Disorders* (*DSM-5*), by the American Psychiatric Association (2013), have been said not to deserve that label. Allan V. Horwitz and Jerome C. Wakefield (2007) have made such an argument in relation to certain forms of depression that they regard as normal responses to distressing life circumstances—something strongly reminiscent of Elliott's (1998) idea of "good" alienation, alienation bound up with authenticity.

Finally, it has been suggested that some people with mental disorders find the concept of a true or authentic self useful when coping with their conditions. For instance, Hope and colleagues (2011, 23) have reported that some patients with anorexia nervosa find it helpful to conceptualize their authentic self as the healthy, non-anorexic one, viewing by contrast their anorexia as an inauthentic part of themselves, against which they are struggling. Such observations raise the question whether the concept of a true self can be of use to clinical practitioners trying to help their patients get better. Another question is whether, even when the concept does appear to help a patient in his or her process of recovery, his or her use of that concept might still in principle conflict with the actual truth about who he or she "really" is—assuming of course there is such a truth.

CONCLUSION

Although it is commonly accepted that authenticity is a significant moral value, there are different ways of thinking about the concept, leading to conflicting positions on certain issues in bioethics. On the one hand, the self-creation approach, with its emphasis on autonomy, seems most relevant to questions about regulation and respect for people's decisions, whether to refuse treatment or to use some neuroenhancer. It is commonly agreed that if these decisions are authentic, they should be respected, provided they do not harm others. The self-discovery model of authenticity, on the other hand, might be more relevant to how we should live our lives and how we should encourage people to live theirs, either directly or by influencing the general social ethos. It also suggests some important concerns about technological interventions into the brain, whether for treatment or enhancement purposes, that the self-creation approach tends to neglect. That said, supporters of the self-discovery model have typically not spelled out their views as fully as those on the other side of the debate. There clearly remains room for further discussion on the question whether the idea of an authentic self can be construed in a plausible manner, as opposed to being merely studied from a sociological perspective, and if it can be so construed, what its exact nature is and how—if at all—the technological interventions previously discussed might threaten a person's proper relation to that self.

SEE ALSO *Emotions; Law and Morality; Natural Law*

BIBLIOGRAPHY

American Psychiatric Association. 2013. *Diagnostic and Statistical Manual of Mental Disorders*. 5th rev. ed. Washington, DC: Author.

"Authenticity." 2012. In *Oxford English Dictionary*, 2nd ed., edited by John Simpson. http://www.oed.com/view/Entry/13325

Bolt, Ineke, and Maartje Schermer. 2009. "Psychopharmaceutical Enhancers: Enhancing Identity?" *Neuroethics* 2 (2): 103–11.

DeGrazia, David. 2005. *Human Identity and Bioethics*. Cambridge, UK: Cambridge University Press.

Elliott, Carl. 1998. "The Tyranny of Happiness: Ethics and Cosmetic Psychopharmacology." In *Enhancing Human Traits: Ethical and Social Implications*, edited by Erik Parens, 177–86. Washington, DC: Georgetown University Press.

Elliott, Carl. 2003. *Better Than Well: American Medicine Meets the American Dream.* New York: Norton.

Erler, Alexandre. 2012. "One Man's Authenticity Is Another Man's Betrayal: A Reply to Levy." *Journal of Applied Philosophy* 29 (3): 257–65.

Frankfurt, Harry G. 1988. *The Importance of What We Care About: Philosophical Essays.* Cambridge, UK: Cambridge University Press.

Hope, Tony; Jacinta Tan; Anne Stewart; et al. 2011. "Anorexia Nervosa and the Language of Authenticity." *Hastings Center Report* 41 (6): 19–29.

Horwitz, Allan V., and Jerome C. Wakefield. 2007. *The Loss of Sadness: How Psychiatry Transformed Normal Sorrow into Depressive Disorder.* Oxford: Oxford University Press.

Jeffries, Stuart. 2002. "The Quest for Truth." *Guardian*, November 29. http://www.guardian.co.uk/books/2002/nov/30/academicexperts.highereducation

Karp, David A. 2006. *Is It Me or My Meds? Living with Antidepressants.* Cambridge, MA: Harvard University Press.

Kraemer, Felicitas. 2009. "Picturing the Authenticity of Emotions." In *Emotions, Ethics, and Authenticity*, edited by Mikko Salmela and Verena Mayer, 71–90. Amsterdam: Benjamins.

Kramer, Peter D. 1993. *Listening to Prozac.* New York: Viking.

Levy, Neil. 2011. "Enhancing Authenticity." *Journal of Applied Philosophy* 28 (3): 308–18.

Mulligan, Kevin. 2009. "Was sind und was sollen die unechten Gefühle?" In *Das Authentische: Zur Konstruktion von Wahrheit in der säkularen Welt*, edited by Ursula Amrein, 225–42. Zurich: Chronos Verlag.

Parens, Erik. 2004. "Kramer's Anxiety." In *Prozac as a Way of Life*, edited by Carl Elliott and Tod Chambers, 21–32. Chapel Hill: University of North Carolina Press.

President's Council on Bioethics. 2003. *Beyond Therapy: Biotechnology and the Pursuit of Happiness.* New York: Dana.

Sartre, Jean-Paul. 1980 [1946]. *Existentialism and Humanism.* Translated by Philip Mairet. London: Methuen.

Singh, Ilina. 2005. "Will the 'Real Boy' Please Behave? Dosing Dilemmas for Parents of Boys with ADHD." *American Journal of Bioethics* 5 (3): 34–47.

Taylor, Charles. 1992. *The Ethics of Authenticity.* Cambridge, MA: Harvard University Press.

Trilling, Lionel. 1972. *Sincerity and Authenticity.* Cambridge, MA: Harvard University Press.

Williams, Bernard A. O. 2002. *Truth and Truthfulness: An Essay in Genealogy.* Princeton, NJ: Princeton University Press.

Alexandre Erler
Research Associate, Oxford Uehiro Centre for Practical Ethics, University of Oxford

AUTHORITY IN RELIGIOUS TRADITIONS

Each of the world's religious traditions must make moral decisions that are both responsive and responsible: responsive to new challenges, and responsible to the moral values that are grounded in the faith and life of its community. Each tradition has different understandings of the sources, vectors, and authority of its teachings. Thus the question, "What does X believe about Y?"—as in, "What does Catholicism believe about contraception?"—is a commonly heard construct in bioethics discussions, but its apparent simplicity masks a multilayered and challenging reality.

A simple way of constructing the inquiry is to ask four questions: (1) What are the sources of authority? (2) What is the method of interpreting those sources? (3) Who are the accepted interpreters? (4) How does the religious community receive those interpretations? Within the traditions, questions of authority are often the focus of the most serious debate. For conservative Protestants, for example, the question of biblical inerrancy is the primary dividing line between conservative and liberal denominations. In addition, the question of belief itself is often posed in an unclear fashion: the questions of what a religion teaches, what its members profess, and what its members practice can yield radically different answers. The question, "What is the Catholic stance on contraception?" could be taken to address what the church hierarchy teaches about the subject, or what the church as a whole (including its lay members) believes, or what members actually practice. Much depends on who is asking the question and for what purpose. The question of authority is especially salient for bioethics, because medical advances are constantly raising new questions. How does a tradition whose founding sources may go back thousands of years respond to issues such as stem cell research or withdrawal of a ventilator?

A nuanced and comprehensive account of sources of authority in even the major religious traditions is beyond the scope of this essay. The question of authority is a circular one in almost any religious tradition because the question of who or what is authoritative is itself a matter for debate. What follows by necessity is a brief overview—not, it is to be hoped, veering toward caricature—of a few traditions that have been chosen for their dissimilarity. The goal is to show how the locus of authority differs among various traditions: in other words, to explicate why the statements "Catholicism teaches …", "Judaism teaches …", and "Buddhism teaches …" are not parallel in terms of the sources and vectors of authority or the expected responses of each faith's adherents.

JUDAISM

All three of the Abrahamic traditions (Judaism, Christianity, Islam) are grounded in an ultimate source of morality, that is, the Word of God as enunciated in Scriptures, or holy texts. However, the three traditions differ sharply as to what counts as "scripture," how it is interpreted, and by whom.

The majority of religious Jews identify with one of three main branches of the tradition: Orthodox, Conservative, and Reform. The primary distinction among these branches is their relationship to halakhah, Jewish law. Halakhah is the compendium of Jewish jurisprudence that begins with the first five books of the Hebrew Bible (said to contain 613 precepts for behavior) and continues with rabbinic commentaries on the Bible, collected in the Mishnah and the Talmud. Among Orthodox Jews, halakhah is the unchanging will of God, not subject to historical development (but needing interpretation, nonetheless, to respond to new questions). Conservative Judaism takes halakhah as decisive but views it as a human rather than divine body of work; Conservative Jews are also more likely to use non-halakhic sources (such as science) as additional grounds for decision. Reform Judaism may use halakhah as one resource for understanding its history, values, and tradition, but does not consider it normative, relying instead on Enlightenment notions of personal autonomy, justice, and individual rights, grounded in divine warrant. Within these broad categories, rabbis, *posek*s (experts), and lay scholars, even when referring to the same texts, may disagree vigorously on practical topics such as when abortion is permissible. Although groups of Jews, especially among the ultra-Orthodox, may follow a particular rabbi, there is no one overarching authority. Thus in *Contemporary Jewish Ethics*, Menachem M. Kellner observes: "One must not ask today, 'What is the Jewish position on such and such?' but rather, 'What is the Orthodox, Conservative, or Reform interpretation of the Jewish position on such and such?'Although many writers persist in presenting *the* Jewish position on various subjects, it very often ought more correctly to be characterized as *a* Jewish position" (1978, 15).

A further complication arises from Judaism's being both an ethnic and a religious category. In both Israel and America, perhaps half the people who check "Jewish" on a hospital admittance form or opinion survey observe few if any religious traditions and are usually referred to as "secular Jews." It would be quite strange to speak of a parallel category of, for instance, "secular Presbyterians." As Ronald M. Green points out in a 1999 essay, secular Jewish perspectives on bioethical issues may still be heavily influenced by the "bioethical sensibility" of Judaism (including, for example, respect for medicine and an activist approach to healing) (166).

CHRISTIANITY

The three largest categories within Christianity are the Eastern Orthodox Church, Roman Catholicism, and Protestantism in its many forms. In large part, the differences that led to these divergences were focused on issues of authority as well as on theology. The schism that led to separate Catholic and Anglican Churches was caused primarily by disagreement over the authority and jurisdiction of the Pope in Rome.

All Christian authority is rooted in Christ and the Gospels. An important difference between Protestant and Roman Catholic Christianity is the former's emphasis on the accessibility of truth directly to the individual layperson, without the mediation of a priest. Thus Martin Luther, the seminal figure of the Protestant Reformation, is known for the slogan *solo scriptura*, or "only Scripture," meaning that the individual can understand the truth by prayerful encounter with the Bible. Although few Protestant sects dispensed entirely with ministers, the movement emphasized lay literacy and Bible reading in the vernacular, and it cannot be separated from Gutenberg's invention of the printing press in the mid-fifteenth century. In contrast, Roman Catholicism, at least until the Second Vatican Council (1962–65), located the power to proclaim and interpret God's word primarily in the bishops and priests, with the laity as relatively passive recipients. The discussion here focuses on Roman Catholicism because it is one of the most hierarchical and (ostensibly) univocal religious traditions, with a relatively clear set of official positions. Yet it is important to understand, first, how much room nonetheless remains for debate, and second, how unusual it is for a tradition to have such an official process that claims to discern the truth for all adherents. (The Church of Jesus Christ of Latter-day Saints [Mormons] is another example.)

James Gustafson points out that Catholicism is like Judaism in possessing a code of law (canon law): "Writings in moral theology are used not only to teach persons what principles ought to guide their conduct and what actions are judged morally illicit, they also provide the priest … with criteria by which he can enumerate and judge the seriousness of various sinful acts in order to assign the appropriate penance" (1978, 1–2). In Protestant church life this juridical role quickly withered (though one could certainly have witnessed it in the Massachusetts Bay Colony), rendering Protestant theological ethics more "pedagogical than juridical" (Gustafson 1978, 3). Because one can hardly expect Scripture alone to answer directly such questions as the morality of organ transplants or sperm banks, all Christian denominations, as Margaret Farley explains in her 2006 book on Christian sexual ethics, have relied on some combination of Scripture, tradition, contemporary experience, and secular disciplines.

Catholic moral theology is pursued in the context of the teaching authority of the Church, which remains "a supreme court of appeals to adjudicate what is morally right and wrong" (Gustafson 1978, 5). In the second half of the twentieth century, after the liberalizing reforms of the Second Vatican Council, and in the beginning of the twenty-first century, during the conservative papacies of John Paul II and Benedict XVI, the outlines of Church authority have been very much contested. "Non-Catholics, as well as many Roman Catholics, often presume that the Catholic Church's teaching authority is clearer and simpler than it actually is either in principle or in practice" (Gustafson 1978, 5). Despite a certain amount of debate, however, the Catholic church makes a claim to monolithic institutional authority that is lacking in Protestantism; one consequence is a greater diversity in Protestant than in Catholic ethics.

A commonly misunderstood element of Roman Catholic teaching is the doctrine of infallibility, which states that the Pope is immune from error when speaking *ex cathedra* ("from the chair") on matters of faith and morals, with the intention of binding the Church. The bishops share in this infallibility when they define a dogma in union with the Pope (e.g., at an ecumenical council). Defined only relatively recently, at the First Vatican Council (1868–70), infallibility appears to refer to a very few doctrines, specifically the Immaculate Conception and Assumption of Mary. Nonetheless, debate continues over the functional infallibility of other teachings, such as *Humanae Vitae* (the 1968 encyclical on birth control) or John Paul II's 1998 pronouncement (*Ad Tuendam Fidem* [To Defend the Faith]) that the ordination of women is a topic closed to discussion. Of great moment is the tension between the obligation of individual conscience and the obligation of obedience, a tension Charles Curran (1986) terms "faithful dissent."

ISLAM

The Arabic term for Islamic law, *sharia*, literally means a path or way to a water hole in the desert. For the desert dwellers living in the time of the Prophet Muhammad, water and direction were essential to life. Sharia is theoretically comprehensive, and Islam, meaning the way of submission to the will of God, is a complete way of life. Thus, as John Kelsay (1994) explains, there is no aspect of life that is not addressed in sharia.

Sharia rests on four sources. The Koran is the compilation of verses revealed orally to Muhammad through an angel, over a twenty-three-year period, and is believed by traditional Muslims to be the verbatim word of God. In addition to the Koran, there are three supplemental sources of Islamic law. The most important is the hadith ("narration"), the accounts of the sayings and doings of the Prophet that embody the Sunna, or normative prescriptions. Not all hadith are considered canonic by all Islamic denominations and legal schools; furthermore, some hadith are considered more authoritative than others. The degree to which a particular hadith is accepted can depend on its coherence with the teachings of the Koran and also with the degree of reliability of its sources and "chain of transmission." The next source of law is *ijtihad*, analogical, case-oriented reasoning whose method closely parallels that of the Jewish and Roman Catholic casuistic traditions. *Ijtihad* comes from the root *jihad*, meaning to struggle (in this case, the religious scholar's struggle to implement God's law in human institutions). *Fiqh*, or Islamic jurisprudence, applies these resources to problems of the day, such as proper observance of ritual, medical issues, social legislation, and so on. Among Sunni Muslims, who comprise about 85 percent of Islam, there are four major schools of *fiqh*.

Finally, there is *ijma*, or consensus. According to Eric Winkel, consensus as the concept of the "informal agreement of the community" has an overriding authority, and yet "there is no consensus on the definition of consensus" (1995, 3). Consensus could include literally the whole community, or could apply only to the community of *ulama* (interpreters) or only to *ulama* of a certain age.

> The legal discourse of Islam may be conceived of as a more or less flexible superstructure erected over the shari'ah, which in turn may be defined as the set of injunctions emanating from the Qur'an and Sunnah. … Those who deal with this superstructure, and help it flex and bend to meet new circumstances, may be loosely defined as the *ulama*, those who have knowledge. This amorphous people, women and men, are recognized in their communities by their knowledge. (Winkel 1995, 3)

Prominent religious leaders issue religious opinions in the form of a fatwa, but there is no one authority, even within the different branches of Islam. In that sense, Islam is much like Judaism, with adherents clustering around one or several leaders, who may issue differing fatwas on such bioethical issues as the permissibility of organ donation.

BUDDHISM

Buddhism is a religious and philosophical tradition based on the teachings of a historical figure, Siddhartha Gautama, who lived in the Indian subcontinent sometime during the fifth century B.C.E. and is commonly called the Buddha, or "awakened one." After his death, Buddhism split into two large schools, Mahayana and Theravada, and each of those schools into many subtraditions. The casual observer would be hard put to connect the simplicity of Zen with the polychromatic exuberance of Tibetan Buddhism. Yet, at the level of moral teachings, there is much common ground, namely the principles and precepts originally expounded in the Four Noble Truths, the Eightfold Path, and other teachings of the Buddha. Our knowledge of the Buddha's teachings is based on several canons of scripture, which derived from oral transmission by early Buddhist religious orders. "These canons gradually diverged as different floating oral traditions were drawn on, and systemizing tests peculiar to each school were added" (Harvey 2000, 4).

Buddhist ethics seeks to apply the Buddha's teachings to worldly concerns, and it is those teachings that are the ultimate authority. The foundation of Buddhist ethics lies in the concept of Dharma, the universal law that governs the universe, and with which human actions should be in harmony. The ultimate goal is complete spiritual liberation, traditionally framed as freedom from rebirth; one attains this through morality, meditation, and insight.

Actions are judged to be good or bad largely by the intent and character of the actor, a view not unlike Western virtue ethics. "An analysis of the mental process of the decision maker is as important as the analysis of available information regarding the issue" (Taniguchi 1994, 38). But actions are also characterized by good results: "right actions are those that are wholesome and do no harm to either oneself or others" (Keown 2005, 6). Right behavior can be summed up by the Five Precepts, which all Buddhists formally accept: refraining from violence, stealing, lying, sexual immorality, and intoxicants.

Buddhism never developed a detailed code of conduct for laypeople, although there are very specific codes of discipline for those in monastic orders. Thus modern Buddhists attempting to shape a Buddhist response to such issues as in vitro fertilization find themselves thrown back on the original precepts and example of the Buddha himself, without a dense layer of mediating structures.

The vectors of authority in Buddhism are diffuse, varying among sects, branches, and countries. A questioner would go to her local priest, and the priest would work his or her way up an institutional hierarchy. For Tibetan Buddism, the Dalai Lama is the ultimate authority, meaning not merely the current person, but the whole tradition that stands behind him.

Buddhism's focus on personal spiritual development and its lack of theistic claims allow it to coexist easily with other religious traditions. In Asia, Buddhism has joined with Shintoism and Confucianism; in North America, some informal counts show that as many as a third of adherents are Jewish. These people may not think of themselves as "converts" to Buddhism but as adding Buddhism to existing belief and practice. Thus an individual's code of ethics may be a personal mix of Buddhist precepts and principles and practices from other traditions.

RECEPTION

Bioethics is an applied field of study that can never lose its grip on real-world questions, responses, and behaviors. Thus it is important for bioethicists not to lose sight of the final source of religious authority: reception by the faith community. There are very few nations left in the modern world where religious authorities can dictate the attitudes and behavior of their community of adherents.

An interesting example in the United States is the reaction by a number of Roman Catholic organizations to a feature of the Affordable Care Act, signed into law by President Barack Obama in 2010. The health care law requires almost all employers to cover the cost of contraceptives as part of employee health insurance plans. Roman Catholic dioceses, schools, and other institutions protested that paying for their employees' contraceptives would force them to go against Church doctrine, which forbids artificial contraception. Public discussion of this issue in 2012 commonly cited a 2011 survey by the Guttmacher Institute that found that Catholic women were as likely as other American women to make use of artificial contraception. What the official spokespersons say and what self-identified Catholics actually do are not necessarily the same thing. To use another example, formal Jewish teaching, which embraces the value of life, including at life's end, entails some of the most restrictive and vitalist teachings of any major religion. It leaves little room for withdrawal of life support, much less active assistance in hastening the dying process. And yet, in surveys of physicians cited by Green (1999), those who identified as Jewish were among the most open to accepting some form of physician-assisted death. Thus the way a faith community receives religious authority is mediated by numerous other factors, such as socioeconomic status, personal experiences, and the surrounding culture.

SEE ALSO *Autonomy; Body: II. Cultural and Religious Perspectives; Buddhism, Bioethics in; Christianity, Bioethics in; Coercion; Consensus, Role and Authority of; Embryo and Fetus: V. Religious Perspectives; Ethics: V. Religion and Morality; Islam, Bioethics in; Judaism, Bioethics in; Population Ethics: III. Introduction to Religious Traditions*

BIBLIOGRAPHY

Cahill, Lisa. 1990. "Can We Get Real About Sex?" *Commonweal* 117 (15): 497–503.

Curran, Charles. 1986. *Faithful Dissent*. Kansas City, MO: Sheed and Ward.

Davis, Dena S. 1994. "Method in Jewish Bioethics." In *Religious Methods and Resources in Bioethics*, edited by Paul F. Camenisch, 109–26. Dordrecht, Netherlands, and Boston: Kluwer.

Davis, Dena S. 1999. "It Ain't Necessarily So: Clinicians, Bioethics, and Religious Studies." In *Notes from a Narrow Ridge: Religion and Bioethics*, edited by Dena S. Davis and Laurie Zoloth, 9–19. Hagerstown, MD: University Publishing Group.

Farley, Margaret. 2006. *Just Love: A Framework for Christian Sexual Ethics*. New York: Continuum.

Green, Ronald M. 1999. "Religions' 'Bioethical Sensibility': A Research Agenda." In *Notes from a Narrow Ridge: Religion and Bioethics*, edited by Dena S. Davis and Laurie Zoloth, 165–82. Hagerstown, MD: University Publishing Group.

Gustafson, James M. 1978. *Protestant and Roman Catholic Ethics: Prospects for Rapprochement*. Chicago: University of Chicago Press.

Harvey, Peter. 2000. *An Introduction to Buddhist Ethics: Foundations, Values, and Issues*. Cambridge, UK, and New York: Cambridge University Press.

Kellner Menachem Marc, ed. 1978. *Contemporary Jewish Ethics*. New York: Sanhedrin Press.

Kelsay, John. 1994. "Islam and Medical Ethics." In *Religious Methods and Resources in Bioethics*, edited by Paul F. Camenisch, 93–108. Dordrecht, Netherlands, and Boston: Kluwer.

Keown, Damien. 1992. *The Nature of Buddhist Ethics*. New York: St. Martin's.

Keown, Damien. 2005. *Buddhist Ethics: A Very Short Introduction*. Oxford, UK, and New York: Oxford University Press.

McBrien, Richard P. 1980. *Catholicism*. Vol. 2. Minneapolis, MN: Winston Press.

Newman, Louis E. 1994. "Text and Tradition in Contemporary Jewish Ethics." In *Religious Methods and Resources in Bioethics*, edited by Paul F. Camenisch, 127–43. Dordrecht, Netherlands, and Boston: Kluwer.

Taniguchi, Shoyo. 1994. "Methodology of Buddhist Biomedical Ethics." In *Religious Methods and Resources in Bioethics*, edited by Paul F. Camenisch, 31–66. Dordrecht, Netherlands, and Boston: Kluwer.

Winkel, Eric. 1995. "A Muslim Perspective on Female Circumcision." *Women Health* 23 (1): 1–7.

Dena S. Davis
Professor, Religion Studies, Lehigh University

AUTONOMY

The concept of autonomy in moral philosophy and bioethics recognizes the human capacity for self-determination, and puts forward a principle that the autonomy of persons ought to be respected. At this level of generality, there is not much with which to take issue; a full account of autonomy must further define self-determination and state how and to what extent autonomy should be respected. Autonomy as a capacity of persons must be distinguished from autonomy as a property of actions and decisions, for a person with the capacity for autonomy may act non-autonomously on particular occasions, for example, when coerced to do something. Autonomy as a fundamental value and a basic right is part of the moral and political theory of liberal individualism. According to this view, autonomous individuals are the ultimate source of value: The basis for an action, social practice or government policy to be right or good lies in the values, preferences or choices of autonomous individuals. In social philosophy, individual autonomy as a basic value and a fundamental right may be in tension with community values, such as caring for others, promoting the good of society, and preserving and enhancing the moral practices of society. In clinical bioethics, the right to autonomy of individual patients exists in tension with health care professionals' obligations to benefit patients. These conflicts will be examined in what follows.

AUTONOMY AS CAPACITY

According to Stanley Benn in *A Theory of Freedom* (1988) and Lawrence Haworth in *Autonomy: An Essay in Philosophical Psychology and Ethics* (1986), there are three elements to the psychological capacity of autonomy: agency, independence, and rationality. Agency is awareness of oneself as having desires and intentions and acting on them. (Desire includes inclinations, aversions, wants, and similar terms.) When people have a desire for some state of affairs, they form an intention to do what they believe will bring about the desired state of affairs; further, they want their desire to determine their action.

The capacity for agency distinguishes persons from inanimate objects and from nonhuman animals. Inanimate objects can be affected by objects and conditions external to them, as can persons, but unlike persons, inanimate objects cannot be said to act on desires. Nonhuman animals have desires, but there is no (noncontroversial) reason to believe that they have the capacity for self-consciousness that is manifest in having an awareness of desires and wanting them to be effective in action. Agency does not imply that persons are never influenced by external forces or that persons never act impulsively. It is an account of how persons are able to act and not how they always act.

Independence is the absence of influences that so control a person's behavior that it cannot be said that he or she wants to act as he does. This may seem a feature of an autonomous action rather than an element of psychological capacity. Cases exist, however, in which a person's course of life is under constant threat of violence from others, and the person always acts to avoid harm: war, poverty, abusive relationships, police states. When the whole of a person's beliefs, plans, self-image, and ways of relating to others are the result of unrelenting coercion and manipulation, then that person has little or no capacity for autonomy.

According to the 1986 book *The Morality of Freedom* by Joseph Raz, autonomy also requires that persons have an adequate range of options. Coercion and manipulation limit options, but options are also limited by social and physical environments. If a person's options are numerous and noncoerced, but are trivial in relation to what is valued by the person, then there is no capacity for autonomy in a significant sense. This would be the case in a totalitarian, caste, or slave society where a combination of coercion and ideology suppress the aspirations and real options of a segment of society. A full account of the conception of autonomy must distinguish external influences that defeat autonomy from external influences that are consistent with being autonomous. The former includes coercion and manipulation, and the latter includes persuasion and the normal limitations of physical and social environments.

The third element of the capacity for autonomy is means-end rationality, or rational decision making. In addition to the self-consciousness of agency, the capacity for rational decision making requires a person:

1. whose beliefs are subject to standards of truth and evidence;
2. with ability to recognize commitments and to act on them;
3. who can construct and evaluate alternative decisions;
4. whose changes in beliefs and values can change decisions and actions; and
5. whose beliefs and values yield rankings of action commitments.

Gerald Dworkin, in his 1976 article "Autonomy and Behavior Control," and James Childress, in his 1990 article "The Place of Autonomy in Bioethics," argue that another way to understand rationality as an element of the capacity for autonomy is as the capacity for reflection on desires. A rational person can have a desire for or fear of something, such as a desire for food or a fear of surgery, and also have the wish that he or she not have that desire or not be moved by that fear. Persons who lack the psychological capacity for rational decision making are those who are severely mentally ill—paranoiacs, compulsive neurotics, schizophrenics, and psychopaths. Such persons have the capacity for agency, that is, they are aware of acting on their desires, but they fail to meet one or more of the above conditions. Benn (1988) gives the example of a paranoid patient who persists in a delusion that the health care professionals are Martians attempting to capture him as unable to adjust beliefs and actions to a reality confirmed by evidence.

PRINCIPLE OF RESPECT FOR AUTONOMY

Principles that support autonomy can be directed at the everyday relationships and encounters between persons; at the constitution, laws, and regulations of a nation-state; and at the policies of institutions such as hospitals, insurance companies, schools, and corporations. What ought to be done to respect autonomy will not be the same at all these levels and will be a function of a broad social ideology.

The minimal content for a principle of respect for autonomy is that persons ought to have independence, that is, be free from coercion and other similar interferences. John Stuart Mill made this the main principle in *On Liberty* (1947): No one should interfere with the liberty of action of another except to prevent harm to others. This obligation not to coerce others is defensible as an obligation binding on individuals, private organizations, and governments. Mill defended his principle of liberty, not because he believed that there is a fundamental right to autonomy nor that autonomy is valuable in itself, but because the recognition of liberty is supported by the principle of utility. This principle is that an action or policy is right to the extent that it promotes the greater happiness for the greater number. Securing negative liberty, however, does not establish autonomy as fundamental in moral theory. Other philosophers have gone further than Mill in their defense of autonomy.

The most widely quoted principle of respect for autonomy is one of Immanuel Kant's versions of the categorical imperative: "Treat others and oneself, never merely as a means, but always at the same time as an end in himself" (Kant 1956, 101). This is frequently expressed as treating others as persons, and its distinctive Kantian claim is that others should be treated as rational beings who have their own ends. A further explanation of this principle is that persons should be seen as having interests in two senses. First, persons have interests in those things that are a benefit to nearly everyone, for example, being free of pain, not being killed, being saved from dying. A physician can treat a patient without that person's consent and still protect these interests. Second, autonomous persons "take an interest" in things, that is, have preferences, projects, and plans. Acting only with concern to serve interests in the first sense, as is sometimes alleged against uses of the principle of utility, is insufficient for respecting another's autonomy; we must also discover and take into account the individual's values and objectives (Benn 1988). For example, a physician may believe that a surgical procedure is an effective treatment to relieve the pain of a patient's ulcer, but the patient may have a greater aversion to the risks of surgery than the physician does, and would prefer a restricted diet and medication. To not solicit, or to ignore, the patient's preferences in this matter would not respect his or her autonomy.

AUTONOMY, RIGHTS, AND LIBERTY

The concept of rights presupposes that right-holders are beings with the capacity for autonomy, who make choices and can use discretion whether or not to exercise a right. Basic liberties in a liberal democracy are protected by constitutional and other legal rights. The idea of a right has three elements: the right-holder (the person who has the right); the object of the right (the activity or thing to which the right-holder has a right); and the duty-bearer (the person or institution who must do what the right requires). Negative rights are rights not to be interfered with; for example, everyone has the right not to be given medical treatment without consent, and all health care providers must respect this right. Positive rights are rights that a person be provided with something—for example, the right of all senior citizens in the United States to Medicare payment for health care, a right binding on government agencies and health care providers.

Recognizing the negative right to autonomy imposes on everyone the obligation not to coerce or otherwise interfere with the action of another. This protection of autonomy is not as costly to social institutions as recognizing positive rights to autonomy. If there is a positive right to *X*, this means that someone is under an obligation to provide *X* to the right-holder(s). For example, if every citizen has a fundamental positive right to the best quality medical care, then the state must provide full access to medical care to all citizens. While there cannot be a positive right to autonomy per se—for autonomy as capacity is not something that can simply be given to persons who do not have it—there can be rights to other things required for, or supportive of, autonomy. Among them are rights to a decent minimum of health care and education, a decent standard of living, political participation, freedom of inquiry and expression, and equal opportunity to compete for positions in society. These goods contribute to autonomy in two ways: first, they make possible the development of the capacity for autonomy; second, they make autonomy meaningful by establishing the personal and social powers and range of options for autonomously chosen projects and plans. Discrimination against minorities and women decreases their autonomy by explicitly excluding them from desirable positions in society and by implicitly agreeing to the limited range of options offered to minorities and women.

AUTONOMY AS AN IDEAL

There is no sharp line separating accounts of autonomy as an ideal from autonomy as an actual capacity of persons. Autonomy can be described as a high level of self-determination few persons will actually achieve, and yet it can still be regarded as a capacity for all persons, if it is believed that all persons under suitable conditions could acquire it and use it to direct their lives. Views that describe autonomy at a level that nearly all normal adult persons can and do exercise are views of autonomy as capacity, and views that describe it at a higher level are accounts of autonomy as an ideal.

Autonomy as an ideal will center on a person's use of the capacity for deliberation and reflection. The person who realizes the ideal of autonomy is, first, one who is consciously aware of having the capacity, someone who believes that he or she can use it to shape his or her life. Second, the autonomous person will make particular decisions with a sense of control—creating and evaluating options. That person will also reflect on how values, preferences, attitudes, and beliefs received in the socialization process function in his or her own decision making, examine the kind of person this makes him or her, consider alternatives, and make a commitment to accept or try to alter who he or she is. This is, of course, a matter of degree; like every virtue, it can be realized well and thoroughly or in some small measure. The ideal of autonomy does not require individuals to make conscious, deliberate decisions before every action. A person who has accepted a set of preferences, beliefs, and attitudes can respond without much thinking to common situations that fall into recognized patterns.

AUTONOMY OF ACTIONS

In a clinical setting, it is often important to determine whether a patient's decision regarding treatment, or the decision of a proxy in the case of an incompetent patient, is autonomous. A person who has the capacity for autonomy may, for a variety of reasons, not act autonomously on a particular occasion. Determining whether a particular action or decision is autonomous is a matter of how the three elements of the capacity for autonomy (agency, independence, and rationality) are involved in the process of deciding. The autonomy of actions is a matter of degree because independence and rationality are matters of degree, though agency is not.

Ruth Faden and her colleagues Tom Beauchamp and Nancy King, in their book *A History and Theory of Informed Consent* (1986), describe the three elements of autonomy as intentionality, freedom from controlling influence, and understanding. They point out that controlling influences and understanding can be seen on two independent continua. An action can be performed within the range of full understanding to full ignorance, and within the range of completely uncontrolled to completely controlled.

Bruce Miller in his 1981 article "Autonomy and the Refusal of Lifesaving Treatment," views the autonomy of actions and decisions on four levels: (1) as free action (agency and independence); (2) as authenticity (the decision is consistent with what is known about the person's values, preferences, and plans); (3) as effective deliberation (rationality); and (4) as moral reflection (deliberation about one's values, preferences, and plans). The decision of a patient may be autonomous at one or more but not all levels. For example, a patient who accepts a recommended treatment without reflecting much about the decision, acted autonomously at the level of free action, and perhaps authenticity, but not at the levels of rationality and moral reflection.

The legal concept of competence is closely related to the concept of autonomy. A competent person is one who has the capacity for autonomy, and a competent decision is one that is autonomously made.

David Jackson and Stuart Youngner present six cases of decision making in an intensive-care unit that "illustrate specific situations in which superficial preoccupation with the issues of patient autonomy and death with dignity could have led to inappropriate clinical and ethical decisions" (Jackson and Youngner 1979, 407). In one of the cases, a patient with multiple sclerosis appeared autonomously to refuse further lifesaving treatment following a suicide attempt. Psychiatric evaluation, however, showed that the patient had become depressed and withdrawn at the time his wife and sons began spending time with his mother-in-law, who had been diagnosed with inoperable cancer.

Jay Katz in his book *The Silent World of Doctor and Patient* (1984) has said that insufficient attention has been given to the unconscious and irrational motivations of behavior. It is not only patients' motivations that should be examined, but physicians' as well, for example, their denial of uncertainty. Whether a patient's decision to consent to or refuse treatment is autonomous depends on more than the patient's statement of decision and reasons. Physicians and patients must engage in conversations; physicians are obligated to facilitate patients' opportunities for reflection to prevent ill-considered decisions, and patients are obligated to participate in the process of thinking about their choices. The US President's Commission (1982) echoes this view in its discussion of the importance of communication between patient and health professional to attain shared decision making based on mutual trust.

PRIVACY, INFORMED CONSENT, AND PATERNALISM

Autonomy as a fundamental right is used to justify rights to privacy, confidentiality, refusal of treatment, informed consent, and a decent minimum of health care. The legal right to privacy has two components. The right to control information about oneself is protected in medicine as the patient's right to confidentiality of information gained by health professionals. The right not to be interfered with and to make one's own decisions is protected in medicine as a competent patient's right to refuse recommended treatment and as the obligation of health professionals to obtain a patient's informed consent to treatment. Informed consent requires that a patient be informed of a recommended treatment and of the options for treatment and their likely consequences, and that the patient give express permission for a treatment (often in writing). The right to autonomy also requires that patients be told the truth about their medical status and prognosis, that their questions be answered, and that they receive assistance from health care providers in making rational decisions. Meaningful exercise of the right to autonomy in living requires that individuals possess physical and psychological capacities within the normal, human range. So the positive right to autonomy supports a right to a level of health care that will return a person to and maintain him at the normal range of functioning. This includes acute care, for example, repair of a broken bone; chronic care, for example, treatment of diabetes or heart disease; and supportive care for permanent disability, for example, wheelchairs for paraplegics.

Paternalism in health care is treating a patient against his or her wishes on the grounds that the health care provider is professionally obligated to provide care that will benefit patients, and that the health care provider knows better than the patient what is good for the patient. When paternalism is justified, it overrides patient autonomy, at least partially. An example of justified paternalism could be when a physician does not accede to a patient's refusal of emergency treatment because the patient believes he or she will surely die.

CRITICISMS OF AUTONOMY

Some authors have criticized the centrality of autonomy in medical decision making (Clements and Sider 1983; Callahan 1984; Thomasma 1984). Their argument states that the primary obligation of health care providers is to maintain and restore health. There are two aspects to this claim. First, if patient autonomy is given primacy over the obligations of health professionals, physicians and other providers may violate their obligation to maintain and restore the health of patients; for example, a patient may refuse a treatment that will save his or her life or prevent a serious illness. These conflicts between autonomy and patient benefit have often been decided by courts, usually in the form of a request by a terminally ill patient's family member or other agent that life-preserving treatments such as respirators be withdrawn, a request denied by physicians who cite their obligation to preserve life.

A second aspect of the criticism of autonomy recognizes the centrality of patients' values and wishes in cases of deciding whether to forgo life-preserving treatment for a terminally ill patient, but other sorts of medical care decisions depend less on respecting patients' rights to autonomy and more on the value of restoring and maintaining the capacity for living a meaningful life. In this sort of case, autonomy is secondary to principles of beneficence, compassion, and caring.

Defenders of autonomy can make several replies to this critique. (1) Some of the attacks on autonomy wrongly assume that it is simply a principle of negative freedom, that is, the right not to be interfered with. (2) The claim of the centrality of patient autonomy in medicine does not imply that it is the only value. The principles of beneficence or non-maleficence may, in some circumstances, justify paternalism. (3) Autonomy cannot be ignored in medical decision making. Knowing what will be most beneficial for a patient often requires input from the patient on values, objectives, and preferences. This is true not only in morally difficult situations that call for a decision about preserving the life of a terminally ill patient, but in less dramatic cases as well, for example, whether a patient should have surgery for a condition that causes minor discomfort and dysfunction but will not develop into something more threatening to health, or whether the patient should simply "live with" the condition. In cases of acute and severe injury or illness where there is clearly a best treatment that will almost certainly restore the patient to health, it can usually be safely assumed that whatever else the patient values, he or she will value the restoration of health, and hence, discussion of the relative value of options and their consequences is not required to respect the autonomy of the patient.

Criticisms of autonomy have also been launched from a broader, communitarian perspective (MacIntyre 1981; Sandel 1982; Callahan 1984). Communitarians charge that the political theory of liberal individualism states that individuals are fully self-determining and that rights to autonomy are the primary or sole standard for individual behavior, institutional practices, and government policy. Communitarians object to liberal individualism on several grounds. First, the socialization process determines, or shapes, the values and preferences of individuals; hence, the idea of autonomously chosen values is factually incorrect. Second, an individual's actions, desires, and objectives are comprehensible only within the context of social conventions and institutions. For example, a person cannot report that he or she is thinking about depositing a check without the conventions of language and the institution of banking. Third, the view that an autonomous individual chooses his or her own values, preferences, and desires presupposes a self that does the choosing. This self will have to have a core of values with which to choose, in which case either there are values not autonomously chosen, or it is inexplicable how individuals come to have a set of values. Communitarians also claim that liberal individualism regards persons as separate from others in the sense that individuals have no obligations to others or to society that are not voluntarily assumed, other than the obligation to respect the individual rights of others. A society that respects only the autonomy rights of all its members is not morally complete. As Daniel Callahan argues in his 1984 article "Autonomy: A Moral Good, Not a Moral Obsession," a good society must recognize obligations to help others; its members must have virtues such as compassion, caring, and love, and they should recognize a commitment to society to maintain social practices and institutions that establish and promote these obligations and virtues.

There may be theories of autonomy that are susceptible to these criticisms, but the fundamental value of autonomy can be defended without embracing such versions of liberal individualism (Sher 1989; Taylor 1985). The conceptions of autonomy presented above recognize that persons are social beings whose values and preferences are shaped by society and that the capacity for autonomy is itself socially determined. Being autonomous requires language and reason, and these abilities are not possible without socially given practices and standards. Reflecting on socially given values and preferences and either accepting them as one's own or changing them in some measure, which is a feature of autonomous persons, cannot be done unless there is a social environment that encourages autonomy. A free society makes autonomy possible.

Amy Gutmann argues, however, in her 1985 article "Communitarian Critics of Liberalism," that a society in which no one does more or less than respect everyone else's liberal rights, in which there is no caring, love, or friendship and no neighborhood associations, political parties, or civic groups, is not one we would want, though it may be a liberal society. Alternatively, a society organized to promote civic virtues and obligations such as beneficence, caring, and compassion, but which does not recognize a right of individuals to be different, to make their own decisions about matters of importance to them or to find a style of life that makes them happy, is also not one we would want. Love and care can be stifling if they do not recognize an individual's own view of what his or her good is. Finally, a defensible theory of the nature and value of individual autonomy will fall between radical individualism and extreme collectivism. It must explain the obligations to create and maintain social and political institutions that support the exercise and flourishing of autonomy. It must explain how the exercise of autonomy depends on the opportunity range and values given in the traditions and structure of society. It will also recognize other fundamental values and explain their place in decision making.

In the early period of contemporary medical ethics, much attention was on medical paternalism in cases of life-and-death decision making for terminally ill patients and on what can be called "medical opportunism" in research on human subjects. Critics of these practices brought the rights of patients and subjects to the forefront of medical ethics. In a climate of concern for allocation of health care resources and other issues of social policy, autonomy appears less frequently in medical ethics literature than do moral concepts such as justice, fairness, equality, economic efficiency, and cost-containment. This shift in issues should not lead to the view that autonomy has lost its importance in moral and social theory and in bioethics.

BIBLIOGRAPHY

Benn, Stanley I. 1988. *A Theory of Freedom*. Cambridge, UK: Cambridge University Press.

Berg, Jessica; Paul Appelbaum; Charles Lidz; and Lisa Parker, eds. 2001. *Informed Consent: Legal Theory and Clinical Practice*. 2nd ed. New York: Oxford University Press.

Callahan, Daniel. 1984. "Autonomy: A Moral Good, Not a Moral Obsession." *Hastings Center Report* 14 (5): 40–42.

Childress, James F. 1990. "The Place of Autonomy in Bioethics." *Hastings Center Report* 20 (1): 12–17.

Clements, Colleen D., and Roger C. Sider. 1983. "Medical Ethics' Assault upon Medical Values." *Journal of the American Medical Association* 250 (15): 2011–15.

Davies John K. 2002. "The Concept of Precedent Autonomy." *Bioethics* 16 (2): 114–33.

Donchin, A. 2001. "Understanding Autonomy Relationally: Toward a Reconfiguration of Bioethical Principles." *Journal of Medicine and Philosophy* 26 (4): 365–86.

Dworkin, Gerald. 1976. "Autonomy and Behavior Control." *Hastings Center Report* 6 (1): 23–28.

Dworkin, Gerald. 1988. *The Theory and Practice of Autonomy*. Cambridge, UK: Cambridge University Press.

Ells, C. 2001. "Shifting the Autonomy Debate to Theory as Ideology." *Journal of Medicine and Philosophy* 26 (4): 417–30.

Faden, Ruth R.; Tom Beauchamp; and Nancy M. P. King. 1986. *A History and Theory of Informed Consent*. New York: Oxford University Press.

Gaylin Willard. 1996. "Worshiping Autonomy." *Hastings Center Report* 26 (6): 43–45.

Gutmann, Amy. 1985. "Communitarian Critics of Liberalism." *Philosophy and Public Affairs* 14 (3): 308–22.

Haworth, Lawrence. 1986. *Autonomy: An Essay in Philosophical Psychology and Ethics*. New Haven, CT: Yale University Press.

Kant, Immanuel. 1964. *Groundwork of the Metaphysics of Morals*. Translated and edited by Herbert James Paton. New York: Harper & Row.

Katz, Jay. 1984. *The Silent World of Doctor and Patient*. New York: Free Press.

Jackson, David L., and Stuart Youngner. 1979. "Patient Autonomy and 'Death with Dignity.'" *New England Journal of Medicine* 301 (8): 404–8.

MacIntyre, Alasdair C. 1981. *After Virtue: A Study in Moral Theory*. Notre Dame, IN: University of Notre Dame Press.

Mill, John Stuart. 1947. *On Liberty*. Edited by Aubrey Castell. New York: Appleton-Century-Crofts.

Miller, Bruce L. 1981. "Autonomy and the Refusal of Lifesaving Treatment." *Hastings Center Report* 11 (4): 22–28.

Pantilat, Steven Z. 1996. "Patient-Physician Communication: Respect for Culture, Religion, and Autonomy." *Journal of the American Medical Association* 275 (2): 107–10.

Raz, Joseph. 1986. *The Morality of Freedom*. Oxford: Clarendon Press.

Sandel, Michael J. 1982. *Liberalism and the Limits of Justice*. Cambridge, UK: Cambridge University Press.

Schneider, Carl E. 1998. *The Practice of Autonomy: Patients, Doctors, and Medical Decisions*. New York: Oxford University Press.

Sher, George. 1989. "Three Grades of Social Involvement." *Philosophy and Public Affairs* 18 (2): 133–57.

Taylor, Charles. 1985. "Atomism." *Philosophical Papers: Philosophy and the Human Sciences* 2. Cambridge, UK: Cambridge University Press.

Taylor, Charles. 1991. *The Ethics of Authenticity*. Cambridge, MA: Harvard University Press.

Thomasma, David C. 1985. "Freedom, Dependency, and the Care of the Very Old." *Journal of the American Geriatrics Society* 32 (12): 906–14.

US President's Commission for the Study of Ethical Problems in Medicine and Biomedical and Behavioral Research. 1982. *Making Health Care Decisions: A Report on the Ethical and Legal Implications of Informed Consent in the Patient-Practitioner Relationship*. Washington, DC: Government Printing Office.

Wear, Stephen; Tristam H. Engelhardt; and Kevin W. Wildes, eds. 1998. *Informed Consent: Patient Autonomy and Clinician Beneficence within Health Care*. 2nd ed. Washington, DC: Georgetown University Press.

Bruce L. Miller (1995)
Professor Emeritus, Department of Philosophy, Michigan State University

AUTONOMY [ADDENDUM]

The previous entry conceives of autonomy mainly (but not completely) in thin, procedural terms, marked by *inter alia* agency, independence, and rationality or intentionality, voluntariness (freedom from controlling influence), and understanding. Over the last several years, there have been vigorous debates about whether thicker and more substantive conceptions of autonomy are more defensible conceptually, empirically, and ethically. These debates have spawned a huge literature in both bioethics and philosophy (see, e.g., Taylor 2005; Taylor 2009; Christman 2011). Moreover, in contrast to some of their predecessors who opposed autonomy as a masculinist value, many recent feminist philosophers and bioethicists have sought to reconceive autonomy as relational rather than individualistic (Mackenzie and Stoljar 2000; Stoljar 2013). Relational autonomy has received broad and positive attention. However, despite some shared themes among conceptions of relational autonomy, there is considerable variety, and several conceptions include aspects of other thick, substantive notions of autonomy. (For a depiction of the variety of feminist thought on autonomy, see Stoljar 2013; for a perspective on autonomy from non-western cultures, see Traphagan 2013.)

In relational autonomy—also called "autonomy in a relational context," "situated autonomy," "contextual autonomy"—attention is not limited to the immediate decision, "the moment of medical decision making," but rather encompasses the broader context of relations that shape those decisions (Sherwin 1998, 19, 32). Proponents of relational autonomy, particularly (but not only) feminist thinkers, have criticized common individualistic interpretations and applications of the principle of respect for autonomy. Relational autonomists view as very problematic the dominant picture of the self they find—and sometimes exaggerate—in descriptions of autonomy, especially in bioethics: individualistic, self-made, self-interested, independent, atomistic, isolated, insulated, disembodied, rationalistic, emotionless, and the like.

Of course, very few proponents of thin and procedural conceptions of autonomy accept all of these characteristics, which represent tendencies in some conceptions. These tendencies have evoked several criticisms. Autonomy, understood as self-rule or self-governance, does not mean self-creation. The independence emphasized by proponents of personal autonomy need not deny interdependence in community and the emergence and expression of the self in relationships. For relationalists, individuals' autonomous choices are not given, individualistically achieved, or unchangeable. Instead, we need to recognize, in the words of feminist philosopher Susan Sherwin, "the importance of supportive social conditions for fostering autonomous action." According to Sherwin, "Relational autonomy redefines autonomy as the social project it is, but it does not deny that autonomy ultimately resides in individuals" (Sherwin 1998, 39).

The self is frequently an oppressed self, as many feminist critiques emphasize. Hence, it is important to examine critically the constraints and limitations under which many persons exercise—or attempt to exercise—their autonomy. Some of these conditions may be forms of social injustice that thwart autonomy by limiting options.

Proponents of relational autonomy also stress that we are "temporally extended selves" (Baumann 2008, 445). "Under relational theory," Sherwin writes, "selfhood is seen as an ongoing process, rather than as something static or fixed" (Sherwin 1998, 35). Hence, it is essential to consider the self over time as well as in relation. We have to put a person's current consents and dissents in a broad temporal context that includes the past and the future as well as the present. This complicates respect for autonomy if a person's choices at T2 or T3 differ from those at T1. Sometimes physicians and other caregivers must determine whether to override a person's present choices and actions in light of his or her past or anticipated future choices and actions. Questions of authenticity noted in passing in the above entry become very important at this juncture, but it is critical not to rule out the possibilities either of subtle shifts or of dramatic changes in a person's framework of values.

Some proponents of relational autonomy build moral responsibility into their conception of autonomy. For them, autonomous persons recognize and act on their responsibilities to others, including the society (McLean 2010). This move appears in Onora O'Neill's (2002) Kantian-influenced substitution of "principled autonomy" for personal or individual autonomy in bioethics. From these standpoints, we are not being autonomous if we do not attend to the impact of our decisions and actions on others. A different approach holds that people's decisions may still be autonomous even when they are unethical in failing to attend to relational responsibilities (Beauchamp and Childress 2013). In such circumstances, their actions may be justifiably overridden even though they satisfy thin and procedural conditions for autonomy. That some choices are unethical does not indicate that they are non-autonomous. Take, for instance, a person's refusal to follow a governmental order for quarantine in a public health crisis. That refusal could be an autonomous choice but could also be unethical and justifiably overridden in the name of other values. Proponents of autonomy and respect for autonomy need not give it absolute priority.

Thick conceptions of autonomy—this addendum has only focused on selected themes in relational autonomy—direct our attention beyond moments of decision making and conditions such as rationality, intentionality, and voluntariness to the wide range of contexts and factors that surround and influence decision making. For instance, relational perspectives lead caregivers not to assume automatically that what particular patients say or do represents their autonomous choices. Instead, in a caring relationship, it is often important to engage in conversation about and to probe and test persons' decisions and actions. This is an important implication of relational autonomy.

There is a danger that useful aspects of thicker conceptions of autonomy will be turned into necessary conditions for autonomy, conditions that would then ground respect for autonomy. The concern is that this would set a standard for autonomous actions that is too high and too demanding (Beauchamp 2005). It would deprive ordinary decision makers of the protection and support needed for their autonomous choices and actions, as determined by thin, procedural conceptions of personal autonomy (Beauchamp 2005; Beauchamp and Childress 2013).

SEE ALSO *Beneficence; Coercion; Conscience; Ethics: II. Task of Ethics; Expert Testimony; Freedom and Free Will; Human Dignity; Human Rights; Informed Consent: I. History of Informed Consent; Neuroethics and Free Will; Public Health: IV. Ethics; Relativism, Cultural and Ethical; Research Policy: III. Subjects; Shared Decision Making; Subjectivity; Vulnerability*

BIBLIOGRAPHY

Baumann, Holgere. 2008. "Reconsidering Relational Autonomy: Personal Autonomy for Socially Embedded and Temporally Extended Selves." *Analyse & Kritik* 30:445–68.

Beauchamp, Tom L. 2005. "Who Deserves Autonomy, and Whose Autonomy Deserves Respect?" In *Personal Autonomy: New Essays on Personal Autonomy and Its Role in Contemporary Moral Philosophy*, edited by James Stacey Taylor, 310–29. Cambridge, UK: Cambridge University Press.

Beauchamp, Tom L., and James F. Childress. 2013. *Principles of Biomedical Ethics*. 7th ed. New York: Oxford University Press.

Christman, John. 2011. "Autonomy in Moral and Political Philosophy." In *The Stanford Encyclopedia of Philosophy* (Spring), edited by Edward N. Zalta. Accessed November 2, 2013. http://plato.stanford.edu/archives/spr2011/entries/autonomy-moral

Mackenzie, Catriona, and Natalie Stoljar, eds. 2000. *Relational Autonomy: Feminist Perspectives on Autonomy, Agency, and the Social Self.* New York: Oxford University Press.

McLean, Sheila. 2010. *Autonomy, Consent and the Law*. London: Routledge-Cavendish.

O'Neill, Onora. 2002. *Autonomy and Trust in Bioethics*. Cambridge, UK: Cambridge University Press.

Sherwin, Susan. 1998. "A Relational Approach to Autonomy in Health Care." In *The Politics of Women's Health: Exploring Agency and Autonomy*, edited by Susan Sherwin and the Canadian Feminist Health Care Research Network, 19–47. Philadelphia: Temple University Press.

Stoljar, Natalie. 2013. "Feminist Perspectives on Autonomy." In *The Stanford Encyclopedia of Philosophy* (Summer), edited by Edward N. Zalta. Accessed November 2, 2013. http://plato.stanford.edu/archives/sum2013/entries/feminism-autonomy

Taylor, James Stacey, ed.2005. *Personal Autonomy: New Essays on Personal Autonomy and Its Role in Contemporary Moral Philosophy*. Cambridge, UK: Cambridge University Press.

Taylor, James Stacey. 2009. *Practical Autonomy and Bioethics*. New York: Routledge.

Traphagan, John W. 2013. *Rethinking Autonomy: A Critique of Principlism in Biomedical Ethics*. Albany: State University of New York Press.

James F. Childress
University Professor,
John Allen Hollingsworth Professor of Ethics,
University of Virginia

B

BENEFICENCE

Beneficence denotes the practice of good deeds. In contemporary ethics, the principle of beneficence usually signifies an obligation to benefit others or to seek their good. It is a principle of major importance in bioethics and has been prominent as a virtue in most moral traditions and in the codes of health professionals since antiquity.

RELIGIOUS ORIGINS

Long before beneficence was understood as an ethical principle, the duty to benefit others was widely accepted as a basic human behavioral norm. Indeed, thinking of ethics as "principled" is itself a fairly modern idea dating roughly from the European Enlightenment in the seventeenth and eighteenth centuries. Tracing the ur-narrative for the obligation to do good and refrain from harm leads to ancient social and religious teachings. The Jewish Torah is very clear that love of neighbor (and the presumption of benefit from this) is a central value. The well-known Golden Rule—treat others as one would like to be treated—has variants in ancient China, Egypt, and Greece and clear enunciations in Hinduism, Buddhism, Daoism, and the Abrahamic monotheistic religions. Simon Blackburn (2001) observes that there is practically no ethical system, whether religious or secular, that does not have some form of this maxim of imagined reciprocity.

BENEFICENCE AND BENEVOLENCE

Beneficence as a modern ethical principle is best understood as an effort to more carefully define this ancient duty. As such, beneficence as a principle that guides actions should be distinguished from the virtue that motivates actors. The *Oxford English Dictionary* defines *beneficence* as "doing good, the manifestation of *benevolence*, or kindly feeling" (emphasis added). This definition bespeaks the etymology of both *beneficence* and *benevolence*. Beneficence is derived from the Latin *bene* (well, from *bonus*, good) and *facere* (to do), whereas benevolence is rooted in *bene* and *volens* (a strong wish or intention) (Partridge 1983). Philosophers who emphasize a more rationalist approach calculated to guide principled choices tend to endorse beneficence. Those who see ethics as primarily concerned with virtue, character, and the psychological dimensions of the moral life emphasize benevolence.

David Hume (1966 [1777]), for example, conceived of benevolence as one of the instincts implanted in human nature. Like Joseph Butler, Francis Hutcheson, Adam Smith, and other eighteenth-century English-speaking philosophers, Hume was not so much concerned with ethical problem solving as with describing the role and place of benevolence in the moral topography of human beings. Adam Smith used the term *beneficence* but employed it to describe the virtue of goodwill and saw it as a moral passion rather than a principle. Of concern to all these philosophers was a task set for them by Thomas Hobbes a century earlier.

Hobbes (1947 [1651]) set the modern polemical context for discussions not only of beneficence and benevolence but also of ethics more generally. His moral philosophy was determinist, denying any capacity for choice based on values, and relativist, denying any independent reference for the terms *good* and *evil*. Liberty he saw as merely the ability to enact one's desires, not freedom to deliberate and choose. Good and evil simply denoted human appetites and aversions. "Will" was just another desire, not a distinctive moral capacity. Obviously such a philosophy has no place for beneficence as a principle of choice or benevolence as a motivation for the good of others. Ethics devolves into a deterministic egoism. Butler, Hume, Hutcheson, and Smith, in a variety of ways, took as their task a survey of the moral psyche, with special regard for the place of benevolence as something innate or natural to human life. Unless Hobbes's egoistic portrait is correct, any well-rounded view of ethics will include ways of describing and evaluating both the motivational, character-laden aspects and the decisional, action-oriented elements of ethics—that is, both benevolence and beneficence.

MODERN REFINEMENTS

A principle of beneficence can be broadly or narrowly defined. William Frankena (1973) views beneficence as an inclusive principle involving elements of refraining from inflicting harm and preventing or removing evil as well as an obligation actively to promote good. James F. Childress (1982) adopts Frankena's elements but reclassifies them according to two distinct principles: nonmaleficence, the obligation not to inflict harm; and beneficence, the obligations to prevent harm, to remove harm or evil, and positively to promote good. This refinement has the merit of following an intuitive division between refraining and active doing. It elucidates why refraining from harm is usually seen as a universal duty to others, whereas actively promoting good or helping others is typically seen as a less stringent obligation and often as resulting from specific role obligations (being a parent or a doctor) or contractual agreements. A broader-ranging sense of beneficence is, nevertheless, endorsed by some philosophers. For example, in *The Right and the Good*, W. D. Ross (1930, 21) claims that duties of beneficence are incurred because of "the mere fact that there are other human beings in the world whose condition we can make better." Interestingly, the US Department of Health, Education, and Welfare's 1978 *Belmont Report*, which seeks to enumerate the fundamental principles that should guide human subjects research, takes a broad view of beneficence, including under its ambit obligations both to reduce risk and to enhance benefits in research.

RELATION TO UTILITY

Beneficence has natural affinities with a principle of utility. Tom L. Beauchamp and Childress (2009), for example, claim that promoting good always involves a calculation of what harms might also be incurred. A principle of utility is a way to assess harms and benefits. In his *Utilitarianism*, John Stuart Mill 1979 [1863] asserted in 1863 that the measure of "good" by which all actions are to be judged is whether they promote the greatest happiness for the greatest number. Mill saw his principle of utility as a systematic expression of the teachings of Jesus, for example, as embodied in the Golden Rule.

When defined through Mill's utility principle, beneficence becomes vulnerable to two criticisms frequently leveled at utilitarianism. The first is the problem of adequacy. A focus on beneficence as the promotion of happiness to the exclusion of other kinds of goods and obligations seems too narrow. People value things other than happiness, however broadly defined. Promoting the happiness of others can conflict with treating them fairly or respecting them as persons. The second problem is idealism. For Mill (1979 [1863], 16) at least, utilitarianism presented a stringent requirement: "As between his own happiness and that of others utilitarianism requires him to be as strictly impartial as a disinterested and benevolent spectator." To count the good of strangers equally with our own good or that of our families or friends seems saintly and perhaps impossible to achieve.

These problems have led some philosophers to question utilitarianism as a system but also to see beneficence as only one principle among others and as usually (if not always) an imperfect or supererogatory duty. While some principle of utility is necessary to enact beneficence, it need not be Mill's rendition. A utility principle that recognized a variety of goods would at least moderate the force of the criticisms above.

BENEFICENCE AND AUTONOMY

How beneficence is put into practice depends on how it is modified by other principles or circumstances. Especially important in this regard is respect for autonomy or self-determination. Another way to put this is to ask whose notion of good will be definitive. Respect for autonomy means that good will be defined by the recipient of the action rather than the agent. Beneficence not defined by the recipient leads to paternalism, in which the beneficent actor overrides or ignores the recipient's ideas of good and imposes his or her own. The history of medical ethics is largely (but not entirely) a history of paternalist beneficence. In the mid-twentieth century consistent challenges arose to beneficent paternalism through assertions of patient rights. Defenders of simple paternalism in health care relationships are now rare.

Autonomy as a moral principle is historically rooted in freedom as a political principle, to which John Locke's *Second Treatise of Government* (1980 [1690]) gave definitive expression. Freedom, Locke (1980 [1690], 32) asserted, is not license "but a *liberty* [for a person] to dispose, and order as he lists, his person, actions, possessions, and his whole property, within the allowance of those laws under which he is, and therein not to be subject to the arbitrary rule of another, but freely follow his own." The eighteenth-century monument to autonomy is the work of the German philosopher Immanuel Kant (1959 [1785]). Whereas Locke was concerned to protect individuals from the power of the state, Kant focused on freedom of the will. His "practical imperative" requires that others be treated as ends in themselves and never only as a means. For Kant this respect for the moral freedom of others was grounded in recognition of their rational nature. In bioethics this raises the difficult issue of when and to what extent the rational capacities of patients are compromised and in which cases autonomy should give way to medical (or familial) beneficence.

The grounds for limiting beneficence through respect for autonomy were most powerfully stated by Mill. In *On Liberty* (1978 [1859]) he cautioned against supposing that the principle of liberty necessitates a "selfish indifference." Indeed, he asserted, "there is need of a great increase of disinterested exertion to promote the good of others." But, he continued, "disinterested benevolence can find other instruments to persuade people to their good than whips and scourges, either of the literal or of the metaphorical sort" (Mill 1978 [1859], 74).

While advocacy for autonomy as the preeminent principle of medical ethics has been powerful since the 1970s, there are still substantial voices for a beneficence-based theory. Edmund D. Pellegrino and David C. Thomasma (1988, 32) argue that "medicine as a human activity is of necessity a form of beneficence." Rather than espousing the older traditions of paternalism, however, they argue for an enlarged beneficence, "beneficence-in-trust"—a non-rights-based approach that includes respect for autonomy but emphasizes a fiduciary grounding for doctor-patient encounters. This approach has an advantage over single-principle approaches that ground medical obligations in simple beneficence or simple autonomy, conceived as monolithic norms. Beneficence, unleavened by respect for autonomy, can lead to paternalism, whereas autonomy alone obviates trust and often deteriorates into indifference. Still, the feasibility of trust depends on shared values and goals or at least stable role expectations between providers and patients. The greater the pluralism in a society, the more difficult it can be to establish the trust that Pellegrino and Thomasma commend.

HEALTH PROFESSIONAL CODES

While beneficence is important to many philosophical and religious systems of ethics, it is central to the health professions. The Hippocratic oath clearly states that the physician's actions are "for the benefit of the sick." The World Medical Association Declaration of Geneva begins with a pledge to "consecrate" one's life to "the service of humanity" (World Medical Association 2006 [1948]). The principles of the American Medical Association (AMA) (1847) open with the declaration that these principles are established "primarily for the benefit of the patient." The International Council of Nurses (2012 [1973]) devised a code in 1973 that begins with a broad-ranging assertion of beneficence. The "fundamental" responsibility of the nurse, it states, is to promote and restore health, alleviate suffering, and prevent illness. While duties to specific persons are recognized, the obligation to perform beneficent actions is seen as universal, because the need for nursing services is universal.

While all versions of professional ethics agree that the acceptance of a patient or a client creates a specific obligation of beneficence, some codes go further and talk of a general duty to seek the public good in matters of health. Here the 1847 Code of the American Medical Association is notable. Chapter 3 of that code enumerates "duties of the profession to the public." Among those listed are vigilance for the welfare of the community; counsel to the public on health matters; and advice about epidemics, contagion, and public hygiene. Twentieth-century medical codes tend to be more parsimonious in their interpretations of what beneficence entails, although since 2000 there has been a resurgence of interest in what is good for society and not simply for one's patients.

Still, the societal and public policy implications of beneficence in health care are poorly worked out at present. The issues that require attention include general programs of prevention, attention to the social determinants of health and resulting health inequities, and access to health services for the indigent and the uninsured. Most proposals for a more equitable health care system in the United States build on notions of justice as an independent principle rather than deriving their justifications from an extension of duties of beneficence.

LIMITS

If beneficent duties are more than supererogatory or optional, a persistent issue is how to discern their proper scope. Where do obligations to benefit others end? Are we morally required to give away all our surplus income and, beyond that, to chasten ourselves to more modest patterns of consumption? Are physicians obligated never to say no to patients so long as any thread of hope for improvement exists? Would beneficence require acceptance of higher taxes to fund universal health coverage, or does acting for my fellow citizens' good require me to die cheaply and forgo expensive treatments with low probability of benefit?

Beneficent duties may be limited in two ways. The first limiting force consists in duties to oneself. Self-respect and an appropriate attention to one's own well-being will of necessity restrict activities for the good of others unless beneficence is given a preemptive place and is conflated with saintliness. Hume (1966 [1777], 93), for example, believed that persons can be "too good," carrying "attention for others beyond the proper bounds," blunting a due sense of pride and the self-assertive virtues. A second kind of limit involves our psychological capacity for identification of and sympathy with those who could use our help. The press of human suffering that could be alleviated by our actions is immense. To conceive of this larger and seemingly inexhaustible world of suffering as our charge would likely be debilitating. Jonathan Glover (1977) has suggested that a restricted but feasible beneficence may be the price we pay for our sanity. Limits to the duty to promote good restrict us but also orient and direct our finite capacities. But perhaps the greater risk is that we will draw a circle around duties in a niggardly fashion, that our imagination will not be too large, risking paralysis, but too stingy and self-serving. It is this narrow and parochial tendency that concerns the advocates of a robust and extensive beneficence.

RELATIONAL SELVES

The late-twentieth- and early twenty-first-century challenges to ethical theory from psychological studies of moral experience have profound implications for beneficence. In 1982 Carol Gilligan published her research on the moral development of women, *In a Different Voice: Psychological Theory and Women's Development* (1993 [1982]). She claimed that females tend to see moral problems in terms of relationships. They are prone to think of their choices in problem solving as issues of care and responsibility for those relationships. By contrast, males tend to see moral problems in terms of rules and principles and are prone to think of their choices as logical adjudications. Women's moral orientations tend toward valuing and preserving ties among persons, whereas men's tend toward abstract thinking by an agent largely removed from and impartial to the parties involved. Gilligan's claim is not that there are precise gender types for moral experience but that the model of the moral self as an abstract, isolated, principled, and hierarchical thinker is insufficient.

The implications of her research for a principle of beneficence in bioethics and in the ethical codes of health professionals are substantial. Gilligan's research directly challenges the adequacy of thinking of beneficence simply as a principle to be applied to cases and recommends a notion of beneficence grounded in complex, relational understandings of the self. Hence the issues of beneficence can no longer be formulated as if the agent were essentially solitary and could contemplate the scope of his or her duties from afar. The self is already and essentially immersed in a web of mutual responsibilities. The ethical formulations of most health professions exhibit precisely the hierarchical distancing and the assumption of optional relationships depicted in the "male" model. Attending to the different voice in moral experience would mean moving bioethics beyond reliance on applying beneficence, as a principle, to problem cases. Beneficence must also be understood as relevant to and evident in the ongoing, everyday activities of persons in their webs of work, friendship, and family life. A stress on relational selves would also mean taking the ethical codes of health professionals beyond the contract model and into a recognition of a deeper and more integral bond of benefience between healers and the sick and between health professionals and society. Bioethics generally would profit from greater understanding of how social relationships shape concrete moral decision processes.

Interestingly, the neuroscience studies of the first years of the twenty-first century lend support to a more relational understanding of how beneficence and other ethical concepts work. Patricia Churchland's (2011) analysis suggests that our capacity for ethics rests in four interlocking brain processes: caring; recognition of others' psychological states; problem solving in social contexts; and social learning through imitation, trial and error, and analogy. She calls these the "circuitry of caring" and suggests that relational paradigms may be closer to the way we learn moral values and function ethically. This would mean that low-level theories of beneficence—like those of the eighteenth-century Scottish Enlightenment that favor the cultivation of innate moral passions—may be more useful than the high rationalism of Kant. In addition, philosophers of science, such as John Dupré (2012), cite evidence that cooperation is as important as competition in our evolutionary survival, which may underscore the importance of beneficence. Future research in both neuroscience and evolutionary biology will likely sharpen our understandings of the role of ethics and beneficence in human life.

SEE ALSO *Autonomy; Care: III. Care Ethics; Confidentiality; Ethics: IV. Normative Ethical Theories; Harm; Paternalism; Principlism; Relativism, Cultural and Ethical; Utilitarianism*

BIBLIOGRAPHY

American Medical Association. 1847. *Code of Medical Ethics of the American Medical Association.* Chicago: Author. Accessed March 1, 2013. www.ama-assn.org/resources/doc/ethics/1847code.pdf.

Beauchamp, Tom L., and James F. Childress. 2009. *Principles of Biomedical Ethics.* 6th ed. New York: Oxford University Press.

Beauchamp, Tom L., and Lawrence McCullough. 1984. *Medical Ethics: The Moral Responsibilities of Physicians.* Englewood Cliffs, NJ: Prentice-Hall.

Blackburn, Simon. 2001. *Ethics: A Very Short Introduction*. Oxford: Oxford University Press.

Childress, James F. 1982. *Who Should Decide? Paternalism in Health Care*. New York: Oxford University Press.

Churchland, Patricia. 2011. *Braintrust: What Neuroscience Tells Us about Morality*. Princeton, NJ: Princeton University Press.

Dupré, John. 2012. *Processes of Life: Essays in the Philosophy of Biology*. Oxford: Oxford University Press.

Edelstein, Ludwig, 1943. "The Hippocratic Oath: Text, Translation, and Interpretation." *Supplements to the Bulletin of the History of Medicine*, no. 1.

Faden, Ruth, and Tom L. Beauchamp with Nancy King. 1986. *A History and Theory of Informed Consent*. New York: Oxford University Press.

Frankena, William. 1973. *Ethics*. 2nd ed. Englewood Cliffs, NJ: Prentice-Hall.

Fried, Charles. 1978. *Right and Wrong*. Cambridge, MA: Harvard University Press.

Gilligan, Carol. 1993 [1982]. *In a Different Voice: Psychological Theory and Women's Development*. Cambridge, MA: Harvard University Press.

Glover, Jonathan. 1977. *Causing Death and Saving Lives*. London: Penguin.

Hobbes, Thomas. 1947 [1651]. *Leviathan*. Edited by Michael Oakeshott. New York: Oxford University Press.

Hume, David. 1966 [1777]. *An Enquiry concerning the Principles of Morals*. 2nd ed. La Salle, IL: Open Court.

International Council of Nurses. 2012 [1973]. *The ICN Code of Ethics for Nurses*. Geneva, Switzerland: Author. Accessed March 1, 2013. www.icn.ch/about-icn/code-of-ethics-for-nurses/.

Kant, Immanuel. 1959 [1785]. *Foundations of the Metaphysics of Morals*. Translated by Lewis White Beck. New York: Macmillan.

Katz, Jay. 2002 [1984]. *The Silent World of Doctor and Patient*. Baltimore, MD: Johns Hopkins University Press.

Locke, John. 1980 [1690]. *Second Treatise of Government*. Edited by Crawford B. MacPherson. Indianapolis, IN: Hackett.

Loewy, Erich. 1991. *Suffering and the Beneficent Community: Beyond Libertarianism*. Albany: State University of New York Press.

Mill, John Stuart. 1978 [1859]. *On Liberty*. Indianapolis, IN: Hackett.

Mill, John Stuart. 1979 [1863]. *Utilitarianism*. Indianapolis: Hackett.

National Commission for the Protection of Human Subjects of Biomedical and Behavioral Research. 1978. *The Belmont Report: Ethical Principles and Guidelines for the Protection of Human Subjects of Research*. Washington, DC: DHEW and US Government Printing Office.

Partridge, Eric. 1983. *Origins: A Short Etymological Dictionary of Modern English*. New York: Greenwich House.

Pellegrino, Edmund D., and David C. Thomasma. 1988. *For the Patient's Good: The Restoration of Beneficence in Health Care*. New York: Oxford University Press.

Ross, W. D. 1930. *The Right and the Good*. Oxford: Clarendon Press.

World Medical Association. 2006 [1948]. "WMA Declaration of Geneva." Accessed March 7, 2013. http://www.wma.net/en/30publications/10policies/g1/

Larry R. Churchill (1995, 2014)
Ann Geddes Stahlman Chair of Medical Ethics, Center for Biomedical Ethics and Society, Vanderbilt University

BIAS, RESEARCH

In the behavioral sciences, the difficulties of studying complex, changing interactions among living beings led to investigations of possible sources of bias. For example, gender, race, class, and even the presence of a researcher during an interview have been shown to influence the responses of the interviewee. Researchers sought to apply the scientific method to problems in the behavioral sciences, in an attempt to eliminate bias.

HISTORICAL BACKGROUND

Like all scholars, scientists hold, either explicitly or implicitly, certain beliefs concerning their enterprise. Most scientists try to use what they assume to be the best information to collect data and draw theories to elucidate the laws and facts that will be constant, providing that experiments have been done correctly. But the individuals who make observations and create theories are people who live in a particular country at a certain time in a definable socioeconomic condition, and their situations and mentalities impinge on their discoveries. In the fourth century B.C.E. Aristotle "counted" fewer teeth in the mouths of women than in those of men—adding this dentitional inferiority to all the others that he asserted characterized women. In the second century C.E. the Greek physician Galen, having read the biblical book of Genesis, "discovered" that men had one less rib on one side than women did. Neither is true, and both would be refuted easily by observation of what would appear by modern standards to be easily verifiable facts. Although Aristotle and Galen also could count, of course, they took these to be "nonclassical cases," because what we take to be facts can vary depending upon the theory or paradigm—the specific problematics, concepts, theories, language, and methods—guiding the scientist.

Most scientists, feminists, and philosophers of science recognize that no individual can live a life and be entirely neutral or value-free, since science and values are both very important. To some, "objectivity is defined to mean independence from the value judgments of any particular individual" (Jaggar 1983, 357). The paradigms themselves, however, also are far from value-free. The values of a culture, in the historical past and the present society, heavily influence the ordering of observable phenomena into a theory. The worldview of a particular society, time, and person limits the questions that can be asked and thereby the answers that can be given. Therefore, the very acceptance of a particular paradigm that appears to cause a "scientific revolution" in a society may depend at least in part upon the congruence of that theory with the institutions and beliefs of the society.

Elizabeth Potter (2001) documented Robert Boyle's choice of the mechanistic model to explain his law of gases both because it comported well with the data and because it supported the status quo of conservative religion and monarchy of the chemist's seventeenth-century milieu with regard to class and gender compared to the competing animistic model seen as more radical socially. Scholars suggest that Charles Darwin's theory of natural selection in the early nineteenth century was ultimately accepted by his contemporaries (whereas they did not accept similar theories as described by Alfred Russel Wallace and others) because Darwin emphasized the congruence between the values of his theory and those held by the upper classes of Victorian Britain. Social Darwinists used Darwin's theory to base the political and social rights to their wealth and power held by men and the upper classes in biological determinism. In this manner Darwin's data and theories reinforced the natural superiority of wealthy men, making his theories acceptable to the leaders of Victorian English society. Anne Fausto-Sterling's (1999) research revealed how different societies at particular historical periods have also used varying biological and genetic data as determinants for the social construction of gender and race.

Not only what is accepted, but what and how we study, have normative features. Helen Longino (1990, 216) has explored the extent to which methods employed by scientists can be objective, in the sense of not being related to individual values, and lead to repeatable, verifiable results while contributing to hypotheses or theories that are congruent with nonobjective institutions and ideologies, such as gender, race, and class, that are socially constructed in the society: "Background assumptions are the means by which contextual values and ideology are incorporated into scientific inquiry." For example, scientists may calculate rocket trajectories and produce bombs that efficiently destroy living beings without raising the ethical questions of whether the money and effort for this research to support the military could be better spent on other research questions that might be solved by using similar objective methods.

UNINTENDED RESEARCH BIAS

Given the high costs of sophisticated equipment, maintenance of laboratory animals and facilities, and salaries for qualified technicians and researchers, little behavioral or biomedical research is undertaken without governmental or foundation support. The choice of problems for study in medical research is substantially determined by a national agenda that defines what is worthy of study, that is, worth funding. As Marxist (for instance, Bill Zimmerman [1980]), African American (George Campbell Jr.; Ronni Denes; and Catherine Morrision [2000]), and feminist (Sandra Harding [1993, 1998]) critics of scientific research have pointed out, the scientific research undertaken in the United States reflects the societal bias toward the powerful, who are overwhelmingly white, middle or upper class, and male. Members of Congress and the individuals in the theoretical and decision-making positions in the medical and scientific establishments that set priorities and allocate funds for research exemplify these descriptors. The lack of diversity among congressional and scientific leaders may allow unintentional, undetected flaws to bias the research in terms of what we study and how we study it. Some critics have pointed out the way, for instance, scarce resources have been diverted away from public health measures known to prevent diseases for the masses and redirected toward the multibillion-dollar Human Genome Project (and consequently, personalized medicine), characterizing this as an example of placing the interests of the powerful above those of the general public, since gene therapy and designer genes are likely to benefit fewer, wealthier people.

In a relatively short period of time, the definition of what might constitute bias in research and lead to a potential conflict of interest may evolve because of changes in the rate and complexity of translation of basic research into clinical applications. For example, on September 26, 2011, the US Department of Health and Human Services (HHS) implemented a new rule to change the 1995 regulations on this issue ("Responsibility of Applicants for Promoting Objectivity in Research for Which Public Health Service Funding Is Sought and Responsible Prospective Contractors: Final Rule"). These changes occurred because "since the publication of the 1995 regulations, the pace by which new discoveries are translated from the research bench into effective treatment of patients has accelerated significantly, and the biomedical and behavioral research enterprise in the United States has grown in size and complexity. … In addition, these new translational strategies often involve complex collaborations between Investigators and the private sector" (Department of Health and Human Services, 53256). The bias that the HHS guidelines address arises from conflicts of interest (COI). As a result, the HHS guidelines focus on management and transparency of COIs. But research bias takes many other forms.

Examples from research studies demonstrate that unintentional bias may be reflected in at least three stages of application of the scientific method: (1) choice and definition of problems to be studied; (2) methods and approaches used in data gathering, including who is chosen as a subject; and (3) theories and conclusions drawn from the data.

Choice and Definition of Problems to Be Studied. Many diseases that occur in both sexes have been studied in males only, have used a male-as-norm approach, or both. Cardiovascular diseases serve as a case in point. Research protocols for several large-scale studies of cardiovascular diseases failed to assess gender differences. Women were excluded from clinical trials of drugs, researchers said, because of the desire to protect women or fetuses (and fear of litigation) from possible teratogenic effects on fetuses. Exclusion of women from clinical drug trials was so pervasive that a meta-analysis surveying the literature from 1960 to 1991 on clinical trials of medications used to treat acute myocardial infarction found that women were included in less than 20 percent and the elderly in less than 40 percent of those studies. Irving Zucker and Annaliese K. Beery (2011) found that many articles across all science and medical fields failed to report subject sex at all, and two-thirds of the studies that included both males and females failed to analyze the data by sex.

Designation of certain diseases as particular to one gender, race, or sexual orientation not only cultivates ignorance in the general public about transmission or frequency of the disease but also results in research that does not adequately explore the parameters of the disease. Most of the funding for heart disease has been appropriated for research on predisposing factors for the disease (such as cholesterol level, lack of exercise, stress, smoking, and weight) using white, middle-aged, middle-class males. Only in the late twentieth and early twenty-first centuries has research been directed toward elderly women, African American women who have had several children, and other high-risk groups of women. These types of bias raise ethical issues. Health care practitioners treat the majority of the population, which consists of females, minorities, and the elderly, based on information gathered from clinical research in which women and minorities have not been included. Bias in research thus leads to further injustice in health care diagnosis and treatment. Understanding this bias led to changes in policies in the 1990s. Investigators now receiving federal money must give a compelling reason if their studies fail to include both men and women, young and old, and individuals of diverse races. Although this increases the cost of research, since the sample must be larger, cost alone does not stand as a compelling reason.

Approaches and Methods Used in Data Gathering. Using the white, middle-aged, heterosexual male as the "basic experimental subject" not only ignores the fact that females may respond differently to the variable tested but also may lead to less accurate models even for many men. For example, the standard dosage of certain medications is not only inappropriate for many women and the elderly but also for most Asian men because of their smaller body size and weight. Certain surgical procedures, such as angioplasty and cardiac bypass, have resulted initially in higher death rates for women and Asian men, and may require modification for the same reason.

From the Tuskegee syphilis experiment (1932–1972), in which the effects of untreated syphilis were studied in 399 men over a period of forty years, it is clear that men who are black and poor may not receive appropriate treatment or information about the experiment in which they are participating. In a 1999 collection of studies by Adele E. Clarke and Virginia L. Olesen, scholars explore the extent to which gender, race, and class become complex, interlocking variables that may affect access to and quality of health care.

Using only a particular discipline's established methods may result in approaches that fail to reveal sufficient information about the problem being explored. This may be a difficulty for research surrounding medical problems particularly important to the elderly, women, men of color, and homosexual males. Pregnancy, childbirth, menstruation, menopause, lupus, sickle-cell disease, AIDS, and gerontology represent health care issues for which the methods of one discipline are clearly inadequate.

Methods that cross disciplinary boundaries or include combinations of methods traditionally used in separate fields may provide more appropriate approaches. For example, heart disease is caused not only by genetic and physiological factors but also by social or psychological factors, such as smoking and stress.

The biomedical model, although too restricted for an approach to most diseases, remains especially inadequate for women's health, particularly for exploring the causes, treatments, and prevention of events such as menopause that occur as part of the life cycle course and are influenced by both biology and a variety of social, environmental, and other factors. Until 1991 scant research on women's menopausal experience existed. The Women's Health Initiative (WHI), launched by the National Institutes of Health (NIH) that year to study cardiovascular diseases, cancers, and osteoporosis, attempted to raise the priority of women's health and provide baseline data on previously understudied causes of death in women. As the baby boom generation aged, pharmaceutical companies developed an extreme interest in capturing the market of women approaching menopause. These companies redefined menopause as a disease that required hormones to cure it and made large amounts of money by selling hormone replacement therapy (HRT) to women before, during, and after menopause.

Using only the methods traditional to a particular discipline may result in limited approaches that fail to reveal sufficient information about the problem being explored. On July 9, 2002, the NIH announced that the HRT and estrogen-progestin portion of the WHI would be stopped. The study had shown that women taking HRT had a 26 percent increase in breast cancer, a 41 percent increase in strokes, and a 200 percent increase in the rates of blood clots in the legs and lungs. Subsequent studies also revealed that HRT did not improve "quality of life" issues or memory, although women taking HRT did have 37 percent fewer incidences of colon cancer and 34 percent fewer hip fractures than the control group.

Many women expressed outrage against the pharmaceutical companies after the announcement that the HRT portion of the WHI was halted. Before the WHI very little research compared the health of menopausal women who took HRT with those who did not take HRT. Women wanted to know why they had been given HRT before such research had been done.

Theories and Conclusions Drawn from the Data. Emphasis upon traditional disciplinary approaches that are quantitative and maintain the distance between observer and experimental subject supposedly remove the bias of the researcher. Ironically, to the extent that these "objective" approaches are synonymous with a particular approach to scientific phenomena, they may introduce bias. As a corrective to such bias against a science that is too narrow, the scholar Harding (1993, 1998) has proposed the notion of "strong objectivity," which recognizes the cultural, social, and historical forces that shape the questions asked by scientists, their approaches, and the theories and conclusions drawn from their data.

Theories may be presented in androcentric, ethnocentric, or class-biased language. An awareness of language should aid experimenters in avoiding the use of terms such as *tomboyism*, *aggression*, and *hysteria*, for instance, which reflect assumptions about sex-appropriate behavior. Evaluative terms, such as *prostitute*, also require caution. Often the important fact for AIDS research is that a woman has multiple sex partners or is an intravenous drug user rather than that she has received money for sex. The use of a term such as *prostitute* may also induce bias by promoting the idea that women are vectors for transmission to men, when in fact men may have an equal or greater number of sex partners to whom they are transmitting the disease.

Once a bias in terminology is exposed, the next step is to ask whether that terminology leads to a constraint or bias in the theory itself. Theories and conclusions drawn from medical research may be formulated to support the status quo of inequality for oppressed groups. Not surprisingly, the androcentric bias in research that has led to exclusion of women from the definitions and approaches to research problems may result in differences in management of disease and access to health care procedures based on gender. For example, although lesbians are often ignored in studies, when they are recognized, they may be categorized only as women or homosexuals, thereby lumping lesbian health issues with those of heterosexual females or male homosexuals. In fact lesbians may be at higher risk for certain diseases, such as breast and uterine cancer, because many lesbians do not have children, have higher body fat, and limit their access to regular health care checkups relative to heterosexual women because of fear of discrimination. Few studies have focused on lesbians as a separate population for health studies. When lesbians are lumped together with heterosexual women in studies of the incidence or cause of sexually transmitted diseases or other gynecological problems from which they are exempt or for which they are at low risk because they do not engage in heterosexual intercourse, both lesbians and nonlesbians suffer. Defining such studies generally as research on "women's health issues" rather than on "health issues for women engaging in heterosexual sex" leads the general population and some health care workers to think that lesbians are at risk for diseases that they are unlikely to contract while obscuring the true risk behavior for women engaging in heterosexual sex.

CONCLUSION

The newer fields of biomedicine and new media introduce additional opportunities for bias. Biomedicine fuses technology with the biological human body in the form of artificial hips, heart valves, pacemakers, and implants to deliver drugs. Simultaneously, new media technologies explore the reciprocity between science and media by which, in this age of genetics as the life code, culture may become biology. Analyses of metaphors in genome research suggest that, because researchers transpose literature onto biology, it is not possible to critique science without critiquing culture. Since culture emanates from human interactions and creations, culture may introduce further bias.

Recognizing the possibility of bias is the first step toward understanding the difference it makes and combating it. Perhaps white male researchers have been less likely to question or see flaws in biologically deterministic theories that provide scientific justification for their superior status in society because they gain social power and status from such theories. Researchers from outside the mainstream (women, homosexuals, and people of color, for example) are much more likely to be critical of such theories, because they lose power from those theories.

To eliminate bias and recognize the cultural, social, and historical forces impacting their research, the community of scientists needs to include individuals who serve as members on review panels and as leaders of review studies from backgrounds of as much variety and diversity as possible with regard to race, class, gender, and sexual orientation. Only then will it become less likely that the perspective of one group will bias research design, approaches, subjects, and interpretations. Since the scientific method itself is supposed to be "self-correcting," if results are continually tested and subject to critical review, these biases are likely to be exposed.

SEE ALSO *AIDS: II. Health Care and Research Issues; Feminism; Genetic Discrimination; Metaphor and Analogy; Privacy and Confidentiality in Research; Race and Racism; Research, Human: Historical Aspects; Research, Multinational; Research, Unethical; Research Ethics Consultation; Research Methodology; Research Policy*

BIBLIOGRAPHY

Arditti, Rita. 1980. "Feminism and Science." In *Science and Liberation*, edited by Rita Arditti, Pat Brennan, and Steven Cavrak, 350–68. Boston: South End Press.

Campbell, George, Jr.; Ronni Denes; and Catherine Morrision, eds. 2000. *Access Denied: Race, Ethnicity, and the Scientific Enterprise.* Oxford: Oxford University Press.

Campbell, Kristina. 1992. "1 in 3 Lesbians May Get Breast Cancer, Expert Theorizes." *Washington Blade*, October 2.

Chinese Hospital Medical Staff and University of California School of Medicine. 1982. Conference on Health Problems Related to the Chinese in America. San Francisco, May 22–23.

Clarke, Adele E., and Virginia L. Olesen, eds. 1999. *Revisioning Women, Health, and Healing: Feminist, Cultural, and Technoscience Perspectives.* New York: Routledge.

Fausto-Sterling, Anne. 1999. "Gender, Race, and Nation: The Comparative Anatomy of Hottentot Women in Europe, 1815–1817." In *Deviant Bodies: Critical Perspectives on Difference in Science and Popular Culture*, edited by Jennifer Terry and Jacqueline Urla, 19–48. New York: Routledge.

Grobbee, Diederick E.; Eric B. Rimm; Edward Giovannucci; et al. 1990. "Coffee, Caffeine, and Cardiovascular Disease in Men." *New England Journal of Medicine* 323 (15): 1026–32.

Gurwitz, Jerry H.; F. Col Nananda; and Jerry Avorn. 1992. "The Exclusion of the Elderly and Women from Clinical Trials in Acute Myocardial Infarction." *Journal of the American Medical Association* 268 (2): 1417–22.

Hamilton, Jean. 1985. "Avoiding Methodological Biases and Policy-Making Biases in Gender-Related Health Research." In *Women's Health: Report of the Public Health Service Task Force on Women's Health Issues*, vol. 2, edited by Ruth L. Kirschstein and Doris H. Merritt, 54–64. Washington, DC: US Department of Health and Human Services, Public Health Service.

Harding, Sandra. 1993. *The Racial Economy of Science.* Bloomington: Indiana University Press.

Harding, Sandra. 1998. *Is Science Multicultural? Postcolonialisms, Feminisms, and Epistemologies.* Bloomington: Indiana University Press.

Jaggar, Alison M. 1983. *Feminist Politics and Human Nature.* Totowa, NJ: Rowman and Allanheld.

Jones, James H. 1981. *Bad Blood: The Tuskegee Syphilis Experiment.* New York: Free Press.

Kelsey, Sheryl F.: Margaret James; Ann Lu Holubkov; et al. 1993. "Results of Percutaneous Transluminal Coronary Angioplasty in Women: 1985–1986 National Heart, Lung, and Blood Institutes Coronary Angioplasty Registry." *Circulation* 87 (3): 720–27.

Kuhn, Thomas S. 1970. *The Structure of Scientific Revolutions.* 2nd ed. Chicago: University of Chicago Press.

Longino, Helen. 1990. *Science as Social Knowledge: Values and Objectivity in Scientific Inquiry.* Princeton, NJ: Princeton University Press.

Manley, Audrey; Jane S. Lin-Fu; Magdalena Miranda; et al. 1985. "Special Health Concerns of Ethnic Minority Women." In *Women's Health: Report of the Public Health Service Task Force on Women's Health Issues*, vol. 2, edited by Ruth L. Kirschstein and Doris H. Merritt, 37–47. Washington, DC: US Department of Health and Human Services.

Money, John, and Anke Erhardt. 1972. *Man and Woman, Boy and Girl: The Differentiation and Dimorphism of Gender and Identity from Conception to Maturity.* Baltimore, MD: Johns Hopkins University Press.

Multiple Risk Factor Intervention Trial Research Group. 1990. "Mortality Rates after 10.5 Years for Participants in the Multiple Risk Factor Intervention Trial: Findings Related to A Priori Hypotheses of the Trial." *Journal of the American Medical Association* 263 (13): 1795–1801.

National Women's Health Network. 2002. *The Truth about Hormone Replacement Therapy: How to Break Free from the Medical Myths of Menopause.* Roseville, CA: Prima.

Oakley, Ann. 1981. "Interviewing Women: A Contradiction in Terms." In *Doing Feminist Research*, edited by Helen Roberts, 30–61. London: Routledge and Kegan Paul.

Pinn, Vivian, and Judith LaRosa. 1992. *Overview: Office of Research on Women's Health.* Bethesda, MD: National Institutes of Health.

Potter, Elizabeth. 2001. *Gender and Boyle's Law of Gases.* Bloomington: Indiana University Press.

Rose, Hilary, and Steven Rose. 1980. "The Myth of the Neutrality of Science." In *Science and Liberation*, edited by Rita Arditti, Pat Brennan, and Steve Cavrak, 17–32. Boston: South End Press.

Rosser, Sue V. 1994. *Women's Health: Missing from US Medicine.* Bloomington: Indiana University Press.

Rosser, Sue V. 2000. *Women, Science, and Society: The Crucial Union.* New York: Teachers College Press.

Steering Committee of the Physicians' Health Study Group. 1989. "Final Report on the Aspirin Component of the Ongoing Physicians' Health Study." *New England Journal of Medicine* 321 (3): 129–35.

US Department of Health and Human Services. 2011. "Responsibility of Applicants for Promoting Objectivity in Research for Which Public Health Service Funding Is Sought and Responsible Prospective Contractors: Final Rule." *Federal Register* 76 (165): 53256–93.

Webster, Douglas, and Molly Webster. 1974. *Comparative Vertebrate Morphology*. New York: Academic Press.

Worcester, Nancy. 2009. "Hormone Replacement Therapy (HRT): Getting to the Heart of the Politics of Women's Health?" In *Diversity and Women's Health*, edited by Sue V. Rosser, 178–90. Baltimore, MD: Johns Hopkins University Press.

Zimmerman, Bill. 1980. "People's Science." In *Science and Liberation*, edited by Rita Arditti, Pat Brennan, and Steve Cavrak, 299–319. Boston: South End Press.

Zucker, Irving, and Annaliese K. Beery. 2011. "Sex Bias in Neuroscience and Biomedical Research." *Neuroscience and Biobehavioral Reviews* 35 (3): 565–72.

Sue V. Rosser (1995, 2004, 2014)
Provost and Vice President for Academic Affairs, San Francisco State University

BIOCENTRISM VERSUS ANTHROPOCENTRISM

In the context of bioethics, *biocentrism* and *anthropocentrism* carry normative weight as theories of moral considerability, or of what sorts of things morally matter. Unlike the related term, *ecocentrism* (literally, "habitat centered"), both anthropocentrism and biocentrism denote theories seeking to explain the moral worth of individuals, not ecological wholes such as mountains, species, or ecosystems. Anthropocentrism (literally, "human centered") is the view that only human individuals have moral standing—that is, only human beings have a good of their own. Biocentrism (literally, "life centered") is the view that moral standing is properly attributed to the broader domain of all living things: every living organism has a good of its own that makes it deserving of moral consideration. Supporters of both biocentrism and anthropocentrism have argued for stronger and weaker versions of each concept. Generally, anthropocentrism has had an overwhelming historical advantage; that advantage, however, continues to be eroded by contemporary advances in scientific knowledge and a continually developing moral intuition about the place and role of the human being in the natural world.

TAKING A STAND ON VALUE

The distinction between the two terms arose as a result of the development of thought on the nature and extent of moral value. In general, moral worth is described as coming in two forms: instrumental and intrinsic. Instrumental value is that value that a thing has insofar as it is an instrument to some other thing. A doctor, for instance, has instrumental value for a patient insofar as he or she provides that patient with medical treatments and care. An armchair likewise has instrumental value for a person looking to sit down insofar as it provides a place to sit. Accounts of intrinsic value seek to get at the intuitive difference between things such as doctors and armchairs. Common sense would concede that, were one to tear the arms off one's armchair and burn it on the front lawn, that person would be doing nothing morally wrong: he or she would presumably have no moral obligations to the armchair. Of course, were that person to tear the arms off his or her doctor and burn said doctor on the front lawn, that person would have done something morally reprehensible. Doctors, for example, are the sorts of things that have not only instrumental but also intrinsic moral value: they are valuable for more than their usefulness to their patients. Generally, intrinsic value refers to the value a thing has for its own sake. Accounts of both biocentrism and anthropocentrism must take a stand on this distinction: the more weight any account gives to intrinsic value, the more robust that account will be. Generally, the anthropocentrist limits consideration of intrinsic value to human individuals, whereas the biocentrist broadens that consideration to include all living things (with this distinction worked out more carefully below).

ANTHROPOCENTRIC TRAJECTORY

Anthropocentrism can be considered, nonexclusively, in either teleological or normative terms; that is, it might describe either some descriptive fact about the (meta) physical nature of the world, or it might make some ethical claim about the nature of moral value, or both (Attfield 2003). The teleological anthropocentrist claims that the natural world exists for the sake solely of the human individual because of the way the world developed and is structured. Nonhuman individuals exist for use by and for the sake of human individuals. The normative anthropocentrist shifts the claim to the moral realm, asserting that human concerns account for the entire realm of moral considerability: intrinsic value is the stuff of human beings and human beings alone. Historically, the teleological view has been used to support the normative view. Key figures in this history of Western thought include the ancient Greek philosopher Aristotle (384–322 B.C.E.), the medieval theologian Thomas Aquinas (c. 1224–1274), the French philosopher René Descartes (1596–1650), and the German philosopher Immanuel Kant (1724–1804).

Aristotle argued for what has become known as the Great Chain of Being, a teleological taxonomy of increasing species complexity culminating in the human being, differentiated from other living things by unique capacities for language and deliberation. Aristotle applied this teleological view to the further normative claim that it was language that allowed for the human being to form morally important political communities in ways that were impossible for "lesser" species (Aristotle 1984). His metaphysical anthropocentrism set the stage for subsequent developments. Applying Aristotelian logic to Christian cosmology, Thomas Aquinas argued for an anthropocentric view based on divine creation. The human being, made in the image of the Christian God, stood apart—either in dominion over or as steward of—the natural world. Here again, the teleological view grounds the normative, supporting the claim that moral considerability starts and stops at the human individual. This basic view held sway through the medieval era and into the modern age. In modernity, Descartes famously appealed to both Christian cosmology and the current landscape of scientific knowledge to emphasize the dualism between the human individual, as a mind-embodied being, and the nonhuman individual, more akin to a machine than to a human. Descartes's moral outlook was likewise anthropocentric, arguing that humans' obligations began and ended at the minds of human individuals. Kant, too, maintained the basic anthropocentric perspective, but he shifted the criterion of moral considerability to an inherent rational capacity held—presumably, for him—by all and only human individuals. On the more contemporary scene, the hierarchical view of the Great Chain of Being was also supported by early considerations of evolutionary theory. While such hierarchical considerations of the evolution of species are now seen as incorrect interpretations of evolutionary theory (Evogeneao 2013), they were widely used to support the moral superiority claims of, for instance, the social Darwinists of the early twentieth century.

BIOCENTRIC TRAJECTORY

This same distinction between teleological and normative views can likewise be made for biocentrism, the view that moral worth is a property of all living things. Teleological biocentrism claims that the natural world exists for the sake of all living things. Normative biocentrism maintains that the scope of moral considerability encompasses all living things. Early religious perspectives from the East, including the traditions of Buddhism, Jainism, Hinduism, and Japanese Zen, proposed cosmologies that were compatible with biocentrism. According to such views, the human being is seen as an interrelated member of the natural world, rather than a distinct part of it. In the West, Native American religious views likewise tend to share this biocentric view of the interrelatedness of life. So, too, did European philosophers such as Baruch Spinoza (1632–1677) and Friedrich Nietzsche (1844–1900), who both argued along biocentric lines toward normative conclusions that very much differed from their anthropocentric contemporaries. In the contemporary landscape, the animal rights and environmentalist movements have both developed in light of the shifting moral intuitions and developing scientific knowledge concerning the nature of nonhumans, driving away from strict anthropocentrism and toward a biocentric perspective.

STRONG ANTHROPOCENTRISM

Contemporary arguments supporting anthropocentrism are numerous and varied. Weaker and stronger versions of this view have sought out a balance between worldview, moral outlook, and accepted scientific knowledge. In its strongest sense anthropocentrism claims that all and only human beings have inherent value. This position has been championed in the contemporary setting by scholars such as William F. Baxter (1974) and John Passmore (1974). Both Baxter and Passmore maintain that strong anthropocentrism corresponds to the ways humans most commonly think and act, that the application of intrinsic value to nonhumans is meaningless, and that a strictly instrumental account of moral value in nonhumans will offer sufficient protection to them. Whether that instrumental value applies to traditional or intergenerational considerations (Stenmark 2002), strong anthropocentrism maintains a clear line between the intrinsic moral value of the human individual and the mere instrumental worth of the nonhuman.

STRONG BIOCENTRISM

Like anthropocentrism, biocentrism is held in a variety of degrees by its advocates. Strong biocentrism broadens the scope of moral standing to include not just some but all living things. The strong biocentrist supports the view that all living things have intrinsic moral worth. Kenneth E. Goodpaster (1978) exemplifies this view, developing a negative argument against stopping the expansion of moral considerability at anything less than life. Likewise, there are strong biocentrist arguments present in the work of Aldo Leopold (1949) and Arne Naess (1973), although both figures are better known as exemplars of ecocentric perspectives. According to the strong biocentric view, all living things are accorded equal moral considerability or standing but not necessarily equal moral significance.

The strongest biocentric perspective takes a further step: it accords not only equal moral standing but also equal moral significance to all living individuals. Support for this strongest view of biocentrism has been developed by Albert Schweitzer and Paul W. Taylor. Schweitzer's "reverence for life" principle (1923a, 1923b, 1931), building on Christian and Jain religious traditions, refuses to rank or prioritize life-forms and so accords equal moral significance to all living things based on the common property of having a will to live. Taylor's egalitarian biocentrism (1981) works to extend Kant's respect for persons to all living individuals based on their common characteristics as teleological centers of life. Taylor's view proposes an egalitarian respect for nature (1986) that accords equal moral standing and equal moral significance to each and every living individual.

WEAK ANTHROPOCENTRISM AND WEAK BIOCENTRISM

Anthropocentrism can be viewed as compatible with all theories of moral considerability. This weakest view of anthropocentrism is only a nominal view—every theory is human centered insofar as it is human individuals who explore such questions. According to this view, because human moral agents alone are the source of the description or discovery of moral value in the natural world, whether it be intrinsic or instrumental, this description or discovery is necessarily human centered. But such a view does little conceptual work, neither describing the scope of intrinsic value nor justifying ethical perspectives.

A slightly stronger but still weak form of anthropocentrism differs from the strong view in that it accepts that some nonhuman individuals, as well as all human individuals, have intrinsic moral worth. Sentience theorists such as Peter Singer, Mark Bernstein, and Bernard Rollin appeal to weak anthropocentrism to support their views that all and only animals capable of experiencing pain and pleasure are morally considerable. Their views start from the accepted intrinsic moral worth of human individuals and expand outward to account for some subset of nonhuman animals as well: all other nonhuman individuals are accorded merely instrumental worth.

Weak biocentrism mirrors the view of weak anthropocentrism in that both views maintain a similarly broader view of intrinsic value. Weak biocentrism, however, differently prioritizes the relevant moral perspectives. Whereas weak anthropocentrism begins with the assumption that human beings have intrinsic moral value and expands out to include at least some nonhumans, weak biocentrism begins with the view that intrinsic value is the sort of thing that does not expand out from the human but instead includes the human animal as one among the many animals that humans ought to take as morally considerable. Like weak anthropocentrism, it offers an egalitarian perspective on moral standing (see Goodpaster 1978; Stenmark 2002), considering the moral value of human and at least some nonhuman individuals on equal footing. But unlike weak anthropocentrism, weak biocentrism does not suppose that human individuals have higher moral significance than nonhumans. Weak biocentrism thus decenters the human being from a place of moral priority to one of moral equality.

PRACTICAL ADOPTION

Whether taken weakly or strongly, both biocentric and anthropocentric perspectives have been adopted as a justification for a wide range of social and political actions. Biocentrism has supported the continued development of the animal rights and the environmentalist movements by opening space for rethinking teleological and normative relationships in the natural world. It likewise led Van Rensselaer Potter (1971), one of the earliest pioneers of bioethics, to take a broad environmental and evolutionary view of the nascent field of bioethics.

Even while biocentrism has been criticized for justifying "environmental fascism" (Regan 2004) and potentially leading to human harm, it has also been lauded for introducing an alternative to the metaphysical frameworks that have historically supported the merely instrumental use of nonhumans. Anthropocentrism, too, continues to be adopted toward the social and political ends of environmentalism and other ethical fields, driving, for instance, the concerns of André Hellegers (1926–1979) and the early Georgetown University medical bioethicists. Many argue that, given an increased understanding of the vital importance of the natural world and individuals in it for human well-being, an instrumental account of intrinsic moral worth for those nonhuman individuals suffices for their protection. This view can be criticized, however, for ignoring the deeper implications of scientific ecology and evolutionary theory and for having historically led to environmental degradation and maleficent uses of nonhuman individuals. The argument from marginal cases is among the most robustly developed philosophical arguments against the anthropocentric position (Dombrowski 1997; Singer 1990).

CONCLUDING THEMES

The relationship between anthropocentric and biocentric perspectives has important implications for the bioethicist, for the two perspectives are metaphysically incompatible. One's starting point in this debate is contingent on the way one sees the world and the place of the human being in it; that is, it is contingent on one's metaphysical commitments. The anthropocentrist starts his or her consideration of the world—and of moral standing—at the human individual, whereas the biocentrist begins at the living organism. This incompatibility leads to normative and descriptive conflict, resulting in ethical collisions. The resulting impact will have to do partly with future developments in scientific knowledge but also with the continued development of bioethical analysis. Deeper scientific understanding of the natural world seems to drive one toward biocentric conclusions, even while historical intuitions embedded in Western culture push back toward anthropocentrism.

SEE ALSO *Bioethics: IX. Anthropology of; Food; Medicine, Anthropology of; Moral Status*

BIBLIOGRAPHY

Agar, Nicholas. 1997. "Biocentrism and the Concept of Life." *Ethics* 108 (1): 147–68.

Agar, Nicholas. 2001. "Recent Defenses of Biocentrism." In *Life's Intrinsic Value: Science, Ethics, and Nature*, 63–86. New York: Columbia University Press.

Aristotle. 1984. "Politics." In *The Complete Works of Aristotle: The Revised Oxford Translation*, edited by Jonathan Barnes, vol. 2, 1986–2129. Princeton, NJ: Princeton University Press.

Attfield, Robin. 2003. *Environmental Ethics: An Overview for the Twenty-First Century*. Cambridge, UK: Polity Press.

Baxter, William F. 1974. *People or Penguins: The Case for Optimal Pollution*. New York: Columbia University Press.

Biocenticity.net. 2013. "Biocentrism: The Biocentric Universe." Accessed March 18. http://www.biocentricity.net/

Botar, Oliver A. I., and Isabel Wünsche, eds. 2011. *Biocentrism and Modernism*. Farnham, UK: Ashgate.

Dombrowski, Daniel A. 1997. *Babies and Beasts: The Argument from Marginal Cases*. Urbana: University of Illinois Press.

Evogeneao. 2013. "The Great Tree of Life." Accessed March 18. http://www.evogeneao.com/tree-of-life/tree-of-life.htm

Goodpaster, Kenneth E. 1978. "On Being Morally Considerable." *Journal of Philosophy* 75 (6): 308–25.

Lanza, Robert. 2007. "A New Theory of the Universe: Biocentrism Builds on Quantum Physics by Putting Life into the Equation." *American Scholar* 76 (2): 18–33.

Lanza, Robert, and Bob Berman. 2009. "The Biocentric Universe Theory: Life Creates Time, Space, and the Cosmos Itself." *Discover* 30 (5): 52–55.

Leopold, Aldo. 1949. *A Sand County Almanac, and Sketches Here and There*. New York: Oxford University Press.

Naess, Arne. 1973. "The Shallow and the Deep, Long-Range Ecology Movement: A Summary." *Inquiry: An Interdisciplinary Journal of Philosophy* 16 (1–4): 95–100.

Passmore, John. 1974. *Man's Responsibility for Nature: Ecological Problems and Western Traditions*. London: Duckworth.

Potter, Van Rensselaer. 1971. *Bioethics: Bridge to the Future*. Englewood Cliffs, NJ: Prentice-Hall.

Regan, Tom. 2004. *The Case of Animal Rights*. Rev. ed. Berkeley: University of California Press.

Reichmann, James B. 2000. "Anthropocentrism, Biocentrism, and Envirocentrism." In *Evolution, Animal "Rights," and the Environment*, 318–47. Washington, DC: Catholic University of America Press.

Schweitzer, Albert. 1923a. *Civilization and Ethics*. Translated by John Naish. London: A. & C. Black.

Schweitzer, Albert. 1923b. *The Decay and the Restoration of Civilization*. Translated by C. T. Campion. London: A. & C. Black.

Schweitzer, Albert. 1931. *On the Edge of the Primeval Forest: Experiences and Observations of a Doctor in Equatorial Africa*. Translated by C. T. Campion. New York: Macmillan.

Singer, Peter. 1990. *Animal Liberation*. 2nd ed. New York: New York Review of Books.

Stenmark, Mikael. 2002. "The Relevance of Environmental Ethical Theories for Policy Making." *Environmental Ethics* 24 (2): 135–48.

Sterba, James P. 1995. "From Biocentric Individualism to Biocentric Pluralism." *Environmental Ethics* 17 (2): 191–207.

Sterba, James P. 1998. "A Biocentrist Strikes Back." *Environmental Ethics* 20 (4): 361–76.

Sterba, James P. 2011. "Biocentrism Defended." *Ethics, Policy, and Environment* 14 (2): 167–69.

Taylor, Paul W. 1981. "The Ethics of Respect for Nature." *Environmental Ethics* 3 (3): 197–218.

Taylor, Paul W. 1986. *Respect for Nature: A Theory of Environmental Ethics*. Princeton, NJ: Princeton University Press.

Jonathan Beever

Doctoral Student, Department of Philosophy, Purdue University

BIODIVERSITY CONSERVATION

Biodiversity conservation is the coordinated effort to sustain the diversity of life at the genetic, species, and ecosystem levels through the integration of scientific knowledge, philosophical understanding, economic and institutional policies, and management practices. It builds upon earlier historical stages in natural resource protection and management but has as its primary focus not the sustained yield of particular biological resources or the preservation of particular parts of the landscape but the protection, restoration, and maintenance of diversity and functionality in living systems at all levels of the biological hierarchy.

As knowledge of life's diversity—its evolutionary basis, its historical and contemporary distribution, its accelerated loss due to human activity—has grown, the concept of biodiversity has reshaped the aims, assumptions, and methods of conservation. At the same time conservationists have come to emphasize both the intrinsic and the instrumental value of biodiversity (for example, for human health, economic well-being, and ecosystem resilience). These shifts in the foundations of the conservation and environmental movements have recalibrated bioethical perspectives since the mid-nineteenth century. An examination of biodiversity conservation illustrates the significance of bioethics as a field that reaches beyond questions of human health and well-being to embrace the full context of the living world in which humans have evolved and now exist.

THE BACKGROUND OF CONSERVATION

Only since the 1980s have the value and significance of biological diversity become critical to the goals and practice of conservation. As a focus of concerted citizen action, public policy, scientific research, applied management, and professional endeavor, conservation first gained definition in the early 1900s. Over the decades the conservation movement has evolved in response to varied forces: emerging scientific information, shifts in philosophical premises and aesthetic standards, new environmental threats, novel technologies, changing legal mandates, and constantly shifting social, economic, and political conditions. The interplay of these forces has produced a movement that remains in flux and whose goals continue to evolve as the world's ecosystems face increasing challenges to their diversity and integrity.

The Evolving Idea of Conservation. The term *conservation* acquired its modern meaning in the early twentieth century with the rise of the Progressive Era conservation crusade in the United States. However, as an expression of cultural commitment to an enduring and resilient relationship with the natural world, conservation has much deeper prehistoric and historic roots. Prehistoric peoples did not live in a simple or constant state of peaceful coexistence with and within their natural surroundings. Converging lines of evidence from paleontology, paleoecology, archaeology, and anthropology suggest in fact a sobering picture of the human past: that the dispersal of the human population out of Africa over the past 70,000 years has been accompanied by spasms of continental and insular extinction (among other forms of environmental degradation).

In contrast to this record of prehistoric anthropogenic extinction, however, there are countervailing examples of many cultures having achieved relatively sustainable ways of life. Native peoples in landscapes throughout the world developed sophisticated belief systems and resource-use traditions that recognized their connections to and dependence on nonhuman nature. Some of these traditions have survived into the modern era, though they now contend with increasing pressures from population growth, diminished resources, altered land tenure systems, climate change, and rapid economic and technological change. In the past these traditions allowed people to adapt to and sustain themselves in even extreme environments throughout the world. The conservation movement might be characterized as modern society's conscious effort to develop and exercise analogous social practices and restraints to guide its relations with the nonhuman world.

Contemporary environmental dilemmas have prompted modern scholars to reexamine conservation traditions in texts and stories from animist, Native American, Buddhist, Hindu, Judeo-Christian, Islamic, and other faith traditions. In the Judeo-Christian tradition, for example, the biblical injunction to "fill the earth and subdue it, and have dominion over every living thing that moves upon the earth" (Genesis 1:28) has often been cited as providing the justification and rationale for centuries of environmental exploitation in the Western experience. More recently scholars have reinterpreted such textual sources, identifying alternative traditions of stewardship and respect for creation.

Early Western Approaches. Since ancient times, observers have recorded instances of environmental deterioration due to human action. Plato, for example, compared the deforested mountains of Attica to the "bones of a wasted body … the richer and softer parts of the soil having fallen away, and the mere skeleton being left" (Dubos 1980, 3). Evidence of early conservation practices can be found in the history of both Western and non-Western cultures. These include efforts to protect particular species and special lands, to maintain populations of wild plants and animals, and to sustain the productivity of agroecosystems.

European traditions of forestry and game keeping date back to the Middle Ages and beyond. The establishment of royal game preserves and forests on the land estates of feudal Europe led to the development of customs and formalized laws regulating hunting and use of the forests while also giving rise to a venerable tradition of local resentment over centralized resource management. On the continent Germany and France in particular developed silvicultural systems and techniques that prevented wholesale destruction of the forest estate.

Europeans carried these "protoconservation" traditions to their expanding colonial empires. The change in jurisdiction over natural resources from native peoples to colonial and state governments had profound implications for social systems and ecosystems alike. Colonial domination, coupled with rising populations and industrialization, disrupted traditional patterns of land tenure and resource use. In many regions native peoples became increasingly alienated from their landscapes, while Western conservation ideas and practices were slow to adapt to the new environments.

Efforts in North America. In the New World European colonists encountered a landscape of abundance as Native American populations were decimated by disease and displacement. Unchecked resource exploitation was the norm as European settlement of North America proceeded. Despite this record seeds of the later conservation movement were apparent in early efforts to protect wild game populations, forests, soils, waters, and special natural features. Through the 1800s, for example, the new American states intermittently passed laws establishing closed seasons, prohibiting hunting of nongame birds, and placing bounties on predators.

Despite such early resource conservation measures, exploitation of North America's extensive native forests—for conversion to agriculture, for construction and shipbuilding materials, for charcoal and domestic fuel supplies—drove economic development through much of the colonial and early American era. With the exhaustion of the eastern forests and the continuing settlement of interior North America, the focus of forest exploitation shifted to the Great Lakes region. The swift destruction of the Great Lakes pine forests in the latter decades of the 1800s in fact marked a turning point in forest conservation and in the emerging conservation movement generally.

A parallel pattern of resource degradation and early conservation response marked the process of agricultural development in North America. By 1776 the problem of soil erosion was evident to the new nation's leading statesmen. Over the next century destructive agricultural techniques continued to take their toll on native plant and animal diversity in ecosystems across North America (and in other parts of the world as well).

At the same time the preservation impulse in conservation found special expression in the North American setting, as European settlers encountered scenic landscapes and natural features unlike any in their prior experience. Thomas Jefferson, for example, celebrated Virginia's Natural Bridge in his *Notes on the State of Virginia*. The artist George Catlin suggested after his first excursions in the West that portions of the continent's undeveloped lands were "worthy of our preservation and protection" (Nash 2001, 101). Such early expressions of concern were not aimed at conserving biological diversity in the modern sense but sought primarily to protect economically and aesthetically important components of the landscape or ecosystem. Although limited in intent, these early protective measures provided the foundation on which a more coherent conservation movement began to take shape in the latter half of the nineteenth century.

MODERN ORIGINS OF CONSERVATION

Exploration of the world's diverse ecosystems—from the earliest voyages of discovery through the New World scientific expeditions of Alexander von Humboldt, John Bartram and William Bartram, Meriwether Lewis and William Clark, John James Audubon, and others—contributed to a golden age of natural history studies in the eighteenth and nineteenth centuries. Establishment and adoption of the Linnean system of binomial nomenclature in the 1700s allowed for an unprecedented flourishing of taxonomic research. This in turn provided critical foundations for the development of evolutionary theory in the work of Alfred Russel Wallace and Charles Darwin. Although the biological sciences had not yet developed field methods for comprehending the full diversity of life, they had begun to reveal the fundamental processes through which life diversifies and maintains itself.

These gains in systematics, biogeography, and evolutionary theory occurred even as the Industrial Revolution and the expansion of market economies accelerated the progression in scale, pace, and character of human environmental impacts. Through the 1800s the advent of more efficient technologies resulted in increasingly intensive exploitation of forests, game populations, fisheries, agricultural lands, and river systems. Traditional resource management practices and established land tenure systems were abandoned or changed to fit the emerging economies of scale. Industrial pollution and the global spread of invasive species became widespread problems for the first time. The concentration of carbon dioxide and other warming gases in the atmosphere began to increase with the shift to and increasing reliance on fossil fuel energy sources.

Philosophy and Literature. Coincident with these scientific, cultural, and environmental changes, the Enlightenment and romantic movements were altering Western conceptions of order, value, and beauty in the natural world. The natural philosophers of the Enlightenment stressed the smooth workings and stability of a mechanistic natural order. The romantic philosophers and poets emphasized the unity and wholeness to be found in a spontaneously creative organic nature. Although offering fundamentally different conceptions of nature, both encouraged human comprehension of natural objects and processes and so laid the foundation for greater appreciation of human impacts upon the natural world. The writings of Thomas Malthus and other early economic philosophers provided the basic framework for considering the interwoven fate of the human population, human economies, and natural resources.

In Europe the romantic movement drew heavily upon the experiences of New World explorers and settlers, the encounters with native peoples there and elsewhere, and the exposure to wild landscapes. In turn adaptation of the romantic impulse in the North American setting provided important literary and philosophical foundations for conservation. The strong American identification with wild nature found early expression in, for example, the essays of the transcendentalists Ralph Waldo Emerson and Henry David Thoreau, the poetry of William Cullen Bryant and Walt Whitman, and the novels of James Fenimore Cooper.

George Perkins Marsh's *Man and Nature; or, Physical Geography as Modified by Human Action* (1965 [1864]) is widely considered the first great landmark in modern conservation literature. A native Vermonter, Marsh (1965 [1864], 103) saw in the destruction of New England's forests the latest expression of an ancient human tendency to "[derange] the original proportions between different orders of organic life." Drawing on his extensive personal observations of long-term landscape change in New England and the Mediterranean, Marsh argued that human actions had caused widespread disruption of the "harmonies" of the natural world. Marsh's reasoning followed lines that would sound familiar to later generations of ecologists and biodiversity conservationists. "All nature," he wrote, "is linked together by invisible bonds, and every organic creature, however low, however feeble, however dependent, is necessary to the well-being of some other among the myriad forms of life with which the Creator has peopled the earth" (Marsh 1965 [1864], 109).

The publication of Marsh's book provided direction and definition to the nascent conservation movement through the remainder of the 1800s and the first decade of the 1900s. In North America the dispossession of the Native American tribes, the enactment of liberal land distribution policies, and the flow of settlers and capital into "virgin" landscapes resulted in an unprecedented wave of exploitation of natural resources.

Progress in Policy. This period also saw the first concerted efforts to address the causes and consequences of such massive ecological changes. At first these actions tended to focus on particular issues, species, problems, or landscapes. Sportsmen led campaigns to rein in market hunting and to institute stronger game laws at the state and local levels. Exploitation of plume-bearing egrets and other birds for the millinery trade mobilized sportsmen, scientists, and nature lovers to work together for reform. These moves culminated in the passage of the Lacey Act of 1900. The first important piece of modern national wildlife conservation legislation, it barred interstate shipment of wild animal species taken in violation of state laws and soon succeeded in ending the plume trade.

Efforts to reform American land policy proved more difficult. Through the 1800s the nation's land allotment policies had encouraged rapid emigration, immigration, settlement, and land conversion, often accompanied by corruption and land speculation. The lands of the American West presented special challenges to settlement. The geologist and explorer John Wesley Powell attempted in the 1870s and 1880s to devise a more appropriate tenure system that would recognize the inherent environmental limitations and social requirements of the region's arid and semiarid landscape, but the speculative momentum proved intractable. Only decades later did the US government institute more careful land management policies on the nation's remaining public domain. However, Powell's innovations, especially his commitment to a strong role for science in land management, laid important foundations for future private and public conservation planning.

The forestry movement quickly gained momentum in the last decade of the nineteenth century. Forest advocates working through professional scientific and forestry organizations campaigned for national legislation to reform public land laws and prevent further forest destruction. These efforts culminated in 1891 with the adoption of legislation that included a provision allowing the US president to set aside public land forests as forest reserves, the germ of the nation's current system of national forests.

The movement to protect and preserve special scenic landscapes, natural features, and wild spaces likewise gained momentum in the decades following the American Civil War. In 1872 the US Congress established the world's first national park at Yellowstone. In 1885 New York created a state forest preserve in the Adirondack Mountains to protect its wild character and its watershed values. That same year Canada designated Banff National Park, its first. The impetus toward preservation drew heavily upon the enthusiasm of nature writers, such as John Muir, who led the political effort that in 1890 resulted in the designation of an enlarged Yosemite National Park in California and who in 1892 founded the Sierra Club.

At the end of the nineteenth century, the varied strands of conservation concern—over depleted wildlife, widespread deforestation and watershed degradation, inappropriate land development, industrial pollution, and the loss of aesthetic quality—were connected only loosely. In the American experience political corruption and inordinately concentrated wealth had typically accompanied these environmental changes. As the twentieth century began, these overlapping social, economic, political, and environmental concerns brought forth a more consolidated movement that gave new meaning and power to the term *conservation*. However, the growing prominence of conservation also revealed inherent tensions in the emerging movement.

PROGRESSIVE ERA CONSERVATION

When Theodore Roosevelt assumed the American presidency in 1901, the stage was set for a revolution in conservation policy. Roosevelt's partner in political innovation was the forester Gifford Pinchot. Pinchot, the first American to receive formal training in forestry, was a friend of Roosevelt who had been active in the complex politics of the American forestry movement through the 1890s. Their partnership during Roosevelt's presidency resulted in an increase in the total acreage of the forest reserves (renamed national forests in 1905) from 60 million to 151 million acres, the transfer of these lands to the Department of Agriculture under Pinchot's jurisdiction, and the creation in 1905 of the US Forest Service to administer the new national forests.

Pinchot's Forest Service embodied the Progressive Era spirit and its approach to bureaucratic responsibilities. In contrast to Muir and others in the preservationist wing of the conservation movement, Pinchot conceived of the forest in utilitarian terms. The forests were not regarded as "reserves" to be "locked up" but as lands to be worked "for the greatest good of the greatest number for the longest time," as Pinchot's (1967 [1910], 48) formulation of the utilitarian credo put it.

In practice this meant that the forests were to be managed by a trained, professional workforce; that scientific principles were to guide the efficient exploitation and processing of forest resources; and that the wealth derived from the forests was to be equitably distributed for the common good. Applied not only to forests but to natural resources in general, the resource conservation ethic provided the dominant paradigm of the early movement. Absent from many of the Progressive political initiatives were the voices of the increasingly influential preservationists and nature protectors. In contrast to the utilitarian view that Pinchot espoused, adherents of the romantic-transcendental preservation ethic emphasized wild nature's aesthetic and spiritual values and the need to safeguard those values for future generations through strict prohibitions on development and manipulation (Callicott 1990).

The tensions between the utilitarian and preservationist approaches intensified as conservation assumed center stage politically. The schism between the conservation factions came to a head in the bitter political struggle over plans to dam the Tuolumne River in Yosemite National Park's Hetch Hetchy Valley. Waged over a period of six years, the battle culminated in 1913 with the adoption of national legislation providing federal support for the dam. Although Muir and his colleagues lost the battle, they had aroused a national constituency in favor of protection. The growing popular and political acceptance of preservation led directly to the creation of the US National Park Service in 1916.

For all of the profound developments in conservation during the Progressive Era, scant attention was given to the state of the ecological processes and biological diversity characteristic of either wilder or more humanized landscapes. That attention would come only slowly, as conservation science, philosophy, policy, and practice coevolved through the twentieth century.

CONSERVATION THROUGH THE EARLY TWENTIETH CENTURY

As conservation in the United States became institutionalized, it tended to follow the tenets of Pinchot's resource conservation ethic. By the late 1930s the basic principles of utilitarian resource conservation had been applied not only to forests but also to other "useful" components of the biota and the landscape: rangelands, game populations, sport and commercial fisheries, scenic lands and recreational areas, agricultural soils, and river systems. New policies, laws, bureaucracies, academic disciplines, research and training programs, and professional societies arose to promote sustained yields of and from these various "resources."

Internationally the years prior to World War II saw increasing recognition of the global scope of conservation challenges and halting moves to institutionalize a response to those challenges. The Western powers—particularly the United States, Great Britain, France, and Germany—continued to export forestry and national park programs to their colonies and protectorates. Intermittent steps were taken toward greater international cooperation: international conservation conferences in Europe in 1913 and 1923; the establishment in 1928 of an International Office for the Protection of Nature in Brussels; an unprecedented international bird conservation conference in Paris in 1933; the Conference for the Protection of African Fauna and Flora in London also in 1933; the first North American Wildlife Conference in 1936; and the establishment of the Pan-American Union, dedicated largely to conservation issues in the Western Hemisphere, in 1940. These developments set the stage for the expanded international programs that emerged in the aftermath of World War II.

With the outbreak of World War II, conservation issues fell into the background of concerns, proving the difficulty of maintaining mindfulness of human-nature relationships when social crises erupt. As in no other time since the Progressive Era, these years of crisis demonstrated the interwoven nature of social, economic, and environmental problems. However, conservation remained subject to the underlying philosophical rift between the utilitarian and the preservationist approaches. Neither approach adequately addressed the increasingly extensive problems of soil erosion and exhaustion, disruption of hydrological cycles, endangerment and loss of species, and the degradation of biotic communities (both terrestrial and aquatic).

By the 1930s developments in ecology and evolutionary biology over the previous decades had begun to inform conservation issues, even as contemporary problems forced conservationists to reexamine their scientific assumptions. Ecology was revolutionizing scientific understanding of the functioning of biological communities, landscapes, and systems. Evolutionary biology provided new perspectives on, for example, the adaptations, roles, and interactions of all forest species (in contrast to the basic descriptive botany, dendrology, timber physics, and forest mensuration upon which silviculture and forestry had previously rested).

These scientific advances suggested the need to introduce ecological perspectives into the various fields of resource management in the effort to sustain not just the yields of particular commodities but the healthy functioning of ecosystems generally. A key voice in this emerging approach was the American forester and wildlife ecologist Aldo Leopold, who in the course of his career applied ecological principles first to the conservation of forests; then to soils, watersheds, game and wildlife species, agricultural lands; and then ultimately to the land "as a whole."

Writing in 1939, Leopold (1939, 727) noted that ecology provided "a new fusion point for all the natural sciences" and that its emergence

> had placed the economic biologist in a peculiar dilemma: with one hand he points out the accumulated findings of his search for utility, or lack of utility, in this or that species; with the other he lifts the veil from a biota so complex, so conditioned by interwoven cooperations and competitions, that no man can say where utility begins or ends. … The only sure conclusion is that the biota as a whole is useful, and [the] biota includes not only plants and animals, but soils and waters as well.

Leopold's expanded conservation philosophy, as finally expressed in his landmark essay "The Land Ethic" in *A Sand County Almanac* (1949), emphasized the diversity, functional integrity, and beauty of what he called "the biotic community" and rejected the view of nature as merely a collection of disaggregated natural resources. It shifted the role of human beings "from conqueror of the land community to plain member and citizen of it" (Leopold 1949, 204). Leopold's evolutionary-ecological land ethic provided an alternative to the simple economic and utilitarian paradigm, on the one hand, and the strict preservationist approach, on the other (Callicott 1990). This provisional reconciliation would confront continuing challenges in the dramatically altered postwar environment. However, it would also provide those in the conservation movement with new conceptual tools with which to meet those challenges.

BIODIVERSITY: EMERGENCE OF AN IDEA

In the postwar years new tools in the earth sciences provided greater scientific understanding of the interrelations within and among terrestrial, aquatic, marine, and atmospheric systems. In the 1950s and 1960s revolutions in fields ranging from genetics and evolutionary biology to atmospheric chemistry and geology began rapidly to reshape society's understanding of the global biosphere and the human place within it. The publication in 1962 of Rachel Carson's landmark book *Silent Spring* (2002 [1962]) examining the biological impacts of DDT and other pesticides gave rise to the modern environmental movement, distinct from but still connected to the older conservation tradition.

Efforts to protect wildlands in the United States also intensified in the years following World War II. The Wilderness Act in 1964 provided for a strengthened national system of wilderness areas on the public lands of the United States. The Wilderness Act was only one of many laws adopted during this period of environmental awakening. Over the next decade the US Congress enacted a series of important environmental statutes, including the National Environmental Policy Act (1970), the Clean Air Act (1970), the Clean Water Act (1972), and the Endangered Species Act (1973). These far-reaching changes in environmental policy reflected a rising wave of popular support and organized political activism, symbolized by the observance of the first Earth Day on April 22, 1970.

The years following the inception of Earth Day saw increasing acceptance of environmental values. Those values, however, were not easily translated into effective conservation action. Conservation programs tended still to focus on single species, or particular economic resources, or separate jurisdictions within a given landscape. At the international level differences in perspectives between the wealthier, developed countries of the North and the poorer, developing countries of the South likewise proved difficult to overcome. International conservation continued to make important gains through a series of conventions and treaties, including the Convention on Wetlands of International Importance (the Ramsar Convention) (1971), the Convention on International Trade in Endangered Species (CITES) (1975), the International Convention for the Conservation of Migratory Species of Wild Animals (the Bonn Convention) (1978), the United Nations Convention on the Law of the Sea (1982), and the United Nations Convention on Biological Diversity (1992). However, international development policies would incorporate stronger conservation and environmental provisions only gradually, as the need to connect economic development and long-term environmental security became increasingly evident.

As these broad patterns of change in the human dimensions of conservation unfolded in the 1970s and 1980s, the scientific foundations of conservation continued to shift. Taxonomy and systematics provided more robust estimates of the extent of species diversity and of its actual and potential loss. The field of island biogeography revealed principles governing the spatial distribution, relative abundance, persistence, and extinction of species, with important implications for land use and the establishment and management of protected areas. Genetics became an increasingly important component of conservation science as attention focused on the reproductive success of rare and endangered species and the viability of their populations, both in captivity and in the wild. Ecology moved away from its "classical paradigm," which emphasized discrete, stable, determinist equilibria, and toward a view of ecosystems emphasizing flux, uncertainty, and contingency. The emerging field of restoration ecology sought to apply ecological principles to the remediation of species loss and ecosystem degradation. Increasingly, conservation strategies required the integration of knowledge from the many branches of biological and social sciences, involving various levels of biological organization.

The need to rethink conservation across disciplinary lines was driven not only by changes in the foundational sciences but by changes in the environment itself. By the late 1970s scientists and conservationists were alarmed by the escalating loss of genetic, species, and ecosystem diversity at the global scale. Of special concern was the accelerated destruction of the species-rich forests of the humid tropics. The advances in island biogeography revealed that ecosystems of all types were being fragmented by human activity, while even the most effectively protected areas were at risk due to their inadequate size and their isolation. Wildland managers increasingly understood that preservation alone was an inadequate management strategy and that the loss of diversity and the disruption of ecological functions were intimately associated. Agricultural scientists, foresters, and other resource managers too were increasingly concerned about environmental degradation, the breakdown of ecosystem processes, the loss of diversity in humanized landscapes, and the social and economic costs associated with these changes.

These concerns prompted the emergence in the mid-1980s of a new synthetic interdisciplinary field, conservation biology, specifically devoted to the integration of knowledge from the sciences and other disciplines in the effort to understand, maintain, and restore biological diversity (Meine, Soulé, and Noss 2006). Conservation biology has sought to address conservation problems in an evolutionary and ecological context and to stimulate the traditional conservation professions to reassess their management methods and goals accordingly. The compound term *biodiversity* itself was coined in 1986 and has since been widely adopted by conservationists. The concepts of sustainability and sustainable development came into general usage during the same period, reflecting the complex challenge of integrating long-term social, economic, and environmental factors in assessing human demands and impacts on ecosystems.

These concepts gained broader international footing in 1992 at the "Earth summit" in Rio de Janeiro. Among the products of the summit was the Convention on Biological Diversity, which recognizes the conservation of biodiversity as "a common concern of humankind" (United Nations 1992, 1). The convention binds its signatories to undertake conservation efforts in concert with development; to address conservation needs at the genetic, species, and ecosystem levels; and to integrate traditional conservation approaches with the sustainable use of biological resources.

BIODIVERSITY AND BIOETHICS

Since the 1980s the concept of biodiversity has changed the focus in conservation, highlighting the diversity and resilience of living systems and the human effects, positive and negative, on those systems. As such it has reframed the ethical relationship of humans and nonhuman nature. It challenges the traditional utilitarian view of nature as a collection of discrete, economically significant (or expendable) components. Likewise, it challenges the traditional preservationist view that humans can be separated from nature and nature thereby protected from human impacts. By recasting the human role in nature and emphasizing the reality of economic relationships and transeconomic values within ecosystems, biodiversity conservation has inevitably entailed deeper consideration of ethical constructs.

Since the 1980s, the field of biodiversity conservation has matured together with the field of environmental ethics. As the former has sought to expand the purview of conservation to include the diversity of life, the latter has sought to enlarge the scope of ethical inquiry beyond the human sphere. However, the links between biodiversity and bioethics have still to be more fully explored. This has begun to occur more frequently as shared areas of concern have emerged: for example, biodiversity as a source of medicinal compounds; the phenomena of emerging diseases; climate change and human health; water, aquatic ecosystem health, and public health; exploration of the human microbiome; and the links between biodiversity and mental health.

In recognizing these connections to biodiversity, bioethicists are in a sense returning to the roots of their own field. Hans-Martin Sass (2007) credits the German philosopher and educator Fritz Jahr with coining the term *bioethics* in a 1927 article titled "Bio-Ethics: A Review of the Ethical Relationships of Humans to Animals and Plants." The oncologist and biochemist Van Rensselaer Potter introduced the term more broadly in his 1971 book *Bioethics: Bridge to the Future*, which is dedicated to Leopold and in which Potter aimed to address issues at the intersection of biology, ecology, medicine, and ethics. In a later volume, *Global Bioethics: Building on the Leopold Legacy* (1988), he sought explicitly to reclaim the scope of the term from its more restricted meaning of biomedical ethics. The public may anticipate that connections between biodiversity conservation and bioethics will continue to proliferate as understanding grows of the dynamic relationships between levels of biological hierarchy, between humans and nonhuman nature, and between human health and ecosystem health.

CONCLUSION

Although antecedents to conservation can be traced back over centuries, the conservation movement in the modern sense first emerged in the early twentieth century. Since then conservation's aims have steadily evolved beyond the sustained exploitation of particular resources and the protection of particular natural features to address the sustainability and resilience of ecosystems and human communities within them. In the process conservation has come to place greater emphasis on the diversity of life at all geographic scales and all levels of biological organization. In the late twentieth century this shift came to be reflected in the neologism *biodiversity* and in an expanding discourse regarding the ethical significance of biological diversity in human affairs—and conversely the significance of human affairs for the fate of biodiversity. As scientists and ethicists alike come to appreciate more fully the complexity and dynamism of human-nature relationships—physical, psychological, economic, and ecological—the boundaries between environmental ethics and bioethics are likely to dim and the areas of convergence to emerge more clearly.

SEE ALSO *Animal Welfare and Rights: V. Zoos and Zoological Parks; Ecological Bioethics; Environmental Ethics; Food; Synthetic Biology*

BIBLIOGRAPHY

Barrow, Mark V. 2009. *Nature's Ghosts: Confronting Extinction from the Age of Jefferson to the Age of Ecology*. Chicago: University of Chicago Press.

Brennan, Andrew, and Lo Yeuk-Sze. 2011. "Environmental Ethics." *The Stanford Encyclopedia of Philosophy*, edited by Edward N. Zalta. http://plato.stanford.edu/archives/fall2011/entries/ethics-environmental/

Callicott, J. Baird. 1990. "Whither Conservation Ethics?" *Conservation Biology* 4 (1): 15–20.

Callicott, J. Baird. 1997. *Earth's Insights: A Multicultural Survey of Ecological Ethics from the Mediterranean Basin to the Australian Outback*. Berkeley: University of California Press.

Carson, Rachel. 2002 [1962]. *Silent Spring*. New York: Houghton Mifflin Harcourt.

Center for Environmental Philosophy. 2013. Accessed August 21, 2013. http://www.cep.unt.edu

Center for Humans and Nature. 2013. "Biosphere Ethics Initiative." Accessed August 21, 2013. http://www.humansandnature.org/biosphere-ethics-initiative-project-7.php

Daily, Gretchen C., ed. 1997. *Nature's Services: Societal Dependence on Natural Ecosystems*. Washington, DC: Island.

Daly, Herman E., and Kenneth N. Townsend, eds. 1993. *Valuing the Earth: Economics, Ecology, Ethics*. Cambridge, MA: MIT Press.

Dubos, René. 1980. *The Wooing of Earth*. New York: Scribner's.

Ehrenfeld, David W. 1976. "The Conservation of Non-resources." *American Scientist* 64 (6): 648–56.

Ehrenfeld, David W. 1978. *The Arrogance of Humanism*. Oxford: Oxford University Press.

Farnham, Timothy J. 2007. *Saving Nature's Legacy: Origins of the Idea of Biological Diversity*. New Haven, CT: Yale University Press.

Fox, Stephen. 1981. *John Muir and His Legacy: The American Conservation Movement*. Boston: Little, Brown.

Gadgil, Madhav; Fikret Berkes; and Carl Folke. 1993. "Indigenous Knowledge for Biodiversity Conservation." *Ambio* 22 (2–3): 151–56.

Grim, John, and Mary Evelyn Tucker. 2013. *Ecology and Religion*. Washington, DC: Island.

Grove, Richard H. 1995. *Green Imperialism: Colonial Expansion, Tropical Island Edens, and the Origins of Environmentalism, 1600–1860*. New York: Cambridge University Press.

Hays, Samuel P. 1959. *Conservation and the Gospel of Efficiency: The Progressive Conservation Movement, 1890–1920*. Cambridge, MA: Harvard University Press.

International Union for Conservation of Nature. 2010. "Biosphere Ethics Initiative." March 9. http://www.iucn.org/about/union/members/resources/news/?4890/Biosphere-Ethics-Initiative

Leopold, Aldo. 1939. "A Biotic View of Land." *Journal of Forestry* 37 (9): 727–30.

Leopold, Aldo. 1949. *A Sand County Almanac, and Sketches Here and There*. New York: Oxford University Press.

MacPhee, Ross D. E., ed. 1999. *Extinctions in Near Time: Causes, Contexts, and Consequences*. New York: Kluwer Academic/Plenum.

Marsh, George Perkins. 1965 [1864]. *Man and Nature; or, Physical Geography as Modified by Human Action*. Cambridge, UK: Cambridge University Press.

Mayr, Ernst. 1982. *The Growth of Biological Thought: Diversity, Evolution, and Inheritance*. Cambridge, MA: Harvard University Press.

Meine, Curt; Michael Soulé; and Reed E. Noss. 2006. "'A Mission-Driven Discipline': The Growth of Conservation Biology." *Conservation Biology* 20 (3): 631–51.

Miller, Char. 2001. *Gifford Pinchot and the Making of Modern Environmentalism.* Washington, DC: Island/Shearwater.

Moore, Kathleen Dean, and Michael P. Nelson, eds. 2010. *Moral Ground: Ethical Action for a Planet in Peril.* San Antonio, TX: Trinity University Press.

Nash, Roderick. 1989. *The Rights of Nature: A History of Environmental Ethics.* Madison: University of Wisconsin Press.

Nash, Roderick. 2001. *Wilderness and the American Mind.* 4th ed. New Haven, CT: Yale University Press.

Norton, Bryan G. 1987. *Why Preserve Natural Variety?* Princeton, NJ: Princeton University Press.

Pinchot, Gifford. 1967 (1910). *The Fight for Conservation.* Seattle: University of Washington Press.

Potter, Van Rensselaer. 1971. *Bioethics: Bridge to the Future.* Englewood Cliffs, NJ: Prentice-Hall.

Potter, Van Rensselaer. 1988. *Global Bioethics: Building on the Leopold Legacy.* East Lansing: Michigan State University Press.

Rolston, Holmes, III. 2012. *A New Environmental Ethics: The Next Millennium for Life on Earth.* New York: Routledge.

Sass, Hans-Martin. 2007. "Fritz Jahr's 1927 Concept of Bioethics." *Kennedy Institute of Ethics Journal* 17 (4): 279–95.

Taylor, Paul W. 1986. *Respect for Nature: A Theory of Environmental Ethics.* Princeton, NJ: Princeton University Press.

United Nations. 1992. "Convention on Biological Diversity." http://www.cbd.int/doc/legal/cbd-en.pdf

United Nations Educational, Scientific, and Cultural Organization. 2013. "Biodiversity and Culture, Society and Ethics." Accessed August 21, 2013. http://www.unesco.org/new/en/natural-sciences/special-themes/biodiversity-initiative/biodiversity-culture

Whitehouse, Peter J. 2003. "The Rebirth of Bioethics: Extending the Original Formulations of Van Rensselaer Potter." *American Journal of Bioethics* 3 (4): 26–31.

Williams, Michael. 1989. *Americans and Their Forests: A Historical Geography.* Cambridge, UK: Cambridge University Press.

Wilson, Edward O., ed. 1988. *Biodiversity.* Washington, DC: National Academies Press.

Worster, Donald. 2001. *A River Running West: The Life of John Wesley Powell.* New York: Oxford University Press.

Worster, Donald. 2008. *A Passion for Nature: The Life of John Muir.* New York: Oxford University Press.

Curt Meine
Senior Fellow, Center for Humans and Nature
Senior Fellow, Aldo Leopold Foundation

BIOETHICS

This entry consists of the following:

I. HISTORY OF

A tradition of moral discourse has been an integral part of medical theory and practice since the earliest era of literate healing in Western culture. At the origin of this perennial tradition stand the oath of Hippocrates, from the late fifth century B.C.E., and certain maxims, such as "Be of benefit and do no harm," found in the Hippocratic literature from several subsequent centuries. Since that time there has always been a thin stream of reflection about the moral character of those who practice medicine and about certain procedures and styles of practice. Particular attention to the needs of one's patient over the self-interest of the physician and gratuitous care for those who cannot afford to pay for medical attention have been constant themes. Thomas Percival (1740–1804) recapitulated the essence of this tradition in his *Medical Ethics* (1827 [1803]). A similar tradition can be discerned in the history of Chinese, Japanese, Hindu, and Islamic medicine.

The content of these traditions remained relatively stable until the middle of the twentieth century. At that time extraordinary advances in the biological sciences began to bring unprecedented progress into medical practice everywhere in the developed world, making it possible to remedy hitherto lethal conditions by pharmacological and surgical procedures. Infectious diseases were countered by antibiotics; cancer alleviated and sometimes cured by radiotherapy, chemotherapy, and surgery; and mental disease treated by psychopharmacology. The reach of medical care covered far more people than ever before, and for many of them the benefits of treatment were compromised: they lived with reduced quality of life. Deaths from infectious disease were reduced, with the consequence of increased populations in need of sustenance.

A NEW MEDICAL ETHICS

In Western culture from the 1950s onward, thoughtful observers of this new medical world began to wonder whether the traditional Hippocratic ethic—act for the benefit of patients and do them no harm—still provided physicians with adequate guidance. It was no longer clear what constituted a benefit. Were lives extended by antibiotics but marked by years of greater disability, or a reduction in disease-related deaths accompanied by a decrease in food supplies, or highly risky but only rarely successful life-saving surgery to be counted as benefits? Observers of this paradoxical progress wondered whether an ethic wider than traditional medical ethics was needed and whether that ethics should encompass not only the practices of medicine but the goals and application of the biological sciences that propelled medical progress.

This new field of reflection deserved a new name. The neologism *bioethics* was coined in 1971 by the biological scientist Van Rensselaer Potter (1911–2001) (1971, 2), who opened his book, *Bioethics: Bridge to the Future*, by explaining, "I therefore propose the term *Bioethics* in order to emphasize the two most important ingredients in achieving the wisdom that is so desperately needed: biological knowledge and human values." The word, even in so vague a definition, caught on. The *Encyclopedia of Bioethics*, first published in 1978, defined bioethics as "the study of the ethical dimensions of medicine and the biological sciences" (Reich 1978, xix), expanded in 1995 to "a systematic study of the moral dimensions—including moral vision, decisions, conduct and policies—of the life sciences and health care, employing a variety of ethical methodologies in an interdisciplinary setting" (Reich 1995, xxi). The philosopher Daniel Callahan, founder of the Hastings Center, attempted to give this new field some specificity in his 1973 article "Bioethics as a Discipline." With the meaning and content of the field still being debated, scholarly discussion and public controversy has gone on for forty years, creating a large body of thought that can loosely be called a discipline or at least a field of study.

During the 1960s a number of conferences, sponsored by colleges and scientific societies, reflected on the problems arising in this new conjunction of biological science and medicine. The most significant of these was the 1962 Ciba Conference, "Man and His Future," at which leading scientists, such as the molecular biologist Joshua Lederberg (1925–2008), the geneticist Hermann Muller (1890–1967), and the molecular biologist and neuroscientist Francis Crick (1916–2004), expressed their concerns about the very scientific innovations they were themselves creating. Two centers were founded to study these issues—in 1969 the Institute of Society, Ethics, and the Life Sciences (later known as the Hastings Center) and in 1971 Georgetown University's Kennedy Institute of Ethics. These two centers stimulated scholarly research and discussion as well as public awareness of the nascent field of bioethics.

The classic fields of ethical analysis, such as moral philosophy and moral theology, began to glance at the issues of medical ethics. The first notable attempt to do this came even before the era of general concern about bioethical problems. In 1949 the Episcopal theologian Joseph Fletcher (1905–1991) (1954, xix) gave the Lowell Lectures at Harvard on "certain problems of conscience, certain ethical issues, which arise in the course of medical care." Although Fletcher's topics were still conventional matters for medical ethics, such as abortion, contraception, and euthanasia, he stressed a new note that would become a major concern of subsequent bioethics, namely, the right of a patient to determine his or her treatment. However, the first intensive ethical analysis of the new biology in medicine came from the Methodist theologian and Princeton professor Paul Ramsey (1913–1988). In the Yale Beecher Lectures, published as *The Patient as Person* in 1970, he explored the ethical implications, under the conditions of modern medical technology, of the new genetics, transplantation, research, and death and dying. Ramsey laid out careful, often conservative arguments that invited response. A leading Catholic theologian, Richard McCormick (1922–2000), did so in many articles, in which he not only engaged Ramsey and Fletcher in friendly but serious debate but also explored new formulations of Catholic traditional teaching on medical ethics. These and many other scholars formulated a substantive analytic literature about the questions that had puzzled scientists and agitated the public.

THE ROLE OF THE PUBLIC

Public agitation over ethical questions was not theoretical. Actual events shocked the nation, such as the 1972 revelation of the Tuskegee Syphilis Study. Beginning in 1932 the US Public Health Service had enrolled impoverished African American sharecroppers who had syphilis into a research study that withheld standard treatment in order to observe the course of their untreated disease. The research participants were not informed of their diagnosis or of the research project. Public outcry forced the Public Health Service to form a panel of distinguished outsiders, the Tuskegee Syphilis Study Ad Hoc Advisory Panel, which castigated the study as unethical in its beginnings and continuation, recommended compensation for survivors, and called for the establishment of a national research board to regulate all federally funded research with human subjects.

Abuses of human subjects of research had been condemned in 1946–1947 at the Nuremberg trials, military tribunals that tried twenty-three Nazi physicians for performing harmful and often lethal medical experiments on concentration camp prisoners without their consent. The Nuremberg Code, formulated for those trials, listed the principal rules for ethical experimentation;

primary among these was that participation in research should be voluntary and uncoerced. In 1954 the World Medical Association issued similar guidelines, which became known as the Helsinki Declaration. Starting in the early 1960s the expanding National Institutes of Health (NIH), which sponsored research across the nation, began to study how to ensure that the rights and welfare of the human subjects in those studies could be protected. All institutions in which NIH-funded research was conducted were required to have internal committees that reviewed all proposed projects for risks to subjects. In a 1966 article one of the United States' distinguished medical scientists, Henry K. Beecher (1904–1976) of Harvard, indicted the research community for exposing subjects to excessive risk, neglecting consent, and withholding therapies of known efficacy. Beecher's article raised consciousness in the medical research community about the ethics of research. In England the book *Human Guinea Pigs* (1968), by Maurice H. Pappworth (1910–1994), issued a similar, even more detailed indictment—and incidentally marked the field of human research with an indelible moniker, human subjects as guinea pigs.

More than consciousness-raising was needed. The Tuskegee Ad Hoc Panel had urged federal regulations, and the NIH had imposed a process of review, but a broader, firmer public policy was called for. After a series of hearings sponsored by Senator Edward Kennedy, on July 12, 1974, Congress passed the National Research Act (Public Law 93-348) authorizing the establishment of the National Commission for the Protection of Human Subjects of Biomedical and Behavioral Research. Over the next four years the commission investigated many areas of research with human subjects and in 1978 issued the Belmont Report, a broad framework for understanding and applying ethical principles to research. The report and other specific studies, such as "Research Involving Prisoners" (1976), "Research Involving Children" (1977), "Research Involving Those Institutionalized as Mentally Infirm" (1978), and "Institutional Review Boards" (1978), benefited from the input of a wide range of scientists and scholars who were called on to apply their skills to problems, many of which they had never explicitly considered. The result was not only an enforceable public policy about research but the creation of a body of scholarly literature and of a wider community aware of and expert in bioethics.

THE FIRST MAJOR ISSUES

The ethics of research with humans was the first major issue that stimulated bioethics. At the same time, however, a remarkable advance in medical practice created a flurry of ethical questions. Transplantation of human tissue and the replacement of organic functions by mechanical substitutes appeared in the 1950s. Kidney transplantation, pioneered by John Murray in 1954, posed the question whether a surgical operation to remove a viable organ from a healthy person for transplant to another whose kidneys had failed conflicted with the Hippocratic dictum of "do no harm" and violated laws against mutilation. The Ciba Conference of 1966 brought together an international gathering of leading transplant surgeons and other scholars to reflect on this and other ethical problems associated with transplantation. *Law and Ethics of Transplantation* (1966), edited by Gordon E. W. Wolstenholme and Maeve O'Connor, emerged from this conference. Human-to-human transplantation of hearts, first performed by Christiaan Barnard in 1967, aroused widespread astonishment and concern about the very high failure rate of this dramatic procedure. Replacement of lost organic function by machines, first demonstrated in 1960 by Belding Scribner's use of continuous hemodialysis for failed kidneys, garnered public admiration and concern about how to select the tiny cohort of patients who could receive this expensive treatment. A popular magazine article by Shana Alexander, "They Decide Who Lives, Who Dies" (1965), was followed by *Who Shall Live* (Vaux 1970), a collection of reflections by theologians and philosophers on the problem of selecting persons for life and death.

The prospect of developing an artificial heart powered by nuclear energy prompted the director of the National Heart and Lung Institute, Theodore Cooper, to convene an Artificial Heart Assessment Panel in 1972 to advise him on the "economic, ethical, legal, medical, psychiatric and social implications of a totally implantable artificial heart" (National Heart and Lung Institute, Artificial Heart Assessment Panel 1973). The panel, made up of a mix of physicians, lawyers, and one ethicist, discouraged the further development of the nuclear-powered device. This panel and the almost contemporaneous Tuskegee Ad Hoc Study were the first government bodies convened to reflect and recommend on bioethical questions.

Other remarkable advances in medical treatment and diagnosis that appeared in the second half of the twentieth century—such as neurosurgery, antibiotic pharmacology, and chemotherapy for cancer—not only saved lives but extended them. Often extended lives were filled with debility. Successful methods to support compromised respiration pulled patients through critical episodes but sometimes sustained them in sustained comas. The case of Karen Ann Quinlan in 1975 brought the questions of how to define death and when to allow an incurable patient to die to public attention. A broad public debate ensued. Congress reconstituted the national commission as the President's Commission for the Study of Ethical Problems in Medicine and in Biomedical and Behavioral Research (1980–1983), which, among other studies, issued the reports *Defining Death* (1981) and *Deciding to Forego [sic] Life-Sustaining Treatment* (1983). Both documents made important contributions to the legal and ethical understanding of the complex questions surrounding death and dying. A number of well-publicized cases about agonizing decisions to allow newborn babies to die tested this new understanding. The devastating HIV/AIDS epidemic that raged through the 1980s pushed these questions to the forefront of bioethics.

These initial committees on bioethics were followed by many others over the next decades. Appointed at different levels of government, from NIH divisions to congressional and presidential advisory bodies, they were assigned the responsibility of reviewing and recommending policy about a broad range of bioethical issues. Presidents Bill Clinton (1993–2001), George W. Bush (2001–2009), and Barack Obama (2009–) established advisory and investigative bodies by executive order. These bodies were given broad mandates to study ethical issues arising in the biomedical sciences, although several were given specific instructions to explore the growing field of stem cell research, cloning, and genomics. The remarkable expansion of molecular genetics posed new and unique issues about human identity, privacy, and indeed human nature itself. Federal studies of the twenty-first century have concentrated on these questions and their public policy relevance. Bioethicists have served as advisors in public policy development; a dozen were selected to advise President Clinton's Task Force on Health Reform (see Brock 1994).

These government bodies, while having diverse influences, did reveal bioethics as more than a scholarly enterprise carried on in books and debates—it was shown to be a public enterprise. The participants in these commissions and councils came from many professional and public backgrounds and represented a diversity of views about ethical issues. They were scientists, lawyers, clergy, scholars from various disciplines, and citizens at large. Few were experts in academic ethics, although the bodies were supported by persons trained in ethics and were advised by many scholars familiar with ethics and related disciplines. The bodies were given specific mandates to study particular issues, often leading to recommendations about public policy and programs. The unique contributions of these bodies, then, were their focus on an immediate practical problem and policy recommendations. Moral philosophy had never seen such concentrated attention to matters that were to be not simply thought about but acted on.

Bioethics done by committee appeared in other countries. In Great Britain a royal commission led by a distinguished moral philosopher, Mary Warnock, studied the developments in assisted reproduction. A bioethics commission independent of the government and funded by the Nuffield Foundation continued to take up issues as they arose in British society. In France in 1983 President François Mitterrand set up the National Ethics Consultative Committee for the Sciences of Life and Health. The Council of Europe has had a Committee of Experts on Bioethical Issues since 1985, and the United Nations Educational, Scientific and Cultural Organization (UNESCO) has had an International Bioethics Committee since 1993. These groups function in different ways and deal with issues in the national cultures that they serve. In general, they foster investigative and analytic studies as well as international policy.

THE SCHOLARSHIP OF BIOETHICS

Behind this widespread "public bioethics," a scholarly enterprise emerged. A number of philosophers, theologians, lawyers, and social scientists produced books on the general subject or particular topics within it. In addition to the topics surveyed above, the widespread concern for individual rights that swept the United States in the 1970s touched medicine. Physicians were accused of "paternalism," or ignoring their patients' autonomy to decide for themselves about medical treatment. As Robert M. Veatch (1981) explained it, in this view the physician's voice is only one of many that should be heard, and the patient should play a major role in decisions about his or her care. *Principles of Biomedical Ethics*, written by the philosopher Tom L. Beauchamp and the theologian James F. Childress (2013; first published in 1979), both of whom had advised the national commission, set the standard for careful argumentation about the questions of bioethics. In England *Principles of Health Care Ethics* (1994), edited by Raanan Gillon, provided a broad overview of scholarly reflection.

Another form of literature appeared that came to be called *clinical ethics*. The study of bioethics in institutes such as the Hastings Center and the Kennedy Institute was speculative: how were issues to be formulated and what prospects for managing their implications could be discerned? The task of governmental advisory bodies was to provide perspectives about the ways the moral implications of public policy could be articulated and implemented. Clinical ethics, however, arose from the teaching of ethics to medical students, which began in the late 1960s in a few American medical schools and spread throughout medical education over the next several decades. Teachers of ethics who were not physicians learned quickly that a significant part of medical education takes place not in the classroom but at the bedside. The Hastings Center devised a curriculum for the Columbia College of Physicians and Surgeons that covered the four years of medical school, thus including not only didactic lectures but also case conferences. In a 1978 article Mark Siegler used the term *clinical ethics* to describe the practice of teaching ethics in the context of a real case being discussed by physician teachers and medical students. He, together with Albert R. Jonsen and William J. Winslade, published *Clinical Ethics* (2010 [1982]), which became widely used in classroom teaching and clinical consultation. Bioethics in bedside consultation has not flourished in many places outside the United States.

Bioethics has evolved from an expression of moral concern, voiced by a few percipient observers of contemporary science, and from expressions of outrage over abuses of patients and subjects of medical research into a recognized field of study, to which are devoted university departments and degrees, journals, and encyclopedias. It has become a standard feature of institutions where research is done and medicine is practiced. Although the focus on medicine and biomedical science has remained, bioethics has extended to other areas where the human and the biological world interact. The philosopher Peter Singer, professor of bioethics at Princeton University, has been a pioneer in this expansion. He first called attention to the human interaction with animals in *Animal Liberation* (1990). His 2009 volume, *The Life You Can Save*, covers a wide range of issues, from evolutionary biology to world poverty. In the early twenty-first century other important questions about the relationship between human values and biological knowledge, such as the human impact on climate change, had not found their way into the literature of bioethics.

It must be noted that, with the exception of remarks about international bioethics commissions, this summary concerns the United States. However, bioethics has appeared around the world; many scholarly organizations and centers foster its study. The issues surveyed above are found wherever modern medicine is practiced, although perspectives and emphases vary among cultures. Similarly bioethics appears in religious traditions, such as Judaism, Buddhism, and Islam, whose distinctive ethical teachings pose bioethical problems in differing perspectives. In 2002 the International Association of Bioethics initiated an annual conference for bioethicists from around the world. Bioethics has indeed become an international topic (see Green, Donovan, and Jauss 2008).

The historian of medicine David J. Rothman (1991, 189), in his work *Strangers at the Bedside*, observed that "by 1978 … bioethics was a field, would-be ethicists had career lines to follow, and the notion that medical ethics belonged exclusively to medicine had been forgotten by most everyone, except for a cadre of older physicians and a handful of historians." He further noted, "The record … makes a convincing case for a fundamental transformation in the substance as well as the style of medical decision making" (Rothman 1991, 251).

SEE ALSO *Appendix: A History of Medical Ethics; Bioethics Commissions, History of; Care: I. History of the Notion of Care; Ethics: I. History of Ethics; Health and Disease: I. History of the Concepts; Informed Consent: I. History of Informed Consent; Nazi Legacy and Bioethics; Pedagogy of Bioethics; Public Health: I. History; Research, Human: Historical Aspects*

BIBLIOGRAPHY

Alexander, Shana. 1965. "They Decide Who Lives, Who Dies: Medical Miracle and a Moral Burden of a Small Committee." *Life* 53:102–25.

Baker, Robert B., and Laurence B. McCullough, eds. 2009. *The Cambridge World History of Medical Ethics*. Cambridge, UK: Cambridge University Press.

Beauchamp, Tom L., and James F. Childress. 2013. *Principles of Biomedical Ethics*. 7th ed. New York: Oxford University Press.

Beecher, Henry K. 1966. "Ethics and Clinical Research." *New England Journal of Medicine* 274 (24): 1354–60.

Brock, Dan W. 1994. "The Role of Ethics in the Clinton Reform Proposal." *Journal of Health Politics, Policy, and Law* 19 (1): 217–80.

Callahan, Daniel. 1973. "Bioethics as a Discipline." *Hastings Center Report* 1 (1): 66–73.

Callahan, Daniel. 2012. *In Search of the Good: A Life in Bioethics*. Cambridge, MA: MIT Press.

Fletcher, Joseph. 1954. *Morals and Medicine: The Moral Problems of the Patient's Right to Know the Truth, Contraception, Artificial Insemination, Sterilization, Euthanasia*. Princeton, NJ: Princeton University Press.

Gillon, Raanan, ed. 1994. *Principles of Health Care Ethics*. Chichester, UK: Wiley.

Green, Ronald M.; Aine Donovan; and Steven A. Jauss, eds. 2008. *Global Bioethics: Issues of Conscience for the Twenty-First Century*. Oxford: Oxford University Press.

Jonsen, Albert R. 1998. *The Birth of Bioethics*. New York: Oxford University Press.

Jonsen, Albert R. 2000. *A Short History of Medical Ethics*. New York: Oxford University Press.

Jonsen, Albert R.; Mark Siegler; and William J. Winslade. 2010 (1982). *Clinical Ethics: A Practical Approach to Ethical Decisions in Clinical Medicine*. 7th ed. New York: McGraw-Hill Medical.

McCormick, Richard A. 1981. *How Brave a New World? Dilemmas in Bioethics*. Garden City, NY: Doubleday.

National Commission for the Protection of Human Subjects of Biomedical and Behavioral Research. 1978. *The Belmont Report: Ethical Principles and Guidelines for the Protection of Human Subjects of Research*. Washington, DC: DHEW and US Government Printing Office. http://videocast.nih.gov/pdf/ohrp_belmont_report.pdf

National Heart and Lung Institute, Artificial Heart Assessment Panel. 1973. *The Totally Implantable Artificial Heart: Economic, Ethical, Legal, Medical, Psychiatric, Social Implications: A Report*. Bethesda, MD: National Institutes of Health.

Pappworth, Maurice H. 1968. *Human Guinea Pigs: Experimentation on Man.* Boston: Beacon.

Percival, Thomas. 1827 (1803). *Medical Ethics; or, A Code of Institutes and Precepts Adapted to the Professional Conduct of Physicians and Surgeons.* London: Jackson.

Post, Stephen G., ed. 2004. *Encyclopedia of Bioethics.* 3rd ed. 5 vols. New York: Macmillan Reference USA.

Potter, Van Rensselaer. 1971. *Bioethics: Bridge to the Future.* Englewood Cliffs, NJ: Prentice-Hall.

President's Commission for the Study of Ethical Problems in Medicine and in Biomedical and Behavioral Research. 1981. *Defining Death: A Report on the Medical, Legal, and Ethical Issues in the Definition of Death.* Washington, DC: Author.

President's Commission for the Study of Ethical Problems in Medicine and in Biomedical and Behavioral Research. 1983. *Deciding to Forego [sic] Life-Sustaining Treatment.* Washington, DC: Author.

Ramsey, Paul. 1970. *The Patient as Person: Explorations in Medical Ethics.* New Haven, CT: Yale University Press.

Reich, Warren T., ed. 1978. *Encyclopedia of Bioethics.* 4 vols. New York: Free Press.

Reich, Warren T., ed. 1995. *Encyclopedia of Bioethics.* Rev. ed. 5 vols. New York: Macmillan.

Rothman, David J. 1991. *Strangers at the Bedside: A History of How Law and Bioethics Transformed Medical Decision Making.* New York: Basic Books.

Siegler, Mark. 1978. "A Legacy of Osler: Teaching Clinical Ethics at the Bedside." *Journal of the American Medical Association* 239 (10): 951–56.

Singer, Peter. 1990. *Animal Liberation.* New York: New York Review Books.

Singer, Peter. 2009. *The Life You Can Save: Acting Now to End World Poverty.* New York: Random House.

Stevens, M. L. Tina. 2000. *Bioethics in America: Origins and Cultural Politics.* Baltimore, MD: Johns Hopkins University Press.

Tuskegee Syphilis Study Ad Hoc Advisory Panel. 1973. "Final Report of the Tuskegee Syphilis Study Ad Hoc Advisory Panel." Washington, DC: US Public Health Service. http://biotech.law.lsu.edu/cphl/history/reports/tuskegee/tuskegee.htm

Vaux, Kenneth, ed. 1970. *Who Shall Live: Medicine, Technology, Ethics.* Houston Conference on Ethics in Medicine and Technology, 1968. Philadelphia: Fortress.

Veatch, Robert M. 1981. *A Theory of Medical Ethics.* New York: Basic Books.

Warnock, Mary. 1985. *A Question of Life.* Oxford: Blackwell.

Wolstenholme, Gordon E. W., and Maeve O'Connor, eds. 1966. *Law and Ethics of Transplantation.* Ciba Foundation Blueprint. London: Churchill.

Albert R. Jonsen
Senior Ethics Scholar in Residence,
California Pacific Medical Center, San Francisco

II. KEY CASES IN

Many important developments in bioethics have been spurred by cases. The cases summarized below are a heterogeneous group. Some are legal cases, whereas others have only a tangential relationship to law; some received extensive media coverage, whereas others did not. What they share is landmark status and considerable complexity. This overview can only skim the surface, hinting at the stories, histories, and legacies that make these cases "key." At least two book-length treatments of bioethics cases (Johnson et al. 2009; Pence 2010) offer the interested reader more in-depth examination of cases. This entry's bibliography also provides a starting point for further research.

CLINICAL ETHICS

In clinical ethics areas of interest include informed consent, end of life decision making, decision making for children and for individuals with disabilities, and human reproduction.

Informed Consent. In the area of informed consent the influence of case (judge-made) law is particularly extensive, with few cases more influential than *Canterbury v. Spence* (1972). *Canterbury v. Spence* involved a nineteen-year-old patient who underwent an unremarkable laminectomy (removal of the lamina, a vertebral bone) but who suffered major paralysis from a postoperative fall from his hospital bed. According to trial testimony, he and his mother had not been told that a laminectomy carried about a 1 percent risk of paralysis, and there is some discrepancy about whether his mother consented to the procedure prior to the operation.

The historical significance of *Canterbury* is derived from the robust analysis in the 1972 federal appeals court opinion.

1. In holding that the principle of informed consent requires that physicians disclose material risks and information about alternatives that a reasonable patient would wish to know in making treatment decisions (i.e., an objective patient-centered standard), the court in *Canterbury* rejected the professional-discretion standard for disclosure, emphasizing the patient's right to self-determination.
2. The court connected the duty to disclose information to the established duty to treat a patient with reasonable skill.
3. The court refined the scope of obligations by defining "material" risks as those to which a reasonable person would likely attach significance in deciding whether or not to undergo a proposed therapy.
4. The court confirmed that the negligence theory of liability requires that proximate causality be based on

> an objective reasonable patient standard. That is, if "adequate disclosure could reasonably be expected to have caused a [prudent] person to decline the treatment because of the revelation of risk ... causation is shown." (*Canterbury v. Spence* 1972, 791)

In the early twenty-first century most jurisdictions have adopted the reasonable patient standard, but specific applications of the informed consent doctrine continue to create ethical debate. Many bioethicists argue that the goal of informed consent is to empower patients with the information they need to provide their autonomous authorizations for medical interventions and to promote a therapeutic alliance between health care teams and patients through patient engagement (Faden and Beauchamp 1986). Others focus on the practicalities, including whether patients really desire engagement and whether it is worth the additional time and effort (Schuck 1994).

End of Life. The emphasis on self-determination in consent to treatment carried over to the landmark end-of-life cases involving requests to discontinue treatment, beginning with *In re Quinlan* (1976).

In re Quinlan (1976). For unclear reasons, twenty-two-year-old Karen Ann Quinlan ceased breathing for two fifteen-minute periods, resulting in brain damage. She regressed to a chronic persistent vegetative state (PVS). Quinlan's father asked the New Jersey Supreme Court to authorize the discontinuance of "extraordinary medical procedures," namely the use of a ventilator.

The court held that the state's interest in the preservation and sanctity of human life and its defense of the physician's right to administer medical treatment according to professional judgment "weakens and the individual's right to privacy grows as the degree of bodily invasion increases and the prognosis dims" (*In re Quinlan* 1976, 664). The court reasoned that the right to privacy, derived from protections afforded in the Bill of Rights, is broad enough to allow an individual to decline life-sustaining medical treatment. The court's focus then shifted to prognosis and Quinlan's inability to return to cognitive and sapient life and the high degree of bodily invasion by way of intensive twenty-four-hour nursing care and the assistance of the ventilator, antibiotics, a feeding tube, and a catheter. Lacking definitive evidence concerning the patient's wishes, the court deferred to her surrogate decision maker. In doing so the court granted her father's request to withdraw the ventilator. The court's analysis has been heralded as "strikingly prescient and forward-looking" for reasons including its concern for practicalities and its impact on the development of ethics committees (Clark 2006, 393).

Contrary to expectations, Quinlan lived another ten years without ventilator support. The case therefore highlighted a continuing ethical challenge. Decisions about life-sustaining measures are sometimes made with limited or erroneous information (Hall, Bobinski, and Orentlicher 2007).

Cruzan v. Director, Missouri Department of Health (1990). In 1983 twenty-five-year-old Nancy Cruzan lost control of her car and was discovered lying face down in a ditch without respiratory or cardiac function. Cruzan's brain was deprived of oxygen for at least twelve minutes, which resulted in brain damage and regression into a PVS. Cruzan did not need the assistance of a ventilator but required a percutaneous endoscopic gastrostomy (PEG) to receive adequate artificial nutrition and hydration. Her parents requested that hospital employees withdraw the PEG tube and allow Cruzan to die, but they refused to do so without court approval.

The matter eventually reached the US Supreme Court. In a five-to-four decision issued in 1990 the court upheld Missouri's requirement that an incapacitated patient's wish to have life-sustaining measures withdrawn be proven by clear and convincing evidence. Careful reading of the opinion demonstrates that the oft-cited proposition that *Cruzan v. Director, Missouri Department of Health* (1990) creates a "right to die" is inaccurate. Rejecting the right of privacy as the constitutional underpinning for its decision, the majority characterized a capacitated patient's right to refuse life-sustaining measures as a "liberty interest," not a "fundamental" right, and so allowed for more extensive state regulation. Unlike the *Quinlan* court, the majority outlined conceptual difficulties with effectuating a liberty interest for someone unable to claim it, thereby rejecting the claim that incapacitated patients necessarily have the same right to refuse life-sustaining measures as capacitated patients (Clark 2006). According to the majority, Missouri's heightened evidentiary standard furthered a legitimate interest in preserving and protecting human life, ensuring that surrogates' decisions to withdraw life-sustaining measures are in keeping with patients' values, goals, and preferences.

Sandra Day O'Connor, one of the court's associate justices, wrote a separate concurring opinion emphasizing that appropriate procedural safeguards for incapacitated individual's interests should be left to the states. These could range from life-sustaining treatment decision making by surrogates for incapacitated patients without judicial oversight to clear and convincing evidentiary standards with judicial review.

In re Schiavo (2000). After *Quinlan* and *Cruzan* life-sustaining treatment issues seemed settled in law. The legal skirmishes that became known as *In re Schiavo* I, II,

III, and IV, with related developments, tested that supposition.

Theresa "Terri" Marie Schiavo suffered a cardiac arrest from a potassium imbalance, leaving her in a PVS. In *Schiavo* I the patient's husband and legal guardian, Michael Schiavo, asked George Greer, a county circuit court judge, to decide whether Schiavo would have wanted her artificial nutrition and hydration (PEG tube) withdrawn. The Florida Supreme Court had previously interpreted the explicit right to privacy in the Florida Constitution to include the right of an incapacitated patient to refuse artificial nutrition and hydration. Based on the evidence submitted, Greer in 2000 decided that Schiavo would want treatment withdrawn, and the Florida District Court of Appeal agreed (2001). In *Schiavo* II (2001) the appellate court ruled against Schiavo's parents, Robert Schindler and Mary Schindler, with regard to their challenges to the evidence presented at the trial court and the potential conflicts of interest for Michael Schiavo as Terri Schiavo's guardian.

How did a relatively commonplace dispute between family members over a patient's wishes regarding the withdrawal of treatment evolve from a private dispute into a highly publicized and politicized fracas? This change likely occurred around the time of *Schiavo* III (2001), following the Schindlers' shift from attacking Michael's trustworthiness and the sufficiency of evidence about Schiavo's wishes to contesting the credibility of the PVS diagnosis and suggesting that medical treatments were available to restore Schiavo's ability to eat and speak (Goodman 2010). These latter arguments served as the basis for a remand order (*Schiavo* IV [2003]) and attracted media attention and the involvement of disability rights and right-to-life activists. Video clips and images purporting to show that Schiavo was in some other extreme state besides PVS appeared in national and international media.

The anchor in the gale winds of the political furor was the consistency of the judiciary. After numerous motions and appeals, two removals and reinsertions of the PEG tube, attempts by the Florida legislature and the US Congress to intervene (e.g., "Terri's law," which would have allowed the issuance of an executive order requiring the reinsertion of the PEG tube but was ruled unconstitutional), and a refusal of the US Supreme Court to grant certiorari, Schiavo died in 2005 in a hospice after PEG tube removal.

The resolution to this case would seem to suggest the end of end-of-life disputes, but issues remain. Questions may arise concerning decision-making standards for incapacitated patients without advance directives. In the few clinical situations involving patients with living wills, the interpretation of them remains clinically and ethically challenging. Withholding or withdrawing life-sustaining interventions from patients in a PVS or artificial nutrition and hydration interventions from patients in terminal or irreversible condition remains an issue for some religious leaders and organizations (Goodman 2010). Finally, the procedural safeguards articulated by the states are often impractical and largely ignored for everyday end-of-life decision making at patients' bedsides (Clark 2006).

Pediatrics/Disabilities. Disputes involving children, especially children with disabilities, tend to be particularly charged. The Baby Doe and Ashley X cases are representative.

Baby Doe (1982). In 1982 a child was born with Down syndrome and esophageal atresia with tracheaesophageal fistula. The pediatrician consulted recommended immediate transfer to a children's hospital for surgery. The obstetrician told the parents they also had the option of refusing to consent and allowing the child to die. The parents chose the second option. The obstetrician wrote an order (1) permitting oral feeding (with the risk of aspiration), (2) prohibiting intravenous feeding, and (3) directing that the child be kept as comfortable as possible. The pediatrician continued to push for treatment, and the hospital attorney suggested a judicial hearing. The judge ruled that, faced with two divergent medical opinions, the parents had the right to select between them. The county prosecutor took the case to the Indiana Supreme Court, which denied a request for emergency intervention. As the deputy prosecutor was preparing an emergency appeal to the US Supreme Court, the child died (Lyon 1985).

Prior reports of instances of withholding treatment had drawn comment (Pernick 1996; Mercurio 2009), but they had not attracted the same level of media and public attention. Reacting to the controversy, President Ronald Reagan directed the Department of Health and Human Services (HHS) to take action under Section 504 of the Rehabilitation Act. The Rehabilitation Act prohibits recipients of federal funds from discriminating against an otherwise qualified individual solely by reason of his or her handicap. In 1983 the HHS issued interim regulations mandating extensive posting of notices in hospitals with "Baby Doe squads" established to carry out investigations. Ultimately, the US Supreme Court struck down the regulations, finding that Section 504 does not apply to health care providers in situations in which parents refuse to consent to treatment (*Bowen v. American Hospital Association* 1986).

Meanwhile, in 1984 the US Congress sought to address these issues under the rubric of medical neglect through amendments to the Child Abuse Prevention and Treatment Act. Specifically, the amendments require states receiving federal monies for child-protection services to institute programs or procedures for responding to reports of cases in which disabled infants with life-threatening conditions have been denied treatment that, in the treating physician or physicians' reasonable medical judgment, will most likely be effective in ameliorating or correcting all such conditions unless one of three exceptions applies. The first exception is for infants who are irreversibly comatose. The other two exceptions apply only to cases in which treatment would be futile or virtually futile in terms of survival. There is continuing disagreement about how much these regulations matter, given that their requirements fall on states (and via state law on parents) rather than health care providers and given the track record of nonenforcement (Hurst 2005; Kopelman 2005). There is also continuing debate about the substantive ethical issues: whether quality-of-life considerations should factor into decision making for neonates and the amount of discretion to be afforded to parents (Silvers and Francis 2011; Wilkinson 2011). In addition, while the early twenty-first-century legal and professional consensus supports aggressive treatment for children born with Down syndrome with the expansion of prenatal testing, many affected fetuses are being aborted.

Ashley X (2006). Like that of Baby Doe, the case of Ashley X concerned the scope of parental authority in medical decision making and response to disability. Briefly, after birth Ashley was diagnosed with static encephalopathy of unknown origin, leading to marked global developmental deficits. She grew physically, but functionally she continued to resemble a three-month-old infant, unable to sit up, use language, or take food by mouth but able to respond to others. At around age five Ashley began to show signs of precocious puberty. Her parents worried that her accelerating growth and sexual development would make it impossible for them to care for her at home, cause her distress, and increase the potential for abuse by third parties. With physicians at Seattle Children's Hospital, Ashley's parents devised a plan that included growth attenuation via hormonal treatments, a hysterectomy, and breast bud removal. The desired outcome was a height reduction of 13 inches to around 4 feet, 5 inches, with a weight of 75 pounds versus 125 pounds. The hospital's ethics committee reviewed the plan and found it appropriate. Relying on a letter from the parents' attorney stating that no court order was required, the physicians went ahead.

The publication of a case report describing the approach and its ethical justification (Gunther and Diekema 2006) brought sharp criticism from the disability community (e.g., "A Statement of Solidarity for the Dignity of People with Disabilities" 2012) and an investigation. The Washington State agency charged with protecting and advocating for the rights of individuals with disabilities concluded that the sterilization violated state law, because it was carried out without the appointment of a disinterested third party to represent the child's interest and without a court order finding satisfaction of the stringent conditions for involuntary sterilization (Carlson and Dorfman 2007). Seattle Children's Hospital agreed to take a number of corrective actions, including notifying the agency of requests for similar interventions and including a disability rights advocate on the hospital ethics committee. Consensus on the ethical issues remains elusive. Involuntary sterilization has a long history marked by civil rights violations, and commentators debate whether cases such as Ashley's are distinguishable.

Human Reproduction. While US constitutional law has played a critical role in the domain of abortion, most famously and controversially in *Roe v. Wade* (1973), state law has been more significant in domains such as surrogate motherhood, as illustrated by *In re Baby M* (1988).

Roe v. Wade (1973). The woman known by the legal pseudonym "Jane Roe" lacked a story beyond an unwanted out-of-wedlock pregnancy. She was the lead plaintiff in a class-action lawsuit challenging a Texas law criminalizing the performance of an abortion with an exception only for abortions procured or attempted for the purpose of saving the woman's life based on medical advice.

After a federal district court struck down the law, the parties appealed directly to the US Supreme Court. The court held that a right to privacy, grounded in the Fourteenth Amendment's concept of personal liberty and restrictions on state action, encompasses a woman's decision whether or not to terminate a pregnancy. It also recognized important state interests in safeguarding health, maintaining medical standards, and protecting potential life. In exploring the scope of permissible state regulation, the court applied the stringent "compelling state interest" test. It also rejected the argument that a fetus is a "person" under the Fourteenth Amendment and declined to speculate about when "life" begins. It concluded with a three-part framework grounded in contemporary evidence concerning the risks of abortion versus childbirth and the potential for survival ex utero: (1) Prior to the end of the first trimester, the decision and its effectuation "must be left to the medical judgment of the pregnant woman's attending physician"; (2) subsequent to the end of the first trimester, the state may "regulate the abortion procedure in ways that are reasonably related to maternal health"; and (3) subsequent to viability, the state, promoting its interest in the potentiality of human life, may "regulate, and even proscribe, abortion except where it is necessary, in appropriate medical judgment, for the preservation of the life or health of the mother" (*Roe v. Wade* 1973, 164–65).

As reviewed at length in the court's majority opinion written by Harry Blackmun, an associate justice, the history of abortion in the West in general and in the United States in particular had already taken several turns. Since *Roe* the Supreme Court itself has shifted. For instance, in *Planned Parenthood of Southeastern Pennsylvania v. Casey* (1992) the court reaffirmed *Roe*'s essential holding, including treating abortion as a matter of constitutional right and using viability as a significant threshold, but the plurality abandoned the trimester framework and moved to a less demanding "undue burden" test for state regulation. The trend in the early twenty-first century toward more restrictive legislation at the state level has produced a steady stream of judicial opinions working out the implications.

In re Baby M (1988). In February 1985 William Stern and Mary Beth Whitehead entered into a surrogacy contract. According to its terms, Whitehead agreed to be artificially inseminated and to give up her legal claims on any resulting child. Upon surrender of custody, she was to receive $10,000. Following an uneventful pregnancy, Whitehead gave birth to a baby girl. She turned the baby, whom the Sterns named Melissa, over to the Sterns three days later. The next day Whitehead went to the Sterns' home and said she could not live without her baby, but she promised to return the baby in one week. The promise was not honored, and the Sterns filed suit to enforce the surrogacy contract.

The trial court held that the contract was valid, ordered the termination of Whitehead's parental rights, and awarded custody to Stern. On appeal the New Jersey Supreme Court held that the contract was invalid on two grounds. First, it violated state statutes prohibiting payment to a parent to give up a child for adoption, requiring proof of parental unfitness or abandonment before the termination of parental rights, and making an agreement to surrender a child for a private-placement adoption revocable before birth and an offer of counseling. Although the parties tried to structure the contract to skirt these laws, the court was not persuaded. Second, the contract conflicted with public policies of the state. In place of an independent inquiry focused on the best interests of the child, the contractual model allowed custody to be determined by an agreement purchased with money. The court stated that Whitehead's consent, even if fully voluntary and informed (and the court reviewed reasons for skepticism), would not be dispositive: "There are, in a civilized society, some things that money cannot buy" (*In re Baby M* 1988, 440). After disposing of the parties' constitutional claims, the court awarded custody to Stern, citing the converging recommendations of three independent experts.

There is no consensus on the validity of surrogacy contracts. The legal response varies from state to state and country to country. A development that postdates *Baby M* is surrogacy with donated eggs. This can be seen as simplifying matters, because the claims of the parturient are lessened, given that she has no genetic connection to the child, or as making them more complex, because three women can potentially vie for the status of legal mother. Most of the early twenty-first-century bioethics and legal literature is focused on reproductive tourism, especially the use of surrogates from developing countries (e.g., Davis 2012).

RESEARCH ETHICS

In the realm of research ethics, some cases have been critical to the development of consensus, whereas others have sparked debates that have yet to be resolved.

Catalysts for Consensus and Regulation. The development of an international consensus around a set of ethical standards for biomedical research and the ratification of those standards in US policy can largely be attributed to the Nuremberg Doctors' Trial and the scandal surrounding the Tuskegee syphilis study. The Doctors' Trial, which began on December 9, 1946, was the first of twelve sectorial trials held before US military tribunals. The prosecutor reviewed a variety of experiments conducted with prisoners (Taylor 1992), some in connection with the war effort and others tied to the larger Nazi program of "racial hygiene." Experiments involved confinement to low-pressure tanks, drowning, freezing, intentional infection with malaria and typhus, intentional infliction and infection of wounds, poisoning, and chemical sterilization. Of the twenty-three defendants, sixteen were found guilty, and seven were executed. The judges articulated ten principles for the conduct of research involving humans, including informed consent, scientific rationale, acceptable balance of risks and benefits, minimization of risks, and liberty to withdraw. These became known as the Nuremberg Code.

Initially, the code received little attention from the public or the research community (Faden, Lederer, and Moreno 1996), but by the 1950s the code had achieved canonical status. On its fiftieth anniversary in 1997 Evelyne Shuster (1997, 1436) described it as "the most important document in the history of the ethics of medical research."

It is one thing to embrace a code. It is another to translate the principles into provisions of law enforceable by a government agency. The Tuskegee syphilis study was the catalyst for the latter step. The long, sad story of Tuskegee has taken up volumes. What follows is a short summary of key events. In the early twentieth century the

African American educator Booker T. Washington and the philanthropist Julius Rosenwald developed a plan to provide medical treatment, including the treatment of syphilis, in Macon County, Alabama, as part of a larger initiative to promote economic development and self-sufficiency. The preparatory work included a survey conducted by the US Public Health Service (USPHS) to determine the prevalence of syphilis and prospects for mass treatment. The Great Depression put an end to this ambitious plan.

In 1932 the chief of the USPHS Venereal Disease Division became interested in studying the natural course of untreated late latent syphilis. Based on the survey findings and other factors, Macon County was selected as the site. The study was later defended on the grounds that it did not alter the subjects' conditions for the worse. The researchers, however, went to considerable lengths to mislead subjects into believing that they were receiving treatment as part of the study and to block access to treatment. The medical literature at the time supported treating syphilis even in its latent stages despite the toxicities. In addition, the study was not ended in the 1940s and 1950s after penicillin became available. As late as 1969 a committee at the National Communicable Disease Center (later known as the Centers for Disease Control and Prevention) decided to continue the study. The end came only when the media picked up the story in 1972. In 1997 President Bill Clinton issued an official apology and honored the survivors.

Although an initial investigation played down the significance of the study and the associated ethical violations, it spurred passage of the National Research Act of 1974 and the subsequent formation of the National Commission for the Protection of Human Subjects of Biomedical and Behavioral Research. More recent commentators have placed the study in a context of entrenched racism and a history of ethically questionable research involving African Americans.

Vulnerable Populations/Infection-Inducing Experiments. The Guatemala sexually transmitted disease (STD) studies and the Willowbrook hepatitis studies both belong to the history of infection-inducing experiments with vulnerable populations. The Guatemala experiments occurred earliest in time. They received scrutiny, however, only in the early twenty-first century, when the historian Susan M. Reverby, in the course of conducting research on Tuskegee, found a box of relevant documents. A 2011 report of the Presidential Commission for the Study of Bioethical Issues reviews the details. Its title quotes from a 1947 *New York Times* article stating that the reproduction of a promising rabbit-based syphilis prevention study in humans would be "ethically impossible." In fact at the time the USPHS was launching a research effort that would ultimately involve the deliberate exposure of 1,308 Guatemalans to syphilis and other STDs. Subjects included commercial sex workers, soldiers, prisoners, and institutionalized psychiatric patients aged ten to seventy-two. Some earlier STD prophylaxis studies involving intentional exposure conducted with US prisoners incorporated constraints in areas such as consent. For most of the Guatemala subjects, the evidence points in the other direction. For example, documents refer to the budget implications of using volunteers versus the type of subjects being employed and to the use of "double talk" to maintain compliance (Presidential Commission for the Study of Bioethical Issues 2011, 61).

The commission concluded that the experiments involved "unconscionable violations of ethics, even as judged against the researchers' own understanding of the practices and requirements of the medical ethics of the day" (Presidential Commission for the Study of Bioethical Issues 2011, 92). Groups made vulnerable as a result of conscription or institutionalization and situated in a poor country appeared to have been "targeted specifically because of their inability to protect themselves or to have others represent their interests" (Presidential Commission for the Study of Bioethical Issues 2011, 95).

The Willowbrook experiments, while also widely condemned (e.g., Beecher 1966), differed in many important respects. The Willowbrook State School was an overcrowded, underresourced institution for children with mental disabilities located on Staten Island, New York. Given the living conditions, hepatitis was endemic. Saul Krugman, an infectious disease expert, joined the staff in the mid-1950s. Krugman and his colleagues proposed and carried out a research program aimed at distinguishing between strains of hepatitis, possibly leading to the development of a vaccine. The plan involved feeding children local strains of live hepatitis.

Later, in defending his approach, Krugman argued that the children were bound to be exposed to the same strains under natural conditions, that they were admitted to a special well-staffed research unit where they were isolated from exposure to other infectious diseases, and that preliminary epidemiological work had shown that the majority would develop only a subclinical infection followed by immunity. Further, only children of parents who gave informed consent were included; an innovative approach to consent developed after the launch of the experiments included group briefings.

Carefully analyzing Krugman's own data for a study published in 2003, Joel D. Howell and Rodney A. Hayward concluded that infection was far from inevitable, even for children institutionalized from birth. Others have pointed out that the language in a cover letter sent to parents was misleading, suggesting that the goal was to deliver rather than to develop a new mode of prevention. Further, some years into the experiments research participation became the only path to entry into the school. Finally, even though the Willowbrook research (in contrast to the Guatemala research) generated valid and useful science, questions remain about the necessity of using children and the deliberate infection design (Rothman and Rothman 1984; Education Development Center 2009).

Questions continue to arise about infection-inducing experiments (Miller and Grady 2001) and about research in developing countries, especially if the research would be infeasible in the researchers' home country. It is interesting to note that *The Belmont Report: Ethical Principles and Guidelines for the Protection of Human Subjects of Research*, while affirming an order of preference among classes of subjects (e.g., adults before children) and expressing caution about any research use of groups such as the institutionalized mentally infirm and prisoners, failed to provide clear guidance concerning the responsibilities of researchers operating in contexts of social injustice (National Commission for the Protection of Human Subjects of Biomedical and Behavioral Research 1979).

Conflicts of Interest. Debate continues over how to understand and address conflicts of interest in research. Much of what is generally known about the *Moore v. Regents of the University of California* (1990) case comes from an opinion of the California Supreme Court. These facts should be viewed with caution, because as a result of the posture of the case the court was required to treat the allegations in plaintiff John Moore's complaint as true. Moore alleged that when he came to the University of California, Los Angeles, Medical Center for treatment of hairy cell leukemia in 1976, his physician, David Golde, recognized the potential scientific and commercial value of Moore's blood and tissue. Yet in obtaining Moore's consent to the removal of his spleen, blood, and tissue during follow-up visits, Golde failed to inform Moore of his plans for research to exploit this value. Golde then established a cell line from Moore's T lymphocytes. He was later named as the inventor in a patent application on the cell line and pursued various lucrative commercial opportunities.

Moore sought relief on two main grounds—breach of physician disclosure obligations and conversion of personal property. The court held that, as to the first cause of action, the lawsuit could go forward. In California "a physician must disclose personal interests unrelated to the patient's health, whether research or economic, that may affect the physician's professional judgment" (*Moore v. Regents of the University of California* 1990, 129). The majority dismissed the conversion claim, expressing alarm about the policy implications for researchers. An interesting companion case is that of Henrietta Lacks (Skloot 2010).

Moore and Lacks were patients who became unwitting subjects via their physicians' exploitation of the research value of their excised biological materials. The case of Jesse Gelsinger is different in that he knew he was entering a clinical trial; what was obscure was the lead investigator's commercial interest in the trial. The eighteen-year-old Gelsinger suffered from ornithine transcarbamylase deficiency (OTC), a rare metabolic disorder, which he controlled with diet and medication. In the early days of excitement over gene therapy, James Wilson and others at the University of Pennsylvania were exploring the potential contribution of gene therapy to the treatment of OTC. Advised by the well-known bioethicist Arthur L. Caplan to begin with those of age and well enough to consent rather than desperately ill babies who were likely to die anyway, the researchers set out to recruit individuals such as Gelsinger. Gelsinger was infused on September 13, 1999. He died on September 17 following a massive inflammatory reaction.

Gelsinger's father, angered when he learned of Wilson's financial stake, sued, naming Caplan among the defendants, though he was subsequently dropped from the lawsuit. Documents that turned up in subsequent investigations revealed that consent forms were altered to play down risks and that the investigators violated their own protocols. This lawsuit and another filed by attorneys with the US Department of Justice were eventually settled out of court.

Although there has been greater attention in the late twentieth and early twenty-first centuries to financial conflicts of interest in research, here too unresolved questions remain. Do financial conflicts of interest constitute threats to trust that should be tightly restricted and subjected to extensive regulation, or are they necessary adjuncts to socially valuable alliances with industry that can be reconciled with subject welfare through greater transparency? Is there undue emphasis on commercial interests to the neglect of other powerful motivations so that corners are cut in order to move research forward?

SEE ALSO *Law and Bioethics; Nazi Legacy and Bioethics*

BIBLIOGRAPHY

Allen, Arthur. 2000. "Bioethics Comes of Age." *Salon*, September 28. Accessed September 1, 2012. http://www.salon.com/2000/09/28/caplan/

Baby M., In re. 1988. 109 N.J. 396.

Beecher, Henry K. 1966. "Ethics and Clinical Research." *New England Journal of Medicine* 274 (24): 1354–60.

Bowen v. American Hospital Association. 1986. 476 U.S. 610.

Brandt, Allan M. 1978. "Racism and Research: The Case of the Tuskegee Syphilis Study." *Hastings Center Report* 8 (6): 21–29.

Canterbury v. Spence. 1972. 464 F.2d 772 (D.C. Cir. 1972).

Carlson, David R., and Deborah A. Dorfman. 2007. "Investigative Report regarding the 'Ashley Treatment.'" Accessed September 1, 2012. http://www.disabilityrightswa.org/sites/default/files/uploads/Full_Report_InvestigativeReportRegardingtheAshleyTreatment.pdf

Child Abuse Prevention and Treatment Act Amendments of 1984. 2008. Pub. L. No. 98-457, 98 Stat. 1749 (codified as amended at 42 U.S.C. §§ 5101–5106i (2006) and implemented by 45 C.F.R. § 1340.15 (2008)).

Clark, Annette E. 2006. "The Right to Die: The Broken Road from *Quinlan* to *Schiavo*." *Loyola University Chicago Law Journal* 37 (2): 383–403.

Colby, William H. 2002. *Long Goodbye: The Deaths of Nancy Cruzan*. Carlsbad, CA: Hay House.

Cruzan v. Director, Missouri Department of Health. 1990. 497 U.S. 261.

Davis, Erica. 2012. "The Rise of Gestational Surrogacy and the Pressing Need for International Regulation." *Minnesota Journal of International Law* 21 (1): 120–44.

Education Development Center. 2009. "Willowbrook Hepatitis Experiments." In *Exploring Bioethics*. Accessed September 1, 2012. http://science.education.nih.gov/supplements/nih9/bioethics/guide/pdf/teachers_guide.pdf

Faden, Ruth R., and Tom L. Beauchamp. 1986. *A History and Theory of Informed Consent*. New York: Oxford University Press.

Faden, Ruth R.; Susan E. Lederer; and Jonathan D. Moreno. 1996. "US Medical Researchers, the Nuremberg Doctors Trial, and the Nuremberg Code: A Review of Findings of the Advisory Committee on Human Radiation Experiments." *Journal of the American Medical Association* 276 (20): 1667–71.

Goodman, Kenneth W., ed. 2010. *The Case of Terri Schiavo: Ethics, Politics, and Death in the 21st Century*. Oxford: Oxford University Press.

Gunther, Daniel F., and Douglas S. Diekema. 2006. "Attenuating Growth in Children with Profound Developmental Disability: A New Approach to an Old Dilemma." *Archives of Pediatrics and Adolescent Medicine* 160 (10): 1013–17.

Hall, Mark A.; Mary Anne Bobinski; and David Orentlicher. 2007. *Health Care Law and Ethics*. 7th ed. New York: Aspen Publishers.

Howell, Joel D., and Rodney A. Hayward. 2003. "Writing Willowbrook, Reading Willowbrook: The Recounting of a Medical Experiment." In *Useful Bodies: Humans in the Service of Medical Science in the Twentieth Century*, edited by Jordan Goodman, Anthony McElligott, and Lara Marks, 190–213. Baltimore, MD: Johns Hopkins University Press.

Hurst, Irene. 2005. "Baby Doe Rules." *Pediatrics* 116 (6): 1600–1601.

Institute of Medicine. 2009. *Conflict of Interest in Medical Research, Education, and Practice*. Washington, DC: National Academies Press.

Johnson, Sandra H.; Joan H. Krause; Richard S. Saver; and Robin Fretwell Wilson, eds. 2009. *Health Law and Bioethics: Cases in Context*. New York: Aspen Publishers.

Kopelman, Loretta M. 2005. "Are the 21-Year-Old Baby Doe Rules Misunderstood or Mistaken?" *Pediatrics* 115 (3): 797–802.

Krugman, Saul. 1986. "The Willowbrook Hepatitis Studies Revisited: Ethical Aspects." *Reviews of Infectious Diseases* 8 (1): 157–62.

Lyon, Jeff. 1985. *Playing God in the Nursery*. New York: Norton.

Mercurio, Mark R. 2009. "The Aftermath of Baby Doe and the Evolution of Newborn Intensive Care." *Georgia State University Law Review* 25 (4): 835–63.

Miller, Franklin G., and Christine Grady. 2001. "The Ethical Challenge of Infection-Inducing Challenge Experiments." *Clinical Infectious Diseases* 33 (7): 1028–33.

Moore v. Regents of the University of California. 1990. 51 Cal. 3d 120.

National Commission for the Protection of Human Subjects of Biomedical and Behavioral Research. 1978. *The Belmont Report: Ethical Principles and Guidelines for the Protection of Human Subjects of Research*. Washington, DC: DHEW and US Government Printing Office.

Pence, Gregory E. 2010. *Medical Ethics: Accounts of Groundbreaking Cases*. 6th ed. New York: McGraw-Hill.

Pernick, Martin S. 1996. *The Black Stork: Eugenics and the Death of "Defective" Babies in American Medicine and Motion Pictures since 1915*. New York: Oxford University Press.

Planned Parenthood of Southeastern Pennsylvania v. Casey. 1992. 505 U.S. 833.

Presidential Commission for the Study of Bioethical Issues. 2011. *"Ethically Impossible": STD Research in Guatemala from 1946 to 1948*. Washington, DC: Author. Accessed December 30, 2012. http://bioethics.gov/cms/sites/default/files/Ethically-Impossible_PCSBI.pdf

Quinlan, In re. 1976. 355 A.2d 647 (N.J. 1976).

Reverby, Susan M. 2009. *Examining Tuskegee: The Infamous Syphilis Study and Its Legacy*. Chapel Hill: University of North Carolina Press.

Reverby, Susan M. 2011. "'Normal Exposure' and Inoculation Syphilis: A PHS 'Tuskegee' Doctor in Guatemala, 1946–1948." *Journal of Policy History* 23 (1): 6–28.

Roe v. Wade. 1973. 410 U.S. 113.

Rothman, David J., and Sheila M. Rothman. 1984. *The Willowbrook Wars*. New York: Harper and Row.

Schiavo, In re. 2001. 780 So. 2d 176 (Fla. 2d DCA 2001) (*Schiavo* I), review denied, 789 So. 2d 348 (Fla. 2001).

Schiavo, In re. 2001. 792 So. 2d 551 (Fla. 2d DCA 2001) (*Schiavo* II).

Schiavo, In re. 2002. 800 So. 2d 640 (Fla. 2d DCA 2001) (*Schiavo* III), review denied, 816 So. 2d 127 (Fla. 2002).

Schiavo, In re. 2003. 851 So. 2d 182 (Fla. 2d DCA 2003) (*Schiavo* IV), review denied, 855 So. 2d 621 (Fla. 2003).

Schuck, Peter H. 1994. "Rethinking Informed Consent." *Yale Law Journal* 103 (4): 899–905.

Shuster, Evelyne. 1997. "Fifty Years Later: The Significance of the Nuremberg Code." *New England Journal of Medicine* 337 (20): 1436–40.

Silvers, Anita, and Leslie Francis. 2011. "Cloudy Crystal Balls Do Not 'Gray' Babies Make." *American Journal of Bioethics* 11 (2): 36–38.

Skloot, Rebecca. 2010. *The Immortal Life of Henrietta Lacks.* New York: Crown Publishers.

"A Statement of Solidarity for the Dignity of People with Disabilities: A Reaction to the 'Ashley Treatment.'" 2012. Bravenet.com. Accessed September 1. http://pub6.bravenet.com/guestbook/501900445

Stolberg, Sheryl Gay. 1999. "The Biotech Death of Jesse Gelsinger." *New York Times Magazine,* November 28, 136–40, 149–50.

Stossel, Thomas P. 2005. "Regulating Academic-Industrial Research Relationships: Solving Problems or Stifling Progress?" *New England Journal of Medicine* 353 (10): 1060–65.

Taylor, Telford. 1992. "Opening Statement of the Prosecution, December 9, 1946." In *The Nazi Doctors and the Nuremberg Code: Human Rights in Human Experimentation,* edited by George J. Annas and Michael A. Grodin, 67–93. New York: Oxford University Press.

Washington, Harriet A. 2006. *Medical Apartheid: The Dark History of Medical Experimentation on Black Americans from Colonial Times to the Present.* New York: Doubleday.

Wilkinson, Dominic James. 2011. "A Life Worth Giving? The Threshold for Permissible Withdrawal of Life Support from Disabled Newborn Infants." *American Journal of Bioethics* 11 (2): 20–32.

Wilson, Robin Fretwell. 2010. "The Death of Jesse Gelsinger: New Evidence of the Influence of Money and Prestige in Human Research." *American Journal of Law and Medicine* 36 (2–3): 295–325.

Mary A. Majumder
Assistant Professor of Medicine and Medical Ethics, Center for Medical Ethics and Health Policy, Baylor College of Medicine

Courtenay R. Bruce
Assistant Professor of Medicine and Medical Ethics, Center for Medical Ethics and Health Policy, Baylor College of Medicine

III. DISCOURSE IN

The field of bioethics, because of its applications to ongoing and vital moral issues in the public sphere, has become akin to what is referred to in cultural studies as a contact zone, an area where different communities of discourse, which normally do not enter into each other's discursive spheres, are forced to communicate and work with each other (Pratt 1989). Bioethics has brought together an odd assortment of academic, professional, and social groups that are engaged in quite different social and intellectual activities and can be distinguished by their particular forms of discourse: such groups as philosophers, clinicians, economists, theologians, activists, politicians, anthropologists, hospital administrators, journalists, lawyers, and literary critics.

Many of these discourse communities maintain different criteria for membership, symbolic capital, rules of engagement, argument fields, historical context, and speech genres. Conflicts within bioethics can be unusual in the academy, for unlike struggles in a single intellectual field, in which the argument fields tend to be relatively stable, disputes in bioethics can include arguments about exactly which discourse community's rules should judge the debate. For example, in a special issue of the *Journal of Medicine and Philosophy* titled "Literature and Medical Ethics," its editors, K. Danner Clouser, a philosopher, and Anne Hunsaker Hawkins, a literary critic, debate in a series of commentaries whether the very articles they had accepted for publication were qualified to be in the journal. Clouser argues that since philosophy was the first discipline in the scholarly analysis of morality, those in the discipline of literature need to first attend to philosophy's discourse, for otherwise "it is not clear that one is writing about ethics" (1996, 323–24). Hawkins counters Clouser's position by observing that although Plato may have wished to banish the poets, literature has been "a primary source of ethical wisdom though the history of Western civilization" (1996, 341–42). Elsewhere Roland Barthes observes that change in discourse "moves, in its historical impetus, by *clashes,*" through which one discourse struggles against a prior dominant discourse (1977, 199–200). The history of discourse in bioethics could be characterized as a history of continual clashes as various communities of discourse struggle for dominance. Because of this bioethics has become in its discourse a truly interdisciplinary study in which this synthesis, unlike in other multidisciplinary fields, has created an innovative discourse in which a variety of prior discourse traditions have become fused together (cf. Barthes 1977, 155–56).

THEOLOGICAL DISCOURSE ABOUT BIOETHICS BEFORE BIOETHICS

As is often noted, a number of the earliest scholars in bioethics were moral theologians. Such thinkers as Joseph Fletcher, Paul Ramsey, and Richard McCormick responded to the new questions being raised in the public sphere on issues arising from new medical technology. Although the analytic tradition of philosophy, which dominated American philosophy departments, had generally lost interest in the study of ethics (Toulmin 1982), theology departments had through the 1950s been actively engaged in the discussion of moral questions, including a number of subjects that are now considered under the purview of bioethics. Albert Jonsen (1998, chap. 1) has referred to this midcentury period as "medical ethics before bioethics." Although the determining factors that created bioethics in North America have not been agreed upon, these theologians and religious ethicists were a dominant part of the early history of this new field. They were, however, dominant for only a short period of the field's history, although it would be incorrect to argue that they ever became extinct.

The reason for this loss of status was intimately related to the theologians' and religious ethicists' choice of discourse in communicating to the public. As has been often noted, their discourse seemed to many to be curiously nontheological—or perhaps one should say atheological—in nature. As Leon R. Kass observes, "Most religious ethicists entering the public practice of ethics leave their special religious insights at the door and talk about 'deontological vs. consequentialist,' 'autonomy vs. paternalism,' 'justice vs. utility,' just like everybody else" (1990, 7). Martin E. Marty opines that the clearest cause of the secular nature of their discourse is the pluralistic nature of American culture, for theologians normally speak to a particular faith community, and in their attempt to speak to the multitude of faith communities in the United States they spoke to no community, including their own (1992, 274). Stephen E. Lammers echoes Marty's argument when he notes that when religious voices became active in public policy, their drew on "the language of publicly accessible reasons," that is, "the language or languages of liberalism" (1996, 35). Robert Veatch claims that some religious ethicists simply tired of translating their faith's discourse system into a discourse that could be understood by those outside their faith tradition and thus found it more convenient to use secular language as their primary means of thinking through moral issues (Callahan et al. 2000, 83). Carla M. Messikomer, Renée C. Fox, and Judith Swazey suggest that these early religious ethicists were abandoned less because of the particular discourse they used than because they "were regarded more as sages than as clear and clarifying thinkers" (2001, 490).

Although some bioethicists have maintained that a clear separation of liberal discourse and religious discourse needs to be maintained to permit the development of an unbiased public forum for the discussion of bioethics (Engelhardt 1999), there have also been concerns raised that this separation has deprived the public sphere of any language that can provide bioethics with value content beyond legalistic procedural justice. For some—for example, Lammers and Laurie Zoloth—the reintroduction of religious voices into bioethics discourse is necessary for an attention to the larger issues of social justice. Explicitly Christian bioethics centers, such as the Center for Bioethics and Human Dignity at Trinity International University, embody an active attempt in the early twenty-first century to formally place a particular faith tradition's perspective within bioethics debates.

THE HEGELIAN NATURE OF THE DISCOURSE OF PHILOSOPHY

Just as some came to believe that mathematics replaced theology as the queen of the sciences, in bioethics, philosophy was seen as the new headmaster because of its aspiration to appeal to universal values and to draw on rationality, rather than on any particular faith tradition, as the source for its analysis. It is perhaps because of this that philosophy has maintained a strong critical position against ethical and epistemological relativism, for by doing so philosophy's discourse is prevented from becoming simply another instance of local knowledge and thus a victim of the criticisms that were raised against theology's role in public discourse. The discourse of philosophy in bioethics was for a period a battle for dominance between two pivotal post-Enlightenment approaches to moral deliberation: deontology and consequentialism. Although some philosophers in bioethics, such as Peter Singer, continue to hold onto the classic expression of one of the approaches, eventually bioethics in North America came to grant that principle-based bioethics, or principlism, was an approach that could move the conversation beyond a seemingly unending struggle between these two approaches (cf. Evans 2000).

Principlism contended that once one moved past the particular forms of justification in deontology and consequentialism one arrived at a similar set of rules or principles (Beauchamp and Childress 1979, 40). This struggle between two theoretical approaches followed by a discovery of a hidden unity becomes a standard—one might even say Hegelian—narrative for the progress of philosophical theories in bioethics. Virtue ethics is initially viewed as opposed to principlism, but then the two approaches are viewed as complementary (Beauchamp and Childress 1983, 260–68). Casuistry and communitarianism are initially viewed as beginning in very different initial positions when approaching moral problems but then through tracing their roots in Aristotelian ethics are recast as actually having a concealed harmony (see Kuczewski 1997). The voices of care and justice at first demonstrate a fundamental division within human moral perception but are then shown to both be necessary for the construction of a just world (see Sherwin 1992). Narratives and moral rules are eventually seen to need each other to effectively provide a rich analysis of ethical problems.

Philosophical discourse used in bioethics has been generally limited to the Anglo-American analytic tradition. Although there have been notable attempts to introduce the discourse of Continental philosophy, such as Richard M. Zaner's (1988) work in phenomenology, Drew Leder's (1994) and Ronald Carson's (1990) work in hermeneutics, and Arthur W. Frank's work (1995) in postmodernism, philosophical discourse in bioethics has remained generally limited to the analytic tradition in the West.

THE INFLUENCE OF THE PROFESSIONAL DISCOURSES OF MEDICINE AND LAW

Two professional discourse communities have had a profound effect on the construction of the unique discourse of bioethics: medicine and law. Bioethics has had an especially complex relationship with established biomedical practice. Bioethicists have traditionally seen themselves as outsiders to medicine, providing the kind of critique that can come only from a stranger. The title of David J. Rothman's book on the history of bioethics, *Strangers at the Bedside* (1991), is itself an illustration of the way bioethicists have both been framed and frame themselves as outsiders (see Churchill 1978). Bioethics from this perspective provides a counterdiscourse to that of medicine. In many ways the aim of bioethics has been to introduce a discourse that requires that health care professionals self-consciously view patients as strangers instead of as friends or intimates or surrogate children. The explicit introduction of such language as respect for autonomy, patient's rights, informed consent, and advance directives is an attempt to reframe the traditional medical practice from paternalism to patient self-determination.

At the same time bioethics adopted a great deal of the conventional symbols of the medical world. In some instances this was done consciously to rhetorically persuade health care professionals that bioethics should be viewed as a natural part of the clinical environment and in other instances with seemingly little notice to the manner in which bioethics was becoming shaped by medicine's own discourse. Bioethicists have developed methods to "work up" a moral problem similar in format to workups in medicine. These bioethical workups frame the moral problem from the point of view of the clinician. Similarly ethics cases tend to be written in a manner that reproduces clinical case presentations and accentuates the perspective of the physician (Chambers 1999). Some ethicists have adopted the semiotics of the hospital world, engaging in ethics consultations, wearing a white coat, writing notes in medical charts, and doing rounds. A key insight of such thinkers as Frank has been to point out that bioethics has taken the medical perspective to such a degree that it views the patient and the patient's perspective as the other.

The discourse of the law profession has also had a fundamental impact on bioethics. It is not simply that a significant number of the index cases in bioethics have come from the law, such as *Tarasaoff* (1976), *Quinlan* (1976), *Bouvia* (1986), *Cruzan* (1990), *Wanglie* (1991), and *Schiavo* (1998), but also that the courts' various decisions have been taken at times as the final word in some key moral disagreements. Carl E. Schneider notes that the law is at its core "a device for social regulation" and does so by creating a discourse constituting the standards and the resolution when those standards are broken (1994, 17). In doing so the extensive tradition of the law provides bioethics with a systematic, disciplined language for thinking about moral issues in biomedicine, but Schneider also emphasizes that this does not necessarily provide language that is well suited to many moral issues in medicine. Furthermore, Schneider notes, a discourse that has been constructed out of a need for systematic regulation and compensation for the breaking of such regulations does not inevitably constitute a discourse that is ideal for shaping a model for medical relationships. For example, in the discussion of issues in which women do not wish to undergo a cesarean section, bioethics has tended to draft the issue as one between maternal versus fetal rights; this creates a drama that most would judge to be absurd, that is, an adversarial relationship between the mother and the fetus (see Leiberman et al. 1979). As some have noted, the use of rights language, especially negative rights language in the US context, can influence the way moral issues are resolved (Glendon 2008) and frame complex moral issues in terms of simple conflicts of rights.

SOCIAL SCIENCE FOR AND AGAINST BIOETHICS

Perhaps one of the most surprising tensions within bioethics discourse has been with that of the social sciences. Scholars from anthropology, such as Arthur Kleinman, Margaret Lock, Barbara Koenig, and Patricia Marshall, and those from sociology, such as Renée Fox, Charles L. Bosk, Robert Zussman, and Raymond De Vries, have had a profound influence on shaping the discourse of American bioethics. Yet social scientists have tended to argue that their particular methods and discourse have not been taken with adequate earnestness by those in bioethics.

Klaus Hoeyer (2006) has constructed a typology of the various postures that social scientists have taken toward bioethics. They have taken either (1) a deficit model, in which the social sciences provide the contextual richness missing in bioethics analysis; (2) a replacement model, in which taking a social science perspective will make the need for bioethics unnecessary; or a (3) dismissal model, in which bioethics is seen as simply another part of the power structure of health care. The deficit model has been the one most often adopted by bioethicists. In many cases it accepts the traditional role of the social sciences as providing the *is*, the description of how things are, which is the first step toward the next move of constructing the *ought*, which is the normative language that bioethics brings to the issues.

One powerful example of this is the Study to Understand Prognosis and Preferences for Outcomes and Risks of Treatment (SUPPORT) (Support Principal Investigators 1995). This study, supported by the Robert Wood Johnson Foundation, aimed (1) to examine the conditions for end-of-life care in the United States; (2) to provide moral directions and techniques to counter the judgments made on these initial findings; and (3) finally, to study the effectiveness of the interventions. Since the interventions failed to produce the results desired, many have viewed the SUPPORT project as a failure, yet as Ellen H. Moskowitz and James Lindemann Nelson observe, "there seems little room for doubt that the SUPPORT study represents a major watershed in the use of empirical research in bioethics" (1995, S3).

Bioethics has taken into its discourse social science language that has become simply part of the way moral problems in medicine are now described, such as Fox and Harold Lief's use of "detached concern" (1963), Clifford Geertz's employment of "thick description" (1973, 3–30), Bosk's typology of medical errors (1979), and Kleinman's notion of "explanatory models" (1988, chap. 7). The adoption of such language and the use of dialectic methods, such as that of SUPPORT, are viewed by some as evidence of the success of the deficit model.

The replacement model argues that one can essentially exchange such clinical practices of ethics consultations with ethnographic ones. This represents an attempt to abandon traditional bioethics discourse and to replace it with what is considered a more practical form of discourse, which can more accurately define the problems and resolve them. One example of a replacement model is in Daniel F. Chambliss's ethnography of nursing (1996). Chambliss argues that the way bioethics traditionally examines issues, that is, through "abstract logic," provides little assistance in the "social and psychological realities of hospital life" (1996, 7); and his study is itself an example of how empirical investigations can provide a more successful model for resolving moral problems in medicine.

Although the two social science models just discussed criticize bioethics for being either naive or ineffective, the dismissal model characterizes bioethics as itself part of a source of or a contributing factor to the problems bioethicists are trying to resolve. Carl Elliott (2010), for instance, has argued that bioethics has become the very market-driven entity that it originally often criticized of medicine. Nancy Scheper-Hughes (2002) argues that the commodification of the body is explicitly supported by the values promoted by bioethics. But Leigh Turner has noted that many of the descriptions by the social sciences that support such a view tend to create cartoonish characterizations of bioethics practice, so that "we do not just get a 'black and white' sketch of reality; we are offered sociological and anthropological narratives that divide the world into compassionate, discerning social scientists and hard-hearted, shallow bioethicists" (2009, 85).

THE POLITICALIZATION OF BIOETHICS DISCOURSE

One of the most interesting shifts in the late twentieth and early twenty-first centuries within bioethics discourse has been the political redescription of traditional bioethics into an unambiguous expression of left-wing political values. Since the 1990s bioethics has been viewed by neoconservatives as a part of the ongoing culture wars, so traditional bioethicists were described as another part of the dominant liberal ideology in the American academy. The language that was viewed by many in mainstream bioethics as an attempt for a procedural resolution to problems through the promotion of individual interests was seen as an unspoken ideology that devalued certain forms of life. In particular the language of respecting the ability of a person to make decisions about his or her body was argued to have an implicit bias that any lives that could not be classified as capable of fully being persons were not worth protection. Mainstream bioethics in turn viewed the presidential commission appointed by President George W. Bush and headed by Kass as a clear move to promote politically conservative and Christian values in bioethics discourse (Brainard 2004). The controversy over the *Schiavo* case also brought to national attention this division. In 1990 Teresa Schiavo suffered a cardiac arrest and entered a persistent vegetative state. Eight years later her husband, her legally appointed guardian, requested that her tube feeding be stopped. Schiavo's mother and father argued that the feedings should continue. In each stage of the legal proceedings, the courts upheld the husband's position, but the case reached national attention when Florida governor Jeb Bush persuaded the Florida legislature to pass a law (Terri's Law) that gave the governor of the state the power to stay any orders to withhold nutrition and hydration from patients in Schiavo's condition. Conservative members of Congress also attempted to pass legislation in support of the "pro-life" stance taken by Governor Bush. In the national debate over the case, a clear division was seen between traditional bioethicists, who tended to argue on procedural grounds to support the husband's right to be the decision maker, and explicit right-wing politicians and conservative religious groups, who tended to support the parents' view on the grounds of protecting the sanctity of human life. In response to this explicit politicalization of bioethics, some bioethicists began to identify themselves as progressive bioethicists whose language would expressly favor the language and values of the political Left (Check 2005).

FROM PIDGIN TO CREOLE DISCOURSE

Social linguists distinguish between languages that are pidgin and those that are Creole. Pidgin languages arise when two speech communities need to enter into direct and ongoing contact with each other, so that pidgin is a secondary language that has various degrees of complexity and also differing degrees of appropriation from the other languages (Todd 1974; Mühlhäusler 1986). Creole languages are a further development of a pidgin, for it becomes the mother tongue for the generation born into this linguistic contact zone. Bioethics, because of its diversity of discourse communities, clearly initially developed into a metaphoric pidgin language (Andre and Chambers 1997; Andre 2002, 46–54). The question of whether it will develop into a true Creole is still uncertain at this time, but the history of its discourse suggests that it has been moving in that direction.

SEE ALSO *Bioethics Commissions, History of; Casuistry; Continental Philosophy; Ethics; Law and Bioethics; Postmodernism; Pragmatism; Principlism*

BIBLIOGRAPHY

Andre, Judith. 2002. *Bioethics as Practice*. Studies in Social Medicine. Chapel Hill: University of North Carolina Press.

Andre, Judith, and Tod Chambers. 1997. "Bioethics and Pidgin Philosophy." Paper presented at the Annual Meeting of the Society for Health and Human Values, Baltimore.

Barthes, Roland. 1977. *Image/Music/Text*. Translated by Stephen Heath. New York: Hill and Wang.

Beauchamp, Tom L., and James F. Childress. 1979. *Principles of Biomedical Ethics*. New York: Oxford University Press.

Beauchamp, Tom L., and James F. Childress. 1983. *Principles of Biomedical Ethics*. 2nd ed. New York: Oxford University Press.

Bosk, Charles L. 1979. *Forgive and Remember: Managing Medical Failure*. Chicago: University of Chicago Press.

Brainard, Jeffrey. 2004. "A New Kind of Bioethics." *Chronicle of Higher Education* 50 (37): A22–A23.

Callahan, Daniel; Arthur Caplan; Howard Kaye; et al. 2000. "Acadia Institute Project on Bioethics and American Society, Transcript of Advisory Committee Meeting, Sept. 8, 2000." https://repository.library.georgetown.edu/bitstream/handle/10822/557049/AcadiaProjectAdvisoryCommitteeMeeting.pdf?sequence=5.

Carson, Ronald. 1990. "Interpretive Bioethics: The Way of Discernment." *Theoretical Medicine* 11 (1): 51–59.

Chambers, Tod. 1999. *The Fiction of Bioethics: Cases as Literary Texts*. New York: Routledge.

Chambliss, Daniel F. 1996. *Beyond Caring: Hospitals, Nurses, and the Social Organization of Ethics*. Morality and Society. Chicago: University of Chicago Press.

Check, Erika. 2005. "US Progressives Fight for a Voice in Bioethics." *Nature* 437:932–33.

Churchill, Larry R. 1978. "The Ethicist in Professional Education." *Hastings Center Report* 8 (6): 13–15.

Clouser, K. Danner. 1996. "Philosophy, Literature, and Ethics: Let the Engagement Begin." *Journal of Medicine and Philosophy* 21 (3): 321–40.

Elliott, Carl. 2010. *White Coat, Black Hat: Adventures on the Dark Side of Medicine*. Boston: Beacon.

Engelhardt, H. Tristram, Jr. 1999. "Whose Religion? Which Moral Theology? Reconsidering the Possibility of a Christian Bioethics in Order to Gauge the Place of Religious Studies in Bioethics." In *Notes from a Narrow Ridge: Religion and Bioethics*, edited by Dena S. Davis and Laurie Zoloth, 113–28. Hagerstown, MD: University.

Evans, J. H. 2000. "A Sociological Account of the Growth of Principlism." *Hastings Center Report* 30 (5): 31–38.

Fox, Renée C., and Harold Lief. 1963. "Training for 'Detached Concern' in Medical Students." In *The Psychological Basis of Medical Practice*, edited by Harold Lief, 12–35. New York: Harper and Row.

Fox, Renée C.; Judith P. Swazey; and Judith C. Watkins. 2008. *Observing Bioethics*. Oxford: Oxford University Press.

Frank, Arthur W. 1995. *The Wounded Storyteller: Body, Illness, and Ethics*. Chicago: University of Chicago Press.

Geertz, Clifford. 1973. *The Interpretation of Cultures: Selected Essays*. New York: Basic Books.

Glendon, Mary Ann. 1993. *Rights Talk: The Impoverishment of Political Discourse*. New York: Free Press.

Hawkins, Anne Hunsaker. 1996. "Literature, Philosophy, and Medical Ethics: Let the Dialogue Go On." *Journal of Medicine and Philosophy* 21 (3): 341–54.

Hoeyer, Klaus. 2006. "'Ethics Wars': Reflections on the Antagonism between Bioethicists and Social Science Observers of Biomedicine." *Human Studies* 29 (2): 203–27.

Jonsen, Albert R. 1998. *The Birth of Bioethics*. New York: Oxford University Press.

Kass, Leon R. 1990. "Practicing Ethics: Where's the Action?" *Hastings Center Report* 20 (1): 5–12.

Kleinman, Arthur. 1988. *The Illness Narratives: Suffering, Healing, and the Human Condition*. New York: Basic Books.

Kuczewski, Mark G. 1997. *Fragmentation and Consensus: Communitarian and Casuist Bioethics*. Washington, DC: Georgetown University Press.

Lammers, Stephen E. 1996. "The Marginalization of Religious Voices in Bioethics." In *Religion and Medical Ethics: Looking Back, Looking Forward*, edited by Allen Verhey, 19–43. Grand Rapids, MI: Eerdmans.

Lammers, Stephen E. 1999. "Bioethics and Religion: Some Unscientific Footnotes." In *Notes from a Narrow Ridge: Religion and Bioethics*, edited by Dena S. Davis and Laurie Zoloth, 151–63. Hagerstown, MD: University.

Leder, Drew. 1994. "Toward a Hermeneutical Bioethics." In *A Matter of Principles? Ferment in U.S. Bioethics*, edited by E. R. DuBose; R. P. Hamel; and L. J. O'Connel, 240–59. Valley Forge, PA: Trinity.

Leiberman, J. R.; M. Mazor; W. Chaim; and A. Cohen. 1979. "The Fetal Right to Live." *Obstetrics and Gynecology* 53 (4): 515–17.

Lindemann, Hilde. 2001. *Damaged Identities, Narrative Repair*. Ithaca, NY: Cornell University Press.

Marty, Martin E. 1992. "Religion, Theology, Church, and Bioethics." *Journal of Medicine and Philosophy* 17 (3): 273–89.

Messikomer, Carla M.; Renée C. Fox; and Judith P. Swazey. 2001. "The Presence and Influence of Religion in American Bioethics." *Perspectives in Biology and Medicine* 44 (4): 485–508.

Moskowitz, Ellen H., and James Lindemann Nelson. 1995. "The Best Laid Plans." *Hastings Center Report* 25 (6): S3–S5.

Mühlhäusler, Peter. 1986. *Pidgin and Creole Linguistics*. Oxford: Blackwell.

Pratt, Mary Louis. 1989. "Arts of the Contact Zone." In *Negotiating Academic Literacies: Teaching and Learning across Languages and Cultures*, edited by Vivian Zamel and Ruth Spack, 171–85. Mahwah, NJ: Erlbaum.

Rothman, David J. 1991. *Strangers at the Bedside: A History of How Law and Bioethics Transformed Medical Decision Making*. New York: Basic Books.

Scheper-Hughes, Nancy. 2002. "The Ends of the Body: Commodity Fetishism and the Global Traffic in Organs." *SAIS Review* 22 (1): 61–80.

Schneider, Carl E. 1994. "Bioethics in the Language of the Law." *Hastings Center Report* 24 (4): 16–22. doi: 10.2307/3562838.

Sherwin, Susan. 1992. *No Longer Patient: Feminist Ethics and Health Care*. Philadelphia: Temple University Press.

SUPPORT Principal Investigators. 1995. "A Controlled Trial to Improve Care for Seriously Ill Hospitalized Patients." *Journal of the American Medical Association* 274 (20): 1591–98.

Todd, Loreto. 1974. *Pidgins and Creoles*. New York: Routledge.

Toulmin, Stephen. 1982. "How Medicine Saved the Life of Ethics." *Perspectives in Biology and Medicine* 25 (4): 736–50.

Turner, Leigh. 2009. "Anthropological and Sociological Critiques of Bioethics." *Journal of Bioethical Inquiry* 6 (1): 83–98.

Zaner, Richard M. 1988. *Ethics and the Clinical Encounter*. Englewood Cliffs, NJ: Prentice Hall.

Zoloth, Laurie. 1999. *Health Care and the Ethics of Encounter: A Jewish Discussion of Social Justice*. Studies in Social Medicine. Chapel Hill: University of North Carolina Press.

Tod Chambers

Associate Professor of Medical Humanities and Bioethics and of Medicine, Medical Humanities and Bioethics Program, Northwestern University Feinberg School of Medicine

IV. PROFESSIONALISM IN

The concept *professionalism* refers first of all to whatever counts as proper conduct on the part of members of a profession. In other words, the proper conduct of those who are called professionals is the narrowest sense of this term. Some of these standards are common to all professions in a given society (and arguably to any social role in any society if that role can be properly described as an instance of the social institution we call *profession*). But many of these standards are necessarily distinctive for each profession, depending on what counts as the proper exercise of its socially recognized expertise and on the social standards relevant to the kinds of relationships the profession's practitioners have with the individuals or groups it serves and others with whom its practitioners interact. For it is to these two aspects of professional practice, the exercise of expertise and relationships with other persons, that most social standards regarding professions apply.

The conduct of persons in other recognized social roles can also be meaningfully described as professional in a secondary sense, even though these social roles are not professions properly speaking. This means, for present purposes, that the question whether bioethics is a profession does not need to be resolved in order to describe what counts as professionalism in bioethics. But because this is a question of some importance, it is addressed at the end of this entry.

In addition to this focus on a profession's ethics, the concept of professionalism adds the idea of stability, that is, professions' and professionals' conformity to the relevant social standards is socially dependable. Thus to say that some action is unprofessional is not only to claim that it violates or compromises the ethical standards of the relevant profession; it is also affirming that the members of the relevant society are counting on this individual or group to be dependable in conforming to these standards. Therefore, it is also a claim about the practitioners themselves, namely, that they—and not only their actions—are falling short in a socially significant way. However, one cannot expect to be able to stably and therefore dependably exercise expertise and interact with others according to role-specific social standards unless crucial aspects of such conduct—including awareness, judgment, and actual patterns of response to typical practice situations—have become habitual. Thus professionalism in bioethics consists in habitual conformity to the standards of conduct that have been socially accepted for this social role.

It is important to note that the relevant ethical criteria here are specifically social standards, that is, standards that are accepted (through a wide variety of possible social processes) by the relevant society, rather than broader or more foundational moral or ethical norms. If a society is making judgments about the conduct of professions or professionals or the practitioners of other recognized social roles on the basis of broader or more foundational moral or ethical norms, or if a society employs such norms to judge the moral or ethical adequacy of a currently accepted (or a merely proposed or hypothetical) social standard for some aspect of role-based practice, then its judgments of the ethical adequacy of practitioners or practices is based neither on professionalism nor on professional ethics as such. All discussions of professional ethics and of professionalism as criteria for the ethical evaluation of conduct presuppose the existence of relevant social standards that have been accepted in the relevant society.

BIOETHICS AS A RECOGNIZED SOCIAL ROLE

The best way to ask specifically what counts as professionalism in bioethics is to ask two closely related questions about its practice: (1) Whom does it serve? That is, in terms of what characteristics of the individuals or groups it serves, is it responsive to them? (2) What good does it do for them? That is, what categories of benefit does it aim to provide for the persons or groups it serves and/or what kinds of harm does it aim to limit or prevent for them?

Like the practitioners of most social roles, bioethicists do many kinds of good and limit or prevent many kinds of harm for others. For example, they frequently help reduce conflict between parties at odds and/or facilitate communication where there has been misunderstanding or confusion. Many bioethicists hold management or administrative positions, sit on bodies that make policy, and so on. But none of these is a social role for which expertise involves ethics as part of its definition, even though ethics expertise is typically useful in each of them. But there is a reason why the neologism "ethicist" is part of the now current descriptor of practitioners of bioethics. For insofar as bioethics has become a recognized social role in a number of societies (an assumption upon which this entry rests), it is taken for granted in these societies that bioethicists have a distinctive kind of expertise consisting in something that has to do with ethics.

Whom, then, does bioethics serve and what good does it do? Bioethics principally serves people engaged in ethical thinking—trying to determine what ought to be done or not done. Ordinarily people in that mode of thought have moral or ethical judgments to make, and the benefit that bioethicists provide is to assist them in making that determination in the best possible way under the circumstances. Specifically, bioethicists serve such persons in their ethical thinking and judgments in three principal subsidiary roles: as educators; as creators and disseminators of scholarly research; and as providers of what is here called ethics advisory assistance. Practice in one or more of these subsidiary roles constitutes most if not all of the socially acknowledged scope of bioethics as a social role; thus professionalism in bioethics consists in habitual conduct in conformity with the socially accepted standards regarding expertise and relationships for each of these subsidiary roles.

Regarding the first two subsidiary roles, those of educators and scholarly researchers, a number of widely accepted social standards are already in place. Therefore, the important question is whether any additions or adjustments need to be added to the existing standards for educators and scholarly researchers in light of the distinctive kinds of benefit bioethicists aim to provide and harm they aim to limit or avoid for those whom they serve in these roles. With regard to the third of these subsidiary roles, ethics advisory assistance, this social role and the social standards relevant to its proper practice are relatively new in those societies where it is recognized at all. Consequently, bioethicists are debating proposals about what social standards are needed for bioethicists who function in this role.

BIOETHICISTS AS EDUCATORS

In their role as educators, bioethicists serve a wide variety of learners that includes undergraduates, graduate students, students in the health professions, practicing health professionals, practitioners in other professions and other social roles, and the general public. They share the accepted social standards regarding educational expertise, including their understanding of established bodies of relevant knowledge and the direction of relevant new research, with educators in other venues. Additionally, bioethicists in the educator role impart skills in identifying appropriate learning outcomes for various learners, in effective teacher–student communication, in accurate assessment of learning, and in accurate reporting of assessment results when this is part of a credentialing process. Bioethicists also share with other educators certain accepted social standards for relationships, including engaging learners in age-appropriate ways as active rather than passive agents in the learning process, encouraging and being responsive to creativity and originality in their learners, not discriminating and respecting each learner for his or her own sake, and placing a higher priority on benefiting those they serve than on pursuing their own self-interest.

It is widely accepted that ethics education is not indoctrination into a particular view of the correct bases of ethical decision making. No single view of what constitutes correct ethical judgments has yet arisen within cultures or especially cross-culturally, and therefore bioethicists as educators must respect the sincere efforts of others to learn from and contribute to the human dialogue about ethical thinking in the light of their own experience. Understanding and maintaining the difference between indoctrination and the appropriate educator–learner relationship in ethics education is thus an important requirement of professionalism for every bioethics educator.

BIOETHICISTS AS SCHOLAR/RESEARCHERS

In their role as creators and disseminators of scholarly research, bioethicists again share a number of widely accepted social standards regarding both expertise and relationships with scholars/researchers in other fields. These include standards of clarity of exposition, demonstrated awareness of the relevant literature on one's topic, attention to and fairness in discussing alternative views, and transparency about presuppositions and assumptions.

Regarding relationship standards, there are two kinds of interactions that are relevant. Although the ultimate goal of all scholarly research and dissemination is to enhance the understanding and well-being of the larger community, the immediate audience for such research, including in bioethics, is the community of practitioners in the same field. Scholars are well aware of the professional standards of proper relationships within a field, including a refusal to engage in deliberate competition with another scholar, even one whose conclusions or methods one rejects, and a commitment to respect every scholar/researcher who is similarly committed as well as a commitment to contribute to the advancement of understanding for the well-being of everyone.

Much of the work of bioethics scholars has direct implications for health care: it impacts professional practice and policy at many levels, and it influences the ethical decisions made daily in hospitals, clinics, and offices. Thus bioethics scholarship has a significant impact on the lives of a far wider community than that of bioethicists themselves. Professionalism in bioethics therefore entails consideration of the proper relationship between scholars in the field and the larger society that receives their ideas and whose health care their ideas affect. There are, in other words, no "purely academic" issues for bioethicists doing scholarly research.

Scholar/researchers on ethical issues in public policy for health care, in biomedical research, and in clinical medicine tend to write with an express awareness that their proposals might have a direct impact on caregivers' and patients' lives. Renée C. Fox and Judith P. Swazey, in their 2008 book *Observing Bioethics*, for example, explicitly examine what the social standards for the relationship between bioethicists and society ought to be.

ETHICS ADVISORY ASSISTANCE

Ethicists providing ethics advisory assistance serve a variety of individuals and groups. In their roles as members of ethics committees and as individual ethics consultants in hospitals and health care systems, bioethicists provide ethics advice to patients, families, surrogates, and caregiving teams. Bioethicists also offer ethics assistance for various kinds of health care organizations, government bodies, professional societies, and other makers of policy and shapers of health care practice-patterns. The common feature of all such work is that the bioethicist is advising persons or groups who are in the process of making a decision about what ought or ought not to be done, assessing alternative courses of action, policies, or practice-patterns from one or more ethical points of view. In this role the bioethicist aims to help decision makers to do the best ethical thinking they can under the circumstances and thus make the best possible decisions about what ought and ought not to be done.

How is such assistance properly provided? A number of different answers to this question have been proposed. Some believe that the bioethicist's job in this role is to make the final, authoritative decision about what ought to be done in an ethically complex situation, and the decision maker receiving this advice should therefore act accordingly (see Meyers 2007). But this view is disputed and for the same reasons that many bioethicists hesitate to use the expression "ethics consultant." For in clinical settings the term "consultant" ordinarily implies a special expertise that enables the consultant to offer a final, authoritative diagnosis and/or recommendation for action that less expert parties ought to follow. "Ethics advisory assistance" is a more neutral term that carries a less prescriptive connotation.

Many bioethicists voice two objections to the view that their advisory role is to tell those they serve precisely what they ought to do in an ethically complex situation. The first objection concerns ethics expertise. Just as ethics educators eschew indoctrination because of the lack of universal consensus as to the bases of correct moral or ethical judgments, many bioethicists doubt that they have the necessary expertise to provide final, authoritative answers about what ought to be done in ethically complex situations. The ethical decisions that bioethicists are asked to advise about are often matters that cannot be finally decided solely on the basis of accepted social standards regarding the conduct of health professionals or health care institutions. They frequently involve the lives and decisions of patients, and sometimes they concern health care providers who find themselves challenging the moral or ethical adequacy of the social standards that apply to them; in both of these situations, it is in terms of broader and/or more foundational moral or ethical considerations that the decision maker must make a decision.

Bioethicists who provide ethics advisory assistance must attain the same level of expertise as is expected of the bioethics educator regarding the various ways of doing sound ethical thinking and should in addition be well informed as to the accepted social standards for the practice of each of the health professions and for relevant kinds of health care institutions (see American Society for Bioethics and Humanities 2009, 2010). This combined expertise is arguably sufficient to support detailed and situation-specific assistance and coaching of decision makers. Bioethicists in the advisory role can be effective in ensuring that decision makers have all necessary information and an understanding of various approaches to ethical thinking so as to make sound ethical judgments; they can also provide emotional support to people facing difficult decisions. Bioethicists can thus do much good in this role without proposing that their expertise qualifies them to serve as final authorities in ethically complex situations.

The second objection concerns the proper relationship between an ethics advisor and the advisee when the latter is a capable decision maker with adequate information for the decision at hand. Bioethicists must respect the sincere efforts of others to engage in ethical thinking in light of their own experience. Moreover, they must respect the decisions of capable decision makers especially regarding their own health, especially when such persons are regarded as having expertise within their own societies. Bioethicists offering ethics advisory assistance should refrain from presenting themselves as final arbiters as to how capable, well-informed decision makers ought to act. They should also work to diminish the impact on those they serve of the power associated with their socially acknowledged role within the health care setting, especially in their relationships with patients and others who are not themselves in professional or other powerful roles.

IS BIOETHICS A PROFESSION?

Every profession has a distinctive body of expertise. Although the exact nature of bioethical expertise may be subject to debate, the idea that persons having this expertise offer something of genuine social value has attained fairly wide social recognition. But it is important to note that many acknowledged social roles that are not professions have bodies of expertise and that this expertise may be of an esoteric nature that can ordinarily be mastered only with the assistance (and blessing) of practitioners already expert.

The question whether bioethics is a profession revolves more around another essential feature of a profession, social recognition and social authority. Even if bioethics expertise is widely recognized in many societies, the expertise of bioethicists is not necessarily socially authoritative. If it were, that expertise would be socially determining—that is, there would be a stable pattern of conformity to it and additional social institutions to enforce such conformity. But many institutional ethics committees and institutions whose ethics advice is provided by individual bioethicists explicitly state that their advice is to be understood as "optional/optional," that is, no one is institutionally obligated to seek it and no one is institutionally obligated to follow it once given. Legislators and public policy makers who seek bioethicists' advice also clearly view it in the same way; and when the advice of bioethicists has come to be relevant in court cases, the dominant view has been to set aside the liability of those providing it, presumably because no one is socially required to act on it. Although there are some exceptions to this pattern and the future could bring change, as of yet there is no good evidence that bioethics has been accorded the social authority that is typical of a profession.

This does not mean that we speak in vain when we speak of professionalism in bioethics. Professionalism, and its foundation in the existence of socially accepted standards for bioethicists' proper performance of their roles as educators, scholar/researchers, and ethics advisors are matters of genuine social importance in any society that acknowledges bioethics as a social role. And because of this, professionalism in bioethics and the social standards for the proper conduct of bioethicists—both what these standards are in each society and what they ought to be—should be matters of high priority both in the daily lives of bioethicists and in their personal and scholarly reflections on their social role.

SEE ALSO *Ethics: II. Task of Ethics; Health Care, Ethics and Professionalism in; Patients' Responsibilities: II. Co-Relative Rights; Pedagogy of Bioethics; Profession and Professional Ethics*

BIBLIOGRAPHY

Abbott, Andrew. 1988. *The System of Professions: An Essay on the Division of Expert Labor*. Chicago: University of Chicago Press.

American Society for Bioethics and Humanities. 2009. *Improving Competencies in Clinical Ethics Consultation: An Education Guide*. Oakbrook, IL: Author.

American Society for Bioethics and Humanities. 2010. *Core Competencies for Health Care Ethics Consultation*. 2nd ed. Oakbrook, IL: Author.

Bayles, Michael D. 1989. *Professional Ethics*. 2nd ed. Belmont, CA: Wadsworth.

Chambers, Tod. 1999. *The Fiction of Bioethics: Cases as Literary Texts*. New York: Routledge.

Chamblis, Daniel F. 1996. *Beyond Caring: Hospitals, Nurses, and the Social Organization of Ethics*. Chicago: University of Chicago Press.

Davis, Michael, and Andrew Stark, eds. 2001. *Conflict of Interest in the Professions*. Oxford and New York: Oxford University Press.

Elliott, Carl. 1999. *A Philosophical Disease: Bioethics, Culture, and Identity*. New York: Routledge.

Ford, Paul J., and Denise M. Dudzinski, eds. 2008. *Complex Ethics Consultations: Cases That Haunt Us*. Cambridge, UK, and New York: Cambridge University Press.

Fox, Renée C., and Judith P. Swazey. 2008. *Observing Bioethics*. Oxford and New York: Oxford University Press.

Freedman, Benjamin. 2000. *The Roles and Responsibilities of the Ethics Consultant: A Retrospective Analysis of Cases*, edited by Françoise Baylis. Hagerstown, MD: University Publishing.

Freidson, Eliot. 2001. *Professionalism: The Third Logic*. Chicago: University of Chicago Press.

Hester, D. Micah, ed. 2008. *Ethics by Committee: A Textbook on Consultation, Organization, and Education for Hospital Ethics Committees*. Lanham, MD: Rowman and Littlefield.

Jecker, Nancy S.; Albert R. Jonsen; and Robert A. Pearlman, eds. 2007. *Bioethics: An Introduction to the History, Methods, and Practice*. 2nd ed. Sudbury, MA: Jones and Bartlett.

Jonsen, Albert R. 1998. *The Birth of Bioethics*. New York: Oxford University Press.

Meyers, Christopher. 2007. *A Practical Guide to Clinical Ethics Consulting: Expertise, Ethos, and Power.* Lanham, MD: Rowman and Littlefield.

Ozar, David T. 1993. "Building Awareness of Ethical Standards and Conduct." In *Educating Professionals: Responding to New Expectations for Competence and Accountability*, edited by Lynn Curry, Jon F. Wergin, et al., 148–77. San Francisco: Jossey-Bass.

Ozar, David T. 2004. "The Gold Standard for Ethics Education and Effective Decision-Making in Health Care Organizations." *Organizational Ethics: Healthcare, Business, and Policy* 1 (1): 32–42.

Ozar, David. 2007. "The Value of an Ethics Consultation." In *Biomedical Ethics: A Multidisciplinary Approach to Moral Issues in Medicine and Biology*, edited by David Steinberg, 186–89. Hanover, NH: University Press of New England.

Ozar, David T.; Jessica Berg; Linda Emanuel; and Patricia H. Werhane. 2000. *Organizational Ethics in Healthcare: Toward a Model for Ethical Decision-making by Provider Organizations.* Institute for Ethics National Working Group Report. Chicago: American Medical Association.

Parker, Lisa. 2005. "Ethical Expertise, Maternal Thinking, and the Work of Clinical Ethicists." In *Ethics Expertise: History, Contemporary Perspectives, and Applications*, edited by Lisa Rasmussen, 165–207. Dordrecht, Netherlands: Springer.

Rich, John Martin. 1984. *Professional Ethics in Education.* Springfield, IL: Charles C. Thomas.

Rubin, Susan B., and Laurie Zoloth, eds. 2000. *Margin of Error: The Ethics of Mistakes in the Practice of Medicine.* Hagerstown, MD: University Publishing Group.

Schön, Donald A. *The Reflective Practitioner: How Professionals Think in Action.* New York: Basic Books.

Stein, Michael. 2007. *The Lonely Patient: How We Experience Illness.* New York: William Morrow.

Veatch, Robert. 1984. "The Ethics of Institutional Ethics Committees." In *Institutional Ethics Committees and Health Care Decision Making*, edited by Ronald E. Cranford and A. Edward Doudera. Ann Arbor, MI: Health Administration Press.

Wear, Stephen. 2005. "Ethical Expertise in the Clinical Setting." In *Ethics Expertise: History, Contemporary Perspectives, and Applications*, edited by Lisa Rasmussen. Dordrecht, Netherlands: Springer.

Zaner, Richard M. 1988. *Ethics and the Clinical Encounter.* Englewood Cliffs, NJ: Prentice-Hall.

David T. Ozar
Professor, Department of Philosophy, Loyola University Chicago

V. ETHICS OF

An encyclopedia entry on the ethics of bioethics is a signal of the field's coming of age. As the field has grown and developed, its practitioners have begun to cast the same critical eye on their own practices as they have traditionally cast on the disciplines and practices of medicine, the life sciences, and biotechnology. The ethics of bioethics falls into three general and interrelated categories: codes, role and conduct, and conceptual and cultural frameworks.

CODES

Calls for self-examination among bioethicists came as early as 1989, when Benjamin Freedman published his signal article "Bringing Codes to Newcastle." In that article Freedman argued that the time had come to begin thinking about the standards that bioethicists should establish in a code for their own profession. These include minimum standards for ethical conduct that could provide the basis for evaluation and action regarding professional misconduct, guidance for clarifying moral dilemmas, and a basis on which bioethicists could be held accountable by institutions and society.

Early efforts to develop such standards focused on the role of health care ethics consultants, because the specific ethical challenges of this role were not covered in traditional academic or professional codes (Baylis 1994). On the basis of this early work, steps toward the development of codes of ethics for bioethics have been taken by the Canadian Bioethics Society (CBS) and the American Society for Bioethics and Humanities (ASBH), the two major professional societies for bioethics in North America. A helpful chronology by Robert Baker and his colleagues on the ASBH Advisory Committee on Ethics Standards (ACES) in a 2006 report identifies section 5 of the ASBH's 1996 Core Competencies for Health Care Ethics Consultation as the "first code of ethics for clinical ethicists" (Baker et al. 2006, 31). That 1996 code identifies five "special obligations" of clinical ethicists with regard to confidentiality, disclosure and recusal, avoidance of conflicts of interest, autonomy, and nonexploitation, as well as reciprocal obligations of institutions employing them.

In 2000 a working group of the CBS issued a discussion paper titled "Working Conditions for Bioethics in Canada" (MacDonald et al. 2000). The working group's initial effort on working conditions related to the individual moral integrity of the hospital ethics consultant, in particular, "situations or circumstances where an ethics consultant in a Health Care Organisation … encounters serious wrong-doing, significant ethical disagreement, perhaps with an employer, real or potential moral compromise, questions of conscientious objection and/or a felt need to withdraw from a particular situation for moral reasons" (MacDonald et al. 2000, 1). This paper reflected the conflicts of obligation that clinical ethicists were beginning to experience as employees whose organizational role was to explicitly address moral concerns but without clear, established professional standards to define and protect that role. The paper made the case that clinical ethicists—like others whose job is to voice ethical concerns—should be seen as integral to organizational quality management.

This paper was followed in 2003 by the CBS's Draft Model Code of Ethics for Bioethics, which remains in draft form (MacDonald 2003). The draft model code broadens the "Working Conditions" paper beyond ethics consultants to lay out general and special role-related obligations of bioethicists, including obligations "to patients and their families, the public, the 'profession,' students, co-workers/colleagues, and institutions" (MacDonald 2003, 2). The special obligations are written in the form of a pledge or oath to underscore that a bioethicist must make a personal commitment to specific forms of moral conduct. In paraphrase, the special obligations include honesty and integrity, awareness of the limits of one's expertise, confidentiality, avoiding conflict of interest, avoiding exploitation and abuse of power, contributing to the advancement of the field, avoiding actions or statements likely to bring the field of bioethics into undeserved disrepute, continuous learning, and advocating for conditions of employment that are conducive to the effective and ethical pursuit of the goals of the profession.

In 2006 an ACES survey of ASBH members showed that an overwhelming majority of respondents (61%) favored the adoption of a code of ethics, 17 percent opposed it, and 22 percent were neutral (Baker et al. 2006, 13). The seven topics that respondents deemed most important to include in a code were:

1. identifying and managing conflicts of interest,
2. honoring confidentiality and obligations to disclose,
3. reporting serious misconduct,
4. ascribing (co)authorship and crediting contributors to reports and published work,
5. identifying and managing improper pressures and boundary violations by employers and supervisors,
6. presenting incomplete characterizations of complex issues in public venues,
7. reporting problems to employers or supervisors when these are likely to be unwelcome.

On the basis of this response, the ASBH, through its Clinical Ethics Consultation Affairs (CECA) standing committee, moved forward with the development of a draft Code of Professional Responsibilities of Health Care Ethics Consultants. The draft document was made available for public comment at the beginning of 2012, to be followed by an iterative drafting process. In its draft form the code includes the following professional responsibilities: be competent, avoid conflicts of interest, manage conflicts of obligation, protect confidentiality, preserve integrity, make responsible public statements, contribute to the field, and promote just health care. In the call for public comment, ASBH members were specifically encouraged to provide feedback on "promote just health care," as there were different opinions among CECA members about how and whether to include this in the code. To date steps toward a special code of ethics for bioethics seem to be confined to North America.

It is well recognized that bioethics is a field of diverse disciplines and practices. Like other professional codes of ethics, one aim of these proposed codes is to create a shared understanding of bioethical practice and thereby strengthen the identity, integrity, and legitimacy of the field. A related and more straightforward aim is to establish standards of ethical conduct.

ROLE AND CONDUCT

Concerns about ethical conduct among bioethicists became a matter of public discussion in the first years of the twenty-first century, when people within and outside the field questioned whether bioethicists and bioethics centers were compromising their integrity and independent judgment by working for private-sector clients, specifically in the biopharmaceutical industry. The philosopher Carl Elliott was one of the first to raise these concerns in his 2001 article "Pharma Buys a Conscience," in which he pointed out that bioethicists, bioethics centers, and institutional review boards were warning doctors and researchers about financial conflicts of interests even while they themselves engaged in consulting and research activities supported by pharmaceutical money.

In his 2001 article "Throwing a Bone to the Watchdog," Elliott (2001b, 10) observed that because bioethics is "unmoored from a tradition, answerable to a professional code … [it] is fast becoming another cog in the complex machinery of business, entertainment, and politics that controls the shape and direction of American life." Over the next several years this issue became the focus of news reports (Boyce and Kaplan 2001; Stolberg 2001; Blumenstyk 2002; Boyce 2002a, 2002b), scholarly journals, and books in the United States and abroad (Eckenwiler and Cohn 2007; Porz et al. 2007).

During this time a joint ASBH and American Society of Law, Medicine, and Ethics (ASLME) task force led by Baruch Brody and others published the report "Bioethics Consultation in the Private Sector" (Brody et al. 2002), which offered guidance to bioethicists engaging in corporate consultation. The report, which was based on a presumption in favor of private-sector consultation, singled out independence and objectivity as cognitive values worthy of protection in bioethical work. To that end it offered procedural suggestions on how to identify and manage risks to these competencies—leaving it mostly to the discretion of the consultant to determine the best course. These suggestions, which focus largely on negotiating appropriate terms for the consultation, cover such issues as the appropriateness of the client, the process of consultation, whistle-blowing, and disclosure. On the subject of disclosure, the authors, eight of whom indicated that they had been paid corporate consultants, were criticized by two colleagues, Stuart J. Youngner and Robert Arnold (2002), for failing to follow their own guidance by making a meaningful disclosure of the companies that they had worked for and the amount of compensation they had received. In another commentary on the report, Virginia A. Sharpe (2007, 175) noted that one implication of a general endorsement of corporate bioethics consultation is that the conflicts of most concern become "conflicts one might have in addressing similar issues with two competing corporate clients, *not* as conflicts between obligations one might have first as a bioethicist and, second, that as a corporate consultant." Neither the ASBH nor the ASLME adopted the report's recommendations. Since then E. Haavi Morreim (2007, 188), acknowledging the challenge of independence in these relationships, has provided an example of how consultation can be structured to "provide real assistance to a corporation while maintaining a level of integrity essential to good bioethics consultation."

Conflicts of interest and corporate bioethics consultation have, more than any other issue, raised concerns about the credibility of bioethicists and bioethical work and given rise to the expression "ethics of bioethics." Whether and how bioethicists should engage in these consulting relationships are questions about the proper role of bioethics and bioethicists or, to paraphrase Elliott, whether bioethicists will be watchdogs, lapdogs, or show dogs.

Although concerns about bioethicists as "accommodating handmaidens" (Callahan 1996, 3) have been part of bioethical self-reflection since the late twentieth century, as bioethical work has become more institutionalized, some have charged that bioethicists have largely failed to act as whistle-blowers and organizational troubleshooters. Writing about the case of a Canadian scientist who published research findings (about serious drug risks) unfavorable to the economic interests of the pharmaceutical company research sponsor, Françoise Baylis (2004, 49) reflected that "bioethicists in Canada failed Dr. Olivieri and her colleagues" by not defending her against her institution. Baylis based her conclusion in part on her understanding of the proper role for bioethicists. The "duty of bioethicists," she says, "is to speak truth to power" (Baylis 2004, 44). By contrast, John McMillan (2004, 174) has argued that being a moral critic is not an essential role for bioethicists, stating that it is unreasonable to think that "if a bioethicist is not a moral critic then she is not a bioethicist, or at least not a good bioethicist." The business ethicist Thomas Donaldson (2001, 13) has argued that bioethicists must minimally "avoid conflicts of interest *and* remain true to their profession's duty to serve the 'broader good'; granting, however, that it is difficult to identify what that 'broader good' would be." Additional evidence of this difficulty is also found in the efforts of the CBS and the ASBH to articulate a moral identity for the field. In the appendix of the CBS's Draft Model Code, MacDonald notes that how best to characterize the role-related duties and obligations of bioethicists "remains an unresolved issue." Similarly, within the ASBH during the 1990s and the first years of the twenty-first century there was a contentious debate about whether the organization should amend section 4.1 of its bylaws, which prohibits the society from issuing positions on "substantive moral and policy issues" (ASBH 2013). The protracted debate led Steven Miles, a founding ASBH member, to question whether American bioethics has a soul and to publicly resign from the organization in 2004 for its "failure to articulate organizational positions."

The ASBH ultimately retained its general prohibition but established an additional bylaw (section 4.2) permitting the society to "adopt positions on matters related to academic freedom and professionalism in the fields of bioethics and humanities in health care" (ASBH 2013). On the basis of this bylaw, the society's board took action ten times between 2003 and 2011 to advocate on behalf of ethical integrity and freedom of inquiry. The consensus to limit the society's role in taking substantive positions can be seen in a variety of ways, depending on one's point of view. On one hand, it can be seen as a failure to use bioethicists' collective agency and unique expertise to speak out against moral wrongs. On the other hand, it can be seen to reflect, endorse, respect, and protect the diversity of moral opinion among its membership.

CONCEPTUAL AND CULTURAL FRAMEWORKS

A third, related strand in the ethics of bioethics concerns the ethical implications of critiques by feminist scholars, sociologists, race theorists, and others. These analyses address the biases and blind spots inherent in mainstream bioethics' conceptual and cultural frameworks.

The conceptual frameworks of mainstream bioethics are derived from Anglo-American law and moral theories that privilege the norms of autonomy, impartiality, universality, and equality. Important though these norms have been in advancing individual rights, the problem with this grounding in the Western philosophical and legal concept of the person is that it excludes whole domains of human experience, such as relationships of love, care, and trust, and the moral significance of real inequalities and the social determinants of health. As Bruce Jennings (1998, 260) has observed, "Autonomy-centered bioethics emphasizes notions of individual choice and future-oriented planning that are foreign to the lived reality of the poor, the marginalized, and people of color in a multicultural society." Likewise, as Howard Brody (2009, 111) points out in *The Future of Bioethics*, the premise that the "principle of autonomy resolves the problem of power imbalance" is true only in abstract theory and then only for "ideal" individuals who are not actually disempowered, for example, by poverty, homelessness, lack of social support, or violence or certainly by suffering, illness, or disability. Finally, to the extent that autonomous choice is also the guiding value of democratic capitalism, the agenda of mainstream bioethics has found itself, according to Semih Semin and Sahbal Aras (2007) more compatible with the values of the free market than with the values of social solidarity and social justice.

In addition a narrow conception of the person as either an autonomous will (as conceptualized by the eighteenth-century German philosopher Immanuel Kant) or as the locus of utility (classical utilitarianism) has fostered the view that a set of abstract moral principles is the most important moral resource necessary to do bioethical work. In practice this has led to an overemphasis on principlism in mainstream bioethics and an underemphasis on the development of moral character and on rich concepts of moral relationships and moral personality, including communicative skills and a sensitivity to circumstances, to context, and to particular others. As sociologists of bioethics, including Raymond G. De Vries, Lisa Kane Low, and Elizabeth (Libby) Bogdan-Lovis (2009) and Renée C. Fox and Judith P. Swazey (2008), have pointed out, the model of applying bioethical principles is useful in resolving specific dilemmas in health care institutions, but its "inattention to the social facts of bioethical quandaries diminishes the possibility of achieving the goals of bioethics" to inform and improve ethical perception and practice (De Vries, Low, and Bogdan-Lovis 2009, 44).

The cultural frameworks of mainstream bioethics are closely tied to its conceptual foundations. In addition, because bioethics originated and initially developed as a practice in the United States and other developed countries, it reflects the particular concerns of its cultural context. In practice this has meant that mainstream bioethics has focused on individual liberty rather than social justice, the use and abuse of medical technologies rather than on the plight of the poor and others who have no access to health care, the ethics of acute care rather than public health; health care in urban rather than rural settings, ethical issues of importance to developed rather than developing countries, and ethical issues related to biomedicine rather than broader questions concerning health and the biosphere.

As the field has evolved and expanded, many of these limitations have begun to be addressed through the development of diverse and interdisciplinary methodologies, through international and internationalized approaches to bioethics and global health, through important and sustained work on the social and environmental determinates of health and health disparities, and through greater diversity among bioethicists themselves. This broader bioethics agenda has the potential to overcome what Fox and Swazey (2008) have referred to as the inadvertent ethnocentrism and cultural nearsightedness of traditional bioethics. In the process the array of voices, methods, issues, and perspectives in this newest period of the field carries with it the insight that bioethical discourse is situated and contextual, that is, "a culturally specific set of texts and practices produced by individuals and communities in particular places at particular times" (Walker 2009, 4). Given this, the ongoing moral task for bioethicists is to cast a wide net in their thinking, teaching, and practice; to understand and assess the norms at work in moral practice; to understand what the philosopher Amélie Oksenberg Rorty (1988, 21) calls "the daily consequences" of the practices and institutions that these norms recommend; and to subject them to continuous internal critique and reconstruction.

SEE ALSO *Care: III. Care Ethics; Ethics; Eugenics: II. Ethical Issues; Neuroethics; Nursing Ethics; Relativism, Cultural and Ethical; Utilitarianism*

BIBLIOGRAPHY

American Society for Bioethics and Humanities. 2013. "Board Actions." Accessed September 10, 2013. http://www.asbh.org/about/action/board-actions.html

American Society for Bioethics and Humanities, Clinical Ethics Consultation Affairs Standing Committee. 2012. "Code of Professional Responsibilities of Health Care Ethics Consultants." Accessed January 30, 2013. http://www.asbh.org/uploads/files/membership/pdfs/111013%20ceca%20mtg%20minutes.pdf

Andre, Judith. 2002. *Bioethics as Practice*. Chapel Hill: University of North Carolina Press.

Baker, Robert. 2007. "A History of Codes of Ethics for Bioethicists." In *The Ethics of Bioethics: Mapping the Moral Landscape*, edited by Lisa A. Eckenwiler and Felicia G. Cohn, 24–42. Baltimore: Johns Hopkins University Press.

Baker, Robert. 2009. "The Ethics of Bioethics." In *The Penn Center Guide to Bioethics*, edited by Vardit Ravitsky; Autumn Fiester; and Arthur L. Caplan, 9–20. New York: Springer.

Baker, Robert; Robert Pearlman; Holly Taylor; and Kenneth Kipnis. 2006. "Report and Recommendations of the ASBH Advisory Committee on Ethics Standards (ACES)." Accessed

January 30, 2013. http://www.asbh.org/uploads/files/membership/protected/pdfs/acesrprt.pdf

Baylis, Françoise. 1994. *The Health Care Ethics Consultant.* Totowa, NJ: Humana Press.

Baylis, Françoise. 2004. "The Olivieri Debacle: Where Were the Heroes of Bioethics?" *Journal of Medical Ethics* 30 (1): 44–49.

Blumenstyk, Goldie. 2002. "Bioethicists Criticized for Industry Ties." *Chronicle of Higher Education,* July 19.

Boyce, Nell. 2002a. "Code of Conduct for Bioethics Branded 'Soft' on Corporate Ties." *Nature* 417 (6892): 885–86.

Boyce, Nell. 2002b. "A View from the Fourth Estate." *Hastings Center Report* 32 (3): 16–17.

Boyce, Nell, and David E. Kaplan. 2001. "And Now, Ethics for Sale? Bioethicists and Big Bucks; Problem City?" *U.S. News and World Report,* July 20, 18–19.

Brody, Baruch; Nancy Dubler; Jeff Blustein; et al. 2002. "Bioethics Consultation in the Private Sector." *Hastings Center Report* 32 (3): 14–20.

Brody, Howard. 2009. *The Future of Bioethics.* Oxford: Oxford University Press.

Callahan, Daniel. 1996. "Bioethics, Our Crowd, and Ideology." *Hastings Center Report* 26 (6): 3–4.

De Vries, Raymond G.; Lisa Kane Low; and Elizabeth (Libby) Bogdan-Lovis. 2009. "Choosing Surgical Birth: Desire and the Nature of Bioethical Advice." In *Naturalized Bioethics: Toward Responsible Knowing and Practice,* edited by Hilde Lindemann; Marian Verkerk; and Margaret Urban Walker, 42–64. Cambridge, UK: Cambridge University Press.

Donaldson, Thomas. 2001. "The Business Ethics of Bioethics Consulting." *Hastings Center Report* 31 (2): 12–14.

Dula, Annette, and Sara Goering, eds. 1994. *"It Just Ain't Fair": The Ethics of Health Care for African Americans.* Westport, CT: Praeger.

Eckenwiler, Lisa A., and Felicia G. Cohn. 2007. *The Ethics of Bioethics: Mapping the Moral Landscape.* Baltimore: Johns Hopkins University Press.

Elliott, Carl. 2001a. "Pharma Buys a Conscience." *American Prospect* 12 (17): 16–20.

Elliott, Carl. 2001b. "Throwing a Bone to the Watchdog." *Hastings Center Report* 31 (2): 9–12.

Elliott, Carl. 2004. "Six Problems with Pharma-Funded Bioethics." *Studies in History and Philosophy of Biological and Biomedical Sciences* 35 (1): 125–29.

Fox, Renée C., and Judith P. Swazey. 2008. *Observing Bioethics.* Oxford: Oxford University Press.

Freedman, Benjamin. 1989. "Bringing Codes to Newcastle." In *Clinical Ethics: Theory and Practice,* edited by Barry Hoffmaster; Benjamin Freedman; and Gwen Fraser, 125–39. Clifton, NJ: Humana Press.

Jennings, Bruce. 1998. "Autonomy and Difference: The Travails of Liberalism in Bioethics." In *Bioethics and Society: Constructing the Ethical Enterprise,* edited by Raymond G. De Vries and Janardan Subedi, 258–69. New York: Prentice Hall.

MacDonald, Chris. 2003. "Draft Model Code of Ethics for Bioethics." Accessed January 30, 2013. http://www.bioethics.ca/resources/PDF%20documents/draftcode.pdf

MacDonald, Chris; Michael Coughlin; Christine Harrison; et al. 2000. "Draft Discussion Paper: Working Conditions for Bioethics in Canada." Version 8.0. Accessed January 30, 2013. http://www.bioethics.ca/resources/PDF%20documents/workingconditions.pdf

McMillan, John. 2004. "Is Corporate Money Bad for Bioethics?" *Studies in History and Philosophy of Biological and Biomedical Sciences* 35 (1): 167–75.

Miles, Steven. 2002. "Does American Bioethics Have a Soul?" *Bioethics Examiner* 6 (2): 1–2, 5.

Morreim, E. Haavi. 2007. "Ties without Tethers: Bioethics Corporate Relations in the AbioCor Artificial Heart Trial." In *The Ethics of Bioethics: Mapping the Moral Landscape,* edited by Lisa A. Eckenwiler and Felicia G. Cohn, 181–90. Baltimore: Johns Hopkins University Press.

Myser, Catherine. 2003. "Differences from Somewhere: The Normativity of Whiteness in Bioethics in the United States." *American Journal of Bioethics* 3 (2): 1–11.

Porz, Rouven; Christoph Rehmann-Sutter; Jackie L. Scully; and Markus Zimmermann-Acklin, eds. 2007. *Gekauftes Gewissen? Zur Rolle der Bioethik in Institutionen.* Paderborn, Germany: Mentis.

Rorty, Amélie Oksenberg. 1988. *Mind in Action: Essays in the Philosophy of Mind.* Boston: Beacon Press.

Scully, Jackie Leach; Laurel E. Baldwin-Ragaven; and Petya Fitzpatrick, eds. 2010. *Feminist Bioethics: At the Center, on the Margins.* Baltimore: Johns Hopkins University Press.

Semin, Semih, and Sahbal Aras. 2007. "Bioethics and Turkey: Crossroads and Challenges." *Politics and the Life Sciences* 26 (1): 2–9.

Sharpe, Virginia A. 2002. "Science, Bioethics, and the Public Interest: On the Need for Transparency." *Hastings Center Report* 32 (3): 23–26.

Sharpe, Virginia A. 2007. "Strategic Disclosure Requirements and the Ethics of Bioethics." In *The Ethics of Bioethics: Mapping the Moral Landscape,* edited by Lisa A. Eckenwiler and Felicia G. Cohn, 170–80. Baltimore, MD: Johns Hopkins University Press.

Stolberg, Sheryl Gay. 2001. "Bioethicists Find Themselves the Ones Being Scrutinized." *New York Times,* August 2.

Turner, Leigh. 2007. "Global Health Inequalities and Bioethics." In *The Ethics of Bioethics: Mapping the Moral Landscape,* edited by Lisa A. Eckenwiler and Felicia G. Cohn, 229–40. Baltimore: Johns Hopkins University Press.

Walker, Margaret Urban. 2009. "Introduction: Groningen Naturalism in Bioethics." In *Naturalized Bioethics: Toward Responsible Knowing and Practice,* edited by Hilde Lindemann; Marian Verkerk; and Margaret Urban Walker, 1–20. Cambridge, UK: Cambridge University Press.

Youngner, Stuart J., and Robert Arnold. 2002. "Who Will Watch the Watchers?" *Hastings Center Report* 32 (3): 21–22.

Virginia A. Sharpe
National Center for Ethics in Health Care,
Veterans Health Administration
Center for Clinical Bioethics,
Georgetown University Medical Center

VI. RESEARCH METHODS IN

A diverse array of disciplinary approaches and methods are used to conduct work in bioethics, including theology, philosophy, history, law, and the social sciences. Drawing on the prior work of two of the authors (Sugarman and Sulmasy 2010), this entry provides a general framework for methods in bioethics. Because providing a comprehensive treatment of methods in bioethics lies beyond the scope of a single entry (and is itself the subject of several monographs), this framework focuses on the following. First, this entry describes the difference between facts and values; and between empirical and normative research methods in bioethics. Second, these differences are clarified by describing several methods in bioethics, noting their important contributions to the field. Finally, this entry closes by commenting on the possibility of blurring disciplinary and methodological boundaries with interdisciplinary or mixed methods bioethics research.

VALUES, FACTS, AND THE "EMPIRICAL TURN"

Some philosophers divide ethical inquiry into three general types: metaethics, normative ethics, and descriptive ethics (Frankena 1973). Metaethics represents inquiry into the nature and meaning of moral terms, including their semantics, logic, and justification. A metaethical inquiry, for example, attempts to answer questions such as, "Does moral truth exist? What is the logical structure of moral judgment? What is the meaning of the term *justice*?" It refrains from addressing specific moral judgments or specific instances of justice or injustice.

Inquiries in normative ethics involve systematic theorizing and analysis about how individuals and institutions ought to behave, or the virtues they ought to have or develop. Normative ethics explicitly acknowledges specific issues, contexts, and individuals. Normative bioethics attempts to justify answers to questions such as, "Ought we to promote embryonic stem cell research? Should we engage in research with nonhuman primates? Does justice require universal access to health care? Is physician-assisted suicide immoral?" In attempting to answer these questions, normative ethics directly engages *values*, including moral character or virtues, basic principles, duties, and consequences, among others. The source, status, and relative importance of these values occupy much normative work.

In contrast, descriptive ethics attempts to describe what people do or believe (or how organizations and institutions operate) in certain circumstances. Descriptive ethics seeks answers to questions such as, "Do investigators disclose conflicts of interest to potential research participants? Do physicians disclose terminal diagnoses to patients? What do patients believe about embryonic stem cell research?" In short, descriptive ethics tries to discover *facts* about the world.

Because most bioethics scholarship represents either normative or descriptive ethics, clarifying how these relate to one another is important. One can appreciate how descriptive *facts* (what "is") seem to differ from normative *values* (what "ought" to be). To some, this difference amounts to a conceptual distinction referred to as the fact/value distinction or dichotomy. The fact/value distinction, at least as understood in bioethics, is related to the "is/ought distinction" attributed to the philosopher David Hume (2003 [1740]), and to Moore's (1993) naturalistic fallacy. Simply put, the idea is that normative conclusions about what ought to be cannot be derived from mere facts about how the world is.

The range of human judgments over which the fact/value distinction holds remains subject to debate. For example, not all judgments of value are moral, and social values help determine which facts are sought and how much certainty is required. Statisticians and others typically interpret a set of observations as "true" when the probability of a result having occurred by chance is less than 5 percent. If one rejects the distinction between "facts" and values wholesale, the difference between normative and descriptive ethics would fail as well.

Nonetheless, even those otherwise sympathetic to the merging of facts and values are, in bioethics, willing to accept differences between the two for methodological reasons (Leget, Borry, and De Vries 2009). Recognizing this difference, if not a distinction, is critical for at least two reasons.

First, the difference between facts and values helps explain what Sulmasy and Sugarman (2010) consider "illicit inferences" in bioethics. Examples include inferring the morality or immorality of a particular practice from observed facts about history, legality, expert testimony, or popular opinion. The presence of such facts alone does not decide the morality of an issue. For example, neither the fact that most of the public opposed genetic modification of crops nor the testimony of expert scientists in its favor would settle the morality of the issue.

Second, differentiating facts from values helps understand the so-called "empirical turn" in bioethics. After all, if empirical facts are not at least different from values, such a turn would be nonsensical. Sociologists originally observed the "empirical turn" as a result of increasing integration of the empirical social sciences research within and about bioethics starting in the 1990s (Borry, Schotsmans, and Dierickx 2005). Some question, however, what this turn truly represents. On the one hand, studies document a rise in "empirical" research in bioethics, especially during the 1990s (Sugarman, Faden, and Boyce 2010). On the other hand, the concept of introducing empirical facts to normative arguments is hardly novel. Facts have always been assumed or employed in normative arguments. To the extent that an empirical turn occurred in bioethics, if it did at all, it operated at the level of the relationship or integration of facts and values, or of empirical and normative work. Several different models of this relationship have been proposed by Molewijk and colleagues (2004), and they vary in how they integrate facts and values.

Whatever model one chooses, however, normative values and empirical facts interact in a number of ways. Normative values and claims often lead to claims about the world that require empirical verification or might be aided by empirical testing. For example, the idea that there is a universally recognized moral norm requiring informed consent in human subjects research would be undermined if empirical studies demonstrated that no investigators attempted to obtain consent in human research protocols. Only with such studies can bioethicists learn how ideal norms become (or do not become) operationalized in real-world settings.

Similarly, empirical facts, such as those recognized through case studies, frequently inform, motivate, or even correct normative claims and theories. For example, case studies in genomic technology development can inform how patenting and licensing standards ought to be structured (Cook-Deegan and Heaney 2010). Facts can also aid assessment of the likelihood or magnitude of consequences, thereby informing slippery-slope arguments (i.e., arguments where a particular change in norms or policies might lead to negative consequences). Facts might also be used to test normative claims directly; for instance, mathematics might inform whether consensus in ethics consultation leads most often to the "correct" decision (Jansen 2009).

Not all empirical research in bioethics is purely descriptive, if by descriptive one means descriptions of how the world is (i.e., the status quo). For example, a randomized controlled trial of two methods of obtaining informed consent process is different from a questionnaire surveying opinions about informed consent. Whereas the latter is purely descriptive, the former might be used to test different normative theories about informed consent, or even be designed with the normative goal of changing the informed consent process.

In summary, considering methods in bioethics as either normative or empirical is a helpful starting point for understanding how to do and interpret scholarship in bioethics. Maintaining this difference is useful for understanding the feedback of normative values and empirical facts and allowing for normative and empirical work about (not just in) bioethics.

Importantly, the difference between normative and empirical methods does not map directly onto what some consider "disciplines" working in bioethics. Disciplines represent specific communities of scholars connected by shared training, shared assumptions about what knowledge is (or how to discover it), and a shared subject matter. Methods, by contrast, are systematic or agreed upon procedures for answering specific research questions. As such, some disciplines employ multiple methods, both empirical and normative, and the same method might be used by more than one discipline. Characterizing a discipline as purely empirical or normative is therefore impossible, even if some disciplines tend to use more normative or empirical methods. To appreciate this, the following section describes several of the many methods used in bioethics.

SELECTED METHODS IN BIOETHICS

Because a comprehensive review of all methods relevant to bioethics is impossible in an entry of this length, this entry focuses on a few representative examples, in no particular order. In addition, it emphasizes the contribution each has made to bioethics.

Philosophical. Most philosophical bioethics employs normative reasoning and theory as methods for elucidating the right or best course of action. Examples of philosophical "methods" include virtue ethics, duty- or principle-based theories, consequentialism, casuistry, reflective equilibrium, narrative theory, feminism, and pragmatism, among others (Childress 2007).

Philosophical methods contribute much to bioethics, including ways of thinking about personal identity in end-of-life decision making and reproductive choices, genetic causation and biological determinism, the moral standing of nonhuman animals, and so on. The influence of principle-based approaches is perhaps no clearer, however, than in the *Belmont Report* (National Commission for the Protection of Human Subjects of Biomedical and Behavioral Research [US] 1978). This seminal document expresses the basic ethical principles governing human subject research (respect for persons; beneficence; and justice), and according to Beauchamp (2005) it was written in close conjunction with the first edition of *Principles of Biomedical Ethics*. Beauchamp and Childress's *Principles of Biomedical Ethics* (2008) has been arguably the single most influential text for how contemporary bioethics is learned and taught. Nevertheless, philosophical methods alone do not encompass the full spectrum of approaches used in bioethics.

Theological. Theological methods encompass a tremendous diversity of religious traditions and methods (Verhey 1996; Guinn 2006). Broadly speaking, however, theological approaches to bioethics ground normative claims and values within particular religious communities (Cahill 2010). Theologians play important roles in bioethics. This includes work as scholars; as members of national commissions (from the first National Commission for the Protection of Human Subjects of Biomedical and Behavioral Research in 1974 to the most recent one, chartered in 2009, the Presidential Commission for the Study of Bioethical Issues); and as leaders in global efforts for gender equality and health equity, including responses to the AIDS epidemic (Overberg 2006).

Nonetheless, theological approaches face certain challenges in bioethics. Whether norms apply beyond members of a particular religious tradition, for example, or whether certain aspects of religious traditions (such as creation narratives) can or should influence multicultural societies, remains unclear.

Legal. Law and legal scholarship are important to bioethics (Annas 1993; Shapiro et al. 2002; Menikoff 2001). Famous legal cases such as, in the United States, the so-called "right to die" cases of Karen Ann Quinlan, Nancy Cruzan, and Terri Schiavo bring public attention to bioethical issues and motivate further bioethical inquiry. In other instances, legal cases and statutory law outline the bounds of permissible action, even if the legality of an issue does not determine its morality; slavery, for example, was once legal, but this does not mean it was "moral." Among disciplines, legal scholarship in bioethics arguably demonstrates clearly how one discipline can use both normative and empirical methods.

From a normative perspective, legal scholars may develop prescriptive theories of how the law should be or advocate for changes to the law on the basis of normative values. Prominent examples of normative legal scholarship's contributions to bioethics include influence on legislative action, such as the US Genetic Information Nondiscrimination Act of 2008, which prevents certain uses of genetic information by health insurers and employers. Case law has similarly contributed to bioethics, on issues including the ownership of biological specimens (e.g., *Moore v. Regents of University of California* in 1990) and the patentability of genetically modified organisms (e.g., *Diamond v. Chakrabarty* in 1979). Legal expertise is also necessary to help interpret the meaning and scope of legal statutes and cases, and the law is itself the subject of empirical studies, including sophisticated methods of content analysis (Krippendorff 2004).

Historical. History includes both empirical and normative work. How to interpret past events and evidence is at least partly a normative question. History, as a discipline, draws upon different frameworks of interpretation—examples include intellectual and social or cultural histories—and different types of evidence—examples include oral and archaeological evidence—as evidence for arguments and claims about the past (Lederer 2010).

Many issues in bioethics are informed by historical studies. Seminal events in research ethics necessarily require historical analysis: The Tuskegee Syphilis Study (Jones 1981); secret radiation experiments conducted on humans in the United States (Advisory Committee on Human Radiation Experiments 1995); and the more recent revelation of "ethically impossible" studies of sexually transmitted infections conducted by the United States in Guatemala (Presidential Commission for the Study of Bioethical Issues 2011) all illustrate this well. Of course, as Lowenthal (1985) points out, whether "objective" analysis of historical events is possible, and how to interpret the relevance of the past for today, both remain controversial subjects.

Decision Science and Economics. Decision science seeks both to understand descriptively how decisions are made (e.g., by clinicians, patients, ethics committees, and policy makers) and to change prescriptively, if necessary, the decision-making process (Asch 2010). In doing so, decision scientists sometimes employ economic analyses, which focus on, for example, cost-effectiveness analyses or cost-benefit analyses. Common to both is the idea of assigning values and probabilities to the outcomes of proposed actions or changes; economics merely quantifies such actions or changes in monetary terms.

Decision science and economic analyses can contribute much to bioethics to assist evaluation of the likelihood and magnitude of potential consequences arising from particular actions. Sometimes this occurs amid controversy; for example, when considering environmental policies, the US Environmental Protection Agency conducts cost-benefit analyses using the statistical value of a life (recently valued at US$7.4 million, in 2006 dollars) (Copeland 2010). Although conceptually distinct from the value of any particular individual's life, this value can be normatively controversial and yet carries great importance for decision making. Similarly, the use of economic analyses related to abortion, embryonic stem cell research, and financial incentives to improve physician behavior all inform bioethics and policy in instructive, if not controversial, ways.

Qualitative Empirical Methods. Qualitative research, in general, uses nonstatistical methods to analyze particular phenomena through observation, in-depth or semistructured interviews, focus groups, texts, or other sources (Taylor, Hull, and Kass 2010). The goal of qualitative research is to describe and analyze beliefs, attitudes, and circumstances within particular social contexts in a flexible and open-ended manner. This is in contrast to quantitative methods (described below), where the focus is frequently more narrow, the design fixed, and variation minimized. By way of examples, qualitative methods used by sociologists and anthropologists in bioethics have led to greater understanding of decision making at the margins of life in the neonatal intensive care unit (Anspach 1993), of racial identity in the human genome project (Reardon 2005), and of the experiences of research subjects in clinical trials (Fisher 2009).

Researchers in bioethics frequently conduct research using in-depth interviews or focus groups, which involve qualitative techniques. Interview methods vary along a spectrum; on one end, the same questions are posed to all interviewees (i.e., a structured interview), and on the other end, interview content is directed by the interviewee (i.e., an unstructured interview). In-depth interviews can be particularly helpful when examining controversial topics, such as physicians' views of physician-assisted suicide (Emanuel et al. 1998), or issues for which moral ambiguity or subtlety exists, such as decisions about childbearing (Faden and Kass 1996).

Focus groups, by contrast, have certain advantages and disadvantages. Conducting focus groups can be more efficient in terms of time and cost than doing individual interviews. They also create group dynamics and might motivate individuals in the group to consider issues they might not have considered during an individual interview. This same group dynamic, however, can in other circumstances limit individual expression or constrain the discussion, underscoring the importance of having a well-trained moderator. Focus groups have recently been used to examine public perceptions of returning genomic test results (O'Daniel and Haga 2011) and to evaluate potential research participants' views of researchers' financial conflicts of interest (Weinfurt et al. 2006). The results of these and similar qualitative research studies often inform both normative theory and other empirical methods. While they have the advantage of giving so-called "thick descriptions" of morally charged questions, qualitative methods lack generalizability and cannot claim to describe how "all" people think or behave.

Quantitative Empirical Methods. Quantitative survey methods, now commonplace in bioethics, allow measurement of specific variables of interest, often using large or representative sample sizes. In comparison to qualitative methods, quantitative techniques are better able to make claims about a broader or general population, including estimates of the type, prevalence, and relationship among values and demographic variables of interest. Surveys are one commonly used quantitative method. In bioethics, surveys can be employed as a tool for discovery of unrecognized bioethical issues; for assessment of variability in beliefs or practices; or for documenting preferences and moral values (Pearlman and Starks 2010). Some survey methods, such as "discrete choice" experiments, do not survey values directly, but instead elicit them by offering choices among alternatives; such methods have been used to determine public values regarding organ donation, for example (Howard et al. 2011).

Well-designed surveys have the potential to question prevailing dominant views, for example, about beliefs surrounding donation of frozen embryos for research (Lyerly and Faden 2007). Surveys also directly inform policy; the value of a statistical life used in cost-benefit analysis of US federal policy, for example, is calculated through surveys of how much individuals are willing to pay for certain reductions in the risk of death. Quality of life measurements, such as the quality-adjusted life year (or QALY, an attempt to quantify length and quality of life for certain health states), similarly rely on survey methods.

In recent years, quantitative methods in bioethics have moved from surveys and questionnaires to more complex experimental designs. While still representing a small proportion of bioethics research, designing and conducting experimental research can accomplish a number of aims. These range from uncontrolled trials (e.g., prospective studies, such as those demonstrating the relative ineffectiveness of written advance directives [Danis et al. 1991]) to randomized controlled trials (RCTs) of interventions aimed at improving bioethics education and practice. For example, the Study to Understand Prognoses and Preferences for Outcomes and Risks of Treatment (SUPPORT Principal Investigators 1995) tested, but did not find significant efficacy of, an intervention grounded in the ethical principles of autonomy and truth telling. Properly designed and conducted RCTs can therefore provide profound insight to specific questions in bioethics. While quantitative methods can provide great precision and wide generalizability, they can only answer narrow questions, and those questions tend to be shaped by those who ask them.

BIOETHICS: MULTI- OR INTERDISCIPLINARY?

The aforementioned examples describe how a variety of disciplines using diverse methods (both normative and empirical) have contributed to bioethics. A natural question arises as to how these disciplines do, or should, relate. To some scholars, true bioethics involves only "normative" methods, and empirical methods inform, but are not themselves, bioethics.

A more inclusive approach, however, has several advantages. First, many scholars from other disciplines consider themselves "bioethicists," regularly attend bioethics conferences, and work closely with teams doing bioethics scholarship. This is by no means conclusive, but including them within the field of bioethics does legitimize their contributions. Second, and more importantly, from a theoretical standpoint, the line between empirical and normative work (or the "fact/value distinction") is both thin and contested. Separating out only the normative part of bioethics is fraught with difficulties. A number of bioethicists take the approach that bioethics is a field of inquiry that shares a common subject matter, however broad that might be and however fuzzy its boundaries are. Various disciplines, including (though not limited to) the ones above, contribute to our understanding of this field through both normative and empirical methods.

Understanding contemporary bioethics as a "multidisciplinary" field is thus relatively straightforward. Multidisciplinary scholarship is frequently a collective effort where different disciplines address the same question from within their own disciplinary parameters. Sulmasy (2010), for example, details the role of multiple disciplines in examining "substituted judgment." Substituted judgment is the idea that when an individual patient loses decision-making capacity, respect for that patient's autonomy can be met by a surrogate decision maker making the decision he or she thinks the patient would have made. As Sulmasy notes, various disciplines including history, law, medicine, philosophy, and theology, as well as qualitative and quantitative researchers and sociologists, have all contributed expertise to our understanding of substituted judgment. More important, however, is the interplay between normative and empirical methods. Normative theories about substituted judgment, for example, have been undergoing revision because it has been shown empirically that surrogates frequently fail to identify the decision the patient would have wanted, and that patients themselves do not always favor substituted judgment (Sulmasy 2010). Normative theorists have incorporated these empirical data into more robust concepts and theories of substituted judgment.

This type of research thus exemplifies mixed methods research, that is, answering complex and deeply contextual research questions by the use and integration of multiple methods from diverse disciplines and theoretical backgrounds, including empirical (qualitative and quantitative) as well as normative methods. Many questions in bioethics fulfill these criteria, suggesting the importance for scholars to adhere to emerging standards in mixed methods research, such as those proposed by the US National Institutes of Health (Creswell et al. 2011).

Does bioethics research rise to the level of "interdisciplinary" research? Interdisciplinary scholarship might be thought of as the combining of disciplines to address a common question, thereby generating new knowledge not achievable through any one discipline alone. To the extent that this requires shared methods, theories, frameworks, and standards for the creation and interpretation of moral knowledge, some suggest no—Turner (2009) goes so far as to suggest bioethics might not exist. This concern is both theoretical and practical. Theoretically, disciplines with radical foundational differences (about the nature of right and wrong, the nature of personhood, etc.) might be difficult or impossible to combine (Klein 1990). Practically, merging and blurring of disciplinary boundaries might result in poor scholarship standards or the misuse of theory and methods (Jecker 2012).

Others see the effective integration of disciplines as possible or even necessary for bioethics. In such views, many disciplines, particularly the social sciences, generate knowledge about individual human behavior, sociocultural practices, and bioethics itself that is necessary for practicing bioethics (Callahan 1999). Bioethics in the public sphere, including the aforementioned national-level commissions and major institutes and centers, often conducts itself as (and calls itself) "interdisciplinary."

Whether or not criticisms of interdisciplinary bioethics hold, these criticisms do not apply to multidisciplinary research. To the extent that multidisciplinary research retains the foundations and standards of rigor of each disciplinary component, the risk of poor scholarship can be minimized (Adler and Shaul 2012). Moreover, complete theoretical agreement is not prerequisite for multidisciplinary scholarship, as the substituted judgment example suggests.

CONCLUSION

Contemporary bioethics is a multidisciplinary research field whose questions not only allow, but also may require, input from diverse disciplines using a variety of empirical and normative methods. The line between empirical and normative methods can be thin, particularly for normatively guided empirical research and more complex empirical studies. If anything, this underscores the necessity of multidisciplinary teams and mixed methods research to answer certain questions of interest to the field. Whether a truly integrated and interdisciplinary field of bioethics is desirable or even possible remains unclear.

SEE ALSO *Autonomy; Beneficence; Ethics; Law and Bioethics; Law and Morality; Public Health: IV. Ethics; Public Health: VI. Research*

BIBLIOGRAPHY

Adler, Daniel, and Randi Z. Shaul. 2012. "Disciplining Bioethics: Towards a Standard of Methodological Rigor in Bioethics Research." *Accountability in Research* 19 (3): 187–207.

Advisory Committee on Human Radiation Experiments. 1996. *The Human Radiation Experiments: Final Report of the President's Advisory Committee.* New York: Oxford University Press.

Annas, George J. 1993. *Standard of Care: The Law of American Bioethics.* New York: Oxford University Press.

Anspach, Renée R. 1993. *Deciding Who Lives*. Berkeley: University of California Press.

Asch, David A. 2010. "Economics and Decision Science." In *Methods in Medical Ethics*, 2nd ed., edited by Jeremy Sugarman and Daniel P. Sulmasy, 273–93. Washington, DC: Georgetown University Press.

Beauchamp, Tom L. 2005. "The Origins and Evolution of the Belmont Report." In *Belmont Revisited: Ethical Principles for Research with Human Subjects*, edited by James F. Childress, Eric M. Meslin, and Harold T. Shapiro, 12–25. Washington, DC: Georgetown University Press.

Beauchamp, Tom L., and James F. Childress. 2008. *Principles of Biomedical Ethics*. 6th ed. New York: Oxford University Press.

Borry, Pascal; Paul Schotsmans; and Kris Dierickx. 2005. "The Birth of the Empirical Turn in Bioethics." *Bioethics* 19 (1): 49–71.

Cahill, Lisa S. 2010. "Religion and Theology." In *Methods in Medical Ethics*, 2nd ed., edited by Jeremy Sugarman and Daniel P. Sulmasy, 73–90. Washington, DC: Georgetown University Press.

Callahan, Daniel. 1999. "The Social Sciences and the Task of Bioethics." *Daedalus* 128 (4): 275–94.

Childress, James F. 2007. "Methods in Bioethics." In *The Oxford Handbook of Bioethics*, edited by Bonnie Steinbock, 15–45. New York: Oxford University Press.

Cook-Deegan, Robert, and Christopher Heaney. 2010. "Gene Patents and Licensing: Case Studies Prepared for the Secretary's Advisory Committee on Genetics, Health, and Society." *Genetics in Medicine* 12 (4 suppl.): S1–S2.

Copeland, Curtis W. 2010. "How Agencies Monetize 'Statistical Lives' Expected to Be Saved by Regulations." *CRS Report for Congress*, US Congressional Research Service, March 24.

Creswell, John W.; Ann C. Klassen; Vicki L. Plano Clark; and Katherine C. Smith for the Office of Behavioral and Social Sciences Research. 2011. *Best Practices for Mixed Methods Research in the Health Sciences*. Bethesda, MD: National Institutes of Health.

Danis, Marion; Leslie I. Southerland; Joanne M. Garrett; et al. 1991. "A Prospective Study of Advance Directives for Life-Sustaining Care." *New England Journal of Medicine* 324 (13): 882–88.

Emanuel, Ezekiel J.; Elisabeth R. Daniels; Diane L. Fairclough; and Brian R. Clarridge. 1998. "The Practice of Euthanasia and Physician-Assisted Suicide in the United States: Adherence to Proposed Safeguards and Effects on Physicians." *Journal of the American Medical Association* 280 (6): 507–13.

Faden, Ruth R., and Nancy E. Kass, eds. 1996. *HIV, AIDS & Childbearing*. New York: Oxford University Press.

Fisher, Jill A. 2009. *Medical Research for Hire: The Political Economy of Pharmaceutical Clinical Trials*. New Brunswick, NJ: Rutgers University Press.

Frankena, William K. 1973. *Ethics*. 2nd ed. Englewood Cliffs, NJ: Prentice-Hall.

Guinn, David E., ed. 2006. *Handbook of Bioethics and Religion*. New York: Oxford University Press.

Howard, Kirsten; Stephen Jan; John Rose; et al. 2011. "Community Preferences for the Allocation & Donation of Organs—the PAraDOx Study." *BioMed Central Public Health* 11:386.

Hume, David. 2003 [1740]. *A Treatise of Human Nature*. Bk. 3. London: Everyman.

Jansen, Lynn A. 2009. "Consensus and Independent Judgment in Clinical Ethics: Or, What Can an Eighteenth-Century French Mathematician Teach Us About Ethics Consultation?" *Journal of Clinical Ethics* 20 (1): 56–63.

Jecker, Nancy S. 2012. "Applying Ethical Reasoning: Philosophical, Clinical, and Cultural Challenges." In *Bioethics: An Introduction to the History, Methods, and Practice*, 3rd ed., edited by Nancy S. Jecker, Albert R. Jonsen, and Robert A. Pearlman, 127–39. London: Jones & Bartlett Publishers.

Jones, James H. 1981. *Bad Blood*. New York: Free Press.

Klein, Julie T. 1990. *Interdisciplinarity: History, Theory, and Practice*. Detroit, MI: Wayne State University Press.

Krippendorff, Klaus. 2004. *Content Analysis: An Introduction to Its Methodology*. 2nd ed. Thousand Oaks, CA: Sage Publications.

Lederer, Susan E. 2010. "History." In *Methods in Medical Ethics*, 2nd ed., edited by Jeremy Sugarman and Daniel P. Sulmasy, 145–58. Washington, DC: Georgetown University Press.

Leget, Carlo; Pascal Borry; and Raymond de Vries. 2009. "'Nobody Tosses a Dwarf!' The Relation Between the Empirical and the Normative Reexamined." *Bioethics* 23 (4): 226–35.

Lowenthal, David. 1985. *The Past Is a Foreign Country*. New York: Cambridge University Press.

Lyerly, Anne D., and Ruth R. Faden. 2007. "Embryonic Stem Cells: Willingness to Donate Frozen Embryos for Stem Cell Research." *Science* 317 (5834): 46–47.

Menikoff, Jerry. 2001. *Law and Bioethics: An Introduction*. Washington, DC: Georgetown University Press.

Molewijk, Bert; Anne M. Stiggelbout; Wilma Otten; et al. 2004. "Empirical Data and Moral Theory; a Plea for Integrated Empirical Ethics." *Medicine, Health Care and Philosophy* 7 (1): 55–69.

Moore, George Edward. 1993. *Principia Ethica*. New York: Cambridge University Press.

National Commission for the Protection of Human Subjects of Biomedical and Behavioral Research. 1978. *The Belmont Report. Ethical Principles and Guidelines for the Protection of Human Subjects of Research*. Washington, DC: DHEW and US Government Printing Office.

O'Daniel, Julianne, and Susanne B. Haga. 2011. "Public Perspectives on Returning Genetics and Genomics Research Results." *Public Health Genomics* 14 (6): 346–55.

Overberg, Kenneth. R. 2006. *Ethics and AIDS: Compassion and Justice in a Global Crisis*. Lanham, MD: Rowman & Littlefield.

Pearlman, Robert A., and Helene E. Starks. 2010. "Quantitative Surveys." In *Methods in Medical Ethics*, 2nd ed., edited by Jeremy Sugarman and Daniel P. Sulmasy, 233–49. Washington, DC: Georgetown University Press.

Presidential Commission for the Study of Bioethical Issues. 2011. *"Ethically Impossible" STD Research in Guatemala from 1946 to 1948*. Washington, DC: Author.

Reardon, Jenny. 2005. *Race to the Finish: Identity and Governance in an Age of Genomics*. Princeton, NJ: Princeton University Press.

Shapiro, Michael H.; Roy G. Spece; Rebecca Dresser; and Ellen W. Clayton, eds. 2002. *Bioethics and Law: Cases, Materials and Problems.* St. Paul, MN: Thomson West.

Sugarman, Jeremy; Ruth R. Faden; and Alison Boyce. 2010. "A Quarter Century of Empirical Research in Biomedical Ethics." In *Methods in Medical Ethics*, 2nd ed., edited by Jeremy Sugarman and Daniel P. Sulmasy, 21–34. Washington, DC: Georgetown University Press.

Sugarman, Jeremy, and Daniel P. Sulmasy, eds. 2010. *Methods in Medical Ethics.* 2nd ed. Washington, DC: Georgetown University Press.

Sulmasy, Daniel P. 2010. "Research in Medical Ethics." In *Methods in Medical Ethics*, 2nd ed., edited by Jeremy Sugarman and Daniel P. Sulmasy, 295–314. Washington, DC: Georgetown University Press.

Sulmasy, Daniel P., and Jeremy Sugarman. 2010. "The Many Methods of Medical Ethics." In *Methods in Medical Ethics*, 2nd ed., edited by Jeremy Sugarman and Daniel P. Sulmasy, 3–20. Washington, DC: Georgetown University Press.

SUPPORT Principal Investigators. 1995. "A Controlled Trial to Improve Care for Seriously Ill Hospitalized Patients. The Study to Understand Prognoses and Preferences for Outcomes and Risks of Treatments (SUPPORT)." *Journal of the American Medical Association* 274 (20): 1591–98.

Taylor, Holly A.; Sara C. Hull; and Nancy E. Kass. 2010. "Qualitative Methods." In *Methods in Medical Ethics*, 2nd ed., edited by Jeremy Sugarman and Daniel P. Sulmasy, 193–213. Washington, DC: Georgetown University Press.

Turner, Leigh. 2009. "Does Bioethics Exist?" *Journal of Medical Ethics* 35 (12): 778–80.

Verhey, Allen, ed. 1996. *Religion and Medical Ethics: Looking Back, Looking Forward.* Grand Rapids, MI: William B. Eerdmans.

Weinfurt, Kevin P.; Joelle Y. Friedman; Jennifer S. Allsbrook; et al. 2006. "Views of Potential Research Participants on Financial Conflicts of Interest: Barriers and Opportunities for Effective Disclosure." *Journal of General Internal Medicine* 21 (9): 901–6.

Matthew DeCamp
Assistant Professor, Johns Hopkins Berman Institute of Bioethics and Division of General Internal Medicine

Jeremy Sugarman
Harvey M. Meyerhoff Professor of Bioethics and Medicine, Johns Hopkins Berman Institute of Bioethics and Division of General Internal Medicine

Daniel P. Sulmasy
Kilbride-Clinton Professor of Medicine and Ethics, Department of Medicine and Divinity School, University of Chicago
Associate Director, MacLean Center for Clinical Medical Ethics, University of Chicago

VII: EMPIRICAL METHODS IN

The value of empirical data for informing bioethics has emerged over the past twenty years. Concurrently, advances in medicine have rapidly changed the face of medical care, and the sweeping potential of biomedicine has changed the trajectory of human life. While the promise and "threat" of these advances have made bioethics more relevant than ever, they have also highlighted the need for empirical evidence to support underlying assumptions and assertions. Bioethics is now a multidisciplinary field of study where moral philosophy, the medical sciences, and the social sciences intersect. Empirically based studies provide evidence that can guide recommendations for practice and provide a benchmark for evaluating public policies designed to help solve bioethics problems such as the following:

- Patient and family preferences for treatment at the end of life;
- Nature and quality of communication between patients and physicians;
- Attitudes and understanding of informed consent by investigators and research subjects;
- Why policy and legislative initiatives have failed to increase consent rates to organ donation;
- Impact of new genetic information on individuals, families, and society;
- Equity in allocation of scarce resources; and
- Disparities in the provision of care to ethnic minorities.

RESEARCH METHODS

Researchers engaged in the empirical study of bioethics have traditionally used either quantitative or qualitative methods. However, multimethod research that combines the two can provide a richer and more comprehensive understanding of this complex phenomenon. Whereas qualitative research begins by acknowledging that there is a range of different ways of making sense of the world, and approaches its subject matter in a naturalistic, interpretive way, quantitative research overlays hypothesized paradigms on the research phenomena of interest and collects data that can help determine the distributions of characteristics and behaviors in populations and settings. For example, quantitative studies have established how frequently dying patients are treated with futile therapies, but have not been especially successful in explaining why.

Quantitative methods are used to answer hypotheses or to provide generalizable descriptions of populations and the incidence and prevalence of behaviors and problems within a population. Traditional quantitative methods in the social sciences include controlled experiments to compare the effects of an intervention on a sample population and measurement of subject characteristics.

These measurements can include characterizing attitudes, behaviors, or physical characteristics. They are distinguished by the use of measurement tools that can provide reliable and replicable descriptions, usually in the form of numeric signifiers. Examples of such measurements are the use of psychometric tools to measure cognitive traits (e.g., anxiety, coping style, depression) and attitudes (trust in the health care system, fatalism). Secondary sources, such as administrative databases and medical records, are also a major source of quantitative data.

Quantitative methods form the basics of survey research, which has been the bedrock of much of the research conducted in empirical bioethics. In fact, few researchers who conduct empirical research do so without survey research techniques. However, careful attention must be paid to the development of the survey's design, formulating the research question, drawing the sample, and analyzing the data and ensuring its relevance to ethical concepts. Other related methods include the use of hypothetical vignettes. For example, vignettes have been used to explore the ethical implications of paying normal volunteers to participate in research. Hypothetical vignettes provide a less personal and, therefore, less threatening presentation of such issues to research participants. Quantitative methods enable data collection from large samples using standardized procedures that permit comparisons across various populations and time periods. They also allow for controlled interventions or controlled introduction of conditions to subjects.

Bioethics researchers have generally used qualitative methods to generate hypotheses rather than to test hypotheses. Qualitative research is characterized by deduction, whereas quantitative research is characterized by induction. Qualitative methods permit detailed, and sometimes more accurate, observation of behaviors and expand our understanding of the underlying social and cultural characteristics associated with specific patterns of behaviors. Moreover, qualitative methods allow discovery of subjects' perspectives rather than imposing a preexisting framework. Qualitative methods can allow researchers to access areas of investigation that are not amenable to quantitative research, and to explore areas that have been rarely researched in the past. An example is how new genetic technologies are providing the opportunity for personalized medicine but also have implications for patients' privacy that have yet to be studied.

Qualitative methods include not only data collection methods but also analytic approaches. Data can be collected through open-ended interviews and analyzed through a variety of techniques, including close reading of the text and content analysis using either manual approaches or computer programs such as Atlas-TI and SCCAP. Content analysis can provide comprehensive descriptions of phenomena, illuminate processes, and capture beliefs, motivations, and experiences of individuals. It can also explain the meanings that individuals attach to their experiences. For example, exploring how individuals understand the concept of personhood and quality of life, and the implications their conceptualizations have for end-of-life decisions. Focus groups are another method to stimulate discussion and gather data on multifaceted and complex bioethical issues and can be especially useful for obtaining speculative data such as the public's perceptions of biobanking.

Direct observation of health care situations and populations can also provide complex and rich descriptive data. For example, studies of informed consent to clinical trials have included direct observation and audio/video-recording of the consent conversation. Conversations can be examined as narratives and themes explored, or behaviors can be coded to extract quantitative data. For example, a trained observer can use a 0, 1 coding scheme to measure whether certain behaviors (e.g., explaining that trial participation is voluntary) occur or not. Participant observation—in which the observer actually participates in and observes the daily activities of a setting of interest (e.g., observing a primary care setting to understand how or when advance directives are discussed with elderly patients)—can also generate a variety of data types. Personal diaries in which individuals are asked to keep records of activities and behaviors are another qualitative technique that can yield essential data on topics related to bioethics.

Newer methods are also emerging that have utility for bioethics research. One example is meta-analysis or systematic review. Another is deliberative procedures based on theories of democracy, with the aim of providing community members a "voice" in decisions, such as determining priorities for health care spending. This method and others can bring bioethics to the community as part of the movement for community-based and community-engaged research.

CONCLUSION

Ultimately, scholarship in bioethics can benefit from the methodologies of both the humanities and the empirical sciences. Normative bioethics provides a framework and guideposts for suggesting how health care services ought to be delivered, and what the fiduciary responsibilities of clinicians to patients should entail. However, normative bioethics is unable to describe and explain how these play out in real life. Moreover, the value placed in the principles of bioethics and the use of these principles by actors in health care settings can only be illuminated using empirical methods. Applied ethics is certainly the area that will derive the greatest benefit from the addition of empirical, data-driven methods to those of the humanities used in theoretical bioethics. In the clinical arena, health care providers want to know what facts might bear on the ethical questions they confront or how ethical conflicts impact patient care. Policy makers also want data that can guide how health care problems can be understood and resolved. This is not to say that ethical theory is not interesting or important. Ethical theory generated through the methods of the humanities can provide ways of framing the relevant questions or can even help to define what those questions are. Without ethical theory, would we even define the experimentation on human subjects without consent as a problem? Moreover, empirical methods, especially qualitative methods, have much in common with those of the humanities, especially the close reading and interpretation of texts. The divide is perhaps wider in the minds of disciplinary practitioners than is the reality.

In the final analysis, the best empirical research in bioethics will always be based on a sophisticated understanding of the historical, philosophical, and cultural contexts of the delivery and consumption of health care services. Similarly, philosophical debate can often be enriched by an awareness of empirical data. As we move into the future, a more fully articulated merging of these methodologies is much to be desired.

SEE ALSO *Medicine, Anthropology of; Medicine, Sociology of; Organ Transplants, Sociocultural Aspects of; Public Health: V. Methods; Public Health: VI. Research; Public Policy and Bioethics; Research, Unethical; Research Ethics Consultation; Research Methodology: I. Conceptual Issues; Research Policy: I. General Background*

BIBLIOGRAPHY

Appleton, Jane V. 1995. "Analysing Qualitative Interview Data: Addressing Issues of Validity and Reliability." *Journal of Advanced Nursing* 22 (5): 993–97.

Braddock III, H. Clarence, and David Magnus. 2010. "Empirical Methods in Bioethics: A Cautionary Tale." *Annals of Internal Medicine* 152 (6): 396–97.

Frader, Joel. 2008. "The Significance of Empirical Bioethics for Medical Practice: A Physician's Perspective." In *Empirical Methods for Bioethics: A Primer*, Vol. 11, edited by Liva Jacoby and Laura M. Siminoff, 21–36. Oxford, UK: Elsevier.

Joffe, R. Ari; R. Natalie Anton; P. Jonathan Duff; et al. 2012. "A Survey on American Neurologists About Brain Death: Understanding the Conceptual Basis and Diagnostic Tests for Brain Death." *Annals of Intensive Care* 2 (1): 4.

Little, Miles; Jill Gordon; Pippa Markham; et al. 2011. "Virtuous Acts as Practical Medical Ethics: An Empirical Study." *Journal of Evaluation in Clinical Practice* 17 (5): 948–53.

Looker, E. Dianne; Margaret A. Denton; and Christine K. Davis. 1989. "Bridging the Gap: Incorporating Qualitative Data into Quantitative Analyses." *Social Science Research* 18 (4): 313–30.

Loughlin, Michael. 2011. "Criticizing the Data: Some Concerns About Empirical Approaches to Ethics." *Journal of Evaluation in Clinical Practice* 17 (5): 970–75.

Pope, Catherine, and Nick Mays. 1995. "Reaching the Parts Other Methods Cannot Reach: An Introduction to Qualitative Methods in Health and Health Services Research." *British Medical Journal* 311 (6996): 42–45.

Siminoff, Laura A., and Mary M. Step. 2011. "A Comprehensive Observational Coding Scheme for Analyzing Instrumental, Affective and Relational Communication in Healthcare Contexts." *Journal of Health Communication* 16 (2): 178–97.

Smith, Williams; Christine Grady; Benjamin Krohmal; et al. 2011. "Empirical Evaluation of the Need for 'Ongoing Consent' in Clinical Research." *AIDS* 25 (1): 107–14.

Sofaer, Neema, and Daniel Strech. 2012. "The Need for Systematic Reviews of Reasons." *Bioethics* 26 (6): 315–28.

Stunkel, Leanne, and Christine Grady. 2011. "More Than the Money: A Review of the Literature Examining Healthy Volunteer Motivations." *Contemporary Clinical Trials* 32 (3): 342–52.

Laura A. Siminoff (2004, 2014)
Professor and Chair, Department of Social and Behavioral Health, School of Medicine, Virginia Commonwealth University

VIII. SOCIOLOGY OF

There are at least two ways to think about the relationship between the discipline of sociology and the intellectual field and professional practice of bioethics. On the one hand, sociology offers a body of knowledge and a collection of methods that are useful tools for those who are engaged in bioethics. The theories of sociology and the sophisticated techniques for collecting and analyzing data about human behavior developed by sociologists can be (and have been) used to examine the social and cultural features of bioethical quandaries, to measure attitudes—professional and public—about bioethical issues, and to develop and test policies related to ethical problems in health care. On the other hand, bioethics is an interesting area for the further refinement of sociological ideas about medicine, health care, professions, and morality. The field of bioethics is rife with opportunities to deepen our understanding of the social and cultural aspects of human life. Located at the nexus of the moral and the medical, sociologists see in bioethics an occasion to explore the human response to illness; the process by which certain situations come to be defined as "ethical problems"; and the development of health policies intended to promote respect for persons, beneficence, and justice.

These two nearly opposite takes on the relationship between sociology and bioethics can be distinguished as "sociology in bioethics"—the use of sociology to answer bioethical questions—and "sociology of bioethics"—the use of bioethics to answer sociological questions. The range of work done by those who labor at the intersection of these two disciplines extends from "in" to "of." These two approaches also represent conflicting views on the value of sociology for the work of bioethics, views that need not be but often are in tension. The former approach is practical, directly useful in the day-to-day work of bioethicists. The value of the latter approach is less apparent but is equally valuable, because it situates bioethics in its social context, helping its practitioners understand the organizational and cultural limitations on their efforts to promote more ethical behavior. The tension between the two is visible in the way each is regarded by bioethicists. Sociologists using the former approach generally are welcomed by bioethicists, whereas those using the latter approach have been accused of resentment, arrogance, and "baiting bioethics" (see De Vries 2004).

To better understand the place of sociology in the field of bioethics, it is useful to review the history of sociological interest in medical morality. It is no exaggeration to say that sociological interest in matters moral dates to the origin of the discipline. Sociology was born in the nineteenth century, a period of rapid and profound social change. Industrialization, urbanization, secularization, the rise of capitalism, and the advent of mass democracy caused unprecedented physical, social, and psychological dislocation, making visible previously taken-for-granted aspects of social life, raising the questions that became foundational for the new discipline: What is the nature of the moral fibers that hold members of society together? How do changing economic and social situations alter the obligations of humans to each other and to themselves? What are the social and human consequences of the shift from traditional to rational forms of authority?

In their efforts to understand how members of modern societies sorted out how to live together in new social circumstances that altered taken-for-granted ideas of right and wrong, early social scientists studied and wrote about religion, law, politics, the economy, and science. In his *Division of Labor in Modern Society* (1984) Émile Durkheim presented his vision of the social forces that bind individuals together in a society. Responding to Ferdinand Tönnies's (1957) gloomy depiction of the changes wrought by modern life—where small and friendly *gemeinschaft* societies were giving way to the larger and impersonal *gesellschaft*—Durkheim offered a positive view of urbanization and industrialization as a transition from "mechanical" to "organic" solidarity. According to Durkheim, older societies were united in a mechanical, "automatic" way. He found evidence of this in their legal systems, which responded to the violation of norms by lashing out with repressive sanctions: the offender was punished to exact retribution. In modern societies, Durkheim argued, people are connected organically—each dependent on the other in a complex division of labor. This type of society is characterized by a system of restitutive law: when a norm is violated the *conscience collectif* (collective conscience) responds by addressing the imbalance created. The goal is to restore the status quo ante, not to punish the offender. In the work of Max Weber we find an effort to understand how and why values persisted and changed and how these values influenced forms of rationality in modernizing societies. In his classic *Protestant Ethic and the Spirit of Capitalism* (1992 [1930]) Weber showed how Protestant doctrines about the afterlife shaped values and thereby promoted individual behaviors that allowed the flourishing of Western capitalism.

Medical sociology, a field that began to flourish in the 1950s (Bloom 2002), was informed by these classic sociological theories. While medical sociologists of the 1950s, 1960s, and 1970s did not explicitly study the ethics of medicine, much of their work—looking at patterns of diseases, social conceptions of health and illness, the functioning of medical systems, and the health care professions—touched on moral issues in medical care. Talcott Parsons, a social theorist whose work helped define the new field of medical sociology, described medicine as an important system of social control. For Parsons (1951, 428–79), illness was a type of deviance, a threat to the stability of society. Those guilty of deviating from legal norms were sent to legal institutions (courts, prisons, parole offices) intended to rehabilitate them and integrate them back into society; the sick—violators of the norms of health—were treated and rehabilitated by the institutions of the medical system (doctors' offices and hospitals).

Other pioneering studies in medical sociology showed a similar concern with the moral questions that accompany illness and its treatment. Included in this work are:

- studies of medical education that describe the "fate of idealism" and explore how students "negotiate" the demands of course work and examinations (Merton, Reader, and Kendall 1957; Becker et al. 1961);
- ethnographies of work in the hospital that reveal how death is thought about, managed, discussed, and revealed to next of kin and others (Sudnow 1967);
- research on the medical profession that shows an unfavorable balance between the self-interest of professionals and the interest of patients (Freidson 1970);
- studies of stigma and "total institutions" that expose the underside of the treatment given those not seen as "normal" (Goffman 1961, 1963);
- analyses of the medicalization of deviance that describe how the control of certain behaviors moved from legal to medical institutions (Conrad and Schneider 1980).

Each of these now-classic studies in medical sociology focuses on issues important to medical ethics. Although not labeled as such, truth telling, conflict of interest, patient autonomy, and organizational ethics are among the ethically relevant topics explored by these sociologists.

Coincident with the emergence of bioethics as a distinct field in the 1970s, this implicit sociological interest in the morality of medicine gradually became more explicit. Sociologists began more direct study of medical experiments, organ transplantation, and medical errors. In the first half of the decade Bernard Barber and his colleagues (1973) and Bradford Gray (1975) were involved in sociological studies of the treatment of human subjects of medical research. In her study of medical experiments and organ transplantation—described in *Experiment Perilous* (1959) and *The Courage to Fail* (1974, with Judith P. Swazey)—Renée C. Fox touched on matters of ethical import focusing on the uncertainty and stress that accompanied medical research and practice. Although it was self-consciously a study in bioethics, Charles L. Bosk's (1979) investigation of the response to errors in surgery and surgical residency is now widely regarded as one of the first studies to look directly at clinical ethics. Contrary to what most laypeople would expect, Bosk discovered that the "technical" mistakes of surgical residents (e.g., leaving a surgical instrument in the body of a patient) were taken less seriously and were less severely punished (if they were punished at all) than were "normative" errors—violations of the rules governing the relationships between students and their teachers.

These first sociological forays into medical morality set the tone for further work in the sociology of bioethics, studies that used the ethical moments of medicine to further our knowledge of professions, organizations, and societal definitions of infirmity and death. As the twentieth century drew to a close, there emerged a body of sociological and historical research that looked directly and critically at the new interdisciplinary field of bioethics, examining the way bioethicists described and resolved the moral problems of medicine. Fox and Swazey contributed to this work with *Spare Parts* (1992), a critique of the marketing and the high costs of transplant medicine. The medical historian David Rothman (1991) offered a look at "the new moral authority at the bedside," describing how law and ethics transformed medical decision making. Robert Zussman (1992) analyzed decision making in intensive care units; Bosk (1992) watched genetic counselors at work; Jeanne H. Guillemin and Lynda L. Holmstrom (1986), Renée Anspach (1993), and Jessica Mesman (2002) looked at moral deliberations in neonatal intensive care units. Daniel F. Chambliss's (1996) classic study of nursing and ethics offered a slight variation on these studies of moral issues in medical care. Unlike his colleagues, Chambliss did not start out with the intent of exploring medical ethics; instead his ethnography of nursing led him to notice the moral dimensions of hospital life and the many ways "ethics" gets used in organizations. He demonstrates that ethical problems are not discrete, one-at-a-time events occurring between patients, families, and doctors; rather, they are predictable outcomes of social organization.

In the first decade of the twenty-first century, sociological studies of the new profession of bioethics began to appear. In his exploration of the role of bioethicists in the public debate over human genetic engineering, John Hyde Evans (2002) used ideas developed by Weber to call attention to the ways bioethicists conspired with scientists to shrink the debate from a theological one focused on the ends of human life (in Weber's terms, a "substantive rationality"), to a more secular and "thin" debate centered on proper techniques and means ("formal rationality"). According to Evans, "thinning" of the debate was a move made by bioethicists to claim jurisdiction over an area once controlled by theologians. In *Observing Bioethics* (2008) Fox and Swazey detail the social factors associated with the creation of bioethics, showing how the field subtly incorporated American values. They go on to examine the export of bioethics from the United States to other countries (both developed and developing) and to evaluate the politics of bioethics made evident by the ethics "culture wars" associated with former president George W. Bush's council on bioethics.

As work at the intersection of sociology and bioethics matured, it became more difficult to identify research that could be explicitly labeled sociology of bioethics. Rather, we find projects that touch on the social contexts of bioethical issues but bring to bear in their analysis a broader, interdisciplinary approach. In *Better Than Well* (2003) and *White Coat, Black Hat* (2010) Carl Elliott uses philosophical insight to investigate the ethical quandaries associated with technologies of enhancement and the commercialization of medicine. Jill Fisher (2009) employs a science, technology, and society approach to detail the social, cultural, and political conditions that conspired to create the early twenty-first-century (and, according to her, flawed) system for testing and marketing new drugs. In her exploration of the way parents use the moral language of authenticity and personal freedom to justify the use of drug therapy for their children, Illyah Singh (2005) critiques bioethics for its failure to grapple with the social, cultural, and moral context of treatment decisions made by parents. Using the lens of political science, Shobita Parthasarathy (2007) examines international variation in the development and deployment of genetic testing for breast and ovarian cancer, and Adriana Petryna (2009) applies her background in anthropology to analyze the globalization of clinical trials.

Parallel to these studies of bioethics, there has been an "empirical turn" in the field of bioethics itself. First described by Pascal Borry, Paul Schotsmans, and Kris Dierickx (2005, 2006), this shift represents an effort to inform normative arguments with empirical data and to better suit ethical theorizing for practical application in the clinic and in research with humans. Practitioners of sociology in bioethics lend their skills to ethicists, using their discipline to help them solve the dilemmas they face. Sociological methods are ideal for measuring the things bioethicists need measured: Are research subjects and patients really informed after they sign an informed consent? What do research subjects understand (and want to understand) about researchers' conflicts of interest? What does (some section of) the public think about genetic testing? This approach is useful—articles of this type have proliferated—but critics have questioned the use of a methodology shorn of its disciplinary context (Hurst 2010). Divorced from sociological theory, the methods of sociology deliver empty facts—mere descriptions of what others consider to be bioethical issues and/or problems—with no appreciation of the historical and social location of moral decision making. The practical work of sociology in bioethics may help streamline the consent process, for example, but it will miss the opportunity to explain how the interests of a patient/subject are related to cultural ideas about the value of medical therapies or the way health care is organized or paid for.

Like other disciplines, sociology has its own "morality of method," a morality that differs from that which informs the methods of normative philosophers in bioethics. Sociologists are inclined to challenge the "hierarchy of credibility" (Becker 1967, 241), weighing equally the accounts of a social situation given by the disenfranchised (e.g., a poor and uninsured hospital patient) and the enfranchised (e.g., a member of a hospital ethics committee). The methods of philosophy, especially in its Anglo-American version, are morally committed to clarity and logic. When asked to examine conflicts of interest in medical research, for example, the philosophical imagination seeks precision in the meanings and categories of the terms employed (*conflict* and *interest*) and considers the proper application of moral theory to problems created by these conflicts. Given the same task, the sociological imagination begins by exploring the social history of the concept of "conflict of interest," its uses (and abuses), the way the term is operationalized, and who gains and who loses as a result of the policies governing these conflicts.

In *The History and Future of Bioethics* Evans (2012, 170) emphasizes how his distance from bioethics allowed him to examine the field in a way that will help "retain a positive bioethical debate so that we as a society can face the biomedical challenges ahead." There is an irony here. When sociologists begin with questions of their own—questions not given to them by bioethicists or shaped by the field of bioethics—they are more likely to discover social facts useful to the bioethical project of ensuring that health care and the life sciences are done in a way that respects persons and promotes justice.

SEE ALSO *Alternative Therapies: I. Social History; Fertility Control: II. Social and Ethical Issues; Medicine, Sociology of; Public Health: VIII. Social Determinants of Health*

BIBLIOGRAPHY

Anspach, Renée. 1993. *Deciding Who Lives: Fateful Choices in the Intensive Care Nursery.* Berkeley: University of California Press.

Barber, Bernard; John J. Lally; Julia Loughlin Makarushka; and Daniel Sullivan. 1973. *Research on Human Subjects: Problems of Social Control in Medical Experimentation.* New York: Russell Sage Foundation.

Becker, Howard S. 1967. "Whose Side Are We On?" *Social Problems* 14 (3): 239–47.

Becker, Howard S.; Blanche Geer; Everett C. Hughes; and Anselm L. Strauss. 1961. *Boys in White: Student Culture in Medical School.* Chicago: University of Chicago Press.

Bloom, Samuel W. 2002. *The Word as Scalpel: A History of Medical Sociology.* New York: Oxford University Press.

Borry, Pascal; Paul Schotsmans; and Kris Dierickx. 2005. "The Birth of the Empirical Turn in Bioethics." *Bioethics* 19 (1): 49–71.

Borry, Pascal; Paul Schotsmans; and Kris Dierickx. 2006. "Empirical Research in Bioethical Journals: A Quantitative Analysis." *Journal of Medical Ethics* 32 (4): 240–45.

Bosk, Charles L. 1979. *Forgive and Remember: Managing Medical Failure.* Chicago: University of Chicago Press.

Bosk, Charles L. 1992. *All God's Mistakes: Genetic Counseling in a Pediatric Hospital.* Chicago: University of Chicago Press.

Chambliss, Daniel F. 1996. *Beyond Caring: Hospitals, Nurses, and the Social Organization of Ethics.* Chicago: University of Chicago Press.

Conrad, Peter, and Joseph W. Schneider. 1980. *Deviance and Medicalization: From Badness to Sickness.* St. Louis, MO: Mosby.

De Vries, Raymond. 2004. "How Can We Help? From 'Sociology in' Bioethics to 'Sociology of' Bioethics." *Journal of Law, Medicine and Ethics* 32 (2): 279–92.

Durkheim, Émile. 1984. *The Division of Labor in Society.* New York: Free Press.

Elliott, Carl. 2003. *Better Than Well: American Medicine Meets the American Dream.* New York: Norton.

Elliott, Carl. 2010. *White Coat, Black Hat: Adventures on the Dark Side of Medicine.* Boston: Beacon.

Evans, John Hyde. 2002. *Playing God: Human Genetic Engineering and the Rationalization of Public Bioethical Debate.* Chicago: University of Chicago Press.

Evans, John Hyde. 2012. *The History and Future of Bioethics: A Sociological View.* New York: Oxford University Press.

Fisher, Jill. 2009. *Medical Research for Hire: The Political Economy of Pharmaceutical Clinical Trials.* New Brunswick, NJ: Rutgers University Press.

Fox, Renée C. 1959. *Experiment Perilous.* Glencoe, IL: Free Press.

Fox, Renée C., and Judith P. Swazey. 1974. *The Courage to Fail.* Chicago: University of Chicago Press.

Fox, Renée C., and Judith P. Swazey. 1992. *Spare Parts: Organ Replacement in American Society.* New York: Oxford University Press.

Fox, Renée C., and Judith P. Swazey. 2008. *Observing Bioethics.* New York: Oxford University Press.

Freidson, Eliot. 1970. *The Profession of Medicine: A Study of the Sociology of Applied Knowledge.* New York: Dodd, Mead.

Glaser, Barney G., and Anselm L. Strauss. 1968. *Time for Dying.* Chicago: Aldine.

Goffman, Erving. 1961. *Asylums: Essays on the Social Situation of Mental Patients and Other Inmates.* Chicago: Aldine.

Goffman, Erving. 1963. *Stigma: Notes on the Management of Spoiled Identity.* Englewood Cliffs, NJ: Prentice Hall.

Gray, Bradford. 1975. *Human Subjects in Medical Experimentation: A Sociological Study of the Conduct and Regulation of Clinical Research.* New York: Wiley.

Guillemin, Jeanne H., and Lynda L. Holmstrom. 1986. *Mixed Blessings: Intensive Care for Newborns.* New York: Oxford University Press.

Hurst, Samia. 2010. "What 'Empirical Turn in Bioethics'?" *Bioethics* 24 (8): 439–44.

Merton, Robert King; George G. Reader; and Patricia L. Kendall, eds. 1957. *The Student-Physician: Introductory Studies in the Sociology of Medical Education.* Cambridge, MA: Harvard University Press.

Mesman, Jessica. 2002. *Evaren Pioniers: Omgaan met twijfel in de intensive care voor pasgeborenen.* Amsterdam: Aksant.

Parsons, Talcott. 1951. *The Social System.* Glencoe, IL: Free Press.

Parthasarathy, Shobita. 2007. *Building Genetic Medicine: Breast Cancer, Technology, and the Comparative Politics of Health Care.* Cambridge, MA: MIT Press.

Petryna, Adriana. 2009. *When Experiments Travel: Clinical Trials and the Global Search for Human Subjects.* Princeton, NJ: Princeton University Press.

Rothman, David. 1991. *Strangers at the Bedside: How Law and Bioethics Transformed Medical Decision Making.* New York: Basic Books.

Singh, Illyah. 2005. "Will the 'Real Boy' Please Behave: Dosing Dilemmas for Parents of Boys with ADHD." *American Journal of Bioethics* 5 (3): 34–47.

Sudnow, David. 1967. *Passing On: The Social Organization of Dying.* Englewood Cliffs, NJ: Prentice Hall.

Tönnies, Ferdinand. 1957. *Community and Society.* East Lansing: Michigan State University Press.

Weber, Max. 1992 [1930]. *The Protestant Ethic and the Spirit of Capitalism.* New York: Routledge.

Zussman, Robert. 1992. *Intensive Care: Medical Ethics and the Medical Profession.* Chicago: University of Chicago Press.

Raymond De Vries
Professor, Center for Bioethics and Social Sciences and Medicine, University of Michigan Medical School

IX. ANTHROPOLOGY OF

Since the mid-1980s, a growing number of anthropologists have turned their attention to the discipline of biomedical ethics. Bioethics traces its origins as a distinct field to the styles of reasoning and reflection found within analytic philosophy and legal scholarship. Beginning in the 1970s, work in bioethics relied heavily on principle-based analysis, an approach that often led to critiques of the moral dimensions of health care practice divorced from underlying social, cultural, and political context. Often called the "empirical turn" in bioethics, social scientists and others utilizing diverse theoretical and methodological programs have questioned approaches to health care ethics that fail to account for context (Weisz 1990; De Vries and Subedi 1998; Brodwin, 2000; Hoffmaster 2001; Turner 2005, 2009; De Vries et al. 2007; Fox and Swazey 2008; Evans 2012).

Researchers in medical anthropology represent one arm of a strong, and growing, internal critique of bioethics. In addition to social science voices, this critique includes diverse perspectives within philosophy, such as feminist readings of core bioethics dilemmas and a resurgence of interest in the traditions of American pragmatism and casuistry. Even philosophers working within the Kantian tradition have called attention to the need of bioethics to balance the practical realities and diversity of institutions and among professionals with philosophical rigor (O'Neill 2002). Onora O'Neill questions the primacy of autonomy, to the exclusion of a focus on relationships of trust and trustworthiness, in contemporary bioethics discourse.

This entry explores how anthropologists working in the field of bioethics bridge the gap between conceptions of medical morality grounded in local worlds and the universal understandings espoused within the Western philosophical tradition. Ongoing debates about relativism from the perspectives of anthropology and philosophy also are addressed with special attention given to the implications of a "culturally informed" practice of bioethics. Culturally diverse understandings of the meaning and expression of personhood are highlighted in order to illustrate difficulties that emerge when one tries to judge certain practices as good or bad, appropriate or inappropriate. An anthropologically informed bioethics produces a fuller account of health care practices, an account that grounds ethical universals such as respect for persons in local moral worlds.

The body of empirical work reviewed below reveals the thinness of bioethics accounts that disregard social context and that celebrate a particular (often American) version of individual autonomy. Ethical analyses centered exclusively on individual actors create strong barriers to understanding the troubling conflicts that emerge in multicultural worlds, especially in the arena of social justice and human rights. A simplistic application of ethical universals to particular cases discounts the complexity of lived experience and real world dilemmas. In the same way, a naïve and unqualified acceptance of ethical relativism diminishes the potential of negotiating moral consensus across cultural boundaries. An anthropologically grounded framework for bioethics requires a solid recognition of the cultural assumptions that underlie our definition of the "good" in biomedicine. An anthropologically informed bioethics calls attention to the social, political, and structural factors that affect the production of scientific and clinical knowledge and its application in the practice of global biomedicine.

ANTHROPOLOGICAL APPROACHES TO BIOETHICS

The field of bioethics is uniquely multidisciplinary; indeed, it is perhaps best understood as a cultural space in which scholars from many fields interact, joined together by topical interests. However, anthropologists and other social scientists did not play a significant role in the initial development of the field (Evans 2012). In his analysis of medical ethics Richard Lieban (1990, 221–22) suggests two key reasons why anthropologists have been absent. First, given the strong history of cultural relativism in anthropology, studies of health and illness conducted by anthropologists have generally avoided what might be construed as ethnocentric value judgments about other systems. Anthropological focus on documentation and description—as opposed to normative analysis—excludes questions about what is morally "right" or "wrong" about particular health practices. Second, medical anthropologists have often worked in non-Western settings where the technological challenges provided by contemporary biomedicine are less salient. In addition, Patricia Marshall (1992) suggests that bioethicists—unlike anthropologists—have concentrated their attention on the individual rational actor as the primary unit of analysis.

Although bioethics scholars have acknowledged the importance of social milieu—for example, the role of family—in constructing individual choice and shaping decision options, anthropologists, in part because of their traditional subjects, have generally theorized a more complex self, viewing the individual as embedded within a broader social and cultural context. The notion of autonomy, or respect for persons, which many acknowledge has been overcelebrated in bioethics clinical discourse, presumes an individuated self, set apart from the collective experience of family or community, and triumphant over other critical values.

These explanations, however, represent fairly superficial explanations for the lack of anthropological representation within bioethics or interest in it. In fact, the unwillingness of anthropologists to engage with ethics (and for philosophers to reach out to social scientists generally) reflects deep-seated disciplinary boundaries and conflicting epistemologies.

The concept of culture is rarely a starting point in ethics; by contrast, pioneering discussions of comparative medical ethics by anthropologists emphasized the importance of a cultural foundation for framing ethical issues in health care. For example, Peter Kundstadter (1980) addressed ethical challenges associated with development projects in Third World communities, noting the relevance and importance of cultural context for understanding moral dilemmas surrounding beliefs about health and illness and healing roles. Practices such as treatment of less than perfect newborns cannot be adequately understood, much less judged, without detailed local knowledge. Approximately a decade later, Horatio Fabrega (1990) and Richard Lieban (1990) examined the potential of "ethnoethics" for cross-cultural studies of the moral dimensions of health practices. A key starting point is the recognition of variation in the issues that different societies define as morally relevant or problematic. The role of healer is also critical, including the nature of interactions between healers and their patients, interactions among healers themselves, and finally, interactions between practitioners and the larger society.

As engagement with those working in health care ethics increased, anthropologists and others have questioned the fundamental schema underlying bioethics, urging greater attention to cultural context (Muller 1994; Kleinman 1995, 1999; Koenig 1996; Marshall and Koenig 1996, 2000, 2004; Turner 2005, 2009). Cultural interpretation situates the moral dimensions of health care in local ethical practices and local notions of the good. This traditional anthropological orientation to ethics and morality is antithetical to the universalizing discourses of both basic science—which assumes that scientific principles and rules apply to human bodies in all times and places—and the discourse of the philosophical traditions dominant in bioethics—which define a good ethical theory as one that can produce "objective" results that yield rational standards by which to judge actions, irrespective of their history or locality (Marshall and Koenig 2000, 2004).

The medical anthropologist Arthur Kleinman (1995), in his critical analysis of the assumptions and theoretical foundations of bioethics in the 1990s, suggested that the field of bioethics is fundamentally ethnocentric, psychocentric, and medicocentric, and thus shares, rather than moves beyond, biomedicine's fundamental limitations. Kleinman argued that bioethics has failed to engage with the major non-Western moral traditions or to question the "orthodox sources of the self within the western philosophical tradition" (Kleinman 1995, 1669). The medicocentrism inherent in bioethics constrains a practitioner's ability to elicit a complex illness narrative despite the fact that bioethicists are charged with listening to patients and taking account of their perspective and preferences. Although Kleinman maintains optimism that bioethics may open up space in clinical practice for genuine moral reflection and debate, he remains concerned about the limitations of a bioethics devoid of attention to cultural locality: "In the end, then, ethics, once framed as models of moral reasoning championing the reflection and rational choice of autonomous individuals in quest of objective standards, risk irrelevance to the almost always uncertain circumstances and highly contextualized conditions of human experience" (1999, 72).

Anthropologists have the greatest potential to make significant contributions to the field of biomedical ethics in two domains: first, through studies of the cultural production of scientific and clinical knowledge and its translation into medical technology and healing practices and, second, through analysis of the cultural construction of canons of medical morality, including the clinical practices of bioethics itself. Note that this contribution is not linked to the traditional role of anthropology in elucidating the cultural practices of exotic peoples. Ethnographic approaches to ethical questions help clarify the contextual features that are intrinsic to problematic moral issues that arise in medical and research settings throughout the world (Koenig 1988, 1997; Marshall and Koenig 1996, 2010; Hunt 1998; Hogle 1999; Kleinman, Fox, and Brandt 1999; Brodwin 2000; Finkler 2000; Kaufman 2000; Rapp 2000; Farmer 2003, 2006; Hamdy 2012; Roberts 2012).

A broad range of clinical issues and public health concerns have been addressed by anthropologists, including end-of-life decision making, definitions of death, human organ and tissue transplantation therapies, disclosure of medical information, informed consent for medical treatment, reproductive technologies, genetic testing and screening, human rights, and the treatment of human subjects in biomedical research. Scholars working at the boundary of anthropology and the field of science and technology studies have been central to evolving scholarship. A systematic review of the contributions of anthropologists to bioethics, and to our understanding of the moral dimensions of human suffering more generally, is beyond the scope of this entry. Instead, several areas in which anthropologists have focused a cultural lens on moral problems in medicine are highlighted.

ANTHROPOLOGY AND THE STUDY OF BIOMEDICAL TECHNOLOGY

The development of new medical technologies has raised myriad questions at the intersection of culture, morality, and the production and application of scientific discovery (Lock, Young, and Cambrosio 2000; Lock and Vinh-Kim Nguyen 2010). New technologies in biomedicine challenge established meanings of personhood and provide fertile ground for a socially reimagined human body. Does social personhood begin with a fertilized egg, an embryo, at birth, or once the likely survival of an infant is established? How is life's end understood? Anthropological studies can reveal the ambiguous and contested boundaries between nature and culture, boundaries constantly challenged by scientific developments. Anthropological investigations of new reproductive technologies and genetics, in particular, illustrate how understandings of family are necessarily evolving, radically changing traditional notions of kinship and the cultural and biological creation and "production" of children (Ginsburg and Rapp 1995; Becker 2000; Finkler 2000).

New technologies—whether used for life-extending therapy, such as the mechanical ventilator, or diagnosis of death, such as functional brain imaging—may challenge settled understandings of the boundary between life and death (Lock 2002). Liminal states, such as patients existing in persistent coma, are not "natural" entities but are in fact created by new social arrangements, in this case long-term care centers dedicated to the management of those in persistent vegetative state (Kaufman 2000). Bioethical debates about appropriate treatment for those suspended in such liminal states must take account of social forces. Anthropologists have been actively engaged in exploring the moral dimensions of changing definitions of death itself, calling attention to the powerful role that culture plays in shaping beliefs and practices for managing death and dying (Lock and Honde 1990). Perhaps because of its potent emotional valence and symbolic salience, human organ and tissue transplantation has been studied extensively in many parts of the world. The moral questions fundamental to transplantation—whose organs should be replaced, whose may be "harvested," when is a donor "dead enough"—are deeply contingent, varying by beliefs about the location of the soul, the integrity of the physical body and the existence of an afterlife, beliefs which are negotiated within local economies and political arrangements (Lock and Honde 1990; Ohnuki-Tierney 1994; Sharp 1995, 2006, 2013; Ikels 1997; Hogle 1999; E. Gordon 2001, 2013; Joralemon 2001; Lock and Crowley 2008; E. Gordon et al. 2011).

A particular concern of social scientists has been the analysis of organ transplantation and the circulation of organs, characterized initially as an elaborate system of nonmonetary gift exchange, glossed as giving the "gift of life." The sociologist Renée Fox pioneered ethnographic work on transplantation and shares many theoretical and methodological assumptions with that of anthropology. Later analysts have criticized the status of human organs as a source of working capital for poor laborers in developing countries (Cohen 1999), and have documented how a heart can create links of symbolic kinship between donor families and organ recipients (Sharp 2001, 2013). Ethical quandaries stem from the commoditization of bodies that accompanies the marketing of human organs (Marshall and Daar 2000). Most problematic is the exploitation of vulnerable individuals, especially when flows of organs go from poor nations to wealthy ones (Scheper-Hughes 2006). However, allowing individuals the right to sell their organs is justified using a neoliberal market language of rights, a discourse in many ways compatible with bioethics arguments that privilege individual choice and control of one's body. Joralemon (2001) documents the change in discourse about financial incentives for donation (from both living and cadaveric donors) since the origins of US transplantation, showing the impact of a public relations campaign formulated to minimize public resistance to donation.

GENETIC TESTING AND GENOME SCIENCE

Technological advances in genetic testing and genomic science have had a significant impact on the meanings we attach to human identity, the expectations we may have about our vulnerability to disease, and—importantly—on our perception of what we can or cannot control in our own or our children's susceptibility to disease risk (Goodman, Heath, and Lindee 2003). In the arena of prenatal genetic testing, for example, Rapp's (2000) intensive, multiyear ethnographic exploration of the use of amniocentesis for prenatal diagnosis reveals the moral complexity of a seemingly straightforward technology. Ideally, pregnant women should make fully informed, voluntary decisions about undergoing the procedure and continuing a pregnancy if fetal anomalies are discovered. In the city of New York, where Rapp worked, the experience of testing and the eventual decisions made were fundamentally different for women of different social classes and ethnic backgrounds. The exercise of choice can be understood only in light of the social meanings attached to prenatal testing. Rapp warns that if a "new eugenics" emerges, it is unlikely to be imposed by direct state power but rather will be disguised under a rubric of individual choice. Similarly, Nancy Press and Carol Browner's 1998 study of the use of prenatal maternal alpha fetoprotein blood testing (used to predict Down syndrome and other anomalies) illustrates the complex and culturally embedded issues surrounding women's refusal or acceptance of the procedure. Many women accepted the test believing it to be a positive way to assure the health of their baby, much like taking vitamins or other elements of routine prenatal care. In actual practice the only way to avoid the birth of an affected fetus is termination of the pregnancy, but US abortion politics preclude a full and open discussion of the issues, leading to severely truncated communication in the clinic and misapprehension of the usefulness of the prenatal blood test.

Identifying risk for the developing disease represents an important function of genetic testing. Nancy Press, Jennifer Fishman, and Barbara Koenig (2000) demonstrate how cultural context shapes our understanding of the meaning and practice of genetic testing for breast cancer risk, one of the first examples of a genetic test for a common adult-onset disease. Enhancing the decision-making capabilities of individual women is the most commonly suggested bioethical "solution" to the difficult dilemma of disclosing risk for cancer. Cultural analysis suggests two primary reasons for the limitations of this approach: the cultural construction of fear of breast cancer, which has been fueled in part by the predominance of a "risk" paradigm in contemporary biomedicine. The increasing elaboration and delineation of risk factors and risk numbers are in part intended to help women contend with their fear of breast cancer—fears that are inflamed by constant media attention in the form of health education campaigns. However, because there is no known cure or foolproof prevention for breast cancer, risk designation brings with it recommendations for vigilant surveillance strategies and screening guidelines. Thus education about risks exacerbates women's fears of breast cancer, confounding decision making about genetic testing. The volatile combination of the discourses of fear, risk, and surveillance has significant ethical and social consequences for women and their families.

Testing for genetic susceptibility for the occurrence of Alzheimer's disease is another arena in which cultural values are embedded in perceptions of risk and control (Hurley et al. 2005). Genetic testing that reveals susceptibility to disease is cloaked with a scientific objectivity that masks the fundamental truth of uncertainty. Does having a test that reveals genetic susceptibility mean that someone will actually develop a particular disease? Genetic essentialism may play a role in how someone interprets the results of genetic testing, but social realities and environmental influences significantly affect whether and how individuals are actually stricken by illness and disease (Lock et al. 2007; Chilibeck, Lock, and Sehdev 2011). Developments in the area of epigenomics call attention to the complex interactions between social and physical environments and genetics; as Margaret Lock (2013a, 2013b) points out, this represents a "reunification" of the nature versus nurture dichotomy and presents opportunities for anthropological inquiry.

Genetic variation and its implications for human identity is another arena within which anthropologists have contributed and will continue to be engaged. The conceptual categories underlying our understanding of human identity and difference have been of particular concern to anthropology (Gaines 1998; Lee, Mountain, and Koenig 2001; Brodwin 2002; Sankar and Cho 2002; Caulfield et al. 2009). Is the species *Homo sapiens* divided into biologically distinct races? With the advent of new knowledge about human genetic variation, as well as individualized therapies targeted to unique genetic signatures, this issue is of growing moral significance. Given profound health disparities across populations, how are we to tease out the interactions among culture, ethnicity, and, most importantly, of race, in health research and clinical care? Ethnographic studies of the conduct of genetic research reveal how social categories of race inform all domains of biomedical practice. Locating disease etiology in an ethnic group's shared genetic ancestry—potentially excluding consideration of the relevant social determinants of health—may lead to group stigma as well as poor clinical outcomes.

ANTHROPOLOGICAL ANALYSES OF CLINICAL AND RESEARCH ETHICS

In the arena of end-of-life medical care, anthropological studies illustrate how decisions to forgo technological interventions, such as intensive care, are socially negotiated (Slomka 1992; Kaufman 1998). Ethnographic findings allow a useful comparison with decision-making ideals based on abstract principles, providing a critique of models of care that evaluate the success of outcomes using a metric based solely on the exercise of patient choice. A review in 2002 of the empirical literature suggests that the bioethics practices governing end-of-life care (a focus on self-determination, advance care planning, and explicit decisions to forgo life-sustaining treatment) are based on problematic and erroneous assumptions (Drought and Koenig 2002). Studies of bioethics practices applied in culturally diverse clinical settings further illustrate the failure of efforts to enforce universal solutions on complex clinical problems. To fully engage with and respect a patient as a person, what is required is a nuanced understanding of each social environment (Koenig and Gates-Williams 1995; Frank et al. 1998; Long 2000; Crawley et al. 2002; Koenig and Davies, 2003).

Anthropologists have also explored the ethical domain of truth-telling, demonstrating the significant impact of cultural difference on beliefs about disclosure of medical information, especially information relevant to diagnosis and prognosis of cancer and other life-threatening illnesses (Muller and Desmond 1992; Orona, Koenig, and Davis 1994; Carrese and Rhodes 1995; Gordon and Paci 1997; Kaufert 1999; Long 1999). Who decides which facts are truthful, whether that truth harms or helps, and who controls disclosure—all are culturally patterned.

Ethics consultation in hospital settings is a common and highly visible clinical application of bioethics. Anthropological study of the actual practice of ethics consultation reveals the difficulty of simply "applying" bioethics theories in the clinic. A range of issues has been studied, including the nature of clinical disputes that are considered "ethical." In fact, consult requests often stem from nonethical concerns, such as communication failure resulting from the social dynamics of complex hospital environments like intensive care units. Research has also examined actual decision-making processes by institutional ethics committees, power structures within organizational settings and their influence on consultation outcomes, and the potential for conflicts of interests when ethics consultants are institutional employees (Crigger 1995; Orr, Marshall, and Osborn 1995; Kelly et al. 1997; Marshall 2001a).

Voluntary informed consent is considered a universal ethical requirement for good clinical practice and for research with human subjects. However, anthropological studies reveal the ways in which the ideals of informed consent may be constrained in actual practice. The objectives of consent may be undermined by too great a reliance on a narrow conception of the exercise of personal autonomy—one that excludes social relationships, by focus on consent as the articulation of a "legal" contract rather than an ongoing process of communication, and by lack of attention to disparities in knowledge and power between professionals and laypeople (Kaufert and O'Neill 1990; Barnes et al. 1998). Nearly twenty years ago, Pamela Sankar (1996) demonstrated the critical value of classic observational methods by examining the actual practice of informed consent to research participation. Her analysis reveals how the informed consent process shares many characteristics with ritual; actual reflection and active decision making are not part of the dynamic. Rather, research participants offered informed consent had already made up their minds to participate in the study; going through the process of "consenting" served primarily to inaugurate the subjects' participation in the research. Marshall and colleagues (2012) analyzed audio-recordings of informed consent discussions for Phase I pediatric oncology clinical trials. They describe a process of negotiated consent in which discussion between the health care team and the parents of the children used persuasive language to argue for or against participation in the study and to control various aspects of the study treatment and timing.

CROSS-CULTURAL AND INTERNATIONAL CONCERNS

Medical interactions, including discussions of consent, are mediated by language and cultural beliefs about health practices, decisional authority, and professional roles (Marshall 2006). These interactions are complex in any environment; cross-national research projects present particular challenges. Christian Simon, Maghboeba Mosavel, and Debbie van Stade (2007), for example, describe the ethical challenges in designing locally relevant health research in a low-income South African urban community; although they had planned to conduct a study on social factors and the prevention and treatment of cervical cancer in teens, their community collaborators were much more concerned with local violence and issues associated with poverty.

In their study of informed consent to genetic epidemiological studies of hypertension in the United States and Nigeria, Marshall and colleagues (2006) highlight the impact of cultural context on the consent process. Marshall's (2001a) ethnographic work on gene-environment studies of chronic complex diseases in urban and rural Nigeria illustrates challenges in translating difficult scientific concepts in cross-cultural settings; the very idea of consent may be unknown in rural settings where participants are not literate and have little experience of research. Ideal notions of individual consent, as practiced in the United States or other resource-rich countries, do not easily incorporate the significance of family and community relationships for the process of obtaining consent in diverse social environments around the world. In their work on community involvement in genetic research, Richard Sharp and Morris Foster (2000) outline potential strategies for representing the views of the larger community, suggesting that this may be an important component of the overall process of seeking and obtaining consent. Community consultation does not override an individual subject's right to decline or accept participation and may serve to make individual consent more authentic. When working with international research teams, the role of the anthropologist is not simply to facilitate a particular study through in-depth knowledge of the local community but also to tailor the broad objectives of informed consent to fit local needs (Rotimi and Marshall 2010).

CULTURE, MORALITY, AND THE PROBLEM OF RELATIVISM

The landscape of bioethics—in particular the "bedside" practices of clinical ethics and research procedures—is informed by the intellectual and ideological orientations of the analytic philosophers who were key figures in shaping the development of the field. Much work in bioethics reinforces and sustains an Enlightenment preoccupation with the primacy of the individual, "rational" "man." Although theoretically it need not, the field's emphasis on rational decision making and individual autonomy often diminishes the importance of the social realm in ethical analysis. Culture, like emotion, may be viewed as something tangential to the core human, something that might be stripped away to reveal a rational "universal" being underneath. And many bioethics procedures seem designed with that "rational man" in mind. Once practices such as advance care planning or informed consent are enshrined in law and regulation, it becomes increasingly difficult to tailor those procedures to fit local conditions, even though exactly that sort of tailoring may be required to fully observe an ethical principle such as respect for persons. This silencing of culture is confusing to most anthropologists, whereas the anthropologists' "failure" to appreciate the preeminence of universal ethical norms may lead philosophers to the false conclusion that all anthropologists are naïve relativists.

Identifying, defining, and evaluating the nature of morality has been difficult to achieve as a common area of inquiry for bioethicists and anthropologists. Although there is general agreement among the disciplines that the forms and practices of morality are inherently social, the consensus ends there. As Barry Hoffmaster observes, "According to the prevailing positivist approach in Anglo-American philosophy, morality consists of rules and principles, which because they are *normative*, can be articulated and defended only on the basis of rational arguments directed at what *ought* to be the case" (1990, 242). The potential for a meaningful dialogue with anthropologists and other empirical social scientists—who, according to the tenets of moral philosophy, work only at the level of "descriptive" ethics—is thwarted given the normative and metaethical focus of moral philosophy.

Anthropologists and philosophers have approached morality and cultural pluralism from two distinct perspectives. The unique morality expressed in diverse cultural traditions is emphasized in the "cultural relativism" of anthropology. Thus, for anthropologists, morality is viewed as an entity, like other dimensions of culture, that can be empirically described (Hatch 1983; Geertz 1989). It is found in social space, not argued in textbooks. Anthropologists have engaged in prolonged debates about the theoretical and methodological utility of relativism as it relates to cultural context (Herskovits 1972; Hatch 1983; Spiro 1986; Renteln 1988; Fabrega 1990; Shweder 1990).

Indeed, relativism has been foundational in the development of anthropology. The claims of a "moderate" descriptive relativism might be stated as follows: "Because all standards are culturally constituted, there are no available transcultural standards by which different cultures might be judged on a scale of merit or worth" (Spiro 1986, 260). Thus, the only normative judgment that might be possible is one that recognizes the equal worth of moral standards (and this holds for total cultures, single cultural systems such as religion, and specific cultural propositions). A normative claim based on this view is that because universally acceptable evaluative standards do not exist, judgments about cognition, behavior patterns, and emotions of different social groups must be relative to the variable standards of the cultures that produce them (e.g., all logic is ethno-logic or socio-logic). Epistemological relativism, the strongest form of descriptive relativism, is distinguished by its emphasis on the particularist theory of cultural determinism, which holds that because cultures are radically different from each other, each culture produces a unique and culturally particular set of human characteristics (Rosaldo 1993). Epistemological relativism implies the basic incommensurability of moral standards across cultures since panhuman generalizations concerning culture are likely to be untrue; generalizations can be true only if confined to a specific group (Geertz 1973).

The suggestion that it may be impossible to evaluate a moral system because it will always be relative to specific social traditions and historical contingencies is problematic for many philosophers and bioethicists (Tao 2002). From the philosopher's vantage point, the sacredness and primacy of the moral sphere may be threatened by empirical descriptions of cultural variation regarding moral practices. At the heart of this debate is the presumed dichotomy of fact and value. As philosophers have asked: How can an empirical description of what "is" influence the formulation of statements about what "ought" to be? In *Against Relativism,* Ruth Macklin expresses the dominant position within Anglo-American philosophy: "There is no denying that different cultures and historical eras exhibit a variety of moral beliefs and practices. The empirical facts revealed by anthropological research yield the descriptive thesis known as *cultural relativity.* But even if we grant that cultural relativity is an accurate description of the world's diversity, whether anything follows for normative ethics is an entirely different question. Do the facts of cultural relativity compel the conclusion that what is right or wrong can be determined only by the beliefs and practices within a particular culture or subculture?" (Macklin 1999, 4).

Macklin's (1998, 1999) argument for a strong version of antirelativism is based on her adherence to the idea that certain ethical principles are applicable cross-culturally. Macklin does allow that some bioethical practices might need to be compromised in culturally diverse settings. In traditional Navajo society words have enormous symbolic power; thus speaking openly about a poor prognosis is thought to actually bring on death, causing enormous difficulty for clinicians taught to disclose the truth while engaging in advance care planning or explaining the risks of clinical research (Carrese and Rhodes 1995). In her consideration of a clinical compromise about how much information to disclose, a compromise designed to respect Navajo beliefs about the avoidance of discussing negative topics, Macklin (1999, 264) concedes that "a degree of ethical relativism is undeniably present in the less-than-ideal version of informed consent, and it does admittedly constitute a 'lower' standard than that which is usually appropriate in today's medical practice." Although she acknowledges that in some cases it is appropriate to consider cultural difference in the application of ethical standards, Macklin justifies this not by recognizing that morality is culturally embedded, but instead by noting that "flexibility" (in applying ethical rules) is "consistent with adherence to more fundamental ethical principles" (1999, 264).

A fear of unbridled relativism may underlie the deep-seated ambivalence some bioethicists express when weighing the impact of cultural difference on beliefs about the moral. Rorty speaks directly to this concern, "Critics of moral relativism think that unless there is something absolute, something which shares God's implacable refusal to yield to human weakness, we have no reason to go on resisting evil" (Rorty 1999, xxxi). The cultural relativism practiced by most anthropologists, however, is first and foremost a methodological position, a claim that each culture must be approached and judged initially on its own terms. The anthropologist makes every effort not to prejudge practices that are unfamiliar. Note that this methodological stance does not preclude eventual evaluation and judgment.

RELATIVISM, SOCIAL JUSTICE, AND HUMAN RIGHTS

There is an inherent tension between the universalizing discourse of bioethics and the historical celebration of cultural relativism among anthropologists. These two approaches to understanding moral practices in relation to social justice and human rights appear to be antithetical, at least in their most extreme formulations. However, scholars in anthropology and bioethics have begun to explore, once again, the possibility of identifying transcultural or universal dimensions of the social behaviors of human groups. For example, in his attempt to develop a qualified version of ethical relativism, Richard Shweder (1990) identified aspects of moral behavior that are universal and culturally prescribed. Profound differences may exist between the moral codes of different people, but according to Shweder, there is more than one moral code that can be rationally defended. Universal dimensions of morality—justice and fairness, for example—are relatively expressed through discretionary variables such as who is designated as the moral agent, or what behavior and beliefs are judged to be morally relevant.

Alison Renteln (1988) characterizes relativism as a metaethical theory about the nature of moral perceptions. Renteln suggests that relativism is compatible with cross-cultural universals, which could indicate support for particular human rights. It is precisely in the arena of human rights that anthropologists and bioethicists share a common concern for fundamental abuses inflicted on individuals and communities. What is especially troubling for proponents of human rights agendas is the reliance on relativism to justify social and political practices that condone and perpetuate the systematic oppression of individuals and groups based on their gender, ethnicity, religion, or political affiliation. Macklin's (1999) treatise *Against Relativism* provides a good example of the philosophical arguments against a strong form of ethical relativism. Macklin repeatedly calls attention to the dangers of moving from empirical claims about cultural variability to moral justifications in the normative sphere. Robert Baker (1998) offers a model for negotiating value differences relevant to science and health in a multicultural world. In his discussion of bioethics and notions of the "common good" as a foundation for international human rights, David Thomasma (1997) brings us closer to a conception of human rights that acknowledges fundamental human values and, simultaneously, the importance of local context and cultural difference.

Anthropologists studying human rights abuses and structural inequalities clearly differentiate between the documentation of cultural patterns and normative judgments about them. Scheper-Hughes's (2006) work on the global trade in human organs, for example, strongly condemns the organ trade and the dehumanizing practices surrounding it. A culturally informed bioethics must take into account the impact of globalization on social justice, human rights, and public health disparities internationally (Kleinman, Das, and Lock 1997; Das 1999). The anthropologist and physician Paul Farmer, who has addressed a broad range of human rights issues in international health, is especially critical when the "culture argument" is employed to rationalize, excuse, or vindicate suffering and structural violence: "Concepts of cultural relativism, and even arguments to reinstate the dignity of different cultures and 'races,' have been easily assimilated by some of the very agencies that perpetuate extreme suffering. Abuses of cultural concepts are particularly insidious in discussions of suffering in general and of human rights more specifically: cultural difference is one of several forms of essentialism used to explain away assaults on dignity and suffering" (Farmer 1997, 278).

Anthropologists working in bioethics are deeply concerned about global health disparities, including class-based inequities in the United States (Levin and Schiller 1998; Levin and Fleischman 2002). Farmer (2003) levels a harsh critique against the narrow focus of bioethics, arguing strongly for greater attention to structural inequities that maintain health disparities in many areas of the world. The need for broadening the boundaries of bioethics to include the political economy of social suffering is recognized by anthropologists engaged in discussions of global medical morality (Kleinman, Das, and Lock 1997; Das 1999; Kleinman, Fox, and Brandt 1999; Castro and Singer 2004; Farmer 2006; Rylko-Bauer, Whiteford, and Farmer 2009; Alsan et al. 2011; Kim, Farmer, and Porter 2013).

CONCLUSION: THE ROLE OF ANTHROPOLOGY

What, ultimately, will anthropology contribute to the field of bioethics, an increasingly important domain of inquiry in national and international discourses about culture, morality, and health? Whether the question is appropriate care for the dying, the donation and transplantation of human organs, the evaluation of new medical technologies, informed consent in scientific research, or national and international health disparities, the anthropological contribution will be to create carefully researched accounts of how the moral good is located in particular local worlds. Ethnographic methodologies make possible such accounts. Ethnography provides the tools for a robust description of the social dynamics of ordinary moral experience. The application of ethnography in bioethics promises to counter the prevailing policy discourse controlled by economics, decision analysis, and legal procedures, a discourse that often silences social suffering while at the same time providing the illusion of control to individuals (Kleinman 1999, 89).

The paradox of relativism cannot be resolved. Instead, the work of medical anthropologists will enhance our understanding of the moral rendering and interpretation of health practices, scientific discovery, and the various uses and abuses of power in global biomedicine. A single set of universal principles or procedures will be inadequate. Bioethical approaches dominated by a simplistic application of respect for individual autonomy will fail not only in societies with a more nuanced view of the socially embedded nature of personhood, but in the West as well. In health care practice and in scientific research, procedures based on respectful negotiation among competing claims—measures informed by moral pragmatism—are most likely to avoid harm and contribute to the common good. Medical anthropologists have a vital role to play in furthering our understanding of the cultural construction of bioethics practices and their applications throughout the world.

SEE ALSO *Autonomy; Beneficence; Biocentrism vs. Anthropocentrism; Body; Circumcision, Female; Confidentiality; Death; Eugenics; Health and Disease: I. History of the Concepts; Human Nature; Informed Consent: I. History of Informed Consent; Medicine, Anthropology of; Mental Health, Meaning of Mental Health; Mental Illness: I. Definition, Use and Meaning; Population Ethics: I. History of Population Theories*

BIBLIOGRAPHY

Alsan, Marcella M.; Michael Westerhaus; Michael Herce; et al. 2011. "Poverty, Global Health, and Infectious Disease: Lessons from Haiti and Rwanda." *Infectious Disease Clinics of North America* 25 (3): 611–22.

Baker, Robert. 1998. "A Theory of International Bioethics: The Negotiable and the Non-negotiable." *Kennedy Institute of Ethics Journal* 8 (3): 233–73.

Barnes, Donelle; Anne J. Davis; Tracy Moran; et al. 1998. "Informed Consent in a Multicultural Cancer Patient Population: Implications for Nursing Practice." *Nursing Ethics* 5 (5): 412–23.

Becker, Gay. 2000. *The Elusive Embryo: How Women and Men Approach New Reproductive Technologies.* Berkeley: University of California Press.

Brodwin, Paul E., ed. 2000. *Biotechnology and Culture: Bodies, Anxieties, Ethics.* Bloomington: Indiana University Press.

Brodwin, Paul. 2002. "Genetics, Identity, and the Anthropology of Essentialism." *Anthropological Quarterly* 75 (2): 323–30.

Carrese, Joseph A., and Lorna A. Rhodes. 1995. "Western Bioethics on the Navajo Reservation." *Journal of the American Medical Association* 274 (10): 826–29.

Castro, Arachu, and Merrill Singer, eds. 2004. *Unhealthy Health Policy: A Critical Anthropological Examination.* Walnut Creek, CA: AltaMira Press.

Caulfield, Timothy; Stephanie M. Fullerton; et al. 2009. "Race and Ancestry in Biomedical Research: Exploring the Challenges." *Genome Medicine* 1 (1): 8.

Chilibeck, Gillian; Margaret Lock; and Megha Sehdev. 2011. "Postgenomics, Uncertain Futures, and the Familiarization of Susceptibility Genes." *Social Science and Medicine* 72 (11): 1768–75.

Cohen, Lawrence. 1999. "Where It Hurts: Indian Material for an Ethics of Organ Transplantation." *Daedalus* 128 (4): 135–65.

Crawley, LaVera M.; Patricia A. Marshall; Bernard Lo; et al. 2002. "Strategies for Culturally Effective End-of-Life Care." *Annals of Internal Medicine* 136 (9): 673–79.

Crigger, Bette-Jane. 1995. "Negotiating the Moral Order: Paradoxes of Ethics Consultation." *Kennedy Institute of Ethics Journal* 5 (2): 89–112.

Das, Veena. 1999. "Public Good, Ethics, and Everyday Life: Beyond the Boundaries of Bioethics." *Daedalus* 128 (4): 99–133.

De Vries, Raymond, and Janardan Subedi, eds. 1998. *Bioethics and Society: Constructing the Ethical Enterprise.* Upper Saddle River, NJ: Prentice Hall.

De Vries, Raymond; Leigh Turner; Kristina Orfali; and Charles Bosk. 2007. The *View from Here: Bioethics and the Social Sciences.* New York: Wiley.

Drought, Theresa S., and Barbara A. Koenig. 2002. "'Choice' in End-of-Life Decision Making: Researching Fact or Fiction?" *Gerontologist* 42 (Suppl. 3): 114–28.

Edel, May, and Abraham Edel. 1968. *Anthropology and Ethics: The Quest for Moral Understanding.* Cleveland, OH: Press of Case Western Reserve University.

Evans, John H. 2012. *The History and Future of Bioethics: A Sociological View.* New York: Oxford University Press.

Fabrega, Horatio, Jr. 1990. "An Ethnomedical Perspective of Medical Ethics." *Journal of Medicine and Philosophy* 15 (6): 593–625.

Farmer, Paul. 1997. "On Suffering and Social Violence: A View from Below." In *Social Suffering*, edited by Arthur Kleinman, Veena Das, and Margaret Lock, 261–84. Berkeley: University of California Press.

Farmer, Paul. 2003. *Pathologies of Power: Health, Human Rights, and the New War on the Poor.* Berkeley: University of California Press.

Farmer, Paul. 2006. *The Uses of Haiti.* Berkeley: University of California Press.

Finkler, Kaja. 2000. *Experiencing the New Genetics: Family and Kinship on the Medical Frontier.* Philadelphia: University of Pennsylvania Press.

Fox, Renée C. 1990. "The Evolution of American Bioethics: A Sociological Perspective." In *Social Science Perspectives on Medical Ethics*, edited by George Weisz, 201–17. Dordrecht: Kluwer Academic.

Fox, Renée C., and Judith P. Swazey. 2008. *Observing Bioethics.* New York: Oxford University Press.

Frank, Geyla; Leslie J. Blackhall; Vicki Michel; et al. 1998. "A Discourse of Relationships in Bioethics: Patient Autonomy and End-of-Life Decision Making among Elderly Korean Americans." *Medical Anthropology Quarterly* 12 (4): 403–23.

Gaines, Atwood D. 1998. "Culture and Values at the Intersection of Science and Suffering: Encountering Ethics, Genetics, and Alzheimer Disease." In *Genetic Testing for Alzheimer Disease: Ethical and Clinical Issues*, edited by Stephen Garrard Post and Peter Whitehouse, 256–74. Baltimore, MD: Johns Hopkins University Press.

Geertz, Clifford. 1973. *The Interpretation of Cultures: Selected Essays.* New York: Basic Books.

Geertz, Clifford. 1989. "Anti Anti-Relativism." In *Relativism: Interpretation and Confrontation*, edited by Michael Krausz, 12–34. Notre Dame, IN: Notre Dame University Press.

Ginsburg, Faye D., and Rayna Rapp, eds. 1995. *Conceiving the New World Order: The Global Politics of Reproduction.* Berkeley: University of California Press.

Goodman, Alan H.; Deborah Heath; and M. Susan Lindee, eds. 2003. *Genetic Nature/Culture: Anthropology and Science beyond the Two-Culture Divide.* Berkeley: University of California Press.

Gordon, Deborah R., and Eugenio Paci. 1997. "Disclosure Practices and Cultural Narratives: Understanding Concealment and Silence around Cancer in Tuscany, Italy." *Social Science and Medicine* 4 (10): 1433–52.

Gordon, Elisa J. 2001. "'They Don't Have to Suffer for Me': Why Dialysis Patients Refuse Offers of Living Donor Kidneys." *Medical Anthropology Quarterly* 15 (2): 245–67.

Gordon, Elisa J. 2013. "Ethical Considerations in Live Donor Transplantation: Should Complications Be Tolerated?" *Current Opinion in Organ Transplantation* 18 (2): 235–40.

Gordon, Elisa J.; Amna Daud; Juan Carlos Caicedo; et al. 2011. "Informed Consent and Decision-Making about Adult-to-Adult Living Donor Liver Translantation: A Systematic Review of Empirical Research." *Transplantation* 92 (12): 1285–96.

Gordon, Elisa J., and Chris Daugherty. 2003. "'Hitting You Over the Head': Oncologists' Disclosure of Prognosis to Advanced Cancer Patients." *Bioethics* 17 (2): 142–68.

Hamdy, Sherine. 2012. *Our Bodies Belong to God: Organ Transplants, Islam, and the Struggle for Human Dignity in Egypt.* Berkeley: University of California Press.

Hatch, Elvin. 1983. *Culture and Morality: The Relativity of Values in Anthropology.* New York: Columbia University Press.

Herskovits, Melville. 1972. *Cultural Relativism: Perspectives in Cultural Pluralism.* Edited by Frances Herskovits. New York: Random House.

Hoffmaster, Barry. 1990. "Morality and the Social Sciences." In *Social Science Perspectives on Medical Ethics*, edited by George Weisz, 241–60. Dordrecht: Kluwer Academic.

Hoffmaster, Barry, ed. 2001. *Bioethics in Social Context.* Philadelphia: Temple University Press.

Hogle, Linda F. 1999. *Recovering the Nation's Body: Cultural Memory, Medicine, and the Politics of Redemption.* New Brunswick, NJ: Rutgers University Press.

Hunt, Linda M. 1998. "Moral Reasoning and the Meaning of Cancer: Causal Explanations of Oncologists and Patients in Southern Mexico." *Medical Anthropology Quarterly* 12 (3): 298–318.

Hurley, Ann C.; Rose Harvey; J. Scott Roberts; et al. 2005. "Genetic Susceptibility for Alzheimer's Disease: Why Did Adult Offspring Seek Testing?" *American Journal of Alzheimer's Disease and Other Dementias* 20 (6): 374–81.

Ikels, Charlotte. 1997. "Kidney Failure and Transplantation in China." *Social Science and Medicine* 44 (9): 1271–83.

Joralemon, Donald. 2001. "Shifting Ethics: Debating the Incentive Question in Organ Transplantation." *Journal of Medical Ethics* 27 (1): 30–35.

Kaufert, Joseph. 1999. "Cultural Mediation in Cancer Diagnosis and End of Life Decision-Making: The Experience of Aboriginal Patients in Canada." *Anthropology and Medicine* 6 (3): 405–21.

Kaufert, Joseph M., and John D. O'Neil. 1990. "Biomedical Rituals and Informed Consent: Native Canadians and the Negotiation of Clinical Trust." In *Social Science Perspectives on Medical Ethics*, edited by George Weisz, 41–63. Dordrecht: Kluwer Academic.

Kaufert, Joseph M., and Robert W. Putsch. 1997. "Communication through Interpreters in Health Care: Ethical Dilemmas arising from Differences in Class, Culture, Language, and Power." *Journal of Clinical Ethics* 8 (1): 71–87.

Kaufman, Sharon R. 1998. "Intensive Care, Old Age, and the Problem of Death in America." *Gerontologist* 38 (6): 715–25.

Kaufman, Sharon R. 2000. "In the Shadow of 'Death with Dignity': Medicine and Cultural Quandaries of the Vegetative State." *American Anthropologist* 102 (1): 69–83.

Kelly, Susan E.; Patricia A. Marshall; Lee M. Sanders; et al. 1997. "Understanding the Practice of Ethics Consultation: Results of an Ethnographic Multi-Site Study." *Journal of Clinical Ethics* 8 (2): 136–49.

Kim, James Y.; Paul Farmer; and Michael E. Porter. 2013. "Redefining Global Health-Care Delivery." *Lancet*, May 17. [Epub ahead of print.]

Kleinman, Arthur. 1995. "Anthropology of Bioethics." In *Encyclopedia of Bioethics*, edited by William Reich. New York: Macmillan.

Kleinman, Arthur. 1999. "Moral Experience and Ethical Reflection: Can Ethnography Reconcile Them? A Quandary for 'The New Bioethics.'" *Daedalus* 128 (4): 69–97.

Kleinman, Arthur; Veena Das; and Margaret Lock. 1997. *Social Suffering.* Berkeley: University of California Press.

Kleinman, Arthur; Renée C. Fox; and Allan M. Brandt, guest eds. 1999. *Daedalus: Bioethics and Beyond* 128 (4). Cambridge, MA: American Academy of Arts and Sciences.

Koenig, Barbara A. 1988. "The Technological Imperative in Medical Practice: The Social Creation of a 'Routine' Treatment." In *Biomedicine Examined*, edited by Margaret Lock and Deborah R. Gordon, 465–96. Boston: Kluwer.

Koenig, Barbara A. 1996. "The Power (and Limits) of Proximity." *Hastings Center Report* 26 (6): 30–32.

Koenig, Barbara A. 1997. "Cultural Diversity in Decision-Making about Care at the End-of-Life." In *Approaching Death: Improving Care at the End of Life*, edited by Marilyn J. Field and Christine K. Cassel, 363–82. Washington, DC: National Academy of Sciences.

Koenig, Barbara A., and Betty Davies. 2003. "Cultural Dimensions of Care at Life's End for Children and Their Families." In *When Children Die: Improving Palliative and End-of-Life Care for Children and Their Families*, edited by Marilyn J. Field and Richard E. Behrman, 509–52. Washington, DC: National Academy of Sciences. http://books.nap.edu/html/children_die/AppD.pdf

Koenig, Barbara, and Jan Gates-Williams. 1995. "Understanding Cultural Differences in Caring for Dying Patients." *Western Journal of Medicine* 163 (3): 244–49.

Kundstadter, Peter. 1980. "Medical Ethics in Cross-Cultural and Multi-Cultural Perspective." *Social Science and Medicine* 14B (4): 289–96.

Lee, Sandra S. J.; Joanna Mountain; and Barbara A. Koenig. 2001. "The Meanings of 'Race' in the New Genomics: Implications for Health Disparities Research." *Yale Journal of Health Policy, Law, and Ethics* 1 (1): 33–75.

Lee, Sandra Soo-Jin; Joanna Mountain; et al. 2008. "The Ethics of Characterizing Difference: Guiding Principles on Using Racial Categories in Human Genetics." *Genome Biology* 9 (7): 404.

Levin, Betty W., and Alan R. Fleischman. 2002. "Public Health and Bioethics: The Benefits of Collaboration." *American Journal of Public Health* 92 (2): 165–67.

Levin, Betty W., and Nina G. Schiller. 1998. "Social Class and Medical Decisionmaking: A Neglected Topic in Bioethics." *Cambridge Quarterly of Healthcare Ethics* 7 (1): 41–56.

Lieban, Richard W. 1990. "Medical Anthropology and the Comparative Study of Medical Ethics." In *Social Science Perspectives on Medical Ethics*, edited by George Weisz, 221–39. Dordrecht: Kluwer Academic.

Lock, Margaret. 2002. *Twice Dead: Organ Transplants and the Reinvention of Death.* Berkeley: University of California Press.

Lock, Margaret. 2013a. "The Epigenome and Nature/Nurture Reunification: A Challenge for Anthropology." *Medical Anthropology* 32 (4): 291–308.

Lock, Margaret. 2013b. "The Lure of the Epigenome." *Lancet* 381 (9881): 1896–97.

Lock, Margaret; Susan Cox; et al. 2006. "Social, Political, and Epistemological Aspects of Genetics and Genomics." *Community Genetics* 9 (3): 137–41.

Lock, Margaret, and Megan Crowley-Makota. 2008. "Situating the Practice of Organ Donation in Familial, Cultural, and Political Context." *Transplantation Reviews* 22 (3): 154–57.

Lock, Margaret; Julia Freeman; et al. 2007. "Susceptibility Genes and the Question of Embodied Identity." *Medical Anthropology Quarterly* 21 (3): 256–76.

Lock, Margaret, and Christina Honde. 1990. "Reaching Consensus about Death: Heart Transplants and Cultural Identity in Japan." In *Social Science Perspectives on Medical Ethics*, edited by George Weisz, 99–119. Dordrecht: Kluwer Academic.

Lock, Margaret, and Vinh-Kim Nguyen. 2010. *An Anthropology of Biomedicine.* Malden, MA: Wiley-Blackwell.

Lock, Margaret; Alan Young; and Alberto Cambrosio, eds. 2000. *Living and Working with the New Medical Technologies: Intersections of Inquiry.* New York: Cambridge University Press.

Long, Susan O. 1999. "Family Surrogacy and Cancer Disclosure: Physician-Family Negotiation of an Ethical Dilemma in Japan." *Journal of Palliative Care* 15 (3): 31–42.

Long, Susan O. 2000. "Living Poorly or Dying Well: Decisions about Life-Supporting Treatment for American and Japanese Patients." *Journal of Clinical Ethics* 11 (3): 236–50.

Macklin, Ruth. 1998. "Ethical Relativism in a Multicultural Society." *Kennedy Institute of Ethics Journal* 8 (1): 1–22.

Macklin, Ruth. 1999. *Against Relativism: Cultural Diversity and the Search for Ethical Universals in Medicine.* New York: Oxford University Press.

Marshall, Patricia A. 1992. "Anthropology and Bioethics." *Medical Anthropology Quarterly* 6 (1): 49–73.

Marshall, Patricia A. 2001a. "A Contextual Approach to Clinical Ethics Consultation." In *Bioethics in Social Context*, edited by Barry Hoffmaster, 137–52. Philadelphia: Temple University Press.

Marshall, Patricia A. 2001b. "Informed Consent in International Health Research." In *Biomedical Research Ethics: Updating International Guidelines: A Consultation*, edited by Robert Levine. Samuel Gorovitz. and John Gallagher, 101–34. Geneva: Council for International Organization of Medical Sciences, World Health Organization.

Marshall, Patricia. 2006. "Informed Consent in International Health Research." *Journal of Empirical Research on Human-Research Ethics* 1 (1): 25–42.

Marshall, Patricia A.; Clement A. Adebamowo; Adebowale A. Adeyemo; et al. 2006. "Voluntary Participation and Informed Consent to International Genetic Research." *American Journal of Public Health* 96 (11): 1989–95.

Marshall, Patricia A., and Abdallah Daar. 2000. "Ethical Issues in Human Organ Replacement: A Case Study from India." In *Global Health Policy, Local Realities: The Fallacy of the Level Playing Field*, edited by Linda M. Whiteford and Lenore Manderson, 205–30. Boulder, CO: Lynne Rienner Publishers.

Marshall, Patricia A., and Barbara A. Koenig. 1996. "Anthropology and Bioethics: Perspectives on Culture, Medicine and Morality." In *Medical Anthropology: Contemporary Theory and Method*, 2nd ed., edited by Carolyn Sargent and Thomas Johnson, 349–72. Westport, CT: Praeger.

Marshall, Patricia A., and Barbara A. Koenig. 2000. "Bioethiques et anthropologie: Situer le 'bien' dans la pratique medicale [Intersection of Bioethics and Anthropology: Locating the "Good" in Medical Practices]." *Anthropologie et Sociétés* 24 (2): 35–55.

Marshall, Patricia A., and Barbara Koenig. 2004. "Accounting for Culture in a Globalized Bioethics." *Journal of Law, Medicine and Ethics* 32 (2): 252–66.

Marshall, Patricia A., and Barbara A. Koenig. 2010. "Ethnographic Methods." In *Methods in Medical Ethics*, 2nd ed., edited by Jeremy Sugarman and Daniel P. Sulmasy, 215–32. Washington, DC: Georgetown University Press.

Marshall, Patricia A.; Barbara A. Koenig; Paul Grifhorst; and Mirjam van Ewijk. 1998. "Ethical Issues in Immigrant Health Care and Clinical Research." In *Handbook of Immigrant Health*, edited by Sana Loue, 203–26. New York: Plenum Press.

Marshall, Patricia A.; Ruth V. Magtanong; Angela C. Leek; et al., eds. 2012. "Negotiating Informed Consent in Pediatric Phase I Oncology Trials." *Journal of Empirical Research on Human Research Ethics* 7 (2): 51–59.

Muller, Jessica H. 1994. "Anthropology, Bioethics, and Medicine: A Provocative Trilogy." *Medical Anthropology Quarterly* 8 (4): 448–67.

Muller, Jessica H., and Brian Desmond. 1992. "Ethical Dilemmas in a Cross-Cultural Context: A Chinese Example." *Western Journal of Medicine* 157 (3): 323–27.

Ohnuki-Tierney, Emiko. 1994. "Brain Death and Organ Transplantation: Cultural Bases of Medical Technology." *Current Anthropology* 35 (3): 233–54.

O'Neill, Onora. 2002. *Autonomy and Trust in Bioethics.* Cambridge: Cambridge University Press.

Orona, Cecelia J.; Barbara A. Koenig; and Anne J. Davis. 1994. "Cultural Aspects of Nondisclosure." *Cambridge Quarterly of Healthcare Ethics* 3 (3): 338–46.

Orr, Robert; Patricia A. Marshall; and Jamie Osborn. 1995. "Cross-Cultural Considerations in Clinical Ethics Consultations." *Archives of Family Medicine* 4:159–64.

Press, Nancy, and Carol H. Browner. 1998. "Characteristics of Women Who Refuse an Offer of Prenatal Diagnosis: Data from the California Maternal Serum Alpha Fetoprotein Blood Test Experience." *American Journal of Medical Genetics* 78 (5): 433–45.

Press, Nancy; Jennifer R. Fishman; and Barbara A. Koenig. 2000. "Collective Fear, Individualized Risk: The Social and Cultural Context of Genetic Testing for Breast Cancer." *Nursing Ethics* 7 (3): 237–49.

Rapp, Rayna. 2000. *Testing Women, Testing the Fetus: The Social Impact of Amniocentesis in America.* New York: Routledge.

Renteln, Alison D. 1988. "Relativism and the Search for Human Rights." *American Anthropologist* 90 (1): 56–72.

Roberts, Elizabeth F. S. 2012. *God's Laboratory: Assisted Reproduction in the Andes*. Berkeley: University of California Press.

Rorty, Richard. 1999. "Introduction: Relativism: Finding and Making." In *Philosophy and Social Hope*, edited by Richard Rorty, xvi–xxxii. New York: Penguin.

Rosaldo, Renato. 1993. *Culture and Truth: The Remaking of Social Analysis*. Boston: Beacon Press.

Rotimi, Charles N., and Patricia A. Marshall. 2010. "Tailoring the Process of Informed Consent in Genetic and Genomic Research." *Genome Medicine* 2 (3): 20.

Rylko-Bauer, Barbara; Linda Whiteford; and Paul Farmer. 2009. *Global Health in Times of Violence*. Santa Fe, NM: School for Advanced Research Press.

Sankar, Pamela. 1996. "Informed Consent: (W)rituals of Medical Research." Paper presented at the American Anthropological Association Annual Meeting, San Francisco, CA.

Sankar, Pamela, and Mildred K. Cho. 2002. "Toward a New Vocabulary of Human Genetic Variation." *Science* 298 (5597): 1337–38.

Scheper-Hughes, Nancy. 2000. "The Global Traffic in Human Organs." *Current Anthropology* 41 (2): 191–224.

Scheper-Hughes, Nancy. 2006. "The Tyranny of the Gift: Sacrificial Violence in Living Donor Transplants." *American Journal of Transplant (Ethics Corner)*, 7: 1–5.

Sharp, Lesley A. 1995. "Organ Transplantation as a Transformative Experience: Anthropological Insights into the Restructuring of the Self." *Medical Anthropological Quarterly* 9 (3): 357–89.

Sharp, Lesley A. 2001. "Commodified Kin: Death, Mourning, and Competing Claims on the Bodies of Organ Donors in the United States." *American Anthropologist* 103 (1): 112–33.

Sharp, Lesley A. 2006. *Strange Harvest: Organ Transplants, Denatured Bodies, and the Transformed Self*. Berkeley: University of California Press.

Sharp, Lesley A. 2013. *The Transplant Imaginary: Mechanical Hearts, Animal Parts, and Moral Thinking in Highly Experimental Science*. Berkeley: University of California Press.

Sharp, Richard R., and Morris W. Foster. 2000. "Involving Study Populations in the Review of Genetic Research." *Journal of Law, Medicine, and Ethics* 28 (1): 41–51.

Shweder, Richard A. 1990. "Ethical Relativism: Is There a Defensible Version?" *Ethos* 18 (2): 205–18.

Simon, Christian; Maghboeba Mosavel; and Debbie van Stade. 2007. "Ethical Challenges in the Design and Conduct of Locally Relevant International Health Research." *Social Science and Medicine* 64 (9): 1960–69.

Singer, Merrill. 2013. *Global Health: An Anthropological Perspective*. Long Grove, IL: Waveland Press.

Slomka, Jacqueline. 1992. "The Negotiation of Death: Clinical Decision Making at the End of Life." *Social Science and Medicine* 35 (3): 251–59.

Spiro, Melford E. 1986. "Cultural Relativism and the Future of Anthropology." *Cultural Anthropology* 1 (3): 259–86.

Tao, Julia Lai Po-Wah, ed. 2002. *Cross-Cultural Perspectives on the (Im)Possibility of Global Bioethics*. Dordrecht: Kluwer Academic.

Thomasma, David C. 1997. "Bioethics and International Human Rights." *Journal of Law, Medicine and Ethics* 25 (4): 295–306.

Turner, Leigh. 2005. "From the Local to the Global: Bioethics and the Concept of Culture." *Journal of Medicine and Philosophy* 30 (3): 305–20.

Turner, Leigh. 2009. "Anthropological and Sociological Critiques of Bioethics." *Bioethical Inquiry* 6 (1): 83–98.

Weisz, George, ed. 1990. *Social Science Perspectives on Medical Ethics*. Dordrecht: Kluwer Academic.

Patricia A. Marshall (2004, 2014)
Professor of Bioethics and Anthropology, Department of Bioethics, Case Western Reserve University

Barbara A. Koenig (2004)
Professor of Medical Anthropology and Bioethics, Department of Social and Behavioral Sciences, University of California, San Francisco

X. POLITICS OF

As biomedical and biotechnological sciences have advanced in the late twentieth and early twenty-first centuries, questions about what is moral have become part and parcel of questions about what is legal, socially acceptable, and just. Similarly, complex bioethical considerations stand in the background of political questions of whether or not, how, and by whom new biotechnologies should be funded, regulated, and distributed. The resultant public discourse concerns the politics of reproductive technologies, genetics, end-of-life decisions, and new directions in health care. As developments emerge in these areas, traditional boundaries between the natural and the synthetic, life and death, and humans and nonhumans become less clear.

The politics of bioethics describes the ways scientists, physicians, organizations, governments, experts, lay publics, and other participants in the discourse deal with the maintenance of these boundaries and how they balance the approval of biotechnological change with deep-seated worries about precisely what such change might bring. Although the politics of bioethics is often organized around familiar political doctrines, bioethical questions transect the traditional Left-Right spectrum and create alliances of bioconservatives and bioprogressives from both the Right and the Left. Some people may appeal to religious values and insert them into political conversations about bioethics, but at the same time religious perspectives offer a variety of ways to understand and respond to the implications of new biotechnologies. Others may refer to personal and collective events and experiences to shape their political views in bioethics. While the questions presented by new biotechnologies are largely the same across industrialized countries, the nations' varying civic narratives lead them to different conclusions.

BIOETHICS AND BIOPOLITICS

Not only have biology and medicine played an increasingly large role in politics, but bioethical questions have also increasingly become biopolitical. These questions are significantly couched in the ways society attempts to gain control over the power of the life sciences, which are usually accompanied by ethical concerns. For example, the modern abortion controversy encompasses both biology in politics and the politics of biology (or biopolitics). In terms of biology in politics, participants in the abortion discourse organize themselves around pro-choice or pro-life principles. They also engage in biopolitics by attempting to manage the power behind the decision to continue or terminate a pregnancy (Moreno 2011).

Biopolitics was first comprehensively defined by the French philosopher and historian Michel Foucault (1926–1984). He argued that post-Enlightenment modernity is characterized by biopower exerted through the management of bodies and populations by the many institutions that comprise the fabric of society. While states once held power merely over life and death, the objects of governing in modernity are the ways of living, both private and public. The resultant "mentality of government" and the conflicts and negotiations that arise within governmentality constitute Foucault's biopolitics.

Less than two decades after Foucault's death, the world entered what may be called the "biological century"—one characterized by biotechnological advances in genetics, cell biology, and the medical sciences—all of which are new subjects of biopolitics. Biopolitics has moved on to concern control not only of bodies and populations but also of tissues, systems, and genetic information (Rabinow and Rose 2006; Moreno 2011). Conflicts of control over these entities and the technologies that moderate them reflect attempts to reconcile their use for the public good with the maintenance of societal values. Biopolitics therefore is inherently defined by tensions between innovation and tradition, the natural and the synthetic, life and death, and other entrenched values that both guide and bind social action. As people continue to use science to understand the world, new advancements push against these boundaries and make them harder to define. Traditional definitions of what is human and what is not may leave little room to designate the status of clones, hybrids, and chimeras. Similarly, traditional paradigms of life and death may be difficult to negotiate when life-preserving technologies create many possible ways to define what counts as alive and what counts as dead. In her 2005 book *Designs on Nature: Science and Democracy in Europe and the United States*, Sheila Jasanoff contended that a central task of policy making in the life sciences is to ensure that new boundaries for biological entities correspond to society's preexisting social and ethical sensibilities. An inescapable component of policy making and other areas of biopolitics is bioethics; negotiations of control over biotechnology inherently concern negotiations of what is ethical.

BEGINNINGS OF AMERICAN SCIENCE AND POLITICS

The history of science in the United States reflects many themes that are still apparent in the politics of biology: Enlightenment thinking; the relationship between science, progress, power, and prosperity; and the role of government in sponsoring technological innovation. Thomas Jefferson, Alexander Hamilton, Benjamin Franklin, George Washington, and many other Founding Fathers along with the Enlightenment philosophers who influenced them harbored a deep-seated appreciation of science and the experimental methodologies that arose in Enlightenment and post-Enlightenment science. In some cases, they engaged in scientific experimentation of their own, and Jefferson even described the project of establishing a nation in the New World as the "American experiment" (Moreno 2011). By combining these themes into a republican form of government that incorporated both democracy and a constitution, the founders created a nation committed to the pursuit and propagation of knowledge, including science.

Throughout most of the nineteenth century, biology was still largely observational, and most experimental work and technological advances were limited to chemistry, physics, and engineering. Obstacles to investments in science were mostly financial and political rather than moral. The American moral fabric, including its religious Protestant majority, was intellectually compatible with science and the technological innovations that characterized capitalism and the spirit of capturing new frontiers.

As the twentieth century loomed, the United States shifted toward Progressive Era politics. Progressive thought regarded government as an agent of both social and especially economic equality and progress. Evidence, inquiry, consultation with experts, and the belief that progress went hand in hand with moral improvement became important parts of the political process (Moreno 2011). The Progressive Era also ushered in the first and perhaps the most historically prominent instance of biopolitics of the United States: the eugenics movement. Popular throughout the early and mid-twentieth century, eugenic policies sought to manage the heredity and reproductive capabilities of American society (Moreno 2011).

Inspired by Charles Darwin's evolutionary theory, Mendelian genetics, and Herbert Spencer's concept of the "survival of the fittest," eugenicists suggested that criminality, sexual promiscuity, poverty, mental and physical disabilities, "feeblemindedness," and other perceived social ills were prominent, because they were heritable. The responses of eugenics to this took two forms: positive eugenics, which advocated breeding desirable people together to produce desirable offspring, and negative eugenics, which advocated preventing the reproductive capabilities of undesirable people. In the early twenty-first century eugenics is largely discredited as scientifically misguided and morally abhorrent. But in its heyday the scientific bases of eugenics were widely accepted and embraced by progressives as a tool to promote social progress by preventing the decline of the human race through more "scientific" breeding.

In 1914 Harry Laughlin of the Eugenics Record Office at Cold Spring Harbor Laboratory published a "model law" for eugenic sterilization that would ultimately become the basis of government-mandated sterilizations of the "feebleminded." Two prevailing justifications for the program were advanced. The first maintained that public health improvements had interfered with social systems of natural selection and enabled the continuation of parts of society who would not usually survive. The second maintained that the proliferation of these people should be stopped so as not to burden the state. A notable US Supreme Court challenge to the sterilization of a young girl named Carrie Buck, *Buck v. Bell* (1927), resulted in the Virginia sterilization law being upheld on the basis of these concerns.

American attitudes toward eugenics took an about-face after Nazi Germany, which modeled its eugenics policies partly after US sterilization programs, carried the idea to a genocidal extreme. Abuses in Nazi medicine also ushered in many themes that form a significant basis of the bioethical discourse of the present. In 1948 the Second General Assembly of the World Medical Association adopted the Declaration of Geneva, a code of conduct for physicians that embodies the promises outlined in the Hippocratic oath to "do no harm." During the Nuremberg trials (1945–1949), the Nuremberg code was developed to advise the prosecution of Nazi doctors. Its most prominent principle is that the conduct of experimentation and medical treatment requires the voluntary and uncoerced consent of human subjects. In 1964 the World Medical Association adopted the Nuremberg code into the Declaration of Helsinki. While these codes were originally created to protect patients and research subjects, their principles have been used in the late twentieth and early twenty-first centuries to determine the permissible limits of new developments and experimentation in the life sciences (Jasanoff 2005).

THE NEW BIOLOGY

The most cited reason for the emergence of the present biopolitics is the tense cultural politics of the late-twentieth-century United States, but an even more important contributor is the change in the nature of experimental biology and its related disciplines. The discovery of the structure of DNA by James D. Watson and Francis Crick in 1953 was followed in the 1970s by the development of genetic recombination techniques, which scientists use to synthesize chains of genes to create organisms from scratch or alter existing ones. Rather than merely another step in describing the world, the new biology has allowed scientists to physically change it as well. As a result, the late twentieth and early twenty-first centuries have been rife with biopolitical and bioethical questions raised by new developments in synthetic biology, genetics and genetic engineering, stem cell research, and the development of life-extending technologies.

GENETICALLY MODIFIED ORGANISMS AND SYNTHETIC BIOLOGY

The uses of genetically modified organisms are numerous and widespread, ranging from bacteria that can be genetically engineered to produce insulin to the creation of hardier or herbicide-resistant crops. The potentials of these organisms are enormous. They open new avenues in health care, and the possibility of creating more nutrient-rich or higher-yielding crops offers much to resource-poor countries and malnourished populations. At the same time genetically modified crops and foods have elicited societal concerns about unforeseen risks to human health and the environment, about human intervention in nature, and about the growing role of biotechnology corporations in the agriculture and food industries. Questions about whether genetically modified foods are safe for human consumption have underscored policy arguments about whether such foods should be regulated and labeled in supermarkets. Arguments about ethical obligations to the environment, whether they stem from a duty to preserve the earth for future generations or from a duty to care for nature for its own sake, arose for the first time—at least in the context of genetically modified plants—in 1999, when a study found that pollen from Bt corn plants, which are modified to be pesticide resistant, was harming monarch butterflies (Thompson and Hannah 2008).

While scientists have been genetically engineering organisms for some time, the possibility of assembling living organisms entirely from scratch has arisen only in the late twentieth and early twenty-first centuries. In 2010 the J. Craig Venter Institute, a US-based research institution that specializes in the emerging field of "synthetic biology," created the first self-replicating synthetic genome and successfully inserted it into the "shell" of a bacterium of a different species. Whether or not this development represents a major or a minor step in the young field of synthetic biology, concerns about synthesizing genomes date back to several years before this became a real technological possibility. One concern in particular involves the creation of a minimal genome—a genome reduced to only the genes necessary for replication and essential metabolic processes—which is another project being undertaken by the J. Craig Venter Institute. Minimal-genome bacteria could be useful in understanding bacterial evolution and bacterial metabolic processes and could also be deployed as useful starting templates for biological engineering. Yet the implications of intentionally or accidentally releasing synthetic organisms into the environment, concerns about intellectual property in the context of synthetic biology, and the possibility that synthetic biology could be used for nefarious purposes have raised questions about if and how this emerging field should be governed. While synthetic biology in general might strike cultural chords about interventions in nature, minimal genome research in particular evokes cultural and spiritual concerns about reductionist approaches to understanding the basis of life (Cho et al. 1999).

PROPERTY IN THE GENOME: MEDICINE AND AGRICULTURE

New advances in genetics have also raised concerns about property in the genome, highlighting tensions between progress, innovation, and laws written well before new biotechnologies were even imagined. In 1980 the US Supreme Court ruled in *Diamond v. Chakrabarty* that a patent for a genetically modified bacterium could be awarded, because it was considered human made, setting a precedent that allowed biological and eventually gene patents. By 2012 at least 25 percent of the human genome had been patented, as had several plant genes, bacteria, viruses, and plants—a reality that raises questions about the boundary between nature, which is not patentable, and human-made entities, which are patentable.

While patents are designed to encourage innovation by allowing innovators to reap the benefits of their products, numerous challenges to biological patents have arisen in the context of both medicine and agriculture. One notable challenge began in the US court system in 2009, when a group of medical organizations, physicians, and patients sued Myriad Genetics Inc. and the US Patent and Trademark Office. At issue were Myriad's patents on *BRCA1* and *BRCA2* genes, which can determine significant risk factors for breast cancer. Among the reasons for the lawsuit, the plaintiffs held that because Myriad's patents allowed the company to monopolize research and genetic testing for *BRCA1* and *BRCA2*, Myriad was the sole controller of the progress of *BRCA* research and effectively limited patient choice in genetic testing options. In 2010 a New York district court judge ruled that the patents were invalid, because they did not fit the criteria of patentable materials outlined by the US Patent Act of 1790, which permits patents for "any new and useful process, machine, manufacture, or composition of matter, or any new and useful improvement thereof." In 2011 an appeals court overturned the decision, but in March 2012 the US Supreme Court vacated the judgment and turned it back to the appeals court for reconsideration. In August 2012 the federal appeals court upheld patents on the genes but invalidated patents on the processes of comparing gene sequences. The following November the Supreme Court agreed to hear arguments on the patentability of human genes. In June 2013 the court ruled that isolated segments of naturally occurring DNA are not patentable because they are "products of nature," but that cDNA, which is synthesized to contain only the exons, or protein-coding portions, of natural DNA segments, is patentable because exons-only DNA is not naturally occurring.

The Canadian court system dealt with a biological patent case from 2000 to 2004, when Monsanto Canada Inc. (the Canadian division of the US agricultural biotechnology giant Monsanto Company) sued a Saskatchewan farmer, Percy Schmeiser, for infringing on the company's patent for a genetically modified herbicide-resistant variety of canola. Schmeiser claimed that he had never come into contact with Monsanto's transgenic canola plants, arguing that the canola fields on his farm exhibited herbicide resistance because they had been contaminated by "genetic pollution"—cross-pollination with pollen from Roundup Ready canola that was carried to his fields by wind or insects. In 2004 the Supreme Court of Canada ruled in favor of Monsanto, but the case still underscored tensions between the natural and the synthetic and the interests of independent farmers and big corporations. More fundamentally, the use of competing frames of genetic pollution and patent infringement to explain why Schmeiser's fields contained herbicide-resistant canola highlighted the ways genetically modified organisms can push the bounds of political, regulatory, and agricultural conceptions of property (Lezaun 2004).

GENETIC INFORMATION

Genetic screening technologies have opened new possibilities in health care for personalized medicine and decision making but have also raised questions about how individual genetic information should be protected and deployed for individual good and scientific research. One genetic screening technology, preimplantation genetic diagnosis, screens embryos for genetic disorders or other traits before implanting them into a womb and has incited a significant amount of controversy throughout the late twentieth and early twenty-first centuries. This new ability to select embryos for implantation has been vilified by some as a new form of eugenics that creates "designer babies" but praised by others as an important diagnostic tool that can reduce the prevalence of debilitating diseases. While the implications of this technology may hearken back to the eugenics of the earlier part of the twentieth century, its defenders note that this technology is not and would not be deployed by the state but rather by the free choice of individual persons.

In the meantime whole or partial genome sequencing for research and therapeutic purposes has resulted in aggregate collections of individual genetic information. Much of it is found in the private sector, where companies have offered direct-to-consumer genetic testing and genome sequencing at increasingly low costs in the early twenty-first century. Questions about how to best protect the privacy of the individuals whose whole genomes have been sequenced was the subject of a 2012 report by the Presidential Commission for the Study of Bioethical Issues. While the Genetic Information Nondiscrimination Act of 2008 prohibits genetic discrimination in health insurance and employment, the report found that US states' laws vary greatly in the level of privacy protection offered for genetic information.

STEM CELL RESEARCH AND CLONING

The public debate over stem cell research began in 1998, when researchers from the University of Wisconsin and Johns Hopkins University isolated stem cells from a human embryo for the first time. The process of acquiring these stem cells requires the destruction of embryos, and the discovery ushered in an international biopolitical debate that deals with a conflict between the embryo's moral status and progress in medicine. Questions about the status of embryos are not new. Much controversy surrounded and still surrounds the 1973 US Supreme Court decision in *Roe v. Wade*, which legalized abortion subject to regulations. But in the case of embryonic stem cell research, the main question in the United States is whether or not embryonic stem cell research should receive government funding.

In 1994, before the creation of the first human embryonic stem cell line, a federal panel on human embryo research recommended the allocation of government funds because of the potential positive impact embryo research could have on infertility treatments, genetic disorders, and human diseases. President Bill Clinton ultimately rejected these recommendations and determined that federal funding could not be used to create human embryos that would be destroyed in research. This view was codified into law in 1995 through the Dickey-Wicker Amendment, which banned federal funding for research that requires the creation or destruction of embryos.

In 1999, one year after the first embryonic stem cell line was created, Clinton's National Bioethics Advisory Commission (NBAC) recommended that federal funds could be used for research on stem cells derived from embryos discarded after in vitro fertilization (IVF) treatments but not for research involving embryos created specifically for research purposes. In 2000 Clinton changed his policy to reflect the advice of the NBAC. Yet another change in policy occurred in 2001, when, in a famous speech delivered from his ranch in Crawford, Texas, George W. Bush, the newly elected president, announced that federal funding for embryonic stem cell research would be restricted to existing stem cell lines, effectively disallowing the creation of new lines from any and all embryos. While scientists were at first relieved that Bush did not ban the research altogether, they later discovered that only two dozen or so collections of stem cells were usable under the law. In 2009 President Barack Obama issued an executive order lifting Bush's ban on research funding for new embryonic stem cell lines, which allowed federal funding for research on all ethically derived embryonic stem cell lines. In January 2013 the Supreme Court dismissed an appeal for the legal case against the executive order (*Sherley v. Sebelius*).

Because cloning is one way to obtain stem cells that does not require fertilization, much of the uproar over stem cell research has also spilled over into cloning. In 1996, just two years before the creation of the first stem cell line, the cloning of an animal was first successfully performed with the birth of Dolly the sheep. This event invited an array of concerns about the potential of cloned humans, and Clinton immediately placed a ban on human cloning and asked the NBAC to investigate the ethics of research procedures. The NBAC concluded that the physical and psychological risks to mothers and fetuses presented by human cloning were unacceptable, and Clinton agreed.

LIFE-SUSTAINING TECHNOLOGIES

While questions concerning embryonic stem cell research and cloning highlight tensions between what is human and what is not and the natural and the synthetic, the biopolitics of life-sustaining technologies brings into relief serious questions about the point at which life ends and death begins. This tension has been highlighted by a slew of court cases concerning the forced removal or maintenance of feeding tubes, respirators, and other devices for patients for whom consciousness is not physiologically possible. These patients may include those who are comatose, in permanent vegetative states with no hope of recovering, or in persistent vegetative states, a diagnosis that indicates the possibility that they may be able to regain some level of awareness. The line of cases concerning the use of life-sustaining technologies in these cases began in 1975, when a young woman named Karen Ann Quinlan collapsed at a party after consuming alcohol and valium and fell into a persistent vegetative state. When her parents asked the hospital to remove her ventilator, the hospital refused, and the New Jersey Supreme Court later found that Quinlan's parents had the right to act on what were presumed to be her wishes. The 1990 US Supreme Court decision involving Nancy Cruzan enacted a standard of evidence for cases in which patients had previously expressed their wishes to be removed from life-sustaining technologies in the case of being in a permanent or persistent vegetative state.

POLITICS OF BIOPOLITICS

Early bioethicists took notice of the many possibilities of biology soon after Watson and Crick published their findings on the structure of DNA. One of these thinkers, the Christian ethicist Joseph Fletcher (1905–1991), wrote in his 1974 work *The Ethics of Genetic Control: Ending Reproductive Roulette* that the prospect of genetic manipulation might result in a new level of objectification of human beings, but he also thought that the power of the new biology could be and should be harnessed. In contrast, the Princeton University theologian Paul Ramsey (1913–1988) (1970) held reservations about the potentials of the new technology, because he believed that artificial intervention in the process of procreation violated the essence of human nature. Meanwhile, Hans Jonas (1903–1993) (1985), a philosopher at the New School in New York City, advocated "predictive wisdom," the recognition that understanding the collective limits of scientific potentials is important and that control over human biology should be approached with humility.

These varying views about genetics seem to have been a precursor to the ways thinkers, activists, politicians, and laypeople would organize around political values as new biological advances unfolded over the following decades. Many of the same concerns about the ethical implications of modern biology tend to be shared across the political Left–Right spectrum (Moreno 2011). Some on the Left oppose changes in biology as threats to human equality, while some on the Right, especially religious traditionalists and secular neoconservatives, oppose these changes as threats to human dignity. Neoconservatives in particular may also harbor ambivalence toward scientific innovation and its implications for human well-being. Some on the political Left may support these changes in the name of common good or equality, whereas some on the political Right, especially libertarians, do not support intervention in and regulation of biotechnology.

It is possible, then, for political conservatives and political liberals to align together as either bioconservatives or bioprogressives, even if for different ideological reasons (Moreno 2011). Other political groups also find a place on the bioconservative–bioprogressive spectrum. Members of the Green movement may align with bioconservative ideals because of doubts about the implications of science for social justice. Meanwhile, transhumanists embrace technological change as something that can enhance humanity and take a bioprogressive stance to promote the same values bioconservatives try to defend.

EXPERT ADVICE

In addition to the cultural politics of the Right and the Left, the politics of bioethics is also influenced by the political interactions of experts and laypeople. According to Jasanoff (2005), bioethics is at once a disciplinary discourse dominated by experts and a democratic one that involves the participation of lay publics. At the end of the day, people most often first look to government for control of new biotechnologies. Government in turn, along with other social institutions that concern biotechnology, must prove itself to be a legitimate steward of the power of biology. In order to do this, it may turn to government agencies or expert advisory bodies to develop biotechnology policy. These advisory bodies tend to be important places where the borders between science, ethics, and politics come together (Briggle 2009).

Government-mandated bioethics advisory bodies have existed since the 1970s. From 1974 to 1978 Congress mandated the National Commission for the Protection of Human Subjects of Biomedical and Behavioral Research. This commission is best known for its development of the *Belmont Report* in 1978, which outlined informed consent, beneficence, and justice as fundamental principles of ethical human subjects research. In 1978 Congress established another advisory board, the President's Commission for the Study of Ethical Problems in Medicine and Biomedical and Behavioral Research, which produced reports on life-sustaining treatments and gene therapy. In the late 1980s Congress chartered a bioethics advisory board when it created the Biomedical Ethics Advisory Committee.

The responsibility of creating bioethics advisory boards passed from Congress to the White House in 1992, when President Clinton established the NBAC. The NBAC was most noted for producing a report on the ethics of human cloning in 1997 and a 1999 report on ethical issues in stem cell research. In 2001 President Bush established a similar advisory body called the President's Council on Bioethics (PCBE), which was succeeded by the Presidential Commission for the Study of Bioethical Issues when President Obama took office in 2009.

Bioethics commissions are designed to address bioethical questions and bring ethical expertise to biotechnology policies, but they are also subject to democratic legitimation or public acceptance of and trust in the commission's authority (Briggle 2009). Bioethics advisory boards, like any other advisory body, may lose legitimacy in the eyes of the public if their policy recommendations are perceived to discourage innovation or be too overreaching (Moreno 2011). More specifically, advisory boards are regulated by the Federal Advisory Commission Act and are expected to be transparent, fairly balanced, and independent of conflicts of interest (Briggle 2009).

Bush's PCBE was the subject of a significant amount of public and political scrutiny throughout its tenure by seeming to fail many of these expectations. The council's chair, Leon Kass, had been known to advocate bioconservative positions on biotechnology policy outside of his responsibilities to the council. Suspicions of bias arose when the terms of two members, the stem cell biologist Elizabeth Blackburn and the moderate theologian William May, were not renewed and Blackburn claimed that she had been dismissed because she disagreed with Bush and Kass on the ethics of stem cell research and cloning. Kass responded by assuring that the release of Blackburn reflected a change in the council's focus from reproductive and genetic technologies to issues in neuroscience (Briggle 2009). Otherwise the PCBE never publicly stated the reasons for the nonrenewals, but both the council and the Bush administration were publicly criticized for promoting "antiscience" policy (Moreno 2011).

BIOETHICS AND RELIGION

While the traditional US political spectrum dissolves in the face of bioethical questions, entirely different paradigms emerge when bioethics is considered in religious contexts. In the case of embryonic stem cell research, different faiths produce different answers to complex questions about when life begins and the moral status of embryos, resulting in perspectives that range from very permissive to very restrictive. At the same time, religious groups may agree on core issues, including the need for the equitable distribution of beneficial biotechnologies and the obligation to obtain informed consent.

These kinds of bioethical narratives were illuminated in a comprehensive overview of religious perspectives on embryonic stem cell research carried out by Clinton's NBAC as part of its 1999 report *Ethical Issues in Human Stem Cell Research*. The primary aim of this report was to provide Clinton with an overview of the bioethical considerations of stem cell research and to provide recommendations for the allocation of federal funding for such purposes. One part of the report includes perspectives of the Roman Catholic, Protestant, Eastern Orthodox, Jewish, and Islamic faiths. The commission found that these perspectives vary, and they may still vary in the context of other bioethical and policy decisions. For example, a second NBAC report devoted to ethical considerations of human cloning (published in 1997) also solicited input from religious leaders and noted a wide range of responses.

According to the 1999 NBAC report, the Roman Catholic position on embryonic stem cell research is generally restrictive, because blastocysts created through IVF are considered equivalent to human persons. In congruence with the Roman Catholic position on abortion, destroying an embryo for any reason is tantamount to murder. While the moral status of the embryo seems to be independent of whether it was created in vitro or in vivo in Roman Catholicism, in Judaism this difference can determine moral outcomes. The use of IVF embryos for stem cell research is morally permissible, because nonimplanted embryos do not have a legal or moral status in Jewish moral frameworks. In fact Jewish law holds that embryos achieve full human status only after forty days of gestation, and the moral status of IVF embryos is considered to be most similar to that of gametes. Therefore in Judaism, IVF embryos can be discarded, frozen, or used for beneficial research. Jewish tradition also prioritizes saving human life, an attitude that contributes to the high level of permissibility extended to research on potential lifesaving technologies.

Eastern Orthodox perspectives are similar to those of Roman Catholicism, and like Judaism, Islamic traditions place a strong emphasis on saving lives and perceive the personhood of embryos as a process that occurs in stages. In Islam an embryo achieves the moral status of a person around the fourth month of gestation, and the use of blastocysts for research is permissible. Meanwhile, Protestant positions on embryonic stem cell research tend to vary from very restrictive to very permissive. Restrictive perspectives consider the moral status of embryos to be the same as the moral status of persons, whereas less restrictive perspectives offer a more ambiguous consideration of the moral status of embryos. Here it is considered that blastocysts are different from persons and that the perceived lifesaving potential of embryonic stem cell research may sometimes outweigh moral obligations to the embryo. Research may be permissible as long as alternative means are explored and embryos are not created explicitly for research purposes.

While religious perspectives may provide ways of approaching biopolitical questions, such perspectives can become politicized in themselves. The so-called religious Right, also known as the Christian Right, developed as a response to social changes that occurred over the late twentieth and early twenty-first centuries and attempts to bring religious ideals to US policy, including biotechnology policy. This subset of the US public appeals to Christian values to support socially conservative policies; it invokes God and the Bible to strongly oppose abortion and gay marriage while supporting restrictions and regulations on cloning and embryonic stem cell research.

In a 2006 article Barbara Prainsack contends that the bioethical discourse in the United States is largely influenced by these kinds of Christian narratives. She notes that dignity and human life, values that are central to bioconservative agendas, may be viewed as secularized versions of religious ideas of sanctity and God's creation. This in turn seems to perpetuate a divide in the bioethical discourse between those who seek completely secular bioethical inquiries and those whose bioethical ideas are shaped by their religious convictions (Prainsack 2006). National responses to Bush's PCBE's support for restrictions on embryonic stem cell research seemed to embody this tension. Critics accused the council of stacking its membership with conservatives and Christians and of biasing its deliberations toward religious perspectives on biotechnology.

While religion in the American discourse may be characterized by bioethical divides, some scholars suggest that religious perspectives can and should be incorporated into the bioethical discussion. In a symposium on religion and science at the 2011 annual meeting of the American Association for the Advancement of Science, James Childress, who was a member of Clinton's NBAC, explained that inviting religious leaders to engage in bioethical and policy discussions may promote a better understanding of the ideas, inspirations, and methods of reasoning that shape many Americans' attitudes toward biotechnology. Furthermore, learning about areas in which religious perspectives converge with each other and with secular outlooks may be useful in the development of effective biotechnology policy. These were important reasons why the NBAC included religious perspectives in its reports on stem cell research and cloning. The NBAC is the only presidential bioethical advisory body that has explicitly considered religious perspectives on such a large, comprehensive scale in its reports.

BIOETHICS AMONG THE NATIONS

Questions posed by new advances in biotechnology tend to be rather the same across industrialized nations, but the resultant national discourses of these nations can be rather different (Jasanoff 2005). As social, cultural, and political norms, frameworks, and aspirations differ between countries, so do their biopolitical processes and outcomes.

Regulatory styles differ across similarly biotechnologically advanced countries in numerous ways, including the professional positionings of science and medicine, the relationships between the private and public sectors, and the nuances of national politics and legal procedures (Jasanoff 2005). Some of the most marked contrasts in the process and outcomes of biopolitics across nations arise in the distinct civic narratives and national histories they incorporate. For example, Germany's highly restrictive regulations on embryonic stem cell research and cloning speak to its unique post–World War II culture that repudiates anything reminiscent of the abuses of the Nazis. The United Kingdom's biopolitical discourse is characterized by a public sense of uncertainty about the risks that new biotechnologies carry and about the ability of government and industry to manage them. These sensibilities were famously brought into relief during Britain's so-called mad cow crisis in the mid-1990s, when numerous people were infected with bovine spongiform encephalopathy (BSE) after consuming meat. This collective experience may explain why genetically modified foods have been significantly more controversial in Britain than in the United States. For years South Korea was a world leader in stem cell research and cloning until it was learned in 2005 that Hwang Woo Suk, a renowned Korean stem cell scientist, had fabricated research results and bought human eggs from his laboratory employees. Disgraced by his actions, South Korea responded by ending its national stem cell research programs.

While many countries' policies have been formed by particular events or collective experiences, policies of other countries have been strongly informed by entrenched religious narratives. In Iran laws concerning IVF, cloning, and embryonic stem cell research are mainly based on the decrees, or fatwas, of religious Muslim authorities (Aramesh and Dabbagh 2007). Although human reproductive cloning is generally not permitted in Islam or in Iran because of the potential for suffering to be experienced by cloned humans, other forms of cloning and embryo research are permitted. According to a 2007 article by Kiarash Aramesh and Soroush Dabbagh, this is why Iran became the tenth country in the world to produce human embryonic stem cell lines in 2003.

Religion has also played an important role in Italian discourses on biotechnology, which have been characterized by a discord between the country's Catholic tradition and secular laypersons (Testa 2011). In Italy this was especially apparent in discourses surrounding the permissibility of stem cell nuclear transfer as a process of cloning embryos. An advisory body tasked to deal with the question ultimately concluded that there were no ethical problems but only after it successfully cast cloned embryos as not embryos—distinctly artificial and therefore not human.

Biotechnology regulations in other countries may also be shaped by nationalistic goals. Singapore's loose restrictions on biotechnology may be influenced by the nation's aspirations to become a global leader in biotechnology. Prainsack, in her 2006 article, argues that Israeli discourses reflect a combination of both national goals and religious moral frameworks. With its nonrestrictive approaches toward cloning and embryonic stem cell research, Israel boasts one of the most permissive biotechnology policies in the world. Prainsack attributes these outcomes to the distinct Jewish moral reasonings that inform Israeli social paradigms, which not only permit but may even encourage biotechnologies that are controversial in other countries. According to Prainsack, this Jewish ethic also intersects collective and individual nationalistic and pro-natalist cultures that promote biological and especially reproductive technologies.

The Netherlands has historically had strong Christian traditions, yet it is also the only place in the world where both physician-assisted suicide and euthanasia are legal, subject to regulation. This seeming paradox can be explained by cultural emphases on individualization, decreased taboos surrounding death and dying, and a liberal social climate favorable to the introduction of new ideas, all of which led to widespread support for the notion that medicine ought not always focus on prolonging life (Rietjens et al. 2009).

As bioethical questions increasingly deal with governance of new biotechnologies, bioethics has increasingly become biopolitics. A complex interaction between peoples, governments, experts, and other social entities, biopolitics comprises a contentious, multilayered space that is shaped by cultural values, collective histories, personal experiences, and religious beliefs. In the United States participants in the bioethical discourse draw on these social sensibilities to attempt to reconcile a historical appreciation for scientific progress with a concern for the protection of human dignity. As a result, bioprogressives and bioconservatives are represented by both the political Right and the political Left and a wide range of religious beliefs. While most industrialized countries face the same biopolitical questions the United States is dealing with in the twenty-first century, their varying civic narratives cause them to diverge in the way they deal with and ultimately resolve these questions.

At the time of this work, Michelle Spektor was a recent graduate of Cornell University. This article was written by Spektor in her private capacity. No official support or endorsement by the Presidential Commission for the Study of Bioethical Issues or the Department of Health and Human Services is intended, nor should it be inferred.

SEE ALSO *Biopolitics; Health Policy and Politics; Health Policy in the United States*

BIBLIOGRAPHY

Aramesh, Kiarash, and Soroush Dabbagh. 2007. "An Islamic View to Stem Cell Research and Cloning: Iran's Experience." *American Journal of Bioethics* 7 (2): 62–63.

Briggle, Adam. 2009. "The Kass Council and the Politicization of Ethics Advice." *Social Studies of Science* 39 (2): 309–26.

Childress, James. 2011. "Evangelical Christians and Stem Cell Research Policy." Presentation at the annual meeting of the American Association for the Advancement of Science, Washington, DC, February 17–21.

Cho, Mildred K.; David Magnus; Arthur L. Caplan; et al. 1999. "Ethical Considerations in Synthesizing a Minimal Genome." *Science* 286 (5447): 2087–90.

Fletcher, Joseph. 1974. *The Ethics of Genetic Control: Ending Reproductive Roulette.* Garden City, NY: Anchor Press.

Jasanoff, Sheila. 2005. *Designs on Nature: Science and Democracy in Europe and the United States.* Princeton, NJ: Princeton University Press.

Jonas, Hans. 1985. *The Imperative of Responsibility: In Search of an Ethics for the Technological Age.* Chicago: University of Chicago Press.

Lezaun, Javier. 2004. "Pollution and the Use of Patents: A Reading of *Monsanto v. Schmeiser.*" In *Biotechnology: Between Commerce and Civil Society,* edited by Nico Stehr, 135–58. New Brunswick, NJ: Transaction Publishers.

Moreno, Jonathan D. 2011. *The Body Politic: The Battle over Science in America.* New York: Bellevue Literary Press.

National Bioethics Advisory Commission. 1997. *Cloning Human Beings: Report and Recommendations of the National Bioethics Advisory Commission.* Rockville, MD: Author.

National Bioethics Advisory Commission. 1999. *Ethical Issues in Human Stem Cell Research.* Vol. 1, *Report and Recommendations of the National Bioethics Advisory Commission.* Rockville, MD: Author.

National Commission for the Protection of Human Subjects of Biomedical and Behavioral Research. 1978. *The Belmont Report: Ethical Principles and Guidelines for the Protection of Human Subjects of Research.* Washington, DC: DHEW and US Government Printing Office.

Prainsack, Barbara. 2006. "'Negotiating Life': The Regulation of Human Cloning and Embryonic Stem Cell Research in Israel." *Social Studies of Science* 36 (2): 173–205.

Presidential Commission for the Study of Bioethical Issues. 2012. *Privacy and Progress in Whole Genome Sequencing.* Washington, DC: Author.

Rabinow, Paul, and Nikolas Rose. 2006. "Biopower Today." *BioSocieties* 1 (2): 195–217.

Ramsey, Paul. 1970. *Fabricated Man: The Ethics of Genetic Control.* New Haven, CT: Yale University Press.

Rietjens, Judith A. C.; Paul J. van der Maas; Bregje D. Onwuteaka-Philipsen; et al. 2009. "Two Decades of Research on Euthanasia from the Netherlands: What Have We Learnt and What Questions Remain?" *Journal of Bioethical Inquiry* 6 (3): 271–83.

Testa, Giuseppe. 2011. "More Than Just a Nucleus: Cloning and the Alignment of Scientific and Political Rationalities." In *Reframing Rights: Bioconstitutionalism in the Genetic Age,* edited by Sheila Jasanoff, 86–104. Cambridge, MA: MIT Press.

Thompson, Paul B., and William Hannah. 2008. "Food and Agricultural Biotechnology: A Summary and Analysis of Ethical Concerns." *Advances in Biochemical Engineering/Biotechnology* 111:229–64.

Michelle Spektor
Research Associate, Presidential Commission for the Study of Bioethical Issues

Jonathan D. Moreno
Professor of Medical Ethics, History and Sociology of Science, and Philosophy, University of Pennsylvania

BIOETHICS COMMISSIONS, HISTORY OF

In a democracy, one common public policy question is not whether a government can act but how it ought to act. This emphasis upon "ought" in public policy evaluation places the focus on the moral justifications for collective action; however, this moral focus creates a problem. Modern societies have a plurality of conceptions of right action, and therefore there often exists on any given issue a plurality of reasonable, but often incompatible, moral points of view. These differing moral perspectives often lead to different conclusions about what the morally right public policy should be and/or which moral reasons can justify that policy.

Democracies often attempt to find the moral bases for public policy or to resolve disagreements over contentious moral issues through public moral discourse (Brock 1995). These moral deliberations occur within many different institutions, federal bioethics commissions being one of them.

Federal bioethics commissions have been an important source of public bioethics discourse since the 1970s. The discourse within bioethics commissions is conducted by experts who are selected on the basis of their knowledge and skills in various content and technical areas relevant to bioethics. By virtue of their expertise, commission members are granted by political leaders the authority to publicly deliberate about bioethical issues and to recommend which policies and/or practices the government would be morally justified to enact. Federal bioethics bodies in the United States have had a varied history of mandates, results, and impact.

DEFINITION OF FEDERAL BIOETHICS COMMISSIONS

Throughout the modern American history of bioethics, the federal government has been the recipient of the most guidance and policy regarding bioethical dilemmas. As a result of the government's need for information and insight about advances in biomedical science and health care, bioethics commissions have been created as a source of expertise for Congress, the executive bureaucracy, and the president. These commissions, regardless of their locus of origin, mandate, or reporting requirements, shall be termed "federal bioethics commissions."

There exist many competing definitions for what is considered a true federal bioethics commission. Accounts from Mark O. Hatfield and Albert R. Jonsen (1994), the Institute of Medicine (1995), Jonsen (1998), M. L. Tina Stevens (2000), John H. Evans (2001, 2006), and others include or exclude bioethics commissions according to somewhat arbitrary criteria. Some define bioethics commissions according to their governmental location, others by function, and others by composition. To date, no well-established or accepted definition of bioethics commissions exists, probably because these commissions, are so varied in their loci, mandates, composition, and topics. Daniel Wikler (1994a, 1994b) has offered one of the few classification schemes for bioethics commissions, dividing bioethics bodies into one of three categories: populist commissions that sponsor public education and grassroots organization; elite commissions with private meetings, the top scholars and professionals, and a very high national profile; and private commissions in those cases where nongovernmental groups sponsor a commission in lieu of governmental bodies. Wikler's typology, however, is too expansive and would include a vast number of nonfederal bioethics bodies.

Of course, there are many other kinds of bioethics commissions that function at the national level but are not federal in origin. These bodies are part of state governments, professional associations, international bioethics advisory bodies, executive boards, and so forth. Some of these nonfederal bodies have engaged in incredibly important work for bioethics. These are outside the scope of this chapter, however, and will not be discussed in detail here. For the purposes of an overview with regard to US history, a federal bioethics commission shall here be defined as a committee (a) that is impaneled by a federal branch of government and acts under its authority, (b) whose mandate specifically includes ethical inquiry about issues related to biomedical research and health care, and (c) that has interdisciplinary nongovernmental members including scientists, ethicists, physicians, and others.

THE ROLES OF FEDERAL BIOETHICS COMMISSIONS

Federal bioethics commissions are a small subset of commissions within the larger category of federal advisory commissions. Governmental advisory commissions have been common political institutions at the federal level in the United States, particularly through the twentieth century. In general, these advisory bodies are created by presidents (and sometimes Congress) to inform and advise the federal government on matters of public policy. They have gained a certain level of importance as a strategy for dealing with public policy problems and are generally thought to be a permanent fixture in the US government (Dean 1969; Flitner 1986).

Commissions can be created to serve a variety of functions: executive advice, evaluation and review (advisory), fact-finding (investigative), public relations and symbolism (a.k.a. window dressing), public education, agenda setting, organizational restructuring, and policy formulation. The history of federal bioethics commissions suggests that they have served two primary functions—to advise and to investigate (Meslin and Johnson 2008; McGee 2011).

FEDERAL BIOETHICS COMMISSIONS: A HISTORY

The history of federal bioethics commissions typically begins with the National Commission for the Protection of Human Subjects of Biomedical and Behavioral Research. In reality, however, this commission was created two years after the National Institutes of Health (NIH) formed the first federal bioethics advisory panel of any kind. In 1972 the NIH established an advisory panel to assess the ethics of implanting a nuclear-powered heart. The NIH Totally Artificial Heart Assessment Panel ultimately concluded that these devices were not a good idea—arguably a significant impact. However, this was neither a legislative nor a presidential bioethics commission.

As Table 1 suggests, federal bioethics commissions have had widely varied mandates, locations within the federal government, leaders and leadership styles, staffing, and funding. Their relationships with the federal government

Table 1. Federal Bioethics Commissions in the United States, 1974–2012

Commission and Chairs	Creation, Mandate, and Locus	Funding, Staffing, and Reporting
National Commission for the Protection of Human Subjects of Biomedical and Behavioral Research (1974–1979) Chair: Kenneth Ryan	Creation: Title II of the National Research Act of 1974 Mandate: To study the ethical principles underlying biomedical and behavioral research on human subjects and to make recommendations to the secretary of the Department of Health, Education and Welfare (DHEW) and to Congress for the protection of these subjects. Locus: Congressional commission	Members: 11 Appointed by: Secretary Caspar Weinberger, DHEW Funding: DHEW Staff: 16 Reports: 11 in 5 years
President's Commission for the Study of Ethical Problems in Medicine and Biomedical and Behavioral Research (1979–1983) Chair: James A. Gathier, JD	Creation: Public Law 95–622, Executive Order 12184 Mandate: To discuss seven mandated bioethical topics and to report on emerging issues beyond human subjects research. Locus: Independent executive branch commission	Members: 11 Appointed by: President Jimmy Carter Funding: DHEW Staff: 20 (avg.) Reports: 11 in 3 years
Advisory Committee on Human Radiation Experiments (1994–1995) Chair: Ruth Faden, PhD	Creation: Executive Order 12891 Mandate: To investigate human radiation experiments during the period 1944 through 1974 and to identify ethical and scientific standards for past and future government research. Locus: Independent executive branch commission	Members: 14 Appointed by: President William Clinton Funding: Department of Energy Staff: 42 (including full and part-time staff) Reports: 1 in 18 months
National Bioethics Advisory Commission (1995–2001) Chair: Harold Shapiro, PhD	Creation: Executive Order 12975 Mandate: To advise and recommend regarding government policies and practices and to identify general principles to govern ethical conduct in research. Locus: Independent executive branch commission	Members: 15 (amended to 18) Appointed by: President Clinton Funding: Department of Health and Human Services (DHHS) Staff: 16 Reports: 6 in 6 years
President's Council on Bioethics (2001–2009) Chairs: Leon Kass, MD, PhD, and Edmund Pellegrino, MD	Creation: Executive Order 13237 Mandate: To advise the president on bioethical issues emerging as a result of advances in biomedical science and technology. Locus: Independent executive branch commission	Members: 18 Appointed by: President George W. Bush Funding: DHHS Staff: 15 Reports: 7 reports, 1 white paper, and 2 edited volumes in 8 years
Presidential Commission for the Study of Bioethical Issues (2009–) Chair: Amy Gutmann, PhD	Creation: Executive Order 13521 Mandate: To advise the president on bioethical issues emerging as a result of advances in biomedicine and other relevant areas of science and technology. Locus: Independent executive branch commission	Members: 13 Appointed by: President Barack Obama Funding: DHHS Staff: 22 Reports: 5 reports through 4 years

SOURCE: Courtesy of Summer Johnson McGee and Jami Lynn Goodwin. Data compiled from Georgetown University's Compendium of Former Bioethics Commissions and Reports; http://bioethics.georgetown.edu/pcbe/reports/past_commissions; information on President Obama's Presidential Commission for the Study of Bioethical Issues available via www.bioethics.gov.

have also varied as a result of political events as well as scientific advances that have arisen during their terms.

National Commission for the Protection of Human Subjects of Biomedical and Behavioral Research. In the early days of federal bioethics, it was the legislative branch that was most interested in discussing and resolving biomedical ethics issues such as those concerning organ transplantation and human experimentation. Therefore, in a sense, federal bioethics began in the halls of Congress with the Mondale hearings of 1968 (Jonsen 1998). Senator Walter Mondale's legislation proposing the creation of a federal commission on bioethical issues was the first call for a national-level forum to discuss ethical issues in the biomedical and biological sciences. His call was answered nearly five years later when the National Research Act was signed into law by President Richard Nixon, establishing the first federal bioethics commission, the National Commission for the Protection of Human Subjects of Biomedical and Behavioral Research, in 1974.

This commission established the precedent for the creation of bioethics commissions in the United States and arguably throughout the world (Meslin and Johnson 2008). Moreover, the commission, led by Kenneth Ryan, wrote reports on some of the most controversial bioethical topics of the day and did, in fact, help to resolve many of these issues for the government as well as for many bioethicists, who at the time saw the commission as authoritative regarding the prevailing views in bioethics. Not only did the commission produce the *Belmont Report*, still considered one of the most authoritative sources in all of human subjects research, but also its report became the basis for the establishment of the Code of Federal Regulations, human-research regulations which govern all federally funded research in the United States.

President's Commission for the Ethical Study of Problems in Medicine and Biomedical Research. After Congress initiated the first national bioethics commission in 1974 with such great success, five years later a second congressional commission was created: the President's Commission for the Ethical Study on Problems in Medicine and Biomedical Research. The President's Commission, as it is known, similarly tackled the most controversial and important bioethical topics of its time. While some of its reports, as a later Institute of Medicine report went on to conclude, "have gone on the shelf to collect dust" (IOM 1995, 281) such as the commission's report on compensating for research injuries and whistle-blowing in research, some of those topics may have simply been ahead of their time. Meanwhile, other reports, such as *Defining Death*, *Securing Access to Health Care*, and *Deciding to Forgo [sic] Life-Sustaining Treatment*, were incredibly important and widely read, as well as being controversial reports at the time.

Despite the incredible influence of each of the first two bioethics commissions' reports, as would be expected for a presidential or congressional commission, the change of presidential administrations and/or congressional leadership guaranteed their obsolescence. This has been a common theme for federal bioethics commissions: they are subject to dissolution or reconstitution when administrations change because they serve at the pleasure of those who appoint them. The President's Commission was decommissioned immediately—mid-report—as the incoming Reagan administration was incensed upon discovering that the commission was to publish a report on fetal-tissue research.

National Bioethics Advisory Commission. Following the President's Commission, no federal bioethics commission existed in the United States for the remainder of the presidencies of Ronald Reagan and George H. W. Bush. The reason for the lack of attention to or perceived need for a federal bioethics commission through this time involved a number of factors, including the dissatisfaction of the Reagan administration with the President's Commission's slated report on fetal-tissue research, the ascendancy of the religious Right and pro-life politics, and likely the fact that the country went to war with Iraq. All of these events shifted federal bioethics onto the back burner.

This was the case until President William Clinton created the National Bioethics Advisory Commission (NBAC) to advise the federal government, specifically the executive branch, about ethical issues in biomedical research. Notably, within the first six months of the commission's being impaneled, the announcement that a sheep, named Dolly, had been cloned in Scotland hijacked the commission's agenda. President Clinton immediately asked his bioethics commission to drop all of its plans and issue a report within ninety days regarding the implications of this scientific advance. As a result, a number of the commission's stated goals for exploring other pressing issues in biomedical research were sidelined or ignored entirely.

Ultimately, the NBAC did provide President Clinton with a report on time, but its recommendations were largely eclipsed by the president's own recommendations and stated policy, which were issued days before the report was provided to the president. This political problem created somewhat of a tense relationship between the White House and the commission, which they would have to overcome over many years. Still, the NBAC was able to complete six reports in six years—a very productive federal commission by any standard.

Advisory Committee on Human Radiation Experiments. Arguably, the Advisory Committee on Human Radiation Experiments (ACHRE) was the first bioethics commission to diverge from being a solely advisory commission. ACHRE, created by President Clinton in 1994, was commissioned with a dual mandate to conduct an investigation into radiation experiments done by the federal government in the 1950s as well as to produce ethical judgments and policy recommendations about human subjects research in the United States past, present, and future. This commission served in a hybrid role of inquiry and advice giving and issued a single report which consisted of two volumes—one outlining the historical findings from their research and the other outlining the ethics.

President's Council on Bioethics. The President's Council on Bioethics (PCB) was created by President George W. Bush on August 9, 2001, as part of his declarations about stem cell research at the federal level. When President Bush announced that there would be a presidential bioethics council, the PCB became the only federal bioethics commission ever to be announced in a prime-time television broadcast by a sitting president. This immediately elevated the commission, and its first report, *Human Cloning and Human Dignity: An Ethical Inquiry*, was published a year later to national and international prominence.

This commission also took the somewhat unconventional approach of not just producing advisory reports but also creating volumes of readings on bioethics, including selections in the medical humanities. The commission published two different readers on bioethics as well as producing seven reports and one white paper during its eight years of existence.

Yet this commission's auspicious beginnings were met with a rather lackluster end in 2009. Much as with the President's Commission in the early 1980s, the PCB by 2005 found itself subject to a lack of presidential interest. This change within the Bush administration resulted in a change of leadership for the commission: Dr. Leon Kass left as the commission's chair and was succeeded by Dr. Edmund Pellegrino. For three years the commission was moribund, having only a handful of meetings. In the last few months of its existence, the commission did release three reports—but none received much attention from the president, academics, or the media.

President's Commission for the Study of Bioethical Issues. With the President's Commission for the Study of Bioethical Issues (PCSBI), a bioethics commission again took on a dual role as both investigative and advisory when President Barack Obama asked the commission to investigate allegations about research conducted by the US Public Health Service in Guatemala in the late 1940s.

In addition to this report, the PCSBI was asked by the president specifically to explore ethical issues in synthetic biology in response to an announcement by Dr. Craig Venter that he had "created life" in the laboratory. The PCSBI report *New Directions: The Ethics of Synthetic Biology and Emerging Technologies* noted that Venter and his colleagues were in the developmental stages of adapting research biology, technologies, and genetics; called for prudent federal vigilance concerning these emerging sciences and their implications; and advised the administration to create regular, ongoing governance for these technologies while encouraging creativity and innovation from the private sector within ethical boundaries.

The PCSBI was asked to look into research funded by the US Public Health Service in Guatemala from 1946 to 1948, in which prisoners were infected with syphilis without treatment. Chair Amy Gutmann was asked to convene and oversee an international panel to examine global human subjects research, to review the events of the Guatemala trials, and to ensure that current federal and international standards for human subjects research were sufficiently rigorous. The PCSBI published reports on the institutional misconduct in Guatemala and the findings of the international subcommittee and provided suggestions for improvements concerning international human subjects research.

Upon the completion of these investigations, the PCSBI began examining the ethical implications of whole genome sequencing, its potential applications for disease management, and current and future concerns over the privacy of personal and familial genetic information that can be derived from genome sequencing. A report on the commission's findings, along with suggestions on the protection and interpretation of personal genetic information, was released on October 11, 2012.

THE IMPACT OF FEDERAL BIOETHICS COMMISSIONS

Within the field of bioethics there is a perceived prominence for the role of bioethics commissions on the national stage. As one bioethicist has said, "No academic field has been defined more by these government commissions than bioethics" (Moreno 2002). Those who have served on these advisory bodies arguably know them best, and a few have chosen to describe their experiences in the academic literature (Faden 1996; Capron 1997; Childress 1997; Charo 1998; Meslin 1999; Meslin and Shapiro 2002; Meslin 2003). Moreover, some empirical research has been conducted to assess the effects that these commissions have had in various domains, including government, the media, and academia (Office of Technology Assessment 1993; Gray 1995, 261–306; Eiseman 2003). These initial studies were highly informative first looks at bioethics commissions explaining that commissions differ in regard to activity and impact in these domains, both by commission and by report.

Subsequent empirical study has further substantiated the claim that presidential bioethics commissions have a broad and diverse range of impacts upon various domains of government, media, and the professions (Meslin and Johnson 2008). Commissions provide a source of intergovernmental expertise that is often called upon to testify at congressional hearings or consult with governmental officials at the agency level. Moreover, commissions produce reports that can be consulted as authoritative sources of information for journalists, scholars, students, and the general public. Commissions also serve as a venue wherein interest groups and other activist parties can have a voice on matters relevant to their organizations.

Although there is a general sense in which society knows that commissions play an important role in public bioethics, there exist a plethora of anecdotal empirical examples of how commissions perform these roles, both successfully and unsuccessfully. Because presidential bioethics commissions are political institutions that are likely to continue to exist in the future across multiple presidential administrations, it is important that bioethicists and other scholars generate practical theories and usable knowledge that will help to evaluate and possibly guide these advisory bodies in the future.

However, impact is a complex phenomenon dependent upon a variety of factors. Influences on impact often include contextual factors such as presidential commitment, congressional activity, interest group participation, and preexisting social consensus on the public policy problem, but also are likely to include internal factors such as the selection of report topics and a commission's communication and dissemination skills.

Moreover, impact is not a singular thing that can be reduced, although many try, to whether a commission has an impact on changing laws or regulations. Bioethics commissions educate the public as well as individual congresspersons and have members who give congressional testimony or are quoted in the mainstream popular media or local media outlets. All of these are impacts that matter—all of which inform the public policy process and/or the social discourse. Ultimately, the public nature, and thus public accountability, of such commissions is much more complex than anyone has demonstrated to date.

SEE ALSO *America, Bioethics in: I. United States; Bioethics: I. History of; Bioethics Education: IV. Public Education; Nazi Legacy and Bioethics; Organizational Ethics in Health Care*

BIBLIOGRAPHY

Brock, Dan W. 1995. "Public Moral Discourse." In *Society's Choices: Social and Ethical Decision Making in Biomedicine*, edited by Ruth Ellen Bulger, Elizabeth Meyer Bobby, and Harvey V. Fineberg, 215–40. Washington, DC: National Academy Press.

Bulger, Ruth Ellen; Elizabeth Meyer Bobby; and Harvey V. Fineberg, eds. 1995. *Society's Choices: Social and Ethical Decision Making in Biomedicine*. Washington, DC: National Academy Press.

Capron, Alexander M. 1997. "An Egg Takes Flight: The Once and Future Life of the National Bioethics Advisory Commission." *Kennedy Institute of Ethics Journal* 7 (1): 63–80.

Charo, R. Alta. 1998. "The National Bioethics Advisory Commission: Bridging the Tension between Scientific and Public Policy Analysis." *Journal of Biolaw and Business* 1 (2): 84–89.

Childress, James F. 1997. "The Challenges of Public Ethics: Reflections on NBAC's Report." *Hastings Center Report* 27 (5): 9–11.

Dean, Alan L. 1969. "Ad Hoc Commissions for Policy Formulation?" In *The Presidential Advisory System*, edited by Thomas E. Cronin and Sanford D. Greenberg, 101–16. New York: Harper & Row.

Eiseman, Elisa. 2003. *The National Bioethics Advisory Commission: Contributing to Public Policy*. Arlington, VA: RAND.

Evans, John H. 2001. *Playing God? Human Genetic Engineering and the Rationalization of Public Bioethical Debate, 1959–1995*. Chicago: University of Chicago Press.

Evans, John H. 2006. "Between Technocracy and Democratic Legitimation: A Proposed Compromise Position for Common Morality Public Bioethics." *Journal of Medicine and Philosophy* 31 (3): 213–34.

Faden, Ruth R. 1996. "The Advisory Committee on Human Radiation Experiments: Reflections on a Presidential Commission." *Hastings Center Report* 26 (5): 5–10.

Flitner, David. 1986. *The Politics of Presidential Commissions*. Dobbs Ferry, NY: Transnational Publishers.

Gray, Bradford H. 1995. "Bioethics Commissions: What Can We Learn from Past Successes and Failures?" In *Society's Choices: Social and Ethical Decision Making in Biomedicine*, edited by Ruth Ellen Bulger, Elizabeth Meyer Bobby, and Harvey V. Fineberg, 261–306. Washington, DC: National Academy Press.

Hatfield, Mark O., and Albert R. Jonsen. 1994–1995. "The Nation Needs a Bioethics Commission." *Issues in Science and Technology* 11 (2): 5–6.

IOM (Institute of Medicine). Committee on the Social and Ethical Impacts of Developments in Biomedicine, Division of Health Sciences Policy. 1995. *Society's Choices: Social and Ethical Decision Making in Biomedicine*. Edited by Ruth Ellen Bulger, Elizabeth Meyer Bobby, and Harvey V. Fineberg. Washington, DC: National Academy Press.

Jonsen, Albert R. 1998. *The Birth of Bioethics*. New York: Oxford University Press.

McGee, Summer. 2011. "Ideology and Politicization in Public Bioethics." *Cambridge Quarterly of Healthcare Ethics* 20 (1): 73–84.

Meslin, Eric M. 1999. "Engaging the Public in Policy Development: The National Bioethics Advisory Commission Report on 'Research Involving Persons with Mental Disorders That

May Affect Decisionmaking Capacity.'" *Accountability in Research* 7 (2–4): 227–39.

Meslin, Eric M. 2003. "When Policy Analysis Is Carried Out in Public: Some Lessons for Bioethics from NBAC's Experience." In *The Nature and Prospect of Bioethics: Interdisciplinary Perspectives*, edited by Franklin G. Miller, John C. Fletcher, and James M. Humber, 87–111. Totowa, NJ: Humana Press.

Meslin, Eric M., and Summer Johnson. 2008. "National Bioethics Commissions and Research Ethics." In *Oxford Textbook of Clinical Research Ethics*, edited by Ezekiel J. Emanuel, Christine Grady, Robert A. Crouch, et al., 187–97. New York: Oxford University Press.

Meslin, Eric M., and Harold T. Shapiro. 2002. "Some Initial Reflections on NBAC." *Kennedy Institute of Ethics Journal* 12 (1): 95–102.

Moreno, Jonathan D. 2002. "The Brief Career of a Government Advisory Committee: One Member's Perspective." *American Journal of Bioethics* 2 (4): W23.

National Commission for the Protection of Human Subjects of Biomedical and Behavioral Research. 1975. *Research on the Fetus: Report and Recommendations*. Bethesda, MD: Author.

National Commission for the Protection of Human Subjects of Biomedical and Behavioral Research. 1978. *The Belmont Report: Ethical Principles and Guidelines for the Protection of Human Subjects of Research*. Washington, DC: DHEW and US Government Printing Office.

Office of Technology Assessment. 1993. *Biomedical Ethics in U.S. Public Policy*. Washington, DC: Author.

Presidential Commission for the Study of Bioethical Issues. 2010. *New Directions: The Ethics of Synthetic Biology and Emerging Technologies*. Washington, DC: Author.

Stevens, M. L. Tina. 2000. *Bioethics in America: Origins and Cultural Politics*. Baltimore, MD: Johns Hopkins University Press.

White House. 2009. "President Obama Establishes New Presidential Commission for the Study of Bioethical Issues, Names Commission Leadership." November 24. http://www.whitehouse.gov/the-press-office/president-obama-establishes-new-presidential-commission-study-bioethical-issues-nam

Wikler, Daniel. 1994a. "Bioethics Commissions Abroad." *HEC Forum* 6 (5): 290–304.

Wikler, Daniel. 1994b. "Federal Bioethics: Methodology, Expertise, and Evaluation." *Politics and the Life Sciences* 13 (1): 100–101.

Summer Johnson McGee
Associate Professor, Department of Public Management, College of Business, University of New Haven

Jami Lynn Goodwin
Project Manager, Heart and Vascular Center, Barnes Jewish Hospital, University College, Washington University in St. Louis

BIOETHICS EDUCATION

This entry consists of the following:

I. MEDICINE
David Doukas, Michael J. Green, and Robert M. Arnold
II. NURSING
Mila A. Aroskar, Anne J. Davis, and Theresa Drought
II. NURSING [ADDENDUM]
Joy Penticuff
III. OTHER HEALTH PROFESSIONS
Ruth B. Purtilo
IV. PUBLIC EDUCATION
Jacob Moses

I. MEDICINE

Education in medical ethics is as old as medical education itself. The Hippocratic school of medicine of the fourth century B.C.E. Greece is best remembered for the Hippocratic oath, which has provided moral guidance to students of medicine for more than two millennia. Until the latter half of the nineteenth century, efforts to inculcate ethical precepts relied on the apprenticeship model, which guided medical students in the development of knowledge, technical skill, judgment, and a sense of proper professional conduct (Bosk 1979). Direct observation and emulation were the primary methods apprentices used to develop judgment regarding the moral aspects of their actions. With the emergence of medical schools in the nineteenth and twentieth centuries, accelerated by the 1910 Flexner report, the locus of educational control began to shift from the preceptor to the academic medical center (Flexner and Pritchett 1910; Cooke et al. 2006). In the 1920s Abraham Flexner (1866–1959) (1925) advocated enhanced ethics and humanities in medical education, which had implications for the development of how and where ethics was later taught.

In the latter part of the twentieth century, numerous social and political forces precipitated a radical reexamination of the ways students learn and manage ethical issues. Nonphysician humanists—philosophers, theologians, and scholars with interests in applied ethics and the medical humanities—led the initial efforts. In the early 1970s, starting with Pennsylvania State University, medical schools hired these humanists and began to offer elective and later required ethics courses for medical students. Rather than concentrating on the importance of mentorship and role modeling, these courses had a philosophical model emphasizing ethical concepts, such as autonomy and the importance of applying ethical principles to discern the proper course of action. Lectures and seminars became the dominant method of teaching these cognitive skills.

In the early years, with few exceptions, the content of ethics training focused on the extreme ends of life and technological innovations rather than on the day-to-day work of patient care and justice-based concerns. More recently there have been concerted efforts to emphasize everyday ethics (Fox, Arnold, and Brody 1995). There also have been efforts to integrate other aspects of medical humanities into the medical school curriculum, and many schools now teach history, narrative and literature, and visual arts (Doukas, McCullough, and Wear 2010).

Since the late 1990s a trend in ethics education focusing on professionalism has emerged. Professionalism is one of the six outcomes-based general competencies that the Accreditation Council for Graduate Medical Education (ACGME) promulgates in an effort to move toward an outcomes-based curriculum for residents. Although professionalism is often cited as the warehouse for all things ethical in the general competencies, a careful read of all six competencies reveals a wide assortment of expected ethical behaviors and requisite comportment throughout training (Doukas 2003). The ACGME (2011) has moved forward with enhanced measurement of general competency metrics using discrete milestones that demonstrate knowledge and behavioral maturation. Competency-based outcome measures, each specifically citing the necessity of professionalism, are also part of the educational expectations of the Joint Commission (formerly known as the Joint Commission on Accreditation of Healthcare Organizations), the National Board of Medical Examiners, and the US Medical Licensing Examination. These new educational expectations reach beyond traditional modalities of lectures and seminars to include role modeling and team teaching by peers and to involve rigorous assessments with techniques such as 360-degree evaluations, standardized patients, clinical simulation labs, objective structured clinical examinations, and patient surveys.

THE GROWTH OF MEDICAL ETHICS EDUCATION

A series of empirical studies in the 1970s and 1980s documented the rapid growth of teaching programs in the United States and beyond. In a 1974 survey, 97 of 107 responding medical schools reported teaching medical ethics (Veatch and Solitto 1976). Only six of these schools, however, reported a mandatory exposure to medical ethics. In 1982 a majority of physicians reported that they had never received formal education in clinical ethics, and many considered themselves inadequately prepared to address common ethical problems in medicine (Pellegrino et al. 1985). A 1985 study showed that 84 percent of US medical schools had some form of human values curriculum during the first two years (Bickel 1986).

By 1989, 43 of 127 US medical schools reported separate required courses in medical ethics (Miles et al. 1989). By 2000 all responding US medical schools reported "some formal instruction in medical ethics," 78 percent "incorporated ethics into required preclinical courses," 55 percent had a required ethics course, and 74 percent had ethics "studies" during the clinical years of medical school (Lehmann et al. 2004, 682, 686). By 2010 a survey by the Association of American Medical Colleges (AAMC) (2012) showed that 85 percent of graduating medical students felt they had received adequate training in medical ethics, 93 percent believed they learned about fundamental issues in the social sciences of medicine (e.g., ethics, humanism, professionalism, organization, and structure of the health care system), and 97 percent believed they understood the ethical and professional values that are expected of the profession.

Medical ethics in graduate medical education gained traction in the late 1980s, when educators began to advocate explicit teaching of medical ethics during residency training. Residency is a critical formative period, because that is when physicians first have decision-making responsibilities and thus can fully appreciate the relevance of medical ethics to patient care. In 1984 Gail J. Povar and Karla J. Keith found that residents in 40 percent of internal medicine programs had no formal exposure to clinical ethics teaching. Two reports by the American Board of Internal Medicine and American Board of Pediatrics in the 1980s provided strong impetus for the development of teaching programs during the residency years. Residency programs in family medicine, internal medicine, surgery, pediatrics, and obstetrics and gynecology all require education in medical ethics. Reflecting this commitment to ethics training, the ACGME (2011, 9) general competencies require that all residents "demonstrate a commitment to carrying out professional responsibilities and an adherence to ethical principles." Additional expectations are based on both principle-based and virtue-based criteria, translating to humanist and facilitative care for the patient's benefit.

Outside the United States ethics education has taken a slightly different path. There was a long tradition of teaching medical deontology (the study of moral obligation) in both Europe and Latin America, particularly in Catholic medical schools. In the 1980s, however, the focus and quantity of medical ethics programs began to change. In Great Britain the General Medical Council created a committee to study the teaching of medical ethics in British medical schools and to make recommendations. The resulting 1987 Pond Report recommended that the teaching of medical ethics be encouraged in medical school, but no specific guidelines were advocated (Boyd 1987). Although initially little progress was made, a later study showed that most medical schools included ethics education (Goldie 2000).

A 1991 study in Canada showed that fifteen of the sixteen Canadian medical schools provided medical ethics teaching and some sort of examination, the number of required hours ranging from ten to forty-five (Baylis and Downie 1991). Almost all of the schools used physicians as instructors and focused on specific ethical issues (e.g., euthanasia) as opposed to ethical theory and professional codes of ethics. The College of Family Physicians of

Canada and the Royal College of Physicians and Surgeons of Canada require ethics training, and there has been increasing interest in continuing education in bioethics (McKneally and Singer 2001).

In numerous countries medical schools have developed curricula in medical ethics. In 1982 Lagos University in Nigeria initiated two-day workshops at which lawyers, physicians, and patients all participated in lectures and discussions of issues in medical ethics (Olukoya 1984). In Australia medical graduates are required to understand basic medical ethics principles, and in the early 2000s educators promulgated a core curriculum (Working Group on Behalf of the Association of Teachers of Ethics and Law in Australian and New Zealand Medical Schools 2001).

During the period of rapid growth in formal medical ethics education, a wide variety of activities were subsumed under the general heading of ethics programs. There was great variability in the establishment of explicit curricular goals, the identification and support of teaching faculty, the teaching methods employed, and the attempts (if any) at evaluation of educational success. Although a degree of consensus evolved in some areas, important areas of disagreement remained.

EDUCATIONAL GOALS

The goals of medical ethics education have been ambitious and diverse, including increased awareness of ethical issues, cultivation of basic ethical commitments, more humane medical practice, tolerance of conflicting views, development of analytic skill in moral reasoning, enhanced intellectual development in ethics and the humanities, positive attitudes toward patients, less paternalism in clinical practice, and improved clinical decision making (Callahan 1980; Miles et al. 1989). Despite this dauntingly heterogeneous list, a consensus has emerged regarding the following core objectives.

The primary goal is to prepare physicians to deal effectively with ethical issues in clinical practice. Reaching this goal requires that students adopt multiple strategies, including learning to anticipate ethical conflicts before they occur, understanding the values of all parties that can result in conflicts, thinking clearly and critically about ethical issues to inform how to respond to conflicts, and implementing a justified course of action. Each of these objectives requires that students possess specific knowledge, attitudes, and skills. Recognizing ethical issues in patient care requires a receptive attitude concerning the importance of the humanistic and value-laden aspects of medical care. Addressing the ethical aspects of care requires awareness of the patient's values, goals, and preferences and how they affect the patient's wishes regarding treatment options.

The second goal of proficiency in ethics is for students to learn certain behaviors. Even highly motivated students who understand the importance of autonomy and recognize ways patients' values have been ignored or overridden may still have difficulty respecting patient autonomy unless they are skilled in eliciting their patients' personal values, concerns, and goals.

The consensus of core content for medical ethics education originated in the 1985 report of the DeCamp conference (Culver et al. 1985), where leading physicians and ethicists proposed basic curricular goals in medical ethics and emphasized knowledge and ability as the primary educational targets. Among the seven items described in a minimal basic curriculum were the ability to obtain a valid consent to or refusal of treatment, knowledge of how to proceed if a patient refuses treatment, and knowledge of the moral aspects of the care of patients who have a poor prognosis, including those who are terminally ill. Notably absent from this core list were issues related to financial aspects of medical care (including distributive justice and access to health care), physicians' societal obligations, and questions related to abortion. Also, the Decamp goals were primarily knowledge and skill based. The development and cultivation of critical thinking skills was not a primary emphasis.

Building on the earlier reports, subsequent teaching programs emphasized the importance of ensuring that educational goals are appropriate to students' specific levels of training and future career choices. Courses for first- and second-year medical students, who have limited clinical experience, generally focused on developing an awareness of the complex moral issues that arise in contemporary medicine, the importance of patient values, and developing skill in moral reasoning. In contrast, teaching programs for physicians in residency training programs tended to focus on the specific issues that those physicians were already encountering in their fields of practice and the specific knowledge, attitudes, and skills needed to address those problems.

Attempts to teach medical ethics through the lens of professionalism began in the late 1990s. Professional organizations, such as the American Board of Internal Medicine and the ACGME, define professionalism in terms of virtues, such as altruism, respect for others, honor, integrity, accountability, competence, and duty and advocacy. As such, these organizations' statements typically emphasize a physician's public role in promoting health as it relates to quality and access to care as much as it does to individual patient care (American Board of Internal Medicine Foundation; American College of Physicians–American Society of Internal Medicine Foundation; European Federation of Internal Medicine 2002). Other organizations maintain that the critical foundations for professionalism are the beneficence-based duties of caring for patients in concert with a constellation of requisite virtues (Pellegrino 2002). For example, the Liaison Committee on Medical Education (LCME) (2012,

ED-23) requires a medical education program to "include instruction in medical ethics and human values and require its medical students to exhibit scrupulous ethical principles in caring for patients and in relating to patients' families and to others involved in patient care." Educational programs must teach "medical ethics, human values, and communication skills" in a "learning environment [that] promotes the development of explicit and appropriate professional attributes" (Liaison Committee on Medical Education 2012, MS-31-A). The LCME uses a nonprescriptive assessment method without requiring specific content or hours but with the expectation that each medical school identify achievable outcomes that are attainable by a curriculum in medical ethics and humanities of its own choosing.

The 2001 AAMC (2012) "Graduation Questionnaire," available at the AAMC website, assessed professionalism separately from medical ethics, reflecting confusion between the two content areas, and the minority opinion was that too much professionalism was being taught. The problem appears to be rooted in the conflation of professionalism and comportment, whereby surrogate markers, such as a clean white coat, a proper haircut, and penmanship, are substituted for more substantive skills and behaviors. Although such personal choices may have professional implications, particularly with regard to prioritizing patients' interests over personal interest, they are not a meaningful and comprehensive way to assess professionalism in all its complexity. For medical education, the challenge is not only to sensitize students to these superficial expectations of the profession but also to help them appreciate the unique beneficence-based duties of the medical professional in caring for the patient. As such, linking medical ethics and medical humanities to the pedagogical goals of medical professionalism will require more than the application of simple rules about behavior and etiquette; it will also involve reinforcement of the requisite ethical principles and virtues.

EDUCATIONAL METHODS

A variety of methods have been developed to help students attain the knowledge, attitudes, and skills needed to become proficient in dealing with ethical issues in clinical practice. During the preclinical years, teaching methods typically have included large group lectures that present conceptual and historical overviews of issues in medical ethics, small group discussions of cases from readings or experience, and occasionally exposure to ethics consultation, each of these supplemented by readings and videotapes or films. Less commonly, aspects of ethics and professionalism have been enhanced with history, literature, visual arts, and other creative endeavors (Doukas, McCullough, and Wear 2012).

In clinical education there has been a slow but steady increase in the use of practical teaching exercises that emphasize the communication skills necessary for the identification and resolution of ethical problems. Achieving a thorough conceptual understanding of the doctrine of informed consent, for example, is increasingly understood to be of limited value if physicians are not able to explain information clearly to patients. Preparing the trainee for such encounters using standardized patients facilitates how and what to do with feedback provided by the simulated patient. End-of-life ethics education has been highlighted through increased efforts in medical school and residency palliative care education. An example is the website supported by the End of Life/Palliative Education Resource Center (2012).

By the early 1990s there was widespread agreement that much ethics instruction should be case based to enhance the relevance of clinical ethics in patient care. Moreover, empirical findings support the use of case- or problem-based education in promoting students' knowledge of professional judgments regarding ethical issues and suggest that doing so helps integrate moral reasoning with other tasks of patient care (Goldie 2000; Donaldson, Fistein, and Dunn 2010). Some educators, however, have raised concerns about overreliance on case-based teaching (Barnard 1988; Kass 1990).

First, case discussions typically emphasize problem solving in the context of ethical dilemmas but can ignore everyday issues of clinical ethics (e.g., informed consent in routine office care). To the extent that cases deal with either the beginning or the end of life or an exotic use of technology, issues of daily practice or resource allocation are typically overlooked. Second, by concentrating on what should be done in a specific case, learners risk becoming myopic regarding the myriad institutional and interpersonal factors that may have led to the problem (Levine and Zuckerman 1999; Goold, Williams, and Arnold 2000). Third, case-based approaches often ignore the powerful influences of what Fred Hafferty calls the hidden curriculum, which shapes attitudes and behaviors, and often run counter to formal ethics instruction (Hundert, Hafferty, and Christakis 1996). Finally, whereas cases often raise intellectually interesting ethical dilemmas, ethical conflicts in practice are often attributable to communication problems, and the remedy for this lies outside case-based teaching (Blackall, Simms, and Green 2009).

The role of ethical theory in medical education has been subject to considerable debate. Tom L. Beauchamp and James F. Childress (2009), authors of one of the most widely used texts on medical ethics, emphasize the central role of four principles as both a framework for identifying moral issues and as a structure for moral justification: respect for autonomy, nonmaleficence, beneficence, and justice. Others, such as K. Danner Clouser (1989) and Bernard Gert (Culver et al. 1985), argue against this reliance on principles for both theoretical and pedagogical reasons. In addition to intellectual concerns about the nature of proper moral justification, Clouser and others stress the importance of training students to attend to the highly specific biotechnical, psychological, and social complexities of individual cases in their moral reasoning, arguing that through case discussions students often arrive inductively at general precepts that they can then apply to other cases.

For different reasons, feminist theorists, virtue theorists, and casuists have argued for less emphasis on theoretical principles. Rather than viewing cases as ways to illustrate principles, for example, proponents of casuistry argue that they are the primary locus of moral meaning (Jonsen and Toulmin 1988). Instead of using short, theoretically driven hypothetical cases, casuists encourage the use of real cases that illustrate the complexities and uncertainties of clinical practice. John D. Arras (1991, 32) states that these cases "display the sort of moral complexities and untidiness that demand the (non-deductive) weighing and balancing of competing moral considerations and the casuistical virtues of discernment and practical judgment (*phronesis*)." Feminists have argued for greater attention to social, economic, and political factors and their effect on the nature and dynamics of health care (Sherwin 1992). Virtue theorists and feminist theorists suggest that bioethical discussions should address questions such as what kind of person ought I be and what traits and capacities ought I develop rather than what principles should one use to decide how to proceed in a particular situation (Carse 1991).

In an attempt to enhance students' moral imagination and empathy and to emphasize the narrative aspects of medical ethics, educators have also started to include literature and film in teaching bioethics. These resources compel students to critically reflect on the larger context and meaning of their work and, according to William T. Branch (2000, 505), to "conceptualize and generalize their behavioral changes into their mental structure of knowledge, skills and values."

Technological innovations have spawned new approaches to teaching medical ethics. Computers and the Internet allow, for instance, attempts to combine ethics education and communication skills (an example is the MedEthEx [1998] website). Interactive DVDs dealing with difficult issues challenge learners to examine their positions in a structured manner. Telemedicine allows students at distant sites to interact in real time with faculty trained in medical ethics.

The varied approaches to teaching ethics share limitations. First, until the late twentieth century the day-to-day life and behavior of physicians and trainees had received little attention. Curricula are designed by faculty who are often unaware of the issues that students actually confront (student-run programs have focused more attention on issues that students are concerned about, such as abuse and being asked to violate their personal conscience). Similarly, issues not directly applicable to patient care are discussed less frequently. Second, mirroring the paucity of work in philosophy of medicine, there is little discussion of what it means to be a physician in modern society. The integration of ethics, the humanities, and the social sciences into medical education should help with this situation.

FACULTY AND PROGRAM DEVELOPMENT

As in other areas of medical education, the evolution of teaching in medical ethics has been heavily shaped by the availability (or scarcity) of qualified faculty. Throughout the 1970s and the early 1980s a central debate involved the question of whether medical ethics teachers should be physicians or those trained in the humanities, primarily philosophy and religious studies. Mark Siegler (1978), an early proponent of the physician-ethicist model, emphasizes how clinicians' knowledge and professional experience are central to an understanding of the true complexities and realities of ethical problems in the clinical setting.

Whereas respected clinical teachers can be important role models in shaping students' ethical sensibilities, there are strong reasons for using nonphysicians to teach medical ethics. First, many important aspects of the identification, analysis, and resolution of ethical problems in medicine do not fall within a physician's own specialized training or expertise but depend instead on the intellectual background and analytic skills of individuals trained in other disciplines. Second, involving nonphysicians in teaching medical ethics can help sensitize students to the importance of other viewpoints and improve physicians' ability to communicate with nonphysicians—two primary educational goals. A consensus is developing that individuals from a variety of disciplines have important and distinct contributions to make. Counterproductive competition has been obviated at many institutions through team teaching, in which clinicians and nonclinicians play off each other's strengths and bring a broader perspective into the educational arena.

The growth of ethics education has been limited more by a scarcity of trained faculty than by disputes regarding their academic backgrounds. Historically, many programs depended on faculty who, despite an interest in medical ethics, had little formal background in the field. Although this problem has abated with the creation of both short courses and master's programs in medical ethics, faculty who teach ethics nevertheless face barriers to their teaching, including financial and time constraints, students' attitudes toward medical ethics, and a lack of reinforcement by other faculty (Strong, Connelly, and Forrow 1992). Furthermore, ethics teaching programs continue to occupy a tenuous position in most medical schools.

Although the inclusion of ethics test questions in certifying examinations has improved the situation, ethics education rarely achieves parity with the traditional biotechnical basic sciences and clinical training. In part the undervaluing of ethics is a consequence of the culture of medicine, but economic constraints also are a limiting factor. Ethics education conducted in small groups is faculty intensive, and funding for teaching programs and curricular time has decreased. This has happened during a period in which physicians are under increasing pressure to generate income, further limiting the availability of trained facilitators. The early twenty-first-century emphasis on problem-based learning, professionalism, and ethics may result in increased recognition of curricular relevance and the need for teaching resources.

EVALUATION

Evaluation, both of ethics teaching programs themselves and of individual students, remains in flux. Many formal courses use a pass-fail grading system based on class participation and written exercises, either papers or in-class essay examinations. These efforts convey to students the importance of medical ethics in the medical school (as has the addition of questions to the national board examination and many of the specialty board examinations). Although outcomes-based evaluation techniques have evolved with guidance from the ACGME and the LCME, there remains a lack of clarity about which specific teaching goals are most important in ethics and professionalism, about how best to measure whether such goals have been reached, and about realistic expectations of ethics courses (Arnold 2002). Underlying the challenge of evaluating the effect of teaching medical ethics is a deeper debate regarding what the outcome of teaching ethics ought to be.

As an academic discipline, ethics can be taught and has been for centuries. Evaluating the efficacy of that teaching is challenging, however. In medical schools, most efforts have focused on analysis of student essays and/or class participation, but it is by no means clear that such measurement is a meaningful way to determine whether students have the requisite knowledge, attitudes, and skills to deliver effective and appropriate medical care.

In arguing for the importance of formal ethics education, teachers of medical ethics typically have emphasized more ambitious goals, such as improving students' ability to address ethical issues in clinical practice or promoting humanistic qualities and integrity. The ACGME has created an evaluation toolbox for measuring knowledge that includes interactions with standardized patients, objective structured clinical examinations, observed and recorded patient interactions, patient surveys, and 360-degree evaluations (Durning, Hemmer, and Pangaro 2007). Attempts to develop innovative methods of evaluation have included measuring students' skills in moral reasoning and evaluation of students' behavior by nonphysicians, such as nurses and patients. These exercises have attempted to move beyond merely evaluating cognitive skills to analyzing students' actual behavior.

Although the efforts at ethics evaluation show a great deal of promise as formative educational tools, few medical schools use these tools for summative evaluation. Limitations in their psychometric properties and the large number of raters needed for reliable ratings have limited their general use. The numerous potential methodological problems and construct validity issues, particularly in evaluating ethical behavior and character, are compounded in attempts to determine whether improvements are attributable to formal ethics teaching. Nevertheless, with the shift toward outcomes-based education, ethics—along with anatomy, biochemistry, and physiology—will have to prove effective and relevant to patient care.

Whereas formal teaching programs in medical ethics were practically nonexistent in 1970, by the early 2010s there was extraordinary diversity both in the United States and elsewhere with regard to how ethics is taught. Bioethics education in the early twenty-first century is an accepted part of education for students in almost all medical schools and for residents in many programs. The challenge will be to figure out how the profession can articulate outcomes-based goals in medical ethics education, measure them meaningfully, and meet them.

Many questions remain only partially answered. What should be the primary goals of such teaching—analytic ability, behavioral skills, or actual practice? What is the relationship between professionalism and medical ethics? How should those goals vary according to the developmental stage of the health professional and according to the person's specific field of practice within medicine? How can (or should) ethical attention be expanded beyond conflicts at the beginning and the end of life to the day-to-day activities of being a physician? What teaching methods are most effective and efficient in accomplishing curricular goals in each of the various settings? What is the proper role of formal evaluation efforts, both of individual students and of overall teaching programs? What methods of evaluation are both valid and feasible? The challenge of these questions ensures that medical ethics education will continue to evolve.

This is a revised version of the entry that was first written by Robert M. Arnold and Lachlan Forrow in 1995.

SEE ALSO *Casuistry; Conscience, Rights of; Literature and Health Care; Medicine, Anthropology of; Medicine, Profession of; Narrative; Nursing, Profession of; Profession and Professional Ethics*

BIBLIOGRAPHY

Accreditation Council for Graduate Medical Education. 2011. "Common Program Requirements." Approved July 1. http://www.acgme.org/acgmeweb/Portals/0/dh_dutyhoursCommonPR07012007.pdf

American Board of Internal Medicine, Subcommittee on Evaluation of Humanistic Qualities in the Internist. 1983. "Evaluation of Humanistic Qualities in the Internist." *Annals of Internal Medicine* 99 (5): 720–24.

American Board of Internal Medicine Foundation; American College of Physicians–American Society of Internal Medicine Foundation; European Federation of Internal Medicine. 2002. "Medical Professionalism in the New Millennium: A Physician Charter." *Annals of Internal Medicine* 136 (3): 243–46.

American Board of Pediatrics, Medical Ethics Subcommittee. 1987. "Teaching and Evaluation of Interpersonal Skills and Ethical Decision Making in Pediatrics." *Pediatrics* 79 (5): 829–34.

Arnold, Louise. 2002. "Assessing Professional Behavior: Yesterday, Today, and Tomorrow." *Academic Medicine* 77 (6): 502–15.

Arras, John D. 1991. "Getting Down to Cases: The Revival of Casuistry in Bioethics." *Journal of Medical Philosophy* 16 (1): 29–51.

Association of American Medical Colleges. 2012. "Graduation Questionnaire." https://www.aamc.org/data/gq/questionnaires.

Barnard, David. 1988. "Residency Ethics Teaching: A Critique of Current Trends." *Archives of Internal Medicine* 148 (8): 1836–38.

Baylis, Françoise, and Jocelyn Downie. 1991. "Ethics Education for Canadian Medical Students." *Academic Medicine* 66 (7): 413–14.

Beauchamp, Tom L., and James F. Childress. 2009. *Principles of Biomedical Ethics*. 6th ed. New York: Oxford University Press.

Bickel, Janet W. 1986. *Integrating Human Values Teaching Programs into Medical Students' Clinical Education.* Washington, DC: Association of American Medical Colleges.

Blackall, George F.; Steve S. Simms; and Michael J. Green. 2009. *Breaking the Cycle: How to Turn Conflict into Collaboration When You and Your Patients Disagree*. Philadelphia: American College of Physicians Press.

Bosk, Charles L. 1979. *Forgive and Remember: Managing Medical Failure*. Chicago: University of Chicago Press.

Boyd, Kenneth M., ed. 1987. *Report of a Working Party on the Teaching of Medical Ethics*. London: Institute of Medical Ethics.

Branch, William T., Jr. 2000. "Supporting the Moral Development of Medical Students." *Journal of General Internal Medicine* 15 (7): 503–8.

Burling, S. J.; J. S. Lumley; L. S. McCarthy; et al. 1990. "Review of the Teaching of Medical Ethics in London Medical Schools." *Journal of Medical Ethics* 16 (4): 206–9.

Callahan, Daniel. 1980. "Goals in the Teaching of Ethics." In *Ethics Teaching in Higher Education*, edited by Daniel Callahan and Sissela Bok, 61–74. New York: Plenum.

Carse, Alisa L. 1991. "The 'Voice of Care': Implications for Bioethical Education." *Journal of Medicine and Philosophy* 16 (1): 5–28.

Clouser, K. Danner. 1989. "Ethical Theory and Applied Ethics: Reflections on Connections." In *Clinical Ethics: Theory and Practice*, edited by C. Barry Hoffmaster, Benjamin Freedman, and Gwen Fraser, 161–82. Clifton, NJ: Humana.

Cooke, Molly; David M. Irby; William Sullivan; Kenneth M. Ludmerer. 2006. "American Medical Education 100 Years after the Flexner Report." *New England Journal of Medicine* 355 (13): 1339–44.

Culver, Charles M.; K. Danner Clouser; Bernard Gert; et al. 1985. "Basic Curricular Goals in Medical Ethics." *New England Journal of Medicine* 312 (4): 253–56.

De Wachter, Maurice A. M. 1978. "Teaching Medical Ethics: University of Nijmegen, The Netherlands." *Journal of Medical Ethics* 4 (2): 84–88.

Donaldson, Thomas M.; Elizabeth Fistein; and Michael Dunn. 2010. "Case-Based Seminars in Medical Ethics Education: How Medical Students Define and Discuss Moral Problems." *Journal of Medical Ethics* 36 (12): 816–20.

Doukas, David J. 2003. "Where Is the Virtue in Professionalism?" *Cambridge Quarterly of Healthcare Ethics* 12 (2): 147–54.

Doukas, David J.; Laurence B. McCullough; and Steven Wear. 2010. "Reforming Medical Education in Ethics and Humanities by Finding Common Ground with Abraham Flexner." *Academic Medicine* 85 (2): 318–23.

Doukas, David J.; Laurence B. McCullough; and Stephen Wear. 2012. "Perspective: Medical Education in Medical Ethics and Humanities as the Foundation for Developing Medical Professionalism." *Academic Medicine* 87 (3): 334–41.

Drane, James F. 1988. *Becoming a Good Doctor: The Place of Virtue and Character in Medical Ethics*. Kansas City, MO: Sheed and Ward.

Durning, Steven J.; Paul Hemmer; and Louis N. Pangaro. 2007. "The Structure of Program Evaluation: An Approach for Evaluating a Course, Clerkship, or Components of a Residency or Fellowship Training Program." *Teaching and Learning in Medicine* 19 (3): 308–18.

End of Life/Palliative Education Resource Center. "About EPERC." 2012. http://www.eperc.mcw.edu

Flexner, Abraham. 1925. *Medical Education: A Comparative Study*. New York: Macmillan.

Flexner, Abraham, and Henry S. Pritchett. 1910. *Medical Education in the United States and Canada: A Report to the Carnegie Foundation for the Advancement of Teaching*. Bulletin 4. Boston: Merrymount.

Fox, Ellen; Robert M. Arnold; and Baruch Brody. 1995. "Medical Ethics Education: Past, Present, and Future." *Academic Medicine* 70 (9): 761–68.

Goldie, John. 2000. "Review of Ethics Curricula in Undergraduate Medical Education." *Medical Education* 34 (2): 108–19.

Goold, Susan Dorr; Brent Williams; and Robert M. Arnold. 2000. "Conflicts Regarding Decisions to Limit Treatment: A Differential Diagnosis." *Journal of the American Medical Association* 283 (7): 909–14.

Hundert, Edward M.; Fred Hafferty; and Dimitri Christakis. 1996. "Characteristics of the Informal Curriculum and Trainees' Ethical Choices." *Academic Medicine* 71 (6): 624–33.

Jonsen, Albert R., and Steven Toulmin. 1988. *The Abuse of Casuistry: A History of Moral Reasoning*. Berkeley: University of California Press.

Kass, Leon R. 1990. "Practicing Ethics: Where's the Action?" *Hastings Center Report* 20 (1): 5–12.

Lehmann, Lisa S.; Willard S. Kasoff; Phoebe Koch; and Daniel D. Federman. 2004. "A Survey of Medical Ethics Education at U.S. and Canadian Medical Schools." *Academic Medicine* 79 (7): 682–89.

Levine, Carol, and Connie Zuckerman. 1999. "The Trouble with Families: Toward an Ethic of Accommodation." *Annals of Internal Medicine* 130 (2): 148–52.

Levine, Carol, and Connie Zuckerman. 2000. "Hands On/Hands Off: Why Health Care Professionals Depend on Families but Keep Them at Arm's Length." *Journal of Law and Medical Ethics* 28 (1): 5–18.

Liaison Committee on Medical Education. 2012. "Functions and Structure of a Medical School: LCME Accreditation Standards." Accessed May 24, 2012. http://www.lcme.org/connections.htm

McKneally, Martin F., and Peter A. Singer. 2001. "Bioethics for Clinicians: 25; Teaching Bioethics in the Clinical Setting." *Canadian Medical Association Journal* 164 (8): 1163–67.

MedEthEx. 1998. "Exercises in Medical Ethics and Communications Skills." http://webcampus.drexelmed.edu/medethex/index.html

Miles, Steven H.; Laura Weiss Lane; Janet Bickel; et al. 1989. "Medical Ethics Education: Coming of Age." *Academic Medicine* 64 (12): 705–14.

Olukoya, A. A. 1984. "A Workshop on Medical Ethics at the College of Medicine, Lagos University." *Journal of Medical Ethics* 10 (4): 199–200.

Pellegrino, Edmund D. 2002. "Professionalism, Profession, and the Virtues of the Good Physician." *Mount Sinai Journal of Medicine* 69 (6): 378–84.

Pellegrino, Edmund D.; Richard J. Hart Jr.; Sharon R. Henderson; and Gary Edwards. 1985. "Relevance and Utility of Courses in Medical Ethics: A Survey of Physicians' Perceptions." *Journal of the American Medical Association* 253 (1): 49–53.

Povar, Gail J., and Karla J. Keith. 1984. "The Teaching of Liberal Arts in Internal Medicine Residency Training." *Journal of Medical Education* 59 (9): 714–21.

Sherwin, Susan. 1992. *No Longer Patient: Feminist Ethics and Health Care*. Philadelphia: Temple University Press.

Siegler, Mark. 1978. "A Legacy of Osler: Teaching Clinical Ethics at the Bedside." *Journal of the American Medical Association* 239 (10): 951–56.

Strong, Carson; Julia E. Connelly; and Lachlan Forrow. 1992. "Teachers' Perceptions of Difficulties in Teaching Ethics in Residencies." *Academic Medicine* 67 (6): 398–402.

Veatch, Robert M., and Sharmon Solitto. 1976. "Medical Ethics Teaching: Report of a National Medical School Survey." *Journal of the American Medical Association* 235 (10): 1030–33.

Working Group on Behalf of the Association of Teachers of Ethics and Law in Australian and New Zealand Medical Schools. 2001. "An Ethics Core Curriculum for Australasian Medical Schools." *Medical Journal of Australia* 175 (4): 205–10.

David J. Doukas
William Ray Moore Endowed Chair of Family Medicine and Medical Humanism; Professor, Department of Family and Geriatric Medicine; Director, Division of Medical Humanism and Ethics; Codirector, Interdisciplinary Master of Arts: Bioethics and Medical Humanities, University of Louisville

Michael J. Green
Professor, Departments of Humanities and Medicine; Vice Chair for Research, Department of Humanities; Chair, Hospital Ethics Committee, Penn State College of Medicine

Robert M. Arnold
Leo H. Criep Chair in Patient Care, University of Pittsburgh Medical Center Palliative and Supportive Institute; Professor of Medicine, Division of General Internal Medicine, University of Pittsburgh Medical Center Palliative and Supportive Institute
Chief, Section on Palliative Care and Medical Ethics, University of Pittsburgh Medical Center Palliative and Supportive Institute; Chief Medical Officer, University of Pittsburgh Medical Center Palliative and Supportive Institute; Director, Institute for Doctor-Patient Communication, University of Pittsburgh School of Medicine

II. NURSING

Ethics has received increased attention in nursing education programs, but problems remain. This entry provides an overview of nursing ethics education in the United States and in other countries, addressing both the advances made and the issues remaining.

NURSING ETHICS EDUCATION IN THE UNITED STATES

Nursing ethics has been incorporated to some degree in nursing education since the early twentieth century. In the early 1900s ethics was taught as a science necessary to the education of the competent nurse who put patient safety and welfare first (Robb 1900). Ethics teaching, reflecting religious and military influences, focused on the character and ethics of the nurse, the virtues required of nurses (e.g., loyalty and obedience), the duties and obligations nurses owed physicians and the hospitals that employed them, and proper etiquette for nurses. Obligations that nurses have as citizens of the community to participate in public policy and political areas to achieve health care goals first emerged in the *Code of Ethics* proposed by the American Nurses Association (2001) in 1926 and adopted in 1950, as well as in the nursing literature of the first half of the twentieth century (Goodrich 1932; Densford and Everett 1946; Fowler 1997). These wider obligations of nurses as citizens continue to be a very minor theme in nursing ethics education.

Ethics as a distinct part of the nursing curriculum almost disappeared in the 1950s and 1960s, except in programs affiliated with religious traditions and institutions. The 1970s brought renewed attention to nursing ethics education, partly because of the resurgence of medical ethics and the appearance of bioethics in the professional and academic worlds. These were responses to challenges emerging from medical technologies, abuses in research, and changes in the health care environment, challenges for which no ready-made responses were available. Some nursing educators and philosophers recognized, however, that nurses faced ethical issues and challenges different from those faced by physicians, largely because of nurses' positions as employees rather than as independent professionals in health care organizations. Both the National Student Nurses Association and the American Nurses Association passed resolutions calling for more attention to ethics in nursing education programs.

A survey conducted to assess the status of ethics teaching in accredited baccalaureate and graduate nursing programs (Aroskar 1977) disclosed that most schools offered limited opportunities for the study of the ethical aspects of nursing and that these opportunities were often integrated into other nursing courses. Only 7 percent of the programs required work in ethics or medical ethics. Codes of ethics such as the *Code for Nurses* (ANA 1976) were identified as priority content in ethics courses, followed by patients' rights and obligations. No nursing faculty had primary responsibilities for teaching ethics.

Beginning in the late 1970s and early 1980s, nursing ethics education that incorporates values clarification and a more philosophical, principled approach to ethical issues received increased attention in nursing programs. This continuing development, however, depends on administrative support and faculty priorities, interests, and expertise, and the exact approach taken varies greatly from school to school. A few nursing programs have full-time faculty in teaching and research activities devoted to ethics in nursing. Usually these are schools with master's and doctoral programs in nursing that offer studies in ethics, bioethics, and philosophy as electives or as a minor field. Teaching resources such as textbooks and nursing journal articles on ethics have increased significantly. Since 1975, activities to enhance the teaching of ethics in nursing have been supported by the Joseph P. Kennedy, Jr., Foundation, the National Endowment for the Humanities, the Hastings Center, the Fund for the Improvement of Postsecondary Education, and other institutions. There are more than fifty-five academic bioethics centers in the United States offering undergraduate, graduate, or continuing education courses in bioethics. Few, however, have dedicated programs or joint appointments for nursing ethics education.

Baccalaureate education provides the foundations for professional nursing practice that requires knowledge of the ethical obligations of the profession and ethical decision-making skills for the practitioner. Not all baccalaureate nursing programs have required or elective courses in ethics. Ethics education is still not required for program accreditation. Where ethics is a required curriculum component, content may be offered through separate courses or modules (Payton 1980); integrated throughout the curriculum in existing courses (Ryden et al. 1989); or presented in some combination of separate courses and integrated approaches in the classroom and clinical settings. New approaches focus on case discussion, writing portfolios, and web-based interaction to encourage the application of core concepts to clinically encountered situations (Ellenchild Pinch and Graves 2000; Sorrell et al. 1997). An overall goal is to develop morally accountable practitioners who have a clear conceptual framework and the skills for ethical decision making in practice (Cassells and Redman 1989; Fry 1989). Ethics education is required core content for master's education in nursing and for the preparation of advanced practice nurses (AACN 1996; ANA 1996; Kenney 1996).

Sara T. Fry, in a 1989 article, identified the following four models of ethics teaching used in undergraduate and graduate nursing programs and clinical settings:

The *moral-concepts model* incorporates three general areas: the historical foundations of the nursing ethic, including codes of ethics and medical versus nursing ethics; the value dimensions of nursing, such as advocacy, loyalty, and moral obligations; and the skills needed for ethical decision making.

The *moral-issues model* focuses on common moral problems in health care relationships, such as confidentiality and informed consent, and issues of moral concern in health care, such as abortion, termination of treatment, and allocation of health care resources. Course content includes historical and contemporary legal cases that illustrate the legal and ethical aspects of specific issues in patient care.

The *clinical-practice model*, developed by bioethicists and nurse ethicists, incorporates clinical conferences on moral issues in patient care (usually specific to a clinical area), case-study presentations, and ethics rounds that focus on ethical issues pertaining to a patient's care rather than to a patient's clinical condition.

The *ethics-inquiry model*, found primarily at the graduate level, incorporates the forms of traditional philosophical inquiry such as descriptive, normative, and metaethics; explores diverse methods of ethical inquiry; and looks at the relationship of ethical inquiry to other forms of inquiry in science and nursing. Additional topics in ethics education include the role of the nurse as a moral agent; the roles of gender and ethnicity in nursing ethics; the major ethical theories and principles and their application in nursing practice; and the ethics of nursing research.

Since the early 1990s, caring as a foundation of nursing ethics has received a great deal of attention (Bishop and Scudder 1991; Harbison 1992). Curriculum change based on theories of caring has been proposed and, in many places, implemented. Strong critiques of theories of caring and the ethics of care persist, however, and the success of these curricular changes has yet to be established.

The ethics of end-of-life care and pain management have also received much attention since the mid-1990s. Reviews of standard nursing texts found very little content related to pain management, end-of-life care, or the ethical issues at the end of life (Ferrell, Grant, and Virani 1999). Concern over these shortcomings was mobilized into national projects to develop resources for teaching nurses the clinical skills needed for pain and symptom management as well as an understanding of the myriad ethical issues that arise in the provision of end-of-life care. The End-of-Life Nursing Education Consortium project developed a standardized curriculum on end-of-life care and provided train-the-trainer programs for nursing school faculty, continuing education providers, and state boards of nursing across the country (AACN 1996). The Toolkit for Nurturing Excellence at End-of-Life Transition was provided free of charge to all nursing schools (Wells et al. 2002). This computerized learning tool, provided on CD-ROM, contains multimedia components such as audio, video, graphics, photographs, and animation to create an interactive program. Both of these projects contain specific ethics content as a prominent component of the suggested curricula.

Examples of specific outcome objectives for nursing ethics education include the following:

- Identification of ethical dilemmas in the delivery of nursing care
- Identification of the components of an ethical decision-making framework
- Participation in ethical decision making in client care
- Leadership participation in ethics rounds and institutional ethics committees
- Analysis of impediments to the ethical practice of nursing
- Distinguishing the ethical elements of nursing practice from medical or technical elements
- Analysis of nursing codes as they relate to client advocacy.

There are underlying tensions and ongoing debates in nursing ethics education. Argument continues over the question of whether nursing ethics does or should exist as a separate field of inquiry. Differences have arisen between those who teach ethics based on cognitive-moral-development theory and those who teach ethics based on moral philosophy and ethical theory. Evaluation of the effectiveness of ethics teaching has been a continuing challenge. Although research on ethics in nursing education has been expanding, it needs to be developed more systematically if it is to contribute to effective curriculum change (Silva and Sorrell 1991). A shortage of adequately prepared faculty and overcrowded nursing curricula impede ethics teaching in nursing programs.

NURSING ETHICS EDUCATION IN OTHER COUNTRIES

The fact that nursing ethics education in the international arena varies so greatly reflects the state of nursing and nursing education, as well as the priority of health care problems and issues, in many different countries. The lack of systematic, international information about nursing ethics education creates problems in providing a general overview of the topic.

The International Council of Nurses (ICN), based in Geneva, Switzerland, in an effort to address the uneven development of nursing ethics education, has provided ethics education through publications, programs, and conferences. The ICN's code of ethics serves as the nursing code in many countries. The code was revised in 2000. Because these countries have different histories, cultures, and priorities, the question arises as to whether or not all countries have common ethical values and principles regarding nursing and nursing education. In addition, much of nursing ethics education in the United States focuses on the issues that arise from advanced medical technology, whereas the main issue in many other countries is primary health care. More recently, numerous countries have developed their own codes of ethics for nurses.

Since the early 1990s, the ICN has scheduled a special interest group in nursing ethics at its major open international meetings. This has been very successful in identifying nurses around the world with this professional focus.

The *Journal of Nursing Ethics*, which was first published in 1994, provides an arena for information and research from an international perspective. In conjunction with the journal, the editors and editorial board members established an International Centre for Nursing Ethics at the University of Surrey, England, that provides a place for researchers and educators to visit or come for more extended work.

In the United Kingdom nursing education is well developed, and higher education has been available to nurses for many years. In some colleges or departments of nursing, ethics is either taught as a separate course or integrated into other courses. During recent decades, the Royal College of Nursing actively articulated nursing ethics. In addition, nursing educators and others have published numerous papers, research reports, and books focused on nursing ethics. A major British nursing journal includes an ethics column that deals with clinical ethical problems. The Center for Midwifery and Nursing Ethics in London publishes a newsletter, runs educational programs, and serves as a clearinghouse for ethics materials. In 1990 Swansea University, Wales, sponsored the first national conference on nursing ethics and nursing ethics education. Swansea has also sponsored conferences on nursing philosophy, and in 2000 it began publishing a journal with this title that includes ethics articles (de Raeve 2002).

In Canada, numerous conferences have focused on nursing ethics and ethics education. An annual conference to discuss philosophy and nursing touches on many ethical themes. Several schools of nursing have invited visiting professors to teach ethics and have prepared some Canadian nursing professors to teach this subject as well. Canada revised its own nursing code of ethics in 2002.

The ethics committee of the Swiss Nursing Association wrote a code of ethics in the 1980s and has been instrumental in increasing nurses' awareness of the need for more systematic approaches to teaching ethics in nursing programs. The association includes in its annual conference papers on ethics in curriculum content and clinical practice. For some years, one nursing educator has taught courses in Switzerland and France on ethical issues in dying and death, with a special focus on suffering.

Nursing educators in Finland have offered seminars around the country on nursing ethics. One nursing educator has published a book on the topic. Several nursing educators in Finland and other Nordic countries have conducted research on ethical questions and have participated in multinational research projects examining selected ethical issues.

The board of directors of the Center for Medical Ethics at the University of Oslo, Norway, consists of people from diverse health-related professions. It continues to work with nursing educators and nursing researchers in developing educational programs and research focused on ethical issues.

Universities in both Norway and Sweden have invited nursing educators from overseas to lecture on nursing ethics. The annual, weeklong seminar held in Sweden for doctoral students in nursing, which has either a primary or secondary focus on nursing ethics, has been of special interest because of its potential impact on nursing education. Extensive research on the ethics of various clinical problems with elderly patients has been undertaken at the University of Umea, Sweden. In Stockholm, two nursing educators teach and conduct research in nursing ethics.

One nursing educator in Budapest developed an ethics course for nursing students and wrote a textbook to use in this education. Another nursing educator teaches an ethics class at the Academy of Medicine in Lublin, Poland. In the Baltic States and eastern Europe, physicians often are the major or only faculty teaching in nursing schools. For example, Estonia has a shortage of nurses prepared to teach nursing. In this context, emphasis has been placed on the medical model, and little, if any, ethics has been included because the teachers have had limited exposure to ethics content. Nursing leaders in Estonia and other countries with similar problems are developing alternatives to this situation.

Within Latin America, Colombia has been the most active in nursing ethics education. The National Association of Nursing Schools has an ethics committee working with schools of nursing, the Ministry of Health, and the national nursing association to increase ethical content in nursing education. The ethics committee sponsors workshops on nursing ethics and has been involved in research projects on nursing ethics. Chile has a nurse who has dealt with ethical issues working in the national nursing association. Nursing educators in Brazil teach nursing ethics and conduct research on ethics topics. Increasingly, nurses, and colleagues in other professions, are developing collaborative activities in teaching and research in health care ethics. Some of these activities involve Spain.

Australian nursing education throughout the country has supported conferences, seminars, and consultation in nursing ethics. One nursing ethicist in Melbourne has taught in a nursing program and has published several books in the field. The Centre for Human Bioethics, located at Monash University's Clayton campus and established in 1980, examined the state of nursing ethics in Australia and has continued to work with nurses seeking education in ethics. In Queensland, a professor in the university nursing department served as a member of the research ethics committee at her institution. Both Australian and New Zealand nurses contribute regularly to the nursing ethics literature.

Numerous nursing educators present papers at the ongoing World Conference on Bioethics, Medical Ethics, and Health Law, which has also had a Swedish nurse serve on its board. In Israel, Jewish ethics has been taught throughout the nursing curricula, and several educators conduct research in health care ethics.

The High Institute of Nursing at the University of Alexandria, Egypt, held a nursing ethics conference in 1993 on ethics in education and practice. More recently, the Aga Khan University School of Nursing, Pakistan, held a conference and invited a keynote paper on nursing ethics.

In Asia, the People's Republic of China has developed eleven bachelor of science in nursing programs. The curriculum has included an ethics course that combines Confucian and Maoist ethics. The political slogan "serve the people" translates in nursing into respect for patients as persons. One Hong Kong educator conducted extensive research focused on nursing ethics in China. Korean nursing has developed an interest in ethics that manifests the influences of Christian missionary work. At Japan's national and international nursing research conferences, nurses present papers on nursing ethics from a clinical and an educational perspective. The Japanese Association for Bioethics includes nurses as speakers and participants in its conferences. The Japanese Nursing Association has an ethics committee, and, increasingly, the many new colleges of nursing are developing research ethics committees.

This discussion reflects the great differences and many activities in nursing ethics education on the international scene. The lack of teachers and resources to teach nursing ethics remains a serious problem in many countries. Yet one of the most striking developments in nursing ethics education is the amount of international research being conducted. Collaboration among Europeans and among European, Asian, and North and South American nursing colleagues has increased and provides a rich source of data for teaching.

CONCLUSION

The last two decades of the twentieth century saw a significant, worldwide resurgence and expansion of nursing ethics education activities and programs. These efforts varied greatly. Many serious challenges remain for the twenty-first century, including a lack of formal ethics teaching in many programs, inadequate resources such as prepared nursing faculty to teach ethics, and the need for evaluations of the impact of existing nursing ethics education courses and programs on nursing practice.

BIBLIOGRAPHY

AACN (American Association of Colleges of Nursing). 1986. *Essentials of College and University Education for Professional Nursing: Final Report.* Washington, DC: Author.

AACN (American Association of Colleges of Nursing). 1996. *The Essentials of Master's Education for Advanced Practice Nursing.* Washington, DC: Author.

ANA (American Nurses' Association). 1976. *Code for Nurses with Interpretive Statements.* Kansas City, MO: Author.

ANA (American Nurses Association). 1996. *Scope and Standards of Advanced Practice Registered Nursing.* Washington, DC: Author.

ANA (American Nurses Association). 2001. *Code of Ethics for Nurses with Interpretive Statements.* Washington, DC: Author.

Aroskar, Mila A. 1977. "Ethics in the Nursing Curriculum." *Nursing Outlook* 25 (4): 260–64.

Bishop, Anne H., and John R. Scudder Jr. 1991. *Nursing: The Practice of Caring.* New York: National League for Nursing Press.

Blasszauer, Robert, and Elisabeth Rozsos. 1991. "Ethics Teaching for Hungarian Nurses." *Bulletin of Medical Ethics* 69:22–23.

Cassells, Judith M., and Barbara K. Redman. 1989. "Preparing Students to Be Moral Agents in Clinical Nursing Practice: Report of a National Study." *Nursing Clinics of North America* 24 (2): 463–73.

Davis, Anne J.; Bonnie Davidson; Miriam Hirschfield; et al. 1993. "An International Perspective of Active Euthanasia: Attitudes of Nurses in Seven Countries." *International Journal of Nursing Studies* 30 (4): 301–10.

Densford, Katharine J., and Millard S. Everett. 1946. *Ethics for Modern Nurses.* Philadelphia: W. B. Saunders.

de Raeve, Louise. 2002. "Trust and Trustworthiness in Nurse–Patient Relationships." *Nursing Philosophy* 3 (2): 152–62.

Ellenchild Pinch, Winifred J., and Janet K. Graves. 2000. "Using Web-Based Discussion as a Teaching Strategy: Bioethics as an Exemplar." *Journal of Advanced Nursing* 32 (3): 704–12.

Ferrell, Betty R.; Marcia Grant; and Rose Virani. 1999. "Strengthening Nursing Education to Improve End-of-Life Care." *Nursing Outlook* 47 (6): 252–56.

Fowler, Marsha D. M. 1997. "Nursing's Ethics." In *Ethical Dilemmas and Nursing Practice*, 4th ed., edited by Anne J. Davis, Mila A. Aroskar, Joan Liaschenko, and Theresa S. Drought, 17–34. Stamford, CT: Appleton and Lange.

Fry, Sara T. 1989. "Teaching Ethics in Nursing Curricula: Traditional and Contemporary Models." *Nursing Clinics of North America* 24 (2): 485–97.

Goodrich, Annie Warburton. 1932. *The Social and Ethical Significance of Nursing: A Series of Addresses.* New York: Macmillan.

Harbison, Jean. 1992. "Gilligan: A Voice for Nursing?" *Journal of Medical Ethics* 18 (4): 202–5.

International Centre for Nursing Ethics. 2013. Accessed May 8. http://www.surrey.ac.uk/fhms/research/centres/icne/

International Council of Nurses. 2013. "Code of Ethics for Nurses." Accessed May 8. http://www.icn.ch/about-icn/code-of-ethics-for-nurses/

Kenney, Janet W., ed. 1996. *Philosophical and Theoretical Perspectives for Advanced Nursing Practice.* Boston: Jones and Bartlett.

Payton, Rita J. 1980. "A Bioethical Program for Baccalaureate Nursing Students." In *Ethics in Nursing Practice and Education*, 53–65. Kansas City, MO: American Nurses' Association.

Robb, Isabel Hampton. 1900. *Nursing Ethics: For Hospital and Private Use.* Cleveland, OH: Koeckert.

Ryden, Muriel B.; Laura Duckett; Patricia Crisham; et al. 1989. "Multi-course Sequential Learning as a Model for Content Integration: Ethics as a Prototype." *Journal of Nursing Education* 28 (3): 102–6.

Silva, Mary Cipriano, and Jeanne Merkle Sorrell. 1991. *Research on Ethics in Nursing Education: An Integrative Review and Critique.* New York: National League for Nursing Press.

Sorrell, Jeanne Merkle; Hazel N. Brown; Mary Cipriano Silva; et al. 1997. "Use of Writing Portfolios for Interdisciplinary Assessment of Critical Thinking Outcomes of Nursing Students." *Nursing Forum* 32 (4): 12–24.

Wells, Marjorie J.; Diana J. Wilkie; Marie-Annette Brown; et al. 2002. "Technology Available in Nursing Programs: Implications for Developing Virtual End-of-Life Educational Tools." *Journal of Cancer Education* 17 (2): 92–96.

Mila A. Aroskar (1995)
Professor Emerita, Center for Bioethics, University of Minnesota

Anne J. Davis (1995, 2004)
Professor Emerita, School of Nursing, University of California, San Francisco

Theresa Drought (2004)
Bioethics Director, Kaiser Permanente, Woodland Hills, CA

II: NURSING [ADDENDUM]

In the previous edition of this encyclopedia (2004), Mila A. Aroscar, Anne J. Davis, and Theresa Drought described bioethics education in nursing as central to the goal of developing "morally accountable practitioners who have a clear conceptual framework and the skills for ethical decision making in practice." The challenge for nursing bioethics education today is to go beyond the nurse's acknowledgment of moral accountability and capacity for ethical decision making. The challenge is to prepare nurses to successfully integrate ethical decisions into the care of patients. Enacting ethical decisions requires that nurses be able to develop strategies for successful implementation and that they have the legitimate authority to carry out the ethical course of action. Thus, recent theory development and research in nursing ethics education focus on the primacy of educating nurses in ways that prepare them to

- reason about their obligations as professional nurses;
- communicate collaboratively and persuasively in interprofessional care teams; and
- create within complex health care systems the professional authority to practice ethically.

When nurses are able to reason and to communicate persuasively, and when they are full partners in interprofessional decisions about patient care, the stage is set for the next important phase of nursing bioethics education—the development of nursing ethics practice theory that guides the implementation of ethical patient care.

Practice theory produces the outline for practice (Varcoe et al. 2004). A practice theory of nursing ethics would produce guidelines for implementing ethics in everyday practice. Ethics practice theory would set objectives for upholding ethical practice within the specific settings in which nurses and other professionals provide care. Once objectives are set, organizational change theory would be used to identify actions to meet the objectives.

Nursing practice is immersed in context, so practice-level theories of nursing ethics must be developed from the perspective of what transpires between patients and nurses in the daily routines and practice settings of nursing care. This perspective must take into account the particular and specific factors that have ethical relevance within the situations of unique individuals whose constellation of good and harm is absolutely idiosyncratic. Ethical theory developed to the level of practice not only will encompass ideals and standards but also will prescribe the organizational structures, role authorities, and procedures to be followed to ensure that ethical decisions are implemented in patient care.

It is likely that nursing ethics theory, research, and education will be affected profoundly by national and international recognition that safe and high-quality patient care requires the collaborative functioning of a team of multidisciplinary health care professionals (Frenk, Chen, and Bhutta 2010; Interprofessional Education Collaborative Expert Panel 2011). Within the United States, the United Kingdom, Canada, and the World Health Organization, as a part of efforts to improve health care, there is growing attention to the functioning of interprofessional teams. Recommendations of the Institute of Medicine include that nurses should be full partners, with physicians and other health care professionals, in redesigning health care in the United States (see Committee on the Robert Wood Johnson Foundation Initiative 2011). It is likely that other countries will follow this trend as their health care systems change to meet the demands for accessible, affordable high-quality health care.

As nurses increasingly become full partners in interprofessional teams, nursing ethics education will change to accommodate the opportunities full partnership will bring. It is likely that nurses will gain authority to influence interprofessional decisions about patient and community care. Full partnership is likely also to increase the managerial and leadership roles of nurses in the delivery of patient- and population-centered care that is safe, timely, efficient, effective, and equitable. But with this increased authority come requirements for increased education in interprofessional collaboration and organizational leadership, for increased clinical and administrative competence, and for increased responsibility for the safety and quality of the care provided by the entire interprofessional team. Nursing bioethics education will play an important role in preparing nurses to meet these requirements.

SEE ALSO *Narrative; Nursing, Profession of; Nursing, Theories and Philosophy of; Nursing Ethics; Teams, Health Care*

BIBLIOGRAPHY

Banks, Sarah. 2010. "Interprofessional Ethics: A Developing Field? Notes from the *Ethics and Social Welfare* Conference, Sheffield, UK, May 2010." *Ethics and Social Welfare* 4 (3): 280–94.

Benner, Patricia; Molly Sutphen; Victoria Leonard; and Lisa Day. 2010. *Educating Nurses: A Call for Radical Transformation.* San Francisco: Jossey-Bass.

Canadian Interprofessional Health Collaborative. 2010. "A National Interprofessional Competency Framework." Accessed May 9, 2013. http://www.cihc.ca/files/CIHC_IPCompetencies_Feb1210r.pdf

Charles, Grant; Lesley Bainbridge; and John Gilbert. 2010. "The University of British Columbia Model of Interprofessional Education." *Journal of Interprofessional Care* 24 (1): 9–18.

Clark, Phillip G.; Cheryl Cott; and Theresa J. K. Drinka. 2007. "Theory and Practice in Interprofessional Ethics: A Framework for Understanding Ethical Issues in Health Care Teams." *Journal of Interprofessional Care* 21 (6): 591–603.

Committee on the Robert Wood Johnson Foundation Initiative on the Future of Nursing, at the Institute of Medicine. 2011. *The Future of Nursing: Leading Change, Advancing Health.* Washington, DC: National Academies Press.

Edmondson, Amy C., and Kathryn S. Roloff. 2009. "Overcoming Barriers to Collaboration: Psychological Safety and Learning in Diverse Teams." In *Team Effectiveness in Complex Organizations: Cross-Disciplinary Perspectives and Approaches*, edited by Eduardo Salas, Gerald F. Goodwin, and C. Shawn Burke, 183–208. New York: Routledge.

Frenk, Julio; Lincoln Chen; Zulfigar A. Bhutta; et al. 2010. "Health Professionals for a New Century: Transforming Education to Strengthen Health Systems in an Interdependent World." *Lancet* 376 (9756): 1923–58.

Interprofessional Education Collaborative Expert Panel. 2011. *Core Competencies for Interprofessional Collaborative Practice: Report of an Expert Panel.* Washington, DC: Interprofessional Education Collaborative. Accessed May 9, 2013. http://www.aacn.nche.edu/education-resources/ipecreport.pdf

Interprofessional Education Team, Faculty of Health and Wellbeing, Sheffield Hallam University. 2010. "Interprofessional Capability Framework 2010: Mini-Guide." Sheffield, UK: Author. Includes a self-assessment.

Lamb, Gerri; Madeline Schmitt; Paula Edwards; et al. 2008. "Measuring Staff Nurse Care Coordination in the Hospital." Paper presented at the National State of the Science Congress on Nursing Research, Washington, DC, October 2–4.

Rest, James R. 1986. *Moral Development: Advances in Research and Theory.* New York: Praeger.

Rest, James R., and Darcia Narváez, eds. 1994. *Moral Development in the Professions: Psychology and Applied Ethics.* Hillsdale, NJ: Lawrence Erlbaum.

Sargeant, Joan. 2009. "Theories to Aid Understanding and Implementation of Interprofessional Education." *Journal of Continuing Education in the Health Professions* 29 (3): 178–84.

Suter, Esther; Julia Arndt; Nancy Arthur; et al. 2009. "Role Understanding and Effective Communication as Core Competencies for Collaborative Practice." *Journal of Interprofessional Care* 23 (1): 41–51.

Thistlethwaite, Jill, and Monica Moran, on behalf of the World Health Organization Study Group on Interprofessional Education and Collaborative Practice. 2010. "Learning Outcomes for Interprofessional Education (IPE): Literature Review and Synthesis." *Journal of Interprofessional Care* 24 (5): 503–13.

University of British Columbia, College of Health Disciplines. 2008. "The British Columbia Competency Framework for Interprofessional Collaboration." Vancouver, BC: Author. Accessed May 9, 2013. http://www.chd.ubc.ca/files/file/BC%20_Competency%20Framework%20for%20_IPC.pdf

Upenieks, Valda V.; Elizabeth A. Lee; Mindy E. Flanagan; and Bradley N. Doebbeling. 2010. "Healthcare Team Vitality Instrument (HTVI): Developing a Tool Assessing Healthcare Team Functioning." *Journal of Advanced Nursing* 66 (1): 168–76.

Varcoe, Colleen; Gweneth Doane; Bernadette Pauly; et al. 2004. "Ethical Practice in Nursing: Working the In-Betweens." *Journal of Advanced Nursing* 45 (3): 316–25.

Walsh, Claire L.; M. Frances Gordon; Michelle Marshall; et al. 2005. "Interprofessional Capability: A Developing Framework for Interprofessional Education." *Nurse Education in Practice* 5 (4): 230–37.

World Health Organization. 2010. "Framework for Action on Interprofessional Education and Collaborative Practice." Geneva, Switzerland: Author. Accessed May 9, 2013. http://whqlibdoc.who.int/hq/2010/WHO_HRH_HPN_10.3_eng.pdf

Wright, David, and Susan Brajtman. 2011. "Relational and Embodied Knowing: Nursing Ethics within the Interprofessional Team." *Nursing Ethics* 18 (1): 20–30.

Joy Penticuff
Retired Professor and Founding Director,
Concordia Bachelor of Science in Nursing Program,
Concordia University Texas

III. OTHER HEALTH PROFESSIONS

Bioethics education in health professions other than medicine and nursing takes place in professional schools and in both practice and continuing education settings. The group to which "other health professions" refers is so diverse and the organization of health care so varied across national boundaries that no generalizations can adequately embrace the differences. Some major groups in the United States include therapists (e.g., occupational, recreational, respiratory, physical), technologists (e.g., radiological, medical laboratory), physician assistants, pharmacists, dietitians, dentists, and medical social workers. Other countries have organizational structures and areas of training and expertise that, with notable exceptions, affect the depth and content areas of ethics education. This entry relies primarily on trends in the United States, emphasizing major common themes that have emerged in the content and pedagogy of ethics educational offerings.

It also describes common factors that have led to the introduction of bioethics teaching in these fields and how the idea of interprofessional education is breaking down the silos of discipline-specific education.

COMMON THEMES IN CONTENT AND PEDAGOGY

A set of guidelines for professional conduct has been one of the first types of documents produced when a new health field emerges. Up until the 1960s the documents often were called codes of ethics, but they consisted of such topics as dress codes or the importance of good manners and a cheerful disposition, more akin to etiquette guidelines than markers of moral attitudes and conduct. They also emphasized the importance of keeping one's proper place in the bureaucracy, so that all documents except those for dentistry stressed deference to the physician. Dedication to one's tasks was considered essential. The predictable result was that early ethics education was a presentation of a list of "dos and don'ts" that detailed a professional etiquette and morality punctuated by loyalty to one's group.

The educational emphasis and content have evolved as a result both of the maturing of groups other than medicine and nursing into more fully recognized professional areas and of developments in the field of bioethics. Twenty-first-century ethics documents include but go beyond codes of ethics. The codes of ethics themselves have become much more focused on ethical tenets of professional practice, with guides to conduct as adjuncts rather than the major substance. Together with other materials they reflect basic ethical principles and character traits deemed relevant to professional practice. Faculty have adopted these documents as a foundation for education along with a growing clinical journal literature, textbooks, websites, blogs, and other educational materials now available in their fields. Most educational resources are designed around the central notion of ethical responsibility, moral agency, or advocacy on behalf of the patient and society. Some documents also delineate major types of interactions in a given profession and specify principles for each. The predictable result is less focus on indoctrinating students into behaviors and attitudes and more on urging them to a deeper understanding of situations that evoke knowledge of the ethics required for adherence to their professional roles and responsibilities.

The continued development of bioethics and health care ethics as academic and applied areas of study has also profoundly influenced education in these fields. Bioethics draws on insights from philosophy, theology, and a variety of social sciences, thereby providing teacher and learner alike with a broader bandwidth of perspectives on the ethical aspects of professional roles. Teachers can introduce basic theories and methods of ethical analysis and decision making, relating them to the approaches students encounter in other dimensions of clinical practice. The student is exposed to the deeper social significance of behaviors and attitudes that are encountered in the professionalization process, such as compassion, care, honesty, and integrity. Materials from the social sciences also highlight how diversity in ethnic, religious, age, gender, class, and other identities among individuals and groups influence the situations in which ethical challenges arise. Faculty have access to resources that highlight the role that all professional groups play in addressing injustices from the perspective of the larger social-political and organizational environments in which professional services are offered.

There is a growing consensus about the pedagogical methods that should be used to teach bioethics. The case method is especially effective in allowing students to readily recognize key ethical issues as they arise in everyday practice and to grasp the relevance of bioethics to their chosen professions, because the story highlights fine details of their own clinical setting, distinguishing it from others. For instance, a pharmacy student discovers that confidentiality issues are very similar among all professions, but the function of informed consent for the pharmacist providing information about the use of a prescribed medication differs from that of a physician assistant preparing to conduct a pelvic exam on a patient. The dietitian's sporadic but ongoing contact with an ambulatory care patient presents challenges regarding the means of respecting the patient's informed preferences that differ from those of a physical therapist who spends an hour or more every day with an institutionalized patient.

A larger proportion of bioethics instruction is taking place in small group settings where discussion takes place. In addition to case discussions some programs use real or simulated patients and interactive technologies with the goal of integrating ethical aspects of a patient's situation into the diagnostic, treatment, and social aspects of intervention. Much debate continues about where in the curriculum students are the most receptive to integrating relevant ethics dimensions of practice into their formal preparation. A focus on situated learning, or learning in the actual environment of future practice, has many proponents.

Interprofessional educational initiatives are being introduced into many professional preparation settings to instruct students about how their clinical and other functions will be exercised in practice. This trend is receiving attention globally, with several organizations sponsoring meetings to explore common ethical challenges and the need to prepare current students for a globalized health care environment. Understandably this helps close the gap between medical or nursing ethics and those of the other health professions, with the result that the silos of discipline-specific ethics educational offerings are giving way to or are being augmented by those that involve members of the whole health care team.

There is also a variety of positions regarding who should teach bioethics. Some schools of thought favor a stronger emphasis on theory and thus support the idea that persons formally trained in philosophical ethics or moral theology are needed. Others argue that an understanding of the clinical peculiarities and "facts" is most important, resulting in a preference for clinician instructors, especially if they have taken advanced work (or even a short course) in bioethics. Another alternative is a teaching team composed of a bioethicist and a clinician working together. Preferences for one or another of these approaches seem less profession specific than idiosyncratic to particular regions or institutions. In spite of the differences of opinion, the debates revolve around the common goal of effectively integrating the theoretical and practical dimensions of bioethics.

COMMON FACTORS LEADING TO THE NECESSITY OF BIOETHICS EDUCATION

At least three major factors have led to the need for bioethics education with its focus on thoughtful deliberation about complex ethical issues. Underlying each is the age-old understanding that the professionals' loyalty must be patient centered.

The first is the issue of professional autonomy, long on the agenda of medical and in more recent years nursing education. In the United States pharmacists, physical therapists, and others have moved to doctoral-level education and are becoming part of the "doctoring professions," where autonomy is one key criterion. All such emerging groups must gain an understanding of their particular situations and recognize the areas of ethical and clinical accountability that relate to their areas of special expertise and the effects of whether or not they also have ultimate decision-making authority. For example, in some states groups such as physician assistants, nurse practitioners, physical therapists, and social workers have legal license to evaluate or practice independently. But this does not resolve the thorny questions of how to coordinate care for patients or the place of the professional in regard to the physicians' traditional moral-legal role of authority or the regulations hemming in the whole team of providers. The different levels of progress toward full professional status among the groups compound the issue.

A second factor is the way reliance on technology is altering the complexion of the traditional health professional–patient relationship worldwide. Some technology may create a detrimental distance between health professionals and patients. Patients and health professionals alike may place unrealistic expectations on technologies to bring about "miracles," creating dissent and distrust when they fail to do so. And the high cost of many technologies may add undue burdens on patients and families, creating a dilemma of justice for practitioners and teams. The promise of technology cannot be dismissed either. The concepts and methods of ethics are needed for thinking through and acting on technology-related challenges, including the use of robots, simulations, and electronically driven diagnostic and treatment interventions.

A third factor is the presence of persistent inequities in health care systems. The tools of bioethics enable students to understand why inequities are morally unacceptable and provide reasons to support their participation in the advancement of just and fair health-related policies.

Ethics education for all professionals is a lifelong process. Some of this challenge is met through continuing education programs for practitioners offered by various organizations. Courses for persons in specific roles, such as those serving on clinical ethics committees or research committees (institutional review boards), are available as well.

Bioethics education across the professions under discussion in this entry encourages critical thinking, considered ethical action, and the exercise of ethically appropriate character traits. Consequently it will continue to be a powerful resource as new developments in health care and society give rise to ethical issues.

SEE ALSO *Dentistry; Narrative; Nursing, Profession of; Nursing, Theories and Philosophy of; Nursing Ethics; Pastoral and Spiritual Care and Health Care Chaplaincy; Teams, Health Care*

BIBLIOGRAPHY

Flinton, David M., and Nick White. 2009. "Preliminary Findings on the Virtual Environment for the Radiotherapy Training (VERT) System: Simulator Sickness and Presence." *Journal of Radiotherapy in Practice* 8 (4): 169–76.

Golden, David G. 1991. "Medical Ethics Courses for Student Technologists." *Radiologic Technology* 62 (6): 452–57.

Griener, Glenn, and Janet L. Storch. 1994. "The Educational Needs of Ethics Committees." *Cambridge Quarterly of Healthcare Ethics* 3 (3): 467–77.

Haddad, Amy. 2010. "What Health Science Students Learn from Playing a Standardized Patient in an Ethics Course." *Cambridge Quarterly of Healthcare Ethics* 19 (4): 481–87.

Hope, Tony; K. W. M. Fulford; and Anne Yates. 2000. *The Oxford Practice Skills Course: Ethics, Law, and Communication*

Skills in Health Care Education. Oxford: Oxford University Press.

Illingworth, Paul, and Sonja Chelvanayagam. 2007. "Benefits of Inter-professional Education in Health Care." *British Journal of Nursing* 16 (2): 121–24.

Interprofessional Education Collaborative Expert Panel. 2011. *Core Competencies for Interprofessional Collaborative Practice: Report of an Expert Panel.* Washington, DC: Interprofessional Education Collaborative. http://www.aacn.nche.edu/education-resources/ipecreport.pdf

London Deanery Faculty Development. 2013. "Principles of Interprofessional Learning." Accessed May 9, 2013. http://www.faculty.londondeanery.ac.uk/e-learning/interprofessional-education/principles-of-interprofessional-learning

McMillan, John. 2002. "Ethics and Clinical Ethics Committee Education." *HEC Forum* 14 (1): 45–52.

Purtilo, Ruth B. 2000. "A Time to Harvest, a Time to Sow: Ethics for a Shifting Landscape." *Physical Therapy* 80 (11): 1112–19.

Purtilo, Ruth B.; Amy Haddad; and Regina Doherty. 2014. *Health Professional and Patient Interaction*. 8th ed. St. Louis, MO: Elsevier/Saunders.

Purtilo, Ruth B.; Gail M. Jensen; and Charlotte Brasic Royeen, eds. 2005. *Educating for Moral Action: A Sourcebook in Health and Rehabilitation Ethics*. Philadelphia: Davis.

Royeen, Charlotte Brasic; Gail M. Jensen; and Robin Ann Harvah, eds. 2009. *Leadership in Interprofessional Health Education and Practice*. Sudbury, MA: Jones and Bartlett.

Vengler, Mollie, and Michael Theall. 2007. "Case-Based Ethics Education in Physical Therapy." *Journal of Scholarship of Teaching and Learning* 7 (1): 64–76.

Ruth B. Purtilo (1995, 2014)
Professor Emerita, Department of Interdisciplinary Studies, MGH Institute of Health Professions

IV. PUBLIC EDUCATION

Bioethics has long sought to have an influence that reaches outside the academy walls, hospital wards, and research labs to have an impact on the broader public. This aspiration is reflected in the recommendations issued in reports, the mission statements of research centers, and the charters of national bioethics commissions. Bioethics television programs, news stories, web-based forums, and curricula are all tangible manifestations of efforts to educate the public about contemporary bioethical issues, expose it to methods of ethical reasoning, and engage it in dialogue.

THE PUBLIC AND TWO UNDERSTANDINGS OF BIOETHICS EDUCATION

The "public" often invoked in bioethics discourse can be defined broadly as those individuals who do not possess technical or policy expertise in the areas of medicine, science, or technology but who nevertheless have a stake in how biomedical technologies and practices unfold. Sometimes the public's stake is easy to identify, for example, when a state stem cell initiative or physician-assisted suicide provision is up for a referendum vote, but often the public interest is more diffuse.

The possible meaning of public education takes two forms in contemporary bioethics. The first variety, reflecting a general commitment to democratic values of transparency, legitimacy, and participation, understands the role of education as helping members of the citizenry come to informed positions through a deliberate process (Gutmann and Thompson 1997). Drawing on the doctrine of informed consent used with individual patients and research subjects, some have suggested that public education is a core component of stoking a societal debate about matters of shared concern (King and Hyde 2012, xii).

If this view can be criticized as romanticizing the public, others hold a more skeptical or paternalistic stance toward the hoi polloi. In this second view education is a necessary corrective to public ignorance, an anecdote to reactionary opposition to—or uncritical support of—biomedical progress and health policies (Schicktanz, Schweda, and Wynne 2011). For example, bioethicists may call publicly for education about organ transplantation to increase donations or hope that a clearer understanding of the science will quell moral objections to embryonic stem cell research.

Bioethicists thus can serve as both facilitators of and advocates in public debates. These roles reflect two different aims for bioethics education: (1) helping the public develop the reflective capacity needed to engage in ethical deliberation (for example, recognizing an ethical question, identifying stakeholders, respecting differences) and (2) framing the background information (facts, science, and ethical considerations) and arguments specific to a particular issue. A wide range of mechanisms is employed in service of public bioethics education.

BIOETHICS COMMISSIONS

By the start of the twenty-first century more than 100 countries had established bioethics commissions or standing national ethics committees. Although many of these bodies are policy oriented, with little public engagement beyond a requirement that meetings be held in public, some commissions take an active stance in seeking to work with the public. The Nuffield Council of Bioethics in the United Kingdom, the German Ethics Council, and the Bioethics Advisory Council in Singapore, for example, all have mandates to inform the public and encourage discussion in society. Commissions in Europe that have experimented with ways of consulting directly with the public as a part of developing policy recommendations seem particularly committed to education efforts, as it is widely agreed that meaningful public consultation requires a basic comprehension of the relevant scientific and medical facts.

In the United States the President's Council on Bioethics (2001–2009) was chartered by President George W. Bush in part to promote public understanding of bioethics; it published anthologies of essays and short stories to inspire broad public dialogue. These activities (along with the council's membership and style) were heavily criticized for being driven by conservative politics, disconnected from specific policy questions, and colored more by the emotion of fiction than by the hard facts of science (Moreno 2011). As Eric Meslin (2010) notes, "All [bioethics] commissions have faced political pressure of one sort or another." The controversy surrounding Bush's bioethics commission highlights that education efforts originating from the executive branch of government can, at the very least, easily be interpreted as efforts to politically influence public opinion. Though the Presidential Commission for the Study of Bioethical Issues that followed in the administration of President Barack Obama is more oriented to public policy than public pedagogy, this body has included in its reports calls for public education about biotechnology and enhanced ethics education. Examples of the outreach activities of the commissions include generating summaries of commission reports written for the general public, creating guides for instructors, conducting education workshops, and collaborating with performing artists to create works that can provoke public discussion and reflection.

NEWS MEDIA

An editor of *Time* magazine described the role of bioethicists in the media as "laying out the terms of debate, culling the data, stripping the issue bare of superstition or ideology or agenda and inviting us all to walk around the challenges before us, to view them from all angles" (Gibbs 2008, xii). Early scholars in bioethics, though, had little professed interest in communicating with the public through the press.

Through the 1960s and 1970s bioethics public education was achieved primarily through broadcast media—newspapers, magazines, television newscasts—and produced primarily by professional journalists. The general public and early bioethicists alike learned of the atrocities conducted in Tuskegee and the quandaries raised by the rationing of early dialysis machines through the work of reporters (Elliott 2012). As the field grew from infancy, however, it did not take long for reporters to begin to call on bioethicists to provide commentary on the medical dramas and scientific breakthroughs increasingly chronicled in newspaper headlines (Callahan 2012, 150).

By the 1980s and 1990s some in the field began to actively seek out the media, developing documentaries and television specials (such as *Hard Choices*, produced by Seattle Public Television), writing magazine articles for a popular audience, and providing resources to support reporters. Arthur L. Caplan (1993, S14) declared in 1993 that "I've come to believe that there is no point in doing bioethics if, ultimately, some of it doesn't take place in public." Though many scholars remain skeptical of the media—bemoaning, for example, the severe limitations of the sound-bite format that rewards novelty and requires brevity—it is no longer uncommon to find a list of media appearances on a bioethicist's curriculum vitae under the rubric of public service (Fox and Swazey 2008, 107–10).

Documentary series and long journalistic articles that afford the space for an argument or explanation to be laid out—and not merely for the conclusion to be asserted—are more promising media formats for influencing public understanding (Elliott and Kahn 1994). Increasingly, however, these are also the most difficult to find in a fragmented media landscape driven by the twenty-four-hour news cycle. Unlike the universities and teaching medical centers in which bioethicists have gained authority, most media outlets are not educational institutions (Evans 2012), and since the 1990s ideological programming has proliferated, blurring the line between news and editorial content.

INTERACTIVE AND SOCIAL MEDIA

The Internet provides powerful new channels for bioethics education. The public is now just a web search away from reports, commentaries, blog posts, and news items published on bioethics websites. Genuine accessibility, however, requires content to be delivered in plain language that is free of jargon and in a manner lively enough to attract the interest of a general reader.

The vast majority of Internet users seek health information online, and bioethicists are enlisted to produce educational materials for patients and families navigating challenging health care decisions. These guides often are commonly housed on the websites of government health agencies, patient advocacy organizations, and health information services.

Universities and research centers are seeking new ways of employing technology to increase public access to their intellectual resources. Bioethics centers at Georgetown University and the University of Pennsylvania, for example, have developed massive online open courses in bioethics. Such courses and video and discussion boards make the content freely available to a worldwide audience. Questions remain about the viability of virtual interactions replacing those traditionally held face to face.

Social media allow bioethicists and interested members of the public to access and contribute to a constantly changing feed of bioethics news and commentary. The formation of virtual communities can aid in the democratizing of previously elite discussions, though the self-selecting membership of these communities means that ideological echo chambers can also emerge.

SECONDARY AND UNDERGRADUATE EDUCATION

Students often first encounter bioethics in secondary education, where ethical issues are frequently raised in biology courses. Such courses are typically taught by science faculty, who face the challenge of shifting between teaching scientific facts and inquiry to the process of ethical exploration. Programs developed by New York University (2013), the National Institutes of Health (2009), and the Hastings Center (1991) are designed to help instructors by providing case study materials to expose students to bioethics topics and methods. Popular topics include biotechnology, environmental ethics, human subjects research, public health ethics, and experimentation with animals.

Although few colleges and universities offer an undergraduate bioethics major, minors are now common, and courses on bioethical issues are ubiquitous and offered across the humanities and social sciences. Since 1985 the Bioethics Research Library at Georgetown University has maintained a database with hundreds of bioethics course syllabi. Unlike specialized ethics training for medical or research professionals, bioethics education for undergraduate students seeks primarily to prepare young citizens to recognize and grapple with complex questions.

FICTION AND INFORMAL BIOETHICS EDUCATION

Film, novels, plays, and television series can all serve as pedagogical tools. A well-crafted drama contains the key ingredients of dilemmas, conflicts, and emotional appeal required to stir the audience's moral imagination or elicit a sense of ethical tension. Bioethics filmographies (Shapshay 2009; Colt, Quadrelli, and Friedman 2011) demonstrate that there is hardly a bioethical question imaginable—from intersexuality to the challenges of conducting international research on human subjects—that has not received a dramatic treatment.

In debates about the ethics of emerging biotechnology, *Frankenstein, Gattaca,* and *Jurassic Park* have become common shorthand for referencing hubris, discrimination, and unanticipated consequences. Medical dramas on television paint fictional portraits of the dilemmas faced by patients and medical professionals but nevertheless can provide a gateway to thinking about clinical issues in bioethics (Czarny, Faden, and Sugarman 2010).

A danger lies in viewers confusing fact with fiction. Emotional representations can trump the dispassionate weighing of facts and arguments (Guyer and Moreno 2004). Commentaries, courses, and discussions constitute one way to address these problems. To ignore cultural touchstones such as movies and television programs, however, is likely to miss an opportunity for making bioethics accessible and democratic.

CONCLUSION

A major challenge facing public bioethics education is impact assessment. It is simple enough to estimate the number of viewers of a television documentary or monitor the number of visits to a website but much more difficult to measure how bioethics education affects public debate. Advocates can track progress according to opinion polls, but would increased support of industrial applications of synthetic biology following a public outreach be counted as a success or as a failure? And any successes in public bioethics education only raise further questions, such as, what active role should the educated public play in bioethical deliberation?

Much work remains to be done if bioethics is to realize its democratic ambitions and promote public understanding of ethics (Moore 2010). Although the approaches are varied and successes bound to be mixed, experimentation with public education has only increased with the growth of bioethics.

SEE ALSO *Bioethics Commissions, History of; Medical Education; Public Policy and Bioethics*

BIBLIOGRAPHY

Bioethics Research Library at Georgetown University. "Bioethics Syllabus Exchange Repository." http://repository.library.georgetown.edu/handle/10822/556197

Callahan, Daniel. 2012. *In Search of the Good: A Life in Bioethics.* Cambridge, MA: MIT Press.

Caplan, Arthur L. 1993. "What Bioethics Brought to the Public." *Hastings Center Report* 23 (6): S14–15.

Colt, Henri G.; Silvia Quandrelli; and Lester D. Friedman. 2011. *The Picture of Health: Medical Ethics and the Movies.* New York: Oxford University Press.

Czarny, Matthew J.; Ruth R. Faden; and Jeremy Sugarman. 2010. "Bioethics and Professionalism in Popular Television Medical Dramas." *Journal of Medical Ethics* 36 (4): 203–6.

Elliott, Carl. 2012. "An Investigative Bioethics Manifesto." In *Bioethics, Public Moral Argument, and Social Responsibility,* edited by Nancy M. P. King and Michael J. Hyde, 141–53. New York: Routledge.

Elliott, Carl, and Jeffrey Kahn. 1994. "Docs on the Box; or, How We Learned to Stop Worrying and Love the Tube." *Hastings Center Report* 24 (6): 22–23.

Evans, John H. 2012. *The History and Future of Bioethics: A Sociological View.* New York: Oxford University Press.

Fox, Renée C., and Judith P. Swazey. 2008. *Observing Bioethics.* New York: Oxford University Press.

Gibbs, Nancy. 2008. "Why Bioethics Matters Today: A Journalist's Perspective." In *From Birth to Death and Bench to Clinic: The Hastings Center Bioethics Briefing Book for Journalists, Policymakers, and Campaigns*, edited by Mary Crowley, xi–xii. Garrison, NY: Hastings Center. http://www.thehastingscenter.org/Publications/BriefingBook/

Gutmann, Amy, and Dennis Thompson. 1997. "Deliberating about Bioethics." *Hastings Center Report* 27 (3): 38–41.

Guyer, Ruth Levy, and Jonathan D. Moreno. 2004. "Slouching Toward Policy: Lazy Bioethics and the Perils of Science Fiction." *American Journal of Bioethics* 4 (4): W14–17.

Hastings Center. 1991. *New Choices, New Responsibilities: Ethical Issues in the Life Sciences.* Briarcliff, NY: Author.

King, Nancy M. P., and Michael J. Hyde. 2012. "Editors' Introduction." In *Bioethics, Public Moral Argument, and Social Responsibility*, edited by Nancy M. P. King and Michael J. Hyde, ix–xv. New York: Routledge.

Meslin, Eric M. 2010. "Can National Bioethics Commissions Be Progressive? Should They?" In *Progress in Bioethics: Science, Policy, and Politics*, edited by Jonathan D. Moreno and Sam Berger, 143–60. Cambridge, MA: MIT Press.

Moore, Alfred. 2010. "Public Bioethics and Public Engagement: The Politics of 'Proper Talk.'" *Public Understanding of Science* 19 (2): 197–211.

Moreno, Jonathan D. 2011. *The Body Politic: The Battle over Science in America.* New York: Bellevue Literary.

National Institutes of Health. 2009. "Exploring Bioethics: NIH Curriculum Supplement Series." http://science.education.nih.gov/supplements/nih9/bioethics/default.htm

New York University. 2013. "High School Bioethics." http://highschoolbioethics.med.nyu.edu

Schicktanz, Silke; Mark Schweda; and Brian Wynne. 2011. "The Ethics of 'Public Understanding of Ethics': Why and How Bioethics Expertise Should Include Public and Patients' Voices." *Medicine, Health Care, and Philosophy* 15 (2): 129–39.

Shapshay, Sandra, ed. 2009. *Bioethics at the Movies.* Baltimore, MD: Johns Hopkins University Press.

Jacob Moses
New Media Director, The Hastings Center

BIOLOGY, PHILOSOPHY OF

Although it may seem that the philosophy of biology, a field known for its focus on metaphysical, epistemological, and conceptual issues in biology, is far removed from the concerns of bioethics, there is a trend in philosophy of biology toward descriptivism that paradoxically allows for significant bridges with the predominantly normative concerns of bioethics.

About the same time that bioethics was born (the 1960s), the field of philosophy of biology took its first steps. Initially, it looked a lot like the rest of philosophy of science, which often meant focusing on the kinds of concerns that had their roots in physics. David Hull (1974), Michael Ruse (1973), and others created a field that was dominated by formal concerns in evolutionary biology, including the nature and structure of its theories. Questions for the field included the nature of any reductions from the theories of Mendelian and transmission genetics to molecular genetics, whether it was possible to axiomatize evolutionary theory, how to account for the apparent teleology of evolutionary explanations, whether species are classes or individuals, and what the units of selection are. Many of these topics have remained active subfields to the present day.

Over time, philosophy of biology came to include much richer and detailed involvement with both current biology and the history of biology. Many philosophers came to ground their philosophical insights in rich historical accounts of various periods in the history of biology or in contemporary debates of active concern to practicing biologists. This naturalistic turn occurred in many parts of philosophy of science, but seems to have been most acute in philosophy of biology, at least partly for institutional reasons, including the creation of the International Society for the History, Philosophy, and Social Studies of Biology (Callebaut 1993).

Through these developments, the field still largely avoided normative issues and focused on evolutionary biology. Several attempts have been made to move the field to other parts of biology. There are a number of philosophers working on developmental biology and using it as an alternative for framing traditional issues (Oyama, Griffiths, and Gray 2001). Kenneth Schaffner (1993) has made a notable and unusual attempt to discuss the more medical parts of biology. Paul Thagard (1999) has similarly attempted to use work in the biomedical sciences (attempts at explaining the causes of ulcers) to address general philosophical issues in the nature of explanation.

There are a number of topics within philosophy of biology that especially bear on issues within bioethics.

BIOLOGICAL FUNCTION

One of the central concepts in the medical parts of biology, particularly physiology, is the concept of function. It is impossible to understand the way we classify organ systems without this concept. The function of the heart is to pump blood. Hence any blood pump is a heart—even if there are some structural differences between the hearts of different species or (as mechanical hearts demonstrate) differences in the material makeup of the heart. So what makes something a heart is fundamentally its function or purpose. This poses a philosophical problem, because the concept of function is a teleological notion. To say that the function of the heart is to pump blood is simply another way of saying that the heart is designed to pump blood. But who is the designer? Prior to Darwin the answer would have been an appeal to God.

Philosophers have attempted to account for the apparent goal-directed nature of biological science in two different ways. One solution is to accept that functions are goal directed but to appeal to natural selection. Rather than a conscious designer, natural selection designed the heart to pump blood. The etiological view of functions (sometimes called Wright functions) gives an explanation of why a function is there in historical terms: "The function of X is Z means (a) X is there because it does Z and (b) Z is a consequence (or result) of X's being there" (L. Wright 1973). To Larry Wright, "the heart beats *because* its beating pumps blood" (159). In contrast, in 1975 Robert Cummins rejected the goal-directed, historical approach to functions. What matters in thinking of functions is the contribution it makes to a whole system, the role that it plays in bringing about the performance of that system.

Early twenty-first-century commentators have concluded that each approach captures a different notion of function. Where Larry Wright attempts to account for why a function is there (a function as opposed to an accident), Cummins explains what a function does, what it is good for (whether it is an accident or not). Continued debate over whether an etiological account can be developed in the Wright mode and how to overcome various problems continues (Arieu, Cummins, and Perlman 2002).

The concept of function plays an especially important role in medicine since health and disease are often understood as normal (species typical) functioning or dysfunction respectively.

CONCEPTS OF DISEASE AND HEALTH

This is perhaps the most important area of research in philosophy of biology for bioethics. Arthur Caplan explains it as follows:

> It may strain credulity to believe that the analysis of concepts such as *health, disease*, or *normality* can shed light on the ethical and policy issues associated with the vast amounts of new knowledge being generated by the human genome project and related inquiries in biomedicine. However, credulity must be strained. The focus of attention *qua* philosophy tends to be on who owns the genome or whether an insurance company can boot you off the rolls if you are at risk of succumbing to a costly disease. But this is not really where the ethical and philosophical action is with respect to the ongoing revolution in genetics. (Caplan 1992, 128)

There are two important distinctions that must be understood in the debates over concepts of disease. First, there is a distinction between ontological and nominalist concepts of disease. On the ontological (realist) view of disease, diseases are real entities that exist in the world. Nosologies represent a true classification of the world—they carve nature at the joints. The paradigm diseases on this view would be either discrete disease-causing agents that are at the same time identified as the diseases themselves or as discrete lesions. Thus, poliovirus is not the cause of poliomyelitis, it *is* poliomyelitis.

In contrast, the nominalist about disease would appeal to the old saying, "There are no diseases, only sick people." On this view, nosologies are merely conventional systems of classification. They may have a great deal of practical value, but they are not in any meaningful sense true descriptions of reality. In some cases we classify diseases based on the pathogen that causes the disease. In other cases we classify based on the signs and symptoms. In others we focus on the organ system that is damaged, regardless of the causes or the symptoms. Thus, the nominalist would use the current lack of unity in the organization of our taxonomy of diseases as support for the view that it is merely a conventional (and somewhat arbitrary) system. Realists would respond by appealing to the role of disease in medical science and point to similar problems with other taxonomic systems in science that are nonetheless regarded as capturing reality.

One of the arenas where this debate has been most heated has been over the status of the *Diagnostic and Statistical Manual of Mental Disorders* (*DSM*) in all of its versions. The fact that there are so many changes in the different versions of the *DSM* can be interpreted either as an indication that the classification scheme is merely a convention or that the science of psychiatry is progressing (as any science does).

The second related distinction in debates over the concept of disease is that of values in the development of the nosologies. For the nonnormativist, the starting point for understanding disease is to understand the typical functioning in a species. Disease is malfunction of the organism, a failure to function as organisms are designed to do. To understand disease, one needs only to understand physiology. The concepts are the same in humans as in understanding disease in nonhuman organisms. Therefore, nonscientific or epistemological values play no role in the development of the classification and understanding of disease (Boorse 1975).

In contrast, normativists believe that identifying a condition as a disease is a value-laden exercise. To say that a condition is a disease is to say something about what we value. Labeling something as a disease is a way of signaling the undesirability of the state. Normativists appeal to many examples that illustrate the way social values seem to permeate nosology. The early versions of the *DSM* identified homosexuality as a disease. The tendency of some slaves to attempt to escape was identified as a disease in the United States in the nineteenth century. Foot binding in Japan produces a condition that would be recognized as a disease in many parts of the world, but was seen as normal in Japan. Normativists deny that an account of disease solely in terms of typical functioning within a species can work. It is normal in some sense for humans to develop osteoarthritis in old age, normal for teeth to decay, normal to develop many ailments at advanced age. Yet medicine is committed to these things as disease. In fact age itself may be conceived of as both normal and a disease (Caplan, Engelhardt, and McCartney 1981).

Finally, there is a dispute over the meaning of health. Nonnormativists tend to think of health as the absence of disease. In that case, an organism is functioning within the normal parameters of its species at its age. In contrast there are those who adopt a much broader concept of health. On this view health is not the mere absence of disease, but is the full flourishing of a person in multiple dimensions, including psychological, economic, physical, and social well-being. These different conceptions of health and disease lead to very different views about the obligations of medicine toward society, the scope of the medical field, and the nature of medical care.

WHAT COUNTS AS A GENETIC TRAIT?

What does it mean to call something a genetic trait or disease? Clearly, at least part of that judgment rests on some kind of causal assessment. If a disease is genetic, then it is caused by one or more of an organism's genes. Indeed, this seems to fit a more general concept of disease, in which the causal basis of disease is incorporated into our nosologies. As Richard Hull has explained: "In its efforts to understand, control, and avoid disease, modern medicine has incorporated into the very identification of a disease the notion of the cause of the syndrome. This permits the individuation of similar syndromes with distinct causes into different diseases" (1979, 61).

There is a fairly obvious problem with this as a way of distinguishing between genetic and epigenetic diseases. That is because there are genetic and nongenetic factors that are causally relevant to every trait, a fact recognized by virtually all commentators on the concept of genetic disease (see R. Hull 1979; Gifford 1990). So the real issue in deciding that something is a genetic disease is whether the causal factors that are genetic are the most important causes. How do we decide whether genetic factors or environmental factors are more important in the production of various diseases? In response to the selection problem, a number of solutions have been proposed. These can be grouped into a few major categories.

One approach is to try to tease out a notion of genes as direct causes of disease. In 1990 Fred Gifford tried to capture this notion in one of his two definitions: "The trait must be the specific effect of some genetic cause, that the trait must be described or individuated in such a way that it is properly matched to what the gene causes specifically" (Gifford 1990, 329). However, this approach seems hopeless in the face of the actual complexity of development. Quite simply, this definition probably does not identify any diseases or traits as genetic. As Kelly Smith argued in 1990, "Genes do not directly cause anything of immediate phenotypic significance" (338).

Perhaps the most obvious and promising approach to the selection problems is to try a statistical approach. A number of variants on this have been attempted. Gifford writes, "The first and central sense of genetic is this: a trait is genetic if genetic differences in a given population account for the phenotypic differences in the trait-variable amongst members of that population" (Gifford 1990, 334). This seems to exactly capture at least something important about society's concept of genetic disease. It can be put perhaps more precisely in terms of covariance. When some trait is identified as genetic, it can be argued that (in that population) the covariance of the trait with some genetic factor(s) is greater than the covariance of the trait with other (nongenetic) factors. This solves the selection problem neatly by allowing us to pick out which causal factors are irrelevant (the ones that are fixed) and highlight the important ones (the ones that make the difference). In one of the canonical examples of causality, one is inclined to say that the lighting of a match (under normal circumstances) was the cause of the fire, while the presence of oxygen (while a contributing causal factor) was not. In contrast, in an environment where fire was normally present and oxygen was not, one might well pick out the (unusual) presence of oxygen as the cause of a fire.

There are several advantages to this approach to the selection problem. First, it corresponds to the use of analysis of variance that is used by biologists to measure the causal contribution of hereditary and environmental factors in a population. Second, it is capable of clear explication. Third, it has at least some intuitive support. However, this account seems to conflict with common usage in cases where pathogens typically identified as *the* cause of disease are nearly ubiquitous (so that, for example, genetic factors may make the difference between which people exposed to the pathogen become ill).

In spite of its advantages, the statistical approach fails to capture all of the myriad uses of the concept of genetic disease. Another approach has been developed from the way the most important causal factor in an explanation is picked out.

Philosophers have claimed on quite general grounds that the most important cause is chosen in terms of the manipulability of the various factors. Whatever the general virtues of this approach, it is promising when it comes to medicine. In the natural sciences, it could be argued that there is a strong interest in prediction and explanation. In contrast it has been argued that the medical realm is more concerned with the prevention and treatment of disease than with explanation (Engelhardt 1981; Wulff 1984). Instrumentalist interests play a much more central role in medical practice than in science. Hence, the appropriate solution to the selection problem can be formulated in terms of manipulability. The most important cause is the one that is identified as the most easily manipulated to prevent or treat disease. A disease is genetic if it is genes that play this role and epigenetic if it is nongenetic factors that are most easily manipulated.

Like the statistical definition, the manipulability definition captures something important about our usage of the term. In addition it is often an implicit aspect of the justification for the extension of the concept of genetic disease to new cases. However, there are some problems with this approach as well. The obvious problem seems to be that on this analysis, no disease could be classified as genetic. Many of the paradigm genetic diseases (phenylketonuria [PKU], cystic fibrosis [CF]) involve treatments that are not molecular. Indeed, in the case of PKU, the standard treatment involves a change in diet. At the same time the tests for PKU were developed before the actual mutation responsible for the disease had been identified. It is impossible to adhere to the manipulability definition and accept that PKU is a genetic disease. This seems to be a fatal flaw in the manipulability definition. In addition, it is not true that biomedical science is always instrumentally oriented. A great deal of effort is aimed not just at treating and preventing disease, but at understanding it. This may lead to a conflict over which causal factor is most important. The factor most easily manipulated for treating or preventing a disease may not be the most revealing for the purposes of understanding a disease.

It is worth noting that both the statistical approaches and the manipulability approaches seem to imply a relativity in the concept of genetic disease. In the case of the statistical notion, something will count as a genetic disease or not, depending on the population it is a part of. The manipulability definition implies that technological advances will affect what counts as a genetic disease as the reach of our technology is extended. Yet, this result seems to be incompatible with an ontological conception of disease. If diseases are real entities (and independent of values), then the solution to the selection problem should not depend on factors outside of the organism (Boorse 1975). Thus the normativist or constructivist position on disease seems to be supported by these analyses (however inadequate they are as a general account).

EVOLUTIONARY ETHICS

As philosophy has become more naturalized, it is unsurprising that philosophers (and especially philosophers of biology) would attempt to find a way to ground ethics in a biological account of human nature. Perhaps even more significantly, the development of sociobiology and its subsequent incarnation, evolutionary psychology, meant that biologists were looking to explain the origins of morality in an evolutionary account (Wilson 1978; R. Wright 1995; Farber 1998). Michael Ruse has been perhaps the most influential voice on evolutionary ethics (1991, 1993).

Ruse argues that evolutionary theory offers *the* explanation of the origin of altruism and other moral sentiments. He follows the explanatory strategy of the sociobiologists (and evolutionary psychologists) by appealing to the apparent universality of cooperative behaviors and moral sentiments, combined with the obvious adaptive value that cooperative strategies represent. Indeed, there are a number of game theoretic accounts to demonstrate the adaptive value of altruistic behavior in at least some circumstances (J. M. Smith 1982).

Ruse then claims that the fact that evolution explains morality undermines moral realism. He offers two arguments. First, although human moral sentiments evolved, it is quite possible that an alternative set of sentiments could have produced the same effects. The contingency of evolution means that morality itself is contingent. Second, Ruse takes great care in dispelling any teleological interpretation of evolution. Evolution is a directionless process with no end or goal. Since morality is founded on a directionless process, it follows that realism toward ethics is undermined. Evolution is meaningless and without value. Organisms that survived and adapted are not better in a normative sense. Hence there is no normative foundation for ethics.

Critics have attempted a number of strategies, including questioning the extent to which evolution can really account for morality (Lewontin 1992), or denying the relevance of the facts of evolution to normative issues (Nagel 1997). Other critics have argued that a fully naturalized ethics that accepts evolution as the foundation of morality is fully compatible with ethical realism (Maienschein and Ruse 1999).

WHAT IS LIFE?

A research area at the intersection of philosophy of biology and bioethics is over the definition of life. This question has multiple dimensions. National Aeronautics and Space Administration (NASA) scientists wonder about the definition as they pursue research into the question of life on other planets. How will researchers know whether what they find is a living organism or a (nonliving) chemical reaction? Biologists interested in the origins of life similarly strive to understand the demarcation between the living and nonliving as they construct their models. Genomic scientists attempt to better understand gene function by trying to determine the minimal number of genes necessary for life—life's genetic essence. Public policy makers and scientists debate the moral significance of ex vivo fertilized egg cells and the stem cells that can be derived from them. Are the embryos living? Are they alive when they are frozen? Are the stem cells that can be derived from them living beings deserving of respect or are they research tools to be used to help people suffering from disease?

The process of development, from an early embryo to a fully differentiated and functioning organism is a long, complex process. Determining the moral status of that embryo at different stages of the process is a difficult task (Green 2001). Prior to implantation, an embryo's undifferentiated blastomeres are each capable of creating separate and unique individuals (through twinning). Other traits emerge later as the nervous system develops. At what point is there a (human) life? And is life (as opposed to, for instance, personhood) the right concept to be considering? And what is the status of the derived stem cells themselves? As Glenn McGee and Arthur Caplan have argued (1999), the problem of "what's in the dish?" remains one of the key concepts in this policy debate. At heart, though, the issue turns on precisely the kinds of metaphysical and biological issues that philosophy of biology has been exploring for decades. Surprisingly few have weighed in (Maienschein 2003), but more can be expected to do so in the future.

Debates about the origins of life have produced very different approaches to the meaning of life (Rizzotti 1996). Reductionist accounts place a heavy emphasis on genetic features—the ability to replicate is key, and the genes are seen as what make cells alive. In contrast, metabolists have long focused on the interactive elements of living things. Attempts to define the minimal genome represent the latest in the reductionist approach to defining life (Cho et al. 1999).

REDUCTIONISM AND GENETIC DETERMINISM

One of the themes that runs through much of the intersection of philosophy of biology and bioethics is the question of reductionism and its most criticized form, genetic determinism. To what extent are behavior and character dictated by genes? Popular images in magazines hype genes as the new Rosetta stone, the key to unlocking who and what people are (Nelkin and Lindee 1995). Many biologists have defended the view that genes are the primary determinants of key traits (Koshland 1990; Hamer and Copeland 1998).

Philosophically, there are multiple meanings of reductionism that can be distinguished. There is theory reductionism, in which theories at one level are explained by other theories that are seen as more fundamental. Philosophy of science has moved away from traditional views about theories, requiring alternative accounts of formal reductionism that look at models and mechanisms (Sarkar 1998). Reductionism can be epistemological in character—it can be about what provides the epistemological force to claims at different levels. So, for example, the force of rules in psychology could be dependent on the force of genetic rules that would explain the rules in psychology. Ontological reductionism would claim in one way or another that the only real entities are those at lower levels. Ultimately, the ideal reductionist picture would show the unity of science—behavioral accounts can be reduced to population genetics, population genetics can be reduced to molecular genetics, molecular genetics reduced to chemistry, and chemistry to physics. The only real entities are the entities posited by physics.

There have been many criticisms of reductionism (Kitcher 1984; Lewontin 1992; Keller 1995; Sarkar 1998; Kaplan 2000; Moss 2003). These have ranged from technical difficulties with reducing theories from biology to other levels (the only plausible laws in Mendelian genetics are not only false, transmission genetics is a measure of the degree of falsity of the law of independent assortment) to criticisms of specific popular reductions that purport to demonstrate the fundamental importance of genes as the determinants of human characteristics. Reductionism (especially the popular version) is largely a promissory note, one that the critics show is virtually impossible to pay off.

CONCLUSION

Philosophy of biology continues to grapple with conceptual issues that concern bioethicists. The meaning of disease, health, genetics, and even life are all issues that are full of import for normative concerns with how research should proceed, what sorts of science and medicine should be funded, and the moral status of different entities. The turn toward thick descriptions of biology and a growing interest in parts of biomedical science beyond evolution should fuel continued overlap between philosophy of biology and bioethics.

BIBLIOGRAPHY

Arieu, André A.; Robert Cummins; and Mark Perlman, eds. 2002. *Functions: New Essays in the Philosophy of Psychology and Biology*. Oxford: Oxford University Press.

Boorse, Christopher. 1975. "On the Distinction between Disease and Illness." *Philosophy and Public Affairs* 5 (1): 49–68.

Callebaut, Werner, ed. 1993. *Taking the Naturalistic Turn, or How Real Philosophy of Science Is Done, Conversations with William Bechtel, Robert N. Brandon, et al.* Organized and moderated by Werner Callebaut. Chicago: University of Chicago Press.

Caplan, Arthur L. 1992. "If Gene Therapy Is the Cure, What Is the Disease?" In *Gene Mapping*, edited by G. Annas and S. Elias, 128–41. Oxford: Oxford University Press.

Caplan, Arthur L.; Tristram H. Engelhardt Jr.; and James J. McCartney, eds. 1981. *Concepts of Health and Disease: Interdisciplinary Perspectives.* Reading, MA: Addison-Wesley

Cho, Mildred K.; David Magnus; Arthur L. Caplan; et al. 1999. "Ethical Implications of Synthesizing a Minimal Genome." *Science* 286 (5447): 2087–90.

Cummins, Robert. 1975. "Functional Analysis." *Journal of Philosophy* 72 (20): 741–65.

Engelhardt, T. 1981. "The Concepts of Health and Disease." In *Concepts of Health and Disease: Interdisciplinary Perspectives,* edited by Arthur L. Caplan, H. Tristram Engelhardt Jr., and James J. McCartney. Reading, MA: Addison-Wesley.

Farber, Paul. 1998. *The Temptations of Evolutionary Ethics.* Berkeley: University of California Press.

Gifford, Fred. 1990. "Genetic Traits." *Biology and Philosophy* 5 (3): 327–47.

Green, Ronald M. 2001. *The Human Embryo Research Debates: Bioethics in the Vortex of Controversy.* Oxford: Oxford University Press.

Hamer, Dean, and Peter Copeland. 1998. *Living with Our Genes: Why They Matter More Than You Think.* New York: Doubleday.

Hull, David L. 1974. *Philosophy of Biological Science.* Englewood Cliffs, NJ: Prentice-Hall.

Hull, Richard T. 1979. "Why '*Genetic* Disease'?" In *Genetic Counseling: Facts, Values, and Norms,* edited by Alexander M. Capron, Marc Lappé, Robert E. Murray, et al., 57–70. National Foundation–March of Dimes Birth Defects: Original Article Series 15 (2). New York: Alan R. Liss.

Kaplan, Jonathan Michael. 2000. *The Limits and Lies of Human Genetic Research: Dangers for Social Policy.* New York: Routledge Press.

Keller, E. F. 1995. *Refiguring Life: Metaphors of Twentieth-Century Biology.* New York: Columbia University Press.

Kitcher, Philip. 1984. "1953 and All That: A Tale of Two Sciences." *Philosophical Review* 93 (3): 335–73.

Koshland, Daniel E., Jr. 1990. "The Rational Approach to the Irrational." *Science* 250 (4978): 189.

Lewontin, R. C. 1992. *Biology as Ideology: The Doctrine of DNA.* New York: HarperPerennial.

Maienschein, Jane. 2003. *Whose View of Life? Embryos, Cloning, and Stem Cells.* Cambridge, MA: Harvard University Press.

Maienschein, Jane, and Michael Ruse, eds. 1999. *Biology and the Foundations of Ethics.* Cambridge: Cambridge University Press.

McGee, Glenn, and Arthur L. Caplan. 1999. "What's in the Dish?" *Hastings Center Report* 29 (2): 36–38.

Moss, Lenny. 2003. *What Genes Can't Do.* Cambridge, MA: MIT Press.

Nagel, Thomas. 1997. *The Last Word.* New York: Oxford University Press.

Nelkin, Dorothy, and M. Susan Lindee. 1995. *The DNA Mystique: The Gene as a Cultural Icon.* New York: W. H. Freeman Press.

Oyama, Susan; Paul E. Griffiths; and Russell D. Gray, eds. 2001. *Cycles of Contingency: Developmental Systems and Evolution.* Cambridge, MA: MIT Press.

Rizzotti, M, ed. 1996. *Defining Life: The Central Problem in Theoretical Biology.* Padova, Italy: University of Padova.

Ruse, Michael. 1973. *The Philospohy of Biology.* London: Hutchinson.

Ruse, Michael. 1991. "The Significance of Evolution." In *A Companion to Ethics*, edited by Peter Singer. Oxford: Blackwell.

Ruse, Michael. 1993. "The New Evolutionary Ethics." In *Evolutionary Ethics*, edited by Matthew H. Nitecki and Doris V. Nitecki. Albany: State University of New York Press.

Sarkar, Sahotra. 1998. *Genetics and Reductionism.* Cambridge: Cambridge University Press.

Schaffner, Kenneth F. 1993. *Discovery and Explanation in Biology and Medicine.* Chicago: University of Chicago Press.

Smith, John Maynard. 1982. *Evolution and the Theory of Games.* Cambridge: Cambridge University Press.

Smith, Kelly. 1990. "Genetic Disease, Genetic Testing, and the Clinician." *Medical Student Journal of the American Medical Association* 285:327–47.

Thagard, Paul. 1999. *How Scientists Explain Disease.* Princeton, NJ: Princeton University Press.

Wilson, E. O. 1978. *On Human Nature.* Cambridge, MA: Harvard University Press.

Wright, Larry. 1973. "Functions." *Philosophical Review* 82 (2): 139–68.

Wright, Robert. 1995. *The Moral Animal.* New York: Vintage Books.

Wulff, Henrik R. 1984. "The Causal Basis of the Current Disease Classification." In *Health, Disease, and Causal Explanations in Medicine*, edited by Lennart Nordenfeld and Ingemar B. Lindahl, 167–77. Dordrecht, Netherlands: Reidel.

David Magnus (2004)
Thomas A. Raffin Professor in Medicine and Biomedical Ethics, Stanford Center for Biomedical Ethics

BIOLOGY, PHILOSOPHY OF [ADDENDUM]

GENETIC REDUCTIONISM AND BEHAVIORAL GENETICS

The field of behavioral (or behavior) genetics has been much scrutinized by philosophers of biology (Schaffner 1998; Kaplan 2006; Tabery 2007; Tabery and Griffiths

2010). Broadly speaking, behavioral genetics seeks to apply genetic research strategies to the study of behavior (Plomin, De Fries, and McClearn 2008). Philosophers have paid particular attention to claims of a genetic basis for predispositions toward antisocial, aggressive, or criminal behavior (Wasserman and Wachbroit 2001; Kaplan 2006). These debates are part of a much older and larger set of debates over the relative importance of nature and nurture in human development and behavior.

The hypothesis that a predisposition toward a certain kind of behavior may be genetic raises a number of philosophical issues. Perhaps the overarching issue is normative: if an individual's predisposition to some behavior (e.g., alcoholism, violent outbursts, overeating) is genetic, should she or he be held responsible for that behavior? (Kaebnick 2006). Yet philosophers of biology have criticized the genetic reductionism underlying this question. Kenneth F. Schaffner (1998, 233) puts the point succinctly: "We do not find 'traitunculi'—little copies of the traits the genes determine—in the genes themselves."

Methodologically, philosophers of biology have leveled critiques against the technical concept of heritability used in classical population genetics (Sober 2001; Kaplan 2006), most of them echoing or elaborating on the work of Richard Lewontin (1974) in the famed IQ wars with Arthur R. Jensen (Lewontin 1974; Sesardic 1993; Oftedal 2005; Tabery 2007). Heritability is a statistical concept that estimates the proportion of variation in a given trait, be it height, weight, or IQ, in a given population in a given environment that can be attributed to genetic (as opposed to environmental) variation (Sober 2001). Although it may seem that high heritability for a trait would imply that it is "more genetic," this is not necessarily so. This is in part because heritability is a local measure—in a different environment heritability could be lower or higher (Lewontin 1974; Kaplan 2006). Indeed one can plot "norms of reaction" for a given genotype that show the effect of developmental environment on phenotype. Genotypes can give rise to different phenotypes in different developmental environments, a phenomenon known as phenotypic plasticity.

Metaphysically attention to the empirical details of the role of DNA in development at the molecular level has had a deflationary effect on the exalted status of DNA as a "master molecule" or "blueprint" whose instructions are carried out by cellular machinery. Along with the field of behavioral genetics itself (Turkheimer 2000), philosophy of biology has paid increasing attention to the role of gene-environment interactions in the process of human development (Schaffner 1998; Tabery and Griffiths 2010). Adopting a developmentalist stance, Paul E. Griffiths and Robin D. Knight (1998) have put forth a "parity thesis" according to which genes, cellular machinery, environmental inputs, and other contributors to the developmental process are on a par as developmental resources. In addition to undercutting genetic reductionism, the parity thesis has normative implications. If distributive justice demands that developmental resources, such as adequate schooling, nutrition, and shelter (or access to them), be justly allocated, then the parity thesis would imply that should genetic engineering make it possible, genetic material should be added to the list of developmental resources that are candidates for just distribution (Lewens 2002).

Simply put, most complex behavioral traits come about through an interaction between genes and environments, so understanding the normative implications of the genetic contribution involves attending to the empirical details (Boniolo and Vezzoni 2006). An illustration of the importance of gene-environment interaction and the developmentalist perspective can be seen in studies of a possible "gene for antisocial behavior." In the 1990s H. G. Brunner and colleagues (1993) studied a family in the Netherlands in which many of the males exhibited violent and antisocial behaviors. These subjects were found to have low levels of monoamine oxidase A (MAOA) (Brunner et al. 1993). Genetic testing revealed a point mutation in the promoter region for this protein in affected individuals—a gene for antisocial behavior, it would seem. Yet a follow-up study in New Zealand found that low-MAOA individuals were indeed at higher risk for antisocial behavior than high-MAOA individuals but only if they had suffered high levels of childhood abuse (Caspi et al. 2002). In a population without child abuse, the heritability of antisocial behavior would be low or zero. Thus high measures of heritability for a trait can be decoupled from the causal claim that it is genetically determined (Kaplan 2006; but see Jensen 1972; Sesardic 1993).

Whole-genome approaches to behavior have opened new areas for philosophical investigation. For example, genome-wide association studies (GWAS) have revealed that for many traits—not only complex behavioral traits but even such traits as height—genetic variants explain only a small fraction of the heritability, the "missing" or "phantom" heritability problem (Turkheimer 2012; Zuk et al. 2012; Schaffner 2013). Philosophers and behavioral geneticists are recognizing the limitations of purely statistical methods for investigating the genetic basis of complex human behaviors and are paying increased attention to pathways operating at the molecular level (Schaffner 2013). As behavioral genetics enters the molecular area, philosophers are also taking a fresh look at distinct statistical and developmental conceptions of gene-environment interaction (Tabery 2007).

SEE ALSO *Body: II. Cultural and Religious Perspectives; Life; Medicine, Philosophy of; Natural Law; Science, Philosophy of*

BIBLIOGRAPHY

Boniolo, Giovanni, and Paolo Vezzoni. 2006. "Genetic Influences on Moral Capacity: What Genetic Mutants Can Teach Us." In *Evolutionary Ethics and Contemporary Biology*, edited by Giovanni Boniolo and Gabriele De Anna, 77–96. Cambridge, UK: Cambridge University Press.

Brunner, H. G.; M. Nelen; X. O. Breakefield; et al. 1993. "Abnormal Behavior Associated with a Point Mutation in the Structural Gene for Monoamine Oxidase A." *Science* 262 (5133): 578–80.

Caspi, Avshalom; Joseph McClay; Terrie E. Moffitt; et al. 2002. "Role of Genotype in the Cycle of Violence in Maltreated Children." *Science* 297 (5582): 851–54.

Griffiths, Paul E., and Robin D. Knight. 1998. "What Is the Developmentalist Challenge?" *Philosophy of Science* 65 (2): 253–58.

Jensen, Arthur R. 1972. "The IQ Controversy: A Reply to Layzer." *Cognition* 1 (4): 427–52.

Kaebnick, Gregory E. 2006. "Behavioral Genetics and Moral Responsibility." In *Wrestling with Behavioral Genetics: Science, Ethics, and Public Conversation*, edited by Erik Parens, Audrey R. Chapman, and Nancy Press, 199–219. Baltimore: Johns Hopkins University Press.

Kaplan, Jonathan. 2006. "Misinformation, Misrepresentation, and Misuse of Human Behavioral Genetics Research." *Law and Contemporary Problems* 69 (Winter): 47–80.

Lewens, Tim. 2002. "Development Aid: On Ontogeny and Ethics." *Studies in History and Philosophy of Biological and Biomedical Sciences* 33 (2): 195–217.

Lewontin, Richard. 1974. "The Analysis of Variance and the Analysis of Causes." *American Journal of Human Genetics* 26 (3): 400–411.

Oftedal, Gry. 2005. "Heritability and Genetic Causation." *Philosophy of Science* 72 (5): 699–709.

Plomin, Robert; John C. De Fries; and Gerald E. McClearn. 2008. *Behavioral Genetics*. 5th ed. New York: Worth.

Schaffner, Kenneth F. 1998. "Genes, Behavior, and Developmental Emergentism: One Process, Indivisible?" *Philosophy of Science* 65 (2): 209–52.

Schaffner, Kenneth F. 2013. "Can Genes Explain Human Behavior? Doubtful!" Paper presented at the International Society for the History, Philosophy, and Social Studies of Biology conference, Montpellier, France.

Sesardic, Neven. 1993. "Heritability and Causality." *Philosophy of Science* 60 (3): 396–418.

Sober, Elliott. 2001. "Separating Nature and Nurture." In *Genetics and Criminal Behavior*, edited by David Wasserman and Robert Wachbroit, 47–78. Cambridge, UK: Cambridge University Press.

Tabery, James. 2007. "Biometric and Developmental Gene-Environment Interactions: Looking Back, Moving Forward." *Developmental Psychopathology* 19 (4): 961–76.

Tabery, James, and Paul E. Griffiths. 2010. "Historical and Philosophical Perspectives on Behavioral Genetics and Developmental Science." In *Handbook of Developmental Science, Behavior, and Genetics*, edited by Kathryn E. Hood, Carolyn Tucker Halpern, Gary Greenberg, and Richard M. Lerner, 41–60. Malden, MA: Wiley-Blackwell.

Turkheimer, Eric. 2000. "Three Laws of Behavior Genetics and What They Mean." *Current Directions in Psychological Science* 9 (5): 160–64.

Turkheimer, Eric. 2012. "Genome Wide Association Studies of Behavior Are Social Science." In *Philosophy of Behavioral Biology*, edited by Kathryn S. Plaisance and Thomas A. C. Reydon, 43–64. Dordrecht, Netherlands: Springer.

Wasserman, David, and Robert Wachbroit. 2001. *Genetics and Criminal Behavior*. Cambridge, UK: Cambridge University Press.

Zuk, Or; Eliana Hechter; Shamil R. Sunyaev; and Eric S. Lander. 2012. "The Mystery of Missing Heritability: Genetic Interactions Create Phantom Heritability." *Proceedings of the National Academy of Sciences of the United States of America* 109 (4): 1193–98.

John Huss
Associate Professor, Philosophy, University of Akron

BIOPOLITICS

The term *biopolitics* has several overlapping meanings, and the common thread running through them traces the way that biological technologies confer powers to control human bodies, populations, and societies. These power dynamics are not new, but innovations in the life sciences and biotechnologies, especially since the turn of the twenty-first century—sometimes called the biotech century—have given them new currency.

Some observers regard biopolitics as the appearance in the public sphere of issues previously addressed by professional bioethicists and medical ethicists (Pellegrino 2006). According to a broader emerging definition, which guides this entry, biopolitics refers to public understandings, public policies, and public-interest advocacy regarding the social meanings and consequences of a range of human genetic, reproductive, and biological technologies and practices. As such technologies and practices have become more advanced, biopolitics has come to mark important tensions among science, markets, the state, political life, and civil society. Although biopolitics in some contexts includes controversies over genetically modified organisms (GMOs) in the agricultural sector, such issues are not considered in this entry.

The life sciences today are based on techniques of manipulation, in contrast to the emphasis on observation and interpretation that characterized biology in earlier eras. Biotechnologies can alter the workings of cells and entire organisms; they can act directly on human bodies, behaviors, and minds. Another key transformation of the life sciences lies in their fast-growing commercialization:

since the birth of the modern biotechnology industry in the 1970s, the boundary between academic and commercial biology has become more and more blurred. Biotechnology-related products and services provided by laboratories and start-up companies spill out into the marketplace, medical care, the legal and criminal justice systems, pregnancy and family formation, and other realms of daily life. They increasingly shape our imaginations, our values, and our understanding of what it means to be human—now and in the future.

Accordingly, the social and ethical challenges posed by human biotechnologies in the early twenty-first century encompass much broader issues, and capture much greater public attention, than was the case in the early days of the field of bioethics. Biopolitical controversies play out in social realms, including academia, news and online media, and popular culture, and on political stages, including the courts, legislatures, and even national elections. And biopolitics is increasingly a focus for civil-society constituencies and public-interest organizations.

In contrast to bioethics, then, biopolitics focuses on broad social and political dynamics more than on encounters in institutional settings between doctors and patients or between researchers and human subjects. It emphasizes social values and policy proposals more than procedural recommendations and professional guidelines. Though bioethics and biopolitics are in constant conversation with each other, biopolitics is situated largely outside the organizational structures (such as academic departments, hospitals and clinics, institutional review boards, and corporate advisory boards) that are most closely associated with bioethics. Bioethics and biopolitics do, however, share an important affinity in their shared focus on practical responses to ethical questions raised by advances in the life sciences and biotechnology.

This entry sketches the history of the term *biopolitics* in scholarly usage and then turns to its use since the early 2000s by advocates with sharply divergent motivations and views about the preferred biopolitical future. It then comments on a number of biopolitical controversies that have played out in the public sphere.

BIOPOLITICS IN SCHOLARLY USAGE

The term *biopolitics* is used in a number of academic fields, including bioethics, sociology, anthropology, political science, philosophy, and science and technology studies, which examine the power-laden interplay among science, technology, and society. In 1979 two political scientists, Steven A. Peterson and Albert Somit, argued that "the influence of biology seems to have been felt in political science more than in some other social sciences" (Peterson and Somit). Many scholars today associate the term with the work of the French philosopher Michel Foucault (1926–1984), who introduced his theories of "biopower" and "biopolitics" in the mid-1970s (Foucault 2008; Lemke 2011).

Although Foucault's work focused on eighteenth- and nineteenth-century Europe, his ideas about the political powers conferred by biological technologies have had tremendous influence across the social sciences and humanities. Foucault's understanding of biopolitics is situated within his argument for a new way of understanding power: in addition to the top-down control exercised by a sovereign state, he claimed, power is built into our social relationships, norms, and everyday routines. Biopolitics for Foucault represented the means through which populations and individuals are governed in diffuse yet pervasive ways, including those that reach to the level of the body and life itself.

Foucault's post-structuralist approach to biopolitics has been interpreted and expanded upon by many critical theorists, including Donna J. Haraway (1991), Giorgio Agamben (1998), and Michael Hardt and Antonio Negri (2004). In addition, it has motivated similar concepts, such as Paul Rabinow's (1996) "biosociality," Nikolas Rose's (2007) "vital politics," and Adele E. Clarke et al.'s (2010) "biomedicalization." Rose's reworking of biopolitics deserves special attention because it focuses on the twenty-first-century context in which genetics and biotechnology have greatly influenced the politics of what he calls "life itself." In *The Politics of Life Itself*, Rose explains:

> Politics has long been concerned with the vital lives of those who are governed. … But the vital politics of our own century looks rather different. … It is concerned with our growing capacities to control, manage, engineer, reshape, and modulate the very vital capacities of human beings as living creatures. It is, I suggest, a politics of 'life itself.' (2006, 3)

BIOPOLITICS IN SOCIAL AND POLITICAL ADVOCACY

The history of *biopolitics* in social and political advocacy—both as a term and as a set of concerns raised by developments in the life sciences and the biotechnology industry—has been less frequently discussed than has its academic genealogy. A full discussion of this history would be an important contribution to understanding the current landscape of biopolitics. This entry provides just a few landmarks on a rather sketchy map.

Emergence of Issues. Several events in the mid-1970s presaged the emergence of biopolitics in the United States and around the world. The publication in 1975 of Edward O. Wilson's *Sociobiology: The New Synthesis*, which argued that genetics rather than social and environmental conditions are determinant in individual human behavior and in social formations, sparked heated controversy about the politics of biology. Also in 1975 some 140 biologists, physicians, lawyers, and others gathered in California at the "Asilomar Conference on Recombinant DNA" to discuss the potential hazards of biotechnology and to draw up voluntary safety guidelines that many believe were designed to fend off calls for enforceable regulation. The conference and its recommendations pushed the emerging field of biotechnology into public awareness (Berg et al. 1975). In 1976 venture capitalist Robert Swanson and biochemist Herbert Boyer launched a company called Genentech, an event often said to mark the founding of the biotechnology industry.

In 1980, still during the prehistory of biopolitics, a US Supreme Court case, *Diamond v. Chakrabarty*, and a piece of congressional legislation, the Bayh-Dole Act, encouraged the development of the private-sector biotechnology industry and set in motion some of the important economic and political dynamics underlying the emergence of biopolitics. In *Diamond v. Chakrabarty*, the court ruled that genetically engineered organisms could be patented, and the Bayh-Dole Act allowed universities and individual scientists to patent and commercialize technical inventions. In 1983 the first US public-interest organization focusing on the social, ethical, and environmental implications of modern genetic technologies was established in Cambridge, Massachusetts. Called the Council for Responsible Genetics (CRG), the organization has examined biological weapons, worker and community safety in biotechnology laboratories, agricultural biotechnologies, and biomedical developments. It has also developed critiques of genetic reductionism, genetic determinism, and germ-line genetic interventions (Council for Responsible Genetics 2013a).

By the late 1980s and early 1990s a different approach to human biotechnologies in general—and to inheritable genetic modification and other enhancement technologies in particular—began to take shape. This was the futurist ideology, today known as transhumanism, which advocates using genetic and other technologies to enhance (as adherents see it) human capacities and to take control of human evolution. An early transhumanist organization, the libertarian Extropy Institute, was founded in 1990; in 1998 the World Transhumanist Association was established (Hughes 2004).

Developments and Debate. During the 1990s dialogue and debate continued in scholarly publications, bioethical discussions, mainstream media, and popular culture concerning emerging and future applications of human genetic and reproductive technologies. In light of experimental gene-transfer procedures and in anticipation of the completion of a "map" of the human genome, gene therapy was heralded as a miraculous new medical treatment until the tragic death of an eighteen-year-old in a gene-therapy clinical trial in 1999 (Marshall 1999; Nelson and Weiss 1999). Meanwhile, feminist scholars and others examined the growing use of in vitro fertilization (IVF) and its variants, the growth of a market in human eggs and commercial surrogacy (contract pregnancy), and the implications of these developments for women's health and well-being and for the commodification of human reproduction (Rothman 1998).

In the late 1990s a small but influential number of scientists began openly to advocate the development and use of extreme human biotechnologies, including reproductive cloning and inheritable genetic modification for enhancement purposes. The conversation exploded and moved to mainstream news media and popular culture after the 1997 announcement that the first cloned mammal, a sheep called Dolly, had been born. The film *Gattaca*, released the same year (and still exerting strong cultural influence into the twenty-first century), explored the filmmakers' vision of a not-too-distant future of genetic castes and DNA-based discrimination, in which "valids"—those with high-caliber preselected genes—are the ruling elite while "in-valids" labor at menial jobs with no way up or out. In 1998 a conference at the University of California, Los Angeles called "Engineering the Human Germline" drew one thousand participants and was covered on the front pages of the *New York Times* (March 21, 1998) and the *Washington Post* (March 22, 1998). The goal of the conference, said the scientists who organized it, was to make human germline engineering acceptable to the American public (Stock and Campbell 2000).

Even with all this activity the term *biopolitics* was not yet commonly used with its current meaning. An exception was in a volume of collected essays titled *Biopolitics: A Feminist and Ecological Reader on Biotechnology*, published in 1995 by the politically liberal British publisher Zed Books (Shiva and Moser). Its focus was the ecological risks, ethics, and social implications of agricultural biotechnology, but it also included (previously published) essays titled "Human Nature" and "Genes as Causes," both by Ruth Hubbard, professor emerita of biology at Harvard University and a board member of the Council for Responsible Genetics. The publisher's description begins by saying, "Biotechnology is the single most powerful bundle of new technologies currently under development. It is also the most intrusive and determinative technology relating to nature generally and the human body specifically."

Wider Adoption of the Term. In the early 2000s the term *biopolitics* was adopted by writers and advocates with starkly different political and ethical commitments. In 2002 the environmental writer and activist Jeremy Rifkin published "Fusion Biopolitics" in *The Nation*, a left-leaning journal of opinion. Rifkin's news hook was then-pending federal legislation about a research cloning technique, but he went on to note that opposition to creating cloned human beings was found among both progressives and social conservatives. The latter, he said, were motivated by "what they regard as the rights of the unborn," whereas many progressives "argue that with cloning the new progeny become the ultimate shopping experience—designed in advance, produced to specification and purchased in the biological marketplace. … The left also warns that cloning opens the way to a commercial eugenics civilization." Rifkin went on to predict that new and emerging biotechnologies would rearrange traditional political affiliations: "The current debate over cloning human embryos and stem cell research is already loosening the old alliances and categories. It is just the beginning of the new biopolitics."

Transhumanists also began using the term *biopolitics*. According to the World Transhumanist Association founder James Hughes (2004, 55), "at one end of the biopolitical spectrum are the bioLuddites, defending humanity from enhancement technologies, and at the other the transhumanists, advocating for our right to become more than human." Like Rifkin, Hughes argues that biopolitics is becoming "a new dimension" of the "political terrain of the twenty-first century," cutting "across the existing political lines." Hughes distinguishes between what he calls "right bioconservatives" and "left bioconservatives" and describes a "polarization between the transhumanist and bioconservative positions within biopolitics" (Hughes 2011, 165).

The Center for Genetics and Society (CGS), with which both authors of this entry are or have been affiliated, was founded in 2001. Its initial focus was the threat to social justice and equality raised by the prospect of inheritable genetic modifications that could be enabled by cloning, gene transfer, and assisted reproductive technologies. CGS's mission statement, published on the organization's website, signaled its commitments to fundamental progressive principles, including "the equitable provision of health technologies," reproductive rights, disability rights, and a precautionary approach to new technologies (Center for Genetics and Society 2013a). The organization soon adopted the term *biopolitics*; in 2006 it established a blog called *Biopolitical Times*, accessible through its website. For CGS the term *progressive biopolitics* and the phrase *a new biopolitics* connote a commitment to social justice, human rights, and public-interest values. CGS has worked with scholars across a range of disciplines, including law, sociology, anthropology, public health, biology, and science and technology studies, and with advocates promoting various issues, including reproductive health, rights, and justice; racial justice; disability rights; and environmentalism (Center for Genetics and Society 2013b).

BIOPOLITICAL CONTROVERSIES

What does biopolitics look like on the contemporary political landscape? This section offers several brief comments on selected biopolitical issues that have emerged as politically or socially significant in the twenty-first century. This is far from an exhaustive list; the issues discussed here have been chosen because they are widely recognized as politically salient, have triggered legislation or judicial decisions, or have been engaged by public-interest organizations and civil-society constituencies.

Stem Cell Research and Cloning. Research on human stem cells has been one of the most high-profile and fiercely controversial technoscientific issues of the early twenty-first century, especially in the United States. When human embryonic stem cells were first isolated in 1998 at the University of Wisconsin (Devitt 1998), it was immediately evident both that they held significant scientific and medical promise and that they would be politically divisive, primarily because of staunch opposition among social and religious conservatives to research involving human embryos and fetal tissue.

The controversy intensified considerably after President George W. Bush announced a policy in 2001 limiting federal funding for embryonic stem cell research. Stem cell research became a litmus-test issue in the 2004 presidential campaign, with Ron Reagan (b. 1958), the son of the former US president Ronald Reagan, telling the Democratic National Convention that it would produce for each of us a "personal biological repair kit standing by at the hospital" (Reagan 2004). Meanwhile, opponents of embryonic stem cell research proclaimed equally miraculous powers for stem cells derived from adult tissues.

A key aspect of the stem cell debate concerned the use of cloning-based techniques (known as "research cloning" or "somatic cell nuclear transfer") in efforts to create disease-specific and patient-specific stem cell lines. Progressives and liberals who raised concerns about research cloning focused on the enormous numbers of women's eggs it would require and the risks to women this would pose, as well as on the need for rigorous oversight to prevent cloned embryos from being misused in efforts to produce cloned human beings. At the conservative end of the political spectrum, both reproductive cloning and research cloning were objectionable as practices that entail the destruction of (cloned) human embryos (Weiss 2002).

These concerns, and headlines about a few fertility doctors and marginal figures who claimed they were engaged in efforts to clone human beings (Center for Genetics and Society 2004) prompted efforts in state legislatures, in the US Congress, in other countries, and at the United Nations to address human cloning. A handful of US states passed laws against human reproductive cloning (National Conference of State Legislatures 2008), as did dozens of countries (BioPolicyWiki 2009). But legislation at the federal level in the United States (Center for Genetics and Society 2008) and a proposed binding international treaty at the UN (Center for Genetics and Society 2006; United Nations 2005) failed because conservatives refused to support prohibitions on reproductive cloning unless research cloning was included in the same measure.

The stem cell controversy has often been portrayed as a fierce but simple clash pitting scientists, patient groups, and most liberals and progressives against conservatives committed to the full moral status of human embryos—that is, the view that embryos have the same rights as adults and children. But the debate involved additional important issues: irresponsible scientific hyperbole about the certainty and imminence of breakthroughs and cures; the widely agreed-upon need to prohibit the creation of cloned human beings; and the importance of protecting research subjects, starting with the women who at the time were being asked to provide the large numbers of eggs needed for cloning-based stem cell research. In addition, public-interest groups in California raised basic issues of responsible governance concerning that state's stem cell research agency, which was created in 2004 after voters approved a ballot measure for $3 billion in funding (Hayes 2006).

Women's organizations in South Korea, and some women's health advocates in the United States, engaged in the stem cell debate because of concerns about the risks to women undergoing procedures to retrieve the vast quantities of eggs required for cloning-based stem cell research. These concerns played out during the scandal surrounding Hwang Woo Suk, the South Korean researcher whose 2004 announcement that he had created cloned human embryos was revealed to be fraudulent two years later. Hwang had used more than two thousand eggs, many obtained under dubious conditions that sent some twenty women to the hospital (Sample 2006). Two of these women, supported by a coalition of thirty-five Korean women's groups, filed a lawsuit against the South Korean government, but the case was dismissed by the Seoul District Court in 2009 (*Nature* 2009).

The stem cell debate cooled in 2007, when Japanese scientists announced that they had used ordinary skin cells to derive induced pluripotent stem cells, which have properties similar to those of embryonic stem cells (Takahashi et al. 2007). In 2009 President Barack Obama lifted federal funding restrictions on embryonic stem cell research, and in accompanying remarks he called reproductive cloning "dangerous" and "profoundly wrong." By 2009 new controversies had erupted over fraudulent claims made by companies in the United States as well as in countries including Mexico, Ecuador, Japan, Thailand, South Korea, Ireland, and the Netherlands regarding stem cell treatments (Kiatpongsan and Sipp 2009; Cyranoski 2012). Another simmering but not yet widely recognized stem cell issue concerns research into creating human gametes from induced pluripotent stem cells, which could enable experiments with human germline modification (Shanks 2012).

Patents on Human Genes. Although the United Nations and the World Medical Association have stated that human genes are part of the common heritage of humanity, the US Patent and Trademark Office has granted thousands of patents on human genes. About 20 percent of human genes are now patented, and a company or university that holds a patent on a gene can prevent anyone else from studying, testing, or even looking at it (Lovgren 2005).

In 2009 the American Civil Liberties Union (ACLU) and the Public Patent Foundation filed a lawsuit (*Association for Molecular Pathology v. Myriad Genetics*) on behalf of a group of plaintiffs challenging the constitutionality of gene patents, arguing that granting patent protection to genetic sequences is a violation of the First Amendment. The suit named as defendants the US Patent and Trademark Office, as well as Myriad Genetics and the University of Utah Research Foundation, both of which hold patents on the breast cancer genes known as BRCA1 and BRCA2. The twenty plaintiffs included scientific organizations representing 150,000 geneticists, pathologists, and laboratory professionals; women's health groups, including Breast Cancer Action and Our Bodies Ourselves; and individual researchers, genetic counselors, and cancer patients. The scientists said that Myriad had directly prevented some of their work by issuing cease-and-desist letters, thus stifling diagnostic testing and research. The plaintiffs also argued that Myriad had kept the cost of the test for BRCA1 and BRCA2 unreasonably high and that the patents limited women's health care options by disallowing independent medical opinions about particular genetic variants or their interpretation. Friend-of-the-court briefs were filed by women's health, environmental, and scientific organizations, as well as other public-interest groups (Darnovsky and Reynolds 2009). The biotechnology sector was itself divided about the lawsuit.

In June 2013 the US Supreme Court ruled unanimously that human genes may not be patented, a decision greeted with unbridled enthusiasm by the large coalition of plaintiffs and supporters (Liptak 2013).

DNA Police Databases. Police forces around the world are increasingly turning to genetic information to help solve criminal cases. Genetic evidence is being used both to convict perpetrators and to exonerate people who were wrongfully convicted, including many on death row (Handwerk 2005). DNA-based forensic tools are highly accurate when used to compare an unknown DNA sample with another that has already been identified, though they are far from foolproof—serious problems have resulted from human error and sample contamination. The development of massive DNA police databases containing millions of profiles, however, has given rise to new problems and questions. Some concern the accuracy of "cold hits"—searching databases for matches with DNA found at a crime scene when other investigative options have failed. In these cases, and especially when the DNA is incomplete or degraded, reliability plummets. Yet jurors deciding cases involving DNA evidence from cold hits "are often told that the odds of a coincidental match are hundreds of thousands of times more remote than they actually are" (Felch and Dolan 2008).

In many states and countries police are permitted (or required) to obtain and store genetic samples from people arrested for but not necessarily charged with or convicted of crimes. These preconviction sampling practices mean that police databases contain DNA from a large and growing number of innocent people. Furthermore, police are increasingly tapping DNA databases using a technique called familial searching, which brings under surveillance members of extended families, most of whom have never broken the law but whose DNA profiles share commonalities with samples gathered at crime scenes. DNA police databases thus raise significant concerns about civil liberties and the prospect of genetic surveillance. These threats are particularly worrisome for communities that already have disproportionately frequent encounters with criminal justice systems (Obasogie 2009; Krimsky and Simoncelli 2011).

The United Kingdom's national DNA database, which was established in 1995 and is the world's oldest, had by 2008 collected DNA from more than three-fourths of the country's young black men and from more than one-fourth of its entire black population. In 2011, following pressure from civil society organizations and a ruling by the European Court of Human Rights, the government agreed to remove the genetic profiles of an estimated one million innocent people—the first time that any government had rolled back a DNA database and restricted the data that is retained (GeneWatch UK 2013). In the United States, the American Civil Liberties Union has challenged these practices in several jurisdictions.

Direct-to-Consumer Genetic Testing. Dozens of direct-to-consumer (DTC) genetic testing companies, some with significant financial backing, offer to sequence and interpret their customers' genomes. People send in a saliva sample and then receive a report that claims to predict risk for a variety of common diseases and conditions. Most DTC companies test partial genomes, but with prices rapidly plummeting beginning in 2008, whole-genome sequencing is expected to be readily available in the near future (National Human Genome Institute 2013). An investigation by the US Government Accountability Office (2010), however, revealed that the same DNA sent to multiple companies, including those considered most reputable, yielded contradictory results. And the predictions are often highly misleading: many medical professionals are concerned that recipients of these reports will misinterpret them and flood the health care system with requests for consultations or undergo unnecessary medical procedures.

The scientific assumptions underlying genetic testing are also controversial. An increasing number of medical and genetic experts agree that when it comes to predicting common diseases (including most forms of cancer and heart disease) in healthy people, gene tests "have produced little for medicine" (Wade 2010); leading geneticists have begun to acknowledge the "missing heritability" of common traits (Zuk et al. 2011). According to these views, responsible medical practice would limit gene tests to those that are clinically meaningful and useful, and it would temper grand claims about the revolutionary potential of so-called personalized medicine (Dickenson 2010). In 2010 the FDA began considering what kind of regulatory policy and authority it will exercise over DTC gene testing (Singer 2010).

Sex Selection. In China and India sex selection, typically accomplished by abortion after the sex of a fetus has been identified in an ultrasound test, has become staggeringly widespread. Because such abortions mainly affect female fetuses, the practice has created wildly skewed sex ratios: well over 100 million females are statistically missing from these populations (Sen 1990). This imbalance has led to bride migration and bride trafficking and has exacerbated violence against women (Hvistendahl 2011b). Notwithstanding common assumptions by demographers and social scientists that the practice of sex selection would diminish with the spread of modernity and affluence, it is actually growing in popularity, in part because of the increased availability since the early 1980s of cheap and portable ultrasound machines used for prenatal testing. And sex selection is spreading throughout south and east Asia and beyond, to the Caucasus region and even eastern Europe (Hvistendahl 2011b; Hennen 2013). In India women's health groups and feminists have campaigned since the late 1970s against sex selection (Hvistendahl 2011b, 152). India passed a law in 1994 (amended in 2002) prohibiting sex selection through abortion (CHILDLINE India Foundation n.d.), but this legislation has been largely ineffective (Hvistendahl 2011b, 47).

In the United States sex selection has not caused skewed numbers of boys except among second and third children in families of Chinese, Indian, and Korean descent (Almond and Edlund 2008). But sex selection using high-tech methods, such as sperm sorting or embryo screening in conjunction with IVF, has become a $100 million per year industry. A 2006 survey of fertility clinics found that, of the clinics that at that time offered genetic testing of embryos created through IVF, nearly half offered nonmedical sex selection (Genetics and Public Policy Center 2006). Anecdotal evidence suggests that, for the most part, Americans who use these techniques choose to have girls as often as boys. Some argue that this makes sex selection unproblematic; others point out that selecting for boys *or* for girls raises concerns about gender stereotyping, parental expectations, and normalizing selection of other traits. Libertarians have argued that sex selection should be seen as an extension of reproductive choice (Robertson 2001); others see a clear distinction between choosing whether and when to have children and choosing the particular traits of those children (Bhatia et al. 2003).

Antiabortion advocates in the United States have tried to use sex selection as a wedge issue to undermine support for abortion rights, complicating efforts to address the issue by feminists who are in favor of abortion rights but are critical of sex selection. In countries such as Canada, Germany, and the United Kingdom, sex selection has been prohibited without affecting abortion rights (Hvistendahl 2011a).

Noninvasive Prenatal Testing. New techniques for noninvasive prenatal testing (NIPT)analyze fetal DNA that is collected from a woman's blood as early as five weeks into a pregnancy. Already on the market for diagnosing Down syndrome and other chromosomal anomalies, the techniques are being refined to allow identification of fetal genes at thousands of sites. The development of such tests would mean that expecting parents who use NIPT would receive the same kinds of reports about their early-stage fetus as they would get about themselves from a direct-to-consumer genetic testing company. They would face the same kinds of inherent uncertainties in interpreting the results but would be in a position to make a consequential decision about whether to continue the pregnancy.

Because NIPT is less invasive, less risky, and less expensive than the other kinds of fetal gene tests available, and because it relies on a simple blood draw so early in pregnancy, if widely used it would dramatically change the experience of pregnancy and childbearing. Disability rights advocates ask whether health insurers will encourage NIPT, or even require it, in order to avoid the costs of special-needs children. Such advocates are concerned that larger numbers of parents will choose to terminate a pregnancy if the fetus is reported to have any kind of disability, even a type with which many people live full and happy lives. Stanford University bioethicist Henry T. Greely (2011) predicts that the "spectre of eugenics will loom over the whole discussion" of NIPT and that concerns about eugenics "will increase as such testing moves from fatal diseases to less serious medical conditions and then on to nonmedical characteristics" (Greely 290). Meanwhile, reproductive rights advocates, including those disquieted by the prospect of medically irrelevant genetic testing that could carry society into the realm of eugenics, worry that these difficult questions will be swamped by blanket condemnation of the new tests by those who oppose abortion rights under any circumstances (Darnovsky 2011).

Egg Freezing. While techniques to freeze human embryos and sperm have been used for several decades as part of assisted reproduction practices, freezing human eggs has proved more technically challenging. Because of the large amount of water contained in eggs, cryoprotectant chemicals are added to prevent damage when they are frozen and thawed. By the mid 2000s, freezing methods associated with higher survival rates led some fertility clinics to offer egg freezing, though the procedure was considered experimental. In 2012 the American Society for Reproductive Medicine (ASRM) announced that it was removing its "experimental" label from egg freezing (Practice Committee of the American Society for Reproductive Medicine and the Society for Assisted Reproductive Technology 2012).

The move generated a flurry of media coverage, with many news accounts presenting the procedure as an unproblematic path to greater women's freedom and autonomy while omitting or downplaying risks to women's health and social concerns about their lives. In fact, the ASRM's revised guideline is narrowly written; it applies only to women facing infertility as a result of impending medical interventions, typically chemotherapy as a cancer treatment. The ASRM guideline notes that there is inadequate data on the safety and efficacy of egg freezing when used by older women and when eggs are frozen for long periods. In addition, the statement acknowledges that, at the time of publication, the few children born from frozen eggs were still very young and that, therefore, data on long-term risks for these children is limited. Furthermore, there are significant but under-studied health risks of egg extraction that are often not fully explained to women considering undergoing the procedure for any reason (Beeson and Lippman 2006). The risks, over the short term and the long term, are mostly associated with the hormones that shut down and then hyperstimulate the ovaries as part of the procedure.

The prospect of healthy young women with no known fertility problems freezing their eggs as a form of insurance for achieving pregnancy when they are older may be attractive to the fertility industry because it represents a potentially large new customer base. Egg freezing could also trigger another business shift; namely, to an increase in frozen egg banks. This would be more convenient for egg recipients and fertility doctors but could mean lower payments for egg providers in general. It could also mean a new emphasis on recruiting providers from areas of the world where women with traits that are considered desirable may be willing to accept less money, but where the risks of exploitation may be higher.

Some women's rights advocates view egg freezing as a technical fix likely to distract attention from social changes that would address some of the reasons women delay childbearing, such as the dearth of family-friendly workplaces (McCurtis 2008). A related concern is the prospect of women facing additional pressures from employers to postpone childbearing because of the availability of egg freezing (Dana 2012).

Commercial Surrogacy. Commercial surrogacy is a growing sector of the fertility industry. Surrogacy enables gay couples, and some infertile couples who could not otherwise have children, to form families. However, feminist and other critics have long noted the class dimensions of the practice: women who serve as surrogates are invariably less affluent than those who hire them. Concerns about exploitation are heightened when surrogates are poor women in developing countries. The early decades of the twenty-first century have seen a surge in arrangements involving couples looking abroad for surrogates, a practice often referred to as reproductive tourism. India is the most common destination; surrogacy for foreigners is also offered in countries including Mexico, Argentina, Guatemala, and Spain. In India surrogates are often required to live in fertility clinic dormitories away from their own families and to agree to medical procedures, including cesarean sections, for the convenience of those who hire them (Twine 2011; Pet 2012).

Genetic Discrimination. The spread of genetic testing has raised the prospect of discrimination by employers, health insurers, and others against people with genetic variations that may signal increased risk of future disease. Beginning in the 1990s, disease-specific groups, consumer rights organizations, genetic counselors, and others began working to prohibit genetic discrimination. The Coalition for Genetic Fairness, founded in 1997, grew to include more than five hundred organizations by 2008, including industry groups and employers. Legislation to protect against genetic discrimination was first introduced in the US House of Representative in 1995, and a bill called the Genetic Information Nondiscrimination Act was finally signed into law by President George W. Bush in 2008. It covers employment and health care insurance and is widely seen as an important step. But because the legislation does not cover military personnel nor extend to life, disability, or long-term-care insurance, political efforts to prevent genetic discrimination in the United States are sure to continue (Coalition for Genetic Fairness 2013; Council for Responsible Genetics 2013b).

Race-Based Research and Products. Several developments in the biotechnology field threaten to revive discredited notions about race as a scientifically valid biological category, rather than a social and political system. Examples include the misuses of racial categories in genetic and biomedical research, the regulatory approval and marketing of drugs for specified racial groups (most notably the drug BiDil, approved by the FDA in 2005 as a heart medication specifically for African Americans), and representations about racial legacies in genomic ancestry testing (Obasogie 2009). These products and practices obscure the social and political dynamics that shape race, and they divert resources and attention away from identifying and addressing the socioeconomic causes of health disparities (Kahn 2012). As legal scholar Dorothy Roberts (2011) points out, this tendency is particularly disturbing given that many people believe that American society has entered a postracial age. In other words, Roberts says, biological race is being revived at the same historical moment that the social importance of race is being denied or neglected.

BIOPOLITICAL PROSPECTS

The social, ethical, and political challenges posed by human biotechnologies are among the thorniest and most consequential that society faces. As Rifkin (2002) and Jonathan D. Moreno (2011) note, they are already roiling the conventional politics of left and right.

Biopolitical issues are also producing tensions within civil rights and human rights constituencies. Many advocates of gay and lesbian rights, for example, welcome assisted reproductive technologies that expand opportunities to have biologically related children (Mamo 2007), but also worry about the implications of a so-called (and almost certainly spurious) gay gene (*Frontline* 2000). Some racial justice advocates take the advent of race-specific drugs as a sign that the pharmaceutical industry is finally addressing racial health disparities (Winstein 2007); others denounce the drugs as throwbacks to fallacious and dangerous views of racial groupings as biologically determined rather than socially and politically enforced (Roberts 2011; Kahn 2012). Some supporters of reproductive rights believe that reproductive choice should extend to selecting the traits of future children (Robertson 2001); others argue that this is altogether different from a woman's right to decide whether to terminate a pregnancy (Darnovsky 2009; Hvistendahl 2011a).

The biopolitical spectrum is still in formation. Its shape will be determined by several broad political questions: first, the relative weight given to social justice, the public interest, and the common good versus individual liberty and autonomy; second, the extent to which society welcomes responsible public policy and regulation rather than relying on laissez-faire market mechanisms and corporate agendas; and, third, the degree of enthusiasm or caution brought to the assessment of various technologies, practices, and products associated with human genetic and reproductive technologies (Darnovsky 2009).

SEE ALSO *Bioethics: X. Politics of; Cloning; DNA Identification; Embryo and Fetus: III. Embryonic Stem Cell Research; Food; Genetic Discrimination; Genetic Testing and Screening; Health Policy and Politics; Patenting Organisms and Basic Research; Personalized Medicine; Precautionary Principle; Reproductive Technologies; Transhumanism and Posthumanism*

BIBLIOGRAPHY

Agamben, Giorgio. 1998. *Homo Sacer: Sovereign Power and Bare Life*. Translated by Daniel Heller-Roazen. Stanford, CA: Stanford University Press.

Almond, Douglas, and Lena Edlund. 2008. "Son-Biased Sex Ratios in the 2000 United States Census." *Proceedings of the National Academy of Sciences of the United States of America* 105 (15): 5681–82.

Bayh-Dole Act. 1980. 35 U.S.C. § 200–212.

Beeson, Diane, and Abby Lippman. 2006. "Egg Harvesting for Stem Cell Research: Medical Risks and Ethical Problems." *Reproductive Biomedicine Online*. October.

Berg, Paul, et al. 1975. "Summary Statement of the Asilomar Conference on Recombinant DNA Molecules." *Proceedings of the National Academy of Sciences of the United States of America.* 72 (6): 1981–84.

Bhatia, Rajani; Rupsa Mallik; and Shamita Das Dasgupta. 2003. "Sex Selection: New Technologies, New Forms of Gender Discrimination." Committee on Women, Population, and the Environment. October 1. Accessed June 2, 2013. http://www.cwpe.org/resources/healthrepro/sexselnewtech

BioPolicyWiki. 2009. "Reproductive Cloning." Accessed June 2, 2013. http://biopolicywiki.org/index.php?title=Reproductive_ cloning

Center for Genetics and Society. 2004. "Reported Efforts to Clone Human Beings." Accessed June 2, 2013. http://www.geneticsandsociety.org/article.php?id=383

Center for Genetics and Society. 2006. "The United Nations Human Cloning Treaty Debate, 2000–2005." Accessed June 2, 2013. http://www.geneticsandsociety.org/article.php?id=338

Center for Genetics and Society. 2008. "Failure to Pass Federal Cloning Legislation, 1997–2003." Accessed June 2, 2013. http://www.geneticsandsociety.org/article.php?id=305

Center for Genetics and Society. 2013a. "About Us." Accessed May 3, 2013. http://www.geneticsandsociety.org/article.php?list=type&type=10

Center for Genetics and Society. 2013b. "The Tarrytown Meetings." Accessed May 3, 2013. http://www.geneticsandsociety.org/article.php?id=5561

CHILDLINE India Foundation. n.d. "Pre-Natal Diagnostic Techniques Act, 1994." Accessed June 2, 2013. http://www.childlineindia.org.in/Pre-natal-Diagnostic-Techniques-Act-1994.htm

Clarke, Adele E.; Laura Mamo; Jennifer Ruth Fosket; et al., eds. 2010. *Biomedicalization: Technoscience, Health, and Illness in the U.S.* Durham, NC: Duke University Press.

Coalition for Genetic Fairness. 2013. "About the Coalition for Genetic Fairness." Accessed May 3, 2013. http://www.geneticfairness.org/about.html

Council for Responsible Genetics. 2013a. "Accomplishments." Accessed May 3, 2013. http://www.councilforresponsiblegenetics.org/Help/Accomplishments.aspx

Council for Responsible Genetics. 2013b. "Genetic Discrimination." Accessed May 3, 2013. http://www.councilforresponsiblegenetics.org/geneticprivacy/DNA_discrim.html

Cyranoski, David. 2012. "Stem Cell Fraud Hits Febrile Field." *Nature News,* November 12.

Dana, Rebecca. 2012. "The Vitrification Fertility Option: They Save Their Eggs and Thrive at Work. Diane Sawyer's Secret to Resetting the Biological Clock." *Newsweek,* January 23. Accessed May 3, 2013. http://www.thedailybeast.com/newsweek/2012/01/22/the-vitrification-fertility-option.html

Darnovsky, Marcy. 2009. "Political Science: Progressives Can't—and Shouldn't—Remove Politics and Values from Science." *Democracy* 13:36–48. http://www.democracyjournal.org/13/6700.php?page=all

Darnovsky, Marcy. 2011. "One Step Closer to Designer Babies: New Noninvasive Prenatal Genetic Testing Could Change Human Pregnancy Forever." *Science Progress*, April 22. Accessed May 3, 2013. http://scienceprogress.org/2011/04/one-step-closer-to-designer-babies/

Darnovsky, Marcy, and Jesse Reynolds. 2009. "The Battle to Patent Your Genes: The Meaning of the Myriad Case." *American Interest*, September/October.

Devitt, Terry. 1998. "Wisconsin Scientists Culture Elusive Embryonic Stem Cells." *University of Wisconsin-Madison News*, November 6.

Diamond v. Chakrabarty. 1980. 447 U.S. 303.

Dickenson, Donna. 2010. "The Genetic Mystique of 'Me' Medicine." *Globe and Mail*, August 28.

Felch, Jason, and Maura Dolan. 2008. "When a Match Is Far from a Lock." *Los Angeles Times.* May 4. Accessed June 2, 2013. http://articles.latimes.com/2008/may/04/local/me-dna4

Foucault, Michel. 2008. *The Birth of Biopolitics: Lectures at the Collège de France, 1978–1979.* Edited by Michel Senellart. Translated by Graham Burchell. Basingstoke, UK: Palgrave Macmillan.

Frontline. 2000. "The 'Gay Gene' Debate." *Assault on Gay America.* Accessed June 4, 2013. http://www.pbs.org/wgbh/pages/frontline/shows/assault/genetics/

Genetic Information and Nondiscrimination Act. 2008. 42 U.S. C. § 2000ff et seq.

Genetics and Public Policy Center. 2006. "Center Study Probes Preimplantation Genetic Diagnosis." September 20. Accessed May 3, 2013. http://www.dnapolicy.org/news.release.php?action=detail&pressrelease_id=58

GeneWatch UK. 2013. "The UK Police National DNA Database." Accessed May 3, 2013. http://www.genewatch.org/sub-539478

Greely, Henry T. 2011. "Get Ready for the Flood of Fetal Gene Screening." *Nature* 469:289–91.

Handwerk, Brian. 2005. "DNA Frees Death-Row Inmates, Brings Others to Justice." *National Geographic News,* April 8.

Haraway, Donna J. 1991. *Simians, Cyborgs, and Women: The Reinvention of Nature.* New York: Routledge.

Hardt, Michael, and Antonio Negri. 2004. *Multitude: War and Democracy in the Age of Empire.* New York: Penguin.

Hayes, Richard. 2006. *Stem Cells and Public Policy: A Century Foundation Guide to the Issues.* New York: Century Foundation.

Hennen, Claudia. 2013. "More Female Fetuses Aborted in Europe." *Deutsche Welle,* January 7.

Hubbard, Ruth. 1995a. "Genes as Causes." In *Biopolitics: A Feminist and Ecological Reader on Biotechnology,* edited by Vandana Shiva and Ingunn Moser, 38–51. London: Zed Books.

Hubbard, Ruth. 1995b. "Human Nature." In *Biopolitics: A Feminist and Ecological Reader on Biotechnology,* edited by Vandana Shiva and Ingunn Moser, 27–37. London: Zed Books.

Hughes, James. 2004. *Citizen Cyborg: Why Democratic Societies Must Respond to the Redesigned Human of the Future.* Cambridge, MA: Westview Press.

Hvistendahl, Mara. 2011a. "The Abortion Trap: How America's Obsession with Abortion Hurts Families Everywhere." *Foreign Policy,* July 26. http://www.foreignpolicy.com/articles/2011/07/26/the_abortion_trap

Hvistendahl, Mara. 2011b. *Unnatural Selection: Choosing Boys over Girls, and the Consequences of a World Full of Men.* New York: PublicAffairs.

Kahn, Jonathan. 2012. *Race in a Bottle: The Story of BiDil and Racialized Medicine in a Post-Genomic Age.* New York: Columbia University Press.

Kiatpongsan, Sorapop, and Douglas Sipp. 2009. "Monitoring and Regulating Offshore Stem Cell Clinics." *Science* 323 (5921): 1564–65.

Krimsky, Sheldon, and Tania Simoncelli. 2011. *Genetic Justice: DNA Data Banks, Criminal Investigations, and Civil Liberties.* New York: Columbia University Press.

Lemke, Thomas. 2011. *Biopolitics: An Advanced Introduction.* Translated by Eric Frederick Trump. New York: New York University Press.

Liptak, Adam. 2013. "Justices, 9-0, Bar Patenting Human Genes." *New York Times,* June 13.

Lovgren, Stefan. 2005. "One-Fifth of Human Genes Have Been Patented, Study Reveals." *National Geographic News,* October 13.

Mamo, Laura. 2007. *Queering Reproduction: Achieving Pregnancy in the Age of Technoscience.* Durham, NC: Duke University Press.

Marshall, Eliot. 1999. "Gene Therapy Death Prompts Review of Adenovirus Vector." *Science* 286 (5448): 2244–45.

McCurtis, Kiesha. 2008. "Oocyte Cryopreservation: The Next Wave of Assisted Reproductive Technology, or Marketing Ploys for Career-Oriented Women?" *Women's Health Activist* (National Women's Health Network), July/August. Accessed May 18, 2013. http://nwhn.org/oocyte-cryopreservation-next-wave-assisted-reproductive-technology-or-marketing-ploys-career-oriente

Moreno, Jonathan D. 2011. *The Body Politic: The Battle over Science in America.* New York: Bellevue Literary Press.

National Conference of State Legislatures. 2008. "Human Cloning Laws." Accessed June 2, 2013. http://www.ncsl.org/issues-research/health/human-cloning-laws.aspx

National Human Genome Research Institute. "DNA Sequencing Costs." Accessed May 18, 2013. http://www.genome.gov/sequencingcosts/

Nature. 2009. "Korean Egg-Donor Lawsuit Thrown out of Court." March 4. Accessed June 2, 2013. http://www.nature.com/news/2009/090304/full/458020c.html

Nelson, Deborah, and Rick Weiss. 1999. "Hasty Decisions in the Race to a Cure?: Gene Therapy Study Proceeded Despite Safety, Ethics Concerns." *Washington Post,* November 21. Page A01. Accessed June 2, 2013. http://www.washington-post.com/wp-srv/WPcap/1999-11/21/101r-112199-idx.html

Obama, Barack. 2009. "Remarks on Signing an Executive Order Removing Barriers to Responsible Scientific Research Involving Human Stem Cells and a Memorandum on Scientific Integrity." 1 Pub. Papers 199–202. (March 9). Washington, DC: US Government Printing Office.

Obasogie, Osagie K. 2009. *Playing the Gene Card? A Report on Race and Human Biotechnology.* Center for Genetics and Society. Accessed May 3, 2013. http://www.geneticsand society.org/downloads/complete_PTGC.pdf

Pellegrino, Edmund D. 2006. "Bioethics and Politics: 'Doing Ethics' in the Public Square." *Journal of Medicine and Philosophy* 31 (6): 569–84.

Pet, Douglas. 2012. "Make Me a Baby as Fast as You Can: How a California Surrogacy Operation Streamlines Baby Production by Implanting Clients' Embryos in Two Indian Surrogates at the Same Time." *Slate,* January 9. Accessed May 3, 2013. http://www.slate.com/articles/double_x/doublex/2012/01/reproductive_tourism_how_surrogacy_provider_planet hospital_speeds_up_pregnancies_and_lowers_costs_.html

Peterson, Steven A., and Albert Somit. 1979. "Biopolitics: A Preliminary History." *Journal of the History of the Behavioral Sciences* 15 (4): 333–39.

Practice Committees of the American Society for Reproductive Medicine and the Society for Assisted Reproductive Technology. 2012. "Mature Oocyte Cryopreservation: A Guideline." *Fertility and Sterility*. October 22. Accessed May 3, 2013. http://www.fertstert.org/article/S0015-0282%2812%2902247-9/fulltext

Rabinow, Paul. 1996. "Artificiality and Enlightenment: From Sociobiology to Biosociality." In *Essays on the Anthropology of Reason*, 19–111. Princeton, NJ: Princeton University Press.

Reagan, Ron. 2004. Speech at the Democratic National Convention. CSPAN Video Library video, 04:12:48. Filmed July 27. http://www.c-spanvideo.org/program/182718-2 Quotation at 03:13:19–03:13:24.

Rifkin, Jeremy. 2002. "Fusion Biopolitics." *Nation*, February 18. Accessed November 4, 2013. http://www.thenation.com/article/fusion-biopolitics

Roberts, Dorothy. 2011. *Fatal Invention: How Science, Politics, and Big Business Re-Create Race in the Twenty-First Century*. New York: New Press.

Robertson, John A. 2001. "Preconception Gender Selection." *American Journal of Bioethics* 1 (1): 2–9.

Rose, Nikolas. 2007. *The Politics of Life Itself: Biomedicine, Power, and Subjectivity in the Twenty-First Century*. Princeton, NJ: Princeton University Press.

Rothman, Barbara Katz. 1998. *Genetic Maps and Human Imaginations: The Limits of Science in Understanding Who We Are*. New York: Norton.

Sample, Ian. 2006. "Stem Cell Pioneer Accused of Faking All His Research Apart from the Cloned Dog." *Guardian*, January 10.

Sen, Amartya. 1990. "More Than 100 Million Women Are Missing." *New York Review of Books*. December 20. Accessed June 2, 2013. http://www.nybooks.com/articles/archives/1990/dec/20/more-than-100-million-women-are-missing/

Shanks, Pete. 2006. "The Hwang Saga Continues." *Genetic Crossroads*, May 12. Accessed May 3, 2013. http://www.geneticsandsociety.org/article.php?id=2620

Shanks, Pete. 2012. "Induced Pluripotent Stem Cells and Germline Engineering." *Biopolitical Times* (blog), October 16. Accessed May 3, 2013. http://www.biopoliticaltimes.org/article.php?id=6441

Shiva, Vandana, and Ingunn Moser, eds. 1995. *Biopolitics: A Feminist and Ecological Reader on Biotechnology*. London: Zed Books.

Singer, Emily. 2010. "A Turning Point for Genetic Testing: The FDA Plans to Overhaul Its Regulation of the Increasingly Common Diagnostic Tests." *MIT Technology Review*, July 13. Accessed June 2, 2013. http://www.technologyreview.com/news/419814/a-turning-point-for-genetic-testing/

Stock, Gregory, and John Campbell, eds. 2000. *Engineering the Human Germline: An Exploration of the Science and Ethics of Altering the Genes We Pass to Our Children*. New York: Oxford University Press.

Takahashi, Kazutoshi; Koji Tanabe; Mari Ohnuki; et al. 2007. "Induction of Pluripotent Stem Cells from Adult Human Fibroblasts by Defined Factors." *Cell* 131 (5): 861–72.

Twine, France Winddance. 2011. *Outsourcing the Womb: Race, Class and Gestational Surrogacy in a Global Market*. New York: Routledge.

United Nations. 2005. "General Assembly Adopts United Nations Declaration on Human Cloning by Vote of 84-34-37." Press release, August 3. Accessed June 2, 2013. http://www.un.org/News/Press/docs/2005/ga10333.doc.htm

United States Government Accountability Office. 2010. *Direct-to-Consumer Genetic Tests: Misleading Test Results Are Further Complicated by Deceptive Marketing and Other Questionable Practices*. Testimony before the Subcommittee on Oversight and Investigations, Committee on Energy and Commerce, House of Representatives. Statement of Gregory Kutz, Managing Director, Forensic Audits and Special Investigations. July 22. Washington, DC: Author.

Wade, Nicholas. 2010. "A Decade Later, Genetic Map Yields Few New Cures." *New York Times*, June 13.

Weiss, Rick. 2002. "Cloning Creates Odd Bedfellows." *Washington Post*, February 10.

Wilson, Edward O. 1975. *Sociobiology: The New Synthesis*. Cambridge, MA: Belknap Press of Harvard University Press.

Winstein, Keith J. 2007. "NAACP Presses U.S. on Heart Drug." *Wall Street Journal*, January 25.

Zuk, Or; Eliana Hechter; Shamil R. Sunyaeva; and Eric S. Lander. 2011. "The Mystery of Missing Heritability: Genetic Interactions Create Phantom Heritability." *PNAS Early Edition*, December 5. Accessed June 2, 2013. http://www.pnas.org/content/early/2012/01/04/1119675109.full.pdf

Marcy Darnovsky
Executive Director, Center for Genetics and Society

Emily Smith Beitiks
Assistant Director, Paul K. Longmore Institute on Disability, San Francisco State University

BIOTERRORISM

The issues associated with bioterrorism are as broad in their scope and as challenging in their complexity as any in bioethics. These issues engage the resources of basic sciences, history, political philosophy, sociology, health care administration, and public health as well as clinical medicine. In some instances they present unique concerns; in others they are variations on more familiar bioethical problems. In providing a sound bioethical account of these problems this entry will presuppose that the terrorist threat in question is morally unjustifiable because either the cause it represents or the means used to advance this cause cannot be rationally defended.

PUBLIC HEALTH AND CIVIL LIBERTIES

Broad agreement supports the idea that individual liberties of speech, movement, and personal privacy may be abrogated when they present an imminent risk of serious harm to other persons and when no other means of ameliorating this risk is available. This doctrine is familiar in the traditional domain of public health. An additional element presents itself when there is an intentional threat to public safety from persons or states that seek to advance a political agenda.

Whether the political element is in itself sufficient justification for permitting the state to have greater latitude in the abrogation of civil liberties than it would in a naturally occurring public health emergency is a question for debate. One might argue that the intentionality of a terrorist act, expressed through a biological attack, is liable to sow panic in a fashion that differs from the psychological effects of a naturally occurring epidemic. Whether that is the case or not is an empirical matter, and whether the incident justifies a more aggressive response is a matter of political philosophy.

It is clear that the tactics required to minimize the harms of a disease outbreak are not substantially altered by the cause of the contagion. In the case of highly contagious and dangerous diseases like smallpox, public health theory calls for the identification and isolation of primary cases and the creation of a containment ring around plausible secondary cases. This surveillance and containment strategy requires that all those exposed and their immediate contacts be vaccinated, isolated, and quarantined if they become ill. Treatment of all cases within that ring should be sufficient to control the epidemic.

Conceivably a disease might be more likely to appear simultaneously in several distant places as part of a terrorist conspiracy than it would as part of a natural event. There is disagreement among public health experts concerning the point at which a certain number of far-flung individual cases would constitute a dire emergency that would render the ring strategy inadequate.

Although bioethics has emphasized self-determination, the public health context presents demands that are incompatible with strict adherence to individual rights. Some policy experts have argued that, especially in an emergency, effective public health interventions may entail justifiable limitations on civil liberties that would at other times be unacceptable. Limitations on such rights as speech, privacy, and travel should not be excessive or arbitrary, and they must be rationally linked to protection of the public. They may be imposed for a period of time no longer than required by the circumstances.

Not all theorists agree that more stringent restrictions on civil liberties may be required by a bioterrorism event. Some commentators oppose abrogating the right to refuse treatment and any requirement that doctors treat patients against their will. These critics also question the practicality and effectiveness of large-scale quarantine. All these actions tend to undermine the most important defense against panic, which is trust in government authority. Adequate and equitable health care for all would, under this view, go farther than draconian measures to build public trust and elicit cooperation in an emergency.

RESOURCE ALLOCATION IN A RESPONSE TO BIOTERRORISM

Standard accounts of a formal principle of justice require that similar cases be treated similarly, but in an extreme event health care institutions may not have the capacity to absorb large numbers of patients who suddenly present themselves. An important problem is whether the resulting differential treatment is always morally wrong or whether it can be justified in some instances.

The classic approach to sorting battlefield injuries is triage, a nineteenth-century French policy based on the strictly utilitarian principle of the greatest good for the greatest number. Depending on the particular model, triage assessment involves sorting victims into three or five categories that range from urgent to nonurgent to care not needed. Although triage has become a familiar term in the civilian medical world, especially in busy emergency rooms, in its original military context the idea included a criterion of social merit, that the argument for care in any particular case turned on the potential for the individual to return to duty.

Under ordinary circumstances clinical triage differs from battlefield triage. In the former case the most seriously ill are not simply set aside. Rather, resources are made available through such ad hoc means as the temporary diversion of ambulances to other emergency rooms. Under extreme conditions these routine bypass procedures may not be feasible. A social-worth criterion could be transferred to civilians if the circumstances were sufficiently dire that, for example, the very survival of the community was threatened. According to the theologian Paul Ramsey (1970), the comparative social worth of individuals can justifiably be measured in these highly defined circumstances.

First priority must be given to victims who can quickly be restored to functioning. They are needed to bury the dead to prevent epidemic. They can serve as amateur medics or nurses with a little instruction—as the triage officer directs the community's remaining medical resources to a middle group of the seriously injured majority. And among these, one could argue, a physician should be treated first.

A social-worth criterion applied to extreme conditions might appear to be incompatible with respect for each individual person, when the inevitably unsuccessful act of treating some casualties is sacrificed in exchange for the potential survival of a valuable individual whose survival would in turn benefit the larger number. However, James F. Childress (2003) makes the case that the unequal treatment is justifiable precisely because it is respectful in its intention—that is, it is carried out in order ultimately to benefit all of the others, whose survival is made more likely as a result of prioritizing the treatment of a particular person. Respect for all the others who might survive demonstrates respect for each of them as individuals, hence egalitarianism is preserved.

Not all who are possessed of critical skills may be required for the benefit of the community, however. Rather, only a few may be needed, in which case it would be unfair to guarantee all of these individuals a place at the head of the queue. Instead, as Childress outlines, to ensure that at least some of them survive without providing inappropriate advantages to all of them, essential workers may be entered into a weighted lottery in such a way that their selection is more likely, on average, than that of others.

Because the successful management of a bioterrorism event requires a high degree of public trust, criteria for triage and resource allocation should be formulated as part of a public consensus process. Transparency in the development and application of resource-allocation principles under extreme conditions should include their defense and readjustment in light of public reaction. Childress (1997) points to precedent in the case of the allocation of organs. The articulation and adjustment of allocation principles must take place well in advance of the event itself.

THE OBLIGATIONS OF EMERGENCY HEALTH WORKERS

Health care workers are often expected to undergo a degree of discomfort and inconvenience in executing their duties. This expectation is justified by the vulnerability of those under their care, a vulnerability grounded in illness and in the knowledge differential between doctor and patient. Similar role-related obligations apply to other professionals, such as attorneys or securities analysts, whose clientele is inherently vulnerable by virtue of social status or lack of relevant information. Perhaps because of the concreteness and intimacy of their work, no other professional group is held to as high a standard in this regard as are those in health care.

The degree to which health care workers must compromise their own well-being for the sake of others is often unclear. The role-related duties of health care professionals imply at least a modest degree of self-sacrifice for the sake of others who are in need of their services. Ordinarily these sacrifices are limited to brief periods of discomfort or inconvenience, particularly embodied in the rigors of the medical residency. At the extreme, martyrdom and other supererogatory acts spell out the limits of these duties, but detailed guidance is lacking. Although emergency health workers have been designated as a special group with more extensive duties under circumstances that demand urgent attention (for instance, by the World Medical Association [1994] and the Pan American Health Organization [2013]), this designation is not informative about the boundaries of their obligations

One set of considerations has to do with the support that emergency health care workers are given in executing their tasks. Professionals cannot be expected to perform their responsibilities in the absence of adequate materials, much less expose themselves to conditions that put them at risk. Governments must provide "an effective and centralized authority to coordinate public and private efforts" (World Medical Association 1994). As Lisa A. Eckenwiler (2003) points out, in the context of terrorism the society under threat should also provide the material support required for emergency health care workers to do their job, particularly as there is an expectation that their personal welfare is at somewhat greater risk than that of other health professionals. The absence of suitable support is not an excuse for the health care worker to abandon his or her post, but skilled professionals may fairly expect reciprocity in the form of support considering the physical and psychological stresses to which they are exposed.

A consideration of the limits of emergency health care workers' duties also raises a question regarding moral responsibilities to distant others as compared to appropriate concerns for one's own welfare or that of significant persons in one's life. As the victims of catastrophe are less familiar to us and as they become more distant in space or culture, it may become more psychologically challenging to relate to their circumstances, especially if their plight competes for our sympathy with that of someone in greater geographic or social proximity. A presumed feature of health care workers' morality that should in principle set them apart from the rest of society is that their circle of concern knows no distance. But is this presumption of universal concern, of impartiality, always sound when it competes with more local concerns about one's own family, friends, and colleagues? Eckenwiler suggests that partiality is not a vice if it is conceived as one way human beings express their individuality through the uniqueness of their relationships. Health care professionals functioning in emergencies may not be expected and should not be required to subvert justifiable tendencies to place primary value on personal relationships when forced to allocate their caregiving under extreme conditions.

THE ROLE OF PRIVATE SECTOR INSTITUTIONS

Many of the human and material resources that may be required in catastrophic circumstances are in the private sector, especially pharmaceutical manufacturers and managed care organizations. Nonpublic entities are generally agreed to have some responsibilities to the society that provides a stable framework for their business activities, responsibilities that must only increase in the event of social emergency. The contours of these corporate social responsibilities assume a special character in the context of bioterrorism.

Yet private industry cannot be expected or required to resolve all societal problems that are more appropriately considered the province of public entities, such as providing access to medication or health care for all. Rather, these private interests have a duty to participate in the public discourse that seeks the resolution of policy problems and to engage in business practices, such as fair pricing policies, that make solutions practicable. As Evan G. DeRenzo (2003) has pointed out, the rationale for this duty can be expressed in terms of the primary moral purpose of any business, to produce goods or services that contribute to the pursuit of the good life.

In this scheme drug companies can be said to have certain obligations with regard to the bioterror threat. For example, they are obligated to provide security to guard against any potential vulnerabilities in their production activities or storage arrangements. They should make positive efforts to help ensure that medications are available for the treatment of bioweapons injuries with a wide therapeutic range and based on different mechanisms rather than simply produce medications similar to those already available. For cases wherein there is only one patented drug for a certain indication that is related to a bioterror threat, government may consider a "stop the clock" mechanism that permits at least temporarily lifting the patent so that production and distribution can be accelerated.

Managed care organizations (MCOs) have concentrated a large portion of the highly skilled health care workforce in the private sector. This arrangement raises questions, not limited to bioterrorism, about the relationship between corporate responsibilities and threats to the public health. Controlling of costs while also providing excellent health care has proved to be a significant challenge to the industry, and quality improvement efforts have proved disappointing in resolving the cost-quality tension. Ann E. Mills and Patricia H. Werhane (2003) have pointed out that because public health agencies have limited resources, any severe public health problem would further tax the private health care system, and MCOs would be obligated to provide care for victims even if they are not enrolled in some defined health or insurer plan.

In one sense, as the burden of providing care for a potentially large patient population at risk from bioterrorism falls on MCOs—in the form of vaccination, treatment of victims, and planning for attacks—the tension between cost and quality will become still more pronounced. In another sense, however, the requirements of physical survival in extreme circumstances render the cost issue moot, as the best possible care will simply have to be provided. From an economic standpoint the goods and services involved are decommodified, or removed from the marketplace, because market mechanisms are unable to deal with such conditions. Instead MCOs should think of themselves as part of a wider system of health care along with government agencies, the pharmaceutical industry, and academia. Paradoxically the threat of bioterrorism introduces a community perspective into privatized health care in a way that normal economic and political conditions do not.

HUMAN RESEARCH ETHICS AND NATIONAL SECURITY

The development of human research ethics and of biomedical ethics itself has been decisively influenced by experience with the involvement of human subjects in national security experiments. The signal event in this often dispiriting history was the exploitation of concentration camp prisoners in experiments under the cover of World War II, many sponsored by the Nazi German military apparatus. The culmination of the Nazi Doctors' Trial in 1947 was the creation of the Nuremberg Code, which set down rules for human subjects research and is generally considered a landmark document in biomedical ethics.

Subsequent policies regulating human experiments on biological, chemical, and atomic warfare in the US military during the Cold War specifically referenced the Nuremberg Code. However, these policies were not always followed, in some instances because the activity in question was not considered to be a medical experiment but rather was viewed as a training exercise. Secrecy has itself proven to be among the greatest obstacles to developing consistently applied ethical standards in this area.

The populations that have been involved in national security research represent a wide range, including military personnel, conscientious objectors, and institutionalized persons, such as prisoners, mental patients, and medical patients. Military personnel in particular occupy a complex position, because they are expected to subject themselves to risks that would not be required of others and they must accept medical interventions that will preserve or reestablish their fitness for duty. Certain basic ethical standards have been recommended. For instance, a 1996 report from the Advisory Committee on Human Radiation Experiments calls for appropriate security clearance for all parties, including subjects; prior review by an institutional review board; an appeals process; informed consent; and record keeping.

Like the other bioethical issues associated with bioterrorism, the development of ethical standards for the involvement of human beings in national security experiments requires the resources of several disciplines. Still more challenging is the application of these standards, which requires a level of engagement with the political system that clearly identifies bioethics as a practical moral activity.

DUAL-USE RESEARCH OF CONCERN

The US government defines dual-use research of concern (DURC) as life sciences research that, based on current understanding, can be reasonably anticipated to provide knowledge, information, products, or technologies that could be directly misapplied to pose a significant threat with broad potential consequences to public health and safety, agricultural crops and other plants, animals, the environment, materiel, or national security (NIH 2012). Two cases were instrumental in widening public attention to the power of new laboratory techniques with dual-use potential. In 2000 researchers in Australia accidentally created a strain of mousepox virus more powerful than that found in nature. About a year later scientists in New York deliberately synthesized a polio virus. Several other such incidents followed.

National security and public health officials worry that novel pathogens resistant to natural immunity, vaccines, and antibiotics could be developed by state or non-state actors or organizations bent on terrorism. In an era of easy access to biological materials, reagents, and sophisticated equipment, the "barriers to entry" of the production of malign entities appear to be rapidly falling. But suppression of potentially damaging data both cuts against values of open scientific inquiry and conflicts with the conviction popular among scientists that the best defense lies in widespread knowledge. There is as well an inherent conceptual challenge in determining when the dual-use potential of sophisticated basic research can ever be wholly avoided.

In 2010 the US Presidential Commission for the Study of Bioethical Issues considered the possibility that developments in synthetic biology might exacerbate the dual-use security threat. The commissioners concluded that the problem warranted continued scrutiny but had not yet reached a stage that justified specific new measures. The commission called for "prudent vigilance, establishing processes for assessing likely benefits along with assessing safety and security risks both before and after projects are undertaken" (Presidential Commission for the Study of Bioethical Issues 2010, 4). Among the commission's specific recommendations was that federal agencies coordinate and review the adequacy of current regulations. One technical measure that was discussed in the commission's report was that of a "suicide gene," a control mechanism that could be inserted into synthetic organisms that would prevent them from multiplying in the natural environment (Presidential Commission for the Study of Bioethical Issues 2010, 130).

In a reflection of growing concern about dual-use research, in 2012 the World Health Organization (WHO) assembled a group of public health experts to consider whether to extend a temporary moratorium on research with the newly created H5N1 influenza (widely known as the bird flu virus). Sixty percent of people infected with the virus have died, a fatality rate that may exceed even that of the Black Death in fourteenth-century Europe. Precipitating the extraordinary WHO meeting was the creation of a highly virulent strain of the virus by research groups in the United States and the Netherlands. The group recommended both that the moratorium be extended and that publication of the entire manuscripts describing the laboratory process should be delayed (World Health Organization 2012).

SEE ALSO *Coercion; Epidemics; Harm; Hazardous Wastes and Toxic Substances; Immigrants, Access to Health Care; Nazi Legacy and Bioethics; Race and Racism; Warfare: IV. Chemical and Biological Weapons*

BIBLIOGRAPHY

Advisory Committee on Human Radiation Experiments. 1996. *Final Report of the Advisory Committee on Human Radiation Experiments.* New York: Oxford University Press.

Childress, James F. 1997. *Practical Reasoning in Bioethics.* Bloomington: Indiana University Press.

Childress, James F. 2003. "Triage in Response to a Bioterrorist Attack." In *Bioethics after the Terror*, edited by Jonathan D. Moreno, 77–94. Cambridge, MA: MIT Press.

DeRenzo, Evan G. 2003. "The Rightful Goals of a Corporation and the Obligations of the Pharmaceutical Industry in a World with Bioterrorism." In *Bioethics after the Terror*, edited by Jonathan D. Moreno, 149–66. Cambridge, MA: MIT Press.

Eckenwiler, Lisa A. 2003. "Emergency Health Professionals and the Ethics of Crisis." In *Bioethics after the Terror*, edited by Jonathan D. Moreno, 111–32. Cambridge, MA: MIT Press.

Germany (Territory under Allied Occupation, 1945–1955: US Zone). 1949–1953. *Trials of War Criminals before the Nuremberg Military Tribunals under Control Council Law No. 10.* Washington, DC: US Government Printing Office.

Kipnis, Kenneth. 2003. "Overwhelming Casualties: Medical Ethics in a Time of Terror." In *Bioethics after the Terror*, edited by Jonathan D. Moreno, 95–108. Cambridge, MA: MIT Press.

Mills, Anne E., and Patricia H. Werhane. 2003. "After the Terror: Healthcare Organizations, the Healthcare System, and the Future of Organization Ethics." In *Bioethics after the Terror*, edited by Jonathan D. Moreno, 167–82. Cambridge, MA: MIT Press.

Moreno, Jonathan D. 2001. *Undue Risk: Secret State Experiments on Humans*. New York: Routledge.

National Institutes of Health, Office of Biotechnology Activities. 2012. "United States Government Policy for Oversight of Life Sciences Dual Use Research of Concern." March 29. http://oba.od.nih.gov/oba/biosecurity/PDF/United_States_Government_Policy_for_Oversight_of_DURC_FINAL_version_032812.pdf

National Institutes of Health, Office of Biotechnology Activities. 2013. "Dual Use Research." Accessed August 21, 2013. http://oba.od.nih.gov/biosecurity/biosecurity.html

Pan American Health Organization. 2013. Accessed August 21, 2013. http://www.paho.org/usa/

Presidential Commission for the Study of Bioethical Issues. 2010. "New Directions: The Ethics of Synthetic Biology and Emerging Technologies." http://bioethics.gov/cms/synthetic-biology-report

Ramsey, Paul. 1970. *Patient as Person*. New Haven, CT: Yale University Press.

Selgelid, Michael. 2009. "Governance of Dual-Use Research: An Ethical Dilemma." Bulletin of the World Health Organization 87: 720–23.

World Health Organization. 2012. "Public Health, Influenza Experts Agree H5N1 Research Critical, but Extend Delay." February 17. http://www.who.int/mediacentre/news/releases/2012/h5n1_research_20120217/en/

World Medical Association. 1994. "Statement on Medical Ethics in the Event of Disasters." http://www1.umn.edu/humanrts/instree/disasterethics.html

Jonathan D. Moreno (2004, 2014)
David and Lyn Silfen University Professor, Perelman School of Medicine, University of Pennsylvania

BODY

This entry consists of the following:

I: EMBODIMENT IN THE PHENOMENOLOGICAL TRADITION

Philosophical and ethical issues are closely connected with medical and health professional self-understanding, knowledge, research, and practice. The human body occupies a central place in those contexts but especially within medicine—certainly one of the sources for understanding the human body. In this entry, after a brief review of ideas about the body in the history of medicine, its place in philosophical thought since René Descartes (1596–1650) is addressed. This history plays an important role in more recent philosophical reflections on human life, especially in writings directed to the experience of embodiment. After reviewing that history and the understanding of embodiment, some suggestions are made about the relationship between embodiment and the variety of ethical issues presented by medicine, biomedical research, and clinical practice. This discussion is unavoidably difficult, because both that history and the issues raised by efforts to explicate and understand embodiment are complex. Addressing those complexities, however briefly, will be helpful in delineating the specific concepts, terms, and methods used in the phenomenological tradition regarding embodiment.

From the earliest stirrings of human fetal life through old age, individuals are embodied. Whether their bodies are more or less healthy; or are sick, injured, compromised by congenital or genetic defects; or are such that they arouse social prejudice, individuals experience the surrounding world by means of a particular body. Being embodied, furthermore, means having a certain sexuality and thus experiencing the milieu in ways that both structure and are socially structured by that sexuality. Even slight reflection also shows that the human body has aesthetic, economic, political, and other dimensions specific to every cultural time: the body figures prominently in clothing styles, pornography, labor, torture, and the like. The experience of the body by oneself and others plays other important roles in broader terms: in the "body politic," for instance, or in the manufacture of automobiles, or in contexts such as physical examinations in the military.

Underlying all of these, however, is a striking phenomenon: regardless of the state of health, skin coloration, sexuality, or sociopolitical usages, one body is uniquely singled out for a person's experience as "mine," as that sole body through which anything else is experienced. Although any full explication of embodiment must address each of these fascinating dimensions, the first question concerns that core sense of "mineness": How are we to understand that? It is to this that the present entry is devoted. First, however, an equally brief word is needed about the place of the body in medicine.

THE BODY IN MEDICINE

Historically physicians have sought to understand the body's structures (anatomy), functions (physiology), cellular makeup (biology, biochemistry), activating and regulatory mechanisms (neurology, immunology); the several organ systems and their connections (cardiac, pulmonary, renal, hepatic, etc.); and the variety of diseases, injuries, noxious environmental influences, and genetic and congenital conditions that govern the body's development and underlie personal life.

Even with this focus, however, historical medical views of the body have varied over time (Edelstein 1967). For example, the "dogmatic" or "rational" view understood the human body as fundamentally causal in nature—events inside the body were thought to cause outer symptoms (a pathological understanding of the body and disease). By contrast, according to the "empiricist" and "skeptical" traditions, the body and the embodied person form an experiential, temporally developing "whole" in continuous and multiple interactions with the surrounding world (a holistic view). Physicians in later historical times who were convinced of the dogmatic, rational view literally looked inside the body—by dissection and vivisection—and understood its structures and functions. Those who held the empiricist view turned instead to history (the patient's history and the collective histories of other physicians) in treating diseases. These two basic, conflicting models have continued to have an important place in medical understanding (Zaner 1988; Leder 1990).

Although these views continue to be present in medicine, the rationalist tradition (emphasizing the body as a material, causally determined organic system) has been clearly dominant in more recent times. The first major steps in the historical development of a rationalist view of the human body were taken in the early fourteenth century by Mondino de' Luzzi and his student Guido da Vigevano (Singer 1925). By far the most significant steps are found in the seminal work on anatomy by Andreas Vesalius (1514–1564) and later in the important discoveries in physiology by William Harvey (1578–1657), strongly endorsed by Descartes, and continued in the work of seventeenth- and eighteenth-century post-Cartesian physicians, such as Robert Boyle (1627–1691), Friedrich Hoffmann (1660–1742) (King 1978), and Jerome Gaub (1705–1780) (Rather 1965).

In modern times the body was first proposed as a fundamentally causally determined organic system by Giovanni Battista Morgagni (1682–1771) and Xavier Bichat (1771–1802). Before this time, even though abundant autopsy reports had been published, such recorded data had not offered any correlation between clinical and anatomical findings (King 1978). With Morgagni and Bichat, however, this changed profoundly. The introduction of the "clinicopathological correlation" radically altered medical understanding. For the first time what was found at autopsy was taken as "explaining" clinical symptoms observed while the patient was alive. Now disease took on a highly specific form—the "organic lesion" found inside the body—and was no longer associated with a more or less loosely collected set of clinically observed symptoms or patient reports (King 1978; Zaner 1988). Because this "correlation" fundamentally changed the way physicians understood disease, it has been called a "revolution" (Laín Entralgo 1969) comparable to what Copernicus effected in astronomy when he proposed that instead of thinking that the sun moves around the earth, we should perceive it to be the other way around.

The marriage of clinical medicine to biological science, definitively begun in the nineteenth century, was consummated through the work of neurologists such as John Hughlings Jackson (1835–1911) and clinicians such as William Osler (1849–1919) and the educational reforms recommended by Abraham Flexner (1866–1959) in the early twentieth century. Medical thinking then incorporated the idea that the body is a complex system of physiologically interacting structures and mechanisms governed by multiply interrelated controls seated in the neurological system. Some physicians, appreciating that this complex organism (or set of organ systems) serves as the embodied person's means of expression and action, advocated a type of "medical dualism" or "epiphenomenalism"—there must be a place for the "person," whether thought of as a distinct entity or as a causal consequence of the body complex's functional stability across time.

THE BODY IN PHILOSOPHY

Although the history of philosophical and moral deliberations about human life is quite as sophisticated and colorful as medical history, the bulk of reflections have focused on mind (person, self, subjectivity, and related notions) (Zaner 1981). With some notable exceptions, however, there has not been nearly as much reflection about body per se. In large part a basically traditional view of these matters was assumed: that body and soul are distinct (or even separate) realities and that what is essential in human life is to be found in the soul, not the body. The soul (mind, reason) is the pure and unchanging essence of the human; the body, in contrast, is a baser sort of affair, belonging to the changeable, the temporal, and the corrupt. The soul, imprisoned within the corporeal, is subject to the body's peculiar "nature," its appetites and inclinations, but has its true destiny and nature elsewhere—a destiny it must pursue by becoming freed from its worldly, bodily prison.

There have been exceptions to this view of the human body. Descartes (1596–1650), for example, argued that mind (*res cogitans*) and body (*res extensa*) are to be understood as "substances": mutually exclusive, self-subsistent, and ontologically distinct entities, neither of which requires the other to be or to be known. This familiar bifurcation of reality (dualism), often said to be at the basis of modern medicine and modern thought more generally (Eccles 1979; Cassell 1991), led Descartes to the view that mind and body "interact" in some manner, although specifying the form of this interaction proved to be inordinately difficult and highly problematic (Leder 1990).

Hardly satisfied with that, and challenged by Princess Elizabeth (daughter of the exiled king of Bohemia, living at the time in Holland), Descartes's reflections on the body show a surprising turn—one that has not been well appreciated. The mind, he thought, is not "in" the body in the way a boatman is "in" a boat—contingently or accidentally. Rather, the mind is "intimately" connected to the body, an "intimate union" that led him to the view that the human body is intrinsically complex and not at all the simple "extended substance" posited in his metaphysics (Zaner 1988). As Descartes remarked to Princess Elizabeth, neither mathematics nor metaphysics is capable of apprehending this union. It can be known only in "daily conversation" and in clinical encounters—one might say that the union is essentially a matter of concrete experience (Descartes 1963–1973; Lindeboom 1978).

From his early work in anatomy, Descartes had learned that the cadaver does indeed seem to be little more than such an "extension." But from his earnest attempts to provide medical diagnosis, he knew full well that while it is alive, the body is far more than merely a material entity extended in space. For example, writing of the "dropsical patient" in his *Meditations* (Descartes 1955), he took pains to point out that there are in fact two "natures": the one subject to the laws of nature and the other with its own specific characteristics that must be understood in quite different ways than the first (Kennington 1978). Indeed Niels Stenos (1638–1686), a physician who was a younger contemporary of Descartes who specialized in the brain, contended that nature in the first sense was merely heuristic, a "manner of speaking" (*une pure dénomination* is Descartes's phrase), and should not be taken literally (Lindeboom 1978). This intrinsic complexity of the body—as cadaver and as embodying the mind—did not attract the attention of many philosophers (or, for that matter, physicians) (Zaner 1988).

Addressing the Cartesian idea of the "intimate union" of soul and body, Blaise Pascal (1623–1662) argued that one must be able to account for this intimacy. He noted with marked irony that if, like Descartes, one "composes all things of mind and body," surely that mixture would be intelligible—especially to one who so composes all things. Yet not only do we not understand the body, and even less the mind, least of all do we know "how a body could be united to a mind. This is the consummation of [our] difficulties, and yet it is [our] very being" (Pascal 1941, 27–28).

Benedict de Spinoza (1632–1677) thought that Descartes's bifurcation created insuperable difficulties for understanding how the mind could possibly be connected to the body, much less "intimately" connected. Like others at the time, Spinoza's argument is couched in metaphysical terms: he argued that what Descartes termed "substance" (mind and body) could only be "attributes" of the one and only substance, reality itself. Mind and body are essential to one another; the way they are "united," he concluded, then becomes comprehensible. The body is a mirror of the soul; mind, the idea of the body (Spinoza 1951).

Understanding the body continued to preoccupy physicians but did not become a focal issue for philosophers until the early writings of Henri Bergson (1859–1941). Although he did not fully probe the matter, Bergson argued that the human body should be seen as the person's placement or locus in the world. What makes the body, a sui generis phenomenon, unlike any other worldly object is, he believed, that it is experienced as "mine," as "my center" of action and experience. Although it is physical, it is not simply that; it is the "center" of experience, and thus the field of physical objects is spatially organized around it. In addition the human body and its perceptual capacities are in the service of action. The body is fundamentally an actional center. It is that by means of which the embodied person is able to engage in actions in and on the field of objects. Spatial location and the familiar sensory qualities are thus always experienced within specific contexts of action: for the perceiver, "things" are "menacing," "helpful," "handy," "obstacles," and so on (Bergson 1953). Correlated to the body as the center of action, physical things are organized as "poles of action" appearing only within specific activities directed toward them, as Jean Piaget (1896–1980) later emphasized. Because of these characteristics, the human body is a critical factor in the development of language and culture.

In the early days of the twentieth century, Max Scheler (1874–1928) devoted serious reflection to the "lived body" (*Leib*), in particular as regards the performance of "deeds" in moral conduct. Scheler's analysis suggests that both "ego" and the ego's "acts" are distinct from what he terms "lived bodiliness" (*Leiblichkeit*). At the same lived bodiliness must be sharply distinguished from the "thing body" (*Körper*). Although Scheler does not mention it, this idea is a clear echo of the earlier Cartesian insight. The body that embodies the person ("my body") is uniquely singled out for and experienced by the person as "mine" (and in this sense is "intimately connected"). As the person's experiential "center," it is that by means of which the person is, as it were, worlded: in the midst of objects, people, language, culture, and so on. These points, which had also impressed Bergson, came to be regarded as fundamental to embodiment and are crucial for understanding subsequent discussions.

Edmund Husserl (1859–1938) grappled with this phenomenon throughout his career. Its primary feature, he contended, is the experiential relationship of consciousness to its own embodying organism (Husserl 1952b). Granted that this organism (*Leibkörper*) is uniquely singled out (Husserl 1956–1959), the problem of embodiment is to determine in what sense and in what ways it is actually experienced by the person as his or hers, since it is solely by means of that experience that it is at all possible for the person to experience worldly things (physical, biological, cultural).

What had so impressed and troubled Descartes—the "intimate union"—Husserl calls the experiential relationship to the "body-as-mine"; however, he did not appreciate Descartes's insight any more than had Bergson or Scheler. Descartes seems clearly to have recognized that while a person is alive, there is an "intimate union" between body and soul. Yet how are we to understand this "union"—a connection that is all the more peculiar when death occurs and this "alive" body becomes a cadaver that seems no different in kind from any other material thing? Although apparently appreciating this puzzle, Descartes nevertheless obscured matters (as did many others after him) by trying to resolve the very different metaphysical question of the "mind-body" relation.

It is the embodiment phenomenon that Gabriel Marcel (1889–1973) addresses in his analysis of the fundamental opacity (the elemental "feeling," or, as he termed it, *Urgefühl*) at the heart of personal life—my body qua mine (Marcel 1940). It is here too that Maurice Merleau-Ponty (1908–1961) locates the essential ambiguity intrinsic to the body itself (Merleau-Ponty 1945). So "intimate" is this "union," both Marcel and Merleau-Ponty point out, that one is tempted to say, with Jean-Paul Sartre, "I am my body." "My body qua mine" is thus the paradigm of "belonging" or "having": the sense in which things belong to a person is ultimately derived from the ways the "own" body is experienced as belonging to the person. The latter is the condition for the former (Marcel 1935). This existential source of "belonging" becomes apparent especially in instances where mental disturbances occur and the sense of "mineness" becomes severely compromised or remains seriously undeveloped (Bosch 1970). A central issue then emerges: By virtue of what is this one animate organism uniquely singled out to exist in my experience as that whereby everything else in the world is experienced? Which specific processes are there without which this organism would cease to be experienced by me as mine or which give it its sense as mine? (Straus 1958).

The problem is exceedingly complex and subtle and is by no means settled (Zaner 1971, 1981). It is one of those regions where philosophy and medicine can productively learn from one another. Within philosophy, however, there seems at least some agreement that the animate organism becomes and remains an embodying organism solely to the extent that (1) it is not just a physical body but a genuinely animate organism, the sole "object" within which the person's own fields of sensation (that whereon sensations occur) belong; (2) it is the only object "in" which the person immediately "rules and governs," within and from each of its "organs" and the total organism itself; (3) it is that whereby the person's "I can" (walk, perceive, move, grasp, and the like) is most immediately realized and enacted; (4) it is that "by means of which" the person perceives and otherwise experiences the field of worldly objects (things, people, language, etc.) and thus is the person's access to the world and the focus of the actions of the world (objects, people) on the person; and (5) it is not only that whereby the person experiences other things, but it is itself experienced by the person (in health and sickness, and these in specific individual ways)—that is, the person's embodying organism is reflexively related to itself (Husserl 1956–1959).

THE BODY IN MEDICINE AND PHILOSOPHY

It should of course be recognized that, given the uniqueness of each embodiment, individuals experience their bodies (and, correlatively, the surrounding world) in different ways, depending on initial biological endowments, native and cultivated abilities, activities that are available and/or encouraged, and others. Thus a boy who from birth has been unable to walk experiences "I can" in quite different ways from a boy who has that ability. If the latter has an accident that renders him unable to walk, moreover, his inability is experienced quite differently from that of the former—indeed while the one undergoes a "loss," the other may not, except perhaps in the indirect way of realizing that while others can walk, he has never been able to. One who is born blind experiences the surrounding world quite differently from one who goes blind due to an accident—whereas neither experiences a "visual world," the one has "to get used" to the absence of visual space, but the other has never experienced anything else. Even in cases where an individual may from birth lack several bodily capabilities (such as Helen Keller) or loses them through illness or injury, the features suggested above still hold: the embodying organism is that whereby one experiences sensations, which most immediately embody wishes and movements, by means of which one perceives (in whatever ways) and through which other things are experienced. Moreover there are many other meanings the human body acquires—social, political, economic, and others—that a more complete explication of embodiment must address—bodily abilities, stances, comportments, and movements (Buytendijk 1957) that have their sense and place within the spheres of nature, culture, and history.

Embodiment is thus fundamentally connected with various levels and modalities of bodily actions, attitudes, stances, and movements (Buytendijk 1957); personal striving or willing; and perceptual awareness of things (including the body itself). Wishing, desiring, noticing, attending, and the like are or can be actualized (embodied, enacted) by means of corporeal movements (kinesthetic flow patterns correlated with muscle activations) that are functionally correlated with the several perceptual fields and what appears in them (turning one's head and looking at something). Only to that extent can one sensibly say that this organism is "uniquely singled out" from the field of worldly objects as "mine." Involved in embodiment are processes of sensory "feeling"—coenesthetic (of inner body, e.g., of hunger), kinesthetic (of body motion), proprioceptive (of body stance or posture)—and elementary strivings (reaching, squinting, locomotion, etc.). Together, these contribute not only to the sensing of "this" organism as "belonging to me" but also to the forming of the surrounding field of objects as correlated to bodily feelings and movements, positions, and actions.

But it needs to be emphasized that there is quite another dimension to embodiment. Although surprisingly little attention has been devoted to it, it turns out to be quite essential. However tempting it is to say "I am my body" (when, for example, someone strikes me in the face, I say "Don't hit me!"), many cases in psychopathology literature (Binswanger 1958), and situations in daily life, suggest that matters are more complicated. The relation between self and its embodying organism seems as much a matter of "otherness" as of "mineness." However intimate and profound the relation between the person and the person's body, it is equally true that a person experiences his or her body as strange and alien, in ways that can be understood (Leder 1990).

I am my body; but in another sense I am not my body, or not simply that. This otherness is so profound that we inevitably feel forced to qualify the "am": it is not identity, equality, or inclusion. It is "mine," but this means that the person is in a way distanced from it, for otherwise there would be no sense to "belonging"; it would not be characterizable in any sense as "mine." So close is the union that a person's experience of his or her "own" body can be psychologically unnerving (its happy obedience that the person notices for the first time or its hateful refusal to obey his or her wish to do something) (Binswanger 1958). So intimate is it that the person has moments of genuinely feeling "at home" with it. Yet so other is it that there are times when the person treats the body as a mere thing that is other, obsessively stuffing it with food or otherwise mistreating it, or when it is encountered as "having a life of its own" to which the person must willy-nilly attend: like it or not, "my" hair grows and must be trimmed for certain purposes, "my" hands cleaned, "my" bowels moved, "my" cold cured, and so on (Zaner 1981; Leder 1990).

The person finds himself or herself embodied by an animate organism whose peculiar connections to the person (and the person to it) give embodiment its uniquely uncanny character. Nothing is so much "me-myself," yet nothing seems so strange; so deeply familiar (Who else could "I" be?) yet so oddly alien (Who indeed am "I"?). This experience is not indicative of an inability to make up one's mind but, rather, suggests the peculiarity of embodiment. What seems distinctive is this "mineness/otherness" (the most familiar yet the most alien) dialectic that is the core of human body as experienced (Engelhardt 1973; Zaner 1981).

In these terms, to speak of embodiment is to speak of something that "I" am and not something that can be placed over against me (*ob-jectum*) as an object. As embodied, "I" am in a clear sense a fundamental puzzle to myself—precisely what Pascal had appreciated with remarkable insight. What is expressed by "the problem of the body" is precisely the person's "being as embodied," that is, the fundamental sense of being human in the first place. The "self-body" (or "mind-body") problem is therefore a matter of experience: It is enacted at every moment in the ongoing life of the person. These considerations make it easier to appreciate that the human body is essentially expressive. It is that by means of which the person enacts and expresses feelings, desires, strivings, and so on (albeit in culturally and historically different manners) (Merleau-Ponty 1945). This expressiveness signifies that embodiment is valorized, that is, deeply textured with a sense of worth (whether positive or negative, as the case may be). After all, what happens to it happens to me: the person, as that which "rules and governs," is at the same time subject to its conditions. What happens to the person's body, in still different terms, matters to the person whose body it is: The embodying organism lies at the root of the moral sense of inviolability of personhood—of the "privacy," "integrity," "consent," "respect," and "confidentiality" that play such profound roles in research ethics, bioethics, and clinical ethics. Nor does the fact that people can and do dissemble and deceive themselves and others—as in cases of factitious illness when a person is thought to "fake" symptoms (Ford 1983)—belie the body's expressivity. Indeed these are themselves expressive phenomena, however difficult it may be to discover and to interpret them (Burrell and Hauerwas 1974).

This value character of the embodying organism also helps elucidate more fully why the continuing discussions of many bioethical issues—pregnancy, prenatal diagnosis, abortion, psychosurgery, withdrawal of life support, euthanasia—are so highly charged and deeply personal. Likewise the profound moral feelings evoked by certain medical practices (surgery, chemotherapy) and much biomedical experimentation (in particular the Human Genome Project) are understandable, as they are in effect ways of intervening or intruding into that most intimate and integral of spheres: the embodied person. The person is embodied, enacts himself or herself through that specific animate organism that is his or her own, and is thus expressive of that very person. Bodily schemata, attitudes, movements, actions, and perceptual abilities are all value modalities by which one enacts and expresses one's character, personality, habits, goals, moral beliefs—in short, by which the person is alive as such.

To view medical practice and biomedical research from the perspective of embodiment is to appreciate them as planned or potential interventions into the sphere of personal intimacy, whether this sphere be initial (as in infancy) or more developed. Whether such interventions are mainly directed to the body (medicine, surgery) or to the person's mental life or status (psychiatry, psychotherapy), they all unavoidably affect the individual. The person's life as a whole is necessarily affected by surgery no less than by psychotropic medication. Psyche and soma are inextricably bound together as constituents of an integral, contextual whole (Zaner 1981). The expressive and valuative character of this whole, the embodied person, helps explain why every medical intervention falls within the moral order. Recognizing this of course does not of itself settle any of the ethical issues present in research or clinical situations: when it is morally permissible to withdraw life support, for instance, or whether it is right to restrict a retarded person's ability to procreate. However any such issues may eventually be settled, the point here is that medicine is an inherently moral enterprise, in no small way because of the nature of embodiment and the interventional character of medicine (Cassell 1973, 1991).

Clearly the effort to settle the specific ethical issues associated with medical practice and biomedical research requires that the fundamentally ethical nature of any intervention be explicitly recognized and appreciated (Zaner 1988). It can also be appreciated that the ethical issues associated with the medical profession (medical ethics) can be distinguished from those that arise in research (biomedical ethics) as well as from those that occur in clinical settings (clinical ethics). Each set of issues poses important and distinctive problems.

Although embodiment has a place in each of these disciplines, perhaps it is more important in clinical ethics deliberations. Because embodiment is essentially individual, the tasks of identifying, discussing, and (one hopes) settling moral issues that arise in clinical situations require that the specific circumstances of each individual situation be determined. Personal integrity and respect for the unique person are not concerns somehow imported into clinical situations from the outside; they are, on the contrary, intrinsic to the very nature of biomedical research and clinical practice. It might be added that in problematic cases (interventions for an unconscious or incompetent patient, for instance), the decision to intervene in ways that do not or cannot include the patient's own perspective nevertheless requires other ethical grounds and thus must be subject to critical ethical assessment. Other problematic situations—involving mental retardation, disabled infants, and so on—do not escape the necessity to respect the patient, though they do require special ways of taking him or her into account (e.g., consulting family or surrogate) along with the ethical issues involved in decision making (identifying and respecting the moral frameworks of each decision maker).

Medical and other health issues are not only inherently within the moral order but also context specific. No bioethical or clinical ethics issue can be settled in the abstract. Every medical practice, no matter how apparently trivial, is value laden to begin with, which means that it either explicitly or (most often) implicitly expresses some vision of what is, or is thought to be, morally good. The main issue for ethics in clinical situations is to help primary decision makers make explicit what each believes to be most worthwhile, of greatest value, as this is found in ongoing clinical or research situations. Only subsequently does it become possible to make informed judgments about the particular context-specific practices and issues facing people in clinical or research contexts (Zaner 1988).

How one can come to such truly informed judgments is an obvious problem, but it is not within the scope of this entry. It is, one hopes, enough to have delineated the philosophical and ethical dimensions of the human body—in particular the phenomenon of embodiment, its expressive and value character, and consequently the ethical nature of medicine and biomedical research. What remains to be done is also clear: not only to find appropriate ways to incorporate these philosophical and ethical considerations into the teaching and practices of the health professions and the research community but also to study the important aesthetic, political, sexual, and other dimensions of the body in social life more broadly.

BIBLIOGRAPHY

Bergson, Henri. 1953. *Matière et mémoire: Essai sur la relation du corps à l'esprit*. 54th ed. Paris: Presses Universitaires de France.

Bergson, Henri. 1970. *Matter and Memory.* Translated by Nancy Margaret Paul and W. Scott Palmer London: Allen and Unwin, 1970.

Binswanger, Ludwig. 1958. "The Case of Ellen West." Translated by Werner M. Mendel and Joseph Lyons. In *Existence: A New Dimension in Psychiatry and Psychology,* edited by Rollo May, Ernest Angel, and Henri F. Ellenberger, 237–364. New York: Basic Books.

Bosch, Gerhard. 1970. *Infantile Autism: A Clinical and Phenomenological-Anthropological Investigation Taking Language as the Guide.* Translated by Derek Jordan and Inge Jordan. New York: Springer Verlag.

Burrell, David, and Stanley Hauerwas. 1974. "Self-Deception and Autobiography: Theological and Ethical Reflections on Speer's *Inside the Third Reich.*" *Journal of Religious Ethics* 2 (1): 99–118.

Buytendijk, Frederik J. J. 1957. *Attitudes et mouvements: Étude fonctionnelle du mouvement humain.* Paris: Desclée de Brouwer.

Cassell, Eric. 1973. "Making and Escaping Moral Decisions." *Hastings Center Studies* 1 (2): 53–62.

Cassell, Eric. 1991. *The Nature of Suffering and the Goals of Medicine.* New York: Oxford University Press.

Descartes, René. 1955. *Philosophical Writings.* 2 vols. Translated by Elizabeth S. Haldane and George R. T. Ross. New York: Dover.

Descartes, René. 1963–1973. *Oeuvres philosophiques.* 3 vols. Edited by Ferdinand Alquié. 3 vols. Paris: Garner Frères.

Eccles, Sir John. 1979. *The Human Mystery.* New York: Springer Verlag.

Edelstein, Ludwig. 1967. *Ancient Medicine: Selected Papers of Ludwig Edelstein.* Edited by Owsei Temkin and C. Lilian Temkin. Baltimore, MD: Johns Hopkins Press.

Engelhardt, H. Tristram, Jr. 1973. *Mind-Body: A Categorial Relation.* The Hague: Martinus Nijhoff.

Ford, Charles V. 1983. *The Somatizing Disorders: Illness as a Way of Life.* New York: Elsevier Biomedical.

Gurwitsch, Aron. 1964. *Field of Consciousness.* Pittsburgh: Duquesne University Press.

Husserl, Edmund. 1952a. *Allgemeine Einführung in die reinen Phänomenologie.* Vol. 1 of *Ideen zu einer reinen Phänomenologie und phänomenologischen Philosophie.* Vol. 3 of *Husserliana: Gesammelte Werke.* The Hague: Martinus Nijhoff.

Husserl, Edmund. 1952b. *Phänomenologische Untersuchungen zur Konstitution.* Vol. 2 of *Ideen zu einer reinen Phänomenologie und phänomenologischen Philosophie.* Vol. 4 of *Husserliana: Gesammelte Werke.* The Hague: Martinus Nijhoff.

Husserl, Edmund. 1956–1959. *Erste Philosophie (1923–1924).* Vols. 7 and 8 of *Husserliana: Gesammelte Werke.* The Hague: Martinus Nijhoff.

Husserl, Edmund. 1982. *Ideas Pertaining to a Pure Phenomenology and to a Phenomenological Philosophy: First Book; General Introduction to a Pure Phenomenology.* Translated by Fred Kersten. The Hague: Martinus Nijhoff.

Kennington, Richard. 1978. "Descartes and Mastery of Nature." In *Organism, Medicine, and Metaphysics: Essays in Honor of Hans Jonas on His 75th Birthday, May 10, 1978,* edited by Stuart F. Spicker, 201–23. Dordrecht, Netherlands: Reidel.

King, Lester S. 1978. *The Philosophy of Medicine: The Early Eighteenth Century.* Cambridge, MA: Harvard University Press.

Laín Entralgo, Pedro. 1969. *Doctor and Patient.* Translated by Frances Partridge. New York: McGraw-Hill.

Leder, Drew. 1990. *The Absent Body.* Chicago: University of Chicago Press.

Lindeboom, Gerrit A. 1978. *Descartes and Medicine.* Amsterdam: Rodopi.

Marcel, Gabriel. 1935. *Être et avoir.* Paris: F. Aubier.

Marcel, Gabriel. 1940. *Du refus à l'invocation.* Paris: Gallimard.

Merleau-Ponty, Maurice. 1945. *Phénoménologie de la perception.* Paris: Gallimard.

Merleau-Ponty, Maurice. 1962. *Phenomenology of Perception.* Translated by Colin Smith. London: Routledge and Kegan Paul.

Pascal, Blaise. 1941. *Pensées: The Provincial Letters.* Translated by William F. Trotter and Thomas M'Crie. New York: Modern Library.

Piaget, Jean. 1952. *The Origins of Intelligence in Children.* Translated by Margaret Cook. New York: International Universities Press.

Rather, L. J. 1965. *Mind and Body in Eighteenth Century Medicine: A Study Based on Jerome Gaub's "De regimine mentis."* Berkeley: University of California Press.

Sartre, Jean-Paul. 1943. *L'être et le néant: Essai d'ontologie phénoménologique.* Paris: Gallimard.

Sartre, Jean-Paul. 1956. *Being and Nothingness: An Essay on Phenomenological Ontology.* Translated by Hazel E. Barnes New York: Philosophical Library.

Scheler, Max. 1973. *Formalism in Ethics and Non-Formal Ethics of Values: A New Attempt toward the Foundation of an Ethical Personalism.* 5th rev. ed. Translated by Manfred S. Frings and Roger L. Funk. Evanston, IL: Northwestern University Press.

Singer, Charles J. 1925. *Evolution of Anatomy: A Short History of Anatomical and Physiological Discovery to Harvey.* New York: Knopf.

Spinoza, Benedict de. 1951. *Ethics.* In *Chief Works.* Vol. 2. Translated by Robert Harvey Monro Elwes. New York: Dover.

Straus, Erwin W. 1958. "Aesthesiology and Hallucinations." Translated by Erwin W. Straus and Biyard Morgan. In *Existence: A New Dimension in Psychiatry and Psychology,* edited by Rollo May; Ernest Angel; and Henri F. Ellenberger, 139–69. New York: Basic Books.

Straus, Erwin W. 1966. *Phenomenological Psychology: The Selected Papers of Erwin W. Straus.* New York: Basic Books.

Zaner, Richard M. 1971. *The Problem of Embodiment: Some Contributions to a Phenomenology of the Body.* 2nd ed. Phaenomenologica 17. The Hague: Martinus Nijhoff.

Zaner, Richard M. 1981. *The Context of Self: A Phenomenological Inquiry Using Medicine as a Clue.* Athens: Ohio University Press.

Zaner, Richard M. 1988. *Ethics and the Clinical Encounter.* Englewood Cliffs, NJ: Prentice-Hall.

Richard M. Zaner (1995)
Professor of Medicine (Medical Ethics), Emeritus, Vanderbilt University Medical Center

I. EMBODIMENT IN THE PHENOMENOLOGICAL TRADITION [ADDENDUM]

The notion of the body lived in the first person as "mine" and situated in a context of lived meaning is one of phenomenology's most important contributions to biomedical ethics (Nenon 2011). But a further ethical dimension of embodiment arising at the interface between this experiential body and the objectified biomedical body involves the notion of the "inscribed body" (Kirkengen 2001; Kirkengen and Thornquist 2012). Persons who have undergone difficult experiences—including "adverse childhood experiences" (Felitti et al. 1998; Kirkengen 2010) such as abuse and other forms of trauma (rape, torture, etc.)—are often affected, bodily, in ways that go far beyond visible scars from physical injuries (Behnke 2003, 2012). If their experiential reports are not believed, or if there is no context within which their stories can truly be heard, these bodies "into which violation has been inscribed" continue "mutely testifying" to such "socially silenced" violation (Kirkengen 2001, 5), displaying symptoms that may not respond to medical intervention and are eventually marginalized (and perhaps stigmatized) under headings such as "somatization disorders," "medically unexplained symptoms," and other terminological attempts to establish a diagnostic category within the framework of an objectifying attitude (Kirkengen 2010; Eriksen, Kirkengen, and Vetlesen 2012).

For Kirkengen (2001, 2010; Kirkengen and Thornquist 2012), this signals an ethical crisis rooted in a version of Cartesian dualism whereby biomedicine is taken as normative while lived meanings and relationships are rendered invisible or irrelevant to the social production of medical knowledge. Kirkengen accordingly suggests that mainstream medical practice may often contribute—despite the best intentions of its practitioners—to the structural humiliation of human dignity (Margalit 1996). Kirkengen's phenomenological studies of the destructive impact of socially silenced violence/violation resonate with the recognition of the importance of narrative in phenomenologically informed nursing practice (Benner and Wrubel 1989) and clinical ethics (Zaner 1993, 2004; Frank 1995), as well as with the fundamental phenomenological distinction between the "disease state" of an objectified physical body and the "illness" directly lived by the embodied person, expressing a disruption or impairment of the integrity and efficacy of normal embodiment (Toombs 1992; Kirkengen and Thornquist 2012).

Thus even in an age when the personally lived body, with its core sense of "mineness," may sometimes be entirely expropriated by a network of biomedical technologies or "ecotechnics" (Nakhutsrishvili 2012), a phenomenological approach to embodiment finds it ethically imperative not only to respect each patient as an experiencing subject (rather than treating persons solely as medical objects) but also to listen to the story each suffering body has to tell in its uniquely fractured wholeness.

SEE ALSO *Biology, Philosophy of; Feminism; Gender Identity; Human Dignity; Human Nature; Life; Phenomenology; Women, Historical and Cross-Cultural Perspectives*

BIBLIOGRAPHY

Behnke, Elizabeth A. 2003. "Embodiment Work for the Victims of Violation: In Solidarity with the Community of the Shaken." In *Essays in Celebration of the Founding of the Organization of Phenomenological Organizations,* edited by Chan-Fai Cheung, Ivan Chvatík, Ion Copoeru, et al. www.o-p-o.net.

Behnke, Elizabeth A. 2012. "Enduring: A Phenomenological Investigation." In *Body Memory, Metaphor, and Movement,* edited by Sabine C. Koch, Thomas Fuchs, Michela Summa, et al., 83–103. Amsterdam: John Benjamins.

Benner, Patricia, and Judith Wrubel. 1989. *The Primacy of Caring: Stress and Coping in Health and Illness.* Menlo Park, CA: Addison-Wesley.

Eriksen, Thor Eirik; Anna Luise Kirkengen; and Arne Johan Vetlesen. 2012. "The Medically Unexplained Revisited." *Medicine, Health Care and Philosophy* (published online September 29, 2012).

Felitti, Vincent J., et al. 1998. "Relationship of Childhood Abuse and Household Dysfunction to Many of the Leading Causes of Death in Adults: The Adverse Childhood Experience (ACE) Study." *American Journal of Preventive Medicine* 14 (4): 245–58. See also www.cdc.gov/NCCDPHP/ACE and www.acestudy.org.

Frank, Arthur W. 1995. *The Wounded Storyteller: Body, Illness, and Ethics.* Chicago: University of Chicago Press.

Kirkengen, Anna Luise. 2001. *Inscribed Bodies: Health Impact of Childhood Sexual Abuse.* Dordrecht: Kluwer Academic.

Kirkengen, Anna Luise. 2010. *The Lived Experience of Violation: How Abused Children Become Unhealthy Adults.* Translated from the Norwegian by Eugenie Sommer Shaw. Bucharest: Zeta Books.

Kirkengen, Anna Luise, and Eline Thornquist. 2012. "The Lived Body as a Medical Topic: An Argument for an Ethically Informed Epistemology." *Journal of Evaluation in Clinical Practice* 18 (5): 1095–101.

Margalit, Avishai. 1996. *The Decent Society.* Translated by Naomi Goldblum. Cambridge, MA: Harvard University Press.

Nakhutsrishvili, Luka. 2012. "Corps propre et corps technique(s): Jean-Luc Nancy et la phénoménologie." *Studia Phaenomenologica* 12:157–80.

Nenon, Thomas. 2011. "The Limits of Biomedical Ethics and the Specific Role of Phenomenology in Biomedical Ethics." In *Clinical Ethics and the Necessity of Stories: Essays in Honor of Richard M. Zaner,* edited by Osborne P. Wiggins and Annette C. Allen, 45–55. Dordrecht: Springer.

Toombs, S. Kay. 1992. *The Meaning of Illness: A Phenomenological Account of the Different Perspectives of Physician and Patient.* Dordrecht: Kluwer Academic.

Zaner, Richard M. 1993. *Troubled Voices: Stories of Ethics and Illness.* Cleveland, OH: Pilgrim Press.

Zaner, Richard M. 2004. *Conversations on the Edge: Narratives of Ethics and Illness.* Washington, DC: Georgetown University Press.

Elizabeth A. Behnke
Creator, Study Project in Phenomenology of the Body

II. CULTURAL AND RELIGIOUS PERSPECTIVES

Scholarly and popular thought alike have typically assumed that the human body is a fixed, material entity subject to the empirical rules of biological science. Such a body exists prior to the mutability and flux of cultural change and diversity, and is characterized by unchangeable inner necessities. Beginning with the historical work of Michel Foucault and Norbert Elias, the anthropology of Pierre Bourdieu, and phenomenological philosophers such as Maurice Merleau-Ponty, Hans Jonas, Max Scheler, and Gabriel Marcel, however, scholarship in the social sciences and humanities has begun to challenge this notion. Late twentieth-century commentators argue that the body can no longer be considered a fact of nature, but is instead "an entirely problematic notion" (Vernant 1989, 20): "the body has a history" insofar as it behaves in new ways at particular historical moments (Bynum 1989, 171); the body should be understood not as a constant amid flux but as an epitome of that flux (Frank 1991, 40); and "the universalized natural body is the gold standard of hegemonic social discourse" (Haraway 1990, 146).

This scholarly perspective—that the body has a history and that it is not only a biological entity but also a cultural phenomenon—goes hand in hand with the increasing number and complexity of bioethical issues in contemporary society, many of which have strong religious overtones. Some decades ago the only such issue arose in cases where religious and biomedical priorities conflicted in the treatment of illness. Within the majority population, various groups such as Christian Scientists, some Pentecostal Christians, and members of small fundamentalist sects occasionally have created controversy by refusing medical treatment on the grounds that faith in medicine undermines faith in God, in other words, that since healing should occur only at the will and discretion of the deity, human medicine is presumptuous upon divine prerogative. This has been especially problematic when young children suffer and are kept from medical treatment by their parents. In Native American communities it has been, and occasionally remains, the practice for ill people to seek biomedical treatment only after having exhausted the resources of their spiritually based traditional medical systems. This occasionally results in the discovery of serious illness such as cancer or tuberculosis at a very advanced stage and creates a dilemma for health care personnel who are supportive of indigenous traditions yet concerned that their patients also receive timely biomedical treatment.

The number of bioethical issues with religious overtones has recently multiplied. The legality of abortion and the right of access by women to abortion have been defined not only as issues of civil rights and feminist politics but also as religious and moral issues. Surrogate motherhood and donorship of sperm and eggs raise ethical dilemmas regarding the biological, legal, and spiritual connections between parent and child. There is also concern about the apparently godlike ability of biotechnology to determine the genetic makeup of the human species; some see this approaching with the increasing sophistication of genetic engineering and the massive Human Genome Project, which will catalogue all possible human genetic characteristics. At the other end of the life course, the problems of euthanasia, technological prolongation of vital functions by means of life-support machines, and physician-assisted death raise moral and spiritual questions about the prerogative to end the life of oneself or of another. Legal and ethical acceptance of the definition of death as "brain death" has particular significance in that the brain-dead individual's other organs are still viable for transplantation to other persons. In the United States the bioethical dilemma is whether the brain-dead person can morally be considered dead until all other vital functions have ceased or whether removing those organs constitutes killing the patient. In Japan an added dilemma is that a person's spiritual destiny as a deceased ancestor depends in part on maintaining an intact physical body.

Each of these issues has to do with religion, not only because religions often define them as within their moral purview but also because at a profound level each taps into a concern that is at the very core of religious thought and practice: the problem of what it means to be human. More precisely, the problem is the nature of human persons, of what it means to have and be a body, of life and death, and of the spiritual destiny of humankind. In the succeeding sections of this entry these issues are placed in the context of recent thought about the cultural and the historical nature of the human body, about religious conceptualizations of the body, and about religious practices that focus on the body.

THE BODY AS A CULTURAL PHENOMENON

It has been suggested that in contemporary civilization the human body can no longer be considered a bounded entity, in part because of the destabilizing impact of "consumer culture" and its accompanying barrage of images. These images stimulate needs and desires, as well as the corresponding changes in the way the social space we inhabit is arranged with respect to physical objects and other people (Featherstone, Hepworth, and Turner 1991). In this process, fixed "life-cycle" categories have become blurred into a fluid "life course" in which one's look and feel may conflict with one's biological and chronological age; some people may even experience conflict between age-appropriate behavior and subjective experience. In addition, the goals of bodily self-care have changed from spiritual salvation to enhanced health and finally to a marketable self (Featherstone, Hepworth, and Turner 1991; cf. Foucault 1986 and Bordo 1990). As Susan Bordo has observed, techniques of body care are not directed primarily toward weight loss, but toward formation of body boundaries to protect against the eruption of the "bulge" and serve the purposes of social mobility more than the affirmation of social position. Bodily discipline is no longer incompatible with hedonism but has become a means toward it, so that one not only exercises to look good but also wants to look good while exercising. This stands in sharp contrast not only to early historical periods but to other societies such as that of Fiji where the cultivation of bodies is not regarded as an enhancement of a performing self but as a responsibility toward the community (Becker 1994).

This transformation in the body as a cultural phenomenon has been related by Emily Martin (1992) to a global change in social organization. In her view the "Fordist body," structured by principles of centralized control and factory-based production, is on the decline. It is being replaced by a body characteristic of late capitalism, that is, a socioeconomic regime characterized by technological innovation, specificity, and rapid, flexible change. She sees these changes particularly vividly in the domains of reproductive biology, immunology, and sexuality, all of which are increasingly intense loci of bioethical debate.

With respect to immunology in particular, Donna Haraway (1991) understands the concept of the "immune system" as an icon of symbolic and material systematic "difference" in late capitalism. The concept of the immune system was developed in its present form as recently as the 1970s and was made possible by a profound theoretical shift from focus on individual organisms to focus on cybernetic systems. The result has been the transformation of the body into a cybernetic body, one that for Haraway requires a "cyborg ethics and politics" that recognizes radical pluralism, the inevitability of multiple meanings and imperfect communication, and physical groundedness in a particular location.

This groundedness thus extends to biology itself. In addition to immunology, this is evident in recent feminist theory that eliminates "passitivity" as an intrinsic characteristic of the female body and reworks the distinctions between sex and gender, female sexual pleasure, and the act of conception (Jacobus, Keller, and Shuttleworth 1990; Bordo 1990; Haraway 1990). With biology no longer a monolithic objectivity, the body is transformed from object to agent (Haraway 1991). The bioethical implications of the body as experiencing agent are evident in social science work on the experience of illness (Kleinman 1988; Murphy 1987), pain (Good et al. 1992), and religious healing (Csordas 1990, 1994). New disciplinary syntheses grounded in a paradigm of embodiment have also emerged in disciplines such as anthropology (Csordas 1990, 1994), sociology (Turner 1986), and history (Berman 1989).

Many of these new syntheses are predicated on a critique of tenacious conceptual dualities such as those between mind and body, subject and object, and sex and gender (Haraway 1991; Frank, 1991; Ots 1991; Csordas 1990; Leder 1990). Drew Leder, for example, begins his critique of Cartesian mind–body dualism with the observation that in everyday life our experience is characterized by the disappearance of our body from awareness. He contrasts this with a description of *dysappearance*, the vivid but unwanted consciousness of one's body in disease, distress, or dysfunction. He then argues that it is the very sense of disappearance, itself an essential characteristic of our bodily existence, that leads to the body's self-concealment, and thus to a mistaken notion of the immateriality of mind and thought. That such a notion is cultural is evident in the technological domain if one compares Western navigational techniques, which are based on intellectualist mathematical instruments and calculations, with traditional Polynesian navigation, which in contrast relies on concrete sensory information regarding clouds and light, wave patterns, star movement, and the behavior of birds (Leder 1990). Leder further suggests that the Western tradition compounds the error by construing the body as a source of epistemological error, moral error, and mortality. In contrast, based on a phenomenological appreciation of unitary embodiment, he suggests the possibility of a new ethics of compassion, absorption, and communion.

The contemporary cultural transformation of the body can be conceived not only in terms of revising biological essentialism and collapsing conceptual dualities but also in discerning an ambiguity in the boundaries of corporeality itself. Haraway points to the boundaries between animal and human, between animal/human and machine, and between the physical and the nonphysical (Haraway 1991). Michel Feher construes the boundary between human and animal or automaton (machine) at one end of a continuum whose opposite pole is defined by the boundary between human and deity. Cultural definitions of the boundary between human and divine can be significant given the circumstances of corporeal flux and bodily transformation sketched above. This is especially the case when the question goes beyond the distinction between natural and supernatural bodies, or between natural corporeality and divine incorporeality, to the question posed by Feher of the kind of body with which members of a culture endow themselves in order to come into relation with the kind of deity they posit to themselves (Feher 1989). Thus, if the body is a cultural phenomenon in a way that makes its understanding essential to questions of bioethics, religion is an important domain of culture to address in understanding the body.

RELIGIOUS CONCEPTUALIZATIONS OF THE BODY

Perhaps the most vivid example from the domain of religion that the body is a cultural phenomenon subject to cultural transformations is given in the classic work on New Caledonia by Maurice Leenhardt, the anthropologist and missionary. Leenhardt recounts his discovery of the impact of Christianity on the cosmocentric world of the New Caledonian Canaques via a conversation with an aged indigenous philosopher. Leenhardt suggested that the Europeans had introduced the notion of "spirit" to the indigenous way of thinking. His interlocutor contradicted him, pointing out that his people had "always acted in accord with the spirit. What you've brought us is the body" (Leenhardt 1979, 164). In brief, the indigenous worldview held that the person was not individuated but was diffused with other persons and things in a unitary sociomythic domain: "[The body] had no existence of its own, nor specific name to distinguish it. It was only a support. But henceforth the circumscription of the physical being is completed, making possible its objectification. The idea of a human body becomes explicit. This discovery leads forthwith to a discrimination between the body and the mythic world" (Leenhardt 1979, 164).

There could be no more powerful evidence that the body is a cultural and historical phenomenon. Insofar as the objectification of the body has the consequences of individuation of the psychological self and the instantiation of dualism in the conceptualization of human being, it has implications for defining a very different regime of ethical relationships and responsibilities. This is not only a relative difference, but—as is clear in the missionary example of Leenhardt—one that has consequences for relations between different cultures.

Ancient Greek Conceptualizations. There is much more to the cultural and historical variability of the human body, however. For the ancient Greeks, as described by Jean-Pierre Vernant, the distinction between the bodies of humans and the bodies of deities was not predicated on that between corporeality and incorporeality, but on the notion that the divine bodies were complete and human bodies incomplete. Furthermore, this distinction emphasized not bodily features or morphology, but the being's place on a continuum of value and foulness. Bodies were understood as mutable along these dimensions without losing their identity, and thus deities could be simultaneously very heavy and very light, moving over the earth without quite touching it while leaving exceedingly deep footprints (Vernant 1989). The deities thus had bodies that were not bodies, but they had characteristics that never ruptured their continuity with human bodies, and which therefore defined human bodies by their very otherness. The existence of the deities guaranteed that in Greek culture qualities such as royalty and beauty were not abstract concepts or categories, since they were concretely embodied in beings such as Zeus and Aphrodite (Vernant 1989).

Hindu Conceptualizations. In the Hindu worldview *atman*, "self," is understood not as soul in distinction to body, but as the center in relation to an existential periphery, or as the whole in relation to the parts (Malamud 1989). The ritual act of sacrifice is personified and has a body, or in other words the body is both the model for and origin of sacrifice (Malamud 1989). The individual bodies are inherently sexual and are portrayed as couples, or *mithuna*. The masculine is invariably singular and the feminine plural, as in the sun of day in relation to the multiple stars of night, or the singularity of act/mind/silence in relation to the multiplicity of speech. In contrast to the mutable but distinctly individual body of the Greek deities, Hindu ritual portrays a rich "combinatory of the sexes" that constitutes a way of mythically thinking with the body. The *mithunas* achieve cosmic engenderment (begetting) through diverse body operations including dismemberment, multiplication of body parts, replication of bodies, birth, coupling/copulation, merging/incorporation, transformation and transgendering, and the emission of body products/fluids (Malamud 1989).

Jewish and Christian Conceptualizations. If, in Hinduism, engenderment is timeless and instantiated in the cosmos by the sacrificial act, in Judaism it is linear and instantiated in history by the act of procreation. Creation and engenderment are two moments of the same process, a "hiero-history" in which human generation does not imitate a divine process, but is that process (Mopsik 1989). Whereas in the Christian perspective the biblical injunction for man and woman to "become one flesh" is understood to refer to the indissolubility of marriage, in the Jewish perspective it is understood as the production of a child, and the birth of Christ outside the historical chain of engenderments is the basis for the Pauline splitting of the spiritual and carnal individual (Mopsik 1989). This view is elaborated further in the Jewish kabbalistic tradition's notion of the *sefirot*, the engendered emanations of the Infinite that are represented as combining to form a body (Mopsik 1989).

In sharp contrast to the Jewish kabbalistic elaboration of engenderment as life, the Christian gnostic tradition elaborates it as death (Mopsik 1989). Gnosticism sees the corporeal form as the creation of monstrous demiurges or archons, foremost among whom is Ialdabaoth, the equivalent of Jehovah. The human condition is symbolized in the gnostic tale of the archons' rape of Eve, who escapes with her psychic body while her "shadow" or material body is defiled (Williams 1989). The latter is a prison or garment, beastly because humans are created by beasts. Sexuality is an aspect of this beastliness, and hence cannot be part of an embodied sacred process, while the upright posture that distinguishes us from animals is attributed to a separate spark from the authentically spiritual human (Williams 1989).

From a more mainstream Christian perspective, the profound cultural implications of Feher's question of the kind of body people endow themselves with in order to come into relation with the sacred (Feher 1989) can be seen by considering the Eucharist. That the consumption of bread and wine transubstantiated into the body and blood of Christ is essentially a form of ritual cannibalism is emphasized by the story of a miracle in which a priest who doubted the divine reality of the Eucharist was forced to experience the bloody flesh, so that he could come to appreciate God's graciousness in presenting it in the tamer appearance of bread and wine (Camporesi 1989; see also Bynum 1989). In earlier periods of Christianity the spiritual power of the Eucharist extended to the nourishment of the body, and this, not through ingestion but by means of its aroma (Camporesi 1989). Unlike ordinary food, however, it does not become us, but we become it through its sanctifying power (Camporesi 1989). Great anxiety was created among priests with regard to the immense responsibility of transforming something dead into something alive by the utterance of a few words, and among communicants because of the inclusion of such a sacred substance in such a profane terrain as the digestive tract—hence the importance of a fast before communion (Camporesi 1989). Yet because the Eucharist was thought to release its grace only in the stomach, sick people who could not eat were excluded (Camporesi 1989). When later the substantial bread was replaced by thin wafers, it became common to let the wafer melt in one's mouth. Well into the twentieth century, Catholics were taught that biting or chewing the Eucharist was an insult and injury to the deity that could result in divine retribution.

Medieval Conceptualizations. In the 1980s, work on medieval Christian spirituality began to relate to the notion of the body as a cultural phenomenon. Caroline Walker Bynum (1989) has documented the prominence during the years 1200–1500 of a "somatic spirituality" that stands in contrast to gnostic rejection of the body and that reflects a less dualist mentality than has heretofore been attributed to the thought of this period. In general, a great deal of concern with embodiment was evidenced in speculation about whether the final "resurrection of the body" might be a natural consequence of human nature rather than a discrete divine act to occur at the Last Judgment, and whether we will taste and smell heaven as well as see it.

The medieval body was defined less by its sexuality than by notions of fertility and decay, but the contrast between male and female was as important as that between body and soul. Somatic spirituality was especially evident among female mystics, who—in contrast to their more cerebral male counterparts' experience of stillness and silence—tended to blur the boundaries among the spiritual, psychological, bodily, and sexual by cultivating a sensualized relationship of human body with divine body. Bynum draws on the cultural-historical context to understand why the male-dominated ecclesiastical hierarchy allowed this female spirituality to flourish: evidence was needed against the contemporary dualist heresy of the Cathars; because they were denied education in Latin, they wrote in the less linear and more oral style of the vernacular; they were encouraged to act out maternal roles vis-à-vis Christ (Bynum 1989).

In this context the relation between the genders took on remarkable properties. Although ideally a woman would die to defend her holy chastity, it was as likely for a holy man to be resurrected in order to complete a virtuous task. In other ways the genders were blurred, since it was thought that all had both genders within, and that men and women had identical organs with only their internal and external arrangements being different. Because of the powerful symbolic association of the female and the fleshly, while holy women sometimes experienced being the mother or lover of Christ, their nature often allowed them to mystically *become* the flesh of Christ. By the same reasoning, since body is equivalent to female, the incarnate Christ had a female nature, and the image of Christ as mother became a feature of medieval iconography (Bynum 1989).

RELIGIOUS PRACTICES AND THE BODY

Fasting. The cultural-historical transformation of the body is highlighted by comparison of fasting as a technique of the body in the medieval somatic spirituality with the phenomenon of anorexia nervosa in the late twentieth century. In a study of 261 holy women in Italy since the year 1200, Rudolf Bell distinguishes between contemporary anorexia nervosa and what he calls "holy anorexia." Whereas the former is regarded as a syndrome of clinical pathology, in the latter, "the suppression of physical urges and basic feelings—fatigue, sexual drive, hunger, pain—frees the body to achieve heroic feats and the soul to commune with God" (Bell 1985, 13). There are parallels between the two conditions and historical epochs. Bell suggests that the observation that the internal locus of evil as a corrupting force for women in the Middle Ages, in distinction to the external locus of sin as a response to external stimulus for men, corresponds to the Freudian model of anorexia nervosa as a food/sex oral fixation. In addition, in both, "the main theme is a struggle for control, for a sense of identity, competence, and effectiveness" (Hilde Bruch, quoted in Bell 1985, 17). However, there is a critical difference, and "whether anorexia is holy or nervous depends on the culture in which a young woman strives to gain control of her life" (Bell 1985, 20).

Bynum (1987) warns against the assumption that these phenomena are precisely the same, given theological meaning in one epoch and psychiatric meaning in another. She points out that even medieval writers had more than one paradigm for explaining fasting—that it could be supernaturally caused, naturally caused, or feigned—and that there was a clear distinction between choosing to renounce food and the inability to eat. In both historical cases, the behavior "is learned from a culture that has complex and long-standing traditions about women, about bodies, and about food," including what kind of behaviors are in need of cure (Bynum 1987, 198). It is a profoundly cultural fact that in the patristic era miraculous fasting was attributed largely to men, whereas in the medieval period it was characteristic of women; likewise it is cultural that in the medieval period the illnesses of men were more likely thought of as needing to be cured, whereas those of women were to be endured. Furthermore, in the later Middle Ages fasting was associated with a wider array of miracles and practices of somatic spirituality, including subsistence on the Eucharist, stigmata, espousal rings, sweet-smelling bodies, bodily elongation, and incorruptibility. Some of the behavior of these women fits the pattern of nineteenth-century "hysteria"; some is clearly the result of other illnesses; and some follows the thematic of control, altered body concept/perceptions, and euphoria. Yet one cannot be sure whether symptoms are associated with an inability to eat or are the result of freely chosen ascetic fasting. Finally, insofar as psychodynamic explanation can explain only individual cases, Bynum concludes that it is less helpful to know that contemporary labels can in some cases be applied to the medieval phenomenon than to account for cultural symbols that give meaning to the phenomenon, such as body, food, blood, suffering, generativity, or hunger (1987).

Faith Healing. Other contemporary religious practices equally require an appreciation of the body as a cultural phenomenon. How, for example, can we understand the imputed efficacy of "faith healing" among contemporary Christians? An understanding of the body as a cultural phenomenon suggests that ritual healing operates on a margin of disability that is present in many conditions. It is well known, for example, that some people who become "legally blind" are able to engage in a wide range of activities, but others retreat to a posture of near total disability and inactivity. Likewise, persons with chronic pain in a limb may be physically able to move that limb but refrain from doing so for lack of sufficient motivation to make the risk of pain worthwhile. Disability is thus constituted as a habitual mode of engaging the world. The process of healing is an existential process of exploring this margin of disability, motivated by the conviction of divine power and the committed participant's desire to demonstrate it in himself or herself, as well as by the support of the other assembled devotees and their acclamation for a supplicant's testimony of healing. To be convinced of this interpretation one need only consider the hesitant, faltering steps of the supplicant who, at the healer's request, rises from a wheelchair and shuffles slowly up and down a church aisle; or the slowly unclenching fist of the sufferer of chronic arthritis whose hand is curled by affliction into a permanent fist. Ritual healing allows this by challenging the sensory commitment to a habitual posture, by removing inhibitions on the motor tendency toward static postural tone, and by modulating the somatic mode of attention, that is, a person's attention to his or her own bodily processes in relation to others.

Consider also the practice of "resting in the Spirit" or being "slain in the Spirit" among Charismatic and Pentecostal Christians as evidence for the kind of body with which people endow themselves in order to come into relation with the sacred. In this practice, which occurs primarily in healing services, a person is overcome with divine power, and falls into a semi-swoon characterized by tranquility and motor dissociation. Despite its popularity, or perhaps because of it, resting in the Spirit is a controversial phenomenon, and the heart of the issue is its authenticity. More specifically, critics challenge its authenticity, whereas apologists argue for its beneficial effects in terms of healing and spiritual development. Both sides invoke the same biblical scenarios, such as Saul on the road to Damascus and the apostles confronted by the transfiguration of Jesus, and the same religious writers, including the ecstatic mystics Teresa of Ávila and John of the Cross, and both sides draw opposing conclusions about whether these constitute examples of resting in the Spirit. They likewise draw opposing conclusions about the historical prototypes of healers known for similar practices, extending backward in time from Kathryn Kuhlman to Charles Finney, George Jeffreys, George Fox, John Wesley, and the fourteenth-century Dominican preacher John Tauler. To be sure, such analogies and precedents suggest that it would be possible to examine the varying meanings of religious falling or swooning across historical and cultural contexts. In the contemporary context, however, the ideological/theological/pastoral debate about authenticity is predicated on the recurrent, constitutive North American psychocultural themes of spontaneity and control, and on the Charismatic cultural definition of the tripartite person as a composite of body, mind, and spirit.

Spirit Possession. The sacred swoon leads also to the complex issue of dissociation, common to discussions of "spirit possession." Spirits who inhabit people may be regarded either as malevolent, in which case they must be expelled or exorcised, or as benevolent, in which case becoming possessed is an act of worship and devotion. Possession of both types is widely reported in ethnological literature (Bourguignon 1976) and is increasingly common in contemporary Western society. Not only is the negative, or demonic, variant reported among some varieties of Christian religions, but the positive variant of possession by deities is characteristic of rapidly growing African religions. These include religions based on the Yoruba tradition of Nigeria, such as *santeria, candomblé*, and the related *vodun*. The Yoruba religion, in which the possessing deities are called *orixas*, is rapidly aspiring to membership in that select group of "world religions" that once included only so-called civilized faiths such as Christianity, Judaism, Islam, Hinduism, Buddhism, Taoism, and Confucianism. This cultural development requires a more sophisticated understanding of the possession phenomenon not as mental or cognitive dissociation but as physical and existential incarnation; not as a pathological hysterical amnesia to which the devotee becomes abandoned, but as a form of habitual body memory in which the deity's characteristics are enacted in a contemporary form of somatic spirituality.

Abortion Healing Rituals. A final example of the interplay of religion and bioethics with respect to bodily practices pertains to the contemporary cultural debate over abortion. Among participants in the North American Christian religious movement known as the Charismatic Renewal, and in Japan as a facet of what are called the New Religions, healing rituals are conducted both for the removal of guilt presumed to be experienced by the woman, and for the fetus in order to establish its spiritual status. The American practice is largely a private one that takes place within the membership of a discrete religious movement within Christianity and is a specific instance of the healing system elaborated within that movement. The Japanese practice has a relatively public profile not limited to a particular social group and is an instance of a type of ritual common to a variety of forms of Buddhism.

In both societies the affective issue addressed by the ritual is guilt, but whereas in American culture this is guilt occurring as a function of sin, in Japan it is guilt as a function of necessity. For the Americans abortion is an un-Christian act, and both perpetrator and victim must be brought back ritually into the Christian moral and emotional universe; for the Japanese both the acceptance of abortion as necessary and the acknowledgment of guilt are circumscribed within the Buddhist moral and emotional universe. Both rites are intended to heal the distress experienced by the woman, but the etiology of the illness is somewhat differently construed in the two cases. For Charismatics any symptoms displayed by the woman are the result of the abortion as psychological trauma compounded by guilt, along with the more or less indirect effects of the restive fetal spirit "crying out" for love and comfort. In Japan such symptoms are attributed to vengeance and resentment on the part of the aborted fetal spirit that is the pained victim of an unnatural, albeit necessary, act. Finally, not only the etiology but the emotional work accomplished by the two rituals is construed differently. For the Charismatics, this is a work of forgiveness and of emotional "letting go." For the Japanese, in whose cultural context gratitude and guilt are not sharply differentiated, it is a work of thanks and apology to the fetus. Thus, "there is no great need to determine precisely whether one is addressing a guilt-presupposing 'apology' to a fetus or merely expressing 'thanks' to it for having vacated its place in the body of a woman and having moved on, leaving her—and her family—relatively free of its physical presence" (LaFleur 1992, 147).

The contemporary transformation of the human body and scholarly formulations of it, placed alongside the transformative power of religion in its task of defining what it means to be human, offers an important perspective on issues relevant to bioethics. These range from abortion to brain death, from fasting to resting in the Spirit, from consumer culture to dissociation, and bear on the relation between genders, between cultures, and between the poles of dualities such as mind and body. Such phenomena, and new ways of understanding them, will increasingly come to light with continuing elaboration of the body/culture/religion nexus.

BIBLIOGRAPHY

Becker, Anne E. 1994. "Nurturing and Negligence: Working on Others' Bodies in Fiji." In *Embodiment and Experience: The*

Existential Ground of Culture and Self, edited by Thomas J. Csordas. Cambridge, UK: Cambridge University Press.

Bell, Rudolph M. 1985. *Holy Anorexia.* Chicago: University of Chicago Press.

Berman, Morris. 1989. *Coming to Our Senses: Body and Spirit in the Hidden History of the West.* New York: Simon and Schuster.

Bordo, Susan. 1990. "Reading the Slender Body." In *Body/Politics: Women and the Discourses of Science,* edited by Mary Jacobus, Evelyn Fox Keller, and Sally Shuttleworth, 83–112. New York: Routledge.

Bourguignon, Erika. 1976. *Possession.* San Francisco: Chandler and Sharp.

Bynum, Caroline Walker. 1987. *Holy Feast and Holy Fast: The Religious Significance of Food to Medieval Women.* Berkeley: University of California Press.

Bynum, Caroline Walker. 1989. "The Female Body and Religious Practice in the Later Middle Ages." In part 1 of *Fragments for a History of the Human Body,* edited by Michel Feher, 160–219. New York: Zone.

Camporesi, Piero. 1989. "The Consecrated Host: A Wondrous Excess." In part 1 of *Fragments for a History of the Human Body,* edited by Michel Feher, 220–69. New York: Zone.

Csordas, Thomas J. 1990. "Embodiment as a Paradigm for Anthropology." *Ethos* 18 (1): 5–47.

Csordas, Thomas J., ed. 1994. *Embodiment and Experience: The Existential Ground of Culture and Self.* Cambridge, UK: Cambridge University Press.

Featherstone, Mike; Mike Hepworth; and Bryan S. Turner, eds. 1991. *The Body: Social Process and Cultural Theory.* London: Sage.

Feher, Michel. 1989. Introduction. In part 1 of *Fragments for a History of the Human Body,* edited by Michel Feher, 10–17. New York: Zone.

Foucault, Michel. 1986. *The Care of the Self.* Vol. 3 of *The History of Sexuality.* Translated by Robert Hurley. New York: Pantheon.

Frank, Arthur W. 1991. "For a Sociology of the Body: An Analytical Review." In *The Body: Social Process, Cultural Theory,* edited by Mike Featherstone et al., 36–102. London: Sage.

Good, Mary-Jo Delvecchio; Paul E. Brodwin; Byron J. Good; and Arthur Kleinman, eds. 1992. *Pain as Human Experience: An Anthropological Perspective.* Berkeley: University of California Press.

Haraway, Donna J. 1990. "Investment Strategies for the Evolving Portfolio of Primate Females." In *Body/Politics: Women and the Discourses of Science,* edited by Mary Jacobus, Evelyn Fox Keller, and Sally Shuttleworth, 139–62. New York: Routledge.

Haraway, Donna J. 1991. *Simians, Cyborgs, and Women: The Reinvention of Nature.* New York: Routledge.

Jacobus, Mary; Evelyn Fox Keller; and Sally Shuttleworth, eds. 1990. *Body/Politics: Women and the Discourses of Science.* New York: Routledge.

Kleinman, Arthur. 1988. *The Illness Narratives: Suffering, Healing, and the Human Condition.* New York: Basic Books.

La Fleur, William R. 1992. *Liquid Life: Abortion and Buddhism in Japan.* Princeton, NJ: Princeton University Press.

Leder, Drew. 1990. *The Absent Body.* Chicago: University of Chicago Press.

Leenhardt, Maurice. 1979. *Do Kamo: Person and Myth in the Melanesian World.* Chicago: University of Chicago Press.

Malamud, Charles. 1989. "Indian Speculations about the Sex of the Sacrifice." In part 1 of *Fragments for a History of the Human Body,* edited by Michel Feher, 48–73. New York: Zone.

Martin, Emily. 1992. "The End of the Body?" *American Ethnologist* 19 (1): 121–40.

Mopsik, Charles. 1989. "The Body of Engenderment in the Hebrew Bible, the Rabbinic Tradition, and the Kabbalah." In part 1 of *Fragments for a History of the Human Body,* edited by Michel Feher, 48–73. New York: Zone.

Murphy, Robert F. 1987. *The Body Silent.* New York: Henry Holt.

Ots, Thomas. 1991. "Phenomenology of the Body: The Subject-Object Problem in Psychosomatic Medicine and the Role of Traditional Medical Systems Herein." In *Anthropologies of Medicine: A Colloquium on West European and North American Perspectives,* edited by Beatrix Pfleiderer and Gilles Bibeau, 43–58. Brunswick, Germany: Vieweg.

Turner, Bryan. 1986. *The Body and Society: Explorations in Social Theory.* New York: Basil Blackwell.

Vernant, Jean-Pierre. 1989. "Dim Body, Dazzling Body." In part 1 of *Fragments for a History of the Human Body,* edited by Michel Feher, 18–47. New York: Zone.

Williams, Michael A. 1989. "Divine Image—Prison of Flesh: Perceptions of the Body in Ancient Gnosticism." In part 1 of *Fragments for a History of the Human Body,* edited by Michel Feher, 128–47. New York: Zone.

Thomas J. Csordas (1995)
Professor of Anthropology, University of California, San Diego

II. CULTURAL AND RELIGIOUS PERSPECTIVES [ADDENDUM]

Since the 1990s, the sociology of the body has been recognized as an important field within mainstream sociology, especially in the United States and the United Kingdom. Recognition of the theme "the body and embodiment" has consequently had an impact on both the anthropology and sociology of religion. Drawing on the work of Pierre Bourdieu (1990), authors have increasingly emphasized embodiment, religious practice, and experience in terms of his general notion of "habitus." New research focuses study on how people perform and experience religion rather than on religious belief and knowledge. A complementary development has been the notion of "materiality" in religious studies, in which research has examined the connections between body, identity, emotions, place, and objects in religious experience (Keane 2008; Bautista 2012; Pagis 2013). However, one dominant issue in contemporary "body studies" (Turner 2012) has been to consider the impact of technology, especially medical technology, on the human body and its consequences for religion and ethics. The future of the human body is unsurprisingly tied up with technological interventions and how they can transform our embodiment. The potential for redesigning the body has been expressed in the ideas of *transhumance* (Bostrom 2003) and *posthumanism* (Fukuyama 2002). Transhumance and post-humanisn are typically used interchangeably. However, transhumanism is both a social movement and an ideology that seeks to make readily available technologies to eliminate human aging. In addition, it proposes to enhance human intellectual and physical capabilities to bring about a posthuman future.

Technology has obviously been important in the transformation of life expectancy. French women on average enjoy a life expectancy of eighty-one years and Japanese women, eight-five years. It is predicted that the median age of the population in Germany in 2030 will be forty-nine years and in Britain forty-two years (National Intelligence Council 2012). In response, new perspectives on the body and human aging have emerged under the conceptual umbrella of "the life-extension project," namely diverse efforts to promote healthy longevity through the technological enhancement of the human body. In turn, life extension has been promoted by "rejuvenative sciences" that promise to extend life more or less indefinitely.

Standard interventions include cosmetic surgery, dietary management, regular exercise, organ transplants, and intensive medical testing. However, possibilities for the future include cryonics, or techniques to store the body by freezing, the potential use of nanotechnology to conduct microsurgery on failing organs, and the development of computers that could be implanted to replace or upgrade organs. The total effect of these interventions would be to create a posthuman body or hybrid creature. Our bodies have become artifacts that are increasingly manufactured through life-enhancing biomedical technologies (Juvin 2010).

These social changes at one level merely intensify existing ethical issues: For example, how will intergenerational justice play out in a world of active centenarians? In terms of scarce resources, how will international justice be approached when there are major differences in life expectancy across the planet? But there are radically new issues. Transhumance would have the radical consequence of changing the nature of human vulnerability, suffering, and pain (Turner 2006). Religious worldviews, such as Christianity and Buddhism, have typically presupposed the ubiquity of human suffering and finitude. If the life-extension project is successful, existing religious and ethical understanding of life would have to be seriously revised.

SEE ALSO *Authority in Religious Traditions; Bioethics: IX. Anthropology of; Buddhism, Bioethics in; Christianity, Bioethics in; Death: I. Cultural Perspectives; Embryo and Fetus: V. Religious Perspectives; Enhancement Uses of Medical Technology; Judaism, Bioethics in; Medicine, Art of; Native American Religions, Bioethics in; Sexual Ethics; Transhumanism and Posthumanism*

BIBLIOGRAPHY

Bautista, Julius, ed. 2012. *The Spirit of Things: Materiality and Religious Diversity in Southeast Asia.* Ithaca, NY: Southeast Asia Program, Cornell University.

Bostrom, Nick. 2003. "Human Genetic Enhancements: A Transhumanist Perspective." *Journal of Value Inquiry* 37 (4): 493–506.

Bourdieu, Pierre. 1990. *The Logic of Practice.* Translated by Richard Nice. Cambridge: Polity Press.

Fukuyama, Francis. 2002. *Our Posthuman Future: Consequences of the Biotechnology Revolution.* New York: Farrar, Straus and Giroux.

Juvin, Hervé. 2010. *The Coming of the Body.* Translated by John Howe. London: Verso.

Keane, Webb. 2008. "The Evidence of the Senses and the Materiality of Religion." *Journal of the Royal Anthropology Institute* 14 (1): 110–27.

National Intelligence Council. 2012. *Global Trends 2030: Alternative Worlds.* Washington: Author. http://www.dni.gov/index.php/about/organization/national-intelligence-council-global-trends

Pagis, Michael. 2013. "Religious Self-Construction: A Relational Perspective." In *Religion on the Edge: De-Centering and Re-Centering the Sociology of Religion,* edited by Courtney Bender, Wendy Cage, Peggy Levitt, and David Smilde, 92–114. New York: Oxford University Press.

Turner, Bryan S. 2006. *Vulnerability and Human Rights.* University Park: Pennsylvania State University Press.

Turner, Bryan S., ed. 2012. *Routledge Handbook of Body Studies.* Abingdon: Routledge.

Bryan S. Turner
Presidential Professor of Sociology, Department of Sociology, The Graduate Center, The City University of New York

III. COMMODIFICATION OF

The commodification of the human body is an issue of both long-standing and intensifying bioethical concern. Taken as a whole or disaggregated into a dizzying array of parts, the possibilities for generating various forms of clinically useful and commercially valuable products from the human body have grown exponentially since the mid-twentieth century. Such developments raise heated debate about the potential effects on human dignity, identity, liberty, and justice of allowing the human body to be bought and sold.

In trying to account for the practices and ethics associated with "body commodification," both elements of the term must be parsed with care. For the "body" in question may be alive or dead, whole or in parts. And if in parts, such parts may range from vital organs as invested with emotional and cultural weight as the heart; to commonly discarded waste products such as saliva, sweat, and urine; to digitized and patented information, like DNA. Whether such parts are vital or not, renewable or not, easily and safely separable from the body or not, or central to one's sense of personal identity or not—such key forms of differentiation, among others, remind us that "the body" cannot be taken as a unitary, straightforward category.

No more straightforward is the concept of "commodification." Direct payment to the person from whom biological material comes, compensation for costs associated with handling such material, and profits from subsequently developed products are just some of the diverse ways in which bodies and money may get mixed up with one another. Thus the widely used term "commodification" paints with a broad brush, one that encompasses some forms of relation between bodies and the market widely deemed permissible in both legal and ethical terms, as well as others thought by many to be fundamentally and deeply abhorrent.

There is enormous variation and complexity in how the relationship between human biological materials and monetary value has proceeded both across the terrain of the body and across the geography of different nations around the world. Human sperm, for example, has been highly commercialized in many Western countries since the early twentieth century, yet not just the sale but the very use of third-party sperm is banned in many Muslim countries. In contrast, the selling of solid organs is officially illegal in most countries (though such laws are unevenly upheld), but the Iranian government has sponsored a regulated market in live donor human kidneys since 1988. Such diversity makes accounting for the topic of bodily commodification a complex and necessarily incomplete task. By way of offering a strategic, rather than comprehensive, overview, this entry will first provide a basic definition of body commodification and explore the relevant historical and legal context. Next, key bioethical approaches to the question of commodification will be summarized, followed by a more detailed examination of one of the most contentious sites of ongoing bioethical debate: the buying and selling of human organs.

DEFINITION, HISTORY, LEGAL CONTEXT

In its most general meaning, a commodity is understood as something of use or value, at least potentially available for exchange. From Karl Marx, the term takes on a more specific set of meanings related to the production of goods under the alienating conditions of capitalist labor, and the equivalence of those goods with monetary value (Marx 1990 [1867]). In early twenty-first century society, commodification is often used more generally to describe the processes by which things of all kinds are drawn into the market and made available to be bought and sold. Importantly, commodification is not necessarily an irrevocable, irreversible process. Rather, as the anthropologist Arjun Appadurai has argued, things of all sorts—including human bodies—have complex social lives during which they may move into and out of commodity status (Appadurai 1986). Thus the knucklebone of a saint, to take just one historical example, may pass during its own complicated social history from being an integrated part of a living human body, to a disaggregated object available for sale to the highest marketplace bidder, to a sacred relic held in trust and venerated by members of a religious community.

As the example of the saintly knucklebone suggests, there is nothing new about the notion of human bodies—alive or dead, whole or in parts—being subject to market values. Indeed, as the anthropologist Lesley Sharp has described (2000), there is a long global history of brisk markets not just in such religious relics, but in slaves, prostitutes, cadavers for anatomical study, and human body parts for use in a wide variety of healing practices and witchcraft rituals, among other examples. Yet technological advances in medicine in the post–World War II era have dramatically expanded the possibilities for how human bodies may be fragmented and rendered both clinically useful and highly profitable. New techniques for preserving human bodily material (such as liquid nitrogen for storing human ova), for transforming it (such as the ability to fractionate blood into components that can then be amplified into a wide variety of products), and for utilizing it (such as using infant foreskin to grow artificial skin) have contributed to this massive expansion of both utility and profitability. Further extending the possibilities for marketization are not only such scientific techniques but also new legal strategies, so that contracting for the use of a surrogate mother's womb and patenting a patient's DNA, for example, are tools now available to the commodification process

For the tissue banks and pharmaceutical companies that process and provide such human materials, as well as the health care institutions and providers that use them in clinical practice, these human products can generate enormous profits. However, as Catherine Waldby and Robert Mitchell have carefully tracked (2006), this highly lucrative biotechnology industry is built largely on tissues surrendered without recompense by the people from whom they come. This may include tissues drawn from medical procedures performed on living patients, which are then designated as "medical waste" and made available for recycling into a variety of products. Such tissues may also be donated from living or deceased bodies for medical or research use. Or, human tissues may be rendered available for processing into lucrative products through illicit routes, as stolen bodies and their parts are circulated through extensive global black market networks.

Highlighted here is a distinction between what we might call direct and indirect, or downstream, forms of body commodification. A distinction, that is, between cases where payment for a body part goes directly to the person from whom it came (or, in the case of a cadaver, to the person's heirs) and cases where monetary value is generated (and received) at some remove from the person who provided those bodily materials. As shall be taken up in more detail below, there is an entrenched Western tradition of ethical discomfort and legal prohibition surrounding many direct forms of bodily commodification. At the same time, many indirect forms of commodification are flourishing around the world and have become a vital component in one of the most rapidly growing sectors of the global economy.

The legal roots of this distinction between direct and indirect forms of bodily commodification has a long history pertaining to the question of what rights one can have in and over the body. It is a distinction often traced back to John Locke's *The Two Treatises of Government* (1689), in which Locke holds that property rights derive from the mixing of labor with an object, thus creating value and establishing ownership. For Locke, who wrote that "every man has a property in his body," ownership of the living body is the first natural property right and is, through its labor, the source of all other forms of ownership. Yet he holds that the living body is a fundamentally inalienable form of property; like the right to liberty, it cannot be transferred to another. Nor can the dead body be properly construed as salable property: because no labor has gone into its creation, it is *res nullis*, owned by no one. Though subject to diverse readings, Locke's formulation of bodily property rights has shaped common law from the seventeenth century onward in much of the Western world and continues to hold today in what bioethicist Leon Kass has described as the "common-sense and common-law teaching that there is no property in the body, not in my own living body, not in my corpse, and not in my relatives' corpses" (1992, 85).

Despite its powerful sway, however, the historian Ruth Richardson has richly documented (1987) how this particular legal framing of bodily ownership became increasingly problematic as medicine—both as a system of knowledge and as a sought-after service—began to expand through the seventeenth and eighteenth centuries. This expansion stimulated a need for human cadavers that could be dissected in the service of medical research and teaching. Yet existing common law traditions meant that there was virtually no legal source of cadavers to supply this increasing demand. Over time, this demand for anatomical specimens produced a clandestine economy in stolen human cadavers that quietly supplied medical students and anatomists into the early nineteenth century. In the early 1800s, however, a series of public scandals erupted in Britain, culminating in the sensational case of Burke and Hare, two men who were discovered to be murdering people in Edinburgh in order to sell their corpses to a nearby medical school. British Parliament responded to the public horror with passage of the Anatomy Act of 1831, which moved to requisition the unclaimed bodies of the poor from workhouses and hospitals in order to provide a legal—and noncommercialized—source of anatomical specimens. Though the act produced a backlash of fear and fury on the part of the poor who resented being abandoned to such a fate, the legislation held and proved widely influential. Indeed, the original British legislation has come to serve as the basis of modern law on the disposition of human material throughout much of the English-speaking world and beyond.

The essential intent first contained in the Anatomy Act to generate a noncommercial supply of human biological material continues to guide much of modern-day relevant law and policy. In the United States, for example, both the 1968 Uniform Anatomical Gift Act (UAGA) and the 1984 National Organ Transplantation Act (NOTA) established regulations for donating human bodies and their parts—including strong prohibition of payment for these materials. The current version of NOTA, for example, states that "it shall be unlawful for any person to knowingly acquire, receive, or otherwise transfer any human organ for valuable consideration" (1990 [1984], sec. 301a). At a global level, the World Health Organization (WHO) has similarly asserted that "cells, tissues and organs should only be donated freely, without any monetary payment or other reward of monetary value" (2010, 5). Yet as with imprecision of the term "commodification" itself, the exact meaning of terms such as "valuable consideration" or "reward of monetary value" has been subject to debate, leaving the door open to various means by which money may enter the processes of making human tissue available to the many uses to which we now want to put it.

Indeed, despite widespread prohibition of direct commodification of the human body, current law and practice in many places increasingly have come to allow for what is often called "reasonable payment" for the costs associated with removal, transfer, storage, and processing of human materials. This is the means by which hospitals, tissue banks, and organ procurement organizations, for example, are able to receive payment for their work in handling donated human tissues. And following one common reading of Locke's notion of property rights, this also then becomes the means by which the human body may be mixed with labor and thus rendered something that can be "owned" (and hence sold) by such entities as the health care institutions, tissue banks, and pharmaceutical companies that receive them. A similar distinction between paying for the human material itself (which is generally prohibited) and paying for the labor associated with its transfer is sometimes extended to the sources of certain kinds of living human tissue as well. Thus paid egg and sperm donors, for instance, are commonly understood to be compensated, not for the gametes they provide, but for the time and effort required to donate them. Similarly, living kidney donors in many places where organ selling is outlawed may nonetheless be offered recompense for travel expenses, housing, and lost wages associated with the donation process.

Parsing out payment for associated labor from payment for the material itself may be seen as ethically meaningful or as a rhetorical sleight of hand that works to render the buying and selling of human material more palatable. Sleight of hand or not, however, it remains generally true that for those whose bodies provide these materials, receiving payment does not confer legal property rights in the body—nor in the products subsequently generated from them. In contrast, a substantial group of legal decisions in the US courts in fact have granted explicit property rights in bodily materials not to those who provide them, but to those who manipulate and work on them in some way. The production and patenting by scientists of cell lines and DNA sequences derived from tissue surrendered by wholly unaware patients is perhaps the paradigmatic example of this. One early and influential case in this vein involved John Moore, a patient with a rare form of hairy cell leukemia who sued his physicians when he discovered that various patents as well as a proprietary cell line had been developed from his tissue samples without his knowledge. In this case, and in others that have subsequently followed, the court ruled that the patient held no property rights in his own body, and that those rights (and the profits derived from them) resided with the scientists that had worked on the tissue to create a new product.

As the legal scholar Lori Andrews has wryly observed, the Moore case and others that followed created a curious state of policy in which "other people seem to have property rights in our body, but we do not" (1986, 34). There is some evidence that this state of policy may be shifting, as suggested by a June 2013 Supreme Court ruling prohibiting the patenting of isolated breast cancer genes by the biotech company Myriad Genetics (Liptak 2013). Yet the second half of Andrews's observation appears to hold, for refusing to grant property rights to those scientist/entrepreneurs who isolated a gene still does not invest those rights in the patients who provided the biological material on which that work was based.

Ultimately, such rulings over property rights in the body reveal important continuities with the long legal history in this area dating back to the Anatomy Act of 1831. In the Moore decision and similar subsequent rulings, the explicit intent has been to protect and foster the scientific innovation that it was feared would wither without the motivation of proprietary rights and the profits that flow from them. Thus, despite the acknowledged misgivings of some of the involved jurists, the perceived needs of scientific progress have often been largely privileged over the rights of the individual to control what happens to his or her own body. It was, in many ways, a similar privileging of science and its need for bodily material that motivated the move to requisition the bodies of the poor for the needs of medical training and research under the original Anatomy Act nearly two centuries ago.

BIOETHICAL APPROACHES TO COMMODIFICATION

If Locke is often taken as a legal point of departure for considering property rights in the body, the work of Immanuel Kant has played a similarly influential role in moral deliberations about body commodification and its consequences for human dignity (1998 [1785]). The concept of human dignity is a fundamental, if often ambiguous and much-debated moral value in Western bioethics. In discussions of body commodification it is Kant's particular formulation of human dignity as being "above value" that is most commonly evoked. For Kant, there is a fundamental and mutually exclusive opposition between persons (who bear dignity) and things (which may bear a price). One implication of this is that human beings must be treated as having an intrinsic rather than an instrumental value: they must, as Kant would have it, be an end unto themselves, rather than merely a means.

Working from this formulation, many bioethicists have asserted that various forms of body commodification thus threaten fundamental human dignity by treating people as things that can be made equivalent to any other sort of thing through the mechanism of market price. Yet as the array of possibilities for what sorts of bodily material can be rendered alienable and at least potentially profitable has proliferated, it has become harder to discern just where the bright line between "person" and "thing" can and should be drawn. Does the commodification of a substance isolated from urine really threaten dignity and trouble identity to the same degree as the sale of a human embryo, for instance? Moreover, although Kantian concerns about human dignity are most often raised in opposition to body commodification, some have used Kant's privileging of reason and free will in the definition of what it means to be human to argue to opposite effect: that it is restricting a person's ability to do as he or she chooses with his or her own body that limits liberty and thus harms human dignity.

This marshaling of Kantian logic on both sides of the commodification debate is a pattern repeated throughout the extensive bioethical literature, as moral arguments based on each of the core bioethical principles of autonomy, beneficence/nonmaleficence, and justice have been made both to decry and to justify bodily commodification in various forms. Clearly, each particular form of human material raises its own distinctive ethical issues, for the consequential differences between the propositions of paying for the tumorous tissue from a cadaver or for the temporary use of a uterus or for patent rights to the DNA from an entire indigenous population are both considerable and morally significant. Yet the essential arguments for and against various forms of commodification often follow similar paths, disputing what is most likely to hinder or to honor autonomy, to produce more harm or benefit, and to deepen or to ameliorate inequality. Tracking the way such arguments have unfolded around the particular case of solid organs both illustrates these common arguments and engages one of the most contentious, ongoing sites of bioethical debate regarding bodily commodification.

As noted above, direct commodification of human organs for transplantation has been prohibited in almost all nations. Yet active black markets in organs exist in numerous places (most notably India, the Philippines, China, and parts of Eastern Europe), drawing together desperately poor sellers with desperately ill, wealthy buyers from around the world. Only one country in the world, Iran, currently has a government-regulated market in kidneys from living vendors.

The widespread endorsement—if not always enforcement—of the idea that organs for transplantation should be altruistically donated rather than bought and sold is rooted in the history of blood collection and distribution systems developed after World War II. In a celebrated study still centrally cited in current debates over organ commodification, Richard Titmuss compared the social effects and clinical consequences of gift versus commodity systems for blood (Titmuss 1997 [1970]). His analysis painstakingly contrasted the wholly altruistic blood collection system of the United Kingdom with the mixed system employed in the United States, where blood and its components were (and still are) collected from both altruistic donations and commercial transactions. Based on this comparison, Titmuss argued strongly that a commodity system for blood was dangerous and inefficient, primarily because it depended on the participation of the desperate. Those willing to sell their blood, he demonstrated, were more likely to be vulnerable in not only economic but also health terms, and thus more likely to put both themselves and the recipients of their blood at greater risk. Beyond such immediate practical consequences, Titmuss (drawing on classic work on the gift relationship by Marcel Mauss [1967 (1924)]) argued that gift systems for blood donation foster a sense of social connection and mutual commitment among members of a society, whereas commodity systems depend on self-interest in ways that may erode social solidarity and even invite unethical behavior.

Titmuss's essential arguments about the medical and moral risks of commodifying the blood supply were highly influential in the early development of organ transplantation policy and practice in the United States and elsewhere. And they continue to be invoked in the early twenty-first century amid growing calls to reconsider commodification as a means to address the widening gap between supply and demand for organs. For as transplant medicine has expanded, the lists of patients waiting for an organ grow ever longer, and pressure has mounted to find new ways to generate more organs for transplant. The result has been increasingly open debate over whether the gift model ought to give way to what some presume will be the greater efficiencies of a market model. Proposals for various monetized forms of incentivizing organ donation have proliferated, ranging from paying for the funeral costs of deceased organ donors, to setting up a futures market in organs, to establishing a government-regulated system for buying and selling live donor kidneys.

Proponents of a market-based approach, such as the transplant clinicians Arthur Matas (2006) and Benjamin Hippen (2008), the philosopher Janet Radcliffe-Richards (2012), the economists Gary Becker and Jorge Elías (2007), and the bioethicists Charles Erin and John Harris (2003) and Mark Cherry (2005), invariably cite the moral urgency of the dire need of patients awaiting transplantation, arguing that increasing the organ supply is simply an ethical imperative. Given the current inability of the altruistic system to meet demand, commodification is proposed as the most effective means of generating more organs, thus rendering it ethically preferable on grounds of both beneficence and utility. For some, this claim is corroborated by the Iranian experience reported by the transplant surgeon Ahad Ghods (Ghods and Savaj 2006), where the initiation of a regulated kidney market has eliminated waiting lists for kidney transplantation. And not only organ recipients would benefit under a market model, proponents argue, but organ vendors too are thought to benefit from the access to needed resources that the opportunity to sell an organ could provide.

Though its proponents often concede that organ selling is most likely to appeal to the poor, they argue that prohibiting organ sales does not truly protect them from harm, but only further limits their abilities to improve their lives. Further discounting fears about the exploitative potential of commodification, some propose that opening legal, regulated markets in the global North could help eliminate the illegal global markets that currently prey on the most vulnerable in the global South.

Beyond such benefits of legalizing organ sales, however, proponents often see commodification as a fundamental issue of respect for autonomy, of allowing people to make decisions about their own bodies. Implied in this vision of autonomy is an understanding of the body as a vehicle for the self, as objectified property over which the rational self has the right to exert its free will. Interfering with this right on the grounds of potential exploitation, some suggest, constitutes inappropriately paternalistic—even insulting and unjust—treatment of the poor. Further extending this link between autonomy and justice is also the often-posed question: If so many others involved in the transplant process get paid, does requiring organ donors alone to act altruistically truly protect dignity and justice, or does it only further entrench inequality? Ultimately for proponents of organ sales, the compelling ethical good of producing more organs for transplant outweighs the potential—and disputed—harms.

Opponents of organ sales, such as the transplant surgeon Francis Delmonico (Delmonico et al. 2002), the bioethicists Jeffrey Kahn (2003) and Lainie Friedman Ross (2009), the social historians Sheila Rothman and David Rothman (2006), and the anthropologist Nancy Scheper-Hughes (2005) counter each of these claims about the potential benefits and moral justifications of a market in organs. Many simply reject the notion that commodification is likely the most effective means of increasing the organ supply, suggesting that the current level of altruistic donations would almost certainly decline in a marketized environment and might even be wholly destroyed by a backlash of public disgust. Yet even if commodification could produce more organs, many find the risks of exploitation too high to be ethically permissible. Deepening—and legitimizing—the inequitable patterns already observed in the current illegal organs trade, most agree it is the poor who would feel most compelled to sell an organ, while the rich would be most able to purchase them. And although supporters of organ sales see this as a means for the poor to improve their lot in life, opponents point to the research by Lawrence Cohen (1996) and Madhav Goyal (Goyal et al. 2002) in India, Javaad Zargooshi in Iran (2001), and Moazam in Pakistan (2009), which shows that most organ vendors consistently end up significantly worse off, in both economic and health terms. Findings that such vendors start out in more precarious health, that they are often motivated to conceal any health problems in order to be allowed to donate, and that they typically receive little follow-up care echo the concerns first raised by Titmuss about the potential dangers of a commodified system that relies on the desperate. Similarly reminiscent of Titmuss's analysis—and compelling to opponents—is evidence that organ recipients who purchase organs have worse outcomes than those who go through legal, gift-based systems. Taken together, such worrisome effects on both organ sellers and buyers lead many opponents to reject organ sales not just on justice-based grounds of exploitation, but also on utilitarian grounds of producing more harm than good.

Also deeply at stake for opponents are the implications of organ commodification for how we understand what it means to be human. Countering claims that allowing organ sales protects autonomy and hence human dignity is the view that organ markets fundamentally depend on the desperation that will compel vulnerable members of society to sell their organs. As such, selling an organ is seen as a "choice" that is so constrained, perhaps even coerced, that it cannot justly be termed "autonomous." Also challenged is the claim that autonomy implies control by a rational self over an objectified body rendered as property. For many opponents, the body must rather be seen as fundamentally integrated with and constitutive of the self—what Alastair Campbell has called the "embodied self" (2009). This view implies that selling the body cannot be separated off from selling the self, that it fundamentally constitutes (in Kantian terms), treating persons as means, rather than ends. Along such lines, reports from India that moneylenders are increasingly viewing the kidneys of their debtors as collateral that may be called in for repayment seem to illustrate the objectifying dangers to human dignity and solidarity of assigning a price to the human body. Thus, for opponents the overall moral and material harms—for both individual persons and the human collective—of organ commodification clearly outweigh the potential benefits.

Ultimately, the practices and ethics of body commodification—in organs and otherwise—remain highly contested and are still evolving. In the domain of organs, formerly taboo calls for commodification have become increasingly common and subject to serious consideration. Yet substantial opposition remains, and the outcome is not yet clear. Stepping back from this specific case, it is clear that the complexity of possibilities for forms of the body now rendered at least potentially alienable and salable, as well as for forms of direct and indirect commodification, make it no longer possible—or even desirable—to issue blanket proclamations about whether the human body should or should not be commodified.

As the legal scholar Margaret Radin has so compellingly argued over several decades of close observation (1996), the body already *is* commodified, but incompletely so. And as biotechnological practice, legal frameworks, and ethical analyses develop over time, so too—on a case-by-case basis—can we expect the complex relations between bodies and money to continue to shift and change as well.

SEE ALSO *Commercialism in Scientific Research; Genetic Engineering, Human; Organ and Tissue Procurement; Organ Transplants, Medical Overview of; Organ Transplants, Sociocultural Aspects of; Profit and Commercialism; Religious Objections to Medical Care; Reproductive Technologies: V. Gamete Donation; Tissue Banking, Ethical Issues in*

BIBLIOGRAPHY

Andrews, Lori. 1986. "My Body, My Property." *Hastings Center Report* 16 (5): 28–38.

Appadurai, Arjun. 1986. "Introduction: Commodities and the Politics of Value." In *The Social Life of Things: Commodities in Cultural Perspective*, edited by Arjun Appadurai, 3–63. Cambridge: Cambridge University Press.

Becker, Gary S., and Jorge Julio Elías. 2007. "Introducing Incentives in the Market for Live and Cadaveric Organ Donations." *Journal of Economic Perspectives* 21 (3): 3–24.

Campbell, Alastair V. 2009. *The Body in Bioethics*. New York: Routledge.

Cherry, Mark J. 2005. *Kidney for Sale by Owner: Human Organs, Transplantation, and the Market*. Washington DC: Georgetown University Press.

Cohen, Lawrence. 1998. "Where It Hurts: Indian Material for an Ethics of Organ Transplantation." *Daedalus: Journal of the American Academy of Arts and Sciences* 128 (4): 135–66.

Delmonico, Francis L.; Robert Arnold; Nancy Scheper-Hughes; et al. 2002. "Ethical Incentives—Not Payment—For Organ Donation." *New England Journal of Medicine* 346 (25): 2002–5.

Erin, Charles A., and John Harris. 2003. "An Ethical Market in Human Organs." *Journal of Medical Ethics* 29 (3): 137–38.

Ghods, Ahad J., and Shekoufeh Savaj. 2006. "Iranian Model of Paid and Regulated Living-Unrelated Kidney Donation." *Clinical Journal of the American Society of Nephrology* 1 (6): 1136–45.

Goyal, Madhav; Ravindra L. Mehta; Lawrence J. Schneiderman; and Ashwini R. Sehgal. 2002. "Economic and Health Consequences of Selling a Kidney in India." *Journal of the American Medical Association* 288 (13): 1589–93.

Hippen, Benjamin E. 2008. *Organ Sales and Moral Travails: Lessons from the Living Kidney Vendor Program in Iran*. Policy Analysis, no. 614. Washington, DC: Cato Institute.

Kahn, Jeffrey. 2003. "Three Views of Organ Procurement Policy: Moving Ahead or Giving Up?" *Kennedy Institute of Ethics Journal* 13 (1): 45–50.

Kant, Immanuel. 1998 [1785]. *Groundwork of the Metaphysics of Morals*. Translated and edited by Mary Gregor. New York: Cambridge University Press.

Kass, Leon. 1992. "Organs for Sale? Propriety, Property, and the Price of Progress." *Public Interest* 107:85–86.

Liptak, Adam. 2013. "Justices, 9–0, Bar Patenting Human Genes." *New York Times*, June 14, A1.

Locke, John. 1993 [1689]. *The Two Treatises of Government*. London: Dent.

Marx, Karl. 1990 [1867]. *Capital: Volume 1, A Critique of Political Economy*. New York: Penguin.

Matas, Arthur. 2006. "Why We Should Develop a Regulated System of Kidney Sales: A Call to Action!" *Clinical Journal of the American Society of Nephrology* 1 (6): 1129–32.

Mauss, Marcel. 1967 [1924]. *The Gift: Forms and Functions of Exchange in Archaic Society*. New York: Norton.

Moazam, Farhat; Riffat Moazam Zaman; and Aamir M. Jafarey. 2009. "Conversations with Kidney Vendors in Pakistan: an Ethnographic Study." *Hastings Center Report* 3:29–44.

National Organ Transplantation Act. 1990 [1984]. Pub L. 98-507, 98 Stat. 2339–2348.

Radcliffe-Richards, Janet. 2012. *The Ethics of Transplants: Why Careless Thought Costs Lives*. Oxford: Oxford University Press.

Radin, Margaret Jane. 1996. *Contested Commodities: The Trouble with Trade in Sex, Children, Body Parts and Other Things*. Cambridge, MA: Harvard University Press.

Richardson, Ruth. 1987. *Death, Dissection, and the Destitute*. London: Routledge and Kegan Paul.

Ross, Lainie Friedman. 2009. "Con." In "Saving Lives Is More Important Than Abstract Moral Concerns: Financial Incentives Should Be Used to Increase Organ Donation," by Benjamin Hippen, Lainie Friedman Ross, and Robert M. Sade. *Annals of Thoracic Surgery* 88 (4): 1053–61.

Rothman, Sheila M., and David J. Rothman. 2006. "The Hidden Cost of Organ Sales." *American Journal of Transplantation* 6 (7): 1524–28.

Scheper-Hughes, Nancy. 2005. "The Last Commodity: Post-Human Ethics and the Global Traffic in 'Fresh' Organs." In *Global Assemblages: Technology, Politics and Ethics as Anthropological Problems*, edited by Aihwa Ong and Stephen J. Collier, 145–67. Malden, MA: Blackwell.

Sharp, Lesley. 2000. "The Commodification of the Body and Its Parts." *Annual Review of Anthropology* 29:287–328.

Titmuss, Richard. 1997 [1970]. *The Gift Relationship: From Human Blood to Social Policy*. New York: New Press.

Waldby, Catherine, and Robert Mitchell. 2006. *Tissue Economies: Blood, Organs and Cell Lines in Late Capitalism*. Durham, NC: Duke University Press.

World Health Organization. 2010. "Guiding Principles on Human Cell, Tissue and Organ Transplantation." Geneva: World Health Organization.

Zargooshi, Javaad. 2001. "Quality of Life of Iranian Kidney 'Donors.'" *Journal of Urology* 166 (5): 1790–99.

Megan Crowley-Matoka
Assistant Professor, Medical Humanities and Bioethics, Feinberg School of Medicine, Northwestern University

BUDDHISM, BIOETHICS IN

Buddhism originated in India around 500 B.C.E.. In the early twenty-first century Buddhist traditions exist in South, Southeast, and East Asia, as well as Australia, Western and Eastern Europe, and North and South America. The diversity found in these traditions makes it impossible to speak of Buddhism in the singular or to assert an "official" Buddhist perspective. For the purpose of formulating an overview of Buddhist bioethics, however, Buddhist traditions can be categorized into two primary trajectories: Theravada and Mahayana. Theravada traditions are closely identified with the teachings of the historical Buddha, and include both early South Asian Buddhist traditions as well as contemporary South Asian traditions in Sri Lanka, Thailand, and Myanmar (formerly Burma). Mahayana traditions include some later forms of Indian Buddhism, Tibetan and other Himalayan-region Buddhisms (also referred to as Tibetan, Vajrayana, Tantric, and Esoteric Buddhism), and Central and East Asian Buddhist traditions. Both Theravada and Mahayana Buddhism are practiced in such places as Australia, Europe, and North and South America.

Historically, bioethics has been a field of inquiry primarily in Western cultures and thus centers on Western cultural assumptions and moral perspectives. Genetic engineering, cloning, and stem cell research—and the ethical dilemmas they engender—pivot on recent advances in biomedical technology and Western emphases on the value of medical progress. However, moral issues raised by biomedical technology are no longer confined to Western cultural contexts. Predominantly Buddhist countries have begun to confront the ethical implications of biomedicine. Not surprisingly, Buddhist ethical perspectives stem from assumptions that are sometimes very different from Western views, and these concerns affect how Buddhists engage with bioethical issues.

Individuals from North American and European cultural backgrounds may be troubled at the specter of "playing God" in making ethical decisions. From a Buddhist perspective, however, emphasis is placed, for instance, on investigating how the Buddha's exemplary life and compassion might reveal satisfying solutions to problems never envisioned by past Buddhists. After outlining some fundamental Theravada and Mahayana Buddhist ideas, this entry considers ways that Buddhists might respond to bioethical dilemmas and which Buddhist religious ideas could be invoked to make sense of diverse bioethical issues.

THERAVADA BUDDHIST THOUGHT AND PRACTICE

Western interpretations of the Buddhist Dharma—Buddha's law or teaching—often treat it as a philosophy. Although it is possible to view the Dharma this way, Buddha emphasized the centrality of religious practice over philosophy and doctrines. Intellectual understandings merely point at what must ultimately be realized through experience. Buddha posited a religious path attainable through a rigorous tripartite practice of wisdom, morality, and meditation—the foundations of the Noble Eightfold Path, Buddha's outline for how to live the religious life.

Theravada Buddhism focuses particular attention on the life of the historical Buddha (c. 563–483 B.C.E.). Buddha ("The Enlightened One") was a human being who, through assiduous spiritual practices, was able to comprehend the true nature of the universe. The realization of this transcendent wisdom is the achievement of *nirvana*, or enlightenment. Buddha, therefore, is a model for humanity, an example of what is possible by diligent practice of the Dharma.

The biography of the historical Buddha recounts the story of an entitled prince, Siddhartha Gautama of the Sakya clan, who is provided with material comforts and sensual pleasures by the king, his father. Wishing that his son will become a great leader, the king arranges for the prince to be sequestered in the palace, shielded from the pain and suffering that afflicts human beings. Over time, the prince—now grown and married with a young son—becomes curious about the world beyond the confines of the palace. Against his father's wishes, he ventures outside the palace walls on four separate occasions. Each time he encounters an aspect of human experience hitherto unknown to him. The four encounters—a sick person, an elderly person, a corpse, and a religious ascetic—result in the prince's realization of the fundamental suffering of human existence. The encounter with the ascetic prompts Prince Siddhartha's quest to attain an understanding of the world that would end suffering.

Prince Siddhartha subsequently decides to leave the palace and pursue the spiritual life of an ascetic renunciant. Single-minded in his resolve to attain spiritual liberation from the bonds of human existence by denying material needs, he nearly starves to death. As a result, he recognizes that liberation must lie somewhere between extreme hedonism and severe asceticism. He embarks on what becomes known as the Middle Path, a practice that allows sufficient bodily nourishment to carry out meditation and other spiritual practices. Through deep and persistent meditation he attains *nirvana*, thereby becoming Buddha. A reluctant teacher, he eventually accedes to the desire of others that he expound upon what he has learned. Thus begins Buddha's lifelong teaching of the Dharma.

Buddha's teaching centers on wisdom attained through enlightenment, a transcendent awareness of both the problem in the human condition and a means to its solution. This problem finds expression in the Three Marks of Existence, a description of the nature of life within the unenlightened world of *samsara* (the cycle of birth–death–rebirth). Individual status in the samsaric cycle is determined by actions (*karma*) and their moral consequences. Moral behavior leads to a higher spiritual rebirth, while immoral actions result in movement away from enlightenment. Buddha recognized that the samsaric world is fundamentally unsatisfactory and human beings eventually seek escape from it. According to the Three Marks, all existence is characterized by (1) impermanence (*anitya*); (2) suffering (*duhkha*); and (3) absence of a permanent self, soul, or essence (*anatman*).

Impermanence refers to the idea that all aspects of the samsaric world are in constant flux. While the world might appear to have stability and solidity, deeper scrutiny reveals that *samsara* is characterized by perpetual instability. Human beings mistake the temporary coming together of constituent elements (*dharmas*) for permanence. Thus, the world is best characterized not in terms of the atomistic existence of discrete enduring objects, but rather as a state of dependent origination, or interdependence (*pratītya-samutpāada*). Samsaric entities—including human beings—exist as a result of cause and effect. Nothing has an intrinsic foundation or essence that gives rise to its own existence. *Samsara* itself is understood as constituted by conditioned reality, that is, arising from a series of causes and effects.

The second mark of existence is suffering. The Buddhist term *duhkha* refers to both physical and mental suffering—especially the latter. *Duhkha* signifies the anxiety and insecurity prompted by the impermanent, transitory nature of the human condition. Markers of impermanence include the cycle of birth, disease, old age, and death, as well as anticipation of the inevitable loss of happiness and other temporarily pleasant emotions. Buddha did not deny the reality of happiness, but simply noted that it too is fleeting and impermanent. Suffering results from ignorance of the true nature of the samsaric world as transitory, momentary, and subject to constant flux.

The third mark of existence, *anatman* (no-self), refers to the absence of a permanent self or eternal soul that persists after physical death. Human ignorance engenders a misperception of current identity or sense of self as an enduring, independent essence. This idea is illustrated in an Indian Buddhist text that relates a dialogue between King Milinda and the monk Nagasena. In the *Simile of the Chariot*, Nagasena asserts that the self, like a chariot, has no essence. The King protests, so Nagasena describes the process of disassembling a chariot. Once the chariot has been reduced to a pile of parts, the King concedes that there is no essence of the chariot that persists. Like the chariot, human beings consist of constituent elements. These elements coalesce to form both animate and inanimate objects. Upon death, the *dharmas* disperse and re-form due to cause and effect, but no aspect of self, soul, or personality persists. Thus, *anatman* asserts that all existence is causally conditioned. The five aggregates of *dharmas* that constitute human beings are constantly arising and ceasing, but they do not produce a discrete, identifiable self or soul.

In accord with the worldview expressed by the Three Marks of Existence, Buddha taught that liberation from suffering may be attained though the Four Noble Truths:

1. All existence is suffering.
2. Suffering is caused by desire.
3. Cessation of desire results in the cessation of suffering.
4. The Eightfold Path leads to liberation (*nirvana*).

Like a medical analysis of the human condition, the Four Noble Truths mirror the steps of diagnosing a disease (suffering), understanding its cause (desire), identifying the cure for the disease (cessation of desire), and prescribing medicine that effects the cure (Eightfold Path). An outline of attitudes and actions necessary for spiritual advancement and enlightenment, the Eightfold Path offers a foundation for understanding Buddhist ethics in general and Theravada Buddhist bioethics in particular.

Buddha expounded the Eightfold Path as the mental and physical practices necessary to reach liberation from the samsaric world. The Eightfold Path consists of three components:

Wisdom (*prajna*):

- (1) right views
- (2) right intention

Morality (*sila*):

- (3) right speech
- (4) right conduct
- (5) right livelihood

Concentration (*samadhi*):

- (6) right effort
- (7) right mindfulness
- (8) right concentration

Wisdom refers to the fundamental mental states necessary to practice Buddha's Dharma. Right views include knowledge and acceptance of the Four Noble Truths and other aspects of the Dharma. Right intention refers to cultivating qualities such as compassion, benevolence, and detachment from the fruits of actions, and a commitment to harm no living creatures.

Morality is conceptualized in terms of speech, conduct, and occupation. Right speech requires that Buddhists abstain from verbal abuses such as slander, lying, and gossip. Right conduct refers to the avoidance of actions that harm others, such as killing, stealing, and sexual impropriety. Right livelihood extends the ideal of moral actions and prohibits specific occupations. Thus, one must refrain from work that leads—either directly or indirectly—to harming other living beings.

Concentration entails mental practices aimed at purifying the mind of evil and other distracting thoughts and gaining mastery of mental processes and feelings in order to engage in advanced meditation.

The practice of the Eightfold Path is neither linear nor sequential. Rather, all eight aspects must be cultivated simultaneously. Through self-effort these practices eventually effect a spiritual transformation from ignorance to a state of transcendent wisdom (*nirvana*). One who has cultivated the Eightfold Path and achieved liberation is known as an *arhat* (holy one), the model of Theravada Buddhist religiosity that all endeavor to follow.

MAHAYANA BUDDHIST THOUGHT AND PRACTICE

Even a brief survey of Mahayana Buddhism, which arose less than 500 years after the historical Buddha's lifetime, strongly suggests that "Buddhist bioethics" cannot be approached in singular terms. Mahayana refashions Theravada perspectives through the concept of *sunyata* (emptiness), while adding a new soteriological possibility based on faith: birth in a Buddhist paradise as the goal of religious praxis. Thus, Mahayana Buddhism incorporates the ideal of enlightenment achieved through individual self-effort—Zen Buddhism is the most well-known exemplar of this—as well as potential for salvation through birth in a Buddhist paradise. Particularly noteworthy is the Western Paradise, or Pure Land, of Amitabha Buddha, who vows to save all sentient beings that call on him for assistance. Furthermore, anyone—monastic or layperson—could practice devotion to the "other power of Amitabha," emphasizing for the first time nonmonastic practice leading to salvation.

In contrast to Theravada emphasis on the *arhat*, Mahayana focuses on the figure of the *bodhisattva*, a concept that has two primary significances. First, meditation-based Mahayana centers on the *bodhisattva* vow, a pledge to follow the Buddha's Dharma in order to achieve enlightenment and to compassionately assist others in the same quest. Through meditation, the *bodhisattva* aims to perceive the reality of the universe—that all *dharmas* are empty of self-nature. The concept of *sunyata* (emptiness) asserts that all dualistic perceptions are misperceptions and that *nirvana* (enlightenment) and *samsara* (cycle of existence) are the same thing. Otherwise, a duality or opposition between the enlightened and the unenlightened is being expressed. The Mahayana goal is not to transcend *samsara*, but rather to understand—experientially—that dualities result from a mistaken view of *nirvana* as permanent and eternal, existing outside of *samsara*.

Second, in faith-based Mahayana, the term *bodhisattva* describes compassionate figures, like Avalokitesvara (known in China as Guanyin and in Japan as Kannon), who have advanced along the path to enlightenment and gained great spiritual powers. They are called upon for assistance with both spiritual and material difficulties. Faith-based Mahayana recognizes that, for most lay Buddhists, following the Dharma is too difficult. In a degenerate age far removed from the teachings of the historical Buddha, the only hope for release from *samsara* is by calling—single-mindedly and with devotion—on those whose spiritual progress far exceeds one's own. Devotions may be made to Amitabha Buddha for spiritual and material assistance in addition to the intervention of *bodhisattvas*.

Mahayana conceptions of the *bodhisattva* critique the Theravada *arhat* ideal, arguing that in an interdependent world individuals must assume responsibility not only for personal enlightenment, but also for assisting others in the quest. Thus, compassion becomes significant in Mahayana ethics in general, and in bioethics in particular.

APPROACHES TO BUDDHIST BIOETHICS

Buddhist ethical perspectives, unlike some Western views, seldom characterize morality in absolute terms. For Buddhists, ethical behavior is a necessary component of successful adherence to the Dharma rather than an end in itself. Once enlightenment is attained, dualities expressed in ethical problems cease to exist. Action is judged not against an absolute moral standard (such as the Ten Commandments), but rather on the basis of its relative merit in leading toward or away from enlightenment. From an enlightened perspective, actions can no longer be characterized as moral or immoral. Rather, action (*karma*) has a neutral value, transcending moral distinctions. As such, ethics are important to the spiritual practice of human beings, but they have no larger significance.

Historically, Buddhist monastics and laypeople have expressed ethical concern for the poor, the sick, and the elderly. Yet Buddhists differ in their approaches to bioethical dilemmas. In part, competing bioethical interpretations arise from Theravada and Mahayana distinctions. Furthermore, as Buddhism has traveled across Asia and other parts of the world, diverse indigenous cultural traditions have informed Buddhist notions of morality. The divergent views of Buddhist practitioners and scholars of Buddhism add another dimension to understanding Buddhist bioethics. Finally, interpretive concerns arise when contemporary bioethical problems are evaluated using Buddhist texts composed centuries before the advent of current biomedical technologies. Despite these complexities, concepts such as nonharm to living beings (*ahimsa*) in Theravada and compassion (*karuna*) in Mahayana—though they do not posit an explicit bioethics—offer a way to measure the morality of bioethical issues.

THERAVADA BUDDHIST BIOETHICS

Precepts for both monastics and laypersons provide a starting point for investigating Theravada bioethics. Although the number of precepts and issues addressed differs depending on individual religious status, there is nevertheless a core set of values applied to all Theravada practitioners. Buddha's moral conduct serves as a model for those who wish to pursue *nirvana*.

The *sangha*, or monastic community, is bound by a code of moral conduct inscribed in monastic rules (*vinaya*) that were established to promote the rigorous mental and physical discipline required to achieve the Theravada religious goal. These detailed rules regulate monastic life and spiritual practice. The first five of the ten Theravada precepts, which apply to both monastics and laity, are:

1. abstention from causing injury to all living beings;
2. abstention from theft and cheating;
3. abstention from sexual misconduct;
4. abstention from lying and other forms of injurious speech; and
5. abstention from intoxication.

Of these five, injunctions against killing, lying, and sexual misconduct have specific relevance to Theravada bioethics. These precepts carry additional significance when coupled with other Theravada Buddhist concepts. For example, respect for life and noninjury to living beings (*ahimsa*) are linked to the idea of the interdependence of all existence (*pratītya-samutpāada*) and, therefore, a moral responsibility to all beings.

As noted above, Theravada Buddhist traditions assert that the universe is fundamentally impermanent. Given this assumption, Theravada ethics strongly advocate comforting the terminally ill rather than trying to extend life through any means available. The value of life is not commensurate with life span, and death is understood as an inevitable consequence of unenlightened existence in an ephemeral world. Attempts to postpone death are unnatural acts that suggest a morbid (and ignorant) fear of death and an ego-motivated attachment to life.

Buddhist principles both inform and complicate responses to contemporary bioethical dilemmas. For example, in Thailand, Theravada Buddhism is intimately connected to all aspects of life. Advanced medical technology and procedures create confusion over traditional Buddhist moral values that prohibit suicide, killing, and harming other living creatures. Thus, for instance, if a patient requests to be removed from life support, is he or she committing suicide? Similarly, if a doctor takes a patient off life support, is that tantamount to killing the patient? In both instances, there appears to be risk of negative karmic consequence for the patient or the doctor. Though such issues are not addressed in traditional Buddhist texts, actual medical cases have given Thai Buddhists reason to consider morally acceptable responses to these kinds of medical situations.

Bioethics scholar Pinit Ratanakul discusses one such case that has prompted new considerations of Thai Buddhist responses to end-of-life issues, especially euthanasia. Ratanakul (2000) tells the story of Venerable Buddhadasa, a very well-known Buddhist monk and scholar. In 1993, at the age of eighty-six, he suffered a stroke. Although he had clearly expressed a desire to die naturally in keeping with Theravada Buddhist practice, his disciples debated over whether Buddhadasa should remain at the temple or be taken to a hospital. It was decided that Buddhadasa would be hospitalized but that no high-technology means would be used to treat him and that he would be returned to the temple after seven days if his condition had not improved. In the end, Buddhadasa was intubated against his disciples' objections. After a month, the monk was still in a coma. The disciples insisted that he be removed from all life support and allowed to die in peace, but the doctors refused, believing they had a professional obligation to do whatever they could to save this eminent monk's life.

According to Ratanakul, this clash of values, the one medical and the other Buddhist, has led to further reflections by Thai Buddhists on the moral implications of euthanasia. At least some Thai Buddhists now advocate a strict distinction between passive and active euthanasia. Active euthanasia is considered a direct violation of the precept to abstain from causing injury to all living beings. Passive euthanasia, however, is considered acceptable because it allows one to die naturally in accord with Buddhist teachings and avoids the karmic problem of clinging unrealistically to life.

MAHAYANA BUDDHIST BIOETHICS

Mahayana Buddhist bioethics often centers on the ideal of the *bodhisattva*. In devotional Mahayana, *bodhisattvas* such as Avalokitesvara embody compassion and the power to save those in material or spiritual distress—thus serving as ethical exemplars. In meditation-based Mahayana, emphasis is often placed on the ethical implications of a *bodhisattva*'s wisdom and experience of emptiness (*sunyata*). Despite positing different ethical ideals, the moral import of compassion and wisdom are interrelated in faith- and meditation-based Mahayana. Wisdom without compassion is no wisdom at all, and compassion without wisdom is potentially dangerous because action might originate in desire and attachment. Realization of compassion and wisdom results from actualizing attitudes and mental conditions—such as generosity, patience, and diligence—that are among the six perfections that *bodhisattvas* strive to achieve.

In part, the Mahayana *bodhisattva* ideal resulted in an increased emphasis on both monastic and lay concern for the spiritual and material well-being of others. *Bodhisattvas* enact the virtues of compassion and wisdom by striving to alleviate suffering and attending to the sick and elderly, among other selfless activities. When *bodhisattvas* declare the "thought of enlightenment" (*bodhicitta*), they not only vow to attain enlightenment but also pledge to overcome defilements and to utilize compassion and wisdom to save all sentient beings.

For some Mahayana Buddhists, the imperative of compassionate action can override injunctions against harming others, lying, and other apparent violations of Buddhist morality. In essence, precepts may be broken in order to help others. This is possible because of the related notion of *upaya*—an expedient device. According to this important Mahayana concept, the historical Buddha used expedient means to expound the Dharma. That is, he presented his teachings in accord with variations in individual ability to comprehend his religious message. However, these alternate versions of the Dharma ultimately lead to the same truth. Similarly, *bodhisattvas* employ efficacious devices according to the needs of those who seek their aid. Japanese stories, for example, recount instances in which *bodhisattvas* assume the guise of a thief in order to be thrown in jail and thereby gain access to incarcerated individuals in need of spiritual solace. While this expedient device seems to transgress the precepts, the act is justified by virtue of compassion. In this and similar situations, the motivation for a behavior becomes central—a *bodhisattva* can only perform such actions if detached from any idea of self-benefit. As a being liberated from dualistic distinctions such as good and evil, the *bodhisattva* demonstrates action informed by the realization of *sunyata*, and the moral efficacy of integrating compassion and wisdom.

Bodhisattva virtues of compassion and wisdom impact Mahayana views on bioethical issues such as euthanasia. From a Tibetan Buddhist perspective, for instance, medical conditions are directly linked to karmic consequence. One's current life experiences are the result of past actions. A terminal illness, then, is considered the consequences of misdeeds in a previous existence. While it might seem that actively or passively euthanizing a dying patient in a great deal of pain is an act of compassion, Tibetan Buddhists have not usually seen the matter this way. Rather, according to Phillip Lecso (1986), they would say that karmic consequence and the kind of death are more salient considerations.

From a Tibetan Buddhist standpoint, a terminal patient in physical and mental distress is in that condition because of past actions. The patient is the architect of his or her own suffering. The illness is the means whereby the deleterious karmic debt is paid off. As a result, the compassionate act is not euthanasia because killing the patient only postpones—to a future existence—the necessity of paying off the karmic debt. In the end, one cannot circumvent conditions caused by karmic consequence. As Lecso points out, the Mahayana value placed on compassion is expressed by mitigating physical and mental pain through mild, limited, nonlethal medication and the support of family and the Buddhist monastic community.

The kind of death one experiences has significant spiritual implications. Tibetan Buddhists believe that one's state of mind near to and at the time of death can have powerfully good or bad effects on one's rebirth. Euthanasia not only robs the patient of the opportunity of paying off bad karmic consequence but also inhibits the possibility of a better rebirth. Similarly, the use of narcotics to reduce pain has the unwanted side effect of dulling the mind, making the kind of mental states conducive to a better rebirth impossible. To do otherwise, from a Tibetan viewpoint, is to act contrary to wisdom.

BUDDHIST BIOETHICS: PROSPECTS

This entry has offered an overview of the relationship between Buddhist ideas and bioethical issues. The fundamental logic introduced concerning euthanasia, for example, also pertains to Buddhist discussions of other bioethical dilemmas. Most likely, ongoing Theravada and Mahayana debates over the morality of infertility treatments or human cloning will also pivot on concepts of nonharm and compassion.

At least three areas remain for further study that will undoubtedly raise new and important questions about Buddhist bioethics. First, the Buddhist textual record that currently exists represents mostly the views of Buddhist males. What are the ethical perspectives, both past and present, of Buddhist women? Do Buddhist women have different views of bioethical issues than men? Second, as medical technology continues to impact traditionally Buddhist cultures, what new conflicts and challenges will emerge? Finally, in what ways will Western Buddhist (e.g., American Buddhist) understandings of bioethical issues impact traditional Buddhist bioethics?

SEE ALSO *Abortion: VIII. Buddhist Perspectives; Authority in Religious Traditions; China, Bioethics in; Death: II. Eastern Thought; Environmental Ethics: I. Overview; Ethics: V. Religion and Morality; Eugenics: I. Historical Aspects; Hinduism, Bioethics in; Japan, Bioethics in; Population Ethics: X. Buddhist Perspectives; South Asia, Bioethics in; Southeast Asia, Bioethics in*

BIBLIOGRAPHY

Barnhart, Michael G. 1998. "Buddhism and the Morality of Abortion." *Journal of Buddhist Ethics* 5:276–97. http://blogs.dickinson.edu/buddhistethics/files/2010/04/barnh981.pdf

Barnhart, Michael G. 2000. "Nature, Nurture, and No-Self: Bioengineering and Buddhist Values." *Journal of Buddhist Ethics* 7:126–44. http://blogs.dickinson.edu/buddhistethics/files/2010/04/barnhart001.pdf

Becker, Carl B. 1990. "Buddhist Views of Suicide and Euthanasia." *Philosophy East and West* 40:543–56.

Becker, Carl B. 1993. *Breaking the Circle: Death and Afterlife in Buddhism.* Carbondale: Southern Illinois University Press.

Florida, Robert E. 1993. "Buddhist Approaches to Euthanasia." *Studies in Religion Sciences Religieuses* 22 (1): 35–47.

Florida, Robert E. 1994. "Buddhism and the Four Principles." In *Principles of Health Care Ethics*, edited by Raanan Gillon and Ann Lloyd. New York: Wiley.

Florida, Robert E. 1998. "The Lotus Sūtra and Health Care Ethics." *Journal of Buddhist Ethics* 5:170–89. http://blogs.dickinson.edu/buddhistethics/files/2010/04/flori981.pdf

Florida, Robert E. 2000. "Buddhism and Abortion." In *Contemporary Buddhist Ethics*, edited by Damien Keown, 137–68. Richmond, UK: Curzon Press.

Hardacre, Helen. 1994. "Response of Buddhism and Shinto to the Issue of Brain Death and Organ Transplant." *Cambridge Quarterly of Healthcare Ethics* 3:585–601.

Hardacre, Helen. 1997. *Marketing the Menacing Fetus in Japan.* Berkeley: University of California Press.

Harvey, Peter. 2000. *An Introduction to Buddhist Ethics: Foundations, Values and Issues.* Cambridge, UK: Cambridge University Press.

Hughes, James. 2007. "Buddhist Bioethics." In *Principles of Health Care Ethics*, 2nd ed., edited by Richard E. Ashcroft, Angus Dawson, Heather Draper, and John R. McMillan, 127–33. Chichester, West Sussex, UK and Hoboken, NJ: Wiley.

Hughes, James J., and Damien Keown. 1995. "Buddhism and Medical Ethics: A Bibliographic Introduction." *Journal of Buddhist Ethics* 2:105–24. http://blogs.dickinson.edu/buddhistethics/files/2010/04/Buddhism-and-Medical-Ethics.pdf

Keown, Damien. 1992. *The Nature of Buddhist Ethics.* Basingstoke, UK: Palgrave. Reprint, 2001.

Keown, Damien. 1995. *Buddhism and Bioethics.* Basingstoke, UK: Palgrave. Reprint, 2001.

Keown, Damien, ed. 1998. *Buddhism and Abortion.* London: Macmillan.

Keown, Damien. 1999. "Attitudes to Euthanasia in the Vinaya and Commentary." *Journal of Buddhist Ethics* 6:260–70. http://blogs.dickinson.edu/buddhistethics/files/2010/04/keown993.pdf

Keown, Damien, ed. 2000. *Contemporary Buddhist Ethics.* Richmond, UK: Curzon Press.

Keown, Damien. 2005. *Buddhist Ethics: A Very Short Introduction.* Oxford and New York: Oxford University Press.

Keown, Damien. 2008. "Buddhism, Death and Organ Transplantation." *Journal of the International Association of Buddhist Universities* 1:57–70.

Keown, Damien. 2010. "Buddhism, Brain Death, and Organ Transplantation." *Journal of Buddhist Ethics* 17:1–34. http://blogs.dickinson.edu/buddhistethics/files/2010/05/Keown-final1.pdf

LaFleur, William R. 1990. "Contestation and Confrontation: The Morality of Abortion in Japan." *Philosophy East and West* 40 (4): 529–42.

LaFleur, William R. 1992. *Liquid Life: Abortion and Buddhism in Japan.* Princeton, NJ: Princeton University Press.

LaFleur, William R. 2001. "From *Agapé* to Organs: Religious Differences Between Japan and America in Judging the Ethics of the Transplant." In *Ethics in the World Religions*, edited by Joseph Runzo and Nancy M. Martin, 271–90. Oxford, UK: Oneworld Publications.

Lecso, Phillip A. 1986. "Euthanasia: A Buddhist Perspective." *Journal of Religion and Health* 25 (1): 51–57.

Lecso, Phillip A. 1991. "The Bodhisattva Ideal and Organ Transplantation." *Journal of Religion and Health* 30 (1): 35–41.

Lerdmaleewong, Malee, and Caroline Francis. 1998. "Abortion in Thailand: A Feminist Perspective." *Journal of Buddhist Ethics* 5:22–48. http://blogs.dickinson.edu/buddhistethics/files/2010/04/aborti1.pdf

Lock, Margaret. 2002. *Twice Dead: Organ Transplants and the Reinvention of Death.* Berkeley: University of California Press.

Mettanando, Bhikkhu. 1991. "Buddhist Ethics in the Practice of Medicine." In *Buddhist Ethics and Modern Society: An International Symposium*, edited by Charles Wei-hsun Fu and Sandra A. Wawrytko, 195–213. Westport, CT: Greenwood Press.

Meyer, John-Anderson L. 2005. "Buddhism and Death: The Brain-Centered Criteria." *Journal of Buddhist Ethics* 12. http://blogs.dickinson.edu/buddhistethics/files/2010/04/meyer402.pdf

Perrett, Roy W. 1996. "Buddhism, Euthanasia and the Sanctity of Life." *Journal of Medical Ethics* 22 (5): 309–13.

Ratanakul, Pinit. 1986. *Bioethics: An Introduction to the Ethics of Medicine and Life Sciences.* Bangkok: Mahidol University.

Ratanakul, Pinit. 1988. "Bioethics in Thailand: The Struggle for Buddhist Solutions." *Journal of Medicine and Philosophy* 13:301–12.

Ratanakul, Pinit. 1990. "Thailand: Refining Cultural Values." *Hastings Center Report* 20 (2): 25–27.

Ratanakul, Pinit. 1998. "Socio-Medical Aspects of Abortion in Thailand." In *Buddhism and Abortion*, edited by Damien Keown, 53–66. London: Macmillan.

Ratanakul, Pinit. 2000. "To Save or Let Go: Thai Buddhist Perspectives on Euthanasia." In *Contemporary Buddhist Ethics*, edited by Damien Keown, 169–82. Richmond, UK: Curzon Press.

Silva, Padmasiri de. 1991. "Buddhist Ethics." In *A Companion to Ethics: Blackwell's Companions to Philosophy*, edited by Peter Singer, 58–68. Oxford, UK: Blackwell.

Simpson, Bob. 2004. "Impossible Gifts: Bodies, Buddhism and Bioethics in Contemporary Sri Lanka." *Journal of the Royal Anthropological Institute* 10 (4): 839–59.

Slaughter, Bill. 2002. "Animal Use in Biomedicine: An Annotated Bibliography of Buddhist and Related Perspectives." *Journal of Buddhist Ethics* 9:149–58. http://blogs.dickinson.edu/buddhistethics/files/2010/04/slaug021.pdf

Tanida, Noritoshi. 2000. "The View of Religions Toward Euthanasia and Extraordinary Treatments in Japan." *Journal of Religion and Health* 39 (4): 339–54.

Tsomo, Karma Lekshe. 1998. "Prolife, Prochoice: Buddhism and Reproductive Ethics." Feminism and Nonviolence Studies Association. http://www.fnsa.org/fall98/tsomo.html

Tsomo, Karma Lekshe. 2006. *Into the Jaws of Yama, Lord of Death: Buddhism, Bioethics, and Death.* Albany: State University of New York Press.

William E. Deal (2004, 2014)
Severance Professor of the History of Religion,
Department of Religious Studies,
Case Western Reserve University